S0-BRA-486

INTEGRATED MICROSYSTEMS

Electronics, Photonics, and Biotechnology

Devices, Circuits, and Systems

Series Editor
Krzysztof Iniewski
CMOS Emerging Technologies Inc., Vancouver, British Columbia, Canada

Electrical Solitons: Theory, Design, and Applications
David Ricketts and Donhee Ham

Radiation Effects in Semiconductors
Krzysztof Iniewski

Electronics for Radiation Detection
Krzysztof Iniewski

Semiconductor Radiation Detection Systems
Krzysztof Iniewski

Internet Networks: Wired, Wireless, and Optical Technologies
Krzysztof Iniewski

Integrated Microsystems: Electronics, Photonics, and Biotechnology
Krzysztof Iniewski

FORTHCOMING

Nano-Semiconductors: Devices and Technology
Krzysztof Iniewski

Atomic Nanoscale Technology in the Nuclear Industry
Taeho Woo

Telecommunication Networks
Eugenio Iannone

Optical, Acoustic, Magnetic, and Mechanical Sensor Technologies
Krzysztof Iniewski

Biological and Medical Sensor Technologies
Krzysztof Iniewski

INTEGRATED MICROSYSTEMS

Electronics, Photonics, and Biotechnology

Edited by KRZYSZTOF INIEWSKI

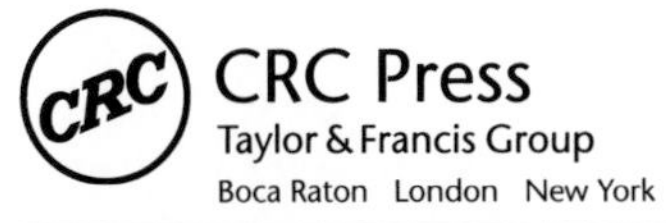

CRC Press
Taylor & Francis Group
Boca Raton London New York

CRC Press is an imprint of the
Taylor & Francis Group, an **informa** business

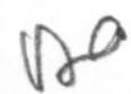

CRC Press
Taylor & Francis Group
6000 Broken Sound Parkway NW, Suite 300
Boca Raton, FL 33487-2742

Printed in the United States of America on acid-free paper
Version Date: 20110719

International Standard Book Number: 978-1-4398-3620-0 (Hardback)

Visit the Taylor & Francis Web site at
http://www.taylorandfrancis.com

and the CRC Press Web site at
http://www.crcpress.com

Contents

Preface

Integrated microsystems are intelligent miniaturized devices and systems, fabricated using processes compatible with CMOS integrated circuits, which combine computation, communications, sensing, and actuation. Integrated microsystems represent a rapidly growing field, embracing developments in electronics, photonics, mechanics, chemistry, and biology. They might include emerging devices fabricated in nanotechnology, microelectromechanical systems (MEMS), or microfluidics. Their presence is widespread in everyday life—although frequently we might not realize that we are dealing with integrated microsystems when using Wii videogames, hearing aids, or pacemakers.

The demand for portable and lightweight microsystems is relentless, filling various needs in consumer electronics, biomedical engineering, or in military applications. Conforming to these small microscale dimensions means that power supplies, processing microelectronics, sensors, wireless transceivers, and other system components must share a common miniaturized platform, frequently in the form of a system-on-chip (SoC) or system-in-package (SiP). Integrating those various components presents myriad diverse thermal, mechanical, and electrical challenges.

One of the most exciting trends in microsystem integration is the inclusion of biosensors. Biosensors can be defined as devices incorporating biological material (tissue, microorganisms, nucleic acids): a biologically derived material intimately associated with or integrated within a microsystem, which may be optical, electrochemical, thermometric, piezoelectric, magnetic, or micromechanical. Biosensors usually yield a digital electronic signal that is proportional to the concentration of a specific agent. Although the signal may in principle be continuous, devices can be configured to yield single measurements to meet specific market requirements. Biosensors have been applied to a wide variety of analytical problems in fields as diverse as medicine, drug discovery, the environment, food process industries, security, and defense.

This book is divided into three parts. Part I deals with microelectronics and biosystems. The first two chapters are devoted to power management and the following eight to various aspects of biosystems and bioelectronics. This part concludes with a chapter on acoustic detection and passive wireless microsystems. Part II is devoted to photonics and imaging. The first two chapters deal with terahertz imaging, the third with x-ray micro-CT systems, and the fourth discusses ultrasound platforms. The following two chapters cover sensing and the remaining six discuss various aspects of photonics subsystems and components. Part III of this book deals with biotechnology and MEMs. The first three chapters are devoted to microfluidic microsystems. Chapters on biosensing, bioimplants, and bionanomaterials follow. The book concludes with chapters on multitransducer systems, MEMs, and piezoelectric and HfO_2 films.

With such a wide variety of topics covered, I hope that the reader will find something interesting to read, and discover the field of integrated microsystems to be both exciting and useful in science and everyday life. Books like this one would not be possible without many creative individuals meeting together in one place to exchange thoughts and ideas in a relaxed atmosphere. I invite you to attend CMOS Emerging Technologies events held annually in British Columbia, Canada, where many topics covered in this book are discussed. See http://www.cmoset.com for presentation slides from the previous meeting and announcements about future ones.

Kris Iniewski

Editor

Krzysztof (Kris) Iniewski manages R&D at Redlen Technologies Inc., a start-up company in Vancouver, Canada. Redlen's revolutionary production process for advanced semiconductor materials enables a new generation of more accurate, all-digital, radiation-based imaging solutions. Kris is also an executive director of CMOS Emerging Technologies (www.cmoset.com), a series of high-tech events covering communications, microsystems, optoelectronics, and sensors.

During his career Dr. Iniewski has held numerous faculty and management positions at University of Toronto, University of Alberta, SFU, and PMC-Sierra Inc. He has published over 100 research papers in international journals and conferences, and holds 18 international patents granted in the United States, Canada, France, Germany, and Japan. He is a frequent invited speaker and has consulted for multiple organizations internationally. He has written and edited several books for Wiley, CRC Press, McGraw-Hill, Artech House, and Springer.

His personal goal is to contribute to sustainability through innovative engineering solutions. He can be reached at kris.iniewski@gmail.com.

Contributors

Altug Akay
Department of Medicine
Brigham and Women's Hospital
Harvard Medical School
Boston, Massachusetts

Miguel V. Andrés
Departamento de Física Aplicada y Electromagnetismo, ICMUV
Universidad de Valencia
Valencia, Spain

Kanna Aoki
Metamaterials Laboratory
RIKEN, the Institute of Physical and Chemical Research
Saitama, Japan

Behraad Bahreyni
School of Engineering Science
Simon Fraser University
Burnaby, Canada

Jean-François Bêche
CEA LETI Minatec
Grenoble, France

Kevin E. Bennet
Division of Engineering
Mayo Clinic
Rochester, Minnesota

Paolo Bifulco
Dipartimento di Ingegneria Elettronica, Biomedica e delle Telecomunicazioni
University of Naples
Naples, Italy

Olivier Billoint
CEA LETI Minatec
Grenoble, France

Charles D. Blaha
Department of Psychology
University of Memphis
Memphis, Tennessee

Kwabena Boahen
Department of Bioengineering
Stanford University
Stanford, California

Rajdeep Bondade
Texas Analog Center of Excellence
University of Texas at Dallas
Richardson, Texas

Stéphane Bonnet
CEA LETI Minatec
Grenoble, France

Rafael A. Calvo
School of Electrical and Information Engineering
The University of Sydney
Sydney, Australia

Gert Cauwenberghs
Department of Bioengineering
Jacobs School of Engineering
and
Institute for Neural Computation
University of California San Diego
La Jolla, California

Mario Cesarelli
Dipartimento di Ingegneria Elettronica, Biomedica e delle Telecomunicazioni
University of Naples
Naples, Italy

Guillaume Charvet
CEA LETI Minatec
Grenoble, France

Hongzhi Chen
Department of Electrical and Computer Engineering
Michigan State University
East Lansing, Michigan

Kyusun Choi
Department of Computer Science and Engineering
The Pennsylvania State University
University Park, Pennsylvania

Lukas Chrostowski
Electrical and Computer Engineering
University of British Columbia
Vancouver, British Columbia, Canada

Cyril Condemine
CEA LETI Minatec
Grenoble, France

Dan P. Covey
School of Biological Sciences
Illinois State University
Normal, Illinois

José L. Cruz
Departamento de Física Aplicada y Electromagnetismo, ICMUV
Universidad de Valencia
Valencia, Spain

Christian Cuadrado-Laborde
CIOp (CONICET La Plata-CIC)
Buenos Aires, Argentina

Utkan Demirci
Department of Medicine
Brigham and Women's Hospital
Harvard Medical School
Boston, Massachusetts

M. Desco
Unidad de Medicina y Cirugía Experimental
Hospital General Universitario Gregorio Marañón
Madrid, Spain

Antonio Diez
Departamento de Física Aplicada y Electromagnetismo, ICMUV
Universidad de Valencia
Valencia, Spain

Ricardo Escolá
CEA LETI Minatec
Grenoble, France

Carmen Kar Man Fung
Department of Electrical and Computer Engineering
Michigan State University
East Lansing, Michigan

Gaetano Gargiulo
School of Electrical and Information Engineering
The University of Sydney
Sydney, Australia

Paul A. Garris
School of Biological Sciences
Illinois State University
Normal, Illinois

Flavio Griggio
The Pennsylvania State University
University Park, Pennsylvania

Régis Guillemaud
CEA LETI Minatec
Grenoble, France

Bhagwati P. Gupta
Department of Biology
McMaster University
Hamilton, Ontario, Canada

Ali Hajimiri
California Institute of Technology
Pasadena, California

Yoshihiko Hirao
Department of Urology
Nara Medical University
Nara, Japan

Alton B. Horsfall
School of Electrical Electronic and Computer Engineering
Newcastle University
Newcastle upon Tyne, United Kingdom

Masaharu Imai
Graduate School of Information Science and Technology
Osaka University
Osaka, Japan

Alexander Chi Fai Ip
Department of Medicine
Brigham and Women's Hospital
Harvard Medical School
Boston, Massachusetts

Hirofumi Iwato
Graduate School of Information Science and Technology
Osaka University
Osaka, Japan

Esmaiel Jabbari
Department of Chemical Engineering
University of South Carolina
Columbia, South Carolina

Thomas N. Jackson
The Pennsylvania State University
University Park, Pennsylvania

Craig Jin
School of Electrical and Information Engineering
The University of Sydney
Sydney, Australia

Isaku Kanno
Department of Micro Engineering
Kyoto University
Kyoto, Japan

T. Kauffmann
Bio-Logic SAS
Claix, France

Yukio Kawano
Department of Physical Electronics
Tokyo Institute of Technology
Tokyo, Japan

Dongsoo Kim
Department of Electrical and Electronic Engineering
Yonsei University
Seoul, South Korea

Hyunsoo Kim
Center for Thin Film Devices and Material Research Institute
The Pennsylvania State University
University Park, Pennsylvania

Insoo Kim
The Center for Neural Engineering
The Pennsylvania State University
University Park, Pennsylvania

F.-M. Kuo
Department of Electrical Engineering
National Central University
Taoyuan County, Taiwan

King Wai Chiu Lai
Department of Electrical and Computer Engineering
Michigan State University
East Lansing, Michigan

Jae-Hoon Lee
GaN Power Research Group
Samsung LED Co., Ltd
Suwon, Korea

Kendall H. Lee
Department of Neurologic Surgery
Mayo Clinic
Rochester, Minnesota

Timothée Levi
CEA LETI Minatec
Grenoble, France

Paul C.H. Li
Department of Chemistry
Simon Fraser University
Burnaby, British Columbia, Canada

Tsung-Hsien Lin
Department of Electrical Engineering
National Taiwan University
Taipei, Taiwan

Jian Liu
PolarOnyx, Inc.
San Jose, California

Yao-Hong Liu
Graduate Institute of Electronics Engineering
National Taiwan University
Taipei, Taiwan

Dongsheng Ma
Texas Analog Center of Excellence
University of Texas at Dallas
Richardson, Texas

Akira Matsuzawa
Graduate School of Science and Engineering
Tokyo Institute of Technology
Tokyo, Japan

Ryan McClintock
Center for Quantum Devices
Northwestern University
Evanston, Illinois

Alistair McEwan
School of Electrical and Information Engineering
The University of Sydney
Sydney, Australia

Bing Miao
School of Electrical Electronic and Computer Engineering
Newcastle University
Newcastle upon Tyne, United Kingdom

Pedram Mohseni
Department of Electrical Engineering and Computer Science
Case Western Reserve University
Cleveland, Ohio

Manijeh Razeghi
Center for Quantum Devices
Northwestern University
Evanston, Illinois

Pouya Rezai
Department of Mechanical Engineering
McMaster University
Hamilton, Ontario, Canada

Gabriel Alfonso Rincón-Mora
Georgia Institute of Technology
Atlanta, Georgia

Joseph Rizzo, III
Department of Ophthalmology
Harvard Medical School
and
Department of Neuro-Ophthalmology
Center of Innovative Visual Rehabilitation
Boston, Massachusetts

Maria Romano
Dipartimento di Ingegneria Elettronica, Biomedica e delle Telecomunicazioni
University of Naples
Naples, Italy

Jean-Pierre Rostaing
CEA LETI Minatec
Grenoble, France

Lionel Rousseau
ESIEE-Paris
Noisy-le-Grand, France

Mariano Ruffo
Dipartimento di Ingegneria Elettronica, Biomedica e delle Telecomunicazioni
University of Naples
Naples, Italy

Daryoosh Saeedkia
TeTechS Inc.
Waterloo, Ontario, Canada

Keishi Sakanushi
Graduate School of Information Science and Technology
Osaka University
Osaka, Japan

Sangeena Salam
Department of Biology
McMaster University
Hamilton, Ontario, Canada

André van Schaik
School of Electrical and Information Engineering
The University of Sydney
Sydney, Australia

P. Ravi Selvaganapathy
Department of Mechanical Engineering
McMaster University
Hamilton, Ontario, Canada

Richard Shephard
School of Electrical and Information Engineering
The University of Sydney
Sydney, Australia

J.-W. Shi
Department of Electrical Engineering
National Central University
Taoyuan County, Taiwan

Sirinrath Sirivisoot
Department of Orthopedics
Brown University
Providence, Rhode Island

Alejandro Sisniega
Unidad de Medicina y Cirugía Experimental
Hospital General Universitario Gregorio Marañón
Madrid, Spain

Nima Soltani
Department of Electrical and Computer Engineering
Ryerson University
Toronto, Ontario, Canada

Mrudula Somu
Department of Medicine
Brigham and Women's Hospital
Harvard Medical School
Boston, Massachusetts

Milutin Stanaćević
Department of Electrical and Computer Engineering
Stony Brook University
Stony Brook, New York

Yoshinori Takeuchi
Graduate School of Information Science and Technology
Osaka University
Osaka, Japan

T. J. Tarn
Department of Electrical and Systems Engineering
Washington University in St. Louis
St. Louis, Missouri

Luke Theogarajan
Department of Electrical and Computer Engineering
University of California
Santa Barbara, California

Susan Trolier-McKinstry
The Pennsylvania State University
University Park, Pennsylvania

Richard L. Tutwiler
The Pennsylvania State University
University Park, Pennsylvania

J. J. Vaquero
Unidad de Medicina y Cirugía Experimental
Hospital General Universitario Gregorio Marañón
Madrid, Spain

Hua Wang
California Institute of Technology
Pasadena, California

Lin Wang
Department of Chemistry
Simon Fraser University
Burnaby, British Columbia, Canada

ShuQi Wang
Department of Medicine
Brigham and Women's Hospital
Harvard Medical School
Boston, Massachusetts

Xu Wang
Electrical and Computer Engineering
University of British Columbia
Vancouver, British Columbia, Canada

Thomas J. Webster
Department of Orthopedics
Brown University
Providence, Rhode Island

Bo Wen
Research Laboratory of Electronics
Massachusetts Institute of Technology
Cambridge, Massachusetts

John Wyatt
Department of Electrical Engineering and Computer Science
Massachusetts Institute of Technology
Cambridge, Massachusetts

Ning Xi
Department of Electrical and Computer Engineering
Michigan State University
East Lansing, Michigan

Feng Xu
Department of Medicine
Brigham and Women's Hospital
Harvard Medical School
Boston, Massachusetts

Lihmei Yang
PolarOnyx, Inc.
San Jose, California

Fei Yuan
Department of Electrical and Computer Engineering
Ryerson University
Toronto, Ontario, Canada

Blaise Yvert
Centre National de la Recherche Scientifique
and
Université de Bordeaux
Bordeaux, France

Jiangbo Zhang
Department of Electrical and Computer Engineering
Michigan State University
East Lansing, Michigan

Xiaohu Zhao
Department of Medicine
Brigham and Women's Hospital
Harvard Medical School
Boston, Massachusetts

Part I

Microelectronics and Biosystems

1 Energizing and Powering Microsystems

Gabriel Alfonso Rincón-Mora

CONTENTS

1.1 MICROSYSTEMS

Considering today's growing demand for and operational needs of portable microelectronics is crucial in drafting a strategy for supplying a derivative application space that is barely emerging, such as wireless microsensors. The challenge is to understand today's market and needs well enough to be able to predict the challenges society will face at the time research reaches the commercialization stage. Equally important is comprehending not only the state of the art of technologies needed to build such systems but also the trends that drive them, so that today's efforts may be able to enhance the future benefits of technologies currently under development. Ultimately, however, predictions of this sort, however good they may be, amount to speculation that scientists and engineers must continually fine-tune with experience and over time.

1.1.1 Market Demand

Consumers continue to enjoy (and consequently demand) smaller and more functionally dense products. Unfortunately, tiny devices necessarily constrain sources to small spaces, limiting the amount of energy they can store and how much power they can supply to impractically low levels. Consider, to cite an illustrative example, that 100 μW, which is drastically below what wireless telemetry requires today to transmit over a distance of 100 m, completely discharges a $5 \times 3.8 \times 0.037$-cm^3 1-mA h thin-film lithium ion (Li ion) battery in 10 h. Adding functionality, as in the case of cellular phones and the applications they now support, only exacerbates the issue because the extra power overhead drains a source that is already easily exhaustible even faster. Although today's efforts aim at reducing the energy that each additional function requires, the cumulative load that wireless transmission and several low-power functions present to a miniature source is nonetheless substantial, reducing the operational life of the system considerably, to the point that consumers lose interest.

Perhaps a more significant application space emerges in the wake of integration in the form of *in situ* but nonintrusive devices, such as biomedical implants. While the motivation for and benefits of monitoring biological activity with *in vivo* contraptions without frequently replacing or recharging batteries are for the most part obvious, the commercial and societal advantages of retrofitting low-overhead, noninvasive intelligence into expensive and difficult-to-replace technologies, such as the power grid, are arguably more economically, sociologically, and ecologically profound. Feeding performance metrics and the use of energy in a factory into a central processor, for instance, to determine the optimal use of power can not only save energy on a grander scale (when applied across a wide region) but also reduce the emission of environmentally harmful by-products and the need for politically charged petroleum. From a commercial standpoint, the potential ubiquity for such miniature sensors across factories, hospitals, airports, farms, homes, subway stations, shopping malls, and other such centers rivals and quite likely exceeds that of cellular phones at maybe 10–100 sensors for every 10×10 m^2 of surface area.

1.1.2 Energy and Power Requirements

Modern microelectronic systems necessarily embed both analog and digital functions. Analog because they must not only manage and process real-life signals, such as, for example, seismic activity, sound waves, motion, temperature, pressure, and others, but also draw energy and condition power from nonideal sources, all of which are continuous in time. State-of-the-art applications, however, also include digital blocks because binary processes enjoy considerably higher noise margins, which is another way of saying that they exhibit higher signal-to-noise ratios (SNRs). The fact is that a small voltage variation, say from 20 to 400 mV, across a 0–1.8-V digital signal has little to no impact on the output word and its bit-error rate (BER), whereas the same variation in a rail-to-rail analog signal swing essentially eradicates more than 1–22% of the data. What all this implies is that the system draws quiescent (DC) and switching (AC) power from the source, as shown in Figure 1.1 [1].

Because the going trend is to incorporate more functionality into a product, a fixed supply voltage is no longer optimal, especially when seeking to extend operational life. While digital-signal processors (DSPs), for example, may draw mW's at 1 V, voltage-controlled oscillators (VCOs) and analog–digital converters (ADCs) can demand considerably less power at maybe 1.8 V and power amplifiers (PAs) significantly more power at 3 V. The end result is a system that, to operate optimally, includes multiple supply voltages capable of feeding diverse power levels.

In the end, irrespective of the supply voltages needed, featuring multiple tasks ultimately burdens a source with additional loads. The problem with a miniature source is that energy is scarce and power levels are low. One way of reducing power (not energy) is to duty-cycle tasks across time so that not more than one set of interdependent functions operate at any given point. Similarly, powering blocks only when absolutely necessary (i.e., on demand) reduces energy that the system would

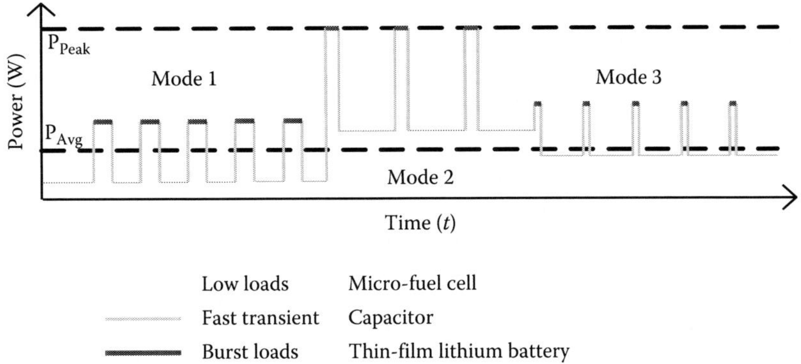

FIGURE 1.1 General loading profile that a modern microsystem presents to a source over time.

otherwise waste. As a result, systems today dynamically change operating modes *on the fly*, as Figure 1.1 also shows, where the DC, peak power, pulse width, and switching frequency change according to the tasks performed.

Extending the operational life of smart microsensors remains a challenge, even after power-moding and duty-cycling functions. The point is that marketable microsystems must draw little to no power. Fortunately, portable and sensor applications naturally call for low duty-cycle operation because devices need not function continuously. The cellular phone, for instance, is for the most part alert, that is, ready to receive calls, and while transmission demands milliwatts, awareness only requires microwatts, which is why radio frequency (RF) PAs are mostly in the light-to-moderate power region of operation, as Figure 1.2 demonstrates in the case of code-division multiple-access (CDMA) applications [2]. Said differently, while talking continuously on the phone for 3–5 h exhausts a fully charged battery, idling might do so in 5–7 days.

While energy and power unavoidably relate, meeting the energy requirements of a microsystem does not necessarily imply that the source can also supply the power needed. As a result, reducing losses to save energy (as in shutting off unused circuit blocks) is as important as duty-cycling tasks over time to decrease power. The source and the circuits that manage the source must therefore account for and respond to various mixed-signal modes whose characteristics (which range from DC and peak power to pulse width, rise and fall times and switching frequency) change over time.

1.1.3 Technology Trends

Trends in technology dictate how and to what extent emerging applications succeed. Not surprisingly, the consumers' affinity to small microelectronic gadgets is motivating scientists and engineers to find innovative ways of confining products into tiny spaces. Accordingly, incorporating as much as possible into the silicon die has been and continues to be increasingly popular. Research and industry are

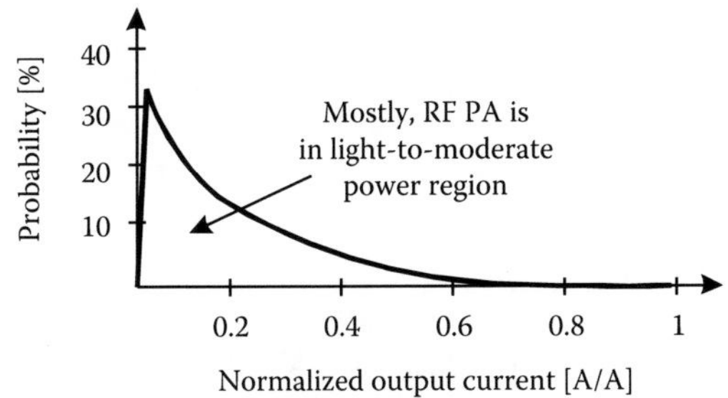

FIGURE 1.2 Probability density curve for RF PAs in CDMA handset applications.

not only building more semiconductor devices on a common substrate but also postprocessing copper layers, microelectromechanical systems (MEMS), and MEMS-like inductors on top.

The problem with system-on-chip (SoC) integration is higher cost, because arbitrarily adding processing steps of increasing complexity to the fabrication process diminishes the commercial appeal of the product. As a result, engineers are also copackaging technologies, such as, for example, high-frequency gallium-arsenide (GaAs) silicon chips with low-cost complementary metal–oxide–semiconductor (CMOS) silicon chips. Power integrated circuit (IC) designers are similarly integrating relatively mature (and consequently lower cost) discrete 1–10-μH power inductors in the $2 \times 2 \times 1\text{-mm}^2$ range with their controlling CMOS and bipolar circuits. SoC and system-in-package (SiP) integration, however, are often insufficient; hence, engineers are also exploring SoP approaches by attaching, for instance, antennae and thin-film Li ions to the external surface of the material encapsulating the silicon die.

Higher SoC integration implies that machinery with finer photolithographic resolutions of, for example, 45 nm necessarily build semiconductor devices with thinner barriers and smaller junctions of increasing doping concentration. The resulting electric fields are more intense and their corresponding breakdown voltages are consequently lower, on the order of 1–1.8 V, constraining circuits to operate with lower supply voltages. While reducing the voltages across charging and discharging parasitic capacitors and DC loads mitigates power losses, a low supply also decreases usable dynamic range, which translates into a lower SNR, and more generally, reduced noise margin.

Unfortunately, while additional on-chip functions inject and cross-couple more noise, SoC, SiP, and SoP designs suffer from diminished filtering capabilities, challenging engineers to design with even lower dynamic ranges. The problem is, unlike in discrete printed-circuit-board (PCB) implementations, on-chip solutions cannot possibly hope to attenuate noise by sprinkling several nF and even μF capacitors across sensitive supplies, input pins, and output pins without increasing the silicon real estate to cost-prohibitive levels. Just to cite an example, consider that capacitance-per-unit-area values of 15–20 $\text{fF}/\mu\text{m}^2$ are typical in state-of-the-art technologies and one 1 nF would occupy roughly 225×225 to $260 \times 260\ \mu\text{m}^2$ of the die, which today probably represents one-quarter to one-eighth of the total area of a relatively complex system. Regrettably, increasing areas beyond, say, $2 \times 2\ \text{mm}^2$, decreases the commercial appeal of the chip because the silicon wafer's die density necessarily decreases, which indicates how many chips (and profits) per 8- or 12-in. wafer, for example, a technology produces. Inductors, incidentally, are even more costly because air-gap inductors do not only occupy considerable space, which limits inductances to maybe 40–100 nH, but also exhibit relatively poor quality factors (i.e., high parasitic series resistances).

The lower filter densities and breakdown voltages that SoC, SiP, and SoP approaches impose shift the burden of attenuating noise to the supply and processing circuits of the system. Functional blocks, such as phase-locked loops (PLLs), ADCs, VCOs, and DSPs, must not only survive more noise in the substrate and supplies but the linear and switching regulators that supply them must also generate less and more effectively suppress switching noise. In other words, higher bandwidth and higher power-supply rejection in supply and interface circuits are necessary to respond quickly enough to offset noise. To add insult to injury, supply voltage variations must also be lower, in the range of 10–50 mV, to maximally extend dynamic range under low breakdown voltages, which is especially difficult without a large on-board capacitor in the presence of fast rising and falling load dumps, and all this with only cost-effective CMOS and maybe bipolar-CMOS (BiCMOS) technologies.

1.2 MINIATURE SOURCES

The fundamental drawback of microscale sources is that limited space constrains energy and power to miniscule levels. What is worse, technologies that store more energy unfortunately suffer from lower power densities, and vice versa. To illustrate this latter point, consider that a capacitor, which responds quickly to changing loads, supplies high power per unit volume, but only for a short while because energy density is low. A fuel cell of equivalent dimensions, on the other hand, which incidentally requires additional time to respond, stores more energy but sources less power, as the Ragone plot of Figure 1.3 corroborates graphically [3]. For this reason, Li ions are popular in cellular phones, laptop computers, digital cameras, and other mobile products, because they represent what amounts to a balanced alternative, with not only moderate energy and power densities but also intermediate speed. Super- or ultracapacitors feature comparable tradeoffs plus additional cycle life. Additionally, the voltage range of supercapacitors extends to zero, below the headroom limit of a circuit under which drawing energy is less probable, which means that the circuit may not leverage some of the energy stored in the capacitor.

Compromising energy, power, and speed for cost is less appealing in small applications such as wireless microsensors where operational life (i.e., energy) is as important as, for example, wireless telecommunication, which demands considerable power. As a result, complementing the relatively higher power levels that inductors, capacitors, ultracapacitors, and Li ions supply with the energy stored in fuel cells, which amass up to 10 times (10×) as much as Li ions, is gathering momentum in industry and research circles alike. Miniature nuclear sources are also garnering attention, even if nuclear energy produces less power, costs more, and poses safety concerns. Energy transducers enjoy more popularity, however, because they are safe (unlike radioactive isotopes), produce little to no by-products (unlike fuel cells), and convert energy from a virtually boundless (infinite) source: the surrounding environment. Ambient energy, unfortunately, is not reliable or consistent, and small transducers produce substantially low power levels. Nevertheless, the promise of extended and perhaps perpetual life is sufficient motivation to fuel research efforts in all directions.

1.2.1 Li Ions

The appeal of Li ion technologies in microscale applications is integration. Rechargeable manganese-based Li ion button cells, for example, that weigh 59 mg, measure 4.8 mm in diameter and are 1.4 mm thick, and feature 1.2 mA h of capacity are already commercially available. Similarly, unpackaged 5 × 5 × 0.31-mm^3 12.5-μA h solid-state thin-film Li ions are also available

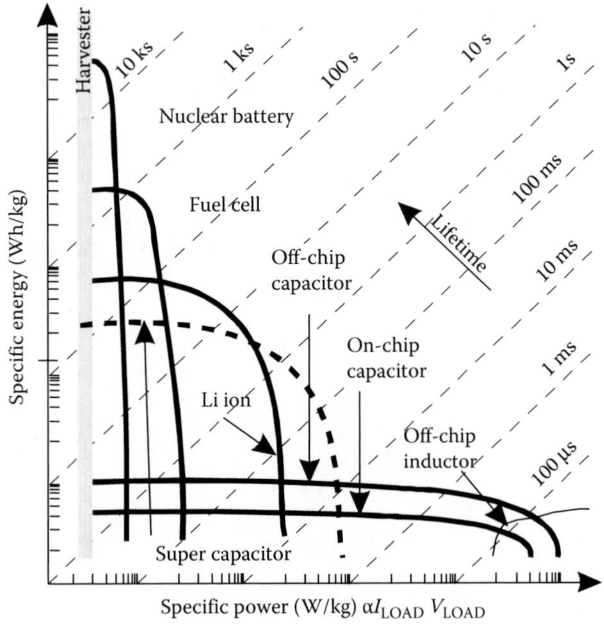

FIGURE 1.3 Ragone plot: relative energy–power performance of various energy-storage devices.

for purchase, although admittedly, not as popular as coin cells because practical applications for them are just now emerging or about to emerge. Nonetheless, the fundamental advantage of Li ions is that, in their solid-state form, they are thin at 0.31 mm and conform to almost any two-dimensional plane; in other words, copackaging or attaching them to a chip is relatively straightforward.

Outside of integration, Li ions also tend to outperform their rechargeable lead–acid, alkaline, nickel–metal–hydride, and nickel–cadmium counterparts in capacity, cycle life, internal resistance, and self-discharge [4]. Cycle life, which refers to the number of discharge–recharge cycles a battery endures before significantly losing capacity (i.e., energy), is typically 10,000 cycles or higher for Li ions and well below 1000 for competing chemistries, except for ultracapacitors, which feature the highest cycle-life performance today. Similarly, internal resistance and self-discharge rates are considerably lower than nickel-based chemistries and relatively constant across cycle life.

Where Li ions falter is in intrinsic cost and management complexity, which lamentably adds cost. The problem is that, to yield the highest possible capacity without suffering irreversible damage, a Li ion charger must (1) carefully precondition the battery when fully exhausted (e.g., at roughly 2.7 V) and (2) accurately charge to but not exceed its maximum rated voltage (e.g., of around 4.2 V). As a result, Li-ion charger circuits usually demand higher power and occupy more silicon area. As stated earlier, however, while compromising performance for cost is acceptable in certain products, such as flash lights, for example, doing so in mobile applications is often impractical because a portable music player, for example, that only plays for 1 h and survives not more than 100 recharge cycles falls short of the three-year average-product-life expectations that modern consumers nowadays demand. Many wireless microsensor applications are even less forgiving, requiring 5–10-year life cycles.

1.2.2 Fuel Cells

Fuel cells are popular in relatively large applications, such as in hybrid electric vehicles, but the question is: Are they feasible at and scalable down to, microscale dimensions? The answer is not obvious, so only time and research will tell. From a practical perspective, passive direct-methanol (DM) proton-exchange membranes (PEMs), a sample of which Figure 1.4 illustrates, enjoy popularity because they do not require mechanical overhead in the form of fuel reformers and (activating) pressure regulators, which would otherwise complicate the structure and impede integration. PEMs are relatively simple and compatible with MEMS technologies, requiring only a PEM, two electrodes and fuel [5]. The membrane, in layman language, is a proton filter in that it only allows protons through. In more chemical terms, the membrane is the medium in which methanol reacts with an oxidant to release carbon dioxide (CO_2) back into the tank and generate, on the other end, water (H_2O) in the vapor phase and ionic charge (i.e., electricity). The truth is that a fuel cell *converts* energy and so it is more like a transducer than a source. Fuel cells become 0.4–0.7-V sources, generally speaking, when fed with fuel and, more specifically, batteries (whose energy eventually depletes under a load over time) when fed from a fuel tank of finite dimensions and therefore limited capacity.

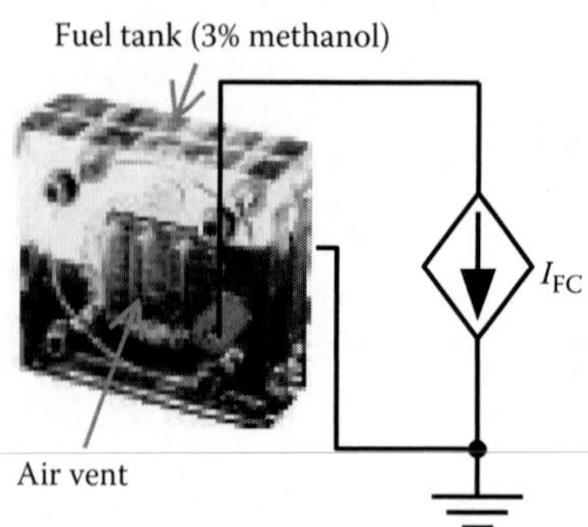

FIGURE 1.4 DM PEM fuel-cell prototype.

Managing by-products is a considerable shortcoming of fuel cells, unfortunately. The system must, for example, seep CO_2 from the tank into the surrounding environment to prevent internal pressure from bursting the structure. The selectivity of the CO_2 filter is also a critical parameter because leaking methanol amounts to losing energy. More challenging is keeping methanol from leaking through the PEM, which is probably the most difficult hurdle research faces today under microscale constraints. To complicate matters, the application must accommodate or somehow absorb the by-products. All the same, at these scales of integration, water and CO_2, in the case of DM PEMs, are relatively benign, and considering that more advances in fuel-cell research will undoubtedly result as time passes, the allure of higher energy densities is difficult to dismiss.

1.2.3 Nuclear Batteries

In the search for higher energy, nuclear batteries outshine most other technologies, albeit at lower power levels. The heat this technology generates at larger scales can fuel thermoelectric generators for a decade, for example. Similarly, the electrons the decaying isotopes emit at micrometer scales can establish a sufficiently strong electric field (and voltage) across parallel and mechanically compliant piezoelectric plates to attract the charged plates and induce current flow upon contact. The emitted electrons can also generate electron–hole pairs in p–n-junction devices, much like photons in photovoltaic cells. Like their photon counterparts, these β-voltaic batteries enjoy the benefits of chip integration. Atomic energy, however, suffers from safety, containment, and cost concerns that may eventually preclude them from ever entering the marketplace. Still, unequaled energy levels continue to propel research, even if the market hesitates.

1.2.4 Ambient Energy

Last but certainly not least in the race for extended operational life is harnessing ambient energy from light, motion, heat, and magnetic fields. Miniature transducers and accompanying microelectronic conditioners are at the forefront of research and, at moderate scales, also at the edge of commercialization. The fact that ambient energy represents a virtually boundless source for a tiny harvester is almost sufficient motivation to drive research forward and entice industry to invest in developing relevant technologies. Lower cost and the absence of by-products further tilt the pendulum of public opinion on the side of harvesters, relegating atomic batteries to special applications that the military, for example, might demand.

1.2.4.1 Light Energy

Solar light is perhaps the most appealing source because, when exposed to the sun, photovoltaic cells can generate 10–15 mW/cm² [6], which is well above those of its counterparts. In effect, incoming photons, as graphically shown in Figure 1.5a, break loosely tied electrons and therefore avail and conduct electron–hole pairs. The voltage that results, however, forward-biases the parasitic

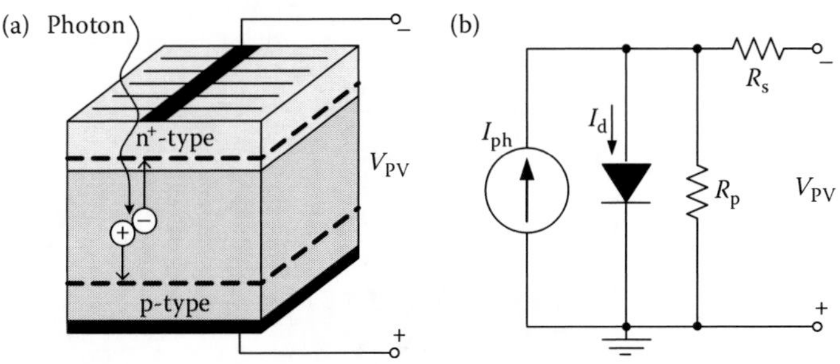

FIGURE 1.5 (a) Photovoltaic cell and (b) corresponding equivalent circuit model.

p–n junction present (Figure 1.5b), which means the diode sinks some of the generated current. The problem with solar energy is that output power falls drastically when direct sunlight is unavailable, down to 10–20 μW/cm^2. These power levels are so low that the act of harnessing, by which is meant the work performed by circuits to transfer energy into a battery, may dissipate most, if not all, of the power available, negating the harvesting objective of the system. Notwithstanding, a few researchers find solace in how often microsystems idle because producing any power whatsoever for extended periods still translates to appreciable energy in the long run.

Industry and research today concentrate most of their efforts either on larger scale systems, where larger surface areas compensate for the lower power densities indoor lighting generates, or on smaller photovoltaic cells that receive direct sunlight, where even 2 × 2 mm^2 generates substantial power (i.e., for a microsystem). Relying on solar energy, however, limits wide-scale adoption because, on one hand, applications may not always place harvesting nodes in places that receive direct sunlight, and on the other, overcast days and evenings interrupt the harvesting process. Many applications, in fact, are not only indoors, such as wireless microsensors in factories, hospitals, and homes, but also mobile, where the host may or may not receive sunlight, as with automobiles, bicycles, airplanes, and people. All this amounts to saying that harnessing indoor lighting is important but challenging under microscale constraints.

1.2.4.2 Kinetic Energy

By definition, mobile products, which represent an increasingly expansive market space, move. And from a commercial standpoint, harnessing kinetic energy from motion is attractive because vibrations are consistent and abundant, be it an engine at 1000–10,000 revolutions per minute or a person at 1–2 strides/s. Kinetic transducers can also generate up to 200 μW/cm^2, providing the onboard harvesting microelectronics more power (when compared to indoor lighting) to operate. Even though power is nowhere near what photovoltaic cells produce when exposed to direct sunlight, harnessing power from dependable 2–300-Hz vibrations over extended periods, as before, accumulates appreciable energy.

One way of drawing power from motion is electromagnetically [7], by allowing vibrations to move a mass attached to a conducting coil about a stationary magnet, as illustrated in Figure 1.6. The electromagnetic field that the magnet generates dampens the kinetic force in the moving mass and decelerates it, thereby transferring the energy in the mass into the coil in the form of a voltage. The role of the spring is to avoid losing remnant energy by temporarily storing and releasing whatever kinetic energy remains so that the mass may once again move back toward the magnet.

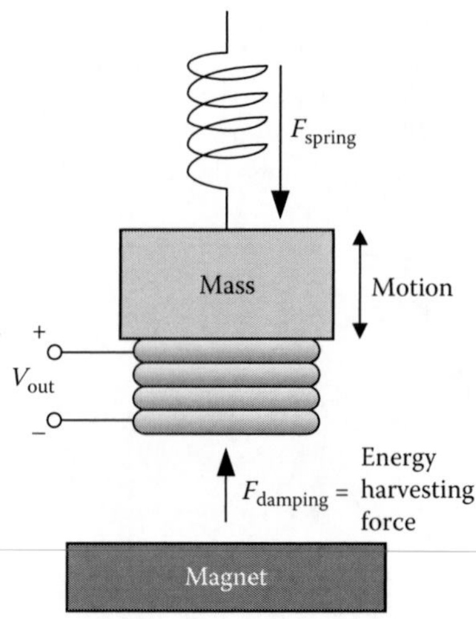

FIGURE 1.6 Transducing kinetic energy in vibrations into the electrical domain electromagnetically.

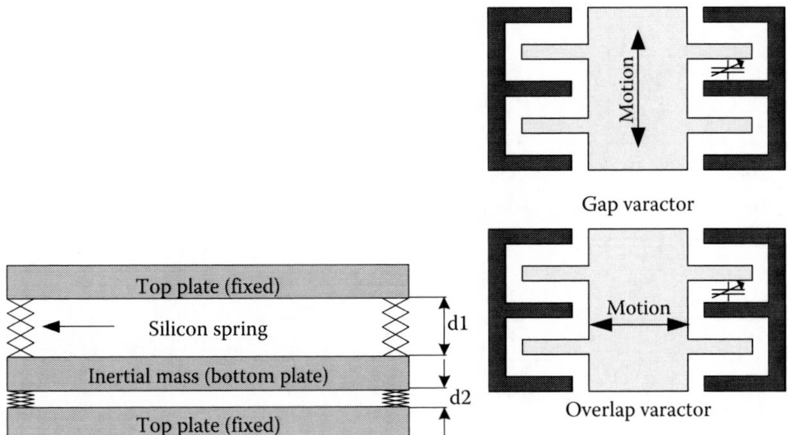

FIGURE 1.7 Vertical profile view and lateral top view of MEMS-compatible variable parallel-plate capacitors (i.e., varactors).

Unfortunately, harnessing energy in this manner is difficult in small volumes because power and voltages are substantially low at approximately 1 μW/cm^3 and tens of mVs. Additionally, conforming and integrating a magnet and a coil into a microsystem also present considerable challenges.

A more effective means of harnessing ambient kinetic energy is by pumping charge electrostatically into a storage device because the power generated is on the order of 50–100 μW/cm^2 and variable capacitors are more easily integrated with MEMS technologies. The idea is for vibrations to vary the vertical or lateral separation distance between two parallel plates of a variable capacitor C_{VAR} (Figure 1.7) so that, when a battery fixes the voltage across C_{VAR}, a reduction in capacitance decreases C_{VAR}'s charge q_C, where

$$C_{VAR} \equiv q_C v_C = q_C V_{BAT}, \tag{1.1}$$

thereby outputting dq_C/dt current [8]. Alternatively, a reduction in capacitance increases v_C when leaving C_{VAR} open-circuited (i.e., fixing q_C), which augments C_{VAR}'s energy E_C, where

$$E_C = 0.5 C_{VAR} v_C^2. \tag{1.2}$$

This latter scenario produces a net energy gain because, while C_{VAR} decreases linearly, E_C's v_C^2 increases quadratically. Allowing v_C to increase to, say, 100–300 V, however, which is not atypical, exceeds the breakdown limits of most vanilla CMOS and BiCMOS process technologies. As a result, at least for the time being, constraining v_C to V_{BAT} seems more practical than fixing q_C.

Although piezoelectric transducers are perhaps more difficult to integrate, they can generate higher power, up to maybe 200 μW/cm^2. Here, a shimmed piezoelectric cantilever, when fastened to a stationary base, as illustrated in Figure 1.8, generates electrical energy in the form of AC charge when mechanical energy in vibrations induces the material to bend and oscillate about its fixed point [9]. The advantages of this approach are that (1) piezoelectric research is relatively mature in its evolution and (2) transducers generate higher power than their electrostatic and electromagnetic counterparts. The disadvantage, of course, is integrating the device, which is why attaching it to the outer surface of a chip is probably one of the best ways of realizing a small SoP platform.

1.2.4.3 Thermal Energy

Temperature represents another source of energy. Thermocouples based on the Seebeck effect, for example, as illustrated in Figure 1.9a, derive thermal energy from a temperature difference. Here,

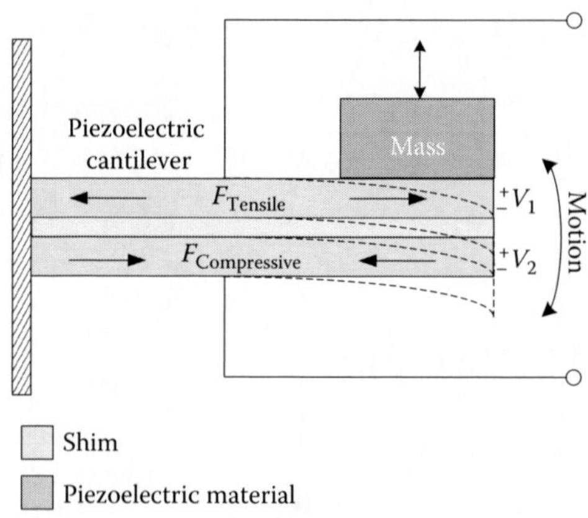

FIGURE 1.8 Shimmed piezoelectric cantilever in response to vibrations.

heat flux carries the dominant charge carriers of each material (i.e., electrons in n- and holes in p-type) from high- to low-temperature regions, much like diffusion would from high- to low-concentration areas. As electrons disappear from the hot end, they leave behind ionized molecules that, instead of attracting holes *from the* n-*type* material itself, attract carriers from the opposite (p-) type rod that is attached (via a low-resistance metallic short). Therefore, as electrons flow from p- to n-type regions to deionize molecules, they absorb (or equivalently, harness) thermal energy, which means electrons jump to a higher energy state. As a result, electrons accumulating at the cold end of the n-type material establish a negative potential with respect to the holes that accrue at the cold end of the p-type rod, generating thermally induced voltages V_1 and V_2 in Figure 1.9a and $V_{Thermal}$ or $V_1 + V_2$ in the corresponding circuit model of Figure 1.9b.

Note that high temperature alone is not sufficient to generate power. In other words, a thermocouple generates a voltage only when a temperature differential exists. Engineers, as a result, usually attach one of the terminals to a cool source via a thermally conducting material (i.e., a heat sink). This requirement impedes integration in two ways. In the first place, not only does a heat sink

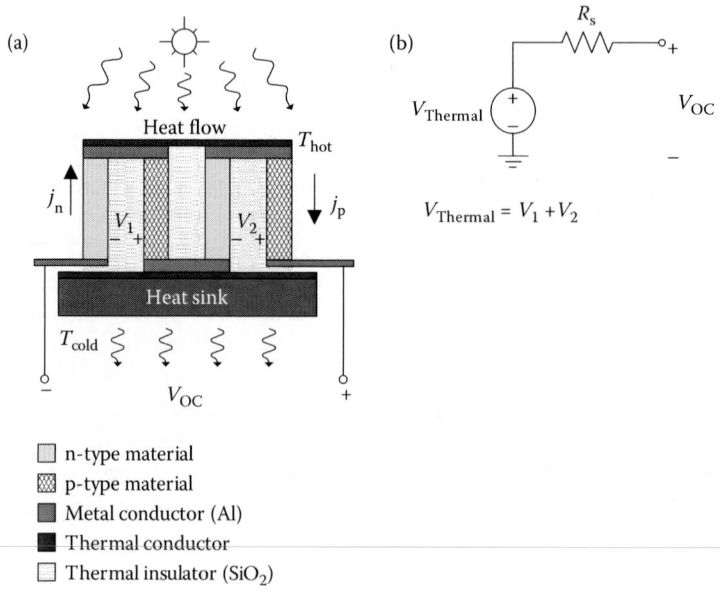

FIGURE 1.9 Seebeck-based thermocouple (a) transducer and (b) corresponding circuit model.

demand space but finding a cool source against which to attach the transducer is not a given for many applications. Second, output power is proportional to the temperature difference across the device and, because microsystems are necessarily small, temperature differentials are correspondingly low, below maybe 10°C. The voltage and power levels they produce are consequently low at about 15 μW/cm^3 [7], which nears the levels produced by indoor lighting and vibrations with an electromagnetic transducer. Power, incidentally, is also proportional to the Seebeck coefficient of the thermoelectric materials used.

1.2.4.4 Magnetic Energy

There is also energy in a magnetic field, such as around an AC power line. Drawing power from such a source inductively, however, is challenging in three respects. To start, like in the case of harnessing kinetic energy electromagnetically, the power levels and voltages generated are substantially low at microwatts and millivolts. While, on one hand, the act of transferring energy already dissipates microwatts and therefore drains most of the little power that is available, on the other, conditioning power in the form of millivolts is, from an integrated circuit's perspective, problematic. As a result, some researchers opt to accumulate and convert magnetic energy into the mechanical domain first, so that a kinetic transducer can then generate power in a more benign form. Unfortunately, each conversion suffers from losses that further reduce what energy was available in the first place.

The second issue with an electromagnetic source is that power decreases drastically with distance: quadratically in the far field and even faster in the near field. As a result, the transducer, to produce useful power, must remain close to a rich source. Such an application exists, as in the case of inductively coupling energy across a near-field separation of, say, 8 mm to wirelessly charge the battery of a portable device, such as a cellular phone. Increasing the distance beyond this point, however, which many wireless microsystems require, decreases system efficiency to such an extent that its commercial appeal loses ground. The third challenge with harvesting magnetic energy is, of course, integration, because the transducer, which reduces to a reasonably good but bulky transformer, is difficult to integrate.

1.2.5 Conclusions

As mentioned earlier, there is no ideal source because, while harvesters, atomic batteries, and fuel cells store appreciable energy, they supply little power. Conversely, inductors and capacitors source high power but stow little energy. And Li ions and supercapacitors are moderate in both respects, sacrificing energy for power and power for energy. Additionally, while filter passives supply power almost instantaneously, Li ions and supercapacitors require time to respond, and fuel cells even more time, whereas atomic batteries and harvesters remain virtually unresponsive to load changes. As a result, systems today normally supply what is close to instantaneous power, which refers to the rising and falling edges of the load shown in Figure 1.1, with capacitors and semisustained bursts with a Li ion.

Relegating the tasks of storing energy and supplying power bursts to a Li ion, however, represents a compromise in energy that is difficult to accept under microscale constraints where both energy- and power-density requirements are severe. Replacing the Li ion with a fuel cell similarly trades power for energy, loading capacitors and inductors with more power and, as a result, increasing either output voltage variations in response to load dumps or space requirements. Further decoupling energy from power is therefore important in microsystems, which is the motivation for classifying technologies into energy sources, energy/power caches, and power supplies.

Harvesters, atomic batteries, and fuel cells fall under the category of energy sources. Of these, atomic batteries are less popular because they are unsafe and costly. Tiny fuel cells, on one hand, source more power (consistently) than harvesters (which are intermittent) but, on the other, produce by-products that are not always easy to manage and so both enjoy popularity in research and industry. Li ions and supercapacitors basically cache energy and power for moderate loads, but while Li ions are perhaps more mature and popular, ultracapacitors survive more charge–discharge cycles, which is why the latter is garnering interest. Finally, capacitors and inductors both supply power, but only capacitors supply instantaneous current, so systems use capacitors to store charge and supply quick load dumps and inductors to supply the collective steady-state needs of the loads and momentary demands of the capacitors.

Of the available ambient sources, solar energy generates the most power, followed by kinetic energy when harnessed by piezoelectric or electrostatic means. Thermal and magnetic energy are less appealing under microscale integration because their power and voltage levels are low. Similarly, indoor lighting also generates low power levels, as does drawing kinetic energy electromagnetically. As a result, some engineers favor solar photovoltaic and vibration-sensitive piezoelectric and electrostatic transducers over their competing counterparts.

1.3 CONDITIONING MICROELECTRONICS

The role of the power-supply circuit in a system is to transfer energy from a source and condition power to supply the needs of its load. Because energy is finite and especially scarce in a microsystem, the overriding measure of success, outside of conditioning, is how much of the available power P_{IN} reaches the output (as P_O). In other words, the power lost (P_L) across the system in relation to P_O determines one of the most important parameters of a power supply: efficiency η or

$$\eta \equiv \frac{P_O}{P_{IN}} = \frac{P_O}{P_O + P_L} \tag{1.3}$$

For example, if the load demands 100 μW and the power supply dissipates 50 μW to generate those 100 μW, then the source supplies 150 μW because the system is 66.7% efficient. Similarly, in the case of harvesters, if a source supplies 100 μW but the system dissipates 50 μW, the output only receives 50 μW at 50%.

Efficiency typically changes with output power P_O because losses do not vary at the same rate. At moderate power, for example, quiescent losses usually become a smaller fraction of a rising load, so efficiency is relatively high [10], such as when losing 75 μW to drive a 1-mW load yields 93%. Unfortunately, because microsystems normally demand lower power levels, losses represent a larger percentage of the load, so efficiency is low, such as when losing 50 μW to drive 50 μW results in 50% efficiency. What is worse, microsystems normally idle and dissipate even less power, such as maybe 1–10 μW. Under these idling conditions, operational life is sensitive to power losses because the lifetime difference of a 1- and a 9-μW loss under a 10-μW load is close to 70% or 1.7× and under a 100-μW load is 10% or 1.1×, and dissipating less than 1 μW is extremely difficult, if not impossible, when powering alert functions and other vital blocks in the system. All this amounts to saying that light load efficiency is probably one of the most difficult challenges to tackle in a microsystem, especially when the act of conditioning, in and of itself, requires work.

1.3.1 LINEAR

Perhaps the most accurate means of conditioning power is linearly because the circuit is always alert, ready to respond to any and all variations in load and source. In other words, in addition to not generating switching noise, a linear conditioner reacts to oppose the effects of transient disturbances injected and coupled into its output. Admittedly, the circuit suppresses noise only up to its bandwidth [11], beyond which the system is unable to respond. Nevertheless, a linear circuit is relatively simple, so it reaps the high-bandwidth benefits that smaller devices and fewer transistors offer.

Architecturally, as shown in Figure 1.10, a controller modulates the conductance of a series switch linearly to conduct whatever current the system demands. In the case shown, a p-channel metal-oxide-semiconductor (MOS) field-effect transistor M_{PS} is only a sample, but nonetheless

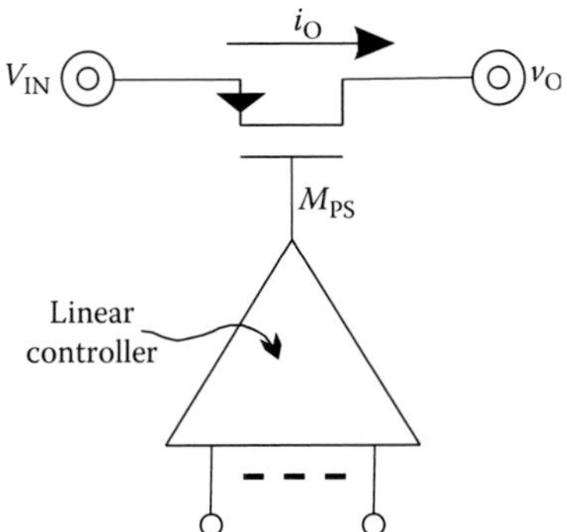

FIGURE 1.10 Basic architecture of a linear LDO conditioner.

popular embodiment of the switch. Low-dropout (LDO) linear regulators, for example, use this topology and sample output voltage v_O to ensure that v_O remains near a user-defined target. Sensing output current i_O, to illustrate another application, and regulating M_{PS}'s conductance (i.e., series resistance R_{PS}) to draw as much i_O as the source allows satisfies the objectives of a harvester.

Irrespective of its conditioning aim, what is ultimately important to conclude is that (1) the circuit does not generate switching noise, (2) DC current I_O only flows to the output (in one direction) and so steady-state input V_{IN} must exceed steady-state output V_O, and (3) the circuit dissipates conduction power across M_{PS} (as P_{PS}) and quiescent power through the controller (as P_C):

$$P_L = P_{PS} + P_C = I_O\left(V_{IN} - V_O\right) + I_Q V_{IN}, \tag{1.4}$$

where $V_{IN} - V_O$ is the voltage across M_{PS} and I_Q is the current V_{IN} supplies to the controller. Although all three points are important, the last one deserves attention because microsystems cannot afford to lose power indiscriminately. Efficiency here, in fact, cannot ever reach the output-to-input voltage ratio V_O/V_{IN} because the voltage across M_{PS} is, by design, $V_{IN} - V_O$ and I_Q is a finite physical requirement for the circuit to operate properly:

$$\eta \equiv \frac{P_O}{P_O + P_L} = \frac{I_O V_O}{I_O V_O + I_O\left(V_{IN} - V_O\right) + I_Q V_{IN}} = \frac{I_O V_O}{I_O V_{IN} + I_Q V_{IN}} < \frac{V_O}{V_{IN}}. \tag{1.5}$$

Consider, for example, that when a 3.6-V Li ion supplies a 1.8-V load, η is no better than 50%, and that is only when I_Q is negligibly smaller than I_O, which is largely not the case in microsystems, particularly when they idle.

1.3.2 Switched Capacitors

Introducing one or more intermediate steps into the energy-transfer process further decouples the needs of the input from those of the output, adding flexibility to the conditioning function. A transitional stage therefore receives, stores, and releases energy when prompted, as a capacitor would when configured accordingly. Charge pumps, as many design engineers refer to them, switch the connectivity of "flying" capacitors in alternate phases across a switching period T_{SW} to first receive energy from a source, be it the actual input or a previous stage, and then release it to a load, which could be just another intermediate stage. The point is charging several flying capacitors in parallel, for instance, from input V_{IN}, as C_{F1} through C_{FN} illustrate in Figure 1.11, and discharging them to a load in series effectively "steps up" or "boosts" the input V_{IN} to a higher voltage v_O, which is an otherwise impossible feat for a linear conditioner to achieve. Similarly, just to show how flexible the

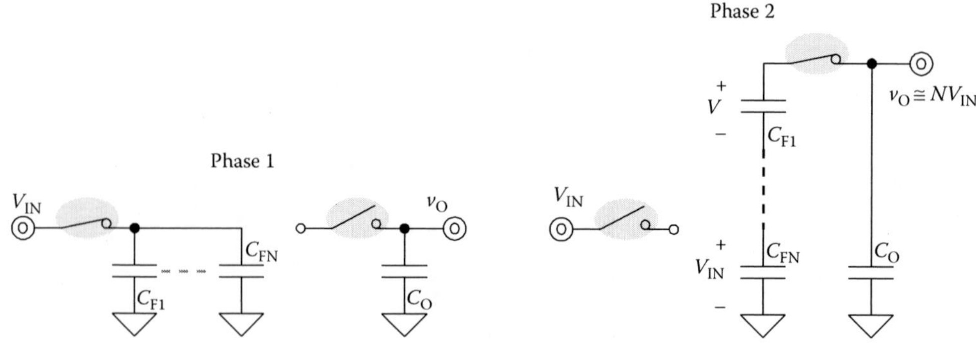

FIGURE 1.11 Switching phases of a boosting two-step charge pump.

architecture can be, charging capacitors from V_{IN} in series and connecting them in parallel with v_O in the alternate phase "steps down" or "bucks" V_{IN} to a lower voltage.

This flexibility, however, results at the expense of noise because decoupling V_{IN} from v_O implies v_O is, at times, disconnected from its source, so the load momentarily discharges whatever output capacitance C_O is present. Allowing C_O to droop this way, before periodically recharging it with the flying capacitors, creates a steady-state ripple in the output Δv_O that amounts to systematic switching noise. To this, the switches, whose task is to reconfigure the connectivity of the network, inject additional noise, because the signals that drive them at switching frequency f_{SW} rise and fall quickly in maybe 10 ns or less, coupling displacement noise energy into sensitive nodes through parasitic devices such as the gate-source and gate-drain capacitors C_{GS} and C_{DG} in CMOS switches.

Because the voltages across conducting switches are dynamic and decrease with time, switched-capacitor circuits do not dissipate the static and often limiting $V_{IN} - V_O$ voltage-drop conduction power that linear conditioners do across M_{PS}. Still, the switches lose momentary switching losses when conducting current with decreasing, but nonetheless finite voltages across them. The initial voltage across the switch that connects V_{IN} to the flying capacitors in Phase 1 of Figure 1.11, for example, is the voltage the load drooped in Phase 2, which is oftentimes not a trivial amount. Similarly, the fully charged flying capacitors and the drooped C_O also present a voltage difference to their connecting switch at the beginning of Phase 2. To help quantify this loss, consider that while V_{IN} in Figure 1.12a loses energy E_{IN} to charge equivalent flying capacitor C_{EQ} from 0 to V_{IN} as

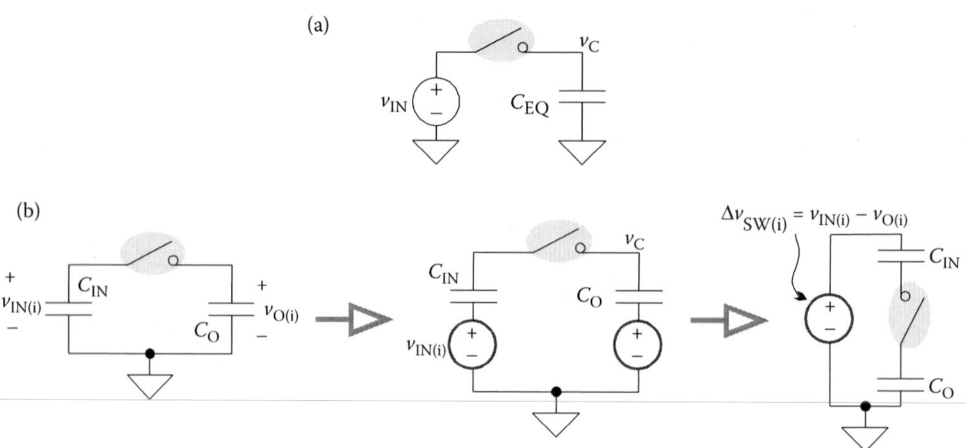

FIGURE 1.12 Charging a capacitor through a switch from (a) an input source and (b) another capacitor.

$$E_{IN} = Q_C V_{IN} = \left(C_{EQ} \Delta v_C\right) V_{IN} \rightarrow C_{EQ} V_{IN}^2, \tag{1.6}$$

C_{EQ} only receives half that energy as

$$E_C = 0.5 C_{EQ} \Delta v_C^2 \rightarrow 0.5 C_{EQ} V_{IN}^2, \tag{1.7}$$

which means the switch used or rather lost the other half [12] as

$$E_{SW} = E_{IN} - E_C = C_{EQ} \Delta v_C V_{IN} - 0.5 C_{EQ} \Delta v_C^2 \rightarrow 0.5 C_{EQ} V_{IN}^2. \tag{1.8}$$

Similarly, because connecting capacitors in parallel, as in Figure 1.12b, equates to charging them in series from a source whose voltage is the initial voltage across the switch $v_{IN(i)} - v_{O(i)}$ or $\Delta v_{SW(i)}$, the switch uses

$$E_{SW} = 0.5\left(C_{IN} \oplus C_O\right)\left(v_{IN(i)} - v_{O(i)}\right)^2 = 0.5 C_{EQ} \Delta v_{SW(i)}^2 \tag{1.9}$$

of the energy that was initially stored in C_{IN} as $0.5 C_{IN} v_{IN(i)}^2$, where C_{EQ} is the series combination of C_{IN} and C_O. In other words, charge pumps generally and necessarily lose switching energy $0.5 C_{EQ} \Delta v_{SW(i)}^2$ in the connecting switches.

Although this fundamental switching loss is by no means negligible, it decreases with reductions in load because all the capacitors droop less (so $\Delta v_{SW(i)}$ is smaller) with lower currents, which is good for microsystems because they demand little to no power when they idle. In practice, however, V_{IN} still supplies the energy that switching noise and leakage currents draw from the capacitors, the quiescent power that energizes the controller, and the switching power that parasitic gate and base capacitors require to charge and discharge every time they switch. So in summary, a charge pump (1) generates switching noise, (2) is able to "buck" or "boost" its input, and (3) dissipates switching power $0.5 C_{EQ} \Delta v_{SW(i)}^2 f_{SW}$ across its connecting switches in proportion to the square of the load (because $\Delta v_{SW(i)}$ is proportional to output current i_O). When compared against its linear counterpart, the output is noisy and less accurate, but also flexible, and the circuit impresses voltages across the switches that not only decrease with load but also decrease with time. Charge pumps also dissipate power to charge and discharge parasitic capacitors that would normally not switch periodically in a linear conditioner.

1.3.3 Switched Inductor

Just as charge pumps employ capacitors to transfer energy, magnetic-based switching converters use inductors to temporarily cache and release input energy to one or several loads [13]. They achieve this by energizing and de-energizing inductors in alternating cycles. In more specific terms, an input source V_{IN} energizes an inductor L_O by inducing L_O to draw current from V_{IN}, that is to say, by connecting the other terminal of L_O to a lower voltage, like ground in Phase 1 of Figure 1.13a. During this time, L_O's current i_L rises linearly, as the graph in Figure 1.13b shows, because L_O's voltage v_L, which equals $L_O di_L/dt$, is positive and constant at, in this case, $V_{IN} - 0$, or more generally, at energizing voltage V_E. Reversing the polarity of v_L to, say, $-v_O$, as shown in Phase 2 of Figure 1.13a, causes L_O to release the energy it received during Phase 1. Because the circuit either regulates the voltage across a load or charges a battery with a well-defined, low-ripple, slow-changing voltage, v_O is, for all practical purposes, a constant, and in this case, also L_O's de-energizing voltage V_{DE}. As a result, i_L generally rises at V_E/L_O when V_{IN} energizes L_O (during Phase 1) and falls at V_{DE}/L_O when L_O delivers energy to v_O (during Phase 2) [14].

A switched-inductor conditioner embodies a few idiosyncrasies worth mentioning. First, L_O conducts DC current, so i_L's ripple Δi_L rides on a steady-state offset $i_{L(avg)}$ or I_L that can also be zero. Conducting current continuously like this places the circuit in what experts call continuous-conduction mode, and inducing L_O to stop conducting current momentarily, which is equivalent to i_L reaching zero and remaining there for a finite fraction of the period, amounts to operating in discontinuous-conduction mode (DCM). What sets $i_{L(avg)}$ is either the power needs of a load or the sourcing capabilities of its source.

Another trait, or rather feature, is that a switched-inductor circuit can buck or boost v_{IN} because L_O can release energy to any output voltage as long as energizing and de-energizing voltages V_E and V_{DE} remain positive and negative, respectively. In fact, permanently attaching L_O's input terminal to V_{IN} is a special embodiment of the general form shown in Figure 1.13a that, to release L_O's energy, requires V_O to exceed V_{IN}. Likewise, connecting L_O's output terminal to v_O directly demands that V_{IN} stay above V_O for L_O to energize. These two special cases, incidentally, implement the well-known boost [15] and buck [16] configurations reported in literature. One last peculiarity to note is that inductors, unlike capacitors, receive *or* deliver energy, not store it statically over time, which is not really a problem in conditioners because the overriding aim is to draw and deliver power, not store it, like rechargeable batteries and large capacitors would.

Within the context of operational life and efficiency, the only elements in a power stage that incur first-order conduction losses are the switches because a capacitor does not conduct DC current and the steady-state voltage across an inductor is zero. Interestingly, while capacitors hold the initial voltage across a switch by sourcing whatever instantaneous currents are necessary, an inductor maintains its current steady by instantly swinging its voltage until it finds a suitable source or sink for the current. In other words, after a connecting switch opens, the inductor induces its terminal voltage to swing instantaneously until it matches the voltage attached to the next switch in the sequence, inducing the small series resistance R_{SW} through the ensuing switch to conduct L_O's average current I_L across time with a voltage and power that is close to zero at $I_L R_{SW}$ and $I_L^2 R_{SW}$. This quasi-lossless property is the driving force behind the commercialization and general adoption of switched-inductor conditioners.

In practice, these conduction losses are small, but nevertheless finite so they reduce efficiency, as do second-order losses similar to those found in linear and charge-pump circuits. The controller, for example, requires sufficient quiescent current to manage the system and deliver a command signal in time before the onset of the next switching cycle. The circuit also dissipates switching power to charge and discharge the parasitic capacitors that the switches present to the controller. When lightly

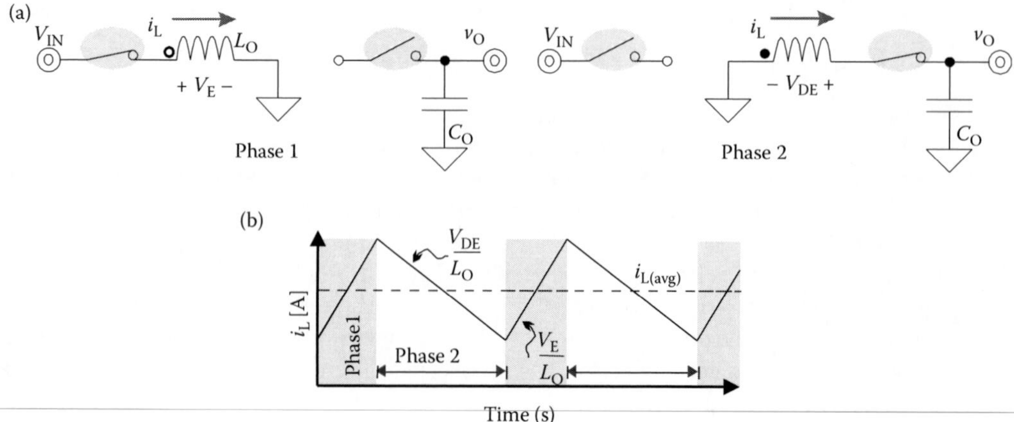

FIGURE 1.13 (a) Switching phases of a switched-inductor converter and (b) the time-domain response of its inductor current.

loaded, in fact, second-order quiescent and switching losses become as important as and in some cases more important than first-order conduction losses because the voltage dropped and power lost across the switches fade with decreasing load levels [17].

Note, however, that good and reasonably sized power inductors are bulky and difficult to integrate [18]. The unfortunate truth is that on-chip inductances typically fall below 100 nH and introduce considerable parasitic equivalent-series resistances that further dissipate conduction power and degrade efficiency. Discrete inductors, on the other hand, are considerably better, and to a certain extent, also relatively small, like for example, a $2 \times 2 \times 1\text{-mm}^3$ 1-μH inductor might saturate at 1.8 A and introduce 0.2 Ω of series resistance. Accordingly, switched-inductor conditioners in microsystems should employ and copackage no more than one power inductor, which is why single-inductor multiple-output (SIMO) strategies are garnering interest in research circles [13]. Using smaller inductances is certainly possible, however, but at the expense of higher conduction losses (because the inductor ripple current Δi_L increases) or switching losses (because the switching frequency f_{SW} increases to keep Δi_L bounded).

Because these magnetic-based circuits switch, they, like charge pumps, introduce switching noise into v_O. If L_O connects directly to v_O via a metallic link, however, like in buck converters, L_O's average current I_L always flows to v_O, which means that I_L matches the DC load and the load in no way discharges output capacitance C_O in steady state. Even so, the ripple inductor current Δi_L never reaches the load, so Δi_L charges and discharges C_O to create a corresponding ripple in v_O. Decoupling v_O from L_O with a switch, unfortunately, as in boost converters, allows the load to discharge C_O when the switch opens, increasing the ripple in v_O. In all, these magnetic conditioners (1) generate switching noise, (2) are able to "buck" or "boost" their inputs, (3) dissipate first-order conduction power $I_L^2 R_{SW}$ across their connecting switches in proportion to the square of the load, and when applied to microsystems, (4) should employ not more than one copackaged inductor.

1.3.4 Conclusions

In comparing performance, the functionality of the conditioners precedes all other parameters, and in the case of microsystems, losses arguably follow because they limit how long a system operates. So on the first count, switching circuits can boost their inputs, while linear circuits cannot, except that a boosting function is not always necessary. Consider, for example, that whereas boosting a 0.4–0.7-V fuel cell to charge a 2.7–4.2-V Li ion requires a switching circuit, bucking a 2.7–4.2-V Li ion to supply a 1.8-V load does not.

From the perspective of power, as summarized in Table 1.1, the switch in a linear circuit drops $V_{IN} - V_O$ continuously, whereas the terminal voltages across the switches in a charge pump decrease with load and across time and those in a magnetic-based converter not only decrease with load but also near zero at $I_L R_{SW}$. In other words, a switched-inductor conditioner is generally the least lossy of the three. Since these losses diminish with load in all three cases, however, when microsystems idle, efficiency is more sensitive to second-order losses, which is where linear circuits might gain an edge, because they do not dissipate switching power P_{SW}. The problem is that miniature devices

TABLE 1.1
Comparing Conditioning Circuits

	V_O	First-Order Losses	Second-Order Losses	Switching Noise in v_O
Linear	Less than V_{IN}	$I_O(V_{IN} - V_O)$	P_Q	None
Switched C	Greater or less than V_{IN}	$0.5 C_{EQ} \Delta v_{SW(i)}^2 f_{SW}$ ($\Delta v_{SW(i)} \propto I_O, t$)	$P_Q + P_{SW}$	$\propto I_O, C_{PAR}, 1/f_{SW}$
Switched L	Greater or less than V_{IN}	$I_L^2 R_{SW}$ ($I_L \propto I_O$)	$P_Q + P_{SW}$	$\propto \Delta i_L$ ($1/L_O, 1/f_{SW}$) and maybe I_O, C_{PAR}

demand both little to no power when idling and moderate to substantial power when transmitting data wirelessly, so a linear circuit is more appealing when idling and less appealing otherwise, and vice versa for a switched-inductor network. In the end, functionality may become the deciding factor, which is why operating in DCM and reducing switching frequency f_{SW} in magnetic-based converters is so important when the load is light, as is decreasing quiescent power P_Q in all three schemes. Note, by the way, that parasitic series resistances in the inductor, capacitors, and board also dissipate Ohmic losses.

Noise in the output may not be a problem for charging a Li ion but is certainly an issue when supplying a functional load like a data converter or sensor-interface circuit whose sensitivity to noise in the supply is often severe. Linear circuits outshine their switching counterparts in this regard because they do not generate noise. In contrast, inductor ripple currents Δi_L in switched-inductor networks produce noise in the output across C_O. Charge pumps are probably the worst because loads momentarily and necessarily discharge C_O. Switched-inductor circuits that decouple the outputs from the inductor also suffer from similar effects, in addition to the Δi_L-induced noise already mentioned. Ultimately, reducing noise in v_O amounts to increasing f_{SW} (to shorten how long v_O floats) and circuit bandwidth (to keep up with f_{SW}), and in the case of inductor circuits, L_O (and f_{SW}) to reduce Δi_L. Raising f_{SW}, however, by and large degrades efficiency, and increasing L_O demands more space, which is the conundrum engineers eventually face when designing these types of circuits: when and how to trade accuracy, efficiency, and integration.

1.4 HYBRID SUPPLIES

The conditioners described in the last section form the foundation from which modern supplies draw inspiration. Since no converter is ideal, engineers first prioritize specifications and then choose one or a combination of approaches according to the most important parameters in the system. In a cellular phone, for instance, battery life is as sensitive to conversion efficiency as a large fraction of the load is to noise in the supply. In such a case, a switched-inductor converter bucks a Li-ion voltage efficiently to a level that minimizes the power lost across a cascaded linear voltage regulator whose purpose is to filter the noise that the switcher generates in the first place and supply the power that the sensitive load demands. In a harvester, saving energy is the chief objective so an efficient switched-inductor charger might fit the bill if power levels are sufficiently moderate for conduction losses to remain significant. Note that supplying a functional load requires a voltage source and feeding a battery a current source or charger, and while circuits may generate these without feedback, shunt- or series-sensed control loops often modulate the conductance or duty-cycle operation of the conducting switches to regulate them [19].

Space in miniature systems is so constricting that using a single sourcing technology represents a sacrifice in energy, power, or both. In these applications, complementing the energy features of fuel cells and ambient energy with the power-generating capabilities of Li ions and ultracapacitors offers appealing qualities that no single source can. Justifying the need for both energy and power, however, is imperative [20] because a hybrid supply is necessarily more complex than a one-source system. From this viewpoint, most microsystems, such as wireless microsensors, idle and communicate information wirelessly and so their power range is vast and as critical as energy, because the latter sets operational life. Hybrid supplies in tiny devices are therefore justifiable.

1.4.1 Fuel Cell–Li Ion Charger-Supply

The main role of a fuel cell in a hybrid system is to store energy and that of a Li ion is to supply power, so the former charges and replenishes the latter. At light loads, however, Figure 1.3 shows that the fuel cell can supply power longer than the Li ion, which means that the fuel cell should also supply power, but only when power is low. As a result, the charger-supply illustrated in Figure 1.14, in addition to recharging a Li ion with fuel-cell power, draws power from both sources to supply the

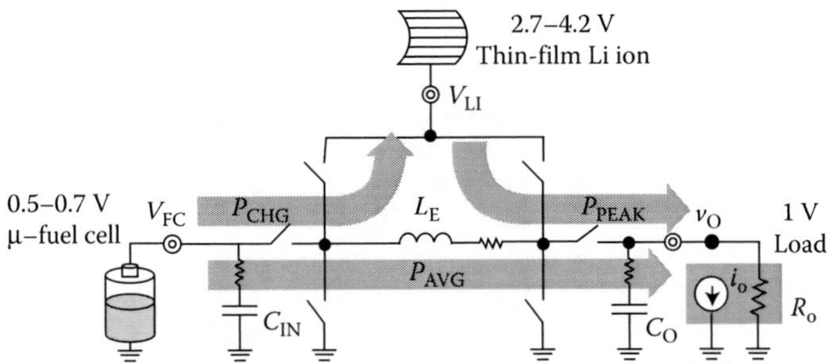

FIGURE 1.14 Single-inductor fuel cell–Li ion charger-supply.

load. As the resulting energy-flow paths indicate, the converter supplies two outputs: the Li ion and the load, and draws energy from two input sources: the fuel cell and the Li ion.

A "passive" DM PEM fuel cell, which is the kind that is best suited for integration, does not include a fuel pump. The surface area of the membrane that the methanol reaches passively, in fact, determines the power rating of the device. Unfortunately, considerable fuel leaks through the membrane as crossover loss, so a fuel cell is particularly lossy when not supplying power. In other words, in addition to not adjusting well to changing loads, fuel cells perform best when supplying constant nonzero currents.

For the fuel cell to source power P_{FC} continuously, the single-inductor multiple-input multiple-output (SIMIMO) conditioner in Figure 1.14 steers whatever P_{FC} fraction the load requires during low-power conditions to output v_O and the remainder to the Li ion. In that way, the portion that reaches v_O as P_O increases with load i_O and the Li ion recharges with what remains, even as the residue decreases with i_O. To this end, inductor L_E energizes from the fuel cell and de-energizes into v_O in alternate cycles for several switching periods ($T_{L.SW}$) until meeting the needs of the load, that is, until v_O reaches its top window target. Once there, L_E draws energy from the fuel cell to recharge the Li ion in similar alternate cycles for several $T_{L.SW}$'s until v_O falls to its lower threshold limit, at which time the converter redirects energy back into the load. This mode of operation persists as long as P_O stays below P_{FC}, which corresponds to the system's light load region of operation.

When P_O surpasses P_{FC}, during heavy loading conditions, the system supplements P_{FC} with Li-ion power P_{LI} to fully sustain the load. Accordingly, L_E energizes from the Li ion and de-energizes into v_O in alternate cycles for several $T_{L.SW}$'s until v_O rises to its top target. Once reached, L_E derives energy from the fuel cell to supply the load, but because P_{FC} is insufficient, v_O falls until it reaches its bottom threshold limit, at which point the converter switches back to drawing energy from the Li ion. Collectively, the system shifts back and forth between two modes: light and heavy, and within each mode, between two power-flow paths, where the prevalence of one path over the other depends on the needs of the load: on i_O.

Nested hysteretic control comparators realize the operation just described by switching between modes and paths according to predefined window limits for v_O [21]. If the load suddenly drops, for example, as Figure 1.15b shows when i_O falls, which means that the system sources more power than needed, v_O rises above the outer window limit $\Delta V_{O.M}$ in Figure 1.15a and b and the mode comparator that senses it sends a command for the system to enter the light mode. Once there, another comparator detects when v_O falls below the smaller window ΔV_O to steer P_{FC} into v_O and when v_O surpasses ΔV_O to redirect P_{FC} into the Li ion. If P_O again exceeds P_{FC}, like after the rising load (i_O) event in Figure 1.15b, v_O drops below the outer window $\Delta V_{O.M}$ and the mode comparator reacts by prompting the system to enter the heavy mode, inducing the switcher to source more power, where the other comparator again controls how often to direct Li-ion power P_{LI} into v_O relative to its fuel-cell counterpart P_{FC}.

The feedback operation hysteretic comparators implement to control v_O includes L_E and C_O, which together introduce a complex-conjugate pair of poles into the frequency response of the

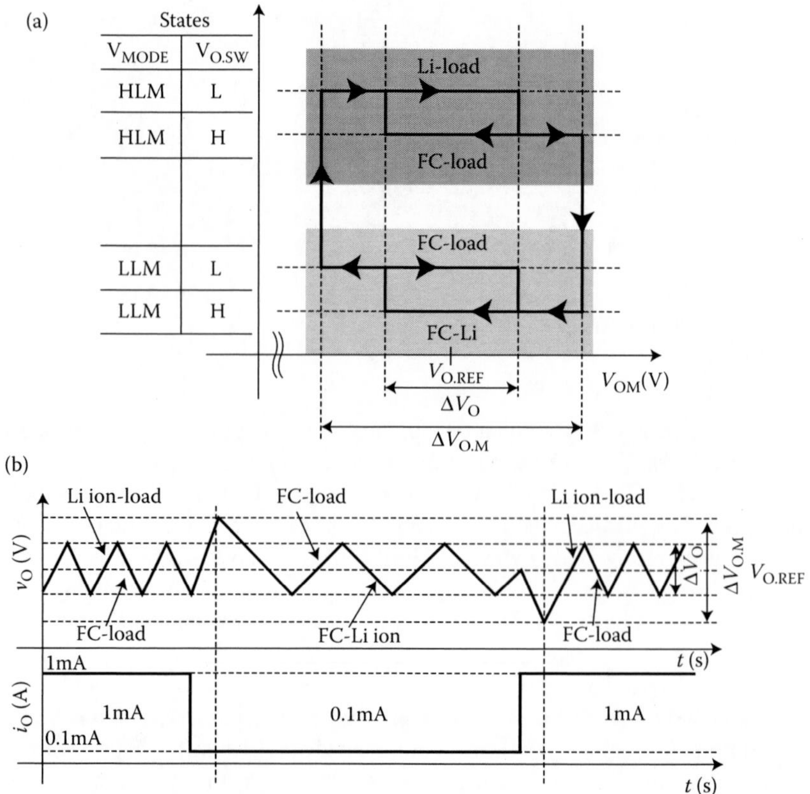

FIGURE 1.15 (a) The nested hysteretic windows that regulate output v_O in light and heavy modes and (b) the corresponding time-domain waveforms.

system. To ensure that the conditioner remains stable, a separate and faster feedback loop at switching frequency $f_{L.SW}$ regulates inductor current i_L so that the system perceives L_E as a current source at frequencies below $f_{L.SW}$. Eliminating L_E's AC effects in this fashion simplifies L_E–C_O's response to that of C_O, which reduces the complex pair of poles into a single C_O-defined pole. This faster loop, incidentally, regulates i_L about a constant lower current I_{FC} when drawing energy from the fuel cell and higher current I_{LI} otherwise.

Note that the fuel cell always sources power when lightly loaded, which is not the case for heavy loads when the Li-ion path intervenes. Since the fuel cell does not respond well to these changes, and even less to L_E's faster energize/de-energize sequence, the input capacitor C_{IN} in Figure 1.14 supplies and sinks whatever transient current the fuel cell does not. Similarly, the output capacitor C_O keeps v_O from changing abruptly by supplying and sinking whatever transient displacement currents the converter is not fast enough to source or sink.

1.4.2 Harvesting Piezoelectric Charger

Ambient power is not only lower but also less reliable than in fuel cells. The advantage, of course, is that energy in the environment is virtually boundless. Nevertheless, drawing power from an intermittent source to supply the needs of an unpredictable and uncorrelated load is problematic. As a result, harvesting and regulation are often separate and distinct functions in a microsystem. While a regulator, for example, supplies a load from a battery, a harvester can charge the battery. So in the more specific case of piezoelectric conditioners, chargers convert and condition rippling AC sources to replenish capacitors, rechargeable batteries, or a combination of both capacitors and batteries.

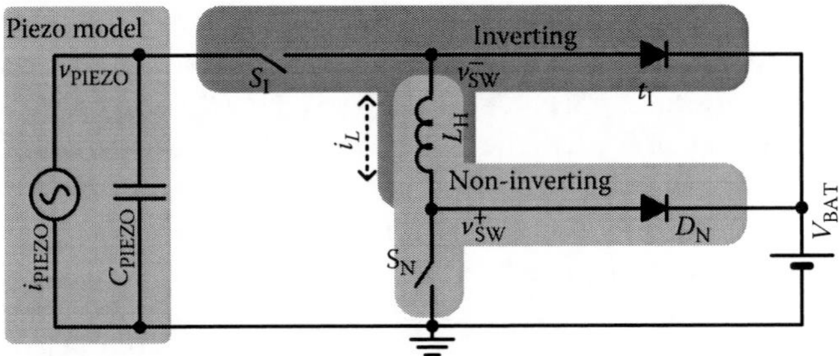

FIGURE 1.16 Single-inductor piezoelectric harvesting charger.

Typical battery-supplied implementations use a diode rectifier to convert an AC signal into a DC voltage that subsequently feeds another converter whose aim is to condition and steer power into a battery. Unfortunately, each conditioning function dissipates power, and collectively, they diminish the gains of a microscale harvester. To minimize this loss, the piezoelectric harvester in Figure 1.16 combines rectification and conditioning into one stage [22]. The underlying aim is to derive power from positive and negative piezoelectric voltages (v_{PIEZO}) with harvesting inductor L_H's forward and reverse current, respectively.

To draw energy from the positive cycle, L_H energizes from positive piezoelectric voltages into ground with switches S_I and S_N and subsequently de-energizes into battery V_{BAT} with S_I and diode D_N. Here, D_N conducts asynchronously because it carries charge only when L_H is ready to release its energy, after L_H's current (in response to S_N opening) induces L_H's positive terminal voltage v_{SW}^+ to rise automatically until forward-biasing D_N. L_H then energizes from negative piezoelectric voltages with S_I and S_N to subsequently source power into V_{BAT} through its inverting terminal v_{SW}^- and D_I. Like D_N, D_I conducts because, after opening S_I, L_H's current induces v_{SW}^- to swing high almost instantly until inducing D_I to offer a path in which to direct its power.

One of the fundamental controlling functions of the foregoing piezoelectric harvester is to synchronize L_H's positive and negative energizing events to v_{PIEZO}'s positive and negative peaks in the vibration period. Comparator CP_{PK} in Figure 1.17 achieves this by comparing v_{PIEZO} to its RD–CD-delayed counterpart v_D, tripping high when v_{PIEZO} surpasses v_D, which happens just after v_{PIEZO} reaches its minimum point on the negative cycle. Similarly, CP_{PK}'s output transitions low just after v_{PIEZO} peaks on the positive cycle, that is, after v_{PIEZO} falls below v_D. The other important role of the controller is to determine the time necessary for L_H to energize. To save energy, the circuit in Figure 1.17 introduces a preprogrammed user-tuned delay τ_{DLY} to ensure that the ensuing AND and NOR gates output an energizing command only for a preset length of time τ_{DLY}.

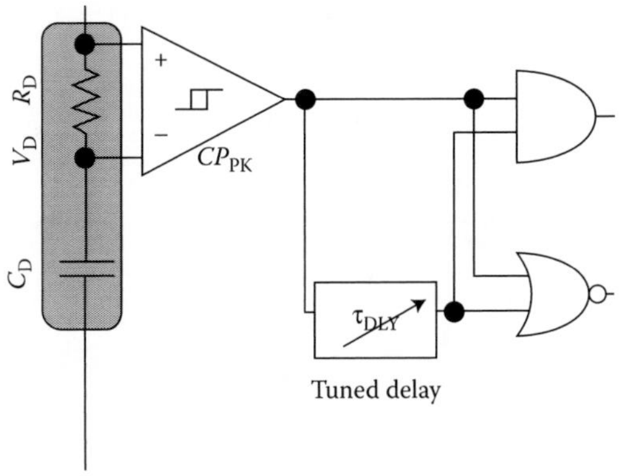

FIGURE 1.17 Peak detector and timed (user-tuned) energize-command generator.

Presetting L_H's energizing time in this fashion is perhaps a crude open-loop approach to controlling L_H. The advantage here is that there is no feedback loop to stabilize or energize. Unfortunately, no two inductors or silicon chips perform exactly the same way, so tuning τ_{DLY} not only adds "test time" to the production cycle (i.e., cost) but also keeps the system from adjusting to variable ambient conditions. Regulating τ_{DLY} with a slow feedback loop would improve the situation, albeit with more power losses. Monitoring how well L_H discharges transducer capacitor C_{PIEZO} (Figure 1.16) for only a short duration immediately after each de-energizing event, for instance, for maybe 100 ns of the 33-ms vibration period, keeps losses down. A digital controller could then store the resulting command until the next energizing event, when the loop can again sample C_{PIEZO}'s remnant energy and tune τ_{DLY}.

1.4.3 Harvesting Electrostatic Charger

Harnessing energy from a variable capacitor C_{VAR} is possible because the work that vibrations exert to separate the conducting plates decreases the device's capacitance. As a result, because charge q_C is the product of C_{VAR} and its voltage v_C (i.e., $C_{VAR}v_C$), reducing C_{VAR} increases v_C, and the quadratic gain that v_C^2 represents in energy $0.5C_{VAR}v_C^2$ overwhelms C_{VAR}'s linear drop. Unfortunately, v_C often rises to 100–300 V, well beyond the breakdown limits of low-cost CMOS process technologies. Alternatively, attaching C_{VAR} to battery V_{BAT} directly constrains v_C and causes q_C to decrease in response to reductions in C_{VAR}, which means that C_{VAR} drives charge (i.e., energy) into V_{BAT}. The cycle-by-cycle progression shown in Figure 1.18 does just this, precharges C_{VAR} to V_{BAT} so that, in connecting V_{BAT} to C_{VAR}, reductions in C_{VAR} pump (i.e., harness) charge into V_{BAT}. The system then disconnects C_{VAR} from V_{BAT} to allow vibrations to reset C_{VAR} to C_{MAX} and v_C to a lower value before allowing the process to repeat [23].

There are two energy-transfer points in the sequence just described. First, the system prepares C_{VAR} for harvesting by precharging it to V_{BAT}. While using a switch to connect C_{VAR} to V_{BAT} is the simplest means of charging C_{VAR} at C_{MAX}, it is also the lossiest because the switch subtracts $0.5C_{MAX}V_{BAT}^2$ from the energy budget. This is the reason why the precharger in Figure 1.19 uses inductor L to charge and invest energy in C_{VAR} [24]. Here, V_{BAT} energizes L when switches S_1 and S_3 close, draining L into C_{VAR} after S_1 and S_3 open and S_2 and S_4 close.

The second energy transfer occurs when C_{VAR} steers charge into V_{BAT}. Now, however, C_{VAR}'s voltage matches V_{BAT} and so the voltage and Ohmic power across a connecting switch are correspondingly low. The harvesting charger in Figure 1.19 therefore employs the asynchronous

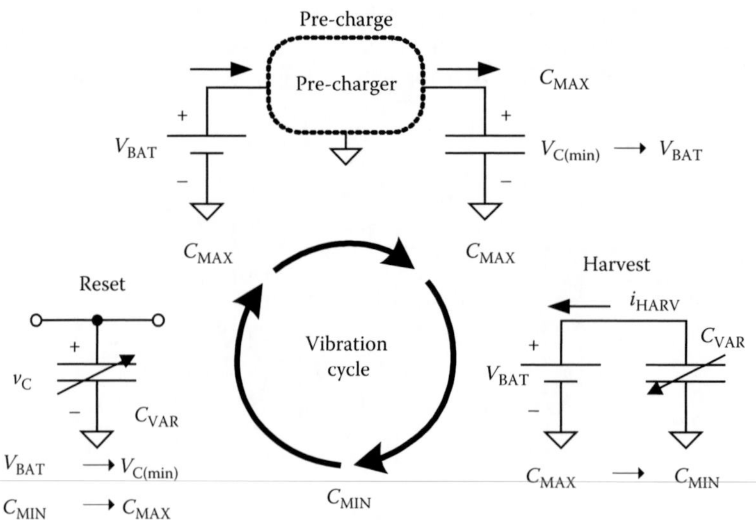

FIGURE 1.18 Battery-constrained electrostatic harvesting sequence.

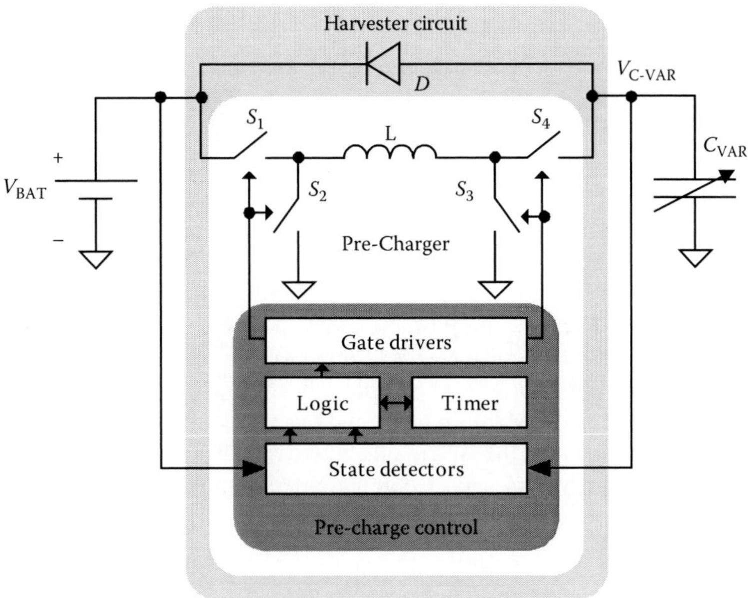

FIGURE 1.19 Battery-constrained electrostatic harvesting charger.

diode switch D for this purpose, which means that the system should precharge C_{VAR} to a diode above V_{BAT}. Diode D drops roughly 0.7 V when conducting harvesting current i_{HARV} into V_{BAT}, so D dissipates more Ohmic power than a synchronous MOS switch would. i_{HARV} in a microsystem is so low, however, that this incremental increase in conduction power is on the same order as the switching power that a synchronous switch might dissipate to charge and discharge its parasitic capacitors. In other words, the area savings and reliability associated with a less complex controller (under equivalent losses) justify using a simple diode switch.

As in the piezoelectric charger described in the previous section, the system's first basic control function is to synchronize L's energizing and de-energizing events to C_{VAR}'s peak capacitance C_{MAX}. Because v_C decreases when vibrations increase C_{VAR} in the reset phase and q_C is constant (i.e., C_{VAR} is open-circuited) and equals $C_{VAR}v_C$, C_{VAR} reaches C_{MAX} just before v_C starts to rise. In other words, monitoring when v_C surpasses its delayed counterpart v_D with a comparator, like CP_{PK} in Figure 1.17, indicates when C_{VAR} reaches C_{MAX} [25]. The second fundamental control task in the system is to determine how long V_{BAT} should energize L to charge C_{VAR} to V_{BAT}. As in the piezoelectric case, a user-defined delay like in Figure 1.17 can set L's energizing time to the appropriate length, and adding a slow correcting loop enables the system to tune and adjust to changing ambient conditions.

As with every harvesting system, the goal is to generate power so as to yield a net energy gain E_{NET}. The problem is that miniature transducers generate little power and conditioning circuits can easily dissipate much of that power. In the electrostatic case presented, the precharger not only dissipates some power in E_{LOSS} but also invests about $0.5C_{MAX}V_{BAT}^2$ in C_{VAR} as E_{INV} to precharge C_{VAR} to V_{BAT} at C_{MAX}. In other words, to produce a net gain, harvesting energy E_{HARV}, which is the energy V_{BAT} receives when C_{VAR} decreases as $\Delta C_{VAR}V_{BAT}^2$, must exceed E_{INV} and all losses in E_{LOSS}:

$$\begin{aligned} E_{NET} &= E_{HARV} - E_{INV} - E_{LOSS} \\ &= \Delta C_{VAR}V_{BAT}^2 - 0.5C_{MAX}V_{BAT}^2 - E_{LOSS} \\ &= 0.5C_{MAX}V_{BAT}^2 - C_{MIN}V_{BAT}^2 - E_{LOSS}. \end{aligned} \tag{1.10}$$

E_{HARV} ultimately depends on C_{VAR}'s total variation, so large C_{MAX}-to-C_{MIN} spreads produce higher gains.

1.4.4 Conclusions

Hybrid supplies in microsystems generally suffer from full-scale integration challenges and poor light load efficiency. Tiny spaces, to start with, constrain energy to such an extent that efficiency concerns overwhelm all other performance metrics, which means that switched-inductor conditioners become almost indispensable. Power inductors, unfortunately, are bulky and difficult to integrate, so hybrid microsupplies cannot afford to use more than one. And even if more efficient than linear and switched-capacitor implementations under moderate to heavy loads, magnetic-based supplies still dissipate conduction, switching, and quiescent power. In fact, a fundamental challenge that designers face in ultra low-power supplies is keeping switching and quiescent losses low, in other words, managing complex systems with little to no power.

Harvesters bear the additional burden of synchronizing circuits to often unpredictable and uncorrelated ambient events and conditions. Not only that, starting and operating a system with no initial energy is especially problematic. Many implementations therefore rely on a battery storing sufficient initial charge to bias and start the system, much like cars depend on charged batteries to ignite their engines. In other words, ultra small solutions often complement a harvesting source with another technology to ensure that the system starts properly.

1.5 SUMMARY

The potential market space for miniature systems such as wireless microsensors is vast. One contributing factor is that adding intelligence to expensive and difficult-to-replace infrastructures nonintrusively has the potential of updating and improving otherwise obsolete and archaic technologies of scale. Not only can power grids manage energy more efficiently with embedded instrumentation, but so can military base camps, space stations, industrial plants, hospitals, farms, and others. Biomedical implants and portable and wearable consumer electronics also reap the benefits of microscale integration. Tiny spaces, however, limit energy and power, and modern mixed-signal systems demand both: energy for operational life and power for functionality (e.g., wireless transmission).

Sadly, no one miniature source is ideal. While capacitors and inductors source high power, for example, they store little energy. Fuel cells and nuclear batteries may store more energy but they supply considerably less power. Li ions and ultracapacitors are moderate in almost every way; however, sacrificing energy for power, or vice versa, for the sake of cost (i.e., of adopting only one technology) is quickly becoming less viable under microscale constraints. From this perspective, harvesting ambient energy is a good way of replenishing and complementing a power-dense device that is easily exhaustible. In fact, harvesters do not release the by-products fuel cells do, nor do they impose the safety hazards or cost infrastructure nuclear batteries do.

Harnessing solar energy generates the most power at several mW/cm^2's; however, direct sunlight is not always available and indoor lighting outputs substantially lower power levels in the μW/cm^2 range. Unfortunately, deriving power from thermal and magnetic energy in small spaces not only produces mV signals that are difficult to condition but also only generates μW/cm^3's. Although kinetic energy cannot generate the mW's solar photovoltaic cells can, vibrations are abundant and consistent, and piezoelectric and electrostatic transducers are capable of yielding moderate power levels from vibrations at around 100–300 μW/cm^3. All the same, research continues and the final verdict on the power capabilities of light, thermal, magnetic, and kinetic transducers is far from certain.

Irrespective of the source, conditioning μW's is difficult because the mere act of transferring energy can dissipate much of the little power that is available. Linear converters, for example, may be noise free, simple, and relatively fast but their conducting switches dissipate Ohmic losses that only decrease linearly with output current. And while losses in switched-capacitor circuits decrease quadratically with load, switched-inductor converters, whose losses also decrease at a similar rate, expose their conducting switches to considerably lower voltages at around 50–150 mV. At μWs, however, quiescent and switching losses become more significant, obscuring the boundary regions where one conditioner's efficiency clearly outperforms that of the others.

Mixed-signal microsystems often reduce losses and increase integration densities by mixing (1) multiple sourcing technologies with (2) magnetic-based converters that only use (3) one inductor. Irrespective of the combination, hybrid supply circuits must carefully manage energy and power flow for maximum life and accurately condition power to fully supply a load and/or replenish a battery. Directing how and where power flows from a miniature DM PEM fuel cell with only a single inductor, for example, is as important as charging a copackaged thin-film Li ion and regulating the voltage across a load. How circuits load transducers, charge batteries, and synchronize to ambient conditions, to cite another application, eventually sets the operational life of a system. Designers must therefore implement these and other basic functions without exhausting or stressing the tiny sources in the microsystem, in other words, perform relatively complex tasks with little to no energy.

REFERENCES

1. G. A. Rincón-Mora and M. Chen, Self-powered chips—The work of fiction, *Power Management Design Line (PMDL)*, 28, 2005.
2. B. Sahu and G. A. Rincón-Mora, A high-efficiency linear RF power amplifier with a power-tracking dynamically adaptive buck-boost supply, *IEEE Transactions on Microwave Theory and Techniques*, 52(1), 112–120, 2004.
3. M. Chen, J. P. Vogt, and G. A. Rincón-Mora, Design methodology of a hybrid micro-scale fuel cell-thin-film lithium ion source, *IEEE International Midwest Symposium on Circuits and Systems (MWSCAS)*, Montreal, Canada, August 5–8, 2007.
4. G.A. Rincón-Mora, *Analog IC Design with Low-Dropout Regulators*. New York: McGraw-Hill, 2009.
5. M. Chen and G. A. Rincón-Mora, A compact electrical model for microscale fuel cells capable of predicting runtime and I–V polarization performance, *IEEE Transactions on Energy Conversion*, 23(3), 842–850, 2008.
6. E. O. Torres and G. A. Rincón-Mora, Energy-harvesting system-in-package (SiP) microsystem, *ASCE Journal of Energy Engineering*, 134(4), 121–129, 2008.
7. E. O. Torres and G. A. Rincón-Mora, Long lasting, self-sustaining, and energy-harvesting system-in-package (SiP) sensor solution, *International Conference on Energy, Environment, and Disasters (INCEED)*, Session A-2, ID 368, 1–33, Charlotte, NC, July 2005.
8. E. O. Torres and G. A. Rincón-Mora, Electrostatic energy-harvesting and battery-charging CMOS system prototype, *IEEE Transactions on Circuits and Systems (TCAS) I*, 56(9), 1938–1948, 2009.
9. D. Kwon and G. A. Rincón-Mora, A rectifier-free piezoelectric energy harvester circuit, *IEEE International Symposium on Circuits and Systems (ISCAS)*, Taipei, Taiwan, May 24–27, 2009.
10. G. A. Rincón-Mora, *Power IC Design—From the Ground Up*. Raleigh: Lulu, 2009.
11. V. Gupta, G. A. Rincón-Mora, and P. Raha, Analysis and design of monolithic, high PSR, linear regulators for SoC applications, *Proceedings of IEEE International System on Chip (SOC) Conference*, pp. 311–315, Santa Clara, CA, 2004.
12. G. A. Rincón-Mora, *Power Management ICs: A Top-Down Design Approach*. Raleigh: Lulu, 2005.
13. D. Kwon and G. A. Rincón-Mora, Single-inductor multiple-output (SIMO) switching DC–DC converters, *IEEE Transactions on Circuits and Systems II (TCAS II)*, 56(8), 957–960, 2009.
14. D. Kwon and G. A. Rincón-Mora, Operation-based signal-flow AC analysis of switching DC–DC converters in CCM and DCM, *IEEE International Midwest Symposium on Circuits and Systems (MWSCAS)*, Cancún, Mexico, August 2–5, 2009.
15. N. Keskar and G. A. Rincón-Mora, A fast, sigma-delta boost DC–DC converter tolerant to wide LC filter variations, *IEEE Transactions on Circuits and Systems (TCAS) II*, 55, 198–202, 2008.
16. H. P. Forghani-zadeh and G.A. Rincón-Mora, An accurate, continuous, and lossless self-learning CMOS current-sensing scheme for inductor-based DC–DC converters, *IEEE Journal of Solid-State Circuits*, 42(3), 665–679, 2007.

17. S. Kim and G. A. Rincón-Mora, Achieving high efficiency under micro-watt loads with switching buck DC–DC converters, *Journal of Low Power Electronics (JOLPE)*, 5(2), 229–240, 2009.
18. G. A. Rincón-Mora and L. A. Milner, How to fully integrate switching DC–DC supplies with inductor multipliers *Planet Analog*, December 18, 2005.
19. G. A. Rincón-Mora, *Analog IC Design: An Intuitive Approach*. Raleigh: Lulu, 2009.
20. M. Chen, J. P. Vogt, and G. A. Rincón-Mora, Design methodology of a hybrid micro-scale fuel cell-thin-film lithium ion source, *IEEE International Midwest Symposium on Circuits and Systems (MWSCAS)*, Montreal, Canada, August 5–8, 2007.
21. S. Kim and G. A. Rincón-Mora, Single-inductor dual-input dual-output buck-boost fbuel cell-Li Ion charging DC–DC converter, *IEEE's International Solid-State Circuits Conference (ISSCC)*, San Francisco, CA, February 2009.
22. D. Kwon and G. A. Rincón-Mora, A single-inductor AC–DC piezoelectric energy-harvester/battery-charger IC converting +–(0.35 to 1.2V) to (2.7 to 4.5V), *IEEE's International Solid-State Circuits Conference (ISSCC)*, San Francisco, CA, February 2010.
23. E. Torres and G. A. Rincón-Mora, Energy budget and high-gain strategies for voltage-constrained electrostatic harvesters, *IEEE International Symposium on Circuits and Systems (ISCAS)*, Taipei, Taiwan, May 24–27, 2009.
24. E. O. Torres and G. A. Rincón-Mora, Electrostatic energy-harvesting and battery-charging CMOS system prototype, *IEEE Transactions on Circuits and Systems (TCAS) I*, 56(9), 1938–1948, 2009.
25. E. O. Torres and G. A. Rincón-Mora, A 0.7 μm BiCMOS electrostatic energy-harvesting system IC, *IEEE Journal of Solid-State Circuits*, 45(2), 483–496, 2010.

2 Power Management IC Design for Efficient DVFS-Enabled On-Chip Operations

Dongsheng Ma and Rajdeep Bondade

CONTENTS

2.1 INTRODUCTION

Over the last few decades, the semiconductor industry has been a harbinger of explosive growth, propelling numerous breakthroughs in almost all fields of science and technology. There have been considerable advancements in a plethora of research domains ranging from high-end medical equipments to sophisticated polymorphic computing architectures. The development of the integrated circuit (IC) industry has resulted in a chip density of over a million transistors per square millimeter, eventually leading to a performance increase by a factor of 1000 within the next 10 years [1]. To satisfy this growth, transistor sizes have continued to shrink, allowing modern very large scale integration (VLSI) systems to be operated at extremely high gigahertz speeds. However, this has caused severe issues related to power dissipation and heat generation. The International Technology Roadmap for Semiconductors (ITRS) forecasts an exponential increase in power dissipation for System-on-Chip (SoC) applications over the next 15 years. This places a tremendous stress on corresponding cooling and packaging solutions, thereby adding to the size, cost and weight of the entire system. This situation is further exacerbated by the maturation of battery technology, which has failed to grow commensurately. Therefore, power dissipation has a considerable impact on the future development of technology and is identified by ITRS as a long-term *Grand Challenge* [2].

To mitigate the urgent power crisis, numerous power management techniques have been developed, which monitor system conditions and optimize their parameters to minimize power dissipation levels. Power management can be performed at various levels of abstraction, and is classified as *device-level, structural-level,* and *system-level* power management.

Device-level power management occurs at the transistor level and involves operation in the weak inversion region, or by applying adjustable body biasing to vary transistors' threshold voltages. Structural-level techniques are component-based, and optimize the power at the circuit level. For example, clock gating principles are used to control leakage in SoC devices. The IBM PowerPC 405LP utilizes clock gating at the IP core and at the register level [3], while the Intel PXA family processors support fine granularity clock gating [4]. Power management is achieved at the highest level of abstraction through system-level optimization techniques. These methods are algorithmic-based and dependent on the type of application being catered to. Numerous techniques exist, for example, vector quantization minimizes the number of operations required to perform a given function [5]. Predictive policies, such as predictive shutdown and wake-up, are techniques that are made use of in commercial processors such as the Transmeta™ Crusoe processor [6]. Among these techniques, the most effective system-level power management technique is recognized as *dynamic voltage/frequency scaling* (DVFS). In this technique, the power delivered to each functional module is varied, based on the instantaneous workload. Optimal voltages and frequencies of operation are supplied, which ensure that all processes in the VLSI system are completed "just-in-time," thereby eliminating any slack periods. This leads to maximized power savings due to the quadratic and linear dependency of voltage and frequency on dynamic power, respectively.

This chapter focuses on the research of DVFS-based cross-layer power management, from the high-level system perspective, to the low-level circuit and device implementation. While there has been considerable effort toward advancing DVFS techniques at the software level, investigation into the development of hardware-based executing platforms has only recently begun. This requires research on hardware–software codesign techniques for synergetic interactions between software-level system operation algorithms and physical layers of device and circuit designs. This chapter discusses the development of these integrated platforms by analyzing state-of-the-art designs and their implementations. This is achieved by examining principles of DVFS and their corresponding hardware implementations, with specific focus on multiple- and variable-output DC–DC converter designs.

2.2 SYSTEM-LEVEL DVFS-BASED POWER MANAGEMENT

One of the most effective system-level power management techniques is DVFS. A significant difference of a DVFS-enabled system to traditional implementations is that it requires a variable or multiple supply voltages as the new control factor in optimizing operation performance and power dissipation. As illustrated in Figure 2.1a, with such a technique, a system is able to continuously monitor individual workloads, and then deliver the most suitable supply voltage and operating frequency accordingly to each module, and thus minimize dynamic power dissipation. Compared to constant-supply systems, a DVFS-based system completes all tasks on the critical path "just-in-time," thereby eliminating any slack periods. Its advantages can be understood by studying the relation between the power dissipated in a system and its workload, as given below.

$$T = \frac{N}{f}, \tag{2.1}$$

$$P_{\text{dyn}} = (\alpha)CV_{\text{DD}}^2 f. \tag{2.2}$$

In this expression, P_{dyn} represents the dynamic power dissipation. N, T, and α are the number of clock cycles, the period of time necessary to complete a particular task, and the switching activity, respectively, the combination of which gives a measure of the workload. The frequency of operation is given by f, while C represents the total gate capacitance. From these parameters and their relationship, a DVFS-based system can be studied. All tasks that are performed by computing systems can

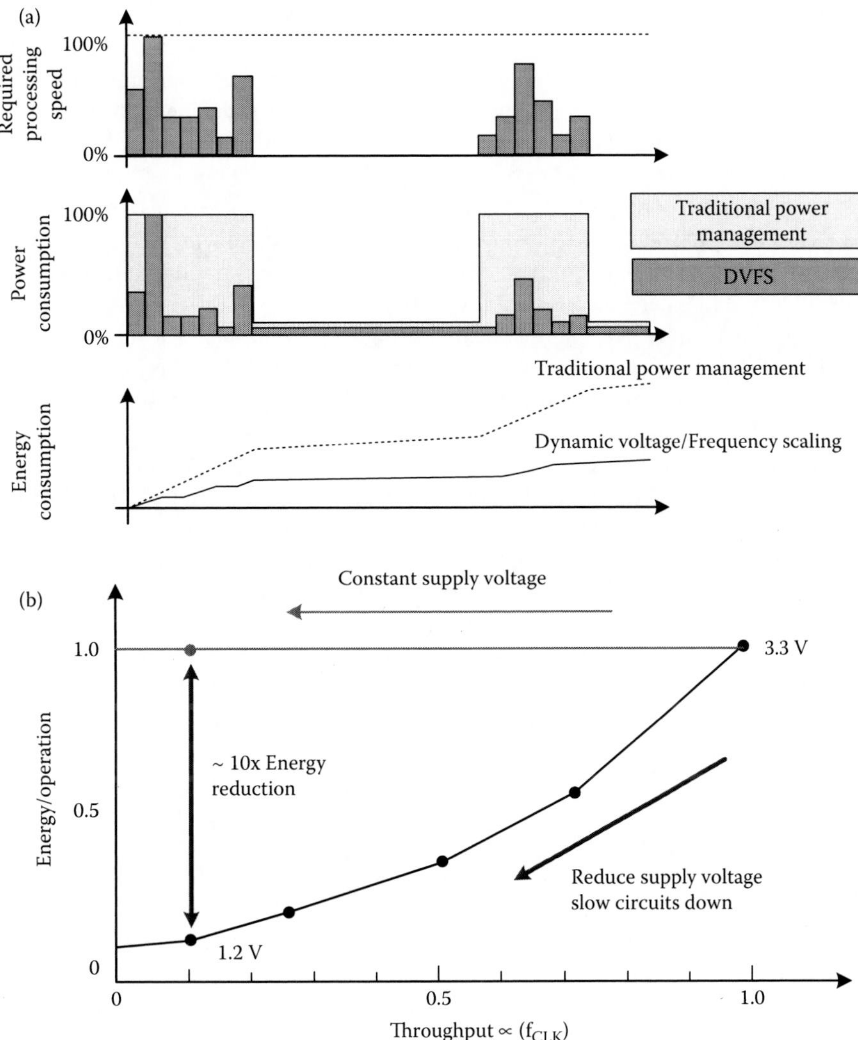

FIGURE 2.1 (a) DVFS versus traditional constant supply power management schemes and (b) their corresponding energy profiles.

be categorized as being either computation-intensive, low-speed or idle, depending on the workload (N, T). For computation-intensive tasks such as video decompression or speech recognition, short latency periods are crucial, causing them to be executed at high frequencies. For low-speed or idle tasks, only a fraction of the throughput is required, as completing them ahead of their timing deadline leads to no discernible benefits. While reducing the operating frequency f decreases dynamic power dissipation, according to Equation 2.2, it does not affect the total energy consumed, since energy consumption E is independent of f, to a first-order approximation, as given by Equation 2.3. Therefore, reducing the frequency alone does not improve battery lifetime, which is especially crucial for portable and embedded applications.

$$E = (\alpha)NCV_{\mathrm{DD}}^{2} \tag{2.3}$$

By reducing the supply voltage along with the frequency, energy savings can also be achieved along with power minimization. Similarly, reducing only the supply voltage of a system, while maintaining constant frequency, improves only the energy efficiency, but compromises the throughput. As a result, to achieve maximized power and energy savings, both clock frequency and supply voltage have to be dynamically varied in response to the instantaneous workload. This is achieved through DVFS algorithms. As shown in Figure 2.1b, by reducing both supply voltage and operating frequency, 10 times energy saving is achieved in digital VLSI systems [7].

To minimize power dissipation, DVFS algorithms determine the optimal operating frequencies at the system level, corresponding to which the supply voltage has to be generated. This voltage is a function of the underlying hardware implementation, process variation, and temperature, apart from just the operating frequency. Therefore, to obtain the instantaneous optimal operating point(s) that minimizes power and energy consumption, different voltage levels are required for DVFS implementation. This is practically implemented using either multiple or a variable power supply. Various practical implementations of multiple supply voltage-based DVFS systems have been realized. For example, it has been shown that with three discrete supply levels, 40.19% of power can be saved in pipelined data paths [8]. More than 47% power savings can be obtained in the media processor presented in [9], which operates with two voltage levels. The study presented in [10] reports a 9-processor Joint Photographic Experts Group (JPEG) application that employs two supply voltages, due to which the overall energy-delay product is reduced by 48%.

DVFS techniques can also operate with the aid of a single variable power supply. Such a supply generates the required voltage value, based on the instantaneous power demands from the load. Variable power supplies have also led to considerable power savings. For example, an embedded CPU system presented in [11] employs a variable power supply, leading to 24.8% power savings. Similarly, with a variable power supply, the DVFS technique is employed in a distributed real-time embedded system to achieve 37.4% reduction in power [12]. In [13], the researchers investigate the use of an adaptive power supply in digital VLSI systems. For example, when 60% of peak performance is sufficient for system needs, it is shown that the power can be reduced by a factor of 3, by lowering the supply voltage by 36%. An adaptive power supply can also be used for high-speed links and is observed to have numerous other advantages, apart from power savings [14]. The adaptive power supply makes the performance more predictable, thereby reducing design margins for uncertainties. The high-speed link would also achieve similar power savings during data transfer. DVFS power management algorithms are ideal in achieving system-level power and energy minimization, by recognizing the necessary performance requirements under various workload conditions. These techniques also utilize global task interdependencies to identify the most optimal supply voltage and operating frequency for achieving a low power profile, thereby improving system efficiency, reliability, performance, and battery lifetime.

2.3 INTEGRATED POWER MANAGEMENT IC DESIGNS FOR DVFS-BASED SYSTEMS

DVFS power management schemes are algorithmic-based and are executed at higher levels of abstraction. Using software processes, these techniques continuously monitor system conditions and determine the optimal operating points for various modules. While they are highly effective in minimizing power dissipation and energy consumption, DVFS techniques still require hardware execution platforms, such as DC–DC converters, in order to provide the required multiple or variable supply voltages. These platforms guarantee that the necessary voltages and frequencies are implemented, distributed, and delivered, irrespective of the variations in the load and undesired battery voltage drops.

DC–DC power converter designs, as hardware-based enabling technologies, are thus crucial in this scenario. State-of-the-art embedded and portable systems are an integrated collection of numerous, highly sophisticated analog and digital modules. Depending upon its function and design, each module operates at an optimal supply voltage that leads to desired operation performance. For example, a typical portable handheld device requires separate voltages to power the liquid crystal display (LCD), processors, input/output (I/O) devices, power amplifier, and so on. Along with the need for separate power supplies, advanced VLSI designs also employ power moding techniques for power management. Each module is operated in one of several functional modes (active, idle, sleep, etc.), depending on its instantaneous workload. Hence, each module not only requires its own power supply, but each supply should be capable of delivering a variable voltage, depending on the instantaneous operating mode. This type of technique is further upgraded through software-based DVFS algorithms that converse with hardware-based DC–DC converters to deliver the required power, while operating at high efficiency. In addition, this is achieved over a large operating range, with a fast transient response to highly dynamic environments.

2.3.1 Overview of Modern Power IC Designs

Driven by perpetual improvements in efficiency and quality of regulation, modern power ICs have undergone several transitions and considerable development. Early power supply designs involved the application of linear regulators to provide a single steady supply voltage. Linear regulators are active linear analog circuits that are used to convert an unstable and noisy DC power source into a well-regulated power output. This is achieved through a simple and low-cost design that is not associated with any magnetic components, making them very desirable for certain noise-sensitive applications. Some popular linear regulator topologies include the standard linear regulator and the low-dropout (LDO) regulator, as illustrated in Figure 2.2. The dropout voltage here refers to the minimum voltage drop required across the linear regulator between input and output voltages to maintain valid output voltage regulation. The fundamental structure of a linear regulator consists of an error amplifier (EA) and a pass power transistor, which operates as a voltage-controlled current source. The EA continuously monitors the output voltage against a bandgap voltage reference. Based on the regulation error, the amount of current delivered to the load is controlled, in order to maintain the output voltage at the desired value. Irrespective of their advantages, the major drawback of linear regulators lies in their topological limitations. Only step-down voltage conversion can be achieved. In the meantime, the efficiency of a linear regulator is highly determined by the dropout voltage. High efficiency is achieved at a low dropout voltage, but drops significantly for higher dropout values. Frequency compensation on such a circuit could be sophisticated and noise/process variation sensitive. Therefore, this type of regulator is not the most efficient hardware implementation for a DVFS-enabled environment, where the ability to provide a large dynamic range of voltages and frequencies is highly preferred.

The drawbacks associated with linear regulators have shifted the researchers' focus to switching and switched-capacitor (SC) DC–DC power converters. These designs aimed to improve the efficiency, transient response, stability, and flexibility for DVFS applications.

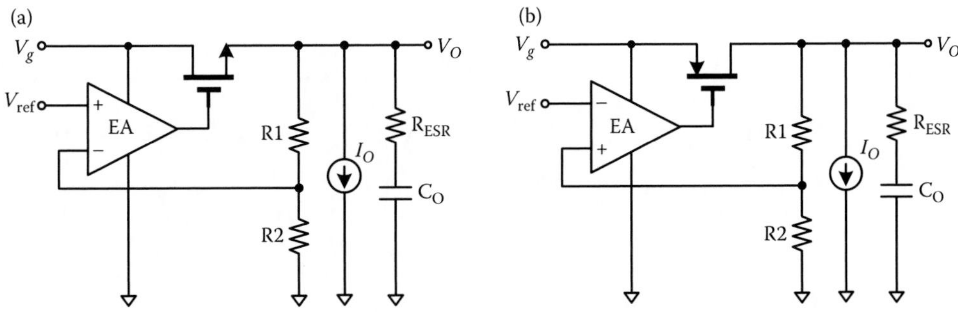

FIGURE 2.2 (a) Standard linear regulator and (b) LDO linear regulator.

First, consider an SC DC–DC converter. It usually consists of two major components: a power stage (also well known as a charge pump (CP)) and a feedback controller. The CP is an array of capacitors, which act as energy storage elements. An example of the voltage doubler CP and of a 2/3 CP topology is shown in Figure 2.3a and b, respectively. The use of power switches and clock control signals leads to appropriate switching actions that cause charge storage on the pumping capacitors in the CP and then charge transference to the output load, with the ultimate goal to maintain a desired voltage value.

The major advantage of SC power converters is their capability for monolithic integration at low power level, since they employ capacitors as energy storage devices, instead of bulky, off-chip inductors. This leads to system miniaturization for certain niche μW-power-level portable and embedded applications. For example, the design in [15] presents a fully on-chip implementation of a step-down SC power converter. Optimized for wireless sensor nodes through the use of a sub-threshold digital pulse-width modulation (DPWM) scheme, the converter is capable of powering loads from 400 μW to 7.5 mW.

Numerous cross-coupled CP topologies have also been proposed for ultra-low-power applications. However, these converters traditionally respond to system dynamics once every half-cycle owing to the inherent clock control schemes, leading to a sluggish transient response. To overcome this, the study in [16] presents two SC DC–DC converter architectures that employ the interleaving regulation scheme. By utilizing multiple sets of clock signals, the interleaving technique ensures that power is continuously delivered to the output load, while significantly reducing output ripple and improving the transient response.

One major drawback of traditional SC DC–DC converters is their ability to provide only a constant gain ratio (GR), which is defined as the ratio of the output voltage to the input voltage of the converter. If the output voltage deviates from this desired level, due to a change in the reference voltage determined by DVFS algorithms, the efficiency of the SC converter drops. If the variation is large, the power loss becomes unacceptably high due to charge redistribution. Hence, to accommodate a large output voltage range and to be capable of powering DVFS-based applications, a SC converter with a fixed GR does not suffice. Based on this challenge, the design in [17] presents an integrated, reconfigurable SC DC–DC converter. It employs 18 power switches in the CP to provide 7 GRs, thereby enabling a variable-output power supply. However, as described above, while the converter is capable of delivering multiple levels of output voltages, it can do so efficiently only at certain discrete levels, depending on the topology of the reconfigurable CP and their corresponding switching actions. For N pumping capacitors, this converter requires $6N$ power switches to provide $4N$–5 GRs. Based on the reference voltage, the closed-loop control scheme involves determining the appropriate configuration of the CP and then generating and routing each clock signal to the corresponding power switches. Therefore, the complexity involved in the power stage and the controller could jeopardize the efficiency of the SC converter. Lastly, if high power levels are desired, due to their limited energy storage capabilities, SC DC–DC converters would require large off-chip capacitors, pins, and pads. The additional requirement for multiple GRs would make such an implementation prohibitively expensive in terms of cost and area.

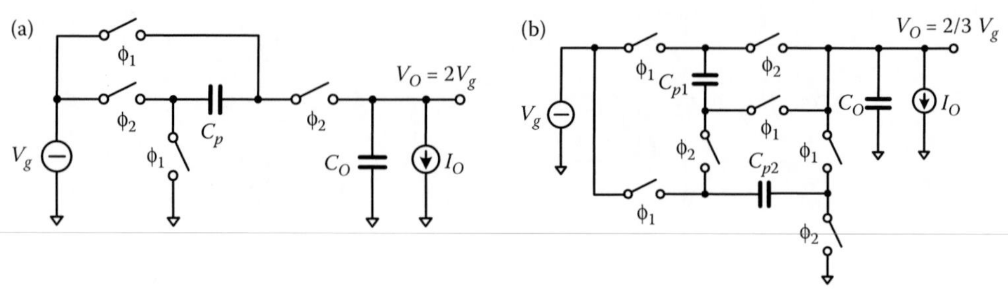

FIGURE 2.3 (a) Voltage doubler CP and (b) a 2/3 CP topology.

As a result, the major focus of this chapter is on the design of switching converters and their applications to DVFS-based power management. Early generations of power management techniques concentrated on the design of switching converters, with a special focus on achieving high efficiency. Initial topologies of switching converters were based on the non-synchronous designs. Compared to earlier linear regulator implementations, these converters had significantly improved performance, and voltage regulation was achieved at higher efficiencies. Boost topologies also allowed for a step-up voltage conversion. However, the disadvantages of higher output noise and power loss due to the use of diodes inspired the need for more efficient converter implementations. This led to the development of synchronous switching DC–DC converters, which are highly sophisticated, multi-mode power delivery modules, capable of operating at efficiencies of over 90% for a wide range of power levels.

While early switching converter designs focused on efficiency improvement, modern works focus on system-level power management with DC–DC converters as the enabling platforms. As mentioned in Section 2.2, DVFS-based techniques assume the availability of either multiple or variable supply voltage levels. Hence, modern converters are designed to provide either a single-variable output or multiple output voltages to load applications. From the system level, the design of modern converters is considerably more involved and complex. These converters should have a fast transient response to minimize latencies and to respond to DVS changes, while ensuring closed-loop system stability. If designed correctly, these DC–DC converters can operate quite effectively as the voltage regulation modules (VRMs) for DVFS-based power management techniques, leading to large power savings and efficient system operation.

2.3.2 DVFS-Compatible Multiple-Output DC–DC Power Converters

Traditionally, a multiple power supply system is implemented by using multiple DC–DC converters. For example, Figure 2.4 illustrates a mobile phone system supplied with multiple discrete voltages, which is implemented using a number of separate single-output DC–DC converters. Each converter is tailored to provide the specific supply voltage required by the corresponding functional module, as discussed earlier. Since each module operates optimally at its characteristic supply, such an implementation leads to reliable and desirable operation performance. However, the main drawback

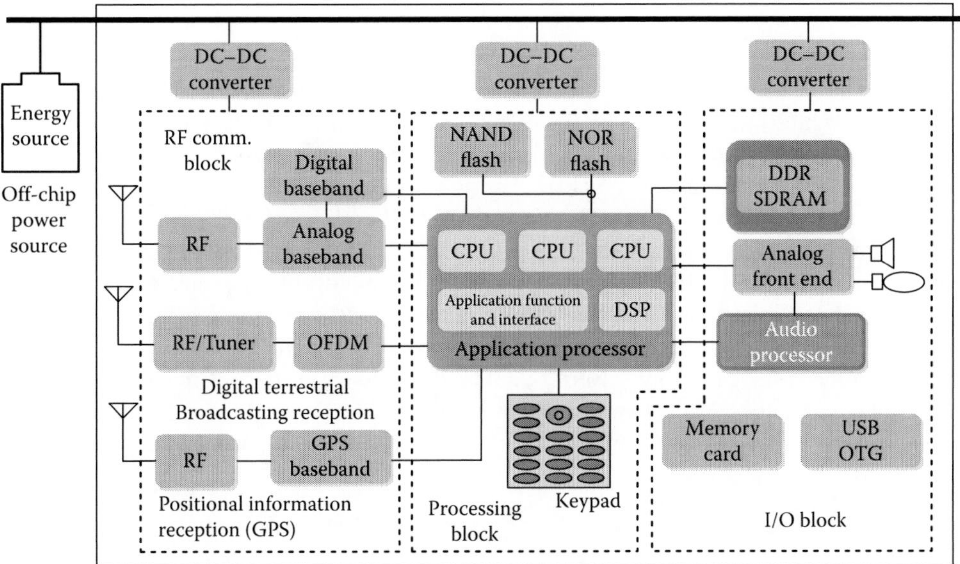

FIGURE 2.4 Block diagram of a typical mobile phone system powered with multiple supply voltages.

of employing separate DC–DC converters is that it drastically increases the system form factor, number of bulky off-chip components, and design complexity. The presence of multiple and bulky power inductors in each converter requires extra system volume, IC pins, and on-chip pads, and introduces severe electromagnetic interference (EMI) noise. To overcome these drawbacks, it would be very appropriate if a single DC–DC power converter could be designed, which provides multiple voltage levels for both regular power delivery and the implementation of DVFS power schemes.

There have been numerous design efforts to develop multiple-output DC–DC converters. Initial implementations presented transformer-based designs that consist of N secondary windings, to distribute energy into various outputs (isolated multiple-output converter) [18]. However, this approach does not allow individual outputs to be precisely controlled and has a severe limitation for the applications of multiple voltage supply scaling. It also leads to significant leakage inductance and cross-coupling among the windings, which causes serious cross-regulation problems. In addition, this method requires at least N inductors or windings, leading to a bulky and expensive system design. A multiple-output converter was proposed in [19], which combines the control loops of N converters into a single loop. Nevertheless, this converter still utilizes multiple inductors, due to which the reduction in external components is minimal.

2.3.2.1 Single-Inductor Multiple-Output DC–DC Converters

2.3.2.1.1 Invention of Single-Inductor Multiple-Output DC–DC Converters

In response to the drawbacks associated with early multiple-output converter designs, single-inductor multiple-output (SIMO) DC–DC converters were developed [20–23]. A converter of this type provides multiple supply voltages while using just a single inductor. As a result, the design complexity is significantly reduced. The use of one inductor considerably lowers the EMI noise, along with system volume, IC pins, and on-chip pads. As required, the converter can be used for both regular power delivery and DVFS applications.

The first integrated SIMO converter was a single-inductor dual-output (SIDO) converter, which employed the time-multiplexing (TM) scheme [20]. The design was inspired by the behavior of two separate converters, with interleaving inductor currents. Consider the operation of two boost converters, A and B, operating with the same switching frequency, as shown in Figure 2.5a. A possible implementation of the power stage and their inductor currents could be as shown in Figure 2.5b. During the first half of the switching cycle, the converter A is active, and power is delivered to its load. During the next half of the switching cycle, from the instant $T/2$ to T, the converter A becomes inactive, while the converter B starts to operate. If it can be ensured that the operation of each converter is restricted to less than half the switching cycle, then the current can be alternatively be assigned to occupy different parts of the switching cycle. Under such conditions, the two separate outputs can time-share the same inductor, resulting in the time-multiplexed operation of a SIMO DC–DC converter.

2.3.2.1.2 Discontinuous Conduction Mode of Operation and Cross Regulation

One of the major challenges during the design of SIMO converters, which is overcome in the converter proposed in [21], is related to cross regulation. For multiple-output converters, each output should be regulated independently. If the output voltage of a sub-converter is affected by changes in the load of another sub-converter, then cross regulation has occurred. This effect is highly undesirable, since in the worst case, the converter could even become unstable. Cross regulation can be further explained by considering two special cases, as shown in Figure 2.6. In Case A (Figure 2.6a), the switching cycles for sub-converters A and B, T_a and T_b, are interdependent, and the expression relating them is given as

$$t_{1b} = \sqrt{\frac{M_b(M_b - 1)R_{oa}}{M_a(M_a - 1)R_{ob}}} \cdot t_{1a} \tag{2.4}$$

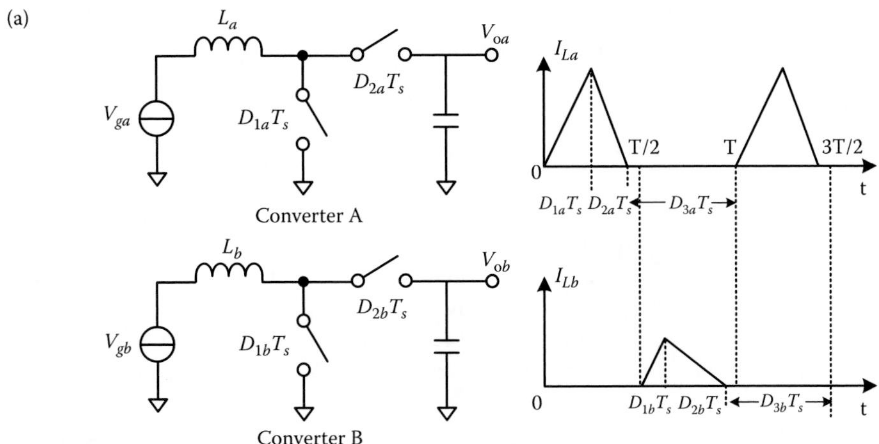

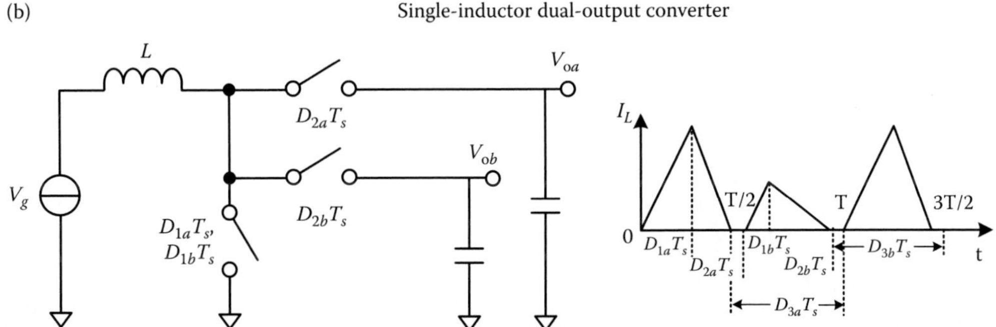

FIGURE 2.5 (a) Two individual boost converters and (b) their assimilation into the SIDO power converter. (Adapted from D. Ma, et al., *IEEE Journal of Solid-State Circuits*, 38(1), 89–100, 2003.)

M_a, M_b and R_{oa}, R_{ob} are the conversion ratios and the equivalent load resistances of outputs A and B, respectively. From Equation 2.4, it can be seen that the duty ratio of output B is dependent on the parameters for sub-converter A. As a consequence, a load change at sub-converter A will affect not only its switching cycle, but the switching cycle of sub-converter B as well. This issue becomes even more serious in the second case (Figure 2.6b). The inductor of the converter is charged to a peak value and then discharged into a sub-converter A for the duration of t_a. The remaining charge is then

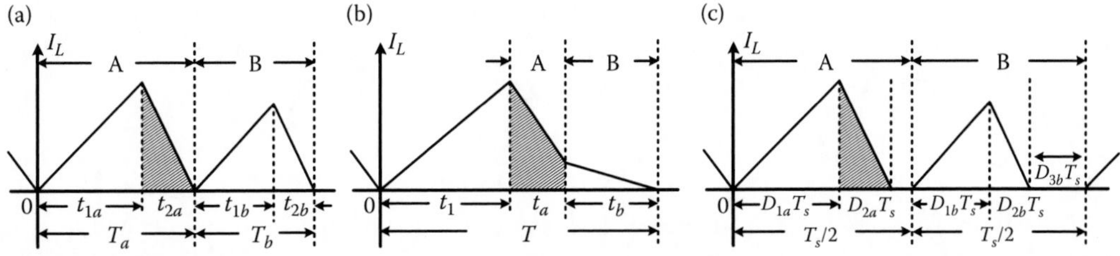

FIGURE 2.6 Cross regulation in SIMO converters in (a) case A, (b) case B, and (c) DCM mode of operation.

transferred to the second sub-converter B, during t_b. Theoretically, t_a and t_b are quadratically proportional, and the expression relating the time durations of each phase is given by

$$t_b = \frac{R_{oa}}{R_{ob}}\left[\frac{M_b(M_a-1)}{M_a(M_b-1)}t_a^2 + \frac{2}{M_a}t_a\right] \tag{2.5}$$

If the sub-converters run at a variable switching frequency according to the loads, then the interdependence of t_a and t_b causes severe cross regulation between the outputs. To overcome the effects of cross regulation, the discontinuous conduction mode (DCM) of operation for SIMO converters was proposed in [21]. As illustrated in Figure 2.6c, a TM control is used to regulate each output separately, with the inductor being charged and discharged distinctly for each sub-converter. To ensure that each sub-converter is independent of the load changes at the other outputs, the TM control ensures that each sub-converter remains operational for a period less than or equal to half the switching period. The converter switches at a fixed frequency and the inductor current goes to zero after discharging into each output. Under these conditions, if $D_{1a}T_s$ is the charging time of the inductor for the output A, then its expression is given by

$$D_{1a}T_s = \sqrt{\frac{2M_a(M_a-1)L}{R_{oa}T}}\cdot T_s \tag{2.6}$$

As the charging time of sub-converter A is dependent only on its load resistance and conversion ratios and not on the parameters related to sub-converter B, cross regulation is avoided.

2.3.2.1.3 PCCM of Operation

While the DCM mode of operation can effectively suppress the effects of cross regulation, at heavy loads it has certain drawbacks. This can be explained by examining the inductor current waveforms for a dual-output converter. Figure 2.7a illustrates the SIMO converter operating in DCM, as explained in Section 2.3.2.1.2. If the power demands at the two outputs increases, so do the duty ratios. However, the time durations of each phase have to be less than or equal to half the switching period, in order to avoid cross regulation (Figure 2.7b). If there is a further increase in the load power demands, operating in DCM will generate large current ripples, thereby leading to a very high peak inductor current, as illustrated in Figure 2.7c. This severely affects the performance of the converter with respect to the ripple voltage, switching noise and the dynamic response. SIMO converters are associated with a maximum peak ripple current ΔI, which places the operating mode at the boundary of DCM and CCM modes. Large power demands can even cause the SIMO converter to operate in continuous conduction mode (CCM) (Figure 2.7d), leading to serious cross regulation effects.

In order to overcome these drawbacks, a novel operating mode for SIMO converters, known as the pseudo-continuous conduction mode (PCCM), was proposed in [22]. In the PCCM mode (Figure 2.7e), the current through the inductor always stays greater than a predetermined DC value I_{dc}. This ensures that the converter is capable of delivering the required high power demand, while still avoiding the effects of cross regulation. The DC current level is determined by corresponding load and current ripple requirements. It can be adjusted to a large value, in order to supply a larger load, and vice versa for light loads.

2.3.2.1.4 Other Modes of Operation of SIMO Converters

Apart from the DCM and PCCM modes of operation, SIMO converters can be operated in other modes. One such mode of operation is known as the single-charge successive-discharge mode of operation. The inductor current profile for this mode is illustrated in Figure 2.8, for a dual-output converter. The inductor is initially charged in the first duty cycle and subsequently discharged into

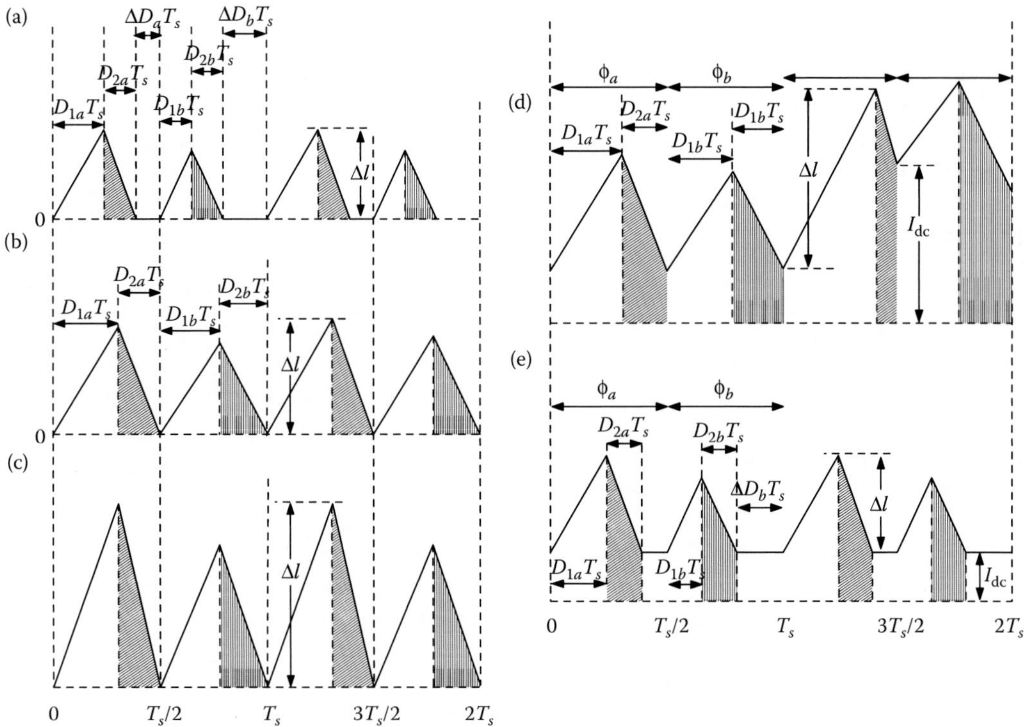

FIGURE 2.7 Inductor current waveforms of a SIMO converter operating in (a) DCM, (b) the boundary of DCM and CCM, (c) the boundary of DCM and CCM with a small inductor, (d) CCM, and (e) PCCM modes of operation.

each of the sub-converters. Similar to the PCCM mode of operation, the inductor is discharged until its value reaches a predetermined DC current I_{dc} and remains at this value for a time duration t_{fw}, that is, the freewheel duration.

However, as discussed in Section 2.3.2.1.2 and illustrated in Figure 2.6b, this mode of operation can be significantly affected by cross regulation. To overcome these drawbacks, the design in [24] presents a charge-control technique for controlling the two sub-converters. In this technique, the power stage of the SIMO converter is controlled based on the charge delivered to each sub-converter. The amount of charge delivered is derived from the inductor current in a cycle-by-cycle manner. This is achieved by employing accurate current sensors to sense I_L, which is scaled down and integrated with the aid of two separate capacitors. The paper describes how charge control is used to effectively eliminate the effects of cross regulation.

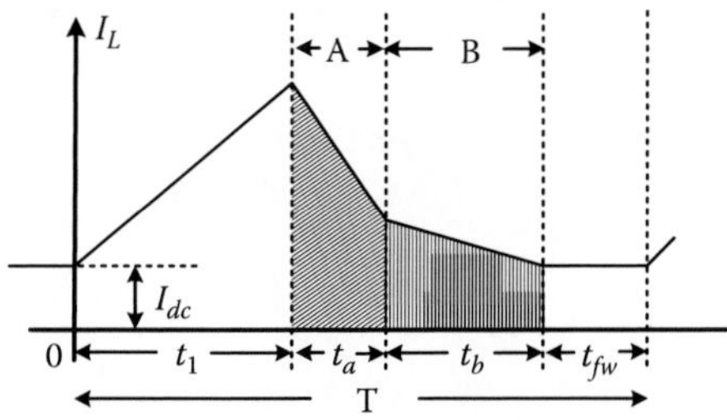

FIGURE 2.8 Single-charge successive-discharge mode of operation. (Adapted from S. C. Koon, Y. H. Lam, and W. H. Ki, *IEEE International Symposium on Circuits and Systems*, Kobe, Japan, pp. 3071–3074, May 2005.)

However, the charge-control technique in [24] has three main drawbacks. First, if the load currents of the sub-converters are small, then a large freewheel duration will lead to excessive conduction losses. Second, current sensing is achieved through a resistor in series with the inductor, leading to excessive power loss, and finally, the step-up/down topology would result in accumulation of current if the power demand of the step-down sub-converter is larger than that of the step-up sub-converter. To overcome these drawbacks, Zhang [25] present an integrated SIDO converter with a non-inverting flyback topology, controlled using the charge-control scheme and a freewheel duration adjustment technique.

2.3.2.1.5 Architectural and Functional Extensions of SIMO Power Converters

SIMO DC–DC converters have been quite beneficial as the hardware-enabling platform for software-based DVFS algorithms. The architectural flexibility of the power stage and corresponding feedback control techniques enables this converter to be tailored to any load application. Extensions in the power stage lead to a family of SIMO converters that can be classified into different categories. Traditionally, the power stage is configured to provide *N* similar-type outputs, leading to a class of converters known as "same-type" converters. Examples of same-type, dual-output converters are boost/boost converters, which were discussed in the previous section, buck/buck converters, and flyback– / flyback– converters or flyback+ /flyback+ converters, the power stages of which are shown in Figure 2.9a–c. Many of the aforementioned converters utilized this conventional type of power stage.

For numerous applications such as LCD displays and charge-coupled devices, both positive and negative power supplies are required. Since a buck converter generates a positive voltage whereas a flyback topology generates a negative output, it is possible to combine these structures to generate a new category of SIMO converters with "bipolar outputs." Examples of such topologies are buck/flyback–, boost/flyback–, and flyback+ /flyback– converters, which are illustrated in Figure 2.9d–f.

SIMO converters can also be extended to generate topologies that produce the same polarity, but having mixed-type outputs. This leads to three more converters, the buck/boost, buck/flyback+, and boost/flyback+ converters, which are illustrated in Figure 2.9g–i.

Apart from topological extensions, SIMO converters can also be modified based on their mode of operation. The PCCM technique can also be applied to any type of power stage, thereby enabling

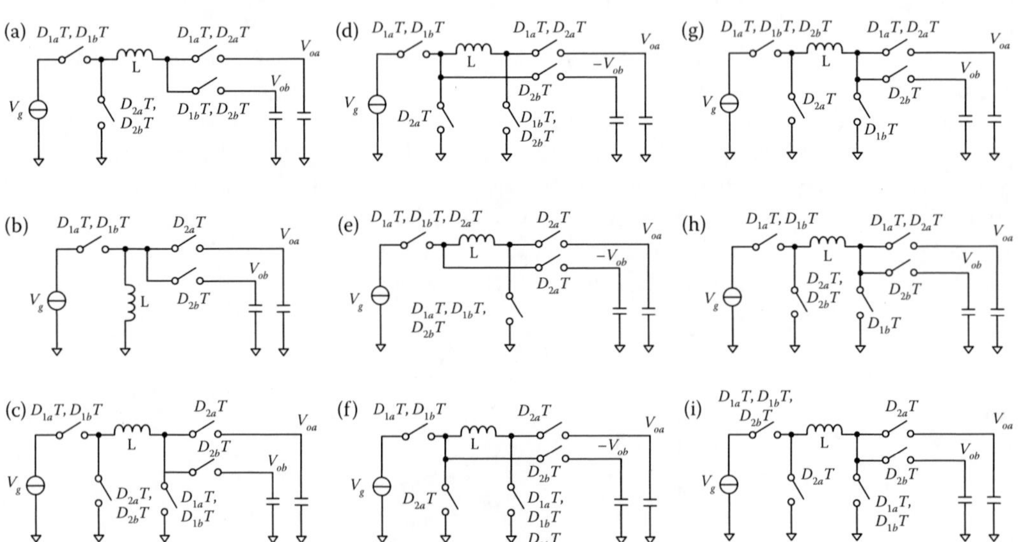

FIGURE 2.9 Power stage of a SIDO (a) buck/buck converter, (b) flyback– /flyback– converter, (c) flyback+ / flyback+ converter, (d) buck/flyback– converter, (e) boost/flyback– converter, (f) flyback+ /flyback– converter, (g) buck/boost converter, (h) buck/flyback+ converter, and (i) boost/flyback+ converter.

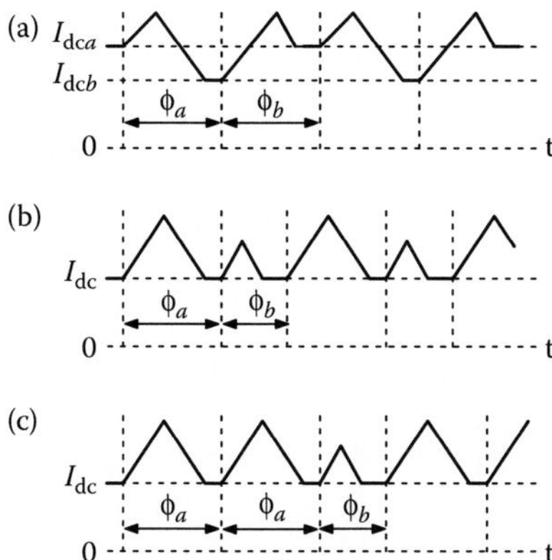

FIGURE 2.10 Inductor current of a SIDO converter with (a) different I_{dc} current levels, (b) switching phases having different durations, and (c) switching phases having consecutive large durations for very large loads.

further design flexibility. While working in the PCCM mode, it is also possible for each sub-converter to operate at different DC current levels, instead of a constant I_{dc}, as shown in Figure 2.10a. This is particularly beneficial when supplying unbalanced loads.

In each N output converter topology discussed so far, it is assumed that the entire switching period T is divided into N equal, non-overlapping phases, with power delivered to a particular output during its corresponding phase. However, the flexibility of the control technique allows for the duration of the switching phases to be modified, in accordance with the output loads. This is depicted in Figure 2.10b, where a longer switch phase is employed for outputs with heavy loads, and vice

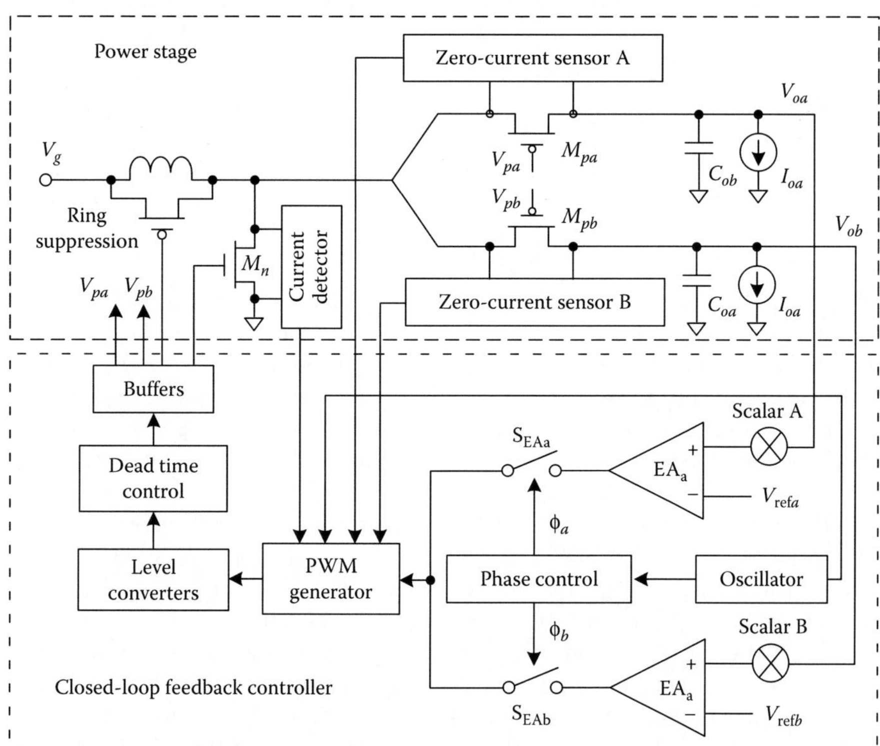

FIGURE 2.11 System block diagram of the closed-loop SIMO converter with TM control. (Adapted from D. Ma et al., *IEEE Journal of Solid-State Circuits*, 38(1), 89–100, 2003.)

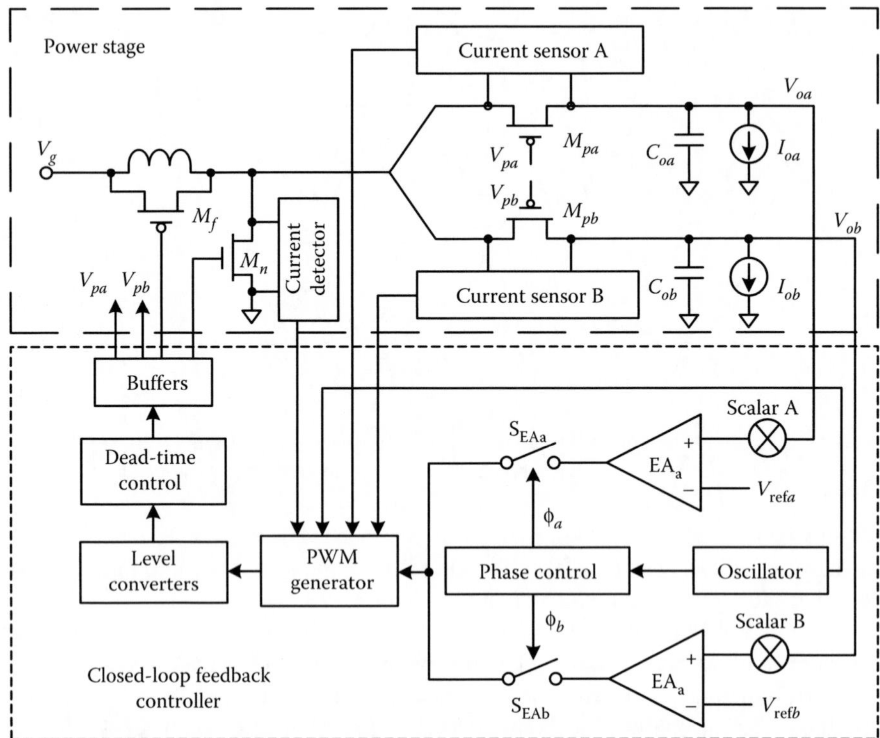

FIGURE 2.12 Block diagram of the SIMO converter capable of operating in the PCCM mode with free-wheel switching. (Adapted from D. Ma, W. H. Ki, and C. Y. Tsui, *IEEE Journal of Solid-State Circuits*, 38(6), 1007–1014, 2003.)

versa. It is also possible to assign consecutive switching phases, having large durations, to large output loads, as shown in Figure 2.10c. Therefore, by appropriately choosing the topology, mode of operation, suitable level of DC currents, and switching phases and durations, it is possible for the SIMO converter to power a wide range of high-end, next-generation VLSI applications.

2.3.2.1.6 Implementations of SIMO DC–DC Converters

The block diagram of the closed-loop SIMO converter operating in the DCM mode [21] is shown in Figure 2.11. It employs a single feedback loop for the control of all the outputs of the converter. The feedback technique is based on the traditional pulse-width modulation (PWM) control scheme, in a time-multiplexed manner to achieve voltage regulation. Based on the voltage regulation error, and with the aid of the inductor current and zero-current sensors, the PWM generator determines the exact duty ratios that control the switching actions of the power stage. The power stage also consists of a ringing suppression circuit that is used to ensure efficient switching actions at the switching node X, in the power stage. By ensuring that the inductor current discharges completely to zero during each phase as discussed in Section 2.3.2.1.2, the effect of cross regulation is avoided.

The architecture of the PCCM-based SIMO converter [22] is shown in Figure 2.12. The power stage is a dual-output boost converter, which employs a freewheeling switch M_f across the inductor to enable the PCCM mode of operation. Current detectors are employed to continuously monitor the inductor current I_L. As illustrated in Figure 2.2e, during the instants of $D_{1a}T_s$, the inductor current ramps up with a voltage across the inductor equal to $V_L = V_g$. From the instants of $D_{1a}T_s$ to $(D_{1a} + D_{2a})T_s$, the voltage across the inductor is $V_L = V_g - V_{oa}$, which is negative and hence the inductor current ramps down. When I_L equals the predetermined dc value, I_{dc} at the instant $(D_{1a} + D_{2a})T_s$, the freewheel switch is turned on and the inductor is shorted. As the voltage across the inductor V_L

equals zero, the inductor does not ramp up or down, and the entire current I_{dc} is carried by the freewheel switch. The feedback still employs the TM-based PWM technique to eliminate the effects of cross regulation. When the converter has to operate under light load conditions, the converter reverts back to the DCM mode of operation.

SIMO converters have been researched considerably, leading to novel control schemes, which are applied for numerous advanced applications. Recently, a SIMO DC–DC converter was presented, which employed an ordered power-distributive control [26]. This converter regulates four main positive boost outputs and one dependent negative output developed by a CP. The design in [27] presents a SIDO DC–DC buck converter design, which shares the magnetic energy stored in the inductor to simultaneously power two independent loads. This converter uses a modified PWM control strategy for output voltage regulation, while dynamically biasing the power transistors' substrate voltages. The TPS65120 SIMO converter presented in [28] is a commercial product, which is designed to offer a power supply solution for small-form-factor thin-film transistor (TFT) LCD panels. The control technique employs two regulation loops, with the first managed through a state machine. The first loop controls the switching actions of the power stage, while the second loop employs a variable peak current control technique for minimizing the inductor current. Finally, the design in [29] proposes a SIMO step-up converter with bipolar outputs, specifically designed for active matrix organic light-emitting diode (OLED) mobile display panels. The positive output voltage is controlled using a modified comparator control technique, while the negative output is regulated using a charge-pump operation with proportional-integral control.

2.3.2.2 Applications of SIMO Converters for System-Level Power Management

SIMO DC–DC converters can also be employed for system-level DVFS-based power management. For example, the work [30] presents a step-up/down single-inductor triple-output (SITO) DC–DC converter, which is illustrated in Figure 2.13. It employs a software-defined adaptive global/local power allocation scheme for multicore/chip multiprocessor systems. The global/local power allocation controller comprises several software algorithms that are implemented digitally and are used for online power sensing and power processing. This is then utilized to deliver the exact supply voltages and frequencies, at the hardware level.

Using hardware–software codesign techniques, the software-defined controller allows the integration of the converter into the processor cores, to give an autonomous and power-aware SoC implementation. Such an implementation allows the SIMO converter to fully exploit the abundance of software resources available in the microprocessor. The hardware–software codesign approach enables the hardware-based DC–DC converter to converse with software-based DVFS algorithms to provide the required voltage levels. Hence, a prompt voltage tracking response is achieved, along with significantly enhanced line/load regulations, while still retaining low cross regulation. Online power processing is used to determine the exact supply voltages that will help achieve joint improvements in power, energy, and performance. The digital implementation of the controller also enables process scalability, therefore ensuring that the design can easily be transferred to future technology generations.

2.3.3 Power Management Using Adaptive-Output DC–DC Converters

2.3.3.1 Digital Control for Adaptive Power Supplies

Sophisticated DVFS-based power management techniques have been devised for modern digital microprocessor systems, which determine the optimal voltages and frequencies of operations based on the instantaneous system workload. While multiple-output DC–DC converters provide a cost-effective solution, these platforms do not completely exploit the capabilities of DVFS algorithms, which require a continuous range of supply voltages. Adaptive power supplies have thus become essential in providing variable power levels, which are defined by the software-based DVFS algorithms during task scheduling by the operating system, and enabling multi-mode operation for the various functional modules.

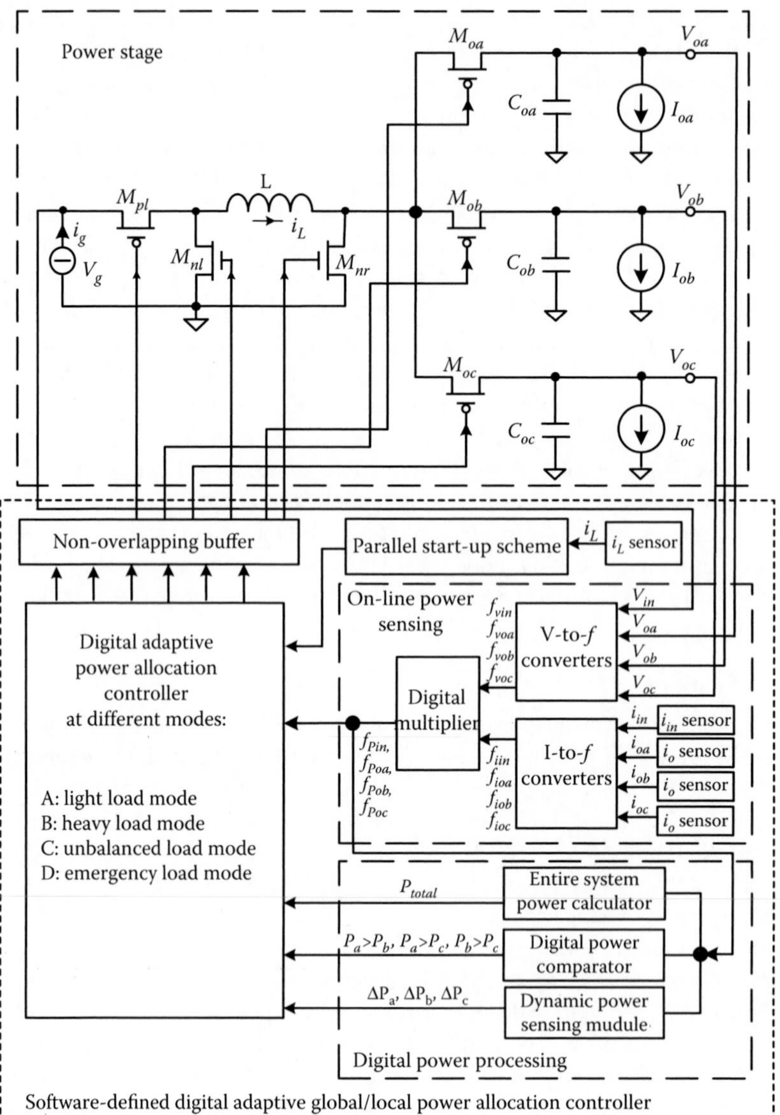

FIGURE 2.13 Circuit implementation of the SITO DC–DC converter with software-defined adaptive global/local power allocation control. (Adapted from R. Bondade and D. Ma, *IEEE International Symposium on Circuits and Systems*, pp. 617–620, May 2010.)

The need for an adaptive power supply for digital microprocessor systems naturally leads to the investigation of digital control techniques for such converters, as it promotes a synergetic power supply–application interface. As described in Section 2.3.2.2, these techniques have the potential to be integrated into future microprocessors, where they can fully utilize abundant on-chip resources for the implementation of circuits such as delay lines, A/D converters, and so on. Digital circuits are also more immune toward noise sources and process variations, thereby enabling a robust DC–DC converter implementation.

However, the design of the adaptive power supply is significantly more challenging than their fixed-output counterparts. These converters should have a fast transient response to minimize latencies and losses to ensure optimal and robust operation of load applications. The tracking speed is required to be significantly enhanced from the state-of-the-art designs, in order to be able to suitably power DVFS applications. Stability issues of adaptive power converters are also considerably more challenging, as the locations of the poles and zeros of the closed-loop system are non-stationary, as they are dependent on the output voltage and load current. Finally, the operating point of the switching converter varies with the voltage levels and load currents, thereby affecting its speed, efficiency, and power-transistor sizing. Thus, the desired adaptive power supply should be capable of maintaining high efficiency, while providing good line and load regulation over a wide range of voltage and load current levels.

Therefore, if designed to overcome the aforementioned challenges, the potential benefits of digital control makes adaptive converters ideal for the development of application-specific, system-aware power supplies.

2.3.3.1.1 DPWM-Based Adaptive-Output DC–DC Converters

Early designs of digitally controlled DC–DC converters were inherited from corresponding analog control schemes, such as traditional PWM techniques. These digital designs employed circuits such as A/D converters, adders/subtractors and digital pulse-width generators, instead of the analog counterparts such as EAs and comparators. For example, pioneer research into the development of a digital control for a buck converter is presented in [31]. This converter employs a voltage-controlled oscillator (VCO), whose frequency is controlled by the supply voltage provided by the DC–DC converter. Output voltage regulation is achieved through the use of counters and adders, to compare the desired reference frequency and the VCO frequency. Based on the voltage regulation error, the switching frequency of the converter is dynamically modulated.

The design in [32] presents a digital PWM-controlled power converter. It achieves voltage regulation through the use of A/D converters. To ensure stability, feedback compensation is implemented digitally and the PWM signals are generated with a hybrid delay line/counter approach. This design leads to low power dissipation and can be used for either supply voltage or processing speed regulation.

The converter architecture presented in [33] describes a complete digital PWM controller designed for high-switching-frequency converters. It employs to A/D converter, compensator, and digital pulse-width modulator, to achieve a high-speed dynamic response and programmability. Another converter is presented in [34], which describes a dual-mode operation for cellular applications. During heavy loads, the converter operates in the PWM mode, to achieve high regulation efficiencies. During standby or idle conditions, the converter switches over to the pulse frequency modulation mode, to extend the battery lifetime. Figure 2.14 illustrates a typical DPWM-based DC-DC converter, to deliver the required power to the output load.

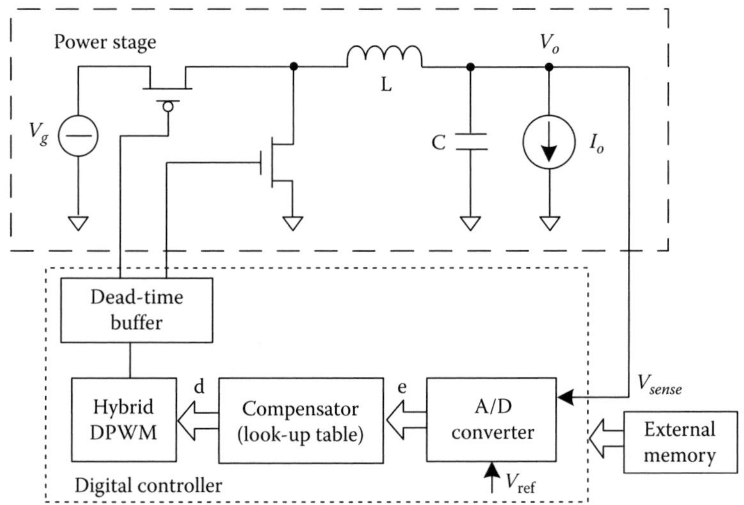

FIGURE 2.14 A typical DPWM DC–DC converter.

Apart from DPWM, there are other control digital control techniques. For example, the adaptive converter presented in [35] achieves both step-up and step-down conversions, by utilizing a triband trimode digital control scheme. The proposed converter employs three control methods, which jointly operate to ensure efficient regulation during start-up, steady state, and during DVS/load transients. The DC–DC converter presented in [36] proposes the use of a digital proportional-integral-derivative (PID)-based regulator. It employs look-up tables, instead of multipliers, to enable a low-power implementation at high switching frequencies. The design in [37] proposes an adaptive power supply with an adaptive pulse-train technique for a low-ripple, fast-response regulation. This converter utilizes a delay-line controller for voltage regulation, thereby reducing ripple voltages by over 50%. The design enables the adaptive pulse-train function for high-resolution regulation in the steady state, while disabling it during dynamic changes, in order to provide a fast transient response. Finally, the digital controller presented in [38] is a programmable, integrated digital PID controller for a buck converter. The design proposes many new features such as a dual-band switching scheme and PWM generator for better output resolution and improved area efficiency, a programmable PID compensator that enhances accuracy and stability and a complex pole–zero cancellation technique to extend the bandwidth of the control loop. The converter has a fast dynamic response, high conversion efficiency, and a wide output voltage range.

As digitally controlled converters are compatible with standard digital complementary metal-oxide semiconductor (CMOS) processes, these control techniques have been uniquely employed to mutually correspond to and control a microprocessor unit (MPU). For example, the design in [39] presents an MPU that is powered by an adaptive-output buck DC–DC converter. The converter converses with the voltage scheduler present in the operating system, which determines the desired clock frequency. Based on the required throughput, the DC–DC converter delivers the required power. Based on this discussion, Figure 2.15 illustrates a typical implementation for the interconnection between a DVS-enabled DC–DC converter and a microprocessor.

2.3.3.2 Nonlinear Control Strategies for Adaptive Power Supplies

While DPWM-based control strategies for adaptive output DC–DC converters provide an intuitive extension to digital microprocessor systems, they traditionally employ intricate circuitry. This

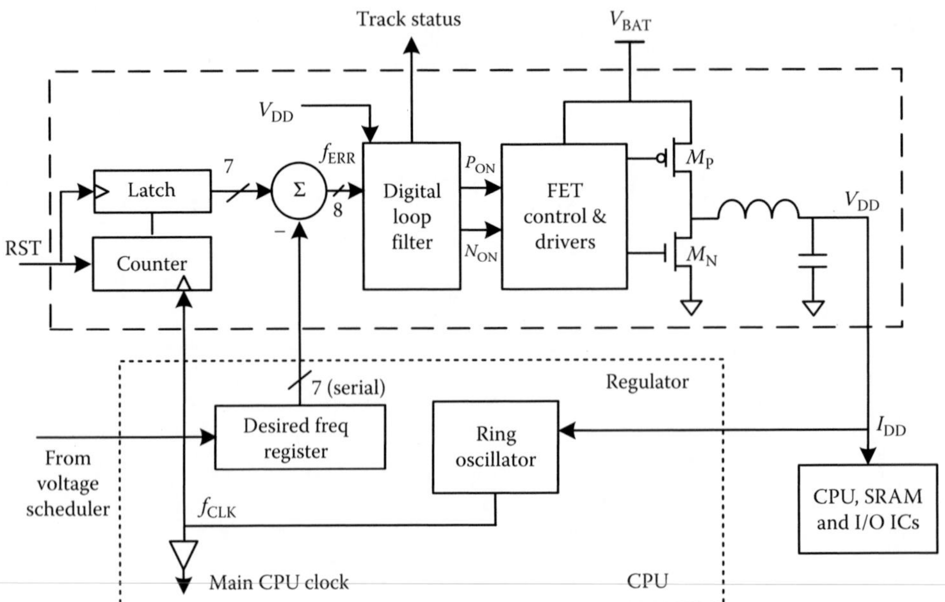

FIGURE 2.15 A typical interconnection between a DC–DC converter and a processor in a DVS-enabled system.

diminishes their transient and voltage tracking speeds, which is desired to be of the order of tens of microseconds or less. To overcome these drawbacks, several nonlinear control techniques have been proposed for adaptive power supplies. These state-of-the-art strategies aim at achieving improved dynamic responses from adaptive power supplies, without compromising any stability margins.

2.3.3.2.1 One-Cycle Control Technique

The rapid growth of technology has resulted in several novel applications such as self-powered devices. These systems employ energy harvesting techniques to harness renewable forms of energy such as solar power, vibration kinetics, and so on. However, the power and voltage generated from energy harvesting mechanisms are associated with large dynamics, due to varying intensities and availability of power sources. Therefore, to ensure efficient and safe operation of target applications, modern DC–DC converters have to be capable of achieving fast line regulation.

This additional criterion has led to further sophistication in the feedback control of switching converters, through the introduction of the dual-loop design. The dual-loop controller achieves both feedback and feedforward control, to ensure that the converter can provide a constant output voltage, irrespective of line or load variations. Based on this concept, the work [40] presents an adaptive buck converter, which is controlled using a one-cycle control technique. As illustrated in Figure 2.16, the one-cycle control is a feedforward nonlinear control technique that is based on extracting voltage information from the switching node of the DC–DC converter, along with the output node. The design also uses dual error correction loops for effective load regulation. The converter is characterized by a very high maximum efficiency and fast up/down DVS-tracking speeds. The adaptive output, one-cycle control-based converter is further extended in [41], which introduces an SC-based controller with dynamic loss control for improved efficiency. This design is considerably more compact and area- and power-efficient, while still retaining the advantages of a fast dynamic response to transient and DVS changes. The SC-based controller in [40] inspired the design of the adaptive switching DC–DC converter presented in [42]. This converter employs a Δ–Σ modulator to perform noise shaping for a well-regulated, variable output voltage, by significantly reducing the noise tones, when compared to conventional PWM-based converters. In order to ensure fast line/

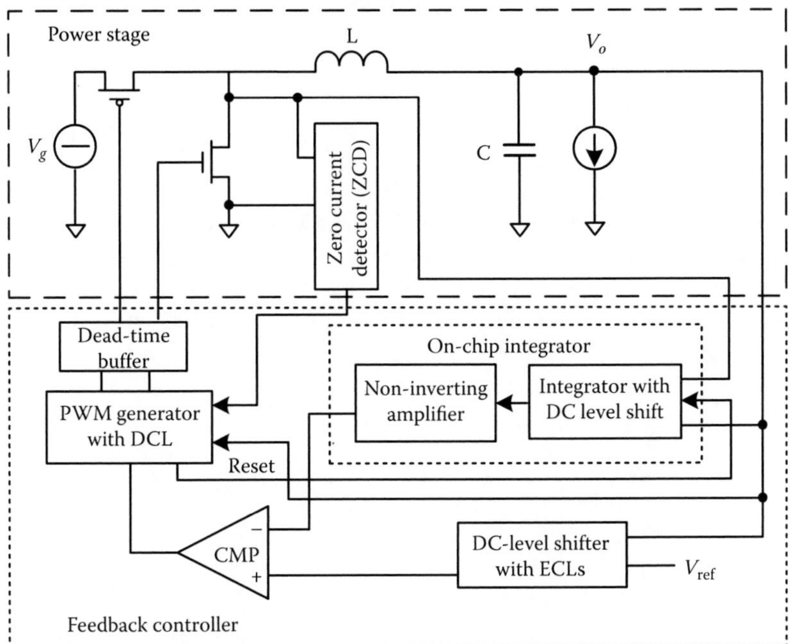

FIGURE 2.16 One-cycle control-based DC–DC converter. (Adapted from D. Ma, W. H. Ki, and C. Y. Tsui, *IEEE Journal of Solid-State Circuits*, 39(1), 140–149, 2004.)

load regulations, this design also introduces an observation-based line and load regulation circuit that helps in determining the switching actions of the power stage.

2.3.3.2.2 Sliding Mode Control Technique

Sliding mode controls were initially introduced to provide a robust control for variable structure systems [43]. The basic principle behind sliding mode control is to design a sliding surface in the control law, which will direct the trajectory of the state variables toward a desired origin. In order to understand the operation principle, the state-space description of a buck–boost converter under sliding mode control, is described. With reference to Figure 2.17, let the voltage regulation error be represented as x_1 and the voltage error dynamics as x_2. For a buck–boost converter, these values are then expressed as

$$\begin{aligned} x_1 &= V_{\text{ref}} - V_{\text{out}} \\ x_2 &= \dot{x}_1 = -\frac{dV_{\text{out}}}{dt} = -\frac{i_{\text{cout}}}{C_{\text{out}}} = \frac{1}{C_{\text{out}}}\left(i_{\text{O}} - \frac{V_{\text{in}}}{V_{\text{ref}} + V_{\text{in}}} \cdot i_{\text{L}}\right) \end{aligned} \tag{2.7}$$

where V_{ref} and V_{out} are the reference and output voltages, and C_{out}, i_{cout}, i_{O}, and i_{L} are the output filtering capacitor, the current flowing through C_{out}, load current, and inductor current, respectively. The sliding surface of the sliding controller is chosen to be a linear combination of x_1 and x_2. The final sliding rule can be expressed as

$$s = k_{\text{v}}(V_{\text{ref}} - V_{\text{out}}) + i_{\text{O}} - k_{\text{i}} \cdot i_{\text{L}} \tag{2.8}$$

The sliding surface serves as a boundary to split the phase plane into two separate regions, as shown in Figure 2.17b. Each region is specified with a switching state to direct the phase trajectory toward the sliding surface. It is only when the phase trajectory reaches and tracks the sliding surface toward the origin that the system is considered to be stable. Ideally, the converter would switch at infinite frequency with its phase trajectory tracking the sliding surface when it enters the sliding mode. However, because of the presence of nonideal switching actions, the discontinuity in the feedback control will produce a particular dynamic behavior in the vicinity of the sliding surface trajectory known as chattering. In order to avoid the chattering and self-oscillating behavior, a hysteresis band is introduced into the control law, with the boundary conditions $s = V_{\text{high}}$ and $s = V_{\text{low}}$. The hysteresis will control the switching frequency and the output ripple voltage of the converter, causing the sliding surface to be split into two lines. The steady state then becomes a limit cycle formed between these two lines, as depicted in Figure 2.17b.

Based on these principles, several sliding-mode adaptive power converters have been developed. For example, a digital controller for adaptive power supplies that uses sliding-mode control is presented in [44]. A buck converter is presented that is capable of providing a fast transient response and robust stability. The design employs a delay line and a ring oscillator as the reference circuit to regulate the

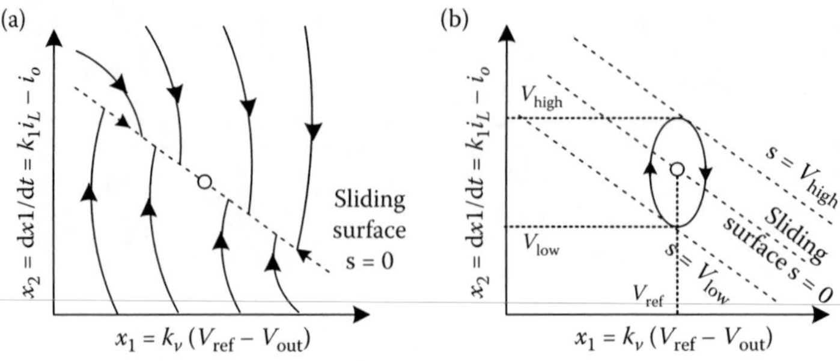

FIGURE 2.17 Phase plane of (a) the sliding rule and (b) the limit cycle.

output voltage from 1.1 to 2.3 V, with a power efficiency varying from 89% to 95%. The paper [45] describes a fast-response sliding mode controller for controlling boost-type converters. It presents novel methods of generating the reference current profile, the sliding surface, and control parameters. The proposed converter is shown to have a faster response, with a lower voltage overshoot, over a wide range of operating conditions when compared to traditional current-mode controls.

2.3.3.3 Application-Aware Adaptive Power Supply Designs

The DC–DC converters hitherto described have focused mainly on improving performance parameters such as power efficiency, line/load regulation, and DVFS tracking speeds. However, compelled by the perpetual increase in scales of integration and the corresponding urgent power crisis, the focus of modern power supply designs has shifted toward a "design-for-system" perspective. Modern DC–DC converters are developed for application-awareness, by analyzing the system needs and instantaneous operating scenarios. On-the-fly reconfiguration at the circuit level then ensures that the power supply dynamically responds to various system-level conditions such as application start-up, local and global transients, and workload variations.

For example, the adaptive power supply described in [46] presents an integrated buck–boost converter with software-defined tri-mode digital control schemes. The DC–DC converter is capable of providing a wide range of output voltages, as determined by DVFS algorithms. The converter is capable of responding to unique system-level operating scenarios by employing three control modes that operate seamlessly during periods of start-up, steady-state operation, and during DVFS or load transient states. The system architecture of the proposed converter is illustrated in Figure 2.18.

To ensure reliable start-up for the buck–boost converter, a tri-band current mode start-up scheme is employed, which divides the inductor current into three different bands, the zero-current band, the low-current band, and the high-current band. By allowing the inductor current to charge up till the

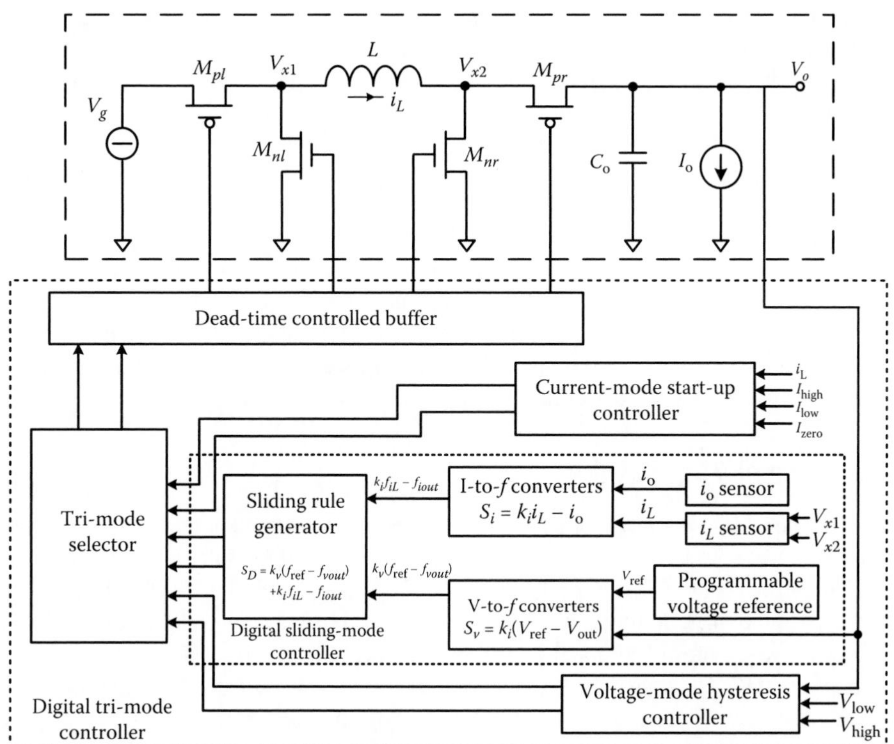

FIGURE 2.18 Block diagram of the buck–boost converter with digital trimode control. (Adapted from F. Luo and D. Ma, *IEEE Transactions on Industrial Electronics*, 57(6), 2151–2160, 2010.)

high-current band and then maintaining it within the high- and low-current bands, the control scheme ensures efficient start-up of the power converter. During steady state, when the output voltage is close to the reference value, to enable fast, robust and accurate voltage regulation, the converter in [46] employs the digital sliding-mode control. The converter can operate in both CCM and DCM, and processes the output voltage, the inductor, the output capacitor, and load currents. Using these processed signals, the control signals for the power switches are generated according to the sliding rule equations, similar to Equations 2.7 and 2.8. During large voltage dynamics, an adaptive digital hysteresis control is employed. The switching actions of the power stage are controlled by containing the output voltage within an adaptively generated hysteresis band of V_{low} and V_{high}.

Another adaptive output DC–DC converter is presented in [47], which introduces a "green-mode" step-up/down converter. As illustrated in Figure 2.19, the proposed converter further enhances the line/load and DVFS transient speeds for application-aware power management. This leads to an inherent design advantage, due to the requirement of smaller inductors and capacitors, thereby leading to a reduction in system volume, printed circuit board (PCB) footprint and cost.

The reconfigurable green-mode adaptive-output converter, illustrated in Figure 2.19a, is a true "design-for-system" power supply. The feedback controller closely monitors and converses with the load application demands to ensure the most optimal configuration of the power stage. Based on the instantaneous power requirements, three green modes of operation are facilitated. The converter automatically reconfigures the power stage into a pseudo-buck, pseudo-boost, or a buck–boost topology to minimize switching power losses, as can be seen from Figure 2.19b. For example, in the pseudo-buck mode of operation, the power transistors M_{p1} and M_{n1} are turned on, while M_{n2} and M_{p2} are turned off. The proposed converter also employs an adaptive power transistor sizing scheme to ensure the optimal size of the power switches, in order to minimize conduction losses and achieve optimal operating performance under all operating conditions.

As mentioned in Section 2.3.3.1, one of the main challenges in modern adaptive power supply design is to achieve fast transient and voltage tracking speeds. The DC–DC converter in [47] achieves this ultrafast response by operating at a switching frequency of 10 MHz, which is implemented through the use of the single-bound hysteresis control (SBHC). This operating scheme is driven by the fact that there exist inherent delays with all comparators and buffer circuits. Hence, instead of a traditional hysteretic operation wherein V_{out} is maintained between two voltage levels, V_{out} is regulated around a single-bound reference voltage. As a result, the delay introduced by the hysteresis ΔT is eliminated, thereby enhancing the closed-loop response considerably. As a result, through the joint and seamless operation of the green-mode scheme and the SBHC control, the converter is capable of achieving a maximum efficiency of 92.1% at a switching frequency of 10 MHz, leading to fast transient and DVS tracking speeds.

With a fast transient/DVS response, a frequency of operation and the capability of providing a large range of supply voltages, the adaptive, single-output DC–DC converter presents a suitable alternative as the hardware-based VRM for modern VLSI applications.

2.4 CONCLUDING REMARKS

As the hardware enabling platform for state-of-the-art power management techniques, variable-/multiple-output DC–DC power converters ensure that each functional module in the system is powered with the most optimal supply voltage and frequency of operation. This ensures that power dissipation and energy consumption are jointly minimized, leading to an improved reliability, efficiency, and battery lifetime. However, most traditional power management designs treat power systems (including power sources and DC–DC converters) as separate modules, isolated from the remainder of the system. In many design cases, such a power system is over-simplified as a constant DC voltage, and the role of power processing is underestimated. As discussed in Section 2.3, DC–DC converters were initially designed from the low-level circuit perspective, with priority given to efficiency enhancement. However, driven by the urgent demands by ever-growing power crisis, the design methodology of such

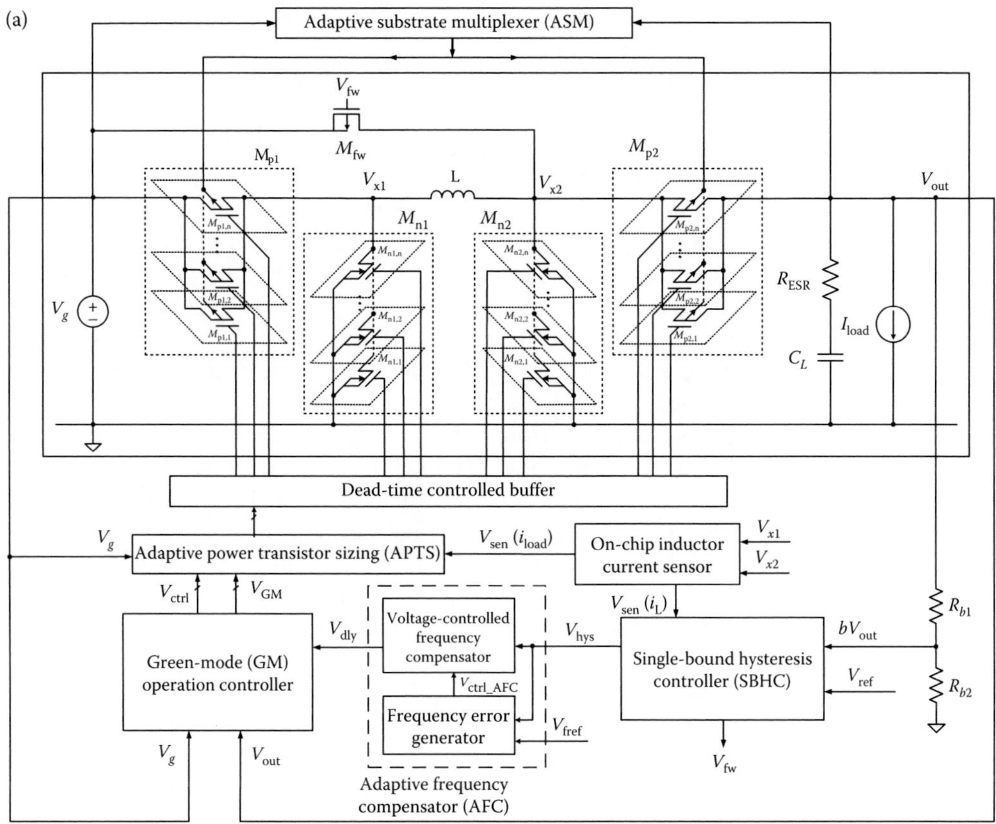

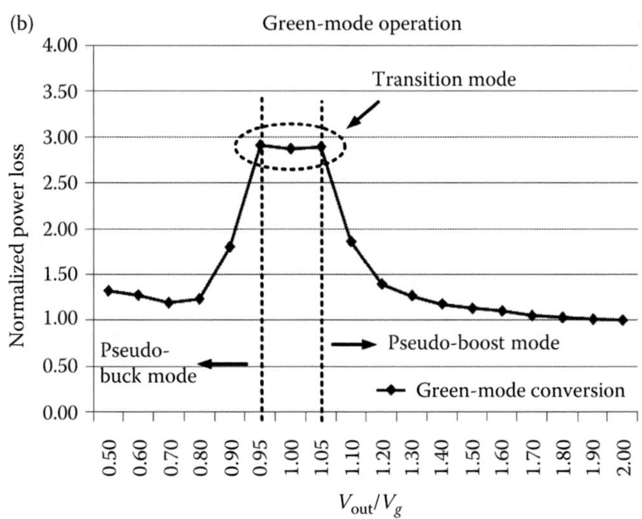

FIGURE 2.19 (a) A green-mode step-up/down switching converter with automatic configuration (Adapted from C. Zheng and D. Ma, *IEEE International Solid-State Circuits Conference*, pp. 204–206, February 2010.) and (b) its operation profile.

converters has shifted toward an application-aware, system-level perspective. State-of-the-art power converters have to be tailored according to their load applications and corresponding operational environments. For example, power converter designs for a self-powerered wireless sensor node would differ considerably from that of a portable multimedia cellular phone.

While 99% of commercial chipsets are digital, future development of DC–DC power converters would heavily engage their integration with digital MPUs, to give a complete SoC implementation, as illustrated in Figure 2.20. This architecture fully utilizes resources available in VLSI systems to ensure efficient closed-loop power regulation. As mentioned before, numerous methods for both feedforward and feedback control of power converters have involved the use of digital techniques. Technically, digital control systems utilize circuits such as delay lines, A/D converters, memories and logics, and so on, which can be easily integrated with low-voltage low-cost CMOS technologies, leading to more area- and power-efficient implementations. Using a complete digital control allows the integration of the entire controller as an integral part of the microprocessor, allowing the available hardware and software resources within the processor to be fully utilized in the converter designs. This has the potential to significantly improve a converter's line/load/DVS transient response, as all hardware–software interactions for voltage tracking and corresponding regulation will occur under online, high-speed, centralized power, and signal processing.

The merging of the DC–DC converter with their corresponding digital load applications also enables the realization of hardware–software codesign techniques. Effective power tracking and power processing carried out at the software level can be directed to generate the most optimal supply voltages and frequencies of operation, at the hardware level. Power processing has the potential to redefine system configuration and design approaches, as it provides a greater degree of design flexibility. Along with power processing, modern power management techniques are also capable of thermal monitoring. This is especially critical for modern computing systems such as multicore processors that can experience sporadic occurrences of thermal hotspots, depending on the operational workload. Hotspots are regions of extremely high temperature (>100°C) and sharp thermal gradients that can often lead to irreparable IC damage. Effective thermal and power management techniques can ensure that the VLSI system always functions within the safe and reliable regions of operation.

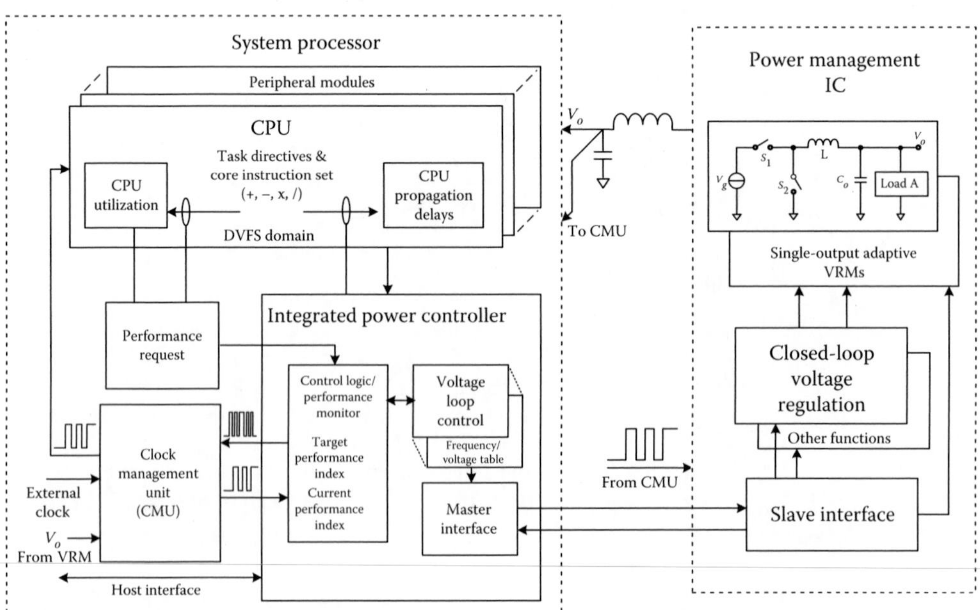

FIGURE 2.20 Integrating power management into SoC with hardware–software codesign.

DVFS-based power management techniques are critical for next-generation VLSI systems. Future research promises to deliver state-of-the-art designs that focus on the integration of hardware–software codesign techniques, to translate local and real-time power and thermal information into the global management platform.

REFERENCES

1. *International Technology Roadmap for Semiconductors: System Drivers*. 2005 edn. Available at: http://www.itrs.net/ Links/2005ITRS/SysDrivers2005.pdf
2. *ITRS, Executive Summary: Grand Challenges*. p. 13. Available at: http://www.itrs.net
3. G. Carpenter, *Low power SoC for IBM's PowerPC appliance platform, IBM Corporation*. Available at: http://www.research.ibm.com/arl/publications/papers/405lp.pdf
4. *Intel PXA250/210 Processor. Intel Incorporated*. Available at: www.intel.com
5. K. Masselos, P. Merakos, T. Stouraitis, and C. E. Goutis, Novel vector quantization based algorithms for low-power image coding and decoding, *IEEE Transactions on Circuits and Systems II: Analog and Digital Signal Processing*, 46(2), 193–198, 1999.
6. A. Klaiber, *The Technology behind Crusoe™ Processors, Transmeta Corporation*. January 2000. Available at: http://pateame.fciencias.unam.mx/arq/proc/crusoetechwp.pdf
7. T. D. Burd and R. W. Brodersen, *Energy Efficient Microprocessor Design*. Norwell, MA: Kluwer Academic Publishers, 2002.
8. J. Chang and M. Pedram, Energy minimization using multiple supply voltages, *IEEE Transactions on Very Large Scale Integration (VLSI) Systems*, 5(4), 436–443, 1997.
9. K. Usami et al., Automated low-power technique exploiting multiple supply voltages to a media processor, *IEEE Journal of Solid State Circuits*, 33(3), 463–472, 1998.
10. W. H. Cheng and B. M. Baas, Dynamic voltage and frequency scaling circuits with two supply voltages, in *IEEE International Symposium on Circuits and Systems*, Seattle, WA, pp. 1236–1239, 2008.
11. Y. Choi, N. Chang, and T. Kim, DC–DC converter-aware power management for low-power embedded systems, *IEEE Transactions on Computer-Aided Design of Integrated Circuits and Systems*, 26(8), 1367–1382, 2007.
12. L. Yan, J. Luo, and N. K. Jha, Joint dynamic voltage scaling and adaptive body biasing for heterogeneous distributed real-time embedded systems, *IEEE Transactions on Computer-Aided Design on Integrated Circuits and Systems*, 24(7), 1030–1041, 2005.
13. J. Kim, Design of CMOS adaptive-supply serial links, PhD thesis, Stanford University, USA, December 2002.
14. G. Y. Wei, J. Kim, D. Liu, S. Sidiropoulos, and M. A. Horowitz, A variable frequency parallel I/O interface with adaptive power-supply regulation, *IEEE Journal of Solid-State Circuits*, 35(11), 1600–1610, 2000.
15. L. Su and D. Ma, Design and analysis of monolithic step-down SC power converter with subthreshold DPWM control for self-powered wireless sensors, *IEEE Transactions on Circuits and Systems-I*, 57(1), 280–290, 2010.
16. D. Ma, L. Su, and M. Somadundaram, Integrated interleaving SC power converters with analog and digital control schemes for energy-efficient microsystems, *Journal of Analog Integrated Circuits and Signal Processing*, 62(3), 361–372, 2009.
17. I. Chowdhury and D. Ma, Design of reconfigurable and robust integrated SC power converter for self-powered energy-efficient devices, *IEEE Transactions on Industrial Electronics*, 56(10), 4018–4025, 2009.
18. R. W. Erickson and D. Maksimovic, *Fundamentals of Power Electronics*, 2nd edn. Norwell, MA: Kluwer Academic Publishers, 2001.
19. A. P. Dancy, R. Amirtharajah, and A. P. Chandrakasan, High-efficiency multiple-output dc–dc conversion for low-voltage systems, *IEEE Transactions on Very Large Scale Integration (VLSI) Systems*, 8(3), 252–263, 2000.
20. D. Ma, W.-H. Ki, C.-Y. Tsui and P. K. T. Mok, Single-inductor dual-output converter for power reduction techniques, *IEEE VLSI Symposium on Circuits*, pp. 137–140, Japan, Jun. 2001.
21. D. Ma, W. H. Ki, C. Y. Tsui, and P. K. T. Mok, Single-inductor dual-output CMOS switching converters in discontinuous conduction mode with time multiplexing control, *IEEE Journal of Solid-State Circuits*, 38(1), 89–100, 2003.
22. D. Ma, W. H. Ki, and C. Y. Tsui, A pseudo-CCM/DCM SIMO switching converter with freewheel switching, *IEEE Journal of Solid-State Circuits*, 38(6), 1007–1014, 2003.

23. W. H. Ki and D. Ma, Single-inductor multiple-output switching converters, *IEEE Power Electronics Specialists Conference*, Vancouver, BC, Canada, 1, 226–231, 2001.
24. S. C. Koon, Y. H. Lam, and W. H. Ki, Integrated charge-control single-inductor dual-output step-up/step-down converter, in *IEEE International Symposium on Circuits and Systems*, Kobe, Japan, pp. 3071–3074, May 2005.
25. Y. Zhang, R. Bondade, D. Ma, On-chip SIMO power converter design with adaptive cross regulation and supply variation control for power-efficient VLSI systems, *Journal of Low Power Electronics (JOLPE) - Special Issue on Low Power Design and Verification Techniques*, 7(1), 71–86, 2011.
26. H. P. Le et al., A single-inductor switching DC–DC converter with 5 outputs and ordered power-distributive control, in *IEEE International Solid-State Circuits Conference*, San Francisco, CA, pp. 534–535, February 2007.
27. E. Bonizzoni, F. Borghetti, P. Malcovati, F. Maloberti, and B. Niessen, A 200 mA 93% peak efficiency single-inductor dual-output DC–DC buck converter, in *IEEE International Solid-State Circuits Conference*, San Francisco, CA, pp. 526–527, February 2007.
28. E. Bayer and G. Thiele, A single-inductor multiple-output converter with peak current state-machine control, in *IEEE Applied Power Electronics Conference and Exposition*, Dallas, TX, pp. 153–159, March 2006.
29. C. S. Chae, H. P. Le, K. C. Lee, G. H. Cho, and G. H. Cho, A single-inductor step-up DC–DC switching converter with bipolar outputs for active matrix OLED mobile display panels, *IEEE Journal of Solid-State Circuits*, 44(2), 509–524, 2009.
30. R. Bondade and D. Ma, Hardware–software co-design of an embedded power management module with adaptive on-chip power processing schemes, *IEEE International Symposium on Circuits and Systems*, Paris, France, pp. 617–620, May 2010.
31. W. Namgoong, M. Yu, and T. Meng, A high-efficiency variable-voltage CMOS dynamic DC–DC switching regulator, in *IEEE International Solid-State Circuits Conference*, San Francisco, CA, pp. 380–381, February 1997.
32. A. Dancy and A. Chandrakasan, A reconfigurable dual output low power digital PWM power converter, in *IEEE International Symposium on Low Power Electronic Devices*, pp. 191–196, August 1998.
33. B. J. Patella, A. Prodic, A. Zirger, and D. Maksimovic, High-frequency digital PWM controller IC for DC–DC converters, *IEEE Transactions on Power Electronics*, 18(1), 438–446, 2003.
34. J. Xiao, A. V. Peterchev, J. Zhang, and S. R. Sanders, A 4-uA quiescent-current dual-mode digitally controlled buck converter IC for cellular phone applications, *IEEE Journal of Solid-State Circuits*, 12(39), 2342–2348, 2004.
35. F. Luo and D. Ma, Design of digital tri-mode adaptive-output buck–boost power converter for power-efficient integrated systems, *IEEE Transactions on Industrial Electronics*, 57(6), 2151–2160, 2010.
36. A. Prodic and D. Maksimovic, Design of a digital PID regulator based on look-up tables for control of high-frequency DC–DC converters, in *IEEE Workshop on Computers in Power Electronics*, Puerto Rico, pp. 18–22, January 2002.
37. C. Zhang, D. Ma, and A. Srivastava, Integrated adaptive DC/DC conversion with adaptive pulse-train technique for low-ripple fast-response regulation, in *International Symposium on Low Power Electronics and Design*, Newport, CA, pp. 257–262, 2004.
38. M. Chui, W. H. Ki, and C. Y. Tsui, A programmable integrated digital controller for switching converters with dual-band switching and complex pole–zero compensation, *IEEE Journal of Solid-State Circuits*, 40(3), 772–780, 2005.
39. T. D. Burd, T. A. Pering, A. J. Stratakos, and R. W. Brodersen, A dynamically voltage scaled microprocessor system, *IEEE Journal of Solid-State Circuits*, 35(11), 1571–1580, 2000.
40. D. Ma, W. H. Ki, and C. Y. Tsui, An integrated one-cycle control buck converter with adaptive output and dual loops for output error correction, *IEEE Journal of Solid-State Circuits*, 39(1), 140–149, 2004.
41. D. Ma, J. Wang, and M. Song, Adaptive on-chip power supply with robust one-cycle control technique, *IEEE Transactions on Very Large Scale Integration Systems*, 16(9), 1240–1243, 2008.
42. M. Song and D. Ma, A fast-transient over-sampled delta-sigma adaptive DC–DC converter for power-efficient noise-sensitive devices, in *IEEE International Symposium on Low Power Electronics and Design*, Portland, OR, pp. 286–291, August 2007.
43. V. Utkin, J. Guldner, and J. X. Shi, *Sliding Mode Control in Electromechanical Systems*, London: Taylor and Francis, 1999.
44. J. Kim and M. A. Horowitz, An efficient digital sliding controller for adaptive power-supply regulation, *IEEE Journal of Solid-State Circuits*, 37(5), 639–647, 2002.

45. S. C. Tan, Y. M. Lai, Chi K. Tse, L. Martinez-Salamero, and C. K. Wu, A fast response fixed-frequency sliding mode controller for boost-type converters with a wide range of operating conditions, *IEEE Transactions on Industrial Electronics*, 54(6), 3276–3286, 2007.
46. F. Luo and D. Ma, Design of digital tri-mode adaptive-output buck–boost power converter for power-efficient integrated systems, *IEEE Transactions on Industrial Electronics*, 57(6), 2151–2160, 2010.
47. C. Zheng and D. Ma, A 10 MHz 92.1%-efficiency green-mode automatic reconfigurable switching converter with adaptively compensated single-bound hysteresis control, in *IEEE International Solid-State Circuits Conference*, pp. 204–206, February 2010.

3 MeSOC-I
A Mixed Signal SOC for Bioinstrumentation in Medical Treatment and Healthcare System

Masaharu Imai, Hirofumi Iwato, Keishi Sakanushi, Yoshinori Takeuchi, Akira Matsuzawa, and Yoshihiko Hirao

CONTENTS

3.1 INTRODUCTION

In recent years, our society has been turning more and more into an aging society. The Japanese are known to have one of the longest life expectancies in the world. On the other hand, some medical issues have arisen. One problem is increasing medical expenses, and another is the dearth of doctors and the uneven distribution of doctors and hospitals all over the country. We believe that the information and communication technology (ICT) system using Large Scale Integration (LSI) technology is a key way of saving Japan or the world from these crucial situations.

Figure 3.1 shows the past and future population pyramids in Japan. In 2005, the total population in Japan is 128 million, and is estimated around 115 million and 90 million in 2030 and 2055, respectively. In 2005, the peaks of population are for around 58- and 28-year-old people, whereas they shift to more than 80-year-old people in 2030. Furthermore, the birth rate in Japan is becoming lower and lower in the last few decades. The aging rate in Japan will become higher and higher in the near future. In fact, such a trend occurs not only in Japan but also in a wide area of the world. Figure 3.2 shows medical care expenses in several countries such as the United States, Canada, France, Germany, Korea, Sweden, United Kingdom, and Japan. As the aging rate becomes higher, the ratio of medical expenses to gross domestic product (GDP) will become higher. If the current situation continues, medical care expenses will occupy a large part of national budgets all over the world.

We started the ubiquitous biomedical information sensing system development project, sponsored by the Ministry of Education, Culture, Sports, Science and Technology (MEXT) of Japan in 2008. This project has three application areas: the urinary disturbance examination system, pregnant

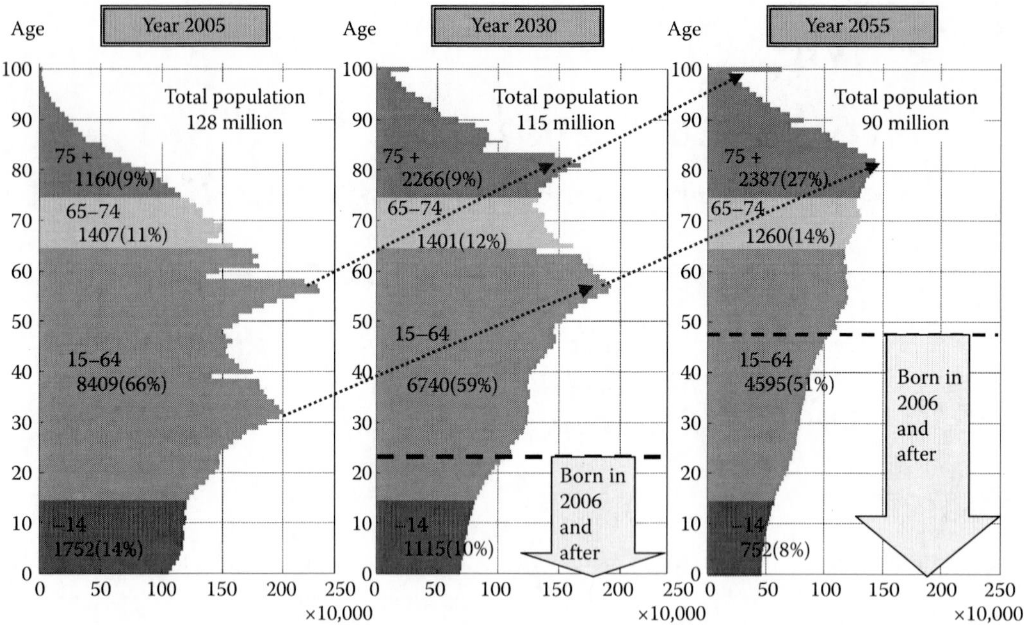

FIGURE 3.1 Past and future population pyramids in Japan.

woman and fetus health check systems, and the lifestyle-related disease detection system. All three systems utilize the ICT system in order to reduce the cost of medical care and strengthen the assurance of human health care. Figure 3.3 shows our proposed urinary disturbance examination system. In this system, a small capsule system implanted in the human bladder measures the bladder's inner pressure and sends measured inner pressure to the data transmitter. The data transmitter receives

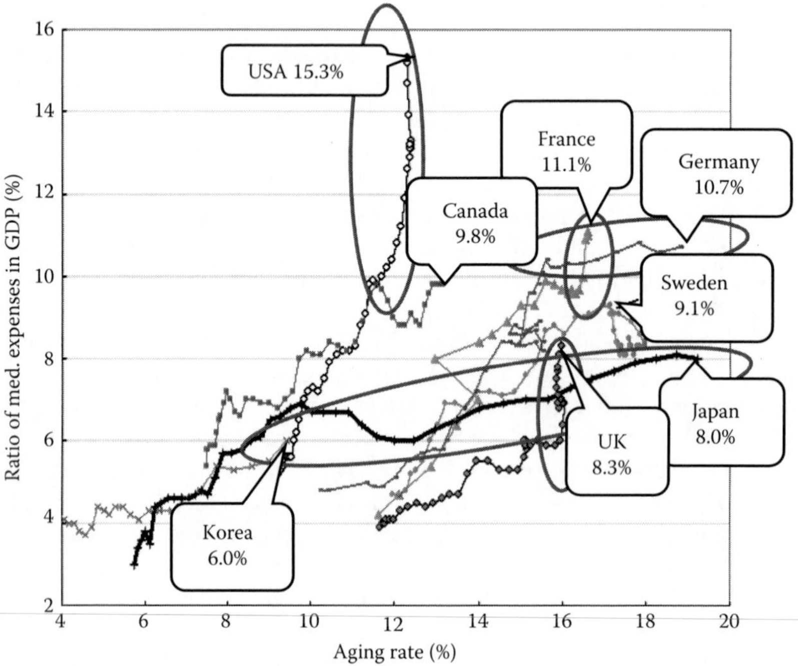

FIGURE 3.2 Medical care expenses in several countries. (Data from WHO core Health Indicators.)

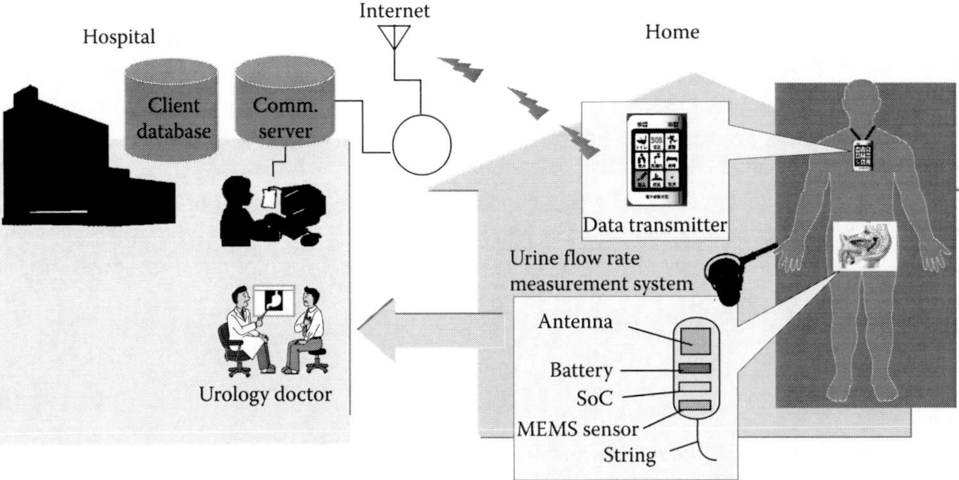

FIGURE 3.3 Urinary disturbance examination system.

sensing data from a small capsule inside the human body and sends its data to the hospital via the Internet. In the hospital, the communication server collects patient data and these are saved into the client database system. Urologists can analyze the data of patients in daily life in the hospital. Figure 3.4 shows our proposed health check system for the pregnant woman and the fetus. In this system, a small sensing system on the human body surface measures the intrauterine pressure and heartbeat of the fetus and sends the data to the hospital. Obstetricians and gynecologists can analyze the physical conditions of the pregnant woman and the fetus in the hospital. These healthcare systems using ICT are the final goals of our project.

3.2 BIOLOGICAL INFORMATION SENSING

3.2.1 Requirements for Biological Information Sensing Systems

In this section, first we will take a brief look at what the targets of biological information sensing are. Then, we will proceed to the requirements for biological information sensing systems.

Figure 3.5 shows some examples of biological information that should be sensed. In Figure 3.5, a lot of sensing information can be listed. For example, brain temperature, brain waves (electroencephalogram

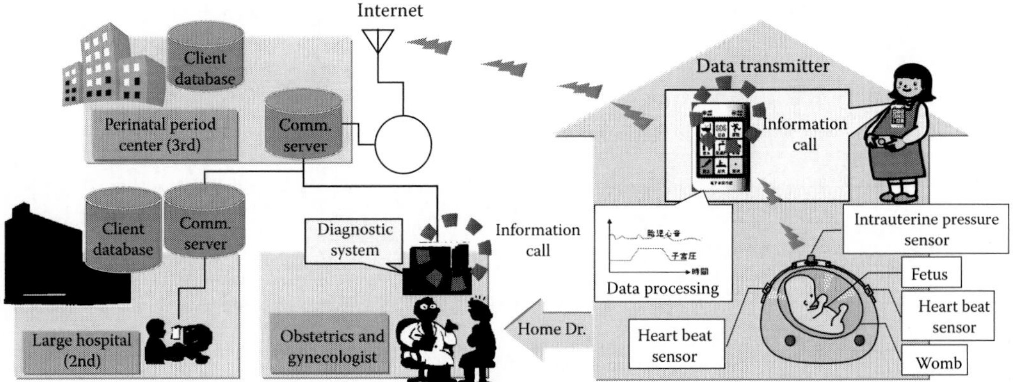

FIGURE 3.4 Health check system for the pregnant woman and the fetus.

(EEG)), and magnetoencephalograms (superconducting quantum interference devices (SQUID)) are indispensable for brain information. For bio-*acousmato* information, a stethoscope, voice, snore, and cardiac sound are important. There is enormous biological information in our body. We are conducting a project for enabling all this information to be scanned by biological information sensing systems in future. In this project, we are developing a system on a chip (SoC) using LSI technology in order to fulfill this goal.

Here, the requirements of SoC for biomedical information sensing are briefly summarized. As functions of SoC, the sensing and transmission of inner body pressure, electric potential, acoustic pressure, and so on are required. Requests from medical doctors for biological information sensing systems are summarized below:

- Lower invasion
- Less restraint
- Less awareness
- Long-term and real-time measurements

From the electrical and electronics points of view, doctors' requirements can be resummarized as follows:

- Smaller size
- Lighter weight
- Lower power consumption

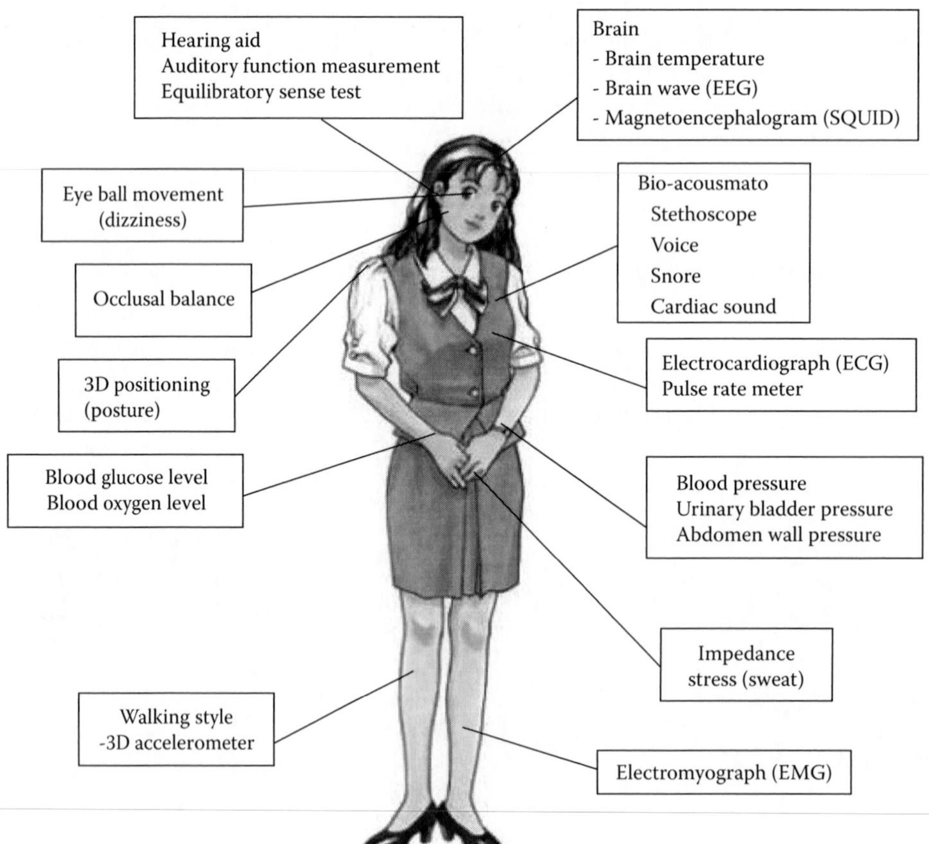

FIGURE 3.5 Biological information sensing. (Copyright IEEE 2010.)

In the next section, we introduce a urinary disturbance examination system as a specific example of biomedical information sensing systems.

3.2.2 Urinary Disturbance Examination System

Conventional urinary disturbance examination systems are very big systems and require long time restraints not only for patients but also for doctors. During measurements, clients suffer from long awareness of measurements and large invasion. The conventional urinary disturbance examination system is shown in Figure 3.6.

This system measures urine flow quantity [1]. Since the system is not so small and is installed in a hospital, patients should visit the hospital for measurements. To measure the conditions of patients, physiological sodium chloride solution is injected into their bladders. Furthermore, this is not the normal daily life situation. The measurement in daily life of the patients is preferred for urine flow measurement and for other kinds of biological information sensing, too. Evaluation of the urination mechanism is conducted using the urine flow rate curve as shown in Figure 3.7.

Healthy people's urine maximum flow rate is higher than that of patients, and their urine flow time is shorter than that of patients. Furthermore, healthy people's urine flow quantity is about 250 ml and after urine flow bladder becomes empty. On the other hand, for example in the prostatic hyperplasia patient case, the maximum flow rate is very low and the urine flow time is very long.

Diagnostics can be carried out by measuring detrusor muscle pressure, too. Detrusor muscle pressure is calculated by subtraction of the inner rectum pressure from the inner bladder pressure as shown in Figure 3.8 [4].

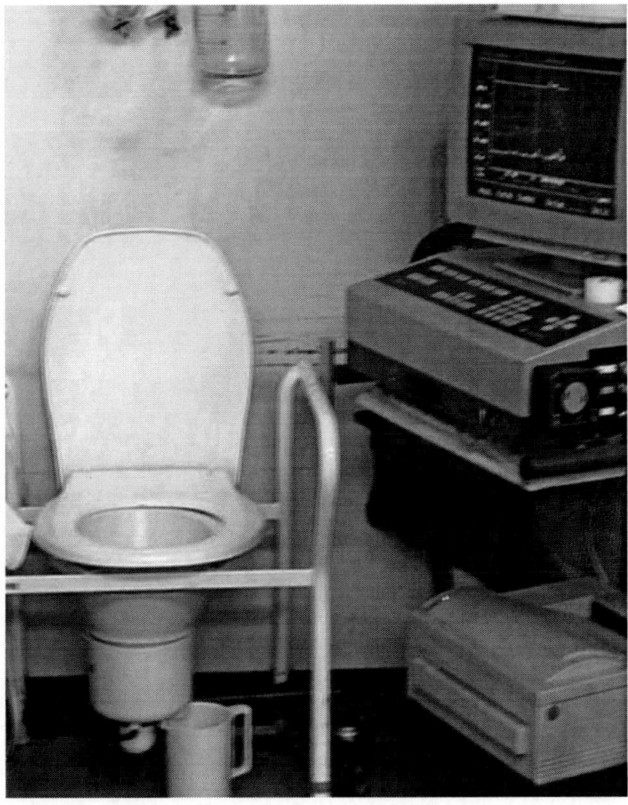

FIGURE 3.6 Conventional urinary disturbance examination system.

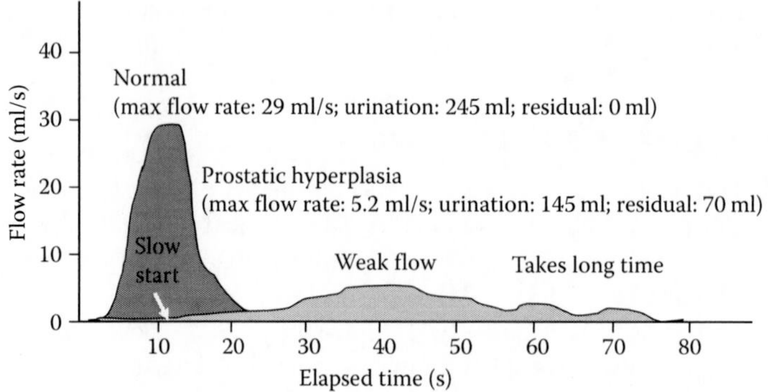

FIGURE 3.7 Evaluation of urination mechanism (urine flow rate curve). (Copyright IEEE 2010.)

Ambulatory urodynamic monitoring (AUM) has become an established method for diagnosing lower urinary tract symptoms (LUTS) attributed to underlying causes such as neurogenic bladder, prostatic hyperplasia, and malignancy [2]. AUM is expected to be able to reduce artifacts and investigate the natural activity of the urinary system in daily life, because AUM releases patients from stressful environments. In AUM, detrusor pressure measurement is indispensable for diagnosing LUTS. Although existing systems for AUM can be used at home, the results are still

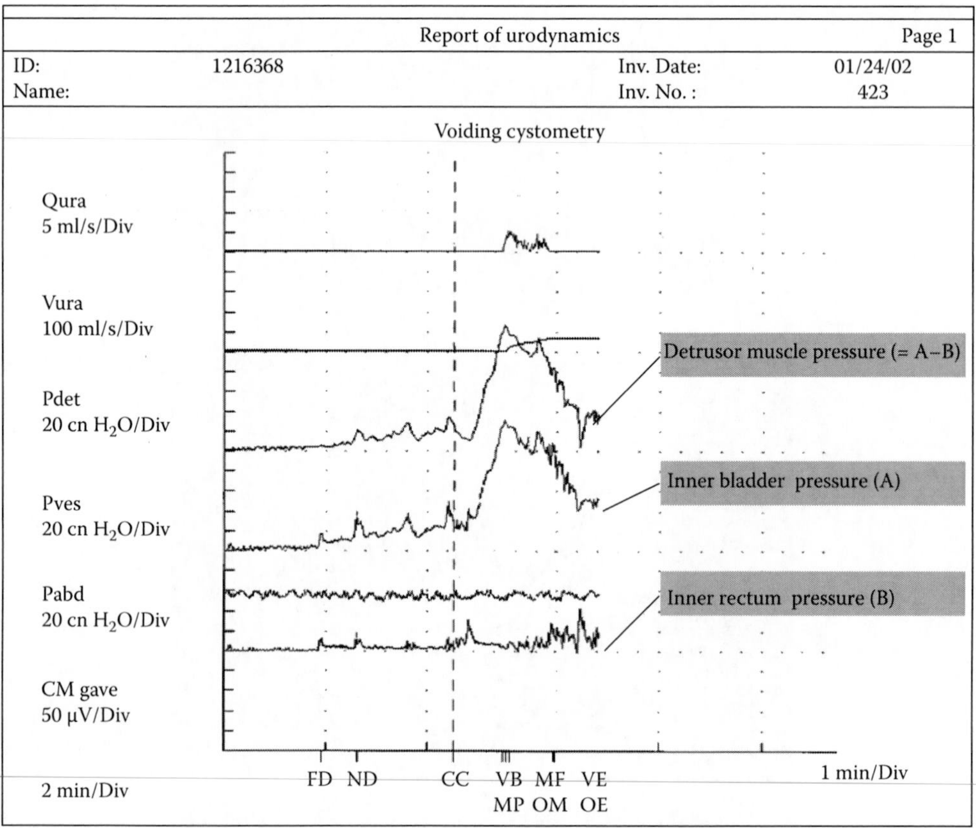

FIGURE 3.8 Diagnostics by measurement of detrusor muscle pressure. (Copyright IEEE 2010.)

supposed to contain artifacts because transurethral catheters adversely affect the test results. To improve the plausibility of the recorded data, the transurethral catheters should be removed for less-invasive pressure measurement. A balloon-type remote pressure sensing system has been proposed in [3]. However, the balloon cannot be used for AUM because the size of 25 mm in diameter is too large to pass through urethra; that is, invasive incision is necessary for inserting the balloon into the bladder.

In our project, we are developing a pressure sensor system for the inner bladder and the inner rectum as shown in Figure 3.9. The diameter of this pressure sensor system is 6.5 mm and the length is 18 mm. This inner pressure sensor is composed of an MEMS sensor for pressure sensing, an antenna coil and a capacitor for data transmission between this system and the transmitter, a small battery as the power source for all of the system, and an SoC for controlling Micro Electro Mechanical Systems (MEMS), data processing, and data transmissions. This SoC is called Medical Domain-Specific SoC, Type I (MeSOC-I). As a data transmission method, this system adopts electromagnetic induction (EMI) transmission, and its frequency is 13.56 MHz. Because transmission characteristics are not good for a small power transmission system, this system uses the error check and correction (ECC) code. The transmission circuit is composed of an antenna coil and a capacitor outside of MeSOC-I. The battery voltage is 1.55 V and its dimension is 4.8 mm in diameter and 2.15 mm in height. The battery's weight is 160 mg and its capacity is 12 mAh. Since this system should work for more than 72 h as a measurement system, all power consumptions of electronic systems in this capsule should be less than 258 μW in power. The MEMs pressure sensor is 1.7 mm wide, 2.21 mm deep, and 0.85 mm high [5].

By implanting this pressure-sensing capsule into the bladder and rectum, patients are freed from going to the hospital and suffering a long time restraint to measure their condition. Furthermore, the long time when doctors should devote to measure is also reduced, and correct biological information on patients in daily life can be gathered for diagnostics. In the next section, details of MeSOC-I are explained.

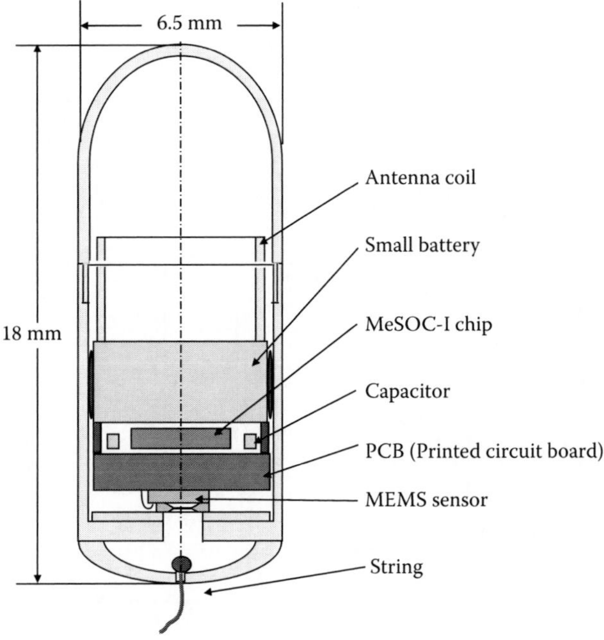

FIGURE 3.9 Inner pressure sensor for implantation. (Copyright IEEE 2010.)

3.3 MEDICAL DOMAIN-SPECIFIC SoC, TYPE I

MeSOC-I is designed for having the following two functionalities: measurement of inner bladder and rectum pressure, and transmission of pressure information [7]. Chip size is limited to 2.5 mm × 2.5 mm through the limitation of the inner pressure sensor capsule size. Since the inner pressure sensor capsule is very small, the size 2.5 mm × 2.5 mm includes the pad region. Since MeSOC-I includes not only the digital circuit block but also the analog circuit block, MeSOC-I uses TSMC 0.18 μm mixed signal CMOS technology as fabrication technology.

The block diagram of MeSOC-I is shown in Figure 3.10. MeSOC-I is composed of a digital circuit block and an analog circuit block. The digital circuit block is composed of Application-Specific Instruction-set Processor (ASIP), static random access memory (SRAM), read only memory (ROM), Timer, and Universal Asynchronous Receiver Transmitter (UART). Embedded ASIP is named Medical Domain-specific Instruction set processor eXtension (MeDIX-I). The size of SRAM and ROM is 8 and 4 kB, respectively. UART is equipped for debugging the MeSOC-I system. The analog circuit block is composed of Capacitance to Digital Converter (CDC), EMI codec circuit [13], clock generator, and power-on reset circuit. Since the output of MEMs is the change of its capacitance, CDC directly converts the change of capacitance into digital data [14].

The chip layout of MeSOC-I is shown in Figure 3.11 and the chip photograph is shown in Figure 3.12.

The analog circuit block occupies less than quarter of the cell layout area without pads. RAM is the largest component in this system. Since this SoC is fabricated for evaluation and testing, it has 100 input/output (I/O) pins. However, since the size limit for SoC is very strict because of the embedded capsule's size, it was difficult to use the normal LSI package. Furthermore, a chip size package was unavailable for this very small size die, and we implemented stacked I/O pins using solder bumps as shown in Figure 3.12. By using these bumps, MeSOC-I is soldered to the printed circuit board without additional space to the real LSI die.

Specifications of MeSOC-I are summarized in Table 3.1. These specifications are based on MeSOC-I revision 3 chip.

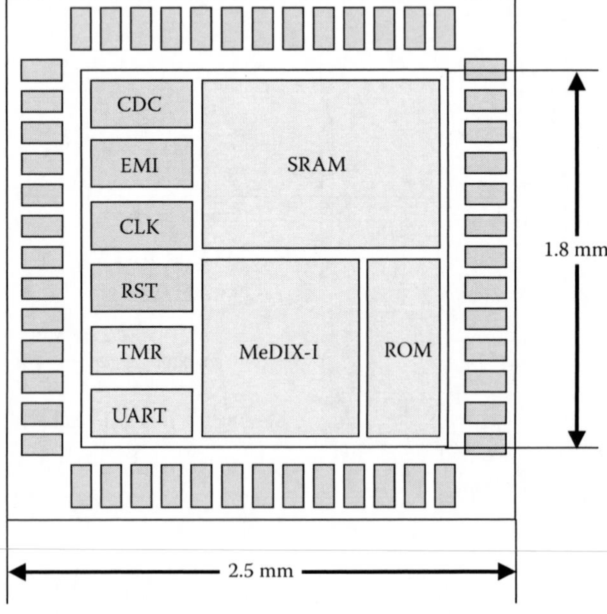

FIGURE 3.10 Block diagram of MeSOC-I. (Copyright IEEE 2010.)

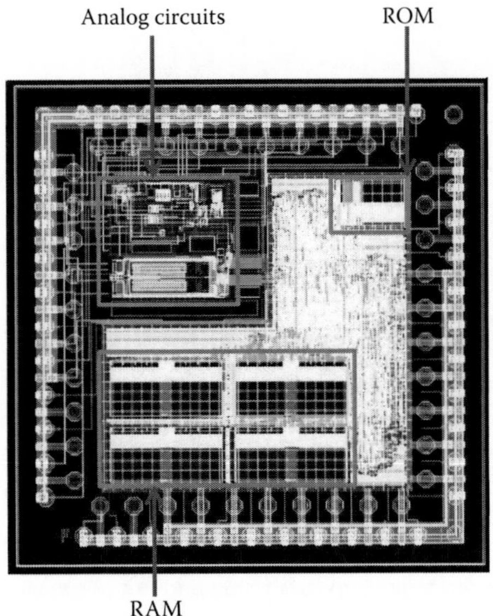

FIGURE 3.11 Chip layout of MeSOC-I.

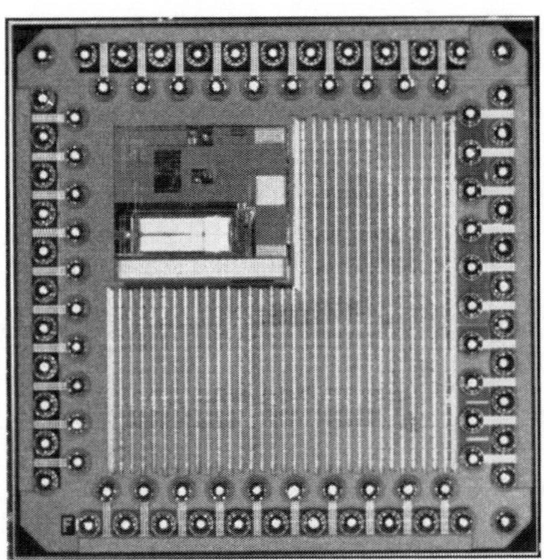

FIGURE 3.12 Photo of MeSOC-I.

TABLE 3.1
Specification of MeSOC-I (Revision 3)

Process	0.18 μm CMOS
Die area	2.5 × 2.5 (mm^2)
Gate count (digital only)	28.2 (kgate)
RAM	8 (kB)
ROM	4 (kB)
Operating frequency	161.4 (kHz)
Operating voltage	1.55 (V)
Power (digital only)	39 (μW)
Life time	Approx. 160 (h)

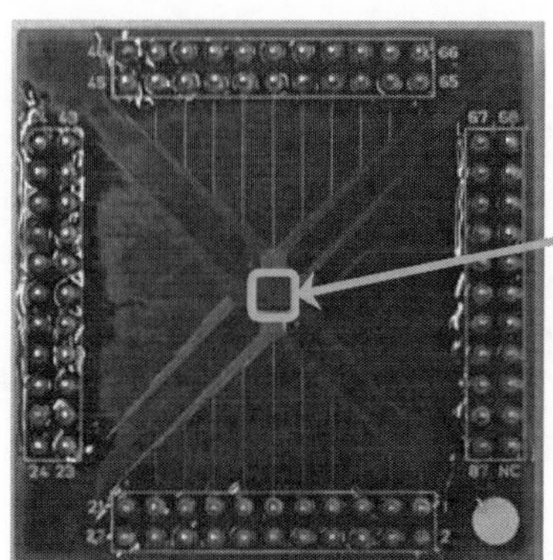

FIGURE 3.13 Chip carrier for chip evaluation.

The specific character of this chip is that the operating frequency is kept very low at 161.4 kHz and this enables the lifetime of the system to be long enough to measure the inner pressure for more than 72 h.

This specification is the same as that of MeSOC-I revision 3 chip and power consumption was measured by revision 3 real chips. We have now fabricated MeSOC-I revision 4 chip, which has larger ROM sizes.

Figure 3.13 shows a chip carrier for MeSOC-I chip evaluation. A chip carrier board is used to enlarge the I/O pitch of MeSOC-I to standard IC pitch for the evaluation board. Figure 3.14 shows the evaluation system for MeSOC-I chip. In this evaluation system, pressure exerted by pushing the cylinder in the syringe is sensed by MEMS, its data are converted into digital data by CDC, its data are filtered, and the processed data are sent to the transmitter.

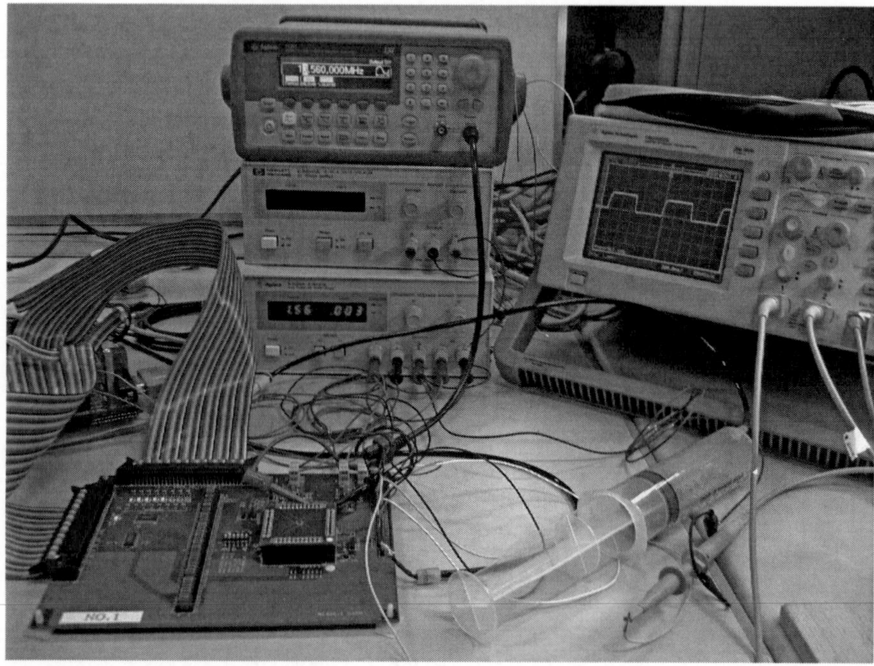

FIGURE 3.14 Evaluation system for MeSOC-I evaluation chip.

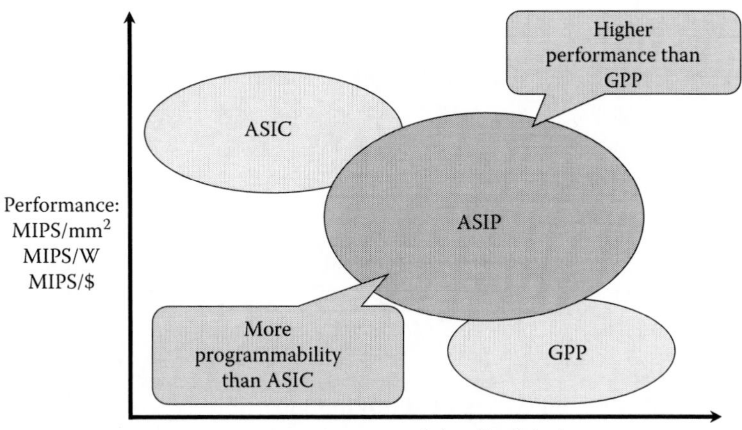

FIGURE 3.15 Advantages of ASIPs.

3.4 MEDICAL DOMAIN-SPECIFIC INSTRUCTION SET PROCESSOR EXTENSION

A specific design feature of MeSOC-I is that MeSOC-I uses an ASIP as its main controller. ASIP is a processor with a custom instruction set for specific applications or domains. Figure 3.15 shows the advantages of ASIP. Application Specific Integrated Circuits (ASICs) can achieve high performance, but their flexibility is not high. On the other hand, the General-Purpose Processor (GPP) can achieve high flexibility, but its performance is not very high. ASIP is the solution for achieving higher performance than GPP and more programmability than ASIC.

MeDIX-I is introduced in MeSOC-I [8]. MeDIX-I is an ASIP for the medical domain. MeDIX-I uses a Brownie micro 16-bit configurable Reduced Instruction Set Computer (RISC) processor [9] as a base processor. Architecture customization of MeDIX-I is conducted by using ASIP Meister [10–12]. ASIP Meister is a developing environment of ASIPs. In this project, ASIP Meister is used for customizing the instruction set of MeDIX-I. MeDIX-I is enhanced by special instructions for Multi-Dimensional Parity Code (MDPC) [6]. ASIP Meister enables easy architecture design space exploration, and MeDIX-I customization could be performed in a short design turnaround time.

Table 3.2 summarizes the architecture of the MeDIX-I processor.

Pipeline stages of the MeDIX-I processor comprise three stages: instruction fetch, instruction decode, and execution (EXE) stages. Instruction and data bit widths are 16 bits. The register file is composed of 16 16-bit registers. The number of instructions is 40, including seven special instructions for MDPC. Of these, 33 instructions are instructions of the base RISC processor. MDPC is a kind of ECC code. MPDC has the following features: 1 bit error correction and 2 bit error detection. MDPC has the feature that it easily extends the bit width of data. In our system, MDPC is used as ECC code. Since MDPC heavily uses bitwise exclusive-or operations, MeDIX-I has special instructions for efficient processing of MDPC.

TABLE 3.2
Architecture Specification of MeDIX-I Processor

Pipeline stages	Three stages
Memory architecture	Harvard architecture
Instruction and data bit width	16 bits
Register file	16 bits × 16
Number of instructions	40

TABLE 3.3
Execution Cycles of Several Implementations of MDPC (Cycles)

Data bit width (bit)	16	64	256
RISC instructions	78	291	1143
Specific HW	25	49	145
	(−68%)	(−83%)	(−87%)
MeDIX-I	13	25	73
	(−83%)	(−91%)	(−94%)

TABLE 3.4
Energy Consumption of Several Implementations of MDPC (nJ)

Data bit width (bit)	16	64	256
RISC instructions	2.69	10.0	39.4
Specific HW	1.43	2.80	8.28
	(−47%)	(−72%)	(−79%)
MeDIX-I	0.57	1.10	3.20
	(−79%)	(−89%)	(−92%)

Execution cycles of several implementations of MDPC are summarized in Table 3.3.

RISC instructions means implementation without special instructions or base processor. Specific Hardware (HW) means implementation of adding special HW for MDPC to MeDIX-I. MeDIX-I means implementation using MDPC special instructions and control instructions appended to the base RISC processor instructions. From Table 3.3, using special instructions, EXE cycles of MDPC achieve from 83% to 94% reduction from those by original RISC instructions. Furthermore, specific HW implementation reduces the EXE cycles compared to the original RISC instructions. However, implementation using specific HW is less efficient than implantation using special instructions. The reason is that the amount of data moved between register files inside the processor and the special registers inside specific HW is enormous. From the EXE cycle point of view, ASIP implementation (special instruction implantation) is the best solution for MDPC code.

Next, we compare the implementations from the energy consumption point of view. Table 3.4 summarizes the energy consumption of several implementations of MDPC.

From Table 3.4, the largest energy is consumed by base processor RISC instructions implementation. From the energy consumption point of view, ASIP implementation (special instruction implantation) is the best solution for MDPC code.

3.5 CONCLUSIONS

In this chapter, we introduce our grappling with the application of ICT using CMOS emerging technology to medical treatment and health care and show the current status of MeSOC design and development in our project. We believe that various biological information sensing systems can be implemented by using MeSOC and they would pave the way for a brighter future with fine medical treatments and better health cares.

ACKNOWLEDGMENTS

This study is partly sponsored by the collaborative research project titled “Development of Healthcare Devices and Systems for Ubiquitous Bioinstrumentation” by the City Area Program of the MEXT of Japan.

REFERENCES

1. W. Schafer, P. Abrams, L. Liao, A. Mattiasson, F. Pesce, A. Spangberg, A. M. Sterling, N. R. Zinner, and P. van Kerrebroeck, Good urodynamic practices: Uroflowmetry, filling cystometry, and pressure-flow studies, *Neurourology and Urodynamics*, 21(3), 261–274, 2002.
2. E. van Waalwijk van Doorn, K. Anders, V. Khullar, S. Kulseng-Hanssen, F. Pesce, A. Robertson, D. Rosario, and W. Schäfer, Standardisation of ambulatory urodynamic monitoring: Report of the standardization sub-committee of the international continence society for ambulatory urodynamic studies, *Neurourology and Urodynamics*, 19(2), 113–125, 2000.
3. C. C. Wang, C. C. Huang, J. S. Liou, Y. J. Ciou, I-Yu Huang, C. P. Li, Y. C. Lee, W. J. Wu, A mini-invasive long-term bladder urine pressure measurement ASIC and system, *IEEE Transactions on Biomedical Circuits and Systems*, 2(1), 44–48, 2008.
4. Damaser, M. S., Andros, G. J., Walter, J. S., Schlehahn, L., Brzezinski, K., Wheeler, J. S., Hatch, D. A., Home monitoring of bladder pressure in pediatric patients with spina bifida, *Proceedings of the 19th Annual International Conference of the IEEE*, Engineering in Medicine and Biology Society, Chicago, IL, 5, 1915–1918, 1997.
5. I. Kimura and T. Itakura, Development of pressure sensor for blood pressure monitors, *Omron Tech*, 41(2), 138–143, 2001 (in Japanese).
6. T. F. Wong and J. M. Shea, Multi-dimensional parity-check codes for bursty channels, *Proceedings of 2001 IEEE International Symposium Information Theory*, Washington, DC, p. 123, 2001.
7. H. Iwato, K. Sakanushi, Y. Takeuchi, M. Imai, A. Matsuzawa, and Y. Hirao, A low power SoC for pressure measurement capsules in ambulatory urodynamic monitoring, in *Proceedings of IEEE Symposium on Low-Power and High-Speed Chips (COOL chips XIII)*, Yokohama, Japan, pp. 441–456, 2010.
8. Y. Takeuchi, H. Ohsawa, T. Kondo, H. Iwato, K. Sakanushi, and M. Imai, Low energy MDPC implementation using special instructions on application domain specific instruction-set processor, in *Proceedings on Asia-Pacific Signal and Information Processing Association Annual Summit and Conference (APSIPA ASC 2010)*, Singapore, PP. 47–52, 2010.
9. http://www.asip-solutions.com/en/products.html
10. M. Imai, Synthesis of application specific CPU core, in *Proceedings of the Synthesis and Simulation Meeting and International Exchange (SASIMI)*, Osaka, Japan, V–I, 1989.
11. M. Itoh, S. Higaki, J. Sato, A. Shiomi, Y. Takeuchi, A. Kitajima, and M. Imai, PEAS-III: An ASIP Design Environment, in *Proceedings of International Conference on Computer Design: VLSI in Computers and Processors (ICCD)*, Austin, TX, pp. 430–436, September 2000.
12. Y. Kobayashi, Y. Takeuchi, and M. Imai, ASIP Meister, *Processor description languages*, P. Mishra and N. Dutt (Eds), Elsevier, Morgan Kaufmann, pp. 163–182, 2008.
13. T. Yamagishi, K. Matsunaga, D. T. N. Huy, M. Miyahara, and A. Matsuzawa, A 6.5 μW inverter based self biasing transceiver, in *Society Conference, 2009, IEICE*, Sapporo, Japan, pp. C–12–21, 2009 (in Japanese).
14. T. M. Vo, Y. Kuramochi, M. Miyahara, T. Kurashina, and A. Matsuzawa, A 10-bit, 290fJ/conv. steps, 0.13 mm^2, zero-static power, self-timed capacitance to digital converter, in *International Conference on Solid State Devices and Materials 2009*, Sendai, Japan, October 2009.

4 Design of a Low-Power Dual-Mode MUX-Based Transmitter for Biomedical Applications

Yao-Hong Liu and Tsung-Hsien Lin

CONTENTS

4.1 OUTLINE

A multimode low-power radio transmitter (TX) designed for implantable biomedical applications is presented in this chapter. The TX support high-data-rate frequency-shift-keying (FSK) and offset-quadrature-phase-shift-keying (O-QPSK) modulations and operates at around 400-MHz band. This chapter begins with an introduction to the target medical applications (Section 4.2) and the design requirements of the radios, with an emphasis on the transmitting devices (Section 4.3). Next, a brief review of the conventional TXs, including mixer- and PLL-based topologies is presented, and their architecture trade-offs are described (Section 4.4). To facilitate low-power and energy-efficient operation for the target applications, two TX architectures are proposed. One is a phase-locked-loop (PLL)-based TX that employs a sigma–delta phase rotator (ΣΔ–PR) to generate G/FSK modulation signals (Section 4.5) and the other is a phase-MUX-based O-QPSK TX (Section 4.6). The circuit implementations and experimental results will be presented in detail (Sections 4.7 and 4.8). Section 4.9 concludes the chapter.

4.2 IMPLANTABLE BIOMEDICAL APPLICATIONS

The physical sizes of many biomedical instruments are scaled down significantly, owing to advances in various areas of technology. The miniaturization of these devices has brought convenience and efficiency in many medical applications. Coupled with the rapid progress of semiconductor and wireless communication technologies, the small form factor also opens up new opportunities for developing implantable medical devices. This implanted device demands bidirectional wireless data telemetry for signal transmission as well as command reception.

The transmission bandwidth of general biomedical signals is typically below several kilohertz. On the other hand, some real-time medical signal transmissions require very high throughput (e.g., several Mbps), such as medical image or multichannel neural signals. The low transmission data rate and the high-power consumption of general consumer low-power radios designed for Bluetooth or Zigbee are not feasible for such applications. This section will introduce these implantable applications that require wideband transmission.

4.2.1 Wireless Capsule Endoscope

One noticeable example is the capsule endoscope system [1], as shown in Figure 4.1. IMD denotes the implant device, whereas EXD denotes the external device. The swallowable device captures a human body's internal images and transmits the data via a wireless interface. Such devices eliminate the need for a cable attached to the medical sensors and thereby greatly improve the patient's comfort level.

One major design challenge associated with these implantable devices is to extend their operation lifetime under a limited energy source (e.g., an Li-cell battery). Therefore, low-power realization is a primary design goal. In particular, the wireless communication module often dissipates a significant amount of power.

4.2.2 Multichannel Neural Recording

The real-time multichannel neural recording system incorporates arrays of miniature *in vivo* Micro-Electrical–Mechanical System electrodes for neural signal detection, as shown in Figure 4.2, for the

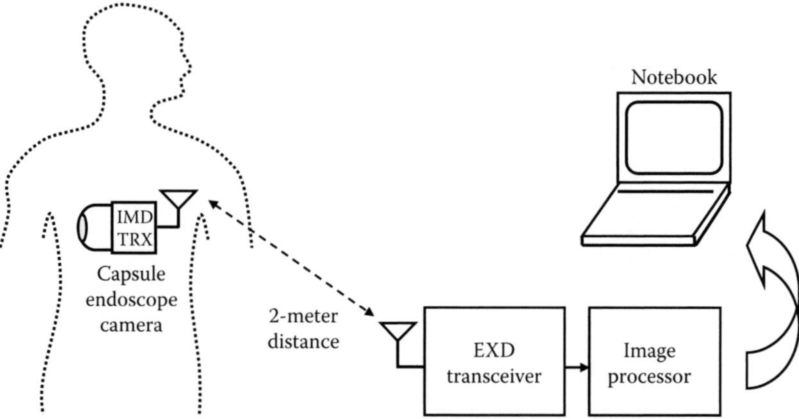

FIGURE 4.1 Wireless capsule endoscope system.

implanted electrodes have the advantages of lower infection risk and less signal interference compared with that of conventional *ex vivo* electrodes [2]. However, the large amount of collected raw data poses great challenges in the design of the implanted transmitters. While various compression or sorting techniques [3,4] can be applied to reduce the amount of neural information, a high transmission data rate is still desirable to support simultaneous multichannel recording. In addition, these transmitters must consume low power and be energy efficient to enable a long operation lifetime.

4.3 REQUIREMENTS OF THE IMPLANTABLE RF TRANSMITTERS

For medical applications requiring wideband transmission, the data communication is typically asymmetrical. The implant device needs to turn-on periodically for listing and receiving "simple" commands to control its operation from the external device, while the collected data to be transmitted outwards are often much larger. A conventional wireless link employing the same uplink and downlink signaling scheme is not energy-efficient in such an application scenario. An asymmetrical wireless link can achieve optimal performance, as depicted in Figure 4.3.

The IMD receiver typically employs an amplitude modulation method—on–off keying—for its low power consumption and fast turn-on time. On the other hand, low power and supporting large data rate are two major considerations in selecting the IMD transmitter signaling approach. In the

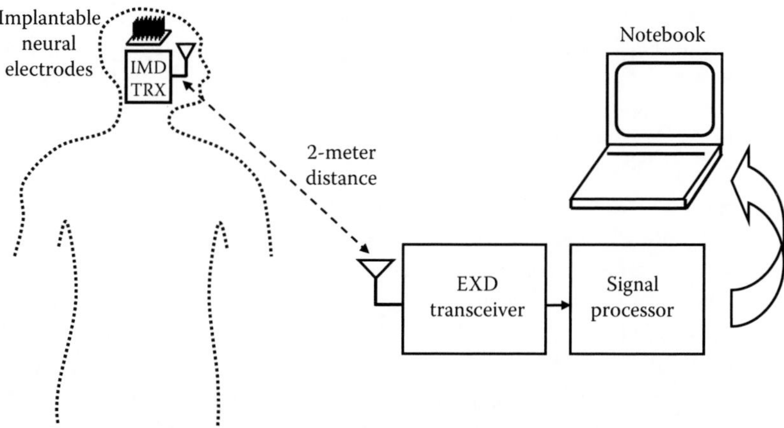

FIGURE 4.2 Implantable multichannel neural recording system.

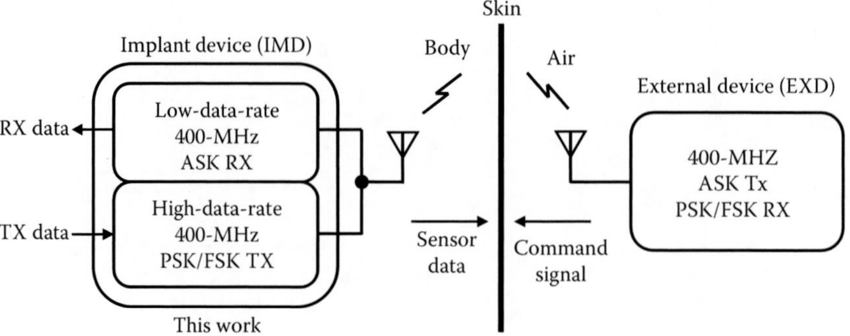

FIGURE 4.3 Asymmetrical transceiver architecture.

proposed system, the frequency-shift-keying (FSK) and phase-shift-keying (PSK) modulation schemes are adopted. Owing to the constant envelope characteristic and the relatively simple modulator designs, FSK and PSK are well suited for a low-power transmitter. This chapter will focus only on the design of a FSK/PSK dual-mode transmitter.

4.3.1 Data Rate Requirements

The transmission data rate, in the capsule endoscope system for example, depends on the image quality, frame rate, and image compression ratio, as expressed in Equation 4.1. Assuming 8-bit 256 × 256-pixel color images with 10 fps (frames/s) and 5:1 image compression ratio, the required IMD transmitter data rate is calculated to be 3.15 Mbps.

$$\text{Data\_rate} = \frac{\text{Bits\_num} \times \text{pixels} \times \text{fps} \times 3(\text{RGB})}{\text{Compression\_ratio}} \quad (4.1)$$

In a neural recording system, the requirement for uncompressed transmission data rate is mainly determined by the number of simultaneous recording channels, and the resolution and sampling rate of the analog-to-digital converter in each channel [2], as expressed below

$$\text{Data rate} = \text{channel num} \times \text{sampling rate} \times \text{bit num} \quad (4.2)$$

In this implementation, it is assumed that the implanted transmitter is designed for a system with a maximum of 64 simultaneous recording channels and each channel is sampled at 8-k samples/s with an 8-bit resolution. Therefore, the transmitter must be capable of delivering a data rate exceeding 4.1 Mbps.

4.3.2 Operation Frequency Band for Implantable Transceivers

The selection of operation frequency for an implanted transmitter must consider the signal propagation characteristics of the human body, circuit power consumption, and implantable antenna size. The proposed wireless transmitter is designed to operate at around 400-MHz frequencies [5]. This frequency range is chosen primarily because the signal propagation characteristics in an implanted environment at 400-MHz band are better than other available frequency bands (e.g., 900-MHz or 2.4-GHz ISM bands) [6], and the circuit power consumption is also likely reduced, while the transmission range is increasing compared to working at the GHz range. On the other hand, compared to the conventional low-frequency magnetic-coupled medical telemetry system [7], operating at a higher radio frequency allows smaller antenna size and larger signal bandwidth.

4.3.3 Modulation Schemes

In many low-power low-data-rate wireless communication systems for biomedical applications, amplitude-shift-keying (ASK) modulation is often used because of its low power consumption and fast turn-on time. However, ASK signal has a poor immunity to channel noise and interferences [8], which makes it impractical for the high-data-rate uplink transmission. In this regard, FSK and PSK signaling schemes are more robust and appropriate even though they require more complicated hardware. Furthermore, the constant-envelope characteristic of the FSK and PSK signals enables the incorporation of a power-efficient nonlinear power amplifier (PA) in the transmitter [9–11]. Even with these benefits, a limited energy source still poses great challenges in the transmitter design.

Figure 4.4 compares the simulated signal-to-noise ratio (SNR) requirements for FSK and PSK demodulators. It shows that the FSK modulators must deliver slightly higher output power than PSK modulation to satisfy a given SNR requirement. For example, to satisfy a 10^{-4} bit-error-rate (BER) requirement, an FSK transmitter needs to provide 3-dB higher output power than a PSK transmitter does. On the other hand, FSK modulation has the advantage of easier demodulation circuit implementation. Therefore, this chapter presents a dual-mode FSK/PSK transmitter for higher flexibility in modulation.

4.3.4 Link Budget Analysis

The radio design requirements are derived and estimated through link budget analysis, as depicted in Figure 4.5. The path loss due to signal propagation can be estimated by the free-space path loss equation shown in Equation 4.3 [12].

$$\text{Path Loss} = \left(\frac{4 * \pi * d}{\lambda}\right)^2 \tag{4.3}$$

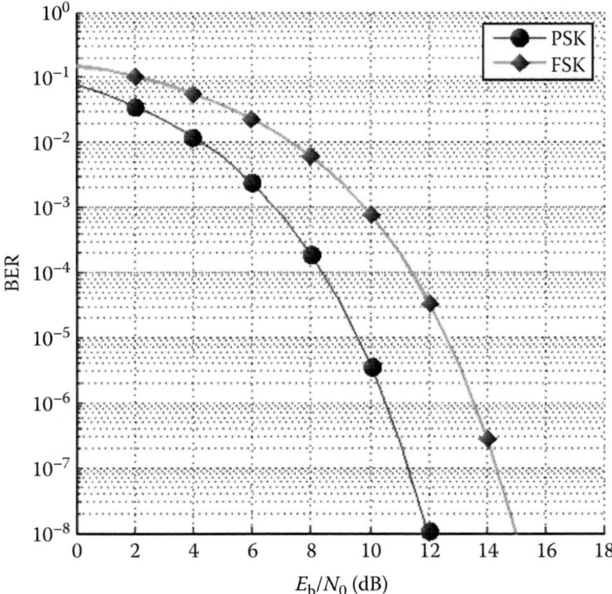

FIGURE 4.4 Simulated BER versus E_b/N_0 for PSK and FSK modulations.

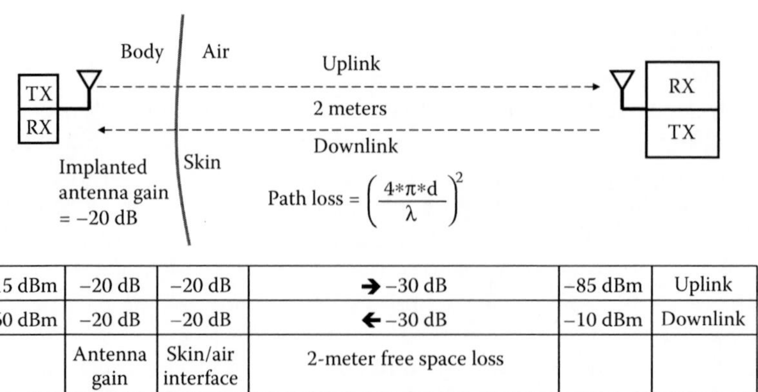

−15 dBm	−20 dB	−20 dB	→ −30 dB	−85 dBm	Uplink
−60 dBm	−20 dB	−20 dB	← −30 dB	−10 dBm	Downlink
	Antenna gain	Skin/air interface	2-meter free space loss		

FIGURE 4.5 Link budget of the proposed wireless interface.

In Equation 4.3, λ is the wavelength. *d* is the distance between the transmitter and the receiver and is specified at 2 m in this study. In addition, assuming an excess loss of 40 dB due to fading, a skin–air interface and a worst-case antenna loss of 20 dB, the total path loss is estimated to be 70 dB.

If the IMD transmitter output power is –15 dBm, then the received power at the external receiver input is calculated to be –85 dBm by using Equation 4.4.

$$P_{\text{RX\_Signal}} = P_{\text{TX}} - \text{Path Loss} - \text{Ant. Loss} - \text{Skin Loss} \tag{4.4}$$

Assuming that the EXD receiver *NF* is 6 dB and the maximum occupied signal bandwidth is 35 MHz at a maximum data rate of 17.5 Mbps, the noise floor of the external receiver can be estimated by using Equation 4.5 (where N_0 is the thermal noise power density, –174 dBm/Hz), which is around –92 dBm.

$$P_{\text{RX\_Noise}} = N_0 + 10 \times \log(\text{BW}) + \text{RX NF} \tag{4.5}$$

Therefore, the SNR at EXD receiver output is around 7 dB. As illustrated in Figure 4.4, a 7-dB SNR (corresponding to 10-dB E_B/N_0 with a bandwidth efficiency of 0.5) is adequate for the G/FSK or O-QPSK demodulator to achieve a bit error rate much lower than 10^{-4}.

4.4 LOW-POWER DIRECT-CONVERSION RF TRANSMITTER ARCHITECTURES

Low-power RF transmitters generally adopt constant-envelope modulation, such as FSK or PSK, to reduce linearity-power trade-off. In addition, direct conversion of the baseband information into RF frequency allows efficient hardware implementation. These direct-conversion transmitters can be realized in either PLL-based or mixer-based architecture. This section will discuss separately these two transmitter architectures.

4.4.1 PLL-Based Direct-Conversion Transmitters

The PLL-based solutions are often favored for low-power applications, for they are more hardware-efficient. There are three major types of PLL-based FSK transmitter architectures [9–11]. For the closed-loop type, as illustrated in Figure 4.6a, the modulation is performed with the PLL closed. The data are applied to modulate the divider or the reference signal. The closed-loop topology is mainly suitable for transmitting narrow-band signals, for the data rate is limited by the loop bandwidth. While an equalizer can be applied to compensate for the loop dynamics and extend the data rate beyond the PLL bandwidth, the gain error of the equalizer degrades FSK modulation performance [9]. The second type of the PLL-based FSK transmitter is based on the open-loop architecture, as

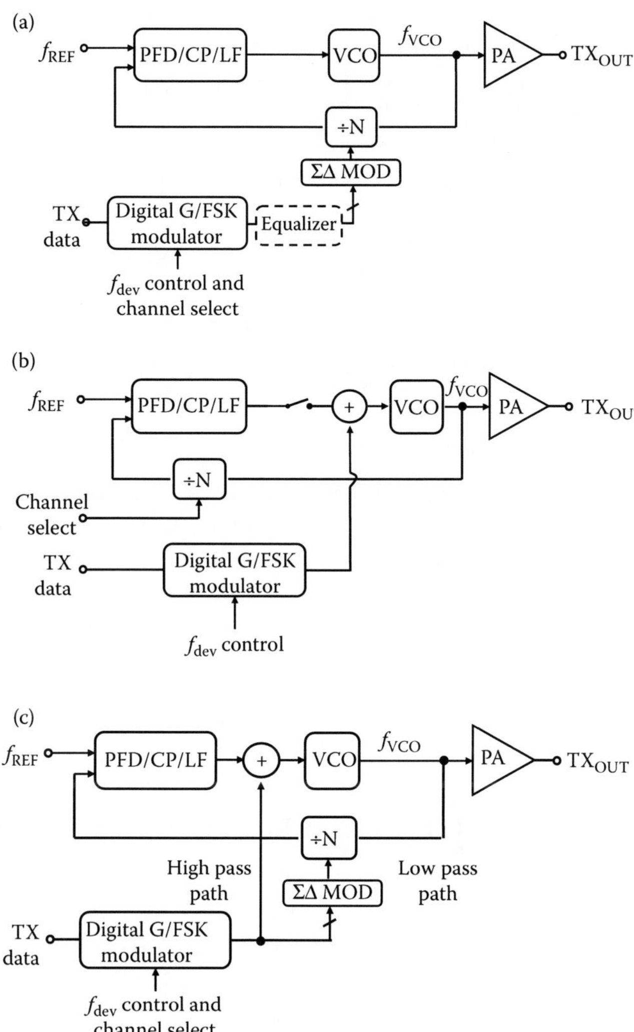

FIGURE 4.6 Conventional PLL-based G/FSK transmitter architectures: (a) closed-loop architecture, (b) open-loop architecture, and (c) two-point architecture. (f_{dev}: deviation frequency.)

depicted in Figure 4.6b. Here, the modulation data are injected to control the voltage-controlled oscillator (VCO) directly. Open-loop topology is free from the bandwidth constraint; however, since the loop is open during data transmission, frequency drift of the unlocked VCO is a major drawback. In practice, the open-loop topology requires periodic relocking of the VCO frequency, thus making continuous operation difficult [10]. In addition, the VCO phase noise is not suppressed by the loop. The third type of the PLL-based FSK transmitter is based on the two-point modulation architecture, as shown in Figure 4.6c. By combining the two previous topologies, the two-point modulation method can overcome the signal bandwidth limitation and the frequency drifting problem occurred in the closed-loop and open-loop topologies. However, this method requires good matching between the high-pass and low-pass paths [11], hence posing some design difficulties.

4.4.2 Mixer-Based Direct-Conversion Transmitters

Mixer-based direct-conversion transmitter architecture, which adopts the Gilbert-cell quadrature mixer as the RF modulator, is very popular for its flexibility in supporting all kinds of modulations.

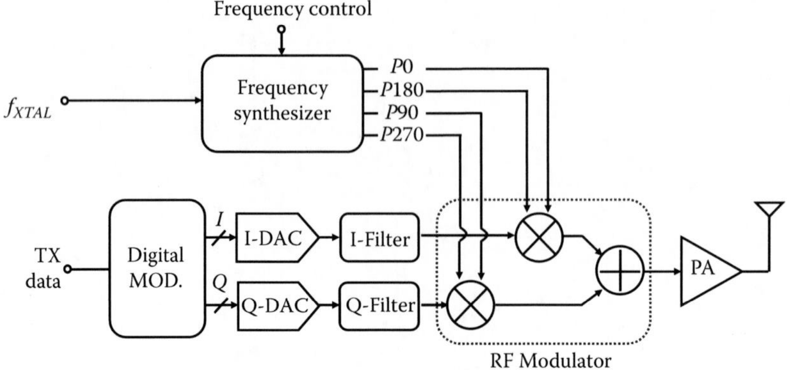

FIGURE 4.7 Block diagram of a conventional mixer-based direct-modulation transmitter.

Figure 4.7 illustrates a direct upconversion design example. It consists of two digital-to-analog converters (DACs), two reconstruction filters, summed-output quadrature mixers, and a linear PA. This architecture is a universal modulator that can modulate all kinds of modulation; however, a higher transmission data rate inevitably leads to higher power consumption of the DACs and filters, presenting a tightly coupled power-bandwidth trade-off. In addition, this transmitter topology is typically sensitive to process, supply voltage, and temperature (PVT) variations and various analog nonidealities, such as offset, IQ mismatch, and nonlinearity effects. Large devices and higher bias currents are required in the analog circuits to overcome these nonideal effects at the cost of increased silicon area and power consumption.

4.5 DUAL-MODE MUX-BASED TRANSMITTER: G/FSK MODE WITH ΣΔ–MODULATED PR

This chapter proposes a MUX-based transmitter that can be adopted as a dual-mode FSK/PSK transmitter for uplink transmission. This section will first discuss the G/FSK transmitter implementation; whereas the PSK transmitter will be separately presented in Section 4.5.

4.5.1 Operation Principle of ΣΔ–Modulated PR

Generally, FSK transmitters can be realized in PLL-based transmitter solutions for they are more hardware-efficient. In order to solve the issues of conventional PLL-based transmitter architectures mentioned in Section 4.4.1, the block diagram of the proposed MUX-based pseudo-open-loop G/FSK transmitter architecture is depicted in Figure 4.8. The proposed G/FSK transmitter consists of a PLL, a proposed sigma-delta-modulated phase rotator ($\Sigma\Delta - \text{PR}$), and frequency dividers. The PLL is designed to lock the VCO at a frequency slightly more than twice the desired transmitter output frequency. The VCO output frequency is then divided by 2 to generate a set of multiphase signals. G/FSK modulation signal is then synthesized by combining these multiphase signals by the proposed $\Sigma\Delta - \text{PR}$. In contrast to the conventional open-loop topology, the VCO remains locked by the PLL continuously. Therefore, the proposed method prevents frequency instability and obviates periodic relocking required in conventional open-loop topology. In addition, since the frequency modulation is performed outside the loop, the data rate is no longer limited by the loop bandwidth, as in the closed-loop architecture.

The core of this architecture lies in the proposed $\Sigma\Delta - \text{PR}$. A phase rotator (PR) takes multiple-phase input signals, and by properly combining these input phases, it can synthesize an output signal at a lower frequency [13–16]. Hence, it can serve as a fractional frequency divider. Its operation is usually based on the edge-combining principle. Figure 4.9a illustrates the block diagram and the operation

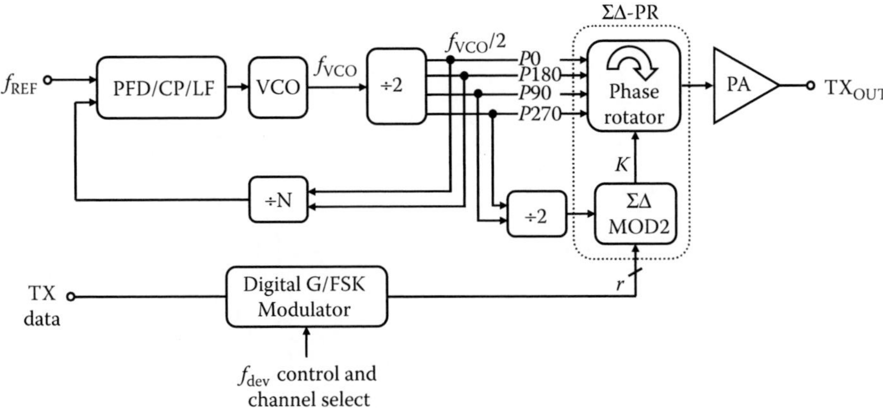

FIGURE 4.8 Proposed MUX-based G/FSK transmitter architecture.

of a conventional edge-combined PR [13], which is composed of a Phase MUX, a resampling stage, and a phase controller. In this circuit, if the input (f_{in}) to the PR is a set of four phase signals in quadrature, fractional frequency division with divide ratios of $1 + (K/4)$ ($K = 0$, 1, 2, or 3) can be realized, with a divide-ratio step size of 1/4. Here, K is the phase control signal. It determines how the phases are selected for edge-combining. The frequency at the PR output can be expressed as

$$f_{out} = \frac{f_{in}}{1+(K/4)} \tag{4.6}$$

Evidently, the output frequency can be changed by selecting a different K value. However, for typical G/FSK applications, the frequency step from the conventional PR is too coarse to produce appropriate modulation signals. Furthermore, in the conventional PR architecture, a resampling circuit triggered by the PR output is often employed to mask out the propagation delay of the phase controller (PC). However, the propagation delay of the Phase MUX and the driving strength of the resampling circuit, which are usually highly sensitive to process–voltage–temperature (PVT) variations, need to be well controlled in order to ensure glitch-free phase transitions [13].

To obtain a finer frequency resolution, this chapter proposes a ΣΔ–PR, where a dithered phase control signal K is applied to control the Phase MUX and produces an effective fractional frequency division step finer than 1/4. As illustrated in Figure 4.9b, the dithering operation is controlled by a sigma–delta modulator. In this study, the dithering operation is controlled by a 1-bit second-order sigma–delta modulator (ΣΔ–MOD2). When a fractional number, $r(0 < r < 1)$, is applied to the ΣΔ–MOD2, a modulated output bit stream K ($K = 0$ or 1) is produced to dither the PR, and generates an average output frequency, f_{out}:

$$\begin{aligned} f_{out} &= r \times \frac{f_{in}}{1+(1/4)} + (1-r) \times \frac{f_{in}}{1+(0/4)} \\ &= f_{in} \times \left(1 - \frac{r}{5}\right) \end{aligned} \tag{4.7}$$

Therefore, a fine-resolution f_{out} is obtained by an appropriate selection of the word length to represent r. As a result, FSK modulation signals with a wide variety of frequency deviations and center frequencies can be conveniently generated.

In the proposed ΣΔ – PR design (Figure 4.9b), the phase controller is triggered by the input multiphase signals to alleviate the propagation delay issue. The phase rotation (i.e., edge combining)

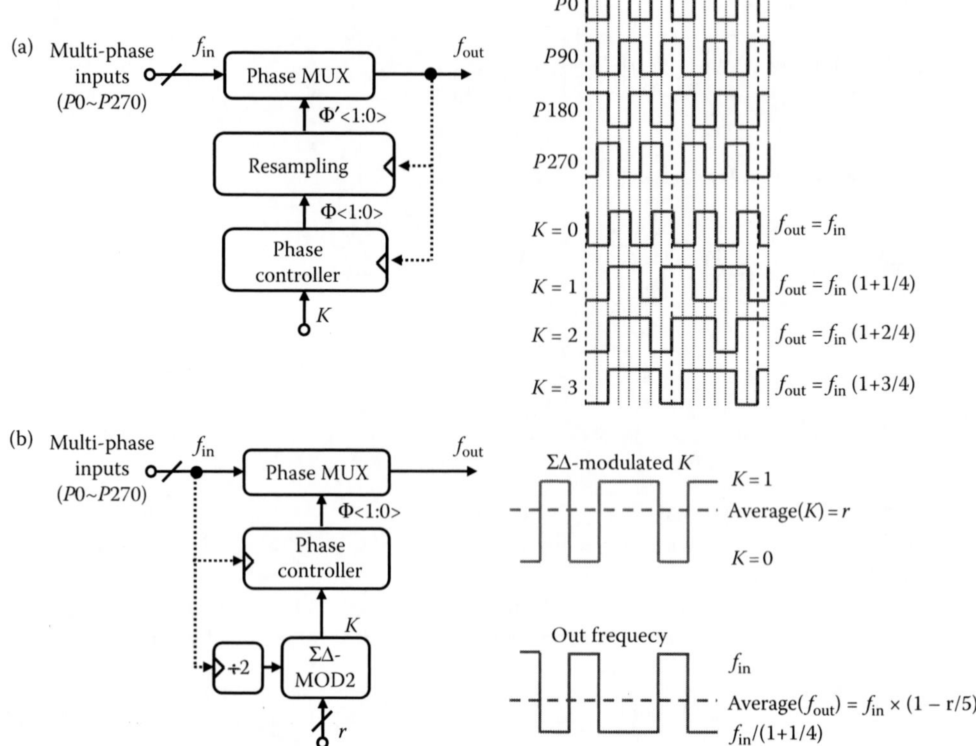

FIGURE 4.9 (a) A conventional PR and the corresponding waveforms with different phase control signals K and (b) the proposed ΣΔ–PR and its operation principle.

operation is therefore synchronized with the input signal. Hence, the timing margin and circuit driving strength requirements are relaxed such that the circuit is less sensitive to PVT variations compared to the conventional implementation.

In short, the main idea of the proposed MUX-based G/FSK transmitter architecture is to generate modulation signals outside the PLL by using a fine-resolution fractional divider. In principle, one can also employ a ΣΔ-dithered divide-by-2/3 [13] frequency divider following the VCO to accomplish this task. In comparison with this approach, the proposed ΣΔ–PR following the divide-by-2 is essentially a ΣΔ-dithered divide-by-2/2.5 frequency divider. Therefore, the proposed implementation achieves a smaller frequency step with better noise performance.

4.5.2 Noise Analysis of the Proposed ΣΔ–PR

Dithering the phase rotator introduces frequency quantization noise to the system. In this section, the noise characteristic of the proposed G/FSK transmitter is investigated. The transmitter output noise power spectrum density (PSD) consists of the phase noise from the PLL (S_{θ_PLL}) and the modulation noise from the ΣΔ–MOD2 ($S_{\theta\_\Sigma\Delta}$). The noise PSD at transmitter output (S_θ) can be expressed as

$$S_\theta(f) = S_{\theta\_PLL} + S_{\theta\_\Sigma\Delta} \tag{4.8}$$

Since the PLL noise has been well investigated in the literature [17,18], this section focuses on the noise due to ΣΔ–MOD2 (i.e., $S_{\theta\_\Sigma\Delta}$).

4.5.3 ΣΔ–PR Noise

The frequency at the ΣΔ–PR output is dithered by the ΣΔ–MOD2 with a frequency step (Δf) of $f_{in}/5$ (see Equation 4.6). Therefore, the output frequency variance is [19]

$$\sigma^2_{f\_\Sigma\Delta} = \frac{\Delta f^2}{12} = \frac{(f_{in} - f_{in}/1.25)^2}{12} = \frac{(f_{in}/5)^2}{12} \tag{4.9}$$

The PSD of this dithered frequency is expressed as the variance divided by the sampling frequency of ΣΔ–MOD2, f_{CLK} (here, f_{CLK} is half of the ΣΔ–PR input frequency $f_{in}/2$), and then multiplied by the noise transfer function of the ΣΔ–MOD2 ($NTF_{\Sigma\Delta}$–MOD2), as expressed below.

$$\begin{aligned} S_{f\_\Sigma\Delta}(f) &= \frac{\sigma^2_{f\_\Sigma\Delta}}{f_{CLK}} \times NTF_{\Sigma\Delta-MOD2} \\ &= \frac{(f_{in}/5)^2}{12} \cdot \left(\frac{1}{f_{CLK}}\right) \cdot \left(2\sin\frac{\pi \cdot f}{f_{CLK}}\right)^4 \\ &= \frac{8}{75} \cdot f_{in} \cdot \left(\sin\frac{2 \cdot \pi \cdot f}{f_{in}}\right)^4 \end{aligned} \tag{4.10}$$

Since the phase noise is the integral of the frequency noise, the phase noise PSD is obtained by dividing the frequency noise PSD by the square of the offset frequency, f, as expressed in

$$\begin{aligned} S_{\theta\_\Sigma\Delta}(f) &= \frac{S_{f\_\Sigma\Delta}(f)}{f^2} \\ &= \frac{8}{75} \cdot \frac{f_{in}}{f^2}\left(\sin\frac{2 \cdot \pi \cdot f}{f_{in}}\right)^4 \end{aligned} \tag{4.11}$$

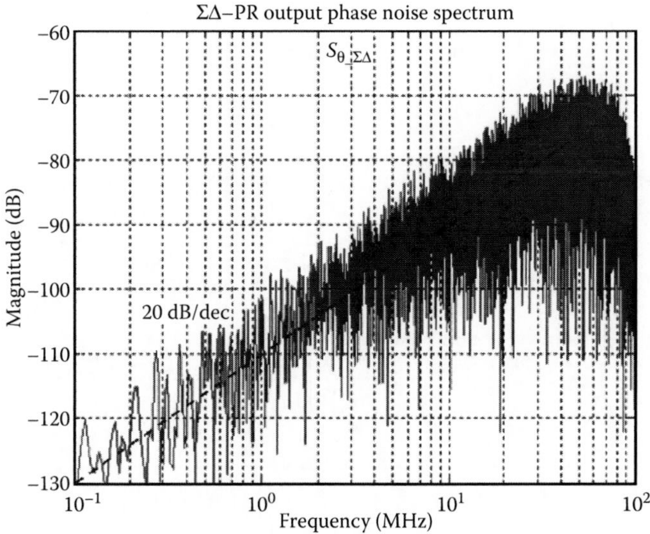

FIGURE 4.10 Simulated phase noise PSD due to ΣΔ-dithering ($S_{\theta\_\Sigma\Delta}$).

Equation 4.11 reveals that the noise $S_{\theta\_\Sigma\Delta}$ is high-pass shaped owing to the sigma–delta modulator operation, and is shifted away from the transmitter output frequency. Figure 4.10 illustrates the simulated high-pass shaping characteristic of $S_{\theta\_\Sigma\Delta}$. The noise due to ΣΔ–MOD2 is increased with a slope of 20 dB/dec. The noise from the ΣΔ–PR will dominate the output noise at higher offset frequencies. A high clock rate modulator and a transmitter output filter help in suppressing the out-of-band noise and other spurious contents to some extent.

4.5.4 Noise Analysis of the Proposed TX with ΣΔ–PR

In order to examine the noise contributions from the ΣΔ–PR and the PLL, and their effects on the total transmitter output noise, a phase-domain noise model is devised. As shown in Figure 4.11a, a white-noise source and a second-order differentiator sampled at a frequency of $f_{VCO}/4$ serve to model the ΣΔ–MOD2 frequency quantization noise ($S_{f\_\Sigma\Delta}$). A scaled accumulator transforms the $S_{f\_\Sigma\Delta}$ into the phase noise PSD ($S_{\theta\_\Sigma\Delta}$). The accumulator is clocked by a four-phase clock with a frequency of $f_{VCO}/2$, which is equivalently sampled at a rate of $2*f_{VCO}$. After summing with the PLL noise PSD (S_{θ_PLL}), the combined output noise PSD (S_θ) can be estimated. The combined noise is then filtered by the transmitter output filter. Figure 4.11b conceptually illustrates the noise contributions from the PLL and the ΣΔ–PR, and the total transmitter noise (S_{θ_TX}). At high offset frequencies, $S_{\theta\_\Sigma\Delta}$ dominates the output noise performance; while at frequencies close to the carrier frequency, PLL dominates.

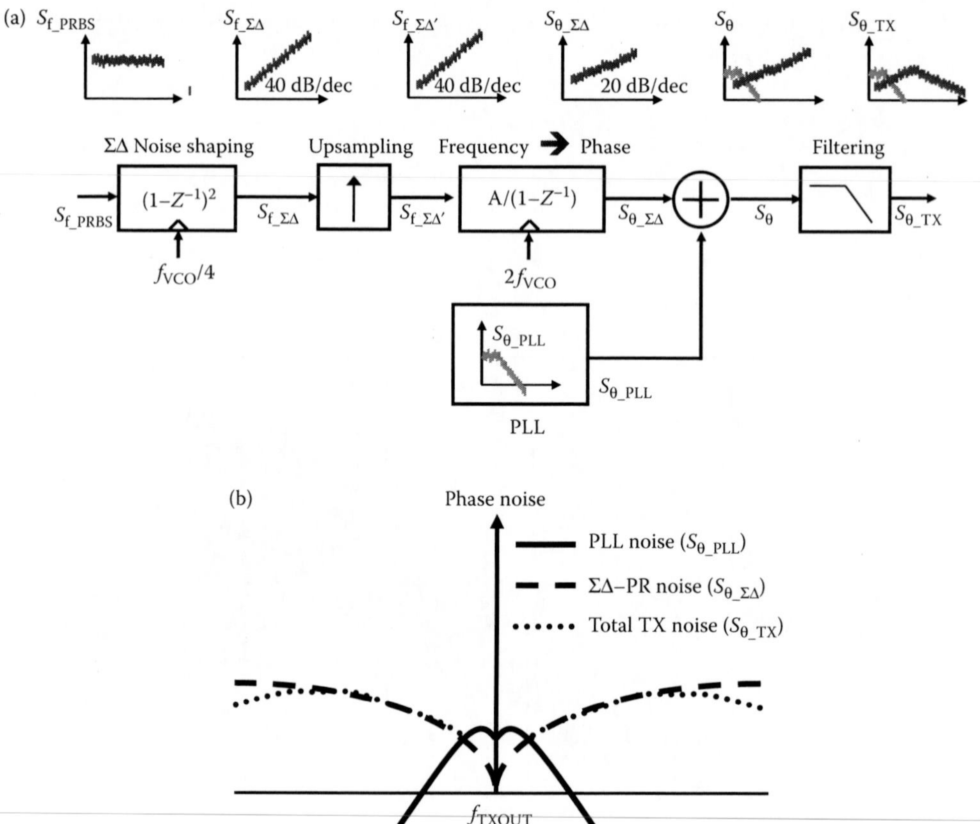

FIGURE 4.11 (a) Noise modeling of the proposed TX. (b) Plot illustrating various noise spectra and total TX output noise.

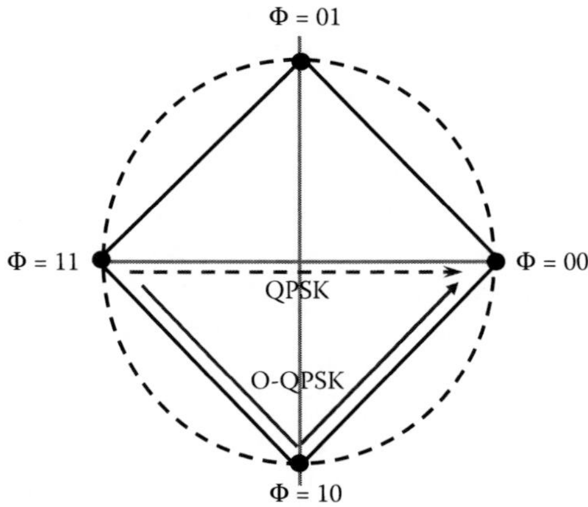

FIGURE 4.12 Constellation of the O-QPSK modulation.

4.6 DUAL-MODE MUX-BASED TRANSMITTER: OFFSET-QPSK MODE WITH PHASE MUX

4.6.1 Operation Principle of Phase-MUX as an Offset-QPSK Transmitter

O-QPSK modulation is a variant form of QPSK modulation. The O-QPSK signal is generated by offsetting one of the data streams by half the symbol period. As a result, a transition between two diagonally opposite phases (e.g., $\Phi = 11$ and $\Phi = 00$) must pass through an intermediate phase (e.g., $\Phi = 10$), as illustrated in the constellation diagram in Figure 4.12. This prevents the signal power from dropping considerably in the presence of finite circuit bandwidth during data transition. Therefore, the O-QPSK signal allows an efficient nonlinear PA to be utilized for low power consumption.

To circumvent the problems of mixer-based transmitters mentioned in Section 4.4.2, a MUX-based (O-QPSK) transmitter is proposed in this section [20]. As shown in Figure 4.13, in this architecture, the quadrature mixers in the conventional transmitter are transformed to the proposed Phase MUX. The Phase MUX selects one of the quadrature phases (*P*0–*P*270) to the PA based on the baseband data (Φ <1:0>). Fundamentally, the proposed Phase MUX directly implements the quadrature phase-shift keying operation, and creates the desired O-QPSK/QPSK

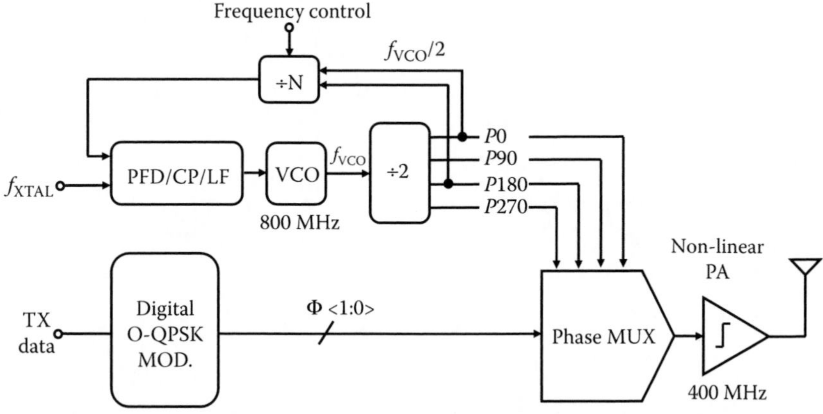

FIGURE 4.13 Block diagram of the proposed Phase-MUX-based O-QPSK transmitter.

modulation signals in a hardware-efficient way. In this architecture, the two power-hungry high-speed DACs and wide-bandwidth filters required in the conventional transmitters are eliminated.

As will be explained in Section 4.7, the Phase MUX consumes low power, and occupies a small chip area, since large on-chip inductors for the mixers are no longer required. The digital O-QPSK modulator implements a compact digital baseband. The digital baseband data are utilized to control the Phase MUX operation. A charge pump frequency synthesizer operating at twice the transmitter output frequency is implemented in the proposed architecture. The VCO output is divided by 2 to generate four phases in quadrature. Since the VCO is operated at twice the carrier frequency, direct pulling from PA is alleviated in this architecture. Furthermore, operating at higher frequency also enables a better inductor quality factor and increases the LC-tank impedance, which facilitates a better oscillation condition.

Before describing the Phase MUX circuit, we first examine a conventional implementation of a quadrature Gilbert-cell up-conversion mixer, as depicted in Figure 4.14a. The input trans-conductance (g_m) stage converts the input analog quadrature voltage signals (V_I, V_Q) into currents. The quadrature current signals are upconverted to the carrier frequency by the switching quads and are then summed together in the current domain. In order to accommodate a large baseband voltage amplitude while minimizing signal distortion, linearization techniques are usually adopted in realizing the g_m stage, which inevitably results in gain reduction. The power consumption of this conventional quadrature mixer is usually high in order to satisfy linearity and gain requirements simultaneously.

Figure 4.14b shows the proposed Phase MUX circuit. The circuit selects a pair of complementary phases based on the data symbol Φ <1:0>. The Phase MUX can be considered as an overdriven

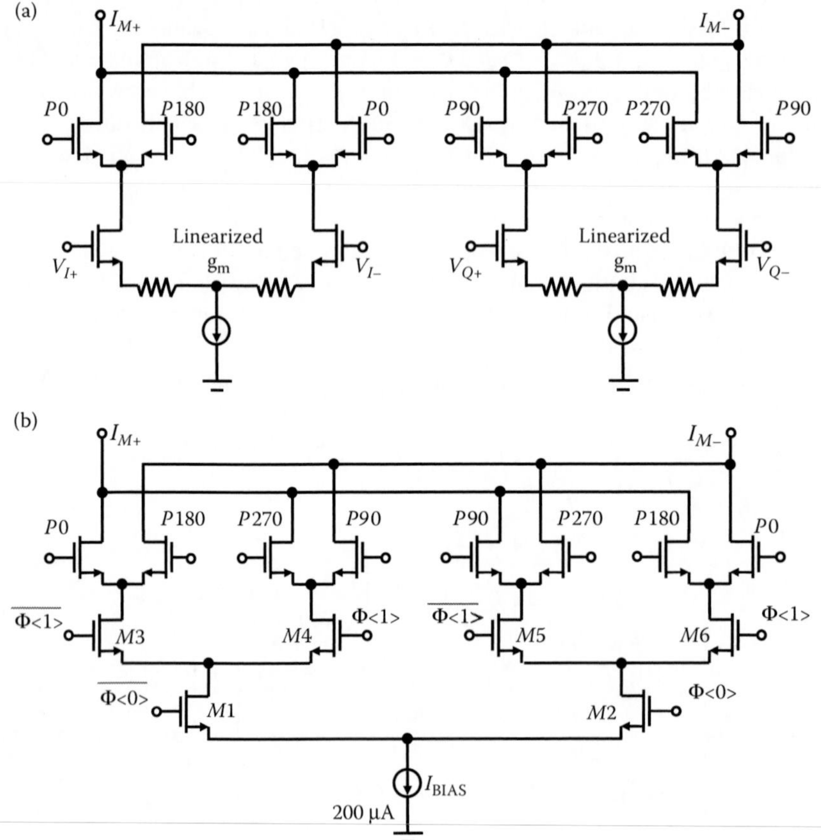

FIGURE 4.14 (a) Schematic diagram of a conventional quadrature Gilbert-cell mixer. (b) Schematic of the proposed Phase MUX.

quadrature Gilbert-cell mixer and is particularly suitable for generating PSK-type modulation signals. The proposed Phase MUX has several benefits. First of all, compared with the conventional mixers, this circuit is less sensitive to PVT variations, because there is no trans-conductance dependence in such a semidigital implementation. Second, since there is no linearized g_m stage employed in this architecture, the Phase MUX avoids the gain and linearity trade-off that exists in a conventional mixer design, thus allowing low power consumption. Finally, large swings from the baseband data Φ <1:0> facilitate a fast circuit operation.

4.6.2 Design Considerations of the MUX-Based O-QPSK Transmitter

The performance of a wireless transmitter is affected by many factors, such as quadrature accuracy, analog offsets, nonlinearity, and phase noise [21]. Although the Phase-MUX-based transmitter is inherently more robust because of its semidigital design, its performance may still be limited by some nonideal effects. This section will discuss the limitation and design considerations of the proposed O-QPSK transmitter.

4.6.2.1 Quadrature Mismatch

The modulation quality of RF transmitters is significantly influenced by the quadrature gain and phase accuracy of the analog baseband and local oscillator (LO) signals. The gain mismatch of a conventional quadrature mixer is dictated by the matching quality between the I-path and Q-path DACs, amplifiers, filters, and mixer trans-conductor stages. In contrast, in the proposed architecture, better gain matching is inherently guaranteed because the same tail current source (I_{BIAS} in Figure 4.14b) is shared between I and Q paths. In addition, the sources of mismatch are reduced since several analog circuits (e.g., DACs, filters, etc.) are removed from the signal paths in the proposed transmitter. The quadrature phase accuracy is ensured by well-balanced LC-VCO and divide-by-2 frequency divider designs.

4.6.2.2 Nonideal Switching of the Data Switches

If the Data Switches of the Phase MUX (M1–M6) are not fully switched, the signal leakage from quadrature phases would degrade the modulation accuracy. Figure 4.15a illustrates the case when M1/M2 are not fully switched, while Figure 4.15b illustrates the case when M3/M4 and M5/M6 are not fully switched. The quadrature phase current will leak to the output and sum with the desired phase current, rotating the I–Q constellation (see Figure 4.15c). Error-vector-magnitude (EVM) degradation due to this phenomenon can be calculated by estimating the phase deviation, as expressed in Equation 4.12, where k is the leakage percentage from the quadrature phase signal.

$$\mathrm{EVM}_{\mathrm{DATA\_SW}} \approx \tan^{-1}\left(\frac{k}{1-k}\right) \tag{4.12}$$

In the proposed transmitter, the input data (Φ <0> and Φ <1>) from the digital O-QPSK modulator are rail-to-rail signals. Incomplete switching of the Data Switches is therefore avoided in this design.

4.6.2.3 Offset of the LO Switches

LO leakage in RF transmitters also significantly affects modulation quality. It is mainly induced by DC offset voltage of the input trans-conductors and LO switches in the upconversion mixers. Compared to a conventional quadrature mixer, the proposed Phase MUX is essentially free from the offset in the Data Switches (M1–M6), since the effects of offset voltage are masked out by fully switching these differential pairs.

However, the offset of the LO switches will alter the duty cycle of output signal and degrade the modulation accuracy. As illustrated in Figures 4.16a and b, assuming that an input-referred offset voltage (V_{OS}) exists at the LO switches M7/M8, this offset voltage changes the duty cycle of the output signal. At the receiver, the altered duty cycle leads to a scaled DC value, thus changing

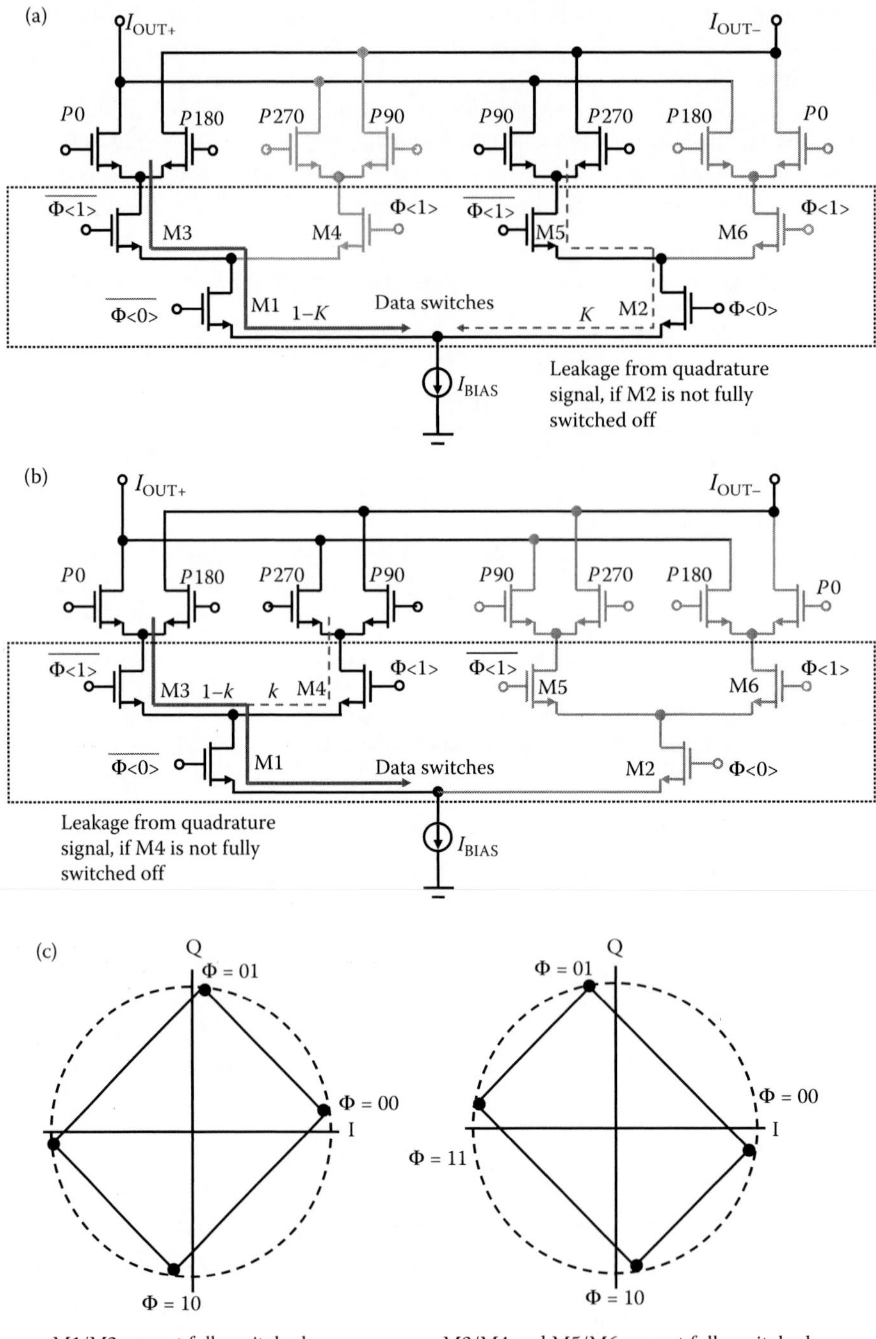

FIGURE 4.15 (a) Nonideal switching of Data Switches M1/M2, (b) nonideal switching of Data Switches M3/M4, and (c) nonideal effects on I–Q constellation.

the magnitude of the receiver demodulated output. Therefore, the modulation accuracy is affected. This nonideality is generated in conjunction with the demodulation process in the external receiver; hence, the limiting action of inverter-type PA does not help in restoring the modulation accuracy. In order to reduce this duty-cycle variation, the slope of the LO signals (i.e., *P*0–*P*270) should be made sharp enough to reduce the sensitivity of the modulation accuracy to LO switches mismatches.

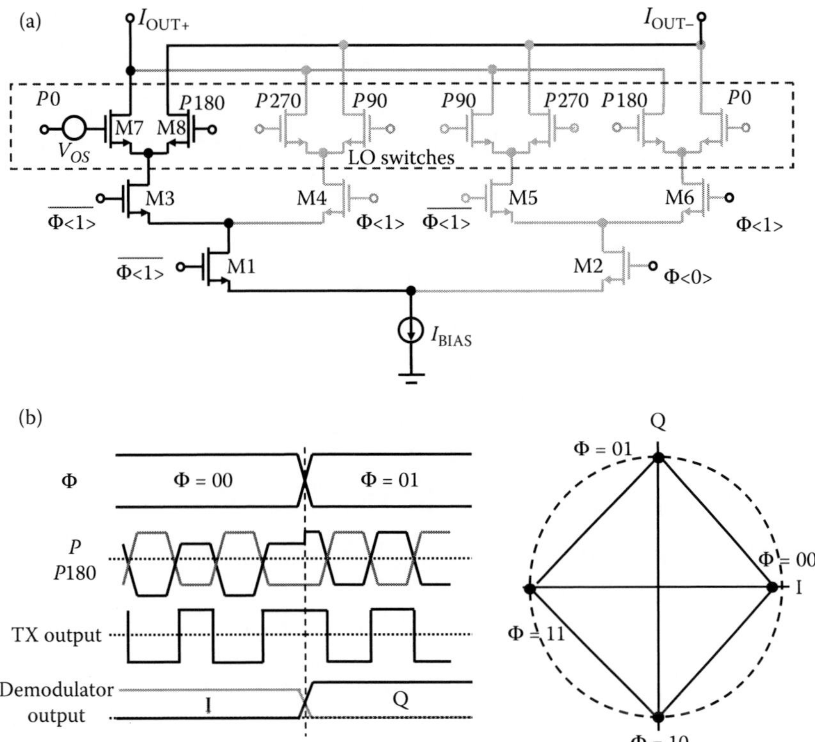

FIGURE 4.16 (a) Offset of the LO switches. (b) Conceptual illustration of the offset effects on the modulation accuracy.

4.6.2.4 Nonlinearity

In a conventional transmitter, the nonlinearity is mainly attributed to the trans-conductor stages of the mixers and the PA. The linearity requirement is more demanding if a high-PAR modulation scheme is employed. In the proposed wireless interface and transmitter design, the linearity issue is relaxed by, first of all, choosing the low-PAR O-QPSK modulation scheme. Furthermore, the operation of the Phase MUX does not rely on linear trans-conductor stages, hence eliminating this source of nonlinearity.

4.7 CIRCUIT IMPLEMENTATION

The proposed dual-mode MUX-based transmitter, which consists of the ΣΔ–PR and a PLL operated at above twice the transmitter output frequency (see Figure 4.17), is demonstrated in the 400-MHz frequency band. In this section, key building blocks are described in detail.

As mentioned in Section 4.6, the proposed ΣΔ–PR can also be adopted as a PSK-type transmitter. This can be achieved by directly selecting one of the quadrature phases through the Phase MUX in the ΣΔ–PR while gating the FSK phase control signal by Data MUX, as shown in Figure 4.17.

4.7.1 High-Speed Glitch-Free PC

The proposed ΣΔ–PR operates on the 400-MHz multiphase input signals and generates a phase-combined output. The "speed" of phase rotation is sigma–delta dithered to produce fractional frequency division with fine resolution. One key component of the ΣΔ–PR is the PC. It determines how the input phases are combined in the Phase MUX. Figure 4.18a shows the block diagram of the

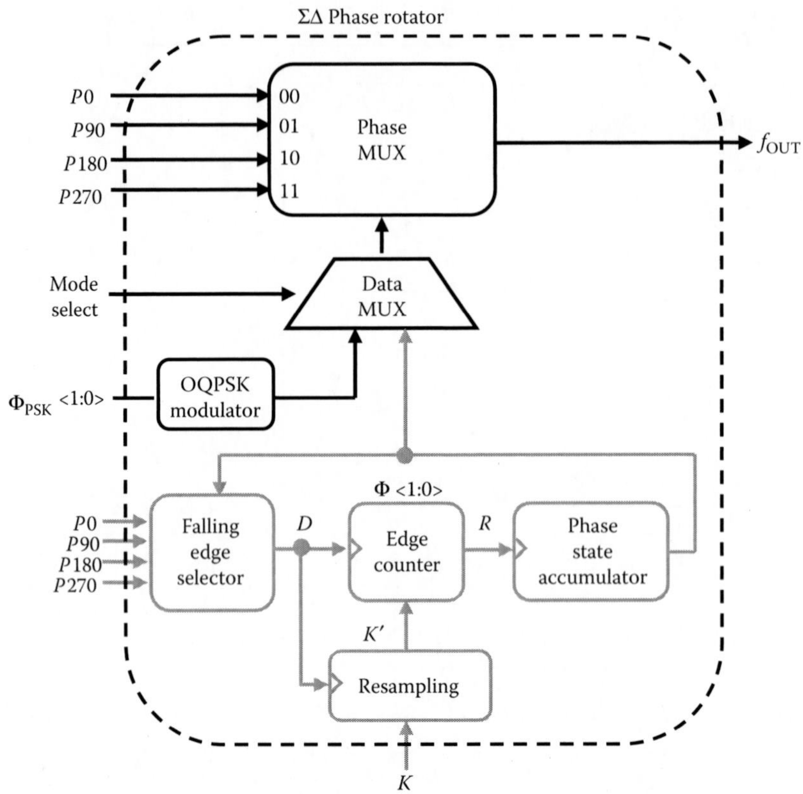

FIGURE 4.17 Implementation of QPSK modulation using Phase MUX in ΣΔ–PR.

PC with Phase MUX. The PC serves to detect and control how the phases are selected, whereas the Phase MUX combines the selected input phase signals (P0–P270) according to the Phase State information (Φ <1:0>) from the PC. The detection and combining functions are implemented separately to relax the circuit timing constrains.

In Figure 4.18a, K is a 1-bit (0 or 1) stream from ΣΔ–MOD2. Depending on K, the frequency division ratio can alternate between 1 and 1.25 (see Equation 4.4). When $K = 0$, the selected phase signal remains unchanged; the output frequency is the same as the input. When $K = 1$, the Phase MUX selects the four phases sequentially, resulting in an equivalent divide-by-1.25 (/1.25) operation. To achieve glitch-free and high-speed operation, the PC must be designed with care to ensure a smooth signal transition.

The PC (see Figure 4.18a) is mainly composed of a falling edge selector (FES), an edge counter (EC), and a phase state accumulator (PSA). The operation timing diagram of the PC is depicted in Figure 4.18b, with the propagation delay ignored for simplicity. When $K = 1$, to achieve seamless transitions between two adjacent phase signals (e.g., $P0 \rightarrow P90$), Phase MUX should change its selection while both phase signals (e.g., $P0$ and $P90$) are at the same logic levels (voltages). (If a transition from $P0$ to $P90$ occurs when $P0 = 0$ and $P90 = 1$, or $P0 = 1$ and $P90 = 0$, an extra pulse will appear at the output in the process of handover.) That is, the PC should update the Phase State Φ and trigger a phase signal transition under such conditions. Furthermore, since the output period is longer than the input period (when $K = 1$), the number of falling (or rising) edges of the input signal can be used as an indicator to signify when the phase transition should occur. Assuming that the output is aligned with the input at the falling edges, if 2 falling edges from a given phase signal are detected, the PC will update the Phase State (Φ) and command the Phase MUX to move its selection to the next phase signal.

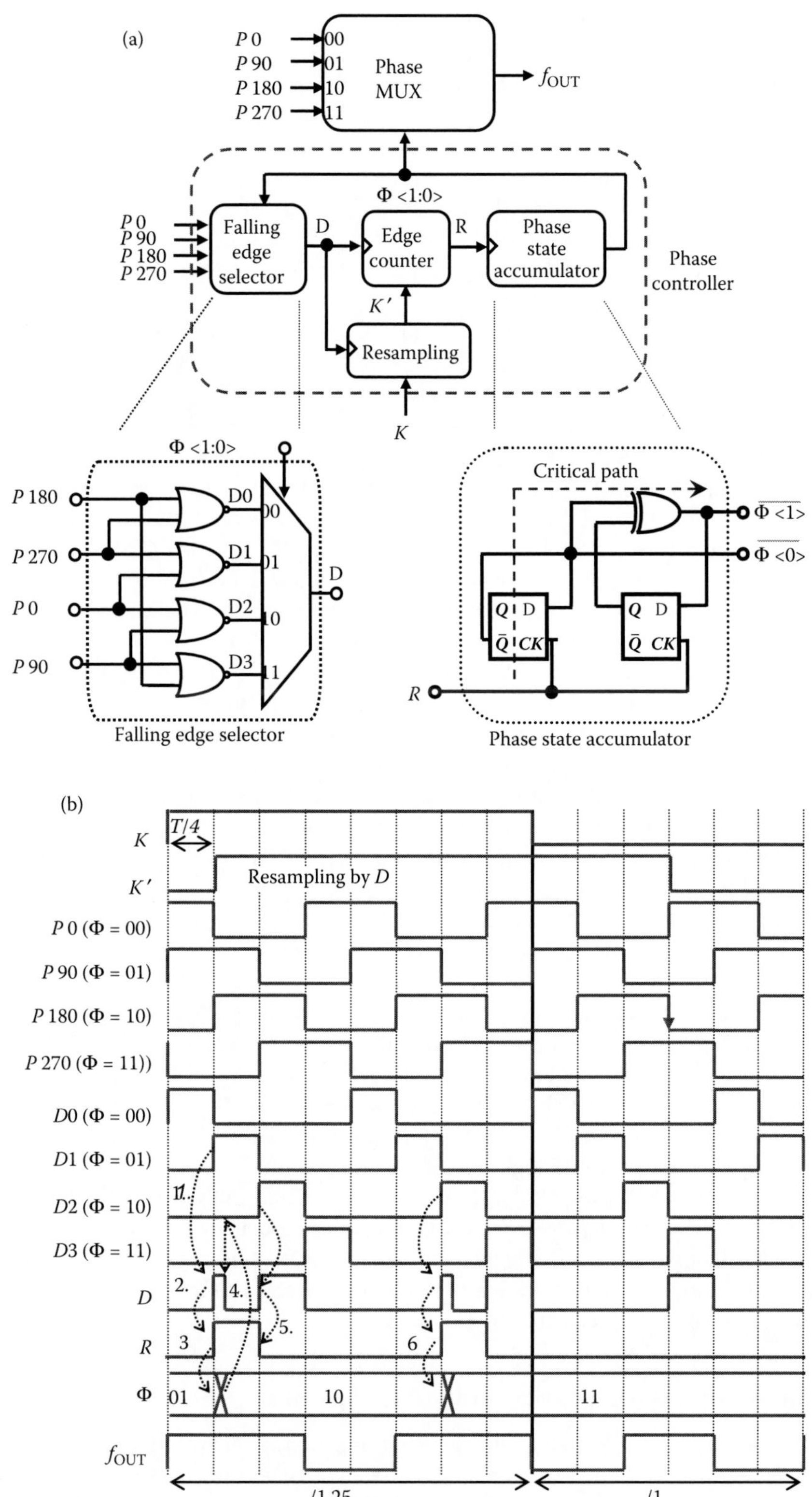

FIGURE 4.18 (a) PC block diagram. (b) Operation timing diagram.

In the FES, before each arrival of the falling edges of the four input phases ($P0$–$P270$), a corresponding pulse signal ($D0$–$D3$) is generated (e.g., a positive pulse at $D0$ is generated before the falling edge of $P0$). According to the 2-bit Phase State (Φ), one of these signals ($D0$–$D3$) is selected as the FES output, D. The signal D then triggers the EC, which is a 1-bit counter. If K' is 1 (K' is the resampled K), the EC records the number of D pulses (hence counting the number of falling edges). Overflow of EC output (R) indicates that a phase transition should take place. The EC output triggers the PSA (a 2-bit counter) to rotate the Phase State (Φ) sequentially. If K' is 0, the counting process is stopped; EC output and subsequently the Phase State remain unchanged. Therefore, the Phase MUX holds its previous phase selection. The resampling circuit is added for timing alignment between K' and D to ensure a proper operation.

Figure 4.18b explains the PC operation in detail. Assume that at a certain instant, the Phase State, Φ <1:0> , is 01; as a result, $D = D1$, and the Phase MUX selects $P90$ as its output. Before the arrival of the falling edge of signal $P90$, a positive pulse $D1$ appears as D (Step 1) and triggers EC. As a result, EC output (R) changes to 1 from 0 (Step 2). The rising transition of R triggers PSA and increases the Phase State Φ <1:0> to 10 from 01 (Step 3). The new Phase State (Φ <1:0> =10) commands the FES to select $D2$ (which is at logic 0 at this instant) as its output D (Step 4), and commands Phase MUX to select $P180$ as its output. At this moment of phase handover, both signals $P90$ and $P180$ are at logic 1; hence the transition from $P90$ to $P180$ during this time interval is glitch-free. Next, before the arrival of the falling edge of $P180$, a $D2$ pulse is generated, causing R to become low (Step 5). Finally, another $D2$ pulse arrives before the next falling edge of $P180$, and it triggers a change in R to update Φ <1:0> to 11 from 10 (Step 6). The Phase MUX then moves on to the next phase signal, $P270$. The above operation constructs a glitch-free edge-combined output signal from the four input phases in a rotary sequence, and effectively divides the input frequency by 1.25. On the other hand, when $K = 0$, the Phase State Φ <1:0> and hence the selected input phase signal remain unchanged. As a result, the divide ratio is 1.

Figure 4.18a also depicts the 2-bit PSA design. The conventional cascaded ripple counter is not suitable to implement this 2-bit accumulator for it has a long propagation delay. On the other hand, a typical 2-bit synchronous accumulator requires two D-Flip-Flop (DFF), three XOR, and two AND circuits [22], thus consuming a large current. The proposed PSA is optimized to achieve high-speed and low-power operation. The critical delay path of the PSA is also identified in Figure 4.18a, and the delay is carefully minimized to ensure an optimum operation of PC.

In Figure 4.18a, it can be observed that the FES, EC, and PSA form a digital feedback loop. Figure 4.19 illustrates the simulated digital timing relationship of this loop when circuit propagation delays are present. T_C is the loop delay from the time signal D triggers the EC, to the next pulse signal ($D0$–$D3$) being selected as the FES output D. To ensure correct function of the high-speed PC, this loop delay (T_C) must be shorter than $T/4$, where T is the period of the input signal. This allows the following EC to record the number of D pulses properly.

In the timing diagram shown in Figure 4.18b, the input multiphase signals ($P0$–$P270$) are illustrated with 50% duty-cycle waveforms. If the signal duty cycle deviates from 50%, the circuit timing margin is reduced. As the duty cycle moves away further, glitches during phase transitions will eventually occur. This will lead to increased spur levels and result in degradation of the modulation accuracy. In this study, the input multiphase signals are generated by the master–slave-type divide-by-2 circuit [13] to ensure a reasonable 50% duty cycle.

4.7.2 High-Speed Digital Second-Order ΣΔ Modulator

The selection of the ΣΔ–MOD2 architecture is an optimization among speed, idle tones, quantization noise, and power consumption. The digital ΣΔ–modulator is implemented in a second-order 1-bit single-loop architecture, as shown in Figure 4.20 [23]. Multibit error-feedback MASH architecture is not adopted here, for it generates multibit output, which is not compatible with the single-bit phase control signal, K. The ΣΔ–MOD2 sampling frequency is chosen high (at half of the input frequency,

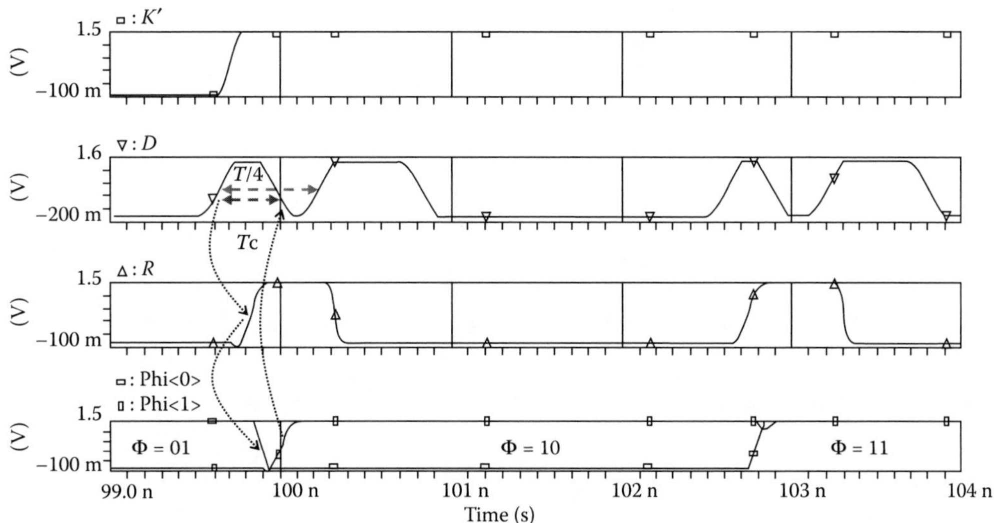

FIGURE 4.19 Simulated digital timing waveforms of the digital loop.

around 200 MHz), in order to effectively shape the quantization noise. The feedback coefficients of the modulator are chosen to allow easy implementation (simply up-shifting the digital words) for reduced circuit complexity and facilitating high-speed operation. The input word length of the ΣΔ–MOD2 is 13 bits, making a frequency resolution of

$$f_{\mathrm{LSB}} = f_{\mathrm{in}} \times \frac{(1 - 1/1.25)}{2^{13}} \cong 10\,\mathrm{kHz} \tag{4.13}$$

4.7.3 Digital Baseband Modulator

Figure 4.21 shows the digital G/FSK modulator, which implements core digital baseband functions. It includes a pseudorandom bit stream (PRBS) generator for characterization purposes, an FSK deviation frequency and data rate controller, and a 16-tape Gaussian FIR filter for GFSK modulation. Data MUX selects either the internal PRBS or external input data as the FSK data.

Figure 4.22 shows the digital O-QPSK modulator. The input 1-bit TX data are sampled by two DFFs with inverted clock phases at half of the clock rate. This circuit produces a 2-bit data stream, with one delayed by half of the symbol period with respect to the other. The data stream is then converted into the differential form for the Phase MUX. The input data can be selected either from the PRBS generator or from an external data source by Data MUX. The PRBS generator is implemented primarily for evaluation purposes.

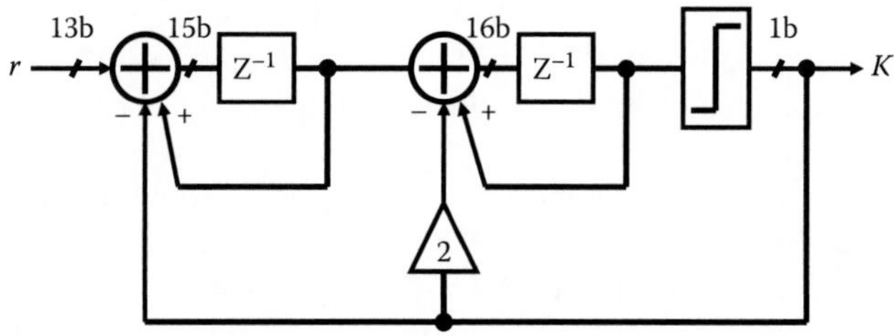

FIGURE 4.20 Architecture of the second-order 1-bit ΣΔ modulator.

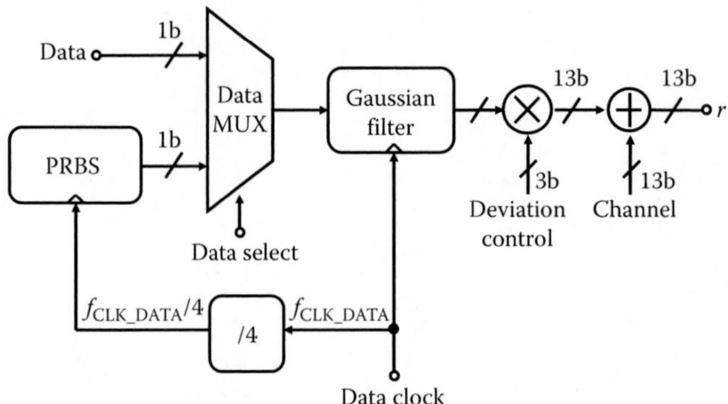

FIGURE 4.21 Digital G/FSK modulator.

4.7.4 Voltage-Controlled Oscillator

Figure 4.23a shows the LC-VCO circuit that utilizes NMOS and PMOS double-switching pairs to reduce power consumption. Compared with the single-switching VCO, the double-switching VCO is easier to start-up and has higher output voltage swing at low bias current, as shown in Figure 4.23b. To further reduce VCO current consumption, a large inductance value (8 nH) is chosen to enhance the LC-tank resonant impedance (R_{Tank}).

The VCO is operated at twice the carrier frequency. In addition to avoiding the pulling effect from PA, a higher operating frequency also allows a smaller inductor with a better quality factor. Moreover, the LC-tank impedance is increased at higher frequency, enabling a better oscillation condition.

The VCO covers frequencies ranging from 710 to 880 MHz, which supports transmitter output from 355 to 440 MHz. To cover the 20% tuning range while keeping a small VCO tuning gain (K_{VCO}), a 2-bit capacitor array is incorporated into the VCO tank circuit.

4.7.5 Frequency Synthesizer and Clock Plan

A frequency synthesizer must have a low-phase noise to achieve a high-quality communication. In addition, a fast-locking frequency synthesizer is also preferable to minimize the energy wasted during the start-up period. This is especially important when the energy source is limited. In this study, the frequency synthesizer is based on a type-II phase-locked loop, as shown in Figure 4.24. A current-mode-logic (CML) divider divides the VCO frequency by two to generate quadrature-phase signals. To ensure balanced loadings among four phases and improve quadrature phase accuracy, signals with 0° and 180° phases are combined via a CML-to-logic buffer and sent to the ΣΔ–MOD2, whereas signals with 90° and 270° are also combined in the same manner before reaching the prescaler of the PLL.

A loop bandwidth of 500 kHz is selected, for it allows fast locking, optimum phase noise, and integration of an area-efficient second-order passive loop filter. This 800-MHz frequency synthesizer consumes only 2.2 mA (including the VCO) from a 1.4-V supply.

The prescaler adopts multimodulus architecture with four stages of divided-by-2/3 cells, as shown in Figure 4.25a. Hence, the dividing ratio can be programmed from 8 to 15. The reference frequency is 19.2 MHz.

The $\Delta\theta \rightarrow I_{\text{CP}}$ linearity of the PFD and charge pump is an important parameter in terms of spurious performance of the frequency synthesizer. Charge injection of switches in the charge-pump circuit is usually one of the dominant effects of $\Delta\theta \rightarrow I_{\text{CP}}$ linearity degradation. Therefore, the spurious suppression technique [24] is adopted in this study to improve the spectrum purity. Figure 4.25b shows the charge-pump implementation and its control timing.

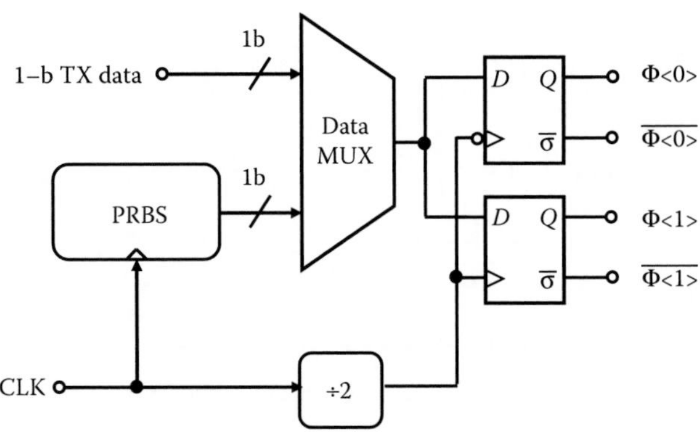

FIGURE 4.22 Digital O-QPSK modulator.

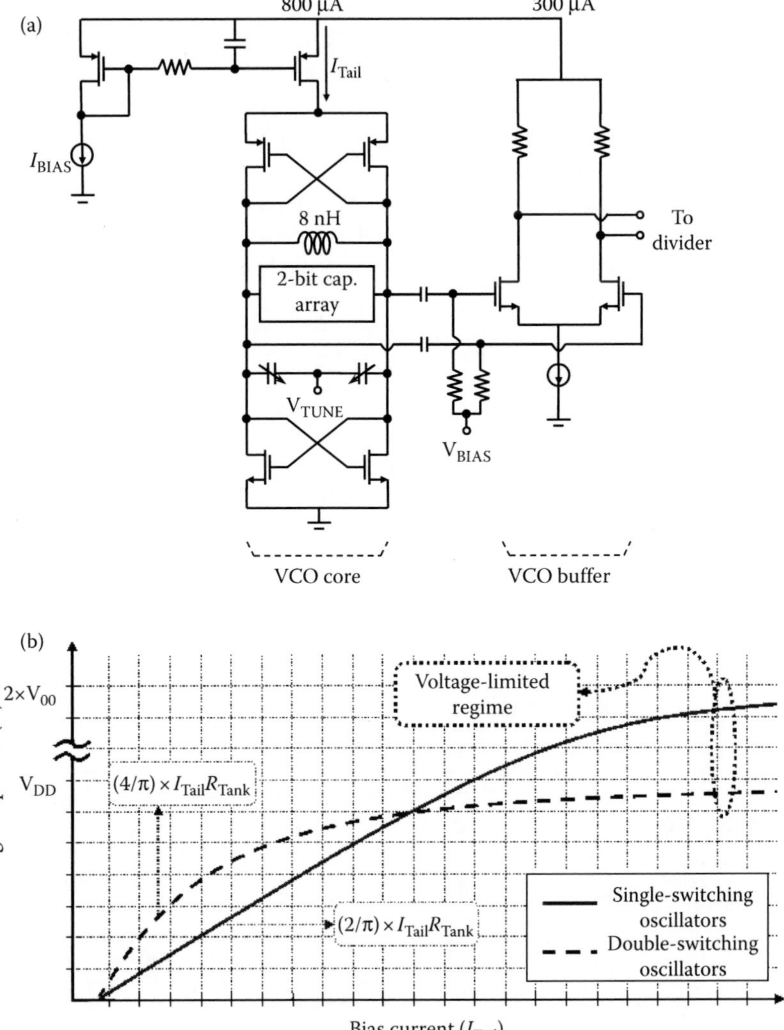

FIGURE 4.23 (a) Simplified schematic of the LC-VCO. (b) Comparison of the single-switching and double-switching VCOs.

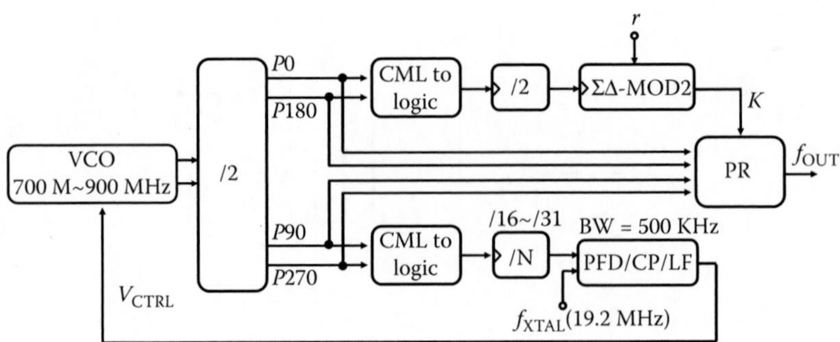

FIGURE 4.24 Block diagram of the PLL implementation and clock generator.

4.7.6 Inverter-Type PA

Figure 4.26a shows the PA circuit implemented in this study. It is based on an inverter-type architecture. The differential currents from the Phase MUX output are first converted into single-ended form by the differential-to-single-ended buffer (M_1–M_6), and then drive two cascaded inverter stages. The first-stage inverter (M_7, M_8) is self-biased to maintain 50% duty-cycle waveforms, reducing the second-order harmonic components. The second-stage inverter (M_9, M_{10}) of the PA drives an external matching network.

This inverter-type PA is compatible with the quasi-constant-envelope nature of the O-QPSK modulation signal and has a better power efficiency. The efficiency is defined as the ratio of the output power to the average DC power consumption of the PA, as expressed in

$$\text{PA efficiency} \equiv \frac{P_{\text{OUT}}}{\text{DC Power}} \approx \frac{2 I_{\text{Avg}}{}^2 R_{\text{L}}}{V_{\text{DD}} \cdot I_{\text{Avg}}} \tag{4.14}$$

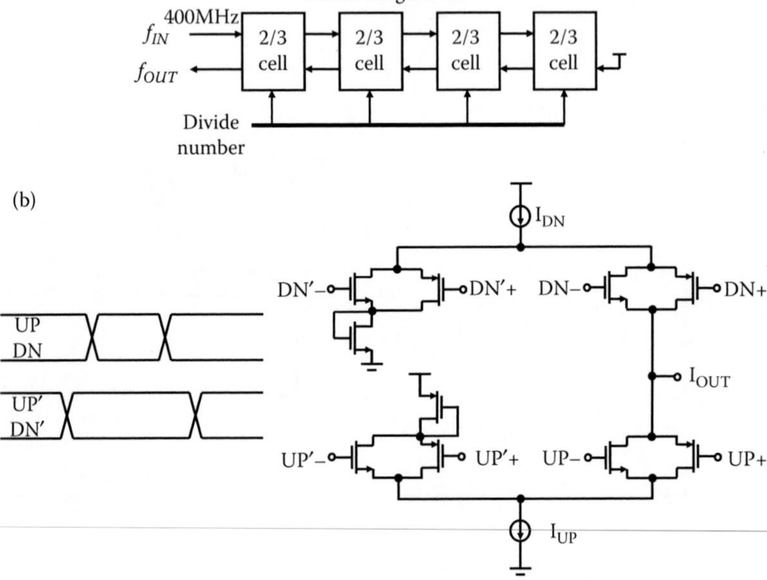

FIGURE 4.25 (a) Multimodulus divider. (b) Charge pump schematic and timing.

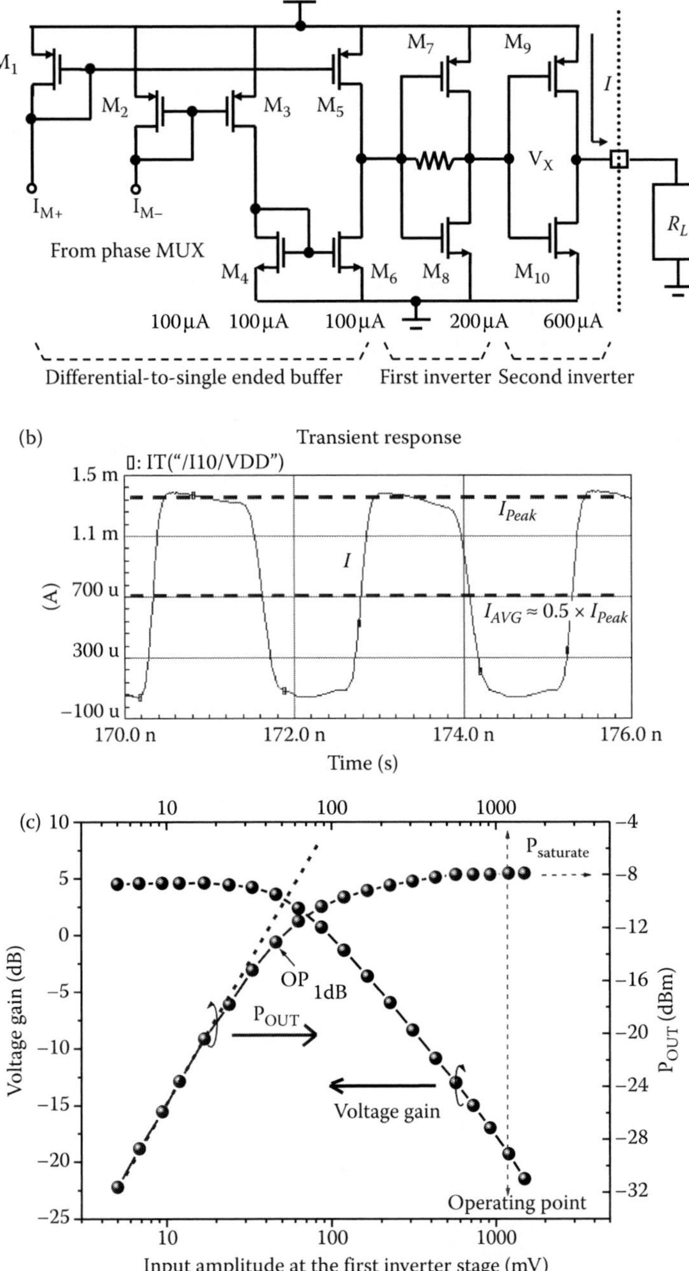

FIGURE 4.26 (a) Inverter-type PA, (b) simulated output driving current of the PA, and (c) simulated output power versus input driving voltage (at 1.5-V supply voltage).

In Equation 4.14, I_{Avg} is determined by the PA supply voltage, load impedance (R_L), device sizes, and the amplitude of the input driving signal. The simulated PA efficiency is around 15% at 1.5-V supply voltage. Figure 4.26b shows the simulated output current waveform of the PA, which illustrates that the current waveform is close to 50%. Figure 4.26c shows the simulated PA characteristics. The saturated output power is around −8 dBm, and the 1-dB compression output power is −12 dBm. This PA is designed to operate at the deep saturation region to achieve a better power efficiency.

4.8 EXPERIMENTAL RESULTS

The proposed dual-mode MUX-based transmitter is implemented in the TSMC 0.18-μm CMOS process. As shown in Figure 4.27, the VCO covers frequencies ranging from 710 to 870 MHz, which supports a transmitter carrier frequency from 355 to 435 MHz. The PLL is measured with a 19.2-MHz reference crystal oscillator and a dividing ratio of 44 ($N = 22$), which locks the VCO frequency (f_{VCO}) to 844.8 MHz. A second-order passive loop filter is integrated on-chip. The PLL loop bandwidth is about 500 kHz.

Close-in phase noise and spurs of LO signals are mainly contributed by the frequency synthesizer. They result in a rotation of the modulation constellation, thus degrading the EVM. Figures 4.28a and b show the LO output spectra with a span of 2 and 50 MHz, respectively. The reference spur level is suppressed to around −69 dBc. The PLL phase noise (measured at transmitter output) is −107.9 dBc/Hz and −110 dBc/Hz at 10-kHz and 100-kHz offset, respectively. The integrated phase error (from 1 kHz to 30 MHz) is only 0.31°. Figure 4.29 shows the measured PLL start-up transient. With a loop bandwidth of 250 kHz, the PLL is settled within 16 μs.

Figure 4.30 shows the measured PA output power (P_{OUT}) and average current (I_{AVG}) versus supply voltage ($V_{DD,PA}$). By changing the supply voltage, the output power can be adjusted to satisfy the up-link transmit distance requirements. The PA delivers around −15-dBm output power at 1.2-V supply voltage, which already can satisfy the 2-m wireless link requirement for the target implantable neural recording applications. The output power can be increased to −8 dBm when the PA supply voltage is raised to 1.8 V. The output power can also be increased by raising the bias current of the Phase MUX, which effectively increases the input amplitude of the PA.

Figure 4.31 shows the dual-mode transmitter chip photo. The whole chip occupies an area of 1.2 mm^2, while the core circuits occupy 0.7 mm^2. The proposed ΣΔ–PR and PA only utilize a very small portion of the chip area since no inductor is required for these two circuits. The whole transmitter only incorporates one inductor, which is employed in the LC-VCO.

4.8.1 G/FSK Modulation Measurement

Figure 4.32a shows the measured single-tone G/FSK transmitter output spectrum with r (see Equation 4.7) around 0.5. The close-in noise is about 30 dB below the carrier under a 1-MHz

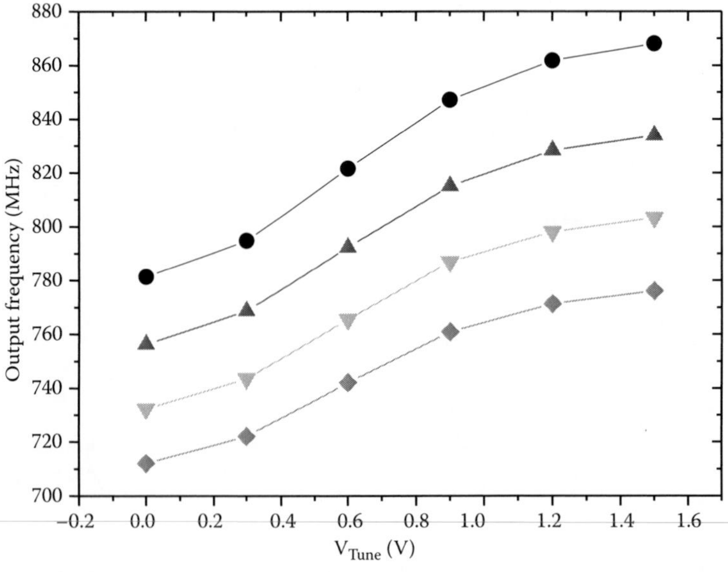

FIGURE 4.27 Measured VCO frequency.

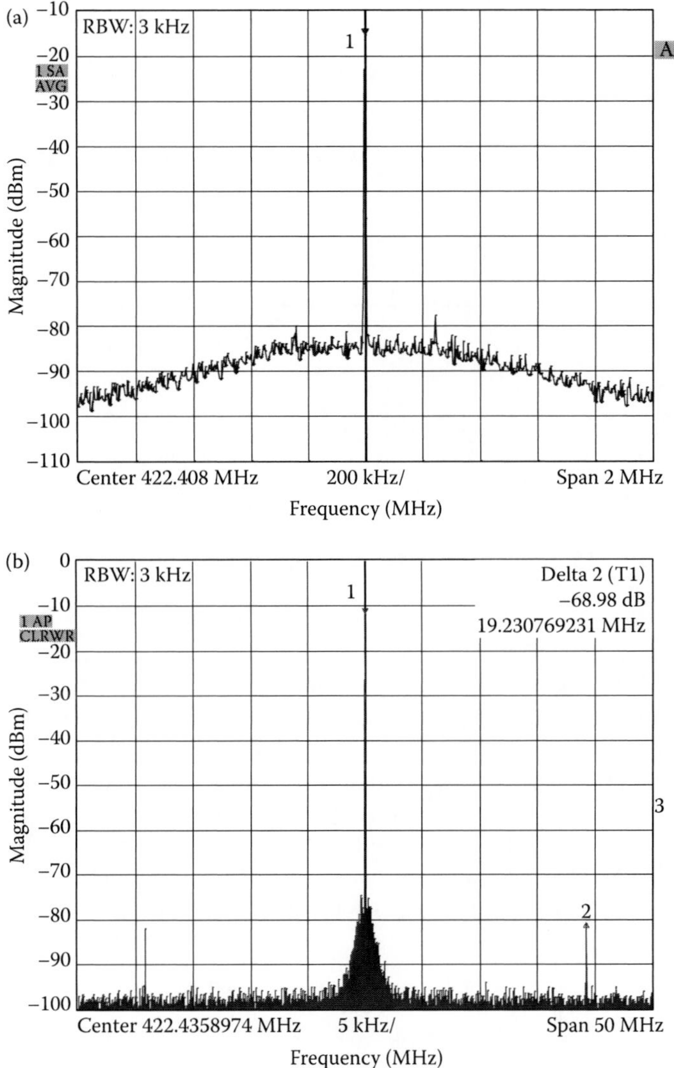

FIGURE 4.28 LO spectra with (a) a 2-MHz span and (b) a 50-MHz span.

resolution bandwidth, which corresponds to a noise level roughly −90 dBc/Hz. The spurious tones at 22-MHz offset frequency and its harmonics at the transmitter output have originated from the idle tones of the ΣΔ–MOD2 and the nonlinearity in the ΣΔ–PR operation. The characteristics of the TX output frequency versus the 13-bit frequency control word (FCW) are plotted in Figure 4.32b. The figure shows a well-behaved characteristic as predicted in Equation 4.6 (K in Equation 4.6 is equal to FCW/2^{13}).

The PLL phase noise (S_{θ}_PLL) measured at the transmitter output (at a frequency of $f_{vco}/2$; when ΣΔ–PR is disabled) is shown in Figure 4.33. This figure also shows the measured and estimated total transmitter output noises (S_{θ}) when ΣΔ–PR is activated. It is observed that the close-in phase noise is dominated by the PLL, while the phase noise at higher offset frequencies (i.e., larger than 10- MHz offset) is mainly contributed by the ΣΔ–modulation noise ($S_{\theta\_\Sigma\Delta}$). The measured total transmitter noise between 100-kHz and 10-MHz offset frequency is higher than that estimated by simulation. Further investigation of this discrepancy reveals that this is attributed to the resampling operation in the ΣΔ–PR. As described in Section 4.7.1, the resampling circuit is added for the

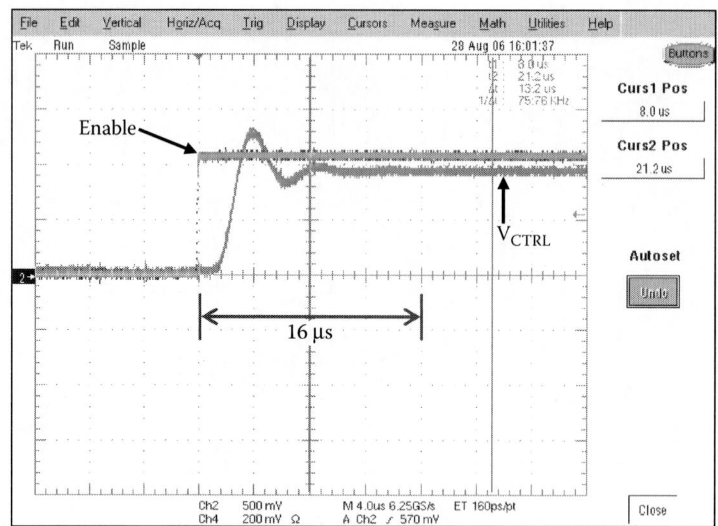

FIGURE 4.29 Measured PLL start-up transient.

purposes of timing alignment. However, this resampling operation deteriorates the noise-shaping characteristics of the ΣΔ–MOD2, resulting in higher noise. When the random modulation data are applied to the ΣΔ–MOD2 input, the magnitude of these spurious tones is lowered and has less impact on the modulation quality. Figure 4.34 shows the measured modulation spectrum of 6-Mbps FSK signal.

While the ΣΔ-dithering allows the phase rotator to achieve fine frequency resolution and wideband operation, the out-of-band emission performance is compromised as in other ΣΔ-dithered transmitter architectures [25]. This unwanted emission is regulated and is specified in various rules (e.g., [8]). Although the off-chip impedance matching network at the transmitter output can help us to lower the unwanted out-of-band noise power, the Q-factor of a low-cost matching circuit is typically limited (around 20). Its effect on noise reduction is also limited. If the

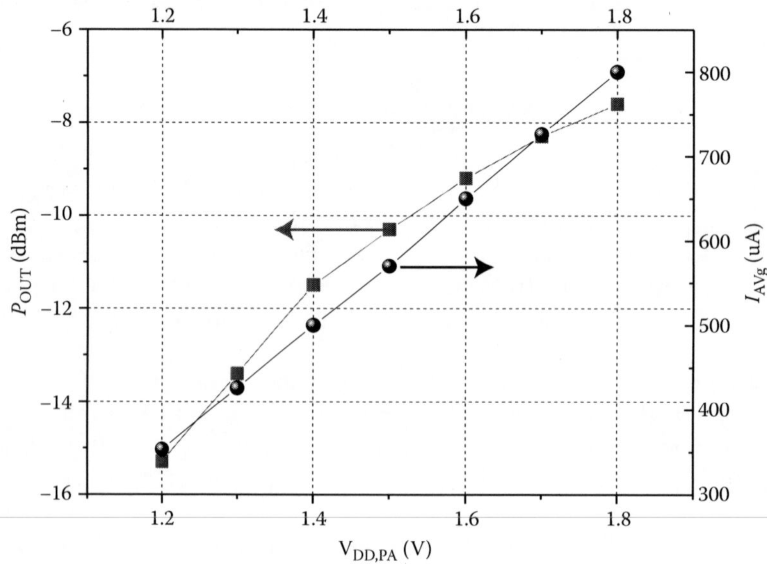

FIGURE 4.30 Measured output power versus supply voltage.

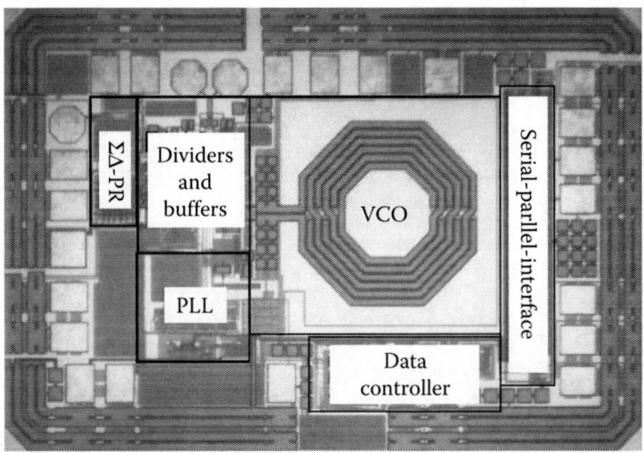

FIGURE 4.31 Chip photo.

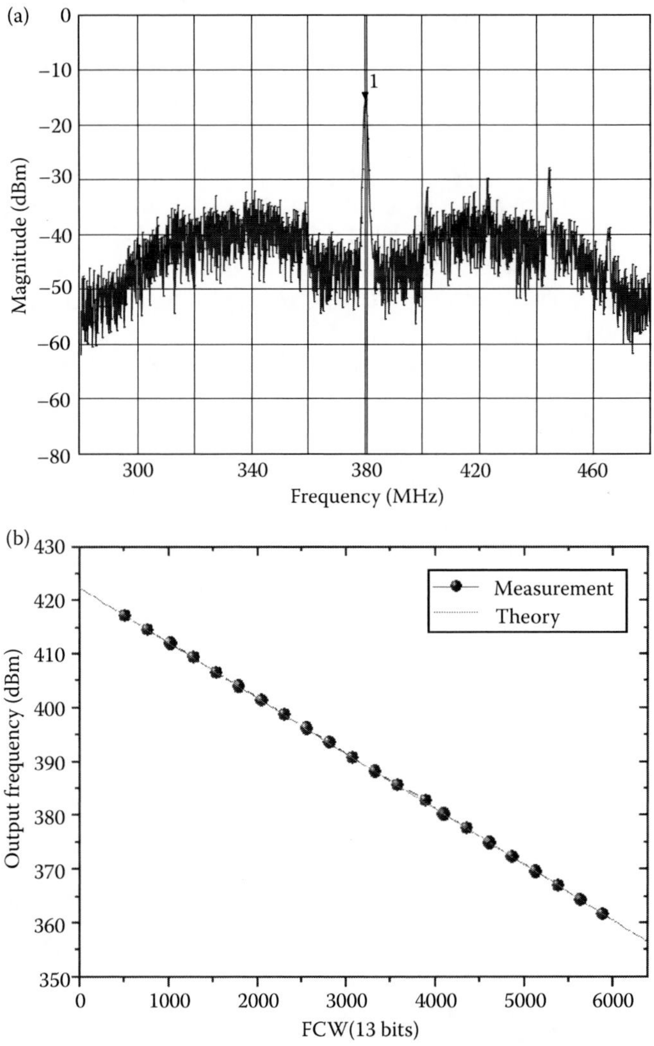

FIGURE 4.32 Measured (a) G/FSK transmitter single-tone output spectrum with a 200-MHz span. (b) Frequency versus FCW (r).

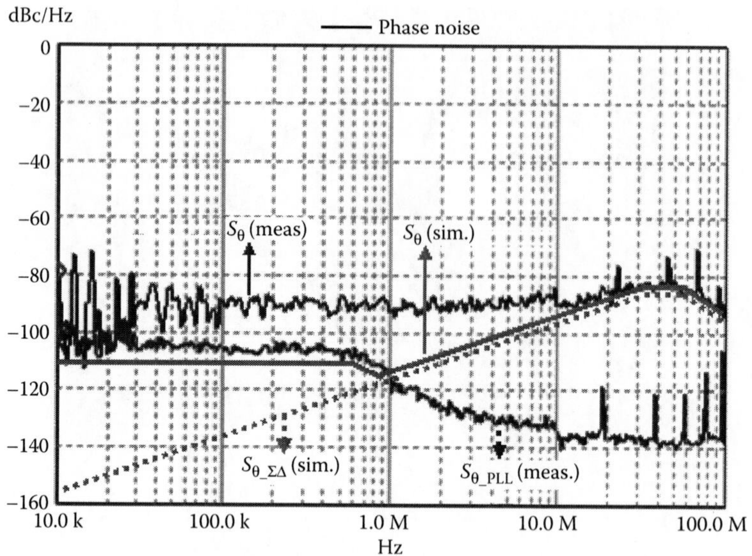

FIGURE 4.33 Overlay of measured and simulated TX phase noise ($S_\theta = S_{\theta\_\Sigma\Delta} + S_{\theta\_PLL}$).

transmitter is required to deliver a large output power, the out-of-band noise power also increases. A high-Q RF band-pass filter with a center frequency tuning circuit [25] is therefore needed to suppress the out-of-band noise power to below a level that satisfies the emission regulations. Since the required output power is low (< −10 dBm) in the targeted short-range wireless medical applications, the noise power and magnitude of spurious emission are also low. The filtering requirement is less demanding.

The proposed transmitter is verified with the 2-FSK and GFSK modulations. Figure 4.35 shows the transmission quality measured at a center frequency of 403.2 MHz, by a vector signal analyzer (VSA), Agilent MXA. The measured FSK errors at 6-Mbps data rate are 4.1% and 11.6% for 2-FSK and GFSK modulations, respectively. FSK error is defined as the ratio of the root mean square frequency jitter to the average FSK deviation frequency, and is a function of phase noise, deviation frequency, and transmission bandwidth [26]. In this architecture, the dominant source of FSK error is the modulation noise due to the ΣΔ-dithering (including the noise degradation caused by the

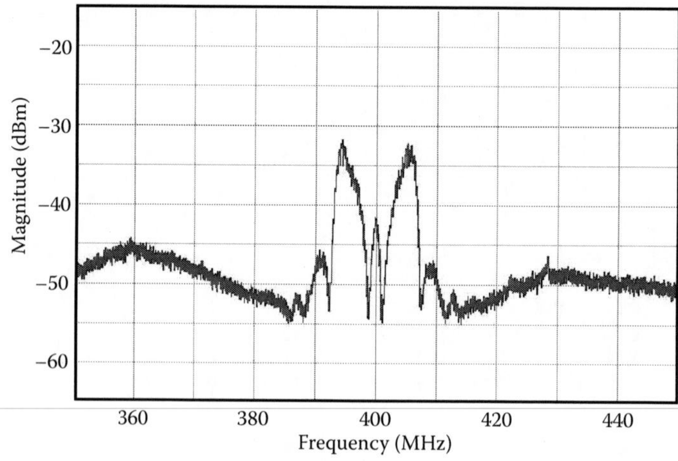

FIGURE 4.34 Measured 6-Mbps FSK modulation spectrum.

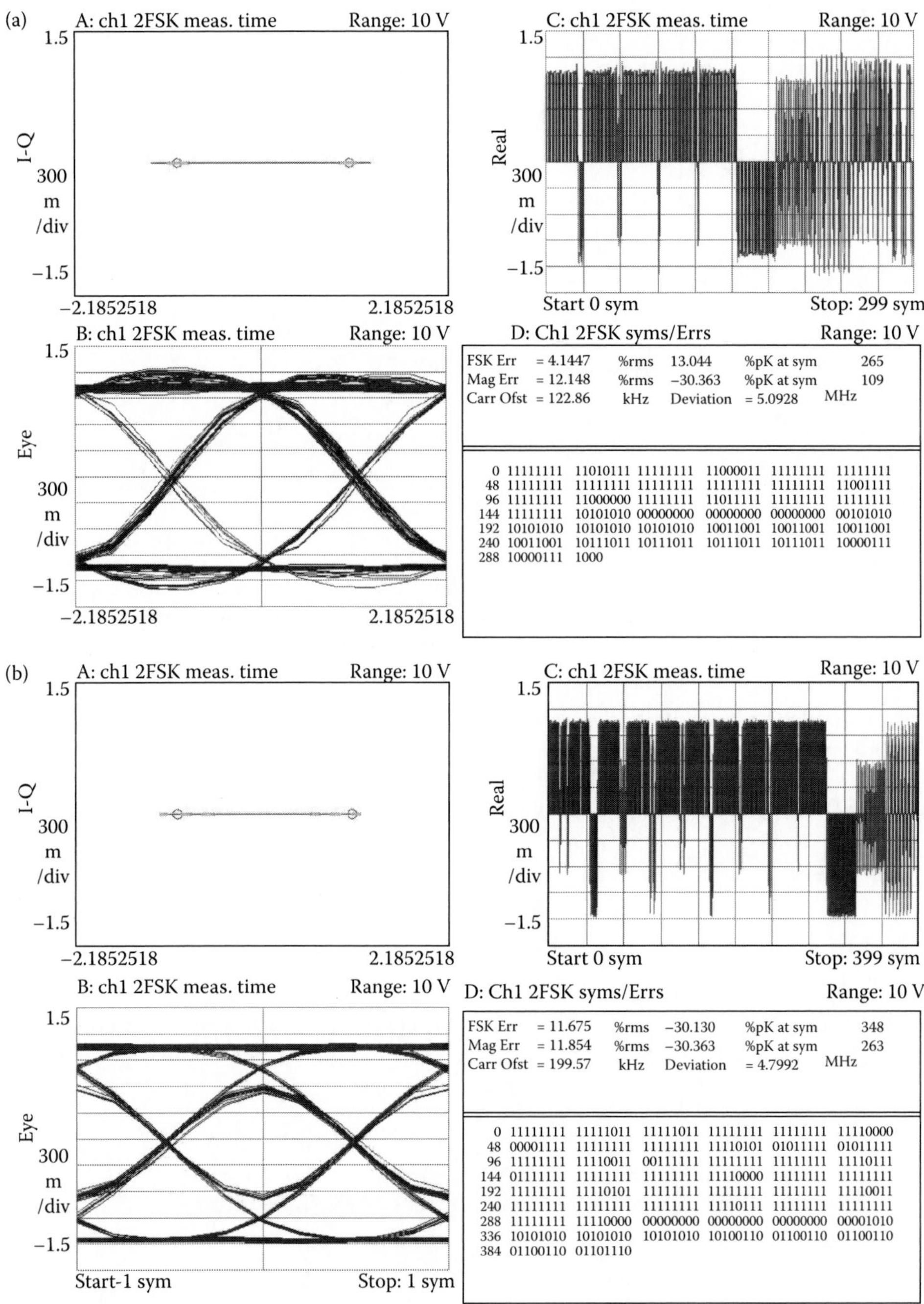

FIGURE 4.35 (a) Measured 6-Mbps FSK modulation characteristics at 403.2 MHz. (b) Measured 6-Mbps GFSK modulation characteristics at 403.2 MHz.

resampling operation). Since this noise component theoretically increases with offset frequency, a higher transmission data rate (i.e., wider noise bandwidth) leads to a higher FSK error. For a given transmission data rate, FSK error can be improved by increasing the frequency deviation. However, this also increases the transmission bandwidth, thus limiting the improvement of the FSK error. Alternatively, employing a more sophisticated ΣΔ–modulator and resampling scheme may reduce

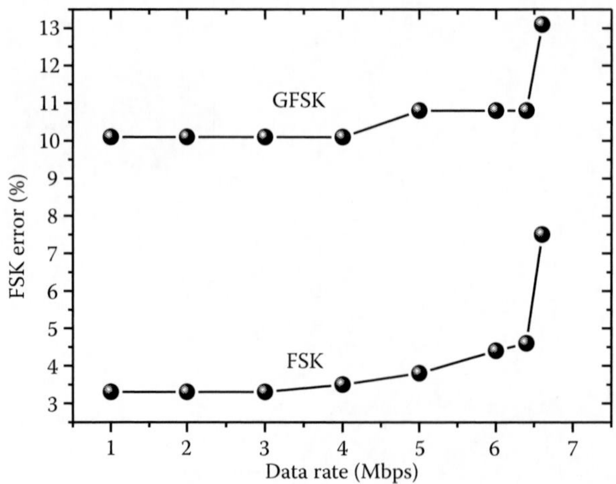

FIGURE 4.36 Measured G/FSK errors versus data rate.

the modulation noise, hence lowering the FSK error. However, this is often at the cost of higher power consumption and design complexity. Figure 4.36 plots the overall FSK and GFSK modulation quality under various transmission data rates (from 1 to 6.5 Mbps). Such a signal quality is adequate for typical G/FSK demodulators to satisfy a BER of better than 10^{-3}.

Operated from a 1.4-V supply, the overall G/FSK transmitter draws 6.3 mA. This fully integrated MUX-based G/FSK transmitter achieves an energy efficiency of 1.5 nJ/bit at 6 Mbps. Table 4.1 summarizes the experimental results. The proposed G/FSK transmitter accomplishes a good energy-per-bit efficiency and delivers a reasonable output power level for short-range high-data-rate wireless applications.

4.8.2 O-QPSK Modulation Measurement

Figures 4.37a and b show the measured O-QPSK eye diagram, constellation, transmitter characteristics, and output spectrum (at 422.4 MHz) at a data rate of 17.5 Mbps. The transmission quality is measured by a VSA with a built-in digital receiver filter. The modulated signal achieves an EVM of

TABLE 4.1
Performance Summary of the G/FSK Transmitter

Supply voltage	1.4 V
Maximum data rate	6 Mbps
TX operating frequency	284 ~ 435 MHz
PLL bandwidth	500 kHz
PA output power (P_{OUT})	–11 dBm
Total G/FSK TX current	6.3 mA
PLL (including VCO)	2.2 mA
$\Sigma\Delta$ – PR	3.5 mA
PA	0.6 mA
Energy/bit (max. data rate)	1.5 nJ/bit

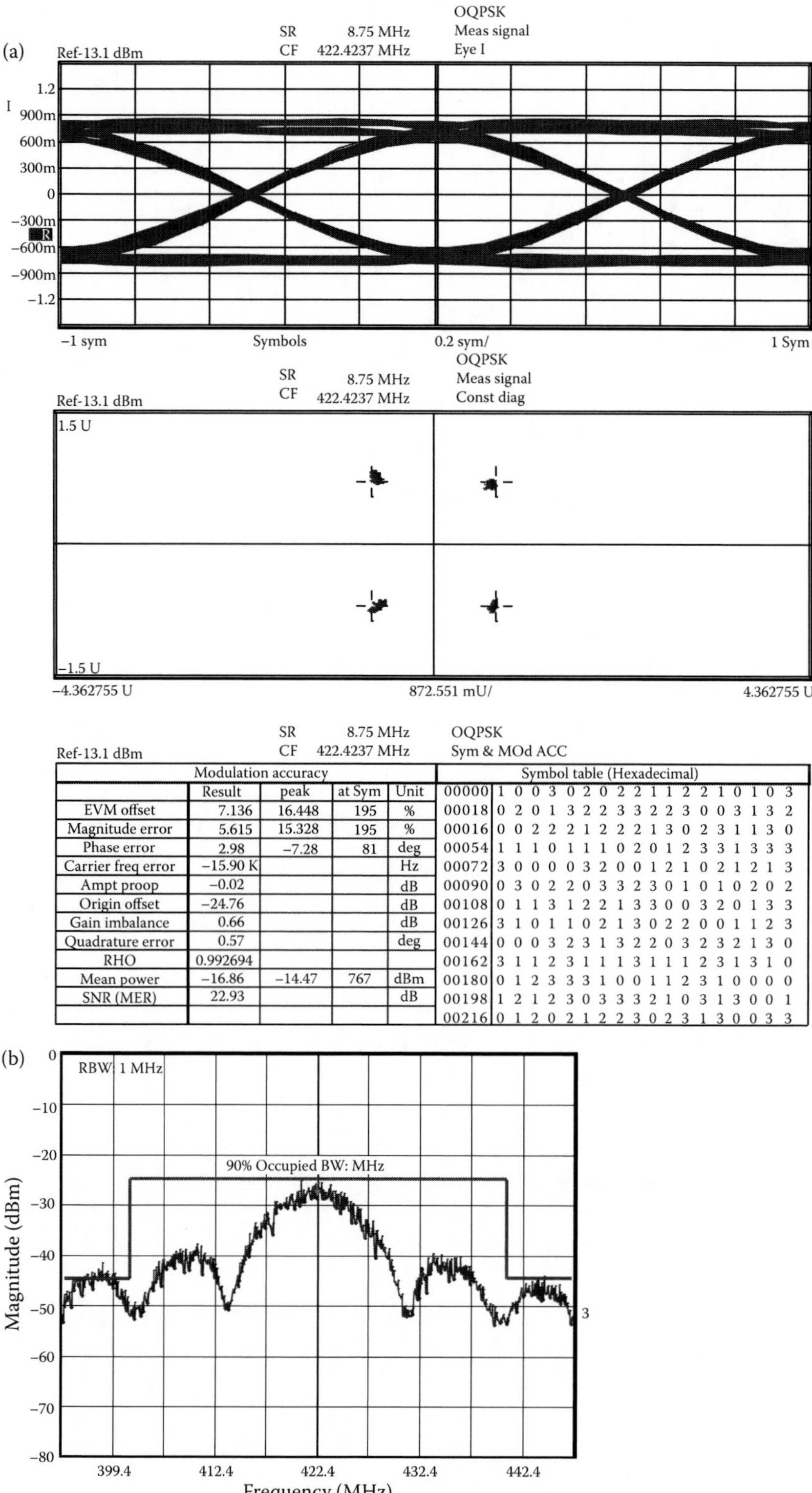

Modulation accuracy				
	Result	peak	at Sym	Unit
EVM offset	7.136	16.448	195	%
Magnitude error	5.615	15.328	195	%
Phase error	2.98	−7.28	81	deg
Carrier freq error	−15.90 K			Hz
Ampt proop	−0.02			dB
Origin offset	−24.76			dB
Gain imbalance	0.66			dB
Quadrature error	0.57			deg
RHO	0.992694			
Mean power	−16.86	−14.47	767	dBm
SNR (MER)	22.93			dB

Symbol table (Hexadecimal)	
00000	1 0 0 3 0 2 0 2 2 1 1 2 2 1 0 1 0 3
00018	0 2 0 1 3 2 2 3 3 2 2 3 0 0 3 1 3 2
00016	0 0 2 2 2 1 2 2 2 1 3 0 2 3 1 1 3 0
00054	1 1 1 0 1 1 1 0 2 0 1 2 3 3 1 3 3 3
00072	3 0 0 0 0 3 2 0 0 1 2 1 0 2 1 2 1 3
00090	0 3 0 2 2 0 3 3 2 3 0 1 0 1 0 2 0 2
00108	0 1 1 3 1 2 2 1 3 3 0 0 3 2 0 1 3 3
00126	3 1 0 1 1 0 2 1 3 0 2 2 0 0 1 1 2 3
00144	0 0 0 3 2 3 1 3 2 2 0 3 2 3 2 1 3 0
00162	3 1 1 2 3 1 1 1 3 1 1 1 2 3 1 3 1 0
00180	0 1 2 3 3 3 1 0 0 1 1 2 3 1 0 0 0 0
00198	1 2 1 2 3 0 3 3 3 2 1 0 3 1 3 0 0 1
00216	0 1 2 0 2 1 2 2 3 0 2 3 1 3 0 0 3 3

FIGURE 4.37 (a) Eye diagram, constellation, and modulation characteristics. (b) Output spectrum.

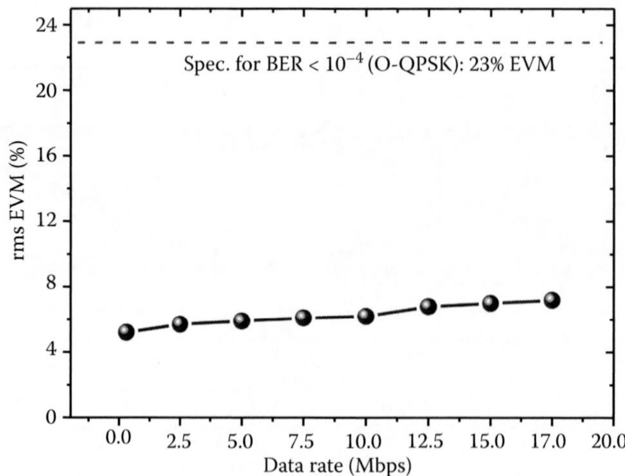

FIGURE 4.38 Measured transmitter OQPSK EVM versus various data rates.

7.2%, which is equivalent to 23-dB SNR. The EVM degradation is mainly attributed to quadrature phase mismatch, nonideal switching of Data Switches, and phase noise of the LO signal. The modulation spectrum shows that 90% of the total output power is confined within 405–440 MHz.

Figure 4.38 plots the overall O-QPSK modulation quality (in measured EVM) versus various transmission data rates (from 1 kbps to 17.5 Mbps). As shown in Figure 4.38, the signal quality up to 17.5 Mbps is more than adequate for typical O-QPSK demodulators to satisfy a BER of better than 10^{-4} (i.e., 23% EVM).

4.8.3 Performance Summary

Table 4.2 summarizes the experimental results of the proposed O-QPSK transmitter. The complete O-QPSK transmitter consumes only 2.9 mA from a 1.2-V supply voltage. It achieves an energy efficiency of 200 pJ/bit at a data rate of 17.5 Mbps. Although the PA is usually the most power-hungry component in a long-range wireless communication system, it is the VCO and PLL that dictate the power consumption in a short-range application as in this study.

TABLE 4.2
Performance Summary of O-QPSK Transmitter

Supply Voltage	1.2–1.8 V
Operation Frequency	355–440 MHz
Data Rate	1 kbps–17.5 Mbps
P_{OUT}	–8 dBm at $V_{DD,PA}$ = 1.8V
	–15 dBm at $V_{DD\cdot PA}$ = 1.2V
Bias Current (Total)	2.9 mA (at V_{DD} = 1.2V)
PLL	1 mA
VCO + Buffer	1.1 mA
Phase MUX + Buffer	0.4 mA
PA	0.4 mA (0.8 mA at $V_{DD,PA}$ = 1.8V)

TABLE 4.3
Performance Comparison with Other Low-Power Transmitter Works

	This Study			
	PSK Mode	**FSK Mode**	**[11]**	**[27]**
Process (CMOS)	0.18 μm		0.13 μm	0.18 μm
Supply Voltage	1.2–1.8 V	1.4–1.8 V	360–600 mV	0.9 V
Modulation Scheme	O-QPSK	G/FSK	FSK	FSK
Operation Frequency	355–440 MHz		2–2.4 GHz	900 MHz
Max. Data Rate	17.5 Mbps	6 Mbps	0.5 Mbps	1 Mbps
P_{OUT}	−15 to −8 dBm	−15 to −8 dBm	−9 to −2 dBm	−4 dBm
Power Consumption	3.5 mW	8.8 mW	1.3 mW	1.8 mW
Energy/bit	0.2 nJ/bit	1.5 nJ/bit	2.6 nJ/bit	1.7 nJ/bit

Table 4.3 compares the performance of the proposed dual-mode MUX-based transmitter with other related works. The proposed O-QPSK transmitter achieves a high data rate with very low power consumption, resulting in good energy/bit performance.

Figure 4.39 compares this study with other low-power transmitters. Although impulse ultra-wide-band transmitters [3] can achieve energy-per-bit performance better than 100 pJ/bit, narrow-band modulation transmitters are more favored for the targeted implantable application because of a simpler demodulator design and better channel characteristics in an implanted environment.

4.9 CONCLUSION

In this chapter, an energy-efficient MUX-based transmitter architecture is proposed for high-data-rate G/FSK and O-QPSK modulations. The G/FSK modulation signals are generated by applying the

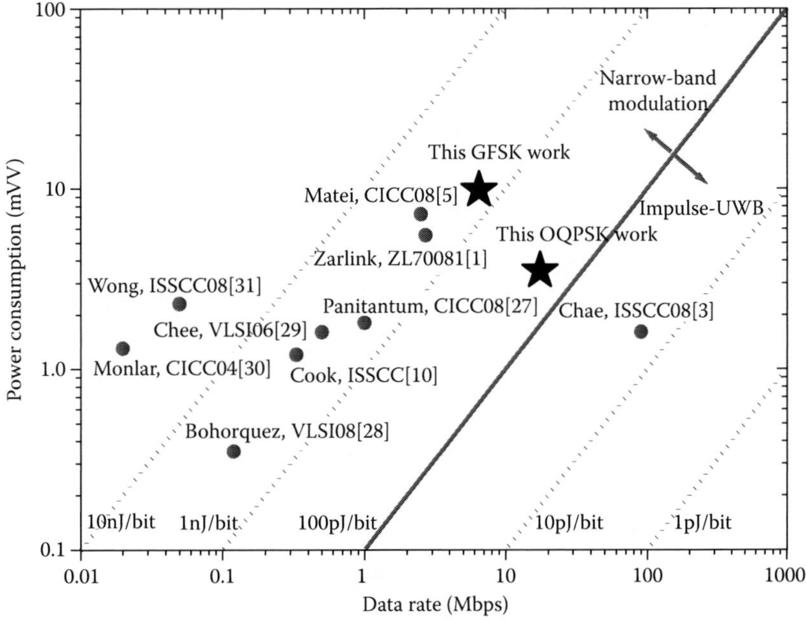

FIGURE 4.39 Energy efficiency comparison of low-power transmitters.

data to modulate the proposed ΣΔ–PR outside the PLL. In the proposed transmitter, the drawbacks of the conventional PLL-based (open-/closed-loop and two-point) architectures, such as VCO frequency drift, unsuppressed VCO phase noise, data rate limitation, accurate path matching requirement, and so on, are avoided. In addition, the decoupling of the modulation and the frequency synthesizer loops allows independent optimization of the PLL for frequency planning, settling time, and phase noise considerations.

For the O-QPSK mode, the proposed Phase MUX efficiently implements the direct phase-shift keying operation. This architecture is insensitive to many analog nonidealities. The high-data-rate transmitter with low power consumption is suitable for wideband implantable medical applications.

The proposed MUX-based transmitter architecture is inherently a digital design. The modulation characteristics, such as modulation schemes, carrier/deviation frequencies, and data rate are easily programmable to adopt for different applications. The digital nature of the proposed architecture enables the transmitter to be less sensitive to analog nonidealities and PVT variations, and may lead to a more energy-efficient operation in advanced deep submicron CMOS processes.

REFERENCES

1. Zarlink Semiconductor, RF integrated circuits for medical applications: ZL70081, http://www.zarlink.com
2. R. Harrison, P. Watkins, R. Jier, R. Lovejoy, D. Black, R. Normann, and F. Solzbacher, A low-power integrated circuit for a wireless 100-electrode neural recording system, in *IEEE Int. Solid-State Circuits Conf. Dig. Tech. Papers*, 454–455, 2006.
3. M. Chae, W. Liu, Z. Yang, T. Chen, J. Kim, M. Sivaprakasan, and M. Yuce, A 128-channel 6 mW wireless neural recording IC with on-the-fly spike sorting and UWB transmitter, in *IEEE Int. Solid-State Circuits Conf. Dig. Tech. Papers*, 146–603, 2008.
4. J. Aziz, R. Genov, M. Derchansky, B. Bardakjian, and P. Carlen, 256-Channel neural recording microsystem with on-chip 3D electrodes, in *IEEE Int. Solid-State Circuits Conf. Dig. Tech. Papers*, 160–161, 2007.
5. E. Matei, E. Lee, J. Gord, P. Nercessian, P. Hess, H. Stover, T. Li, and J. Wolfe, A biomedical implantable FES battery-powered micro-stimulator, in *Proc. IEEE Custom Integrated Circuits Conf.*, 317–324, 2008.
6. J. Ryckaert, P. D. Doncker, R. Meys, A. L. Hoye, and S. Donnay, Channel model for wireless communication around human body, *IEE Electron. Lett.*, 40, 543–544, 2004.
7. T. Akin, K. Najafi, and R. M. Bradley, A wireless implantable multichannel digital neural recording system for a micromachined sieve electrode, *IEEE J. Solid-State Circuits*, 33, 109–118, 1998.
8. L. E. Larson, *RF and Microwave Circuit Design for Wireless Communication*. Boston, MA: Artech House, 1996.
9. M. H. Perrott, T. L. Tewksbury III, and C. G. Sodini, A 27-mW CMOS fractional-*N* synthesizer using digital compensation for 2.5-Mb/s GFSK modulation, *IEEE J. Solid-State Circuits*, 32, 2048–2060, 1997.
10. B. W. Cook, A. D. Berny, A. Molnar, S. Lanzisera, and K. S. J. Pister, An ultra-low power 2.4GHz RF transceiver for wireless sensor network in 0.13 μm CMOS with 400 mV supply and integrated passive RX front-end, in *IEEE Int. Solid-State Circuits Conf. Dig. Tech. Papers*, 370–371, 2006.
11. C. Cojocaru, T. Pamir, F. Balteanu, A. Namdar, D. Payer, I. Gheorghe, T. Lipan et al., A 43 mW Bluetooth transceiver with −91 dBm sensitivity, in *IEEE Int. Solid-State Circuits Conf. Dig. Tech. Papers*, 90–91, 2003.
12. B. Sklar, *Digital Communications*. Upper Saddle River, Englewood Cliffs, NJ: Prentice-Hall, 2001.
13. J. Craninckx, and M. S. J. Steyaert, A 1.75-GHz/3-V dual-modulus divided-by-128/129 prescaler in 0.7-μm CMOS, *IEEE J. Solid-State Circuits*, 31, 890–897, 1996.
14. C.-H. Heng, and B.-S. Song, A 1.8-GHz CMOS fractional-*N* frequency synthesizer with randomized multiphase VCO, *IEEE J. Solid-State Circuits*, 38, 848–854, 2003.
15. C.-H. Park, I. Kim, and B. Kim, A 1.8-GHz self-calibrated phase-locked loop with precise I/Q matching, *IEEE J. Solid-State Circuits*, 31, 777–783, 2001.
16. A. M. Fahim, and M. I. Elmasry, A wideband sigma–delta phase-locked loop modulator for wireless applications, *IEEE Tran. Circuits Syst. II*, 55, 775–785, 2008.

17. M. H. Perrott, M. D. Trott, and C. G. Sodini, A modeling approach for Σ–Δ fractional-*N* frequency synthesizers allowing straightforward noise analysis, *IEEE J. Solid-State Circuits*, 37, 1028–1038, 2002.
18. W. P. Robins, *Phase Noise in Signal Sources*. London: Peter Peregrinus, 1982.
19. R. B. Staszewski, C.-M. Hung, N. Barton, M.-C. Lee, and D. Leipold, A digitally controlled oscillator in a 90 nm digital CMOS process for mobile phones, *IEEE J. Solid-State Circuits*, 40, 2203–2211, 2005.
20. Y.-H. Liu, Cheng-Lung Li, and T.-H. Lin, A 200-pJ/b wireless MUX-based RF transmitter for implantable multi-channel neural recording, *IEEE Trans. Microwave Theory Tech.*, 2009.
21. Q. Gu, *RF System Design of Transceiver for Wireless Communications*. New York, NY: Springer, 2005.
22. S. Brown, and Z. Vranesic, *Fundamentals of Digital Logic with VHDL Design*. Boston, MA: McGraw-Hill, 2000.
23. R. Schreier, and G. C. Temes, *Understanding Delta–Sigma Data Converters*. Chichester: Wiley, 2005.
24. T.-H. Lin, C.-L. Ti, and Y.-H. Liu, Dynamic current matching charge pump and gated-offset linearization techniques for delta–sigma fractional-*N* PLLs, *IEEE Tran. Circuits Syst. I*, 56, 877–885, 2009.
25. A. Jerng and C. G. Sodini, A Wideband ΔΣ Digital-RF Modulator for High Data Rate Transmitters, *IEEE J. Solid-State Circuits*, 42, 1710–1722, 2007.
26. *HP 89440A/HP 89441A Operator's Guide,* Hewlett-Packard Company, Palo Alto, CA, 1996.
27. N. Panitantum, K. Mayaram, and T. S. Fiez, A 900-MHz low-power transmitter with fast frequency calibration for wireless sensor networks, in *Proc. IEEE Custom Integrated Circuits Conference,* 595–598, 2008.
28. J. L. Bohorquez, J. L. Dawson, and A. P. Chandrakasan, A 350 μW CMOS MSK transmitter and 400 μW OOK super-regenerative receiver for medical implant communications, in *Proc. Symp. VLSI Circuits*, pp. 32–33, 2008.
29. Y. H. Chee, A. M. Niknejad, and J. Rabaey, A 46% efficient 0.8dBm transmitter for wireless sensor networks, in *Proc. Symp. VLSI Circuits*, pp. 43–44, 2006.
30. A. Molnar, B. Lu, S. Lanzisera, B. W. Cook, and K. S. J. Pister, An ultra-low power 900 MHz RF transceiver for wireless sensor networks, in *Proc. IEEE Custom Integrated Circuits Conference*, pp. 401–404, 2004.
31. A. C.-W. Wong, D. McDonagh, G. Kathiresan, O. C. Omeni, O. El-Jamaly, T. C.-k. Chan, P. Paddan, A. J. Burdett, A 1V, micropower system-on-chip for vital-sign monitoring in wireless body sensor networks, in *IEEE Int. Solid-State Circuits Conf. Dig. Tech. Papers*, pp. 138–139, 2008.

5 Design of a Frequency Shift–Based CMOS Magnetic Sensor Array for Point-of-Care (PoC) Biomolecular Diagnosis Applications

Hua Wang and Ali Hajimiri

CONTENTS

5.1 INTRODUCTION

Future point-of-care (PoC) molecular-level diagnostic systems require advanced biosensors that can offer high sensitivity, ultra-portability, and a low price-tag. Targeting on-site detection of biomolecules, such as DNAs, RNAs, or proteins, this type of systems is believed to play a crucial role in a variety of emerging applications such as in-field medical diagnostics, epidemic disease control, and biohazard detection [1,2].

Conventionally, microarray technology is used to provide sensing information for biomolecules [3]. However, traditional microarray systems rely on optical detection setups for fluorescent

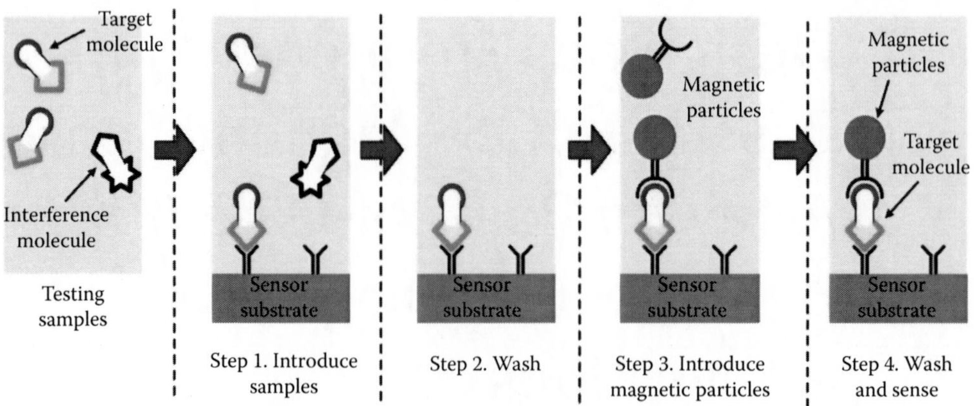

FIGURE 5.1 Typical sensing procedures of a magnetic biosensor using affinity-based sandwich assay.

molecular tags. This requires bulky and expensive optical devices including multiwavelength fluorescent microscopes, which limit the usage of optical microarray for PoC applications.

Another type of sensor modality, electrochemical biosensors, detect target molecules based on their extra electrical charges or dielectric properties. This includes detection schemes, such as impedance spectroscopy [4], amperometric analysis, redox cycling [5], and cyclic voltammetry [6]. However, electrochemical biosensors are subject to excessive noise at the electrode–electrolyte interface induced by drift and diffusion effects [7]. Moreover, this type of modality is sensitive to the offset and background perturbations, which are exacerbated by in-field measurement environments. These issues limit the typical detection sensitivity to several tens or hundreds of nano-Molar [4–6], orders of magnitude higher than the analyte concentrations in typical biochemical tests.

On the other hand, sensor platforms based on magnetic micro/nanoparticle labels have been proposed as a promising biosensing scheme to augment or replace the above sensing modalities for PoC applications. Affinity-based sandwich assays, such as enzyme-linked immunosorbent assay (ELISA) [8], are typically used in magnetic sensing processes, shown in Figure 5.1. The sensor surface is first coated with the desired molecular probes, which have high affinities with the target molecules. Then the test samples are introduced, and the target molecules are captured by the predeposited molecular probes through the surface chemistry. Finally, the surface-activated micro- or nano-magnetic labels are fed into the system and immobilized onto the sensor surface by the captured target molecules. Therefore, by detecting the existence of those magnetic labels, one can infer the presence of the target molecules in the incoming test sample. In comparison with optical microarrays and electrochemical sensors, magnetic biosensors provide the following advantages: First, they directly eliminate bulky and expensive optical devices making a low form-factor and a low-cost system possible. Second, magnetic labels do not have signal quenching or decaying problems often encountered in fluorescence-based optical detection systems, making the magnetic sensing scheme more robust. Moreover, since most biosamples produce negligible magnetic signals compared to the magnetic labels, magnetic biosensing can achieve a very high signal-to-background-noise ratio. In addition, magnetic particle labels provide a powerful and versatile way of micromanipulation on both the cellular and molecular levels. This can be realized by designing and distributing the excitation electrical currents on-chip [9], which create a magnetic field and apply forces on the nearby magnetic labels. Based on the high-integration level and the complex digital control capabilities supported in CMOS processes, this on-chip magnetic manipulation concept can potentially be extended to a reconfigurable microfluidic platform particularly useful for tissue engineering.

Currently reported integrated magnetic sensor schemes include Giant magnetoresistance sensors [10–12], Hall effect sensors [13,14], and NMR relaxometers [15]. However, these magnetic detection schemes require externally generated magnetic fields to bias the immobilized magnetic labels during their sensing processes. Moreover, expensive fabrication processes such as multilayer metal sputtering and deep dry etching on the passivation layers are demanded in those sensor fabrications. Consequently, these issues affect those systems' ultimate form-factors, total power consumption, and manufacturing cost.

In order to address these impediments, we propose an ultrasensitive frequency-shift-based magnetic biosensing scheme that is fully compatible with standard CMOS processes with no need for costly postprocessing steps or any electrical or permanent external biasing magnets [16]. The core of the sensor is an on-chip low-noise inductor-capacitor (LC) oscillator, whose oscillation frequency will experience a down-shift due to the presence of the magnetic labels on the sensor surface during the detection process. This sensor scheme is conducive to implementing a very-large-scaled magnetic microarray without suffering from significant design complexity and manufacturing cost penalty. This can be achieved by integrating more sensor units onto a single chip and tiling the chips to form the entire sensor system [17]. Therefore, the proposed frequency-shift-based magnetic biosensing scheme presents itself as an ideal solution for PoC molecular-level diagnostic applications.

This chapter is organized as follows. Section 5.2 focuses on the sensor mechanism. Theoretical modeling on the sensor transducer gain and the fundamental sensor noise floor is demonstrated to yield the sensor signal-to-noise ratio (SNR). The line-width narrowing effect is also presented to justify the advantage of oscillator-based frequency-shift detection. Section 5.3 demonstrates the design optimization to maximize the sensor SNR under various practical implementation constraints. As a design example, an 8-cell frequency-shift-based sensor array realized in a 130 nm CMOS process is demonstrated [18]. The system architecture and the key building blocks are covered in detail in Sections 5.4 and 5.5 respectively. Section 5.6 presents the measurement results of the sensor system for both electrical performance and magnetic sensing. To the authors' best knowledge, this sensor example achieves the best sensitivity among the CMOS magnetic biosensors reported so far.

5.2 SENSOR MECHANISM

5.2.1 Sensor Operation Principle and Oscillator-Based Frequency-Shift Detection

The core of our proposed sensing scheme is an on-chip LC resonator (Figure 5.2). The current through the on-chip inductor generates a magnetic field and polarizes the present magnetic particles. This polarization leads to an increase in the total magnetic energy in space and thereby the effective

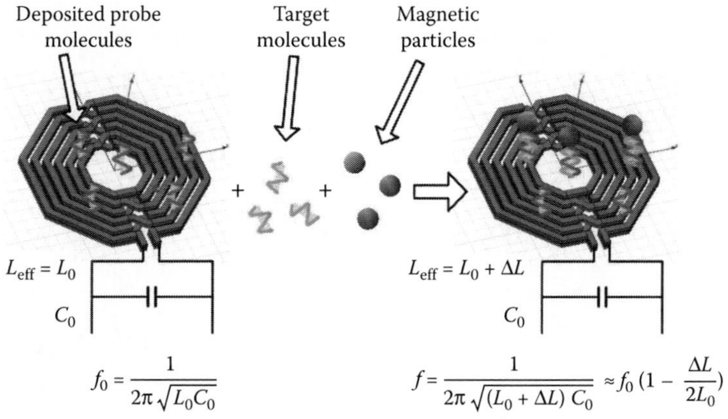

FIGURE 5.2 Proposed frequency-shift-based magnetic sensor scheme.

inductance of the inductor. The corresponding resonant frequency down-shift of the LC tank is given as

$$f = \frac{1}{2\pi\sqrt{LC}} = \frac{1}{2\pi\sqrt{(L_0 + \Delta L)C_0}} \approx f_0\left(1 - \frac{\Delta L}{2L_0}\right), \tag{5.1}$$

where L_0 and C_0 are the nominal inductance and capacitance, while ΔL is the inductance increase due to the magnetic particles. Therefore, this down-shift indicates the existence of the immobilized magnetic particles on the sensor surface, based on which one can infer the presence of the target molecules in the incoming test sample (Figure 5.1).

In order to detect this frequency down-shift, one approach is to directly measure the LC resonator's impedance in its amplitude and/or phase by precision circuits, such as a Wheatstone-Bridge. However, the line width of the tank impedance is fundamentally determined by its quality factor. For a standard CMOS process, this quality factor is often limited by the on-chip inductor quality factor Q (typically 10–20). In contrast, for an on-chip spiral sensing inductor with D_{out} of 100 to~200 μm, a single micron-sized magnetic particle label typical only induces a ppm (part-per-million, i.e., 10^{-6}) or even sub-ppm-level relative frequency-shift. Moreover, to provide a sensitive on-chip impedance measurement solution, the system requires fully integrated high-quality test tone generation, frequency sweeping, and analog-to-digital conversions, which add significantly to the design complexity.

On the other hand, if the same on-chip LC tank is implemented as an oscillator's resonator, based on the virtual damping phenomena, the line-width of the oscillator's phase noise profile will experience a significant line-width compression effect compared with that of with the LC tank impedance function (Figure 5.3) [19]. For a gigahertz-range CMOS oscillator, this line-width compression ratio is typically between 10^{-8} and 10^{-9}. Therefore, oscillator-based frequency detection provides an ultrasensitive measurement platform, which can be readily used to discern the sub-ppm-level relative frequency-shift in sensing the micron- or nanometer-sized magnetic labels. In addition, a simple frequency counter can be implemented locally to the sensor oscillator, and directly provides the digital measurement output of the oscillation frequency. Compared with the aforementioned impedance measurement approach, the oscillator-based frequency sensing provides a much more compact and simplified solution conducive to very-large-scaled sensor array implementations with high pixel density.

5.2.2 Sensor SNR Characterization

In order to fully characterize the proposed oscillator-based frequency-shift magnetic sensing platform, both its signal response (transducer gain) and the measurement noise floor will be discussed in this section. Subsequently, boldface letters denote vectors, and italics denote scalars in the following context.

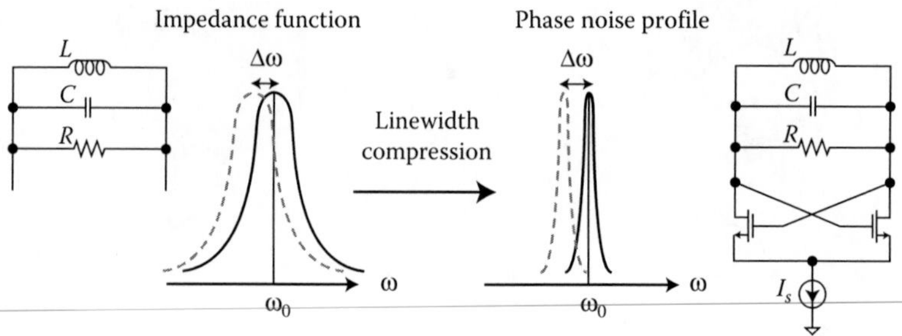

FIGURE 5.3 Line-width compression effect of oscillator phase noise profile compared with passive tank impedance function, assuming the same LC tank is used.

5.2.2.1 Sensor Transducer Gain

Most off-the-shelf magnetic particle labels are superparamagnetic, whose induced magnetization vector M under external polarization magnetic field H can be expressed by a Langevin function and further approximated at room temperature as

$$M \approx \frac{M_{\text{sat}}\mu_0 m_p}{3kT} H = \chi_{\text{eff}} H, \tag{5.2}$$

where M_{sat} is the saturation magnetization; μ_0 is the magnetic permeability in vacuum; m_p is the magnetization factor; and χ_{eff} is the effective susceptibility of the superparamagnetic material [20]. The quantity k stands for the Boltzman constant and T for the temperature. Considering the demagnetization effect [21], based on the χ_{eff} and the demagnetization factor D, the apparent magnetic susceptibility χ_{app} of the label particles can be calculated, which characterizes how their magnetizations respond to the external polarization field. Since both D and χ_{app} depend on the exact shape of the polarized magnetic objects, they are typically three-dimensional vectors even if the object is made of isotropic magnetic material. But, with a spherical shape assumption for the magnetic particles, both D and χ_{app} can be simplified as scalar quantities [21].

Assume that the electrical current I conducting through the sensing inductor generates an excitation magnetic field of H_{ext}. If there are N immobilized magnetic particles each with an equal volume of V_{m} and located at $r_i(x_i, y_i, z_i)$, $i \in [1, N]$ in the vicinity of the sensor surface, the total magnetic energy increase ΔE_{m} in the space due to the particles' magnetic polarizations by H_{ext} is given by

$$\Delta E_{\text{m}} \approx \sum_{i=1}^{N} \frac{1}{2} \iiint_{V_{\text{m}}} \chi_{\text{app}}\mu_0 \, \| H_{\text{ext}}(r_i) \|^2 \, \text{dv} \approx \sum_{i=1}^{N} \frac{1}{2} \chi_{\text{app}}\mu_0 \, \| H_{\text{ext}}(r_i) \|^2 \, V_{\text{m}}, \tag{5.3}$$

if the interactions among the adjacent magnetic particles are negligible and $H_{\text{ext}}(r_i)$ can be treated as a uniform polarization field across the volume V_{m} for the ith magnetic particle. Therefore, the effective inductance change ΔL is given as

$$\Delta L = \frac{2\Delta E_{\text{m}}}{I^2} \approx \frac{\sum_{i=1}^{N} \chi_{\text{app}}\mu_0 \, \| H_{\text{ext}}(r_i) \|^2 \, V_{\text{m}}}{I^2} = \frac{(\chi_{\text{app}} \overline{\| B_{\text{ext}} \|^2} V_{\text{m}}) \times N}{\mu_0 I^2}, \tag{5.4}$$

where $\overline{\| B_{\text{ext}} \|^2}$ is the spatially averaged excitation magnetic flux density for the N magnetic particles. Consequently, the average transducer gain can be defined as

$$\text{Transducer Gain} = \frac{\text{Frequency shift}(\Delta f / f_0)}{\text{No. of magnetic particles}} = \frac{\Delta L}{2L} \cdot \frac{1}{N} = \frac{\chi_{\text{app}}}{2\mu_0} \cdot \frac{\overline{\| B_{\text{ext}} \|^2}}{I^2 L} \cdot V_{\text{m}}. \tag{5.5}$$

The above equation shows that the sensor signal is composed of three factors multiplied together. The first factor $\chi_{\text{app}}/2\mu_0$ is only related to the magnetic property and the particle shape, whereas the last factor V_{m} is determined by the particle size. Both of them can be treated as constant values for a given type of magnetic labels assuming the local magnetic field strength does not saturate the particle's magnetic susceptibility. However, the middle factor stands for an excitation magnetic field factor, which is proportional to the magnitude square of the polarization magnetic field per unit current and normalized by the sensing inductance value. Therefore, to achieve a large sensor transducer gain, the sensor inductor design should maximize the average excitation magnetic field strength per unit current and at the same time minimize its nominal inductance value.

In addition, the spatial "spot" sensor transducer gain at the location $r = (x, y, z)$ is given as

$$\text{Transducer Gain}(r) = \frac{\chi_{\text{app}}}{2\mu_0} \cdot \frac{\| B_{\text{ext}}(r) \|^2}{I^2 L} \cdot V_{\text{m}}, \tag{5.6}$$

where $B_{\text{ext}}(r)$ is the excitation magnetic flux density at the location r.

5.2.2.2 Sensor Noise Modeling

Frequency counting can be used to determine the sensing oscillator's frequency-shift induced by the immobilized magnetic particle labels. During frequency counting, the total number of transitions M for the oscillator transient voltage waveform is measured within a given counting time window T. The measured frequency f is then given by

$$f = \frac{M}{T}. \tag{5.7}$$

The oscillator's accumulated jitter within the window T presents transition errors of its waveform, which lead to total phase error ϕ_{T} and the frequency counting error Δf as

$$\Delta f = \frac{\phi_{\text{T}}}{2\pi} \cdot \frac{1}{T} = \frac{M_{\text{err},T}}{T} \tag{5.8}$$

where $M_{\text{err},T} = \phi_{\text{T}}/2\pi$ stands for the measurement uncertainty for the number of transitions within time T. Therefore, the noise floor for frequency counting can be formulated based on the sensing oscillator's accumulated jitter σ_{T}^2 within the counting window T as

$$\sigma_{\Delta f/f_0}^2 = \frac{(\Delta f)^2}{f_0^2} = \frac{(\phi_{\text{T}})^2}{(2\pi)^2 T^2} \cdot \frac{1}{f_0^2} = \frac{(\phi_{\text{T}})^2}{\omega_0^2} \cdot \frac{1}{T^2} = \frac{\sigma_{\text{T}}^2}{T^2}, \tag{5.9}$$

where Δf is the uncertainty in frequency and f_0 is the nominal frequency. In general, the window T is assumed to be derived from a stable off-chip frequency reference such as an oven-controlled crystal oscillator, whose frequency uncertainty is negligible compared to that of the sensing oscillator.

Assuming that $\phi(t)$ is the excessive noisy phase of the oscillator, the accumulated jitter σ_{T}^2 is fundamentally determined by the sensing oscillator's phase noise as

$$\begin{aligned} \sigma_{\text{T}}^2 &= \frac{1}{\omega_0^2} E\{[\phi(t+T) - \phi(t)]^2\} = \frac{4}{\pi\omega_0^2} \int_0^{+\infty} S_{\phi,\text{DSB}}(\omega) \sin^2\left[\frac{\omega T}{2}\right] d\omega \\ &= \frac{2}{\pi\omega_0^2} \int_0^{+\infty} S_{\phi,\text{SSB}}(\omega) \sin^2\left[\frac{\omega T}{2}\right] d\omega, \end{aligned} \tag{5.10}$$

where $S_{\phi,\text{DSB}}(\omega)$ and $S_{\phi,\text{SSB}}(\omega)$ are the double-side-band (DSB) and single-side-band (SSB) phase noise power spectrum densities (PSDs), respectively [22]. The quantity ω is the phase noise offset-frequency, and ω_0 is the nominal oscillation frequency. In the following discussions, $S_\phi(\omega)$ will be used to denote the SSB phase noise $S_{\phi,\text{SSB}}(\omega)$. Therefore, based on (Equations 5.9 and 5.10) the relative frequency measurement error $\sigma_{\Delta f/f_0}^2$ can be related to the phase noise as

$$\sigma_{\Delta f/f_0}^2 = \frac{\sigma_{\text{T}}^2}{T^2} = \frac{2}{\pi\omega_0^2 T^2} \int_0^{+\infty} S_\phi(\omega) \sin^2\left[\frac{\omega T}{2}\right] d\omega. \tag{5.11}$$

The phase noise $S_\phi(\omega)$ for a CMOS-based oscillator typically contains both $1/f^2$ and $1/f^3$ phase noise components. The former is due to up-conversion and folding of the thermal noise in the oscillator circuit, while the latter is caused by up-conversion of the flicker noise mainly from the oscillator's active devices (Figure 5.4a). This frequency measurement uncertainty $\sigma^2_{\Delta f/f_0}$ can be shown to be a function of the actual counting window T as follows.

For a small T, that is, $T \ll 2\pi/\omega_{1/f^3}$, where ω_{1/f^3} is the $1/f^3$ corner frequency for the phase noise profile $S_\phi(\omega)$, the jitter due to $1/f^2$ phase noise dominates the relative frequency error $\sigma^2_{\Delta f/f_0}$, which becomes inversely proportional to T as

$$\sigma^2_{\Delta f/f_0} = \frac{\sigma^2_T}{T^2} = \frac{k^2 T}{T^2} = \frac{k^2}{T}. \tag{5.12}$$

Here, k is the $1/f^2$ jitter coefficient for the sensing oscillator [22]. Note that $\sigma^2_{\Delta f/f_0}$ decreases when the window T is increased for a longer counting window. This is because the $1/f^2$ phase noise behaves like white frequency noise [23], where the uncertainties in edge transition times are uncorrelated, and as a result, the accumulated jitter power σ^2_T is only linearly proportional to T, shown in (5.12). Thus, the frequency measurement error $\sigma^2_{\Delta f/f_0}$ due to the $1/f^2$ phase noise, as its normalized accumulated jitter (Equation 5.11), can always be reduced using a longer counting time window T.

However, when T is large enough ($T \ll 2\pi/\omega_{1/f^3}$), $1/f^3$ phase noise dominates and results in the frequency error $\sigma^2_{\Delta f/f_0}$ actually independent of T as

$$\sigma^2_{\Delta f/f_0} = \frac{\sigma^2_T}{T^2} = \frac{\zeta^2 T^2}{T^2} = \zeta^2, \tag{5.13}$$

where ζ is the $1/f^3$ jitter coefficient for the sensing oscillator [22]. This is due to the fact that $1/f^3$ phase noise is flicker frequency noise [23], whose edge transitions uncertainties are strongly correlated leading to σ^2_T being proportional to T^2 (14). Since $\sigma^2_{\Delta f/f_0}$ is independent of the window length T for this case, this ζ^2 factor therefore determines the fundamental noise floor for the oscillator-based frequency measurement.

In addition, a measurement error proportional to $1/f_0^2T^2$ due to the uncertainty principle should be superimposed onto the aforementioned two frequency errors. This $1/f_0^2T^2$ error suggests that a frequency resolution of 1 Hz can only be achieved with a counting window longer than one second.

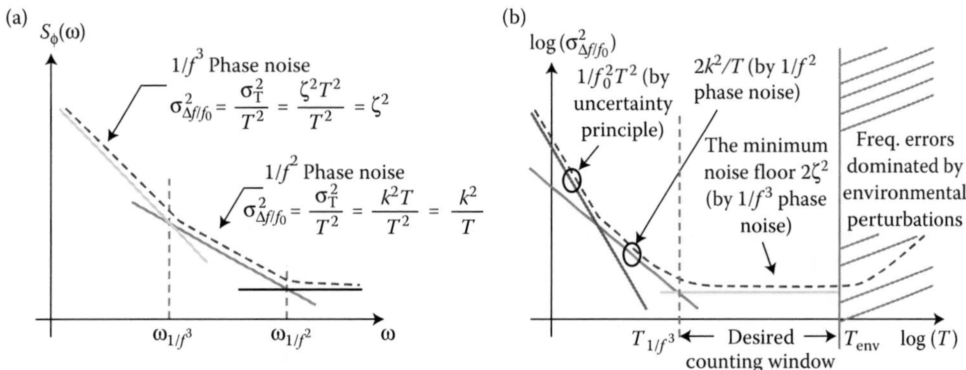

FIGURE 5.4 (a) Typical phase noise profile of an oscillator. (b) Frequency measurement uncertainty versus counting window T in differential operation. The blue curve is the overall frequency counting uncertainty for a given T with the minimum noise floor of $2\zeta^2$.

The total measurement noise with respect to window T is plotted and reveals that the $1/f^3$ phase noise (ζ^2) indeed determines the ultimate sensor noise floor (Figure 5.4b).

In practical implementations, differential sensing can be used to further reject the environmental perturbations, such as temperature drifting and supply variations. This scheme can be implemented as two identical oscillators, one used for sensing and one used as a reference, both being physically placed close to each other and sharing the same electrical supply and biasing circuits, shown as an example in Figure 5.7. Therefore, the environmental variations present themselves as common-mode perturbations to the two oscillators, and can be readily suppressed by differential operations, that is, taking the frequency difference of the sensing and reference oscillators as the sensor output. Note that in this case, since the phase noise is uncorrelated between the two oscillators, the total noise power after the differential sensing actually doubles, if the two oscillators are assumed to have the same phase noise PSD (Figure 5.4b). The extra factor of two accounts for the noise power doubling.

Therefore, the overall sensor SNR in the differential sensing scheme can be formulated as

$$\mathrm{SNR} = \frac{\text{Relative frequency shift}}{\text{Relative frequency error}} = \frac{\Delta f/f_0}{\sqrt{2}\sigma_{\Delta f/f_0}} = \frac{\Delta f/f_0}{\sqrt{2}\zeta}, \tag{5.14}$$

where the frequency shift $\Delta f/f_0$ and error $\sqrt{2}\sigma_{\Delta f/f_0}$ for a given sensing oscillator and magnetic particles distribution can be calculated based on (Equations 5.5 and 5.11), respectively. The factor of two is to account for the noise power doubling due to differential sensing.

5.3 SENSOR DESIGN SCALING LAW

The theoretically derived SNR expression enables sensor design optimization, which will be discussed in detail in this section.

First, for the sensor signal response, the transducer gain equation 5.5 demonstrates that for a given type of magnetic particle labels, the factors related to the magnetic material and the particle volume are both constants. The field factor $\|B_{\text{ext}}\|^2/I^2L$, determined by the sensing inductor geometry, is therefore the only factor subjected to design optimization.

The effect of the sensor noise floor $\sigma^2_{\Delta f/f_0}$ with respect to the sensing inductor design (inductance L and quality factor Q) is discussed next. Since the fundamental noise floor is determined by the $1/f^3$ phase noise, only flicker noise will be considered for the following derivation.

For a given process technology, assuming a fixed biasing current density for the oscillator active-core devices and a constant tank amplitude (limited by the supply V_{DD}), the transistors' DC biasing current I_{d} and width W are related to the tank inductor design as

$$I_{\text{d}} \propto W \propto \frac{V_{\text{DD}}}{R_{\text{tank}}} = \frac{V_{\text{DD}}}{\omega_0 LQ}, \tag{5.15}$$

where R_{tank} is the tank's parallel resistance and Q is its quality factor of the tank (typically dominant by the tank inductance Q in CMOS processes) both at the resonant frequency ω_0. The result of $I_{\text{d}} \propto V_{\text{DD}}/R_{\text{tank}}$ assumes that the oscillator is biased for its optimum operation, that is, the boundary region between the current-limiting and voltage-limiting regime [22]. Moreover, for a fixed biasing current density, the device DC current is proportional to its drain output flicker current noise PSD $i^2_{n,1/f}(\omega) = \beta/\omega$, as

$$I_{\text{d}} \propto W \propto \beta. \tag{5.16}$$

The $1/f^3$ jitter coefficient ζ can be derived using the linear-time-varying phase noise model at a given offset frequency ω [22], and further simplified based on (Equations 5.15 and 5.16) to

$$\zeta^2 \propto S_\phi(\omega)\cdot\omega^3 = \frac{A_0^2}{q_{\max}^2}\cdot\frac{i_{n,1/f}^2(\omega)}{2\omega^2}\cdot\omega^3 = \frac{A_0^2}{q_{\max}^2}\cdot\frac{\beta}{2} \propto \frac{A_0^2}{V_{DD}^2C^2}\cdot\frac{V_{DD}}{\omega_0 LQ} \propto \frac{L}{Q}, \tag{5.17}$$

where A_0 is the DC term of the oscillator's impulse sensitivity function $\Gamma(t)$ and $q_{\max}$ is the tank maximum charge swing [22]. Therefore, assuming differential operation, the relationship between the sensor noise power $\sigma_{\Delta f/f_0}^2$ and the inductor L and Q is given by

$$\sigma_{\Delta f/f_0}^2 = \frac{2\times 2}{\pi\omega_0^2T^2}\int_0^{+\infty} S_\phi(\omega)\sin^2\frac{\omega T}{2}\,d\omega = 2\zeta^2 \propto \frac{L}{Q}. \tag{5.18}$$

This result suggests that the sensor noise floor also depends on the sensor inductor design. Consequently, based on (Equations 5.5 and 5.18), the averaged sensor SNR of a single magnetic particle can be obtained as

$$\mathrm{SNR} = \frac{\Delta f/f_0}{\sigma_{\Delta f/f_0}} \propto \frac{\overline{\| B_{ext} \|^2}}{I^2L}\cdot\sqrt{\frac{Q}{L}} = \frac{\overline{\| B_{ext} \|^2}}{I^2}\cdot\sqrt{\frac{Q}{L^3}}. \tag{5.19}$$

This equation shows that the sensor inductor design is the key to optimize the magnetic sensor performance and maximize its SNR during magnetic sensing.

As an example, the normalized averaged SNR for a 6-turn symmetric inductor detecting a single magnetic bead ($D = 1$ μm) at 1 GHz is shown in Figure 5.5. In this example, both the outer diameter (D_{out}) and the inductor trace width are swept while the trace separation is kept constant at 3.5 μm. For a given D_{out}, the SNR does not vary significantly with the width. This is because for a constant D_{out}, both the inductance L and the averaged $\overline{\|B_{ext}\|^2}/I^2$ scale the same with the inductor width. This leads to a relatively constant SNR for a given outer diameter. On the other hand, for the same trace width, a smaller D_{out} gives a much higher averaged SNR. This is due to both a larger $\overline{\|B_{ext}\|^2}/I^2$

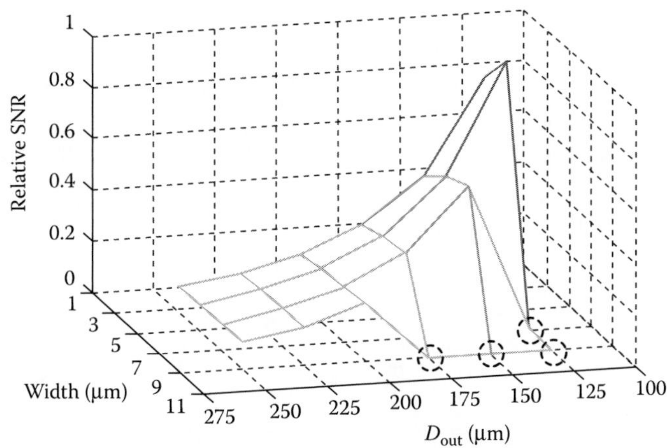

FIGURE 5.5 The simulated averaged SNR for a 6-turn differential symmetric inductor with different geometric sizes at 1 GHz operating frequency. The dotted circles indicate inductor geometries unrealizable due to layout rules.

(i.e., a more concentrated excitation magnetic field) and a smaller inductance value at a smaller inductor footprint, that is, a smaller D_{out}. However, an inductor with an exceedingly small size is practically undesirable for several reasons. First, the LC tank's metal interconnections start to contribute nonnegligible resistances and parasitic inductances comparable to the sensor inductance, which degrades the sensor SNR by lowering both Q and $\Delta L/L_0$ during sensing. Moreover, to maintain the same voltage amplitude at the operating frequency, a low–impedance tank (for a small L) needs to conduct a larger current, which is susceptible to cause magnetic saturation of the particles and yields the decreased detected magnetic signal due to susceptibility χ_{app} degradation as mentioned previously. Furthermore, the frequency-dependent magnetic loss, which degrades the magnetic signal, limits the maximum operation frequency to be around 1 GHz for magnetic beads formed by nanometer-sized magnetic particles suspended in nonmagnetic structures [24,25]. Thus, the inductor size cannot be too small to achieve an acceptable Q at the desired operation frequency. In addition, the design space for the sensing inductor is also limited by other constraints such as the sensor pixel size (footprint) and power consumption.

5.4 A CMOS IMPLEMENTATION EXAMPLE (SYSTEM ARCHITECTURE)

In this section, an 8-cell sensor array implemented in a standard 130 nm CMOS process will be demonstrated as a design example for the proposed frequency-shift magnetic sensing scheme. The system architecture is shown in Figure 5.6.

The differential sensing scheme is implemented for each sensor cell. It is composed of two well-matched sensor oscillators for sensing and reference operations, both operating at a nominal frequency of 1 GHz (Figure 5.7). In the layout, the active cores of the two oscillators are placed in proximity to improve matching and to minimize local temperature differences. The oscillator pair also share the same power supply, biasing and ground lines. As discussed above, these implementation techniques ensure that the environment-related low-frequency noise and drifting appear as the

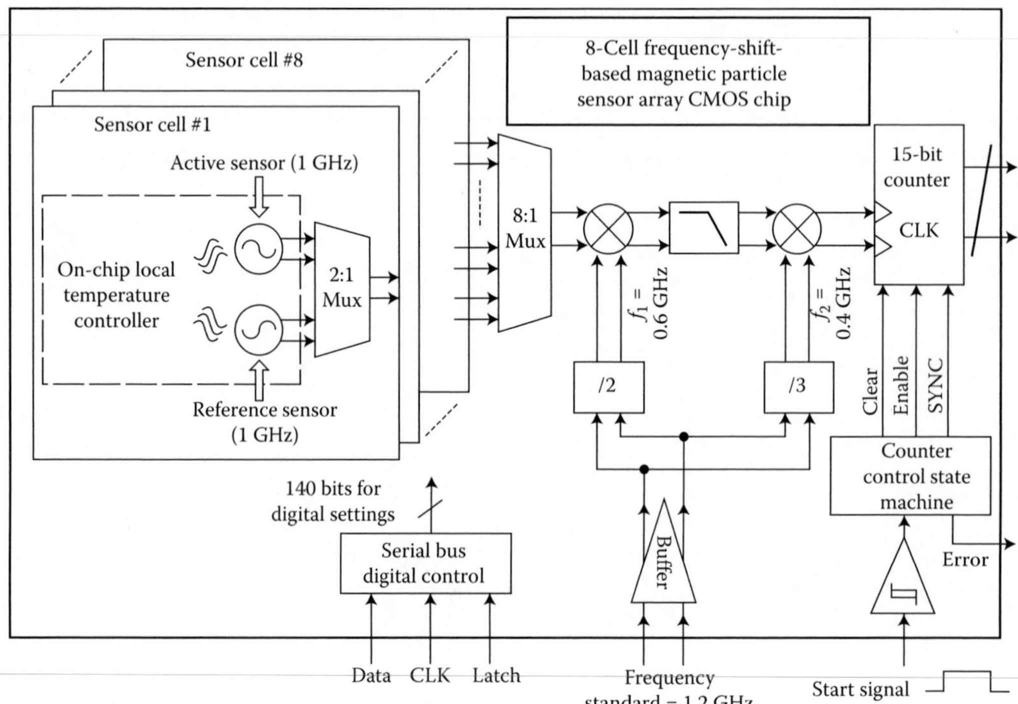

FIGURE 5.6 The 8-cell frequency-shift-based CMOS magnetic biosensor array system architecture.

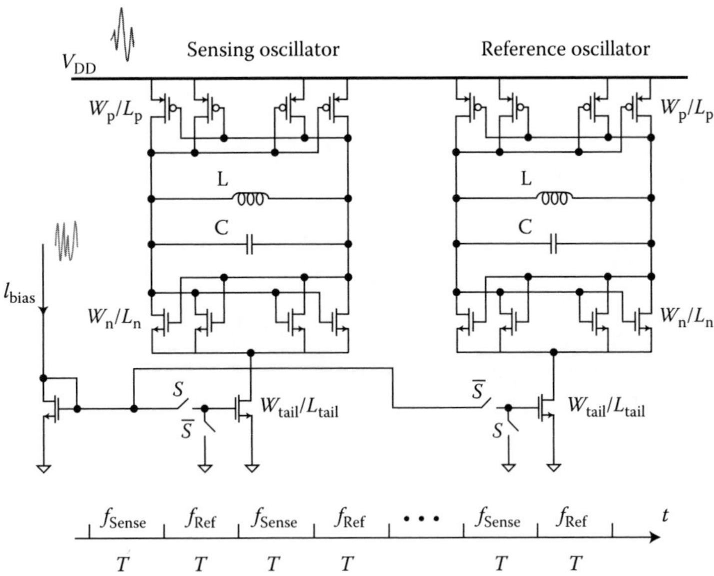

FIGURE 5.7 Schematic of the differential sensing oscillators. The two sensor oscillators are alternatively turned on to perform differential sensing scheme.

common-mode perturbations and are subsequently suppressed by the differential operation. The active and the reference oscillators are turned on alternately in time to avoid parasitic injection locking or oscillator pulling.

On-chip temperature controllers are implemented in this design. They regulate the local temperature for the oscillator active cores through a thermal–electrical feedback loop. This further reduces frequency drifting induced by ambient temperature changes. Instead of regulating the entire chip, the temperature controllers are placed locally at every sensor cell, regulating the differential sensing oscillators' active core temperature to achieve more efficient thermal control with minimal power consumption overhead.

Frequency counters are used to detect the sensing signal's frequency shift and provide direct digital output. In order to facilitate resolving a ppm or sub-ppm-level frequency-shift at 1 GHz, a two-step down-conversion architecture is used to shift the 1 GHz sensor output to a tunable kilohertz-range baseband frequency. Unlike direct down-conversion, this architecture guarantees that the two local oscillator (LO) signals (0.6 and 0.4 GHz) are not close to either the sensor free-running frequency or its dominant harmonics and hence inherently prevents pulling or injection locking on the sensing oscillator pair. By using a 15-bit baseband frequency counter, a maximum counting resolution better than 3×10^{-4}ppm (0.3 Hz at 1 GHz) can be achieved. Note that digital nature of the sensor system's output signal facilitates tiling multiple sensor array chips to form a very-large-scale magnetic microarray for high-throughput applications.

5.5 A CMOS IMPLEMENTATION EXAMPLE (CIRCUIT BLOCKS)

In this section, circuit designs for the major building blocks in the example sensor array system are presented in detail.

5.5.1 Sensing Oscillator

A differential complementary cross-coupled topology is used for the sensing oscillator as shown in Figure 5.7. Switches at the tail current sources control the turning on and off of the oscillators, whose bias current is derived from the same master current source. Common-centroid layout is used to improve matching and design robustness against process gradients. The $1/f^3$ phase noise determines the ultimate noise floor of the sensor. A gate length of 240 μm is used for both the N-channel MOSFET (metal-oxide-semiconductor field-effect transistor) (NMOS) and P-channel MOSFET (metal-oxide-semiconductor field-effect transistor) (PMOS) transistors in the cross-coupled pair to lower the device flicker noise corner. Moreover, the relative weighting between the NMOS active pair and the PMOS active pair is optimized to shape the oscillation transient voltage waveform and minimize the flicker noise up-conversion from the NMOS current tail [26]. Furthermore, to provide frequency tunability of the sensing oscillator, a switched capacitor bank has been adopted to set the desired operating frequency.

Based on the noise analysis described in Section 5.2.2.2, a design goal for the $1/f^3$ phase noise of the sensor oscillator can be obtained, which achieves a given frequency-shift detection sensitivity. For the differential sensing scheme, the frequency counting noise floor $\sigma_{\Delta f/f0,\mathrm{diff}}$ has been shown to be $\sqrt{2}\zeta$, with ζ as the $1/f^3$ jitter coefficient of the oscillator. Numerically, this ζ factor can be obtained from the oscillator's SSB $1/f^3$ phase noise profile $S_\phi(\omega) = c/\omega^3$ based on a close-in corner frequency approximation in [27] as

$$\sigma^2_{\Delta f/f_0} = \frac{2\times 2}{\pi\omega_0^2 T^2}\int_0^{+\infty} S_\phi(\omega)\sin^2\frac{\omega T}{2}\,d\omega = 2\zeta^2 \approx \frac{25c}{2\pi\omega_0^2}. \tag{5.20}$$

Therefore, to achieve a frequency-shift noise floor of less than 1 ppm in a differential operation, the SSB $1/f^3$ phase noise for the sensing oscillator should be below −43.9 dBc/Hz at a 1 kHz frequency offset for a center tone of 1 GHz. For a 0.1 ppm frequency resolution, the phase noise at an offset of 1 kHz should be −63.9 dBc/Hz.

5.5.2 Temperature Regulator

On-chip temperature regulators are implemented locally for each individual differential sensing cells. A temperature controlling system is typically composed of an electrical–thermal feedback loop. This loop senses the difference between the on-chip and the target temperature, and converts it to an electrical signal, which drives an on-chip heater for thermal controlling.

The simplified schematic of our temperature regulator is shown in Figure 5.8. The temperature sensor is implemented as a proportional-to-absolute-temperature (PTAT) voltage and a bandgap

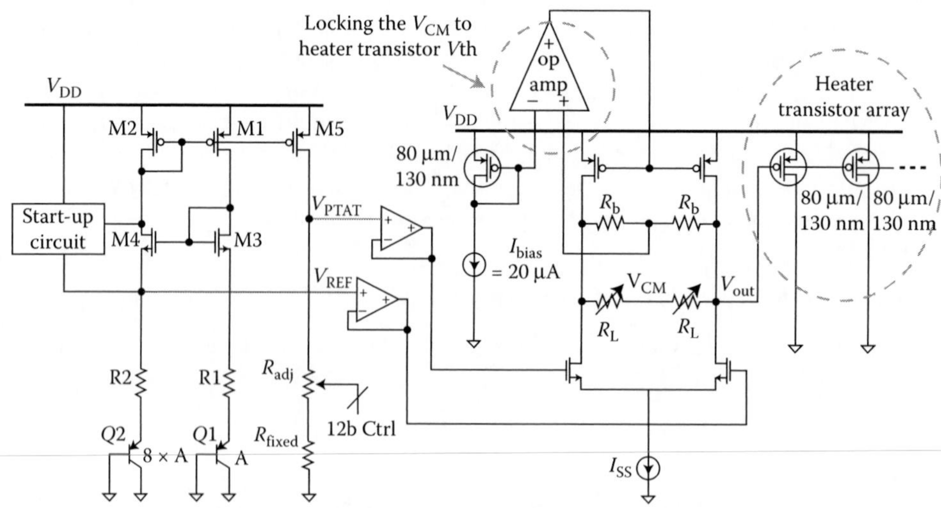

FIGURE 5.8 Simplified schematic for the on-chip temperature regulator.

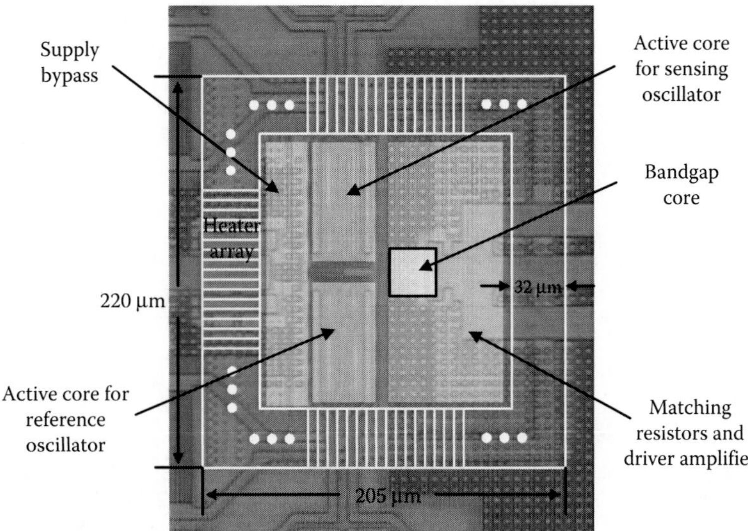

FIGURE 5.9 The layout configuration of the heater structure for one differential sensing cell.

voltage is used as the temperature reference. The PTAT voltage is programmable with 12-bit control on its output resistors that sets the target temperature for thermal regulation. The voltage difference between the two temperature signals is then amplified by a two-stage buffer to drive a heater transistor array. A feedback op-amp is used to lock the common-mode output voltage of the driver to the threshold voltage of a dummy heater transistor. This provides a reliable stand-by driver output voltage to prevent any false turning-on of the heater transistors due to process variations or modeling inaccuracy. The thermal response of the heater array is simulated using Ansoft® Ephysics [28]. Overall, this thermal controller forms a first-order electrical–thermal feedback loop with a typical DC loop gain of 20.5 dB and is stabilized by a dominant pole in the kilohertz range.

The layout configuration of the temperature regulator is shown in Figure 5.9. The bandgap core, including the reference and the PTAT generation, is placed close to the two oscillators' active devices for accurate temperature sensing. The heater array, composed of power PMOS transistors, forms a ring structure, surrounding the oscillator active cores to minimize the spatial temperature difference within the regulator.

5.5.3 Multiplexers and Buffers

Multiplexers and buffer amplifiers together with distribution lines deliver the output signals from the selected sensor cells to a down-conversion block (Figure 5.10). Resistive degeneration is used to linearize the distribution circuit gain. On order to ensure an adequate bandwidth without peaking inductors or excessive power consumption, signals are distributed in current mode through a modified cascode topology [29]. The low impedance at the current summing nodes minimizes the bandwidth penalty due to parasitic capacitances. Since only buffers for the selected branch need to be turned on at any given time, the distribution system overall consumes 10 mA from a 2.5 V supply, and has a –3 dB bandwidth of 2.5 GHz.

5.5.4 Divide-by-2 and Divide-by-3 Frequency Divider

In order to synthesize the down-conversion LO signals, a static divide-by-2 and a divide-by-3 circuit are implemented in current-mode-logic as high-speed digital dividers. Both dividers are composed of feedback D-flipflops (Figure 5.11) and provide divided signals with a 50% duty-cycle to suppress unwanted harmonics. With these dividers, an off-chip 1.2 GHz frequency reference signal is divided

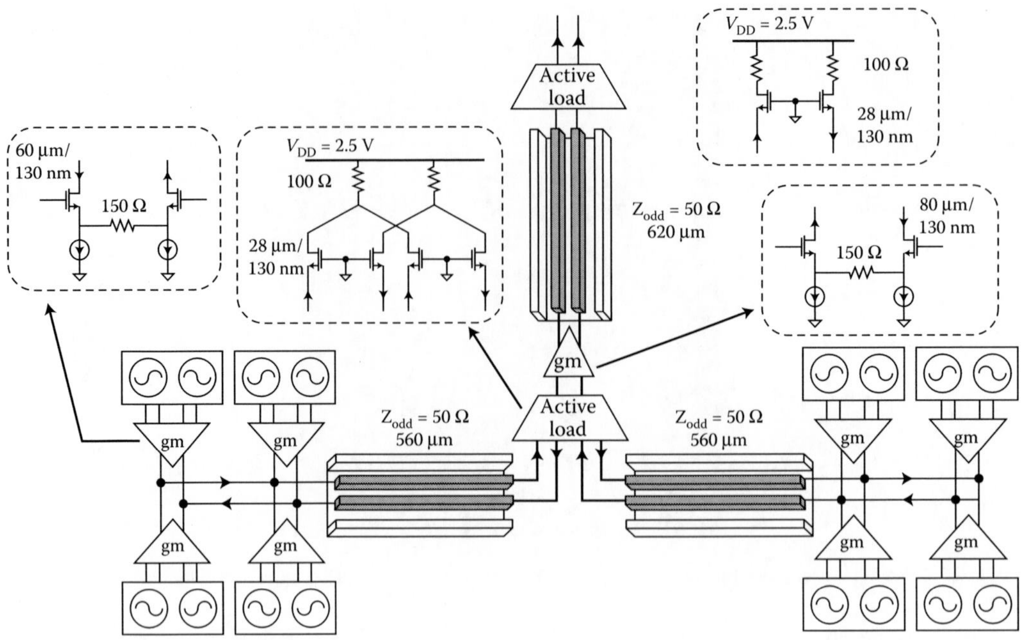

FIGURE 5.10 Schematic for the signal distribution network.

into 600 and 400 MHz LO which down-convert the sensor oscillators' nominal 1 GHz signal. This frequency plan ensures that both LO signals are separated from the fundamental tone and the dominant harmonics of the sensor free-running frequency to prevent oscillator pulling or injection locking on the sensing oscillator pair. Note that although the 1.2 GHz reference signal is fed from off-chip in this implementation, it can also be synthesized on-chip and locked to a megahertz crystal

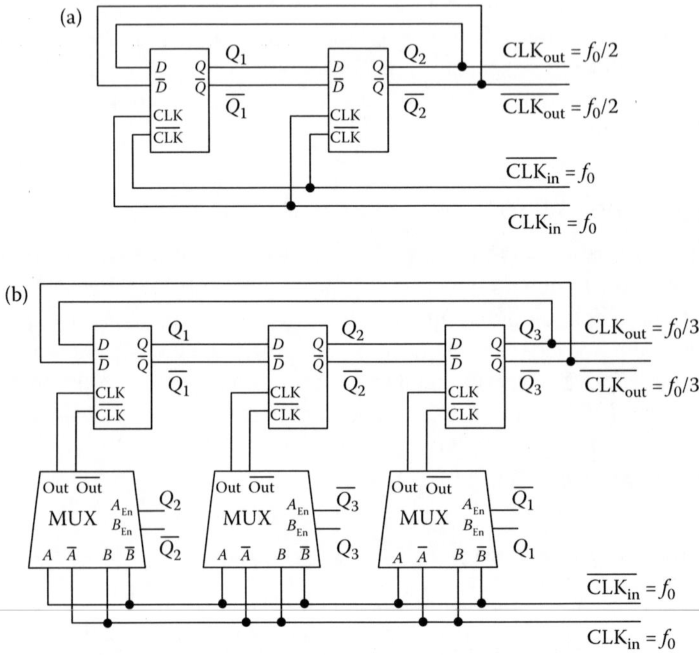

FIGURE 5.11 Schematic for the frequency dividers with 50% duty cycle: (a) Divide-by-2 (b) Divide-by-3.

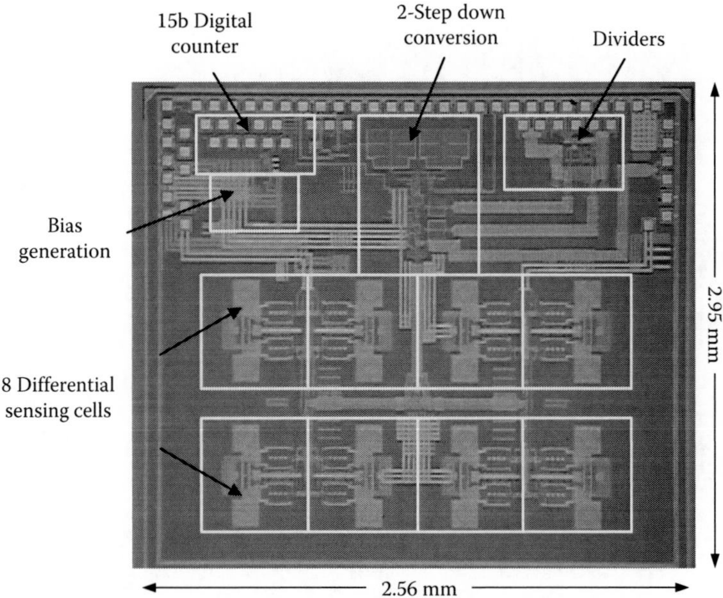

FIGURE 5.12 Chip microphotograph of the CMOS sensor array.

frequency standard. In this case, the presented down-conversion frequency plan also ensures that this 1.2 GHz tone is away from the 1 GHz sensor oscillators. The dividers consume 8 mA from a 1.2 V supply and add negligible noise to the 1.2 GHz reference signal.

5.6 MEASUREMENT RESULTS

The chip microphotograph for the example 8-cell magnetic sensor array is shown in Figure 5.12. The entire chip is implemented in a standard 130 nm 1P8M CMOS process and occupies an area of 3.0×5.2 mm^2. All the critical building blocks are highlighted. Note that the bonding pads are placed along the upper chip edge. This configuration accommodates the integration of the PDMS (polydimethylsiloxan) microfluidic structures for biosample delivery without perturbing the wire-bonds. The wire-bonds can be eventually sealed and protected by the PDMS solution [30]. A minimum distance of 250 μm between adjacent sensing inductors is used, limited by the minimum achievable microfluidic channel width/separation in our in-house PDMS fabrication facilities. This spacing between sensor cells can be substantially reduced by employing more advanced microfluidics processes. The CMOS sensor chip integrated with the PDMS structure is shown in Figure 5.13.

In this section, the electrical performance of the sensor array is first presented. Magnetic sensing measurements are then shown for detecting micron-sized magnetic particles. The results demonstrate the full functionality of our proposed frequency-shift-based magnetic sensing scheme.

5.6.1 Electrical Performance

The measured phase noise performance of the sensing oscillator is shown in Figure 5.14. Consuming 4 mA from a 1.2 V supply, the oscillator has its $1/f^3$ phase noise (at 1 kHz frequency offset) from −59 to −61.8 dBc/Hz for different biasing scenarios with a center tone of 1.04 GHz. Based on the theoretical analysis, this phase noise level provides a frequency measurement uncertainty $\sigma_{\Delta f/f_0}$ between 170.6 and 123.6 ppb (parts-per-billion, i.e., 10^{-9}) in the differential operation scheme, which achieves a sub-ppm sensor sensitivity using frequency-shift detections.

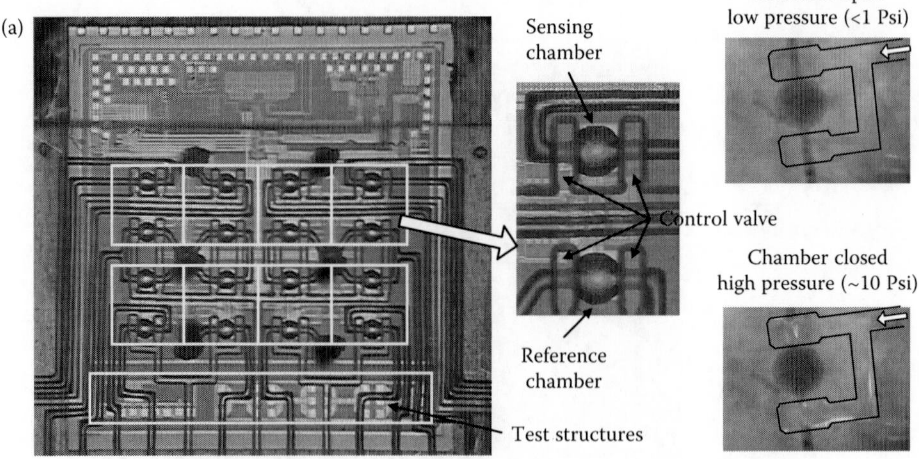

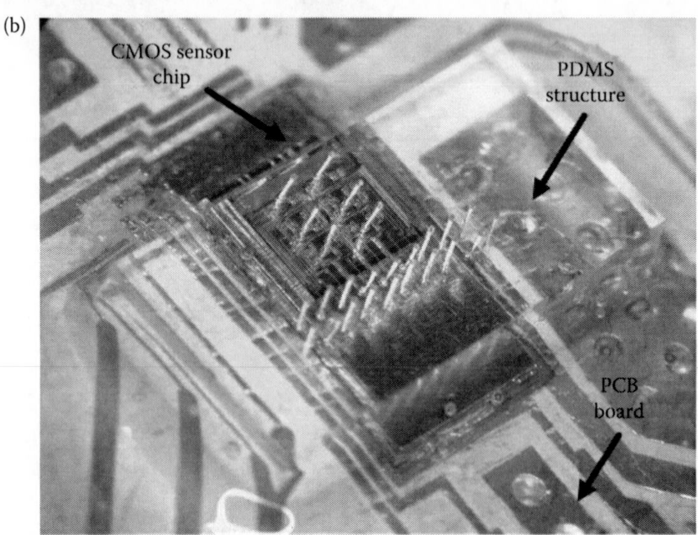

FIGURE 5.13 (a) Chip microphotograph of the CMOS sensor array with PDMS microfluidic structure. (b) Integration of the CMOS sensor chip, PDMS structure, and PCB board for the testing module.

The rejection of environment-related drifting through differential counting is demonstrated in Figure 5.15. The frequency counting results for the sensor and reference oscillators are shown with and without differential operation. A slowly varying common-mode drift of the oscillation frequencies can be observed and is greatly suppressed by the differential operation. Consequently, in the differential operation mode, the measured relative frequency uncertainty $\sigma_{\Delta f/f_0}$ is 130 ppb before averaging, which stays within the theoretical calculated noise range based on the phase noise measurement.

Moreover, the differential frequency counting samples can be averaged to further improve the sensor SNR (Figure 5.16). Let $f_S(i)$ and $f_R(i)$ stand for the frequency measurement in the ith differential counting interval. The total N-sample averaged differential frequency result is

$$\Delta f_{\mathrm{diff},N} = \frac{1}{N}\left[\sum_{i=1}^{N} \Delta f(i)\right] = \frac{1}{N}\left[\sum_{i=1}^{N} f_{\mathrm{s}}(i) - f_{\mathrm{R}}(i)\right]. \tag{5.21}$$

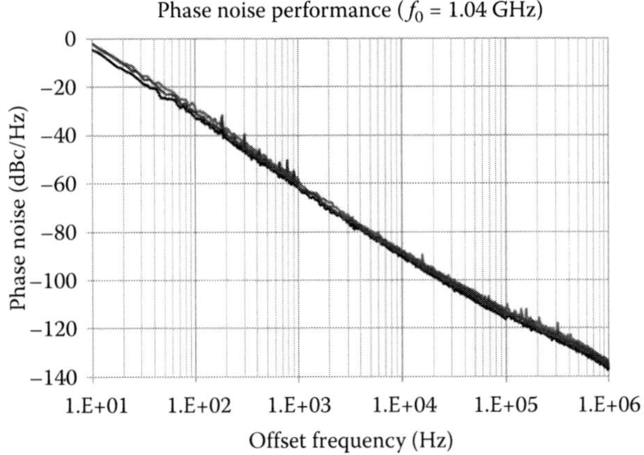

FIGURE 5.14 Measured and simulated phase noise performance of single sensing oscillator at different biasings.

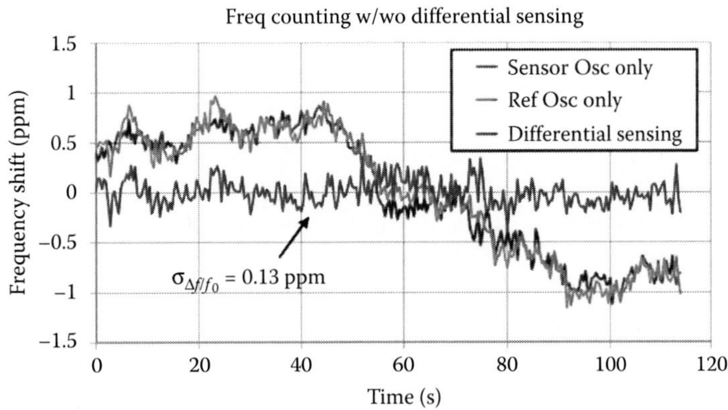

FIGURE 5.15 Suppression of common-mode frequency drifting through differential sensing.

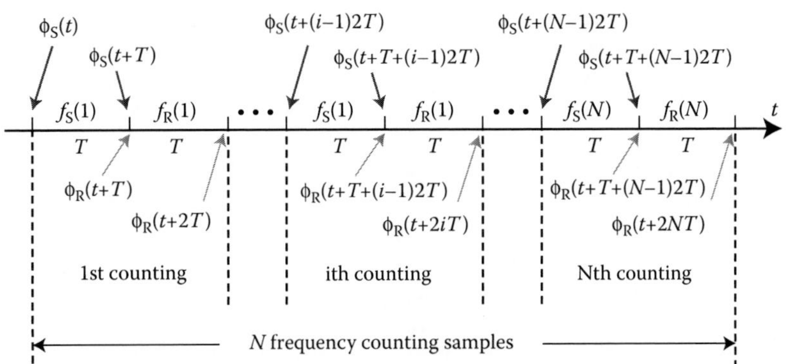

FIGURE 5.16 N-sample averaging on differential frequency counting measurements.

Therefore, using the above noise model and assuming that the sensor and reference oscillators present the same, yet uncorrelated PSD, the frequency measurement noise power after averaging N differential samples can be formulated as

$$
\begin{aligned}
\sigma^2_{\Delta f/f_0,\mathrm{diff},N} &= \frac{1}{T^2\omega_0^2} E\left[\frac{1}{N}\sum_{i=1}^{N}\{\phi_S(t+T+(i-1)2T)-\phi_S(t+(i-1)2T)\}\right. \\
&\qquad \left. -\{\phi_R(t+2T+(i-1)2T)-\phi_R(t+T+(i-1)2T)\}\right]^2 \\
&= \frac{1}{T^2\omega_0^2} E\left[\frac{1}{N}\sum_{i=1}^{N}\{\phi_S(t+T+(i-1)2T)-\phi_S(t+(i-1)2T)\}\right]^2 \\
&\quad + \frac{1}{T^2\omega_0^2} E\left[\frac{1}{N}\sum_{i=1}^{N}\{\phi_R(t+2T+(i-1)2T)-\phi_R(t+T+(t-1)2T)\}\right]^2 \\
&= \frac{2}{T^2\omega_0^2} E\left[\frac{1}{N}\sum_{i=1}^{N}\{\phi_S(t+T+(i-1)2T)-\phi_S(t+(i-1)2T)\}\right]^2 \\
&= \frac{2\times 2}{\pi\omega_0^2 T^2}\int_0^{+\infty} S_\phi(\omega)\cdot\sin^2\left(\frac{\omega T}{2}\right)\cdot\frac{\sin^2(N\omega T)}{\sin^2(\omega T)}\,d\omega \\
&= \mathrm{NPRR}(N)\cdot\frac{2\times 2}{\pi\omega_0^2 T^2}\int_0^{+\infty} S_\phi(\omega)\cdot\sin^2\frac{\omega T}{2}\,d\omega = \mathrm{NRF}(N)\cdot\sigma^2_{\Delta f/f_0,\mathrm{diff}},
\end{aligned}
\tag{5.22}
$$

where ϕ_S and ϕ_R are the excessive noisy phases for the senor and reference oscillators, which are uncorrelated to each other. The ratio between the noise power of the N-sample-averaged differential frequency counting result over the unaveraged one can be defined as a noise-power-reduction-ratio NPRR(N). The simulated NPRR with respect to the averaging sample number N is plotted in Figure 5.17. Note that the noise power for the N-sample averaging is not inversely proportional to the sample number N as the classical averaging scenario for sampled white noise (uncorrelated samples). This is because the waveform transition uncertainties due to $1/f^3$ jitter in the frequency measurement exhibit strong correlations, resulting in a much lower suppression after averaging.

The thermal regulator response is depicted in Figure 5.18 as the total heater current versus on-chip temperature variations. The on-chip temperature is measured through the PTAT voltage. When the temperature deviates from the target settings, that is, 29°C in this measurement, the PMOS

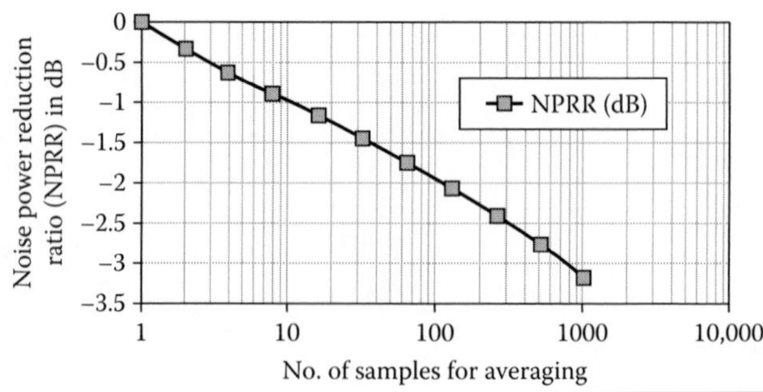

FIGURE 5.17 Simulated Noise Power Reduction Ratio NPRR(N) based on sample averaging, when the $1/f^3$ phase noise is the dominant noise for the sensing oscillators. The x-axis stands for the number of differential frequency counting measurements.

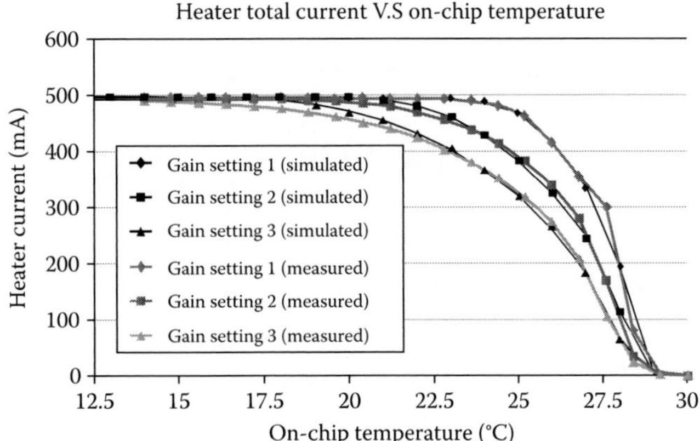

FIGURE 5.18 Simulated and measured heater total current versus on-chip temperature when the target temperature is set at 29°C.

heater ring starts to draw a DC current from the supply and heat up the enclosed differential sensing oscillators' active cores. The measured heater responses for three different loop-gain settings are shown, closely matching the simulated responses.

The electrical performance of the example CMOS sensor array is summarized in Table 5.1.

5.6.2 Magnetic Sensing Measurements

In order to characterize the sensor's magnetic sensing functionalities, two sets of experiments are performed on detecting three types of micron-sized magnetic particles, that is, Dynabeads® M-450 Epoxy, Dynabeads Protein G, and Dynabeads MyOne™ [31]. The first set of experiments is used to verify the sensor's capability of detecting a single micron-sized magnetic particle. The second one is used to characterize the sensor's dynamic range with a wide range of magnetic particles numbers.

In the first experiment, a single magnetic particle is introduced onto the sensor surface for all three bead types. The measurement results are summarized in Table 5.2. The frequency counting window is 0.1 s, and averaging on the sensing data is performed to further improve the SNR. With 160 s used

TABLE 5.1
Measured Electrical Performance of the Sensor Array

Power consumption	Sensor oscillator[a]	4.0 mA–1.2 V
	Downconversion chain, multiplexer[a] and counter	39.6 mA–2.5 V
	On-chip temperature controller[a,b]	24.3 mA–2.5 V
Total power consumption		165 mW
Thermal loop gain (nominal setting)		20 dB
No of differential sensing cells		8
Technology		130 nm CMOS
Chip area		2.95 × 2.56 mm
Sensor inductor size (D_{out})		140 μm

[a] At any given time, only one sensor oscillator with its temperature controller and buffer will be turned on to avoid pulling and/or injection-locking between oscillators.

[b] Here the target chip temperature is set at 29°C with the ambient temperature of 27°C. The 20 dB loop gain ensures the actual on-chip temperature is at 28.8°C.

TABLE 5.2
Typical Sensor Response to Off-the-Shelf Magnetic Bead

Bead Type	Bead Size (Diameter, μm)	Recorded $\Delta f/f$ per Bead (ppm)	Sensitivity (No of Beads)	SNR	Averaging Time (Seconds)[a]
Dynabeads®M-450 Epoxy	4.5	9.6	1	40.0 dB	90
Dynabeads®Protein	2.4	2.6	1	28.6 dB	90
Dynabeads®MyOne™ carboxylic acid	1	0.23	1	8.0 dB	160
Polystyrene bead (Non-magnetic)	1	0.0035[b]			

[a] The counting window T is 0.1 s for these measurements.

[b] This $\Delta f/f$ per bead is a calculated average value for a measured frequency shift of 100 polystyrene beads sensed at the same time.

for averaging, an SNR of 8.0 dB is achieved for detecting a single 1 μm magnetic particle (Dynabeads MyOne). After 90 s of averaging, the achieved SNR for a single 2.4 and 4.5 μm magnetic particle (Dynabeads® Protein G or Dynabeads M-450 Epoxy) are 28.6 and 40.0 dB, respectively. As a control sample, polystyrene beads ($D = 1$ μm) are tested. Polystyrene is the nonmagnetic structure material used to hold the nanomagnetic grains and form most off-the-shelf micron-size magnetic bead products. The polystyrene beads show significantly lower frequency-shift responses compared with the 1 μm magnetic beads. This verifies that our sensor's frequency shifts for the presented magnetic beads are mainly due to the inductance (magnetic) rather than the capacitance (dielectric) changes. Typical measurement results for a single magnetic bead of 2.4 μm and 1 μm are shown in Figure 5.19. The traces representing the cumulative averaging on the data are also shown.

In the second experiment, different numbers of magnetic beads for all three bead types are separately applied onto the sensor surface, and their corresponding frequency shifts are recorded respectively. Since the excitation magnetic field amplitude $\|B_{ext}(r)\|$ is generally not a constant across the sensor surface for a 6-turn symmetric sensing inductor layout, the local transducer gain will consequently be spatially nonuniform based on Equation 5.6. Therefore, in this experiment the distribution of the beads are first recorded by a high-magnification camera. Then their measured frequency shifts are normalized by their corresponding spatially averaged transducer gain factors, which are obtained through theoretical calculations based on the transducer gain model in Equation 5.6. Note that the normalized frequency-shift results assume that all the beads' responses are normalized to the center of the sensing inductor. The normalized and raw frequency-shift results versus bead numbers are plotted in Figure 5.20. The total bead count is limited to around 200–400. This is because beyond this number, the beads start to aggregate on the sensor surface, which significantly prevents accurate bead identifications under the microscope. Nevertheless, the linear sensor responses after normalization prove the validity of our spatial sensor transducer gain modeling in Equations 5.5 and 5.6. Moreover, this measurement demonstrates a sensor dynamic range of greater than 81 dB.

A sensor performance comparison among state-of-the-art CMOS–based biosensors is summarized in Table 5.3. Sensor testing results based on actual DNA samples are reported in [18]. The frequency-shift magnetic sensor array example presents the best sensitivity among the reported magnetic biosensors in CMOS and achieves a competitive performance compared to the reported CMOS biosensors.

5.7 DISCUSSION AND CONCLUSION

As an extension to the presented oscillator-based magnetic sensor array, a correlated-double-counting (CDC) frequency-shift sensor scheme is introduced in [33,34] to further decrease the

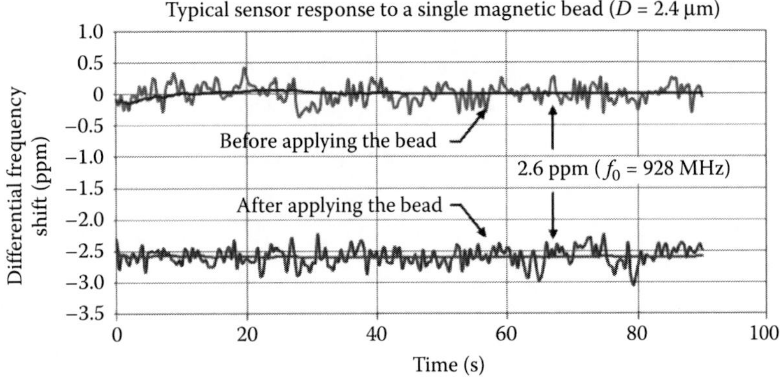

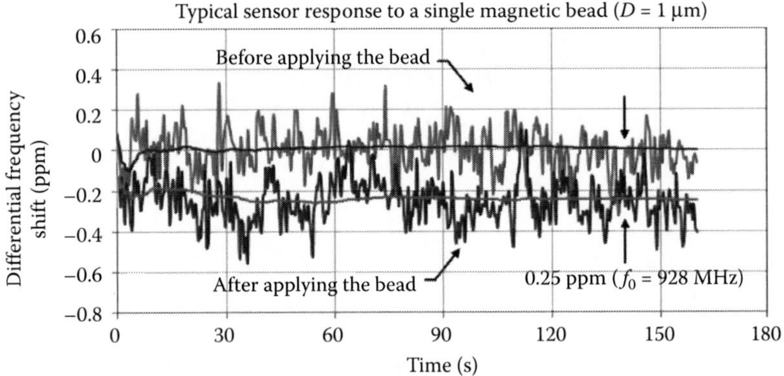

FIGURE 5.19 Typical sensor response of a single Dynabeads® Protein G ($D = 2.4$ μm) and MyOne™ ($D = 1$ μm).

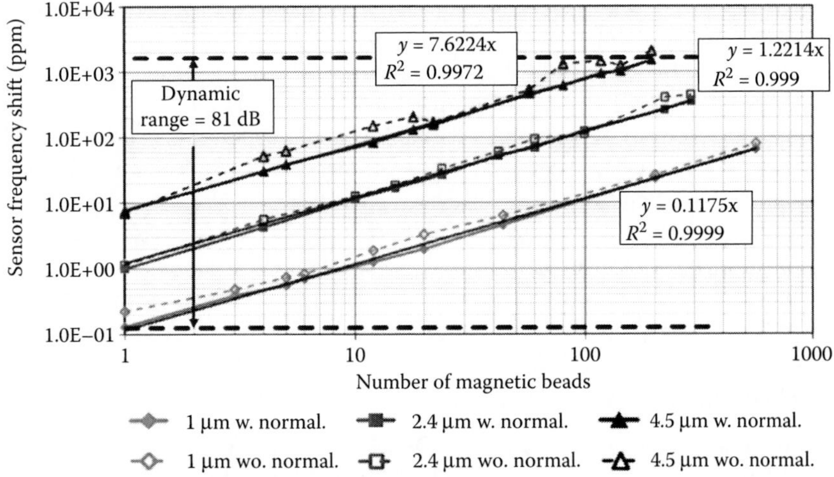

FIGURE 5.20 Measured sensor response w./wo. spatial transducer gain normalization. The counting window T is 0.1 s.

TABLE 5.3
Performance Comparison With Published CMOS Biosensors

Sensor Type	Sensitivity (Magnetic Beads)	Sensitivity (Molecules)	External Magnets	Costly Post-Processing	Optical Device
		Magnetic Sensor			
Frequency-shift-based sensor (this work)	1 ($D = 1$ μm)	1 nM[18]	No	No	No
GMR sensor [8]	1 ($D = 2.8$ μm)		Yes	Yes	No
GMR sensor [10]		10 nM	Yes	Yes	No
Hall effect sensor [12]	1 ($D = 2.8$ μm)		Yes	Yes	No
NMR relaxometer [13]		4 nM	Yes	No	No
		Optical Sensor			
CMOS image sensor [32]		0.125 nM	No	Yes	Yes
		Electrochemical Sensor			
Electrochemical sensor [4]		100 nM	No	No	No
Electrochemical sensor [5]		1 μM	No	No	No
Electrochemical sensor [6]		100 nM	No	Yes	No

minimum sensor noise floor below $2\delta^2$, for the basic differential sensing case shown in (Equation 5.19). Through oscillator active core sharing, this scheme physically establishes $1/f^3$ phase noise correlation between the sensing and the reference oscillators. Similar to the common-mode environmental noise for the oscillator pair, the correlated $1/f^3$ phase noise is then largely suppressed via subsequent differential sensing. This significantly reduces the overall sensor noise for the frequency-shift measurements without requiring either low $1/f^3$ phase noise or power overhead. Moreover, averaging the CDC frequency counting data can be shown to present a much more effective noise suppression effect, that is, a lower NPRR(N), compared to a standard differential scheme shown in 5.19, which further boosts the sensor SNR. In parallel, the issue of transducer gain uniformity is addressed in [35] and [36]. In this study, a two-layered stacked coil is proposed as the sensing inductor, which provides an equalized excitation magnetic field (in magnitude) across the sensor surface. In addition, floating shimming metal pieces are introduced to further enhance the transducer spatial gain uniformity. Therefore, the frequency-shift magnetic sensor achieves a linear sensor response versus the particle numbers without any postnormalization steps.

In summary, a novel frequency-shift-based magnetic biosensing scheme is introduced for future PoC molecular diagnosis applications. Fully compatible with standard CMOS processes, the sensor scheme achieves high sensitivity, hand-held portability, and low power consumption without using any external magnetic biasing fields or expensive postprocessing steps. Theoretical limits on sensor SNR and design optimization techniques have been presented. An 8-cell sensor array implemented in a standard 130 nm CMOS process has been demonstrated as a design example. Both electrical and magnetic sensing measurement results have been presented to verify the sensing scheme's functionality. To the authors' best knowledge, this presented magnetic sensor array example achieves the best sensitivity among the CMOS magnetic sensors reported so far.

ACKNOWLEDGMENTS

The authors would acknowledge Dr. Yan Chen, Dr. David Wu, and Mr Constantine Sideris for their technical supports during the sensor testing. The authors would also like to thank Professor Axel Scherer, Sander Weinreb, Azita Emami, and the members of Caltech high-speed–integrated circuit group (CHIC) for their helpful discussions.

REFERENCES

1. N. K. Tran and G. J. Kost, Worldwide point-of-care testing: Compendiums of POCT for mobile, emergency, critical, and primary care and of infectious diseases tests, *J. Near-Patient Testing and Technology*, 5(2), 84–92, 2006.
2. G. J. Kost, *Principles and Practice of Point-of-Care Testing*, Philadelphia, PA: Lippincott Williams & Wilkins, 2002.
3. D. Stekel, *Microarray Bioinformatics,* Cambridge: Cambridge University Press, 2003.
4. A. Hassibi and T. H. Lee, A programmable 0.18 μm CMOS electrochemical sensor microarray for biomolecular detection, *IEEE Sensors J.* 6(6), 1380–1388, 2006.
5. M. Schienle, C. Paulus, A. Frey, F. Hofmann, B. Holzapfl, P. Schinder-Bauer, and R. Thewes, A fully electronic DNA sensor with 128 positions and in-pixel A/D conversion, *IEEE J. Solid-State Circuits*, 39 (12), 2438–2445, 2006.
6. F. Heer, M. Keller, G. Yu, J. Janata, M. Josowicz, and A. Hierlemann, CMOS electro-chemical DNA-detection array with on-chip ADC, in *IEEE ISSCC Dig. Tech. Papers*, February 2008, pp. 168–169.
7. A. Hassibi, R. Navid, R. W. Dutton, and T. H. Lee, Comprehensive study of noise processes in electrode electrolyte interfaces, *J. Appl. Phy.*, 96(2), 1074–1082, 2004.
8. B. Alberts, D. Bray, K. Hopkin, A. Johnson, J. Lewis, M. Raff, K. Roberts, and P. Walter, *Essential Cell Biology*, 2nd Edn, Garland Science/Taylor & Francis Group, New York, 2003.
9. H. Lee, Y. Liu, D. Ham, and R. M. Westervelt, Integrated cell manipulation system—CMOS/microfluidic hybrid, *Lab Chip*, 7(3), 331–337, 2007.
10. G. Li, V. Joshi, R. L. White, S. X. Wang, J. T. Kemp, C. Webb, R. W. Davis, and S. Sun, Detection of single micron-sized magnetic bead and magnetic nanoparticles using spin valve sensors for biological applications, *J. Appl. Phys.,* 93(10), 7557–7559, 2003.
11. G. Li, S. Sun, R. Wilson, R. White, N. Pourmand, and S. X. Wang, Spin valve sensors for ultrasensitive detection of superparamagnetic nanoparticles for biological applications, *IEEE J. Sensors and Actuators A,* 126, 98–106, 2006.
12. S. Han, H. Yu, B. Murmann, N. Pourmand, and S. X. Wang, A high-density magnetoresistive biosensor array with drift-compensation mechanism, in *IEEE ISSCC Dig. Tech. Papers*, February 2007, pp.168–169.
13. T. Aytur, P. R. Beatty, and B. Boser, An immunoassay platform based on CMOS Hall sensors, *Solid-State Sensor, Actuator and Microsystems Workshop,* Hilton Head Island, SC, June 2002, pp. 126–129.
14. P. Besse, G. Boero, M. Demierre, V. Pott, and R. Popovic, Detection of a single magnetic microbead using a miniaturized silicon Hall sensor, *Appl. Phys. Lett.*, 80(22), 4199–4201, 2002.
15. Y. Liu, N. Sun, H. Lee, R. Weissleder, and D. Ham, CMOS mini nuclear magnetic resonance system and its application for biomolecular sensing, *IEEE ISSCC Dig. Tech. Pap*, February 2008, pp. 140–141.
16. H. Wang, A. Hajimiri, and Y. Chen, Effective-inductance-change based magnetic particle sensing, U.S. Patent (No. 20090267596 A1), March 7, 2008.
17. H. Wang and A. Hajimiri, Ultrasensitive magnetic particle sensor system, U.S. Provisional Patent CIT-5224-P, September 15, 2008.
18. H. Wang, Y. Chen, A. Hassibi, A. Scherer, and A. Hajimiri, A frequency-shift CMOS magnetic biosensor array with single-bead sensitivity and no external magnet, *IEEE ISSCC Dig. Tech. Papers*, February 2009, pp. 438–439.
19. D. Ham and A. Hajimiri, Virtual Damping and Einstein Relation in Oscillators, *IEEE J. Solid-State Circuits*, 38(3), 407–418, 2003.
20. K. H. J. Buschow and F. R. de Boer, *Physics of Magnetism and Magnetic Materials*, Springer, New York, 2003.
21. D. E. Bray and R. K. Stanley, *Nondistructive Evaluation*, Taylor & Francis Group, London, UK, 1997.
22. A. Hajimiri and T. H. Lee, *The Design of Low Noise Oscillators*, Springer, Norwell, Massachusetts, 1999.
23. D. A. Howe, D. W. Allan, and J. A. Barnes, Properties of signal sources and measurement methods, *Proc. 35th Annual Symp. Frequency Control*, Philadelphia, Pennsylvania, 1981.
24. P. Talbot, A. M. Konn, and C. Brosseau, Electromagnetic characterization of fine-scale particulate composite materials, *J. Magn Magn Mater.*, 249, 2002, pp. 481–485.
25. C. Brosseau, J. B. Youssef, P. Talbot, and A. M. Konn, Electromagnetic and magnetic properties of multicomponent metal oxides heterostructures: Nanometer versus micrometer-sized particles, *J. Appl. Phys.*, 93(11), 9243–9256, 2003.
26. A. Hajimiri and T. H. Lee, Design issues in CMOS differential LC oscillators, *IEEE J. Solid-State Circuits*, 34(5), 717–724, 1999.

27. C. Liu and J. A. McNeil, Jitter in Oscillators with 1/f noise sources, *IEEE ISCAS Dig. Tech. Papers,* May 2004, pp. 773–776.
28. http://www.ansoft.com
29. A. Babakhani, X. Guan, A. Komijani, A. Natarajan, and A. Hajimjri, A 77-GHz phased-array transceiver with on-chip antennas in silicon: Receiver and antennas, *IEEE J. Solid-State Circuits*, 41(12), 2795–2806, 2006.
30. H. Wang and A. Hajimiri, Low cost bounding technique for integrated circuit chips and PDMS devices, U.S. Provisional Patent CIT-5320-P, February 25, 2009.
31. http://www.invitrogen.com.
32. B. Jang, P. Cao, A. Chevalier, A. Ellington, and A. Hassibi, A CMOS fluorescent-based biosensor microarray, *IEEE ISSCC Dig. Tech. Papers*, February 2009, pp. 436–437.
33. H. Wang, A. Hajimiri, and S. Kosai, Noise suppression techniques in high-precision long-term frequency/timing measurements, U.S. Provisional Patent CIT-5318-P, February 20, 2009.
34. H. Wang, S. Kosai, C. Sideris, and A. Hajimiri, An ultrasensitive CMOS magnetic biosensor array with correlated double counting (CDC) noise suppression, *IEEE MTT-S Int. Microwave Symp. (IMS)*, Anaheim, California, May 2010.
35. H. Wang and A. Hajimiri, Effective-Inductance-Change Magnetic Sensor with Spatially Uniform Transducer Gain, *U.S. Provisional patent CIT-5108-P*, March 7, 2008.
36. H. Wang, C. Sideris, and A. Hajimiri, A frequency-shift based CMOS magnetic biosensor with spatially uniform sensor transducer gain, *IEEE CICC Dig. Tech. Papers*, September 2010.

6 System Architecture for Neural–Electrical Interface and Processing

Jean-François Bêche, Timothée Levi, Guillaume Charvet, Olivier Billoint, Lionel Rousseau, Jean-Pierre Rostaing, Cyril Condemine, Stéphane Bonnet, Ricardo Escolá, T. Kauffmann, Blaise Yvert, and Régis Guillemaud

CONTENTS

6.1 INTRODUCTION

Advances in multielectrode array (MEA) fabrication technology have led to the development of new system architectures for both *in vitro* and *in vivo* neurological applications. High-density MEA and application-specific integrated circuits (ASIC) can now be associated in compact implantable devices to provide a means of recording brain activity and stimulating neurons' networks for applications ranging from basic neurosciences studies, to the study and treatment of chronic diseases, and to the brain–computer interface. The ultimate goal is to provide fully autonomous and implantable wireless devices that will be able to interface with the brain for either recording or stimulation or both. The development of these devices requires the integration of many functions, either on the same substrate or on different ones. System-level design becomes crucial for optimization of performance, modules' assembly, and power consumption. While *in-vivo* stimulation devices are already available, one of the current challenges is to provide high-resolution recording capabilities on a large number of channels for cortical implants. Because of the large number of recording electrodes provided by MEA probes, systems' architectures must now include some level of low-power embedded digital signal processing to reduce the large number of data to match the wireless data transmission bandwidth [1,2].

An ASIC, which is presented in the first part, has been specifically developed for *in vitro* neuroscience applications and has been integrated into a dedicated hardware instrument, the BioMEA instrument [3,4], presented in the second part. The analog characteristics of this system allow the recording of both local field potential (LFP) and action potential (AP or spike) signals simultaneously. Bipolar current stimulation can also be performed by the system [5].

6.2 FIRST-GENERATION ASIC DEVELOPMENT: AGNES

Asic for General Neurons Electrical Study (AGNES) is a 64-channel CMOS ASIC for MEA-based *in-vitro* applications and is capable of performing either waveform recording or current stimulation or both simultaneously [6]. The MEA probes are connected to the ASIC's bidirectional ports. The recording channels are each made of a low-noise gain-selectable amplifier followed by a sample-and-hold circuit operated simultaneously on every channel. Readout of this analog sampling memory is then performed through a 64-multiplexer coupled to an output buffer. For stimulation operations, externally digital stored patterns can be routed through a channel-level multiplexer to a voltage-to-current converter to deliver the current stimulation signal to the corresponding MEA probe (Figure 6.1). Due to its adjustable gain and its wide bandwidth, AGNES can record electrochemical potentials, LFPs, and AP signals or spikes.

The analog output signal of the amplification channel is buffered and is digitized by an off-chip analog-to-digital converter. Sampling rates up to 50 kSps (kilo samples per second) per channel can be achieved.

6.2.1 Low-Noise Amplification and Selectable Gain

The AGNES ASIC offers the possibility of independently setting the gain of each channel. The low-noise continuous-time amplifier has two stages with maximal gains of 75 (preamplifier) and 10 (amplifier). The gain of each channel can be set to 1 by closing the feedback switch (Figures 6.2 and 6.3), thus offering four gain settings: 1, 10, 75, and 750. The input-referred voltage noise over the full bandwidth of the AGNES ASIC has been measured to be 4.3 μV_{RMS}.

Both the preamplifier and the amplifier are built around the same operational transconductance amplifier (OTA) architecture with positive metal oxide semiconductor (PMOS) inputs and with independent biasing circuits (Figure 6.4).

The power consumption of each stage is 125 μW. Diode clamps have been purposely placed between the differential inputs of each amplifier to prevent saturation.

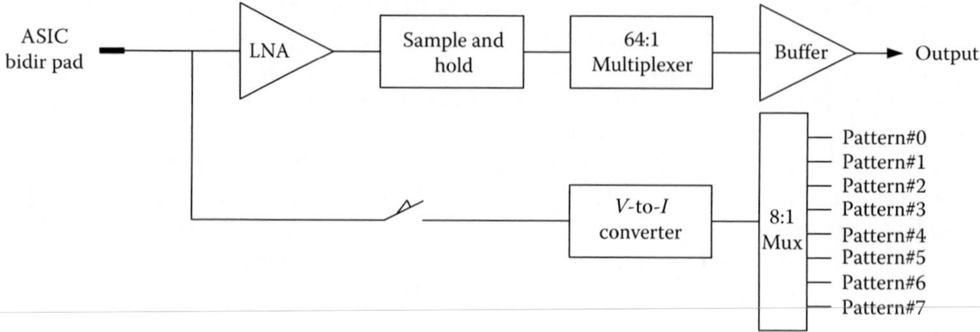

FIGURE 6.1 AGNES amplification and stimulation architecture.

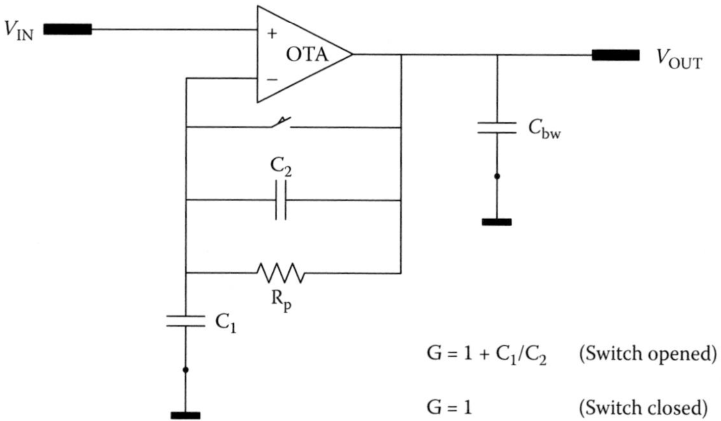

FIGURE 6.2 Single stage amplifier (preamplifier or amplifier).

6.2.2 Bandwidth

The bandwidth of the amplifier is 0.08 Hz–3 kHz. The low-frequency cutoff was purposely set low to allow the recording of electrochemical potentials. The large time constant associated with this cutoff is obtained using diode-connected PMOS transistors using the technique described in [7]. On the preamplifier stage, two transistors are used; this number is increased to five in order to reduce large signal distortion on the amplifier stage.

The high-frequency cutoff is given by the roll-off associated with the gain of the OTA and the value of the bandwidth-setting capacitor (C_{bw}). The frequency response of the low-noise amplifier is illustrated in Figure 6.5.

6.2.3 Sample and Hold, Multiplexer, and Readout Amplifier

The channels' amplified signals are simultaneously sampled onto capacitors (C_H) in a snapshot-like mode (Figure 6.6). The sampled signals are then read out through a multiplexer and an output buffer

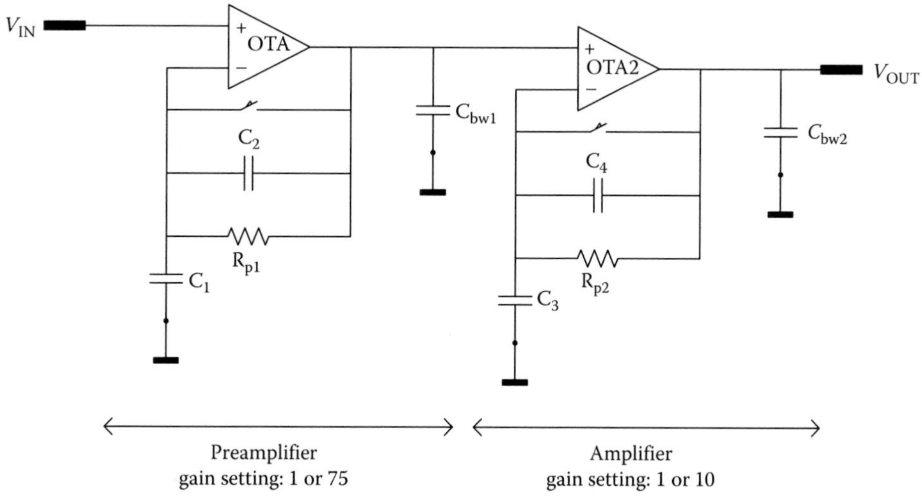

FIGURE 6.3 The low-noise amplifier's architecture.

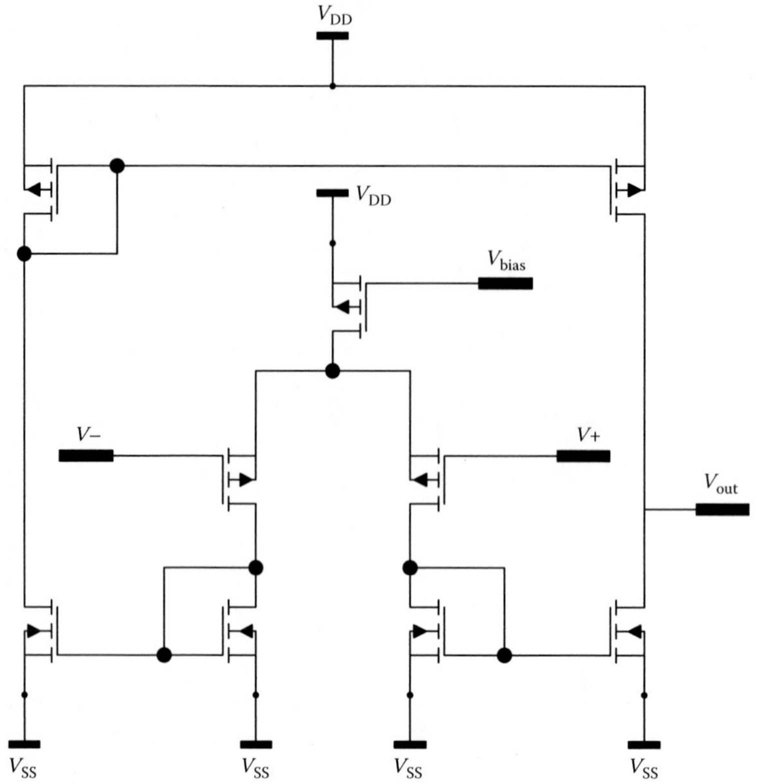

FIGURE 6.4 OTA architecture.

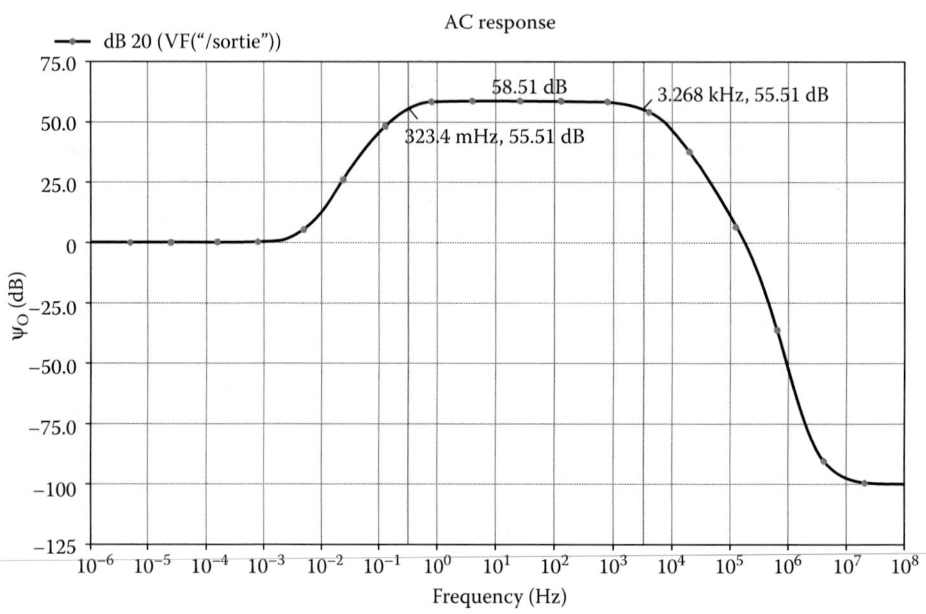

FIGURE 6.5 Simulated AC response of the low-noise amplifier (gain setting = 750).

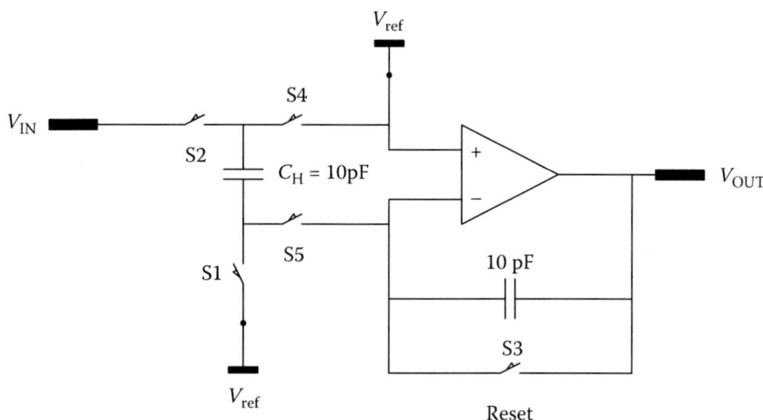

FIGURE 6.6 Sample-and-hold circuit and readout amplifier.

for off-chip digitization. These elements have sufficient bandwidth characteristics to allow sampling rates up to 65 kSps on each channel. An on-chip digital controller delivers all the control timing signals for both the sampling and the multiplexed readout operations.

The sample-and-hold and readout sequence is the following. All switches are considered open to start with. The C_H capacitor is first connected to the reference voltage (S1 closed). Second, the input voltage is applied to C_H (S1 and S2 closed). Both switches are then opened, leaving C_H floating. During the readout, the reset switch (S3) is activated and released and then both transfer switches (S4 and S5) are closed for the charge transfer onto the amplifier's feedback capacitor. The reference voltage sets the DC value at the output of the amplifier, typically the midpoint between V_{DD} and V_{SS}.

The complete multiplexer's architecture is depicted in Figure 6.7. The readout timing sequence is depicted in Figure 6.8 and is implemented by an on-chip controller using a bit shift register to successively address each sample-and-hold cell.

The readout amplifier is a rail-to-rail amplifier, with a topology described in Figure 6.9. The amplifier has an output dynamic range of (0.5 V, 4.5 V) for a total power consumption of 3 mW. The maximum readout rate achievable is 65 kSps per channel with a capacitive load of 20 pF.

6.2.4 Stimulation Circuit Architecture

Electrical stimulation delivered in the form of a current can trigger or alter neural activity. The current stimulation must be charge-balanced in order not to modify the DC value of the neural tissues. The architecture we implemented is built around an input 8-to-1 multiplexer and a voltage-to-current converter. Eight digital stimulation patterns stored off-chip are individually selectable for each channel to allow the user to apply any of the eight possible patterns. The voltage-to-current converter can deliver up to ±400 μA (Figure 6.10). The bandwidth of the converter is sufficient to handle a sampling rate of 1 MSps. Switches have been inserted in series with the converter output to prevent any DC residual from leaking into the probes. Those are closed only during the stimulation phase. The stimulation function can be entirely disabled by powering down the associated section of the circuit.

6.2.5 Power Supplies and Physical Size

Each section of the circuit is powered through individual power blocks (one for the preamplifiers, one for the amplifier, etc.). To get rid of the random, slowly varying DC offset potential that exists at the electrode–electrolyte interface, the ASIC can be supplied with floating V_{SS}, V_{DD} ($V_{DD} - V_{SS} = 5$ V). The circuit size is 2.4×11.2 mm^2 (0.35 μm CMOS process) and its power consumption is about 125 mW (Figure 6.11).

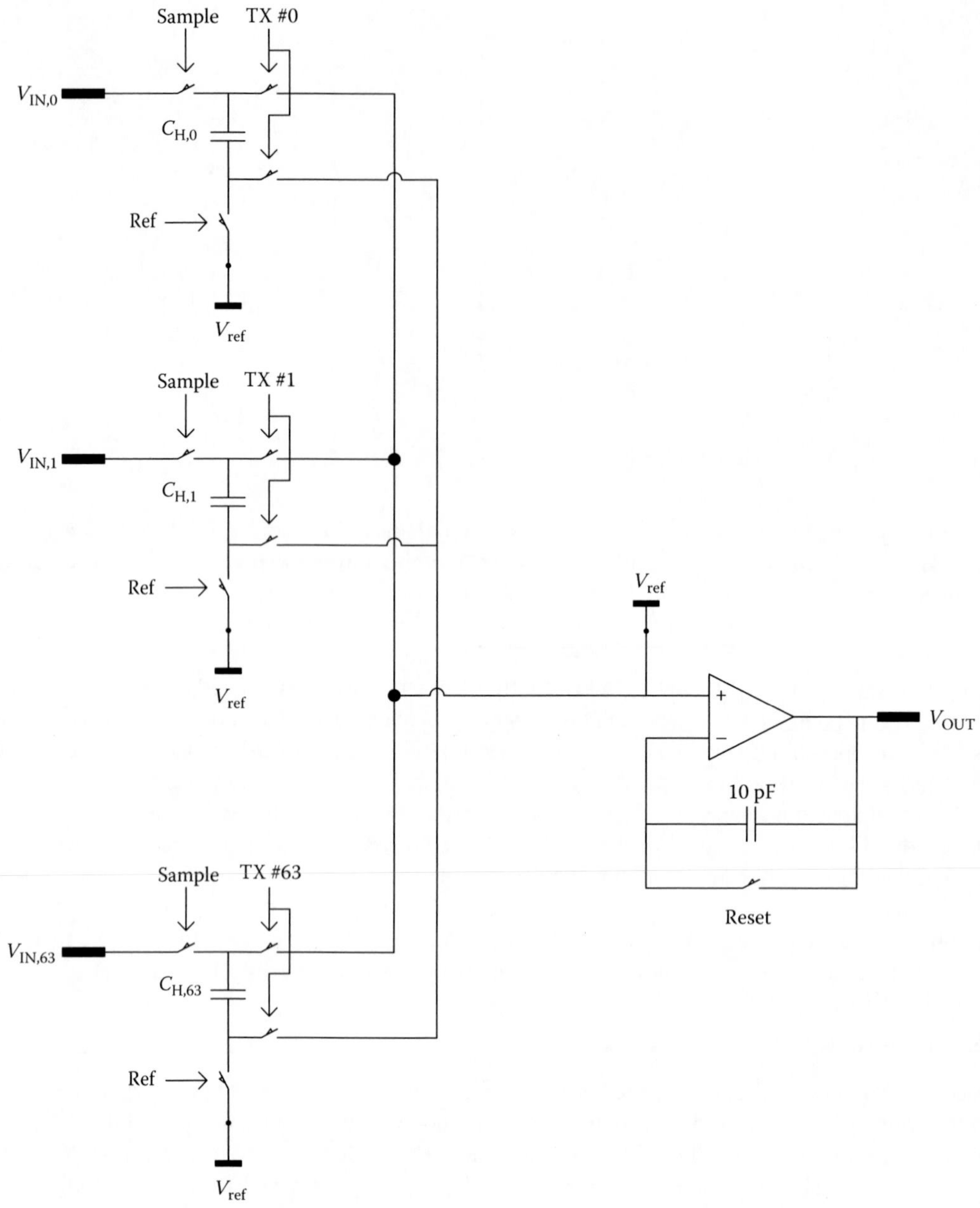

FIGURE 6.7 Sample-and-hold circuit, multiplexer and readout amplifier (64 channels).

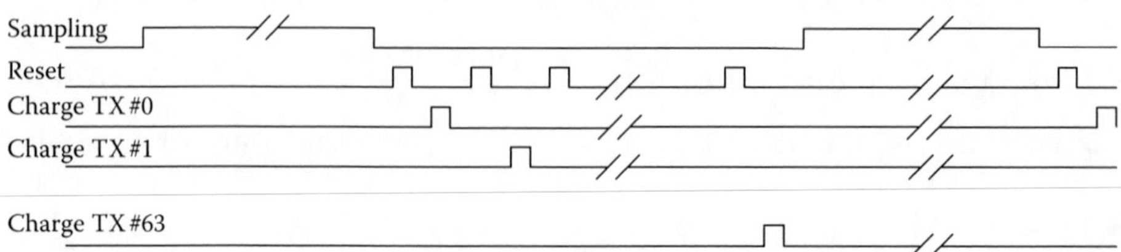

FIGURE 6.8 Sample-and-hold and readout timing diagram.

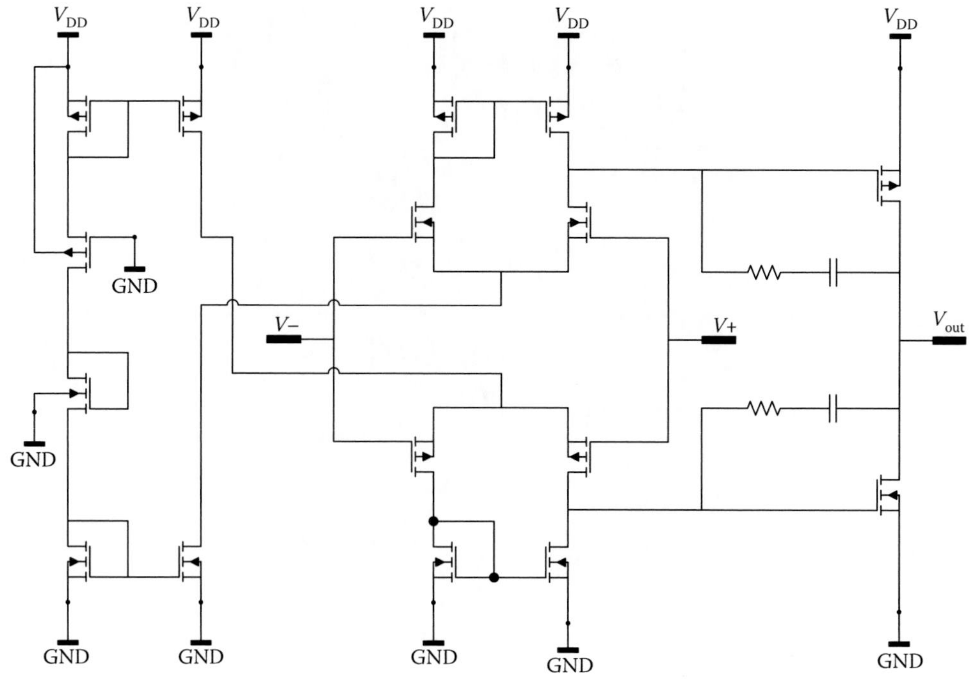

FIGURE 6.9 Rail-to-rail readout amplifier topology.

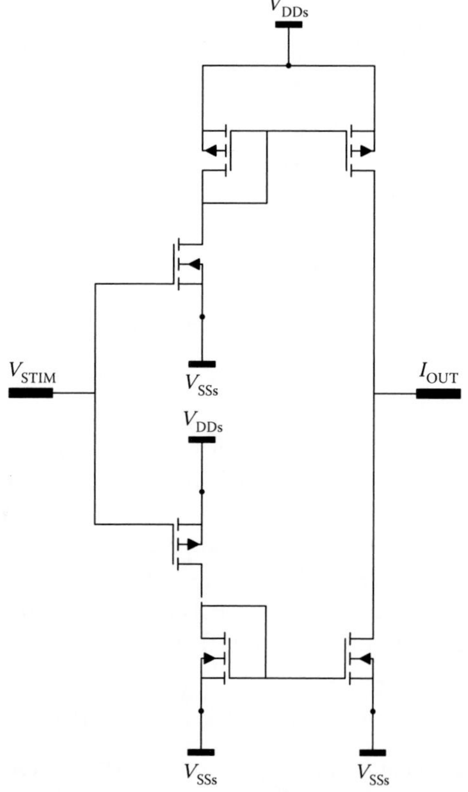

FIGURE 6.10 Voltage-to-current converter.

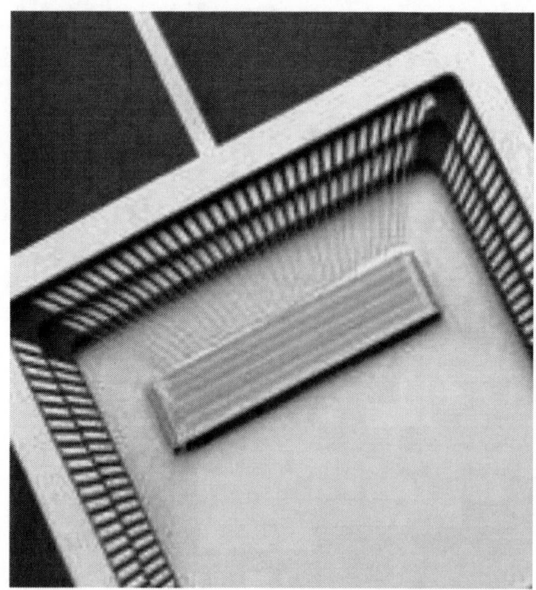

FIGURE 6.11 AGNES die.

6.2.6 AGNES Characteristics Summary

Parameter	**Result**
Power consumption	125 mW
Input-referred noise	4.3 μV rms
Signal bandwidth	0.08 Hz–3 kHz
Maximum sampling frequency	50 kHz
Maximum multiplexing frequency	3.2 MHz
Input impedance	>1012 Ω
Variable gain	1, 10, 75, 750
Maximum stimulation current	±400 μA
Area (in 0.35 μm CMOS)	27 mm^2

6.3 THE BioMEA SYSTEM

The AGNES ASIC has been integrated in a complete data acquisition system for *in vitro* applications, called the BioMEA system [8]. The modular architecture of the system allows using up to four AGNES ASICs offering 256 channels for simultaneous waveform recording and up to 32 stimulation patterns (eight per ASIC). Four subsystems operate under the supervision of a controller implemented in a Field Programmable Gate Array.

The BioMEA system has been successfully interfaced with several types of MEA from different manufacturers such as ESIEE, Ayanda, or Neuronexus.

6.3.1 Digitizing, Recording, and Storing Signal Waveforms

Each AGNES ASIC provides an analog 64-multiplexed signal controlled by the on-chip sequencer, itself synchronized with the FPGA-embedded data acquisition controller (Figure 6.12). The multiplexed signal is fed into an ADC driver for offset and gain adjustments prior to digitization. The data from the

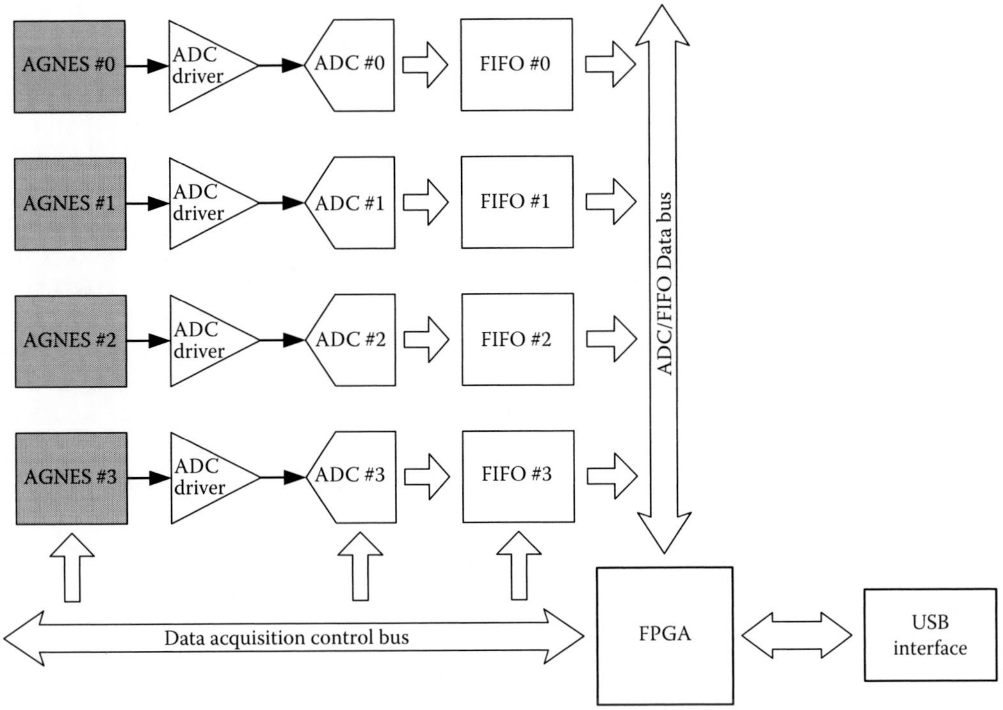

FIGURE 6.12 BioMEA, waveform digitizing and storage architecture.

14-bit 10 MSps pipeline ADC (AD9240 from Analog Devices [9]) is then stored in a first in first out (FIFO) memory, used as a buffer for the USB data transfer to the data acquisition computer.

6.3.2 Stimulation Patterns Storage and Delivery

The AGNES ASIC has eight dedicated stimulation pattern inputs and each channel has an internal 8-to-1 multiplexer to select the appropriate pattern. The patterns are externally loaded from the software interface through the USB port into onboard 64 k × 16 static random access memory (SRAM) memories. Those patterns are then transformed into analog waveforms using eight 14-bit digital-to-analog converters (Figure 6.13) (AD9764 from Analog Devices [9]). Although the throughput rate of this converter can exceed 100 MSps, the bandwidth of the on-chip voltage-to-current converter does not allow rates higher than 1 MSps.

6.3.3 Control Electronics, USB Interface, and Data Acquisition

An Altera EP1C20 Cyclone FPGA [10] is at the core of the digital backend, controlling both the data acquisition and the stimulation, and interfacing with the computer through the USB interface. We developed a specific and dedicated software application that allows configuring the entire system and retrieving the data for real-time display on the computer. The retrieved data are tagged, channel-sorted, and stored in the computer after demultiplexing and processing. The USB interface is built around the Cypress CY7C68013AFX2LP microcontroller and data transfers can be performed in high-speed mode at 480 Mbit/s.

6.4 EXPERIMENTAL RESULTS OF THE BioMEA SYSTEM

The BioMEA system has been used for *in vitro* [5] and *in vivo* [11] experiments, both in recording and in stimulation modes.

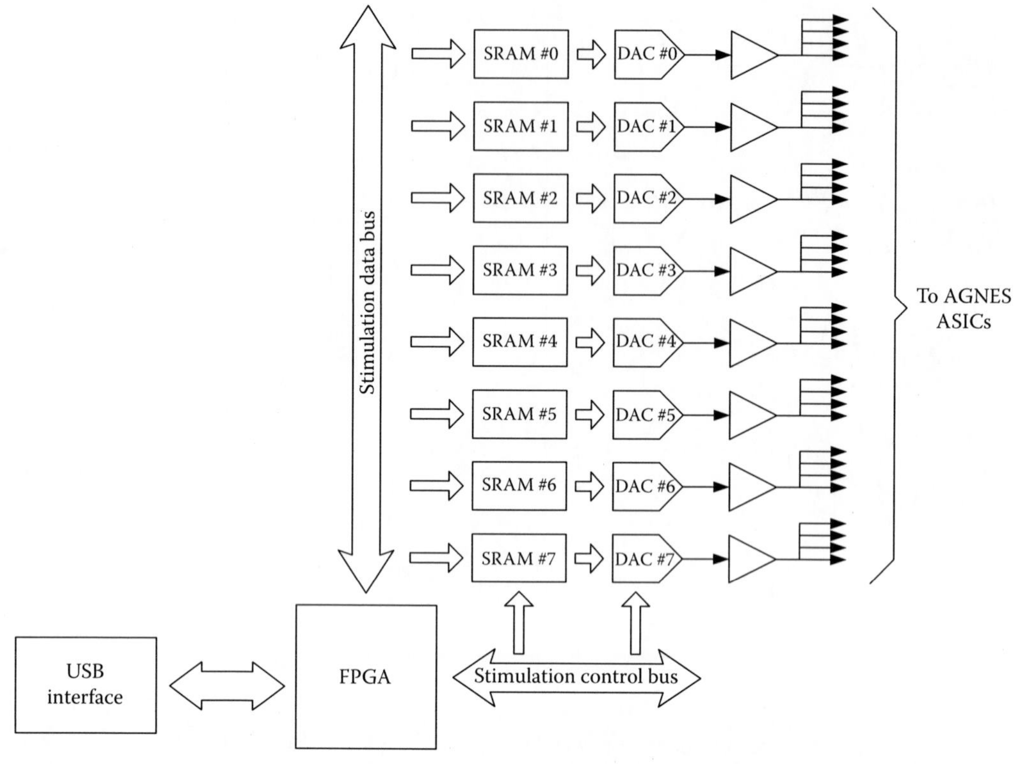

FIGURE 6.13 BioMEA, stimulation patterns storage and digital-to-analog conversion.

An example of *in vitro* experiments is given in Figures 6.14 and 6.15. A complete embryonic mouse hindbrain and spinal cord preparation was positioned on an 8 × 32 electrode array developed by ESIEE-Paris [5] fitting the size of the preparation (electrode spacing 250 × 450 μm^2). Such immature neural networks exhibit rhythmic activity propagating through the structure.

A propagating wave of activity is shown on 18 channels, with both LFPs in the hindbrain and bursts of spikes in the thoraco-lumbar region of the spinal cord (Figure 6.15, panel A2). A close-up view of a recorded burst is shown in A3. Isolated spikes of rather small amplitudes (20–40 μV) could also be clearly detected out of the background noise (A4). An example of propagating wave triggered by electrical stimulation on another preparation (stage E14.5) is shown in B. A cathodic-first biphasic pulse of 100 μA and 500 μs/phase was delivered through an electrode in the medulla (filled dot in B1). The response to the stimulation is shown here for three other electrodes (open circles in panel B1) and also for the stimulation electrode, which can be switched back to recording mode rapidly after stimulation. Here, data were high-pass filtered to reduce the stimulus-induced saturation artefact. Activity recorded by electrode 1 shows spontaneous bursts (spont) and bursts elicited by electrical stimuli (stim, B2). Every stimulus in the medulla triggers a wave of activity propagating rostro-caudally along the spinal cord (B3).

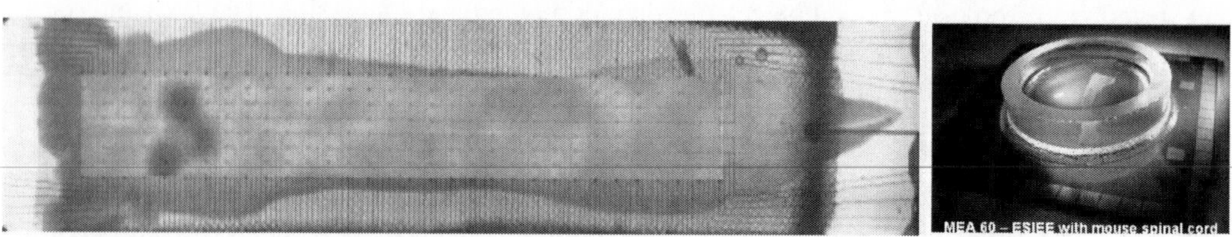

FIGURE 6.14 Mouse spinal cord on ESIEE 256-probe MEA.

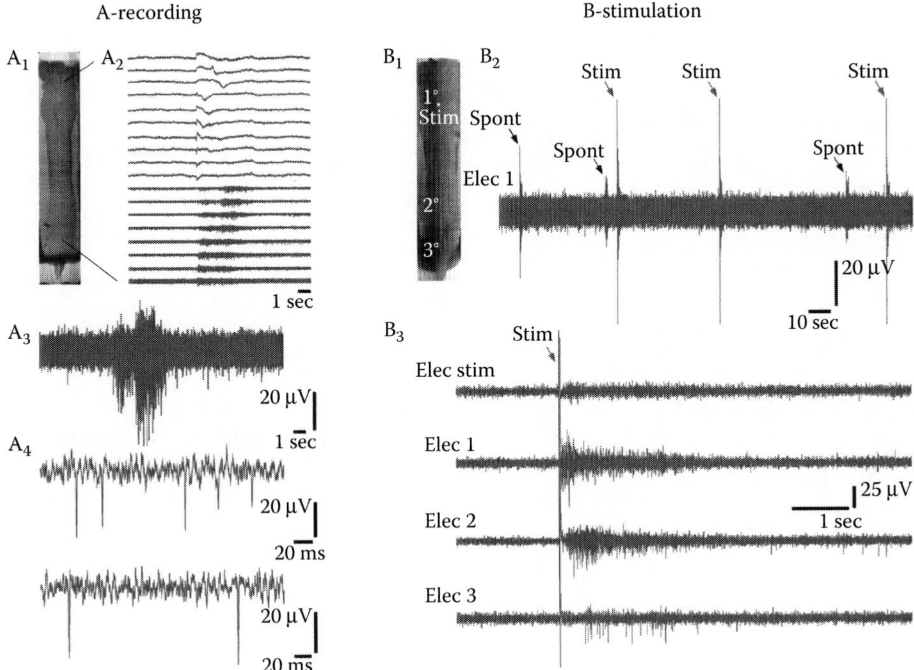

FIGURE 6.15 Mouse spinal cord recordings and stimulation using the BioMEA system (From B. Yvert, CNRS, University of Bordeaux. With permission.)

6.4.1 Conclusions and Perspectives

This chapter presented the architecture and performances of the AGNES ASIC integrated into the BioMEA system. Experimental validations have provided results beyond the proof-of-principle barrier.

High-performance ASICs targeting brain implants are currently under development at LETI. Such developments require a multidisciplinary approach dealing with the different aspects of the system architecture. Although the analog processing performances are generally determined by the power budget, as it is commonly expressed with the NEF figure of merit, power management is becoming the main issue for implants. Novel low-power analog and digital architectures need to be put in place to optimize both the performances and the power budget associated with those functions. Low-power analog-to-digital converters must be developed and integrated into the design to enable embedded digital signal processing to optimize the data content transmitted through the RF transceivers. The wireless capability of the implantable devices is a core issue because of the dual functionality it must provide. On the one hand, data must be transferred between the implant to the base station for configuration, data collection, and system monitoring. On the other, the implant must be capable of harvesting its powering energy from the wireless signal. Low-power communication solutions are required to provide a short-range wireless link between the implanted devices and the external terminal providing control, monitoring and human interface, using the Medical Implant Communication Services standard (MICS) [12,13]. Remote inductive power techniques are already used to recharge implanted batteries and could potentially be used for brain implants as long as the battery is implanted in a readily accessible location. Real-time signal processing is also essential to the development of implants with a large number of channels because of the low power budget and the narrow data bandwidth of the transmission channel. Low-power, low-complexity and yet high-performance real-time algorithms must then be developed [14–21] to effectively process the large number of incoming data without losing any relevant information. An example of real-time spike detection and sorting, that is, determining which neuron has produced this spike classification of signals, is shown in Figure 6.16.

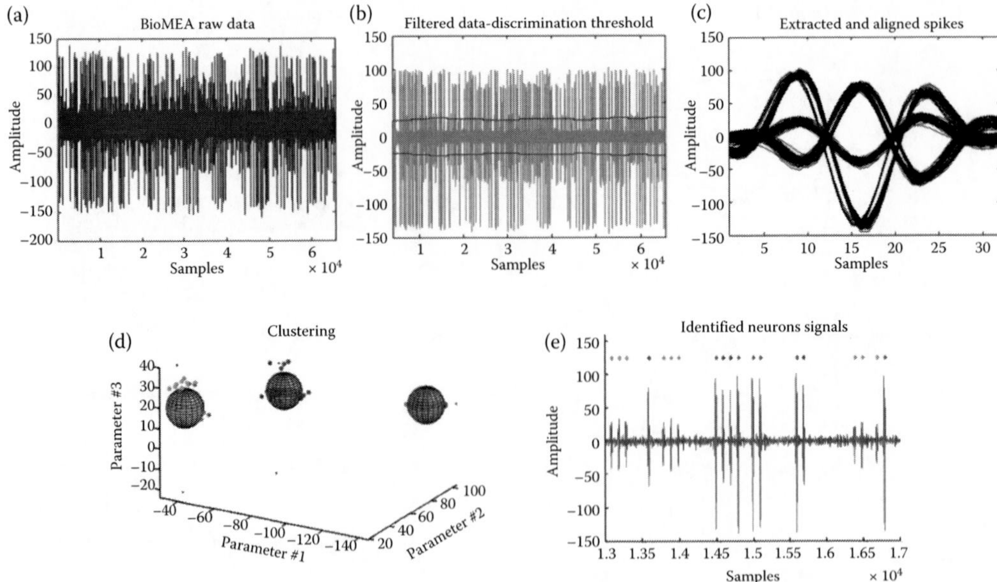

FIGURE 6.16 Real-time detection and association of signals with neurons or clusters; (a) raw data, (b) real-time threshold computation and detection, (c) spike extraction, (d) clustering, and (e) postanalysis identification associating spikes with their clusters or neurons of origin.

Finally, system integration and assembly issues might play an important role in the optimization of the engineering solutions for implants, requiring complex multichip module architectures. Today's systems in package are limited by the classic wire bonding techniques (Figure 6.17) in terms of cost, size, and performance. Neural interface including analog recording, symmetrical stimulation, digital signal processing, RF, and power management will require a three-dimensional (3D) assembly in order to reduce packaging costs and dimensions [22,23].

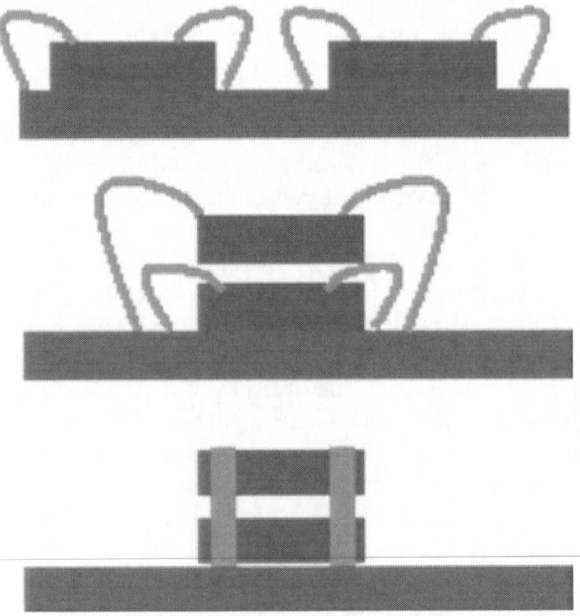

FIGURE 6.17 3D integration principle.

REFERENCES

1. R. R. Harrison et al., A low-power integrated circuit for a wireless 100-electrode neural recording system, *IEEE Journal of Solid-State Circuits,* 42(1), 123–133, 2007.
2. Y. Perelman and R. Ginosar, An integrated system for multichannel neuronal recording with spike/LFP separation, integrated A/D conversion and threshold detection, *IEEE Transactions on Biomedical Engineering*, 54(1), 130–137, 2007.
3. http://www.leti.fr
4. Biologic SAS, http://www.biologic.info.
5. G. Charvet et al., B BioMEA: A versatile high-density 3D microelectrode array system using integrated electronics, *Biosens Bioelectron*, January 13, 2010.
6. O. Billoint et al., A 64-channel ASIC for *in-vitro* simultaneous recording and stimulation of neurons using microelectrode arrays, *29th International Conference of the IEEE Engineering in Medicine and Biology Society*, Lyon, France, 2007.
7. R. R. Harrison and K. D. Wise, A low-power low-noise CMOS amplifier for neural recording applications, *Journal of Solid-State Circuits*, **38**, 958–965, 2003.
8. G. Charvet et al., BioMEA: A 256-channel MEA system with integrated electronics, *29th International Conference of the IEEE Engineering in Medicine and Biology Society*, Lyon, France, 2007.
9. http://www.analog.com/
10. http://www.altera.com/
11. S. Saillet et al., Closed-loop control of seizures in a rat model of absence epilepsy using the BioMEATM system, *Proceedings of the fourth International IEEE EBMS Conference on Neural Engineering*, Antalya, Turkey, April 29–May 2, 2009.
12. FCC Rules and Regulations, *MICS Band Plan*, Table of Frequency Allocations, Part 95, January 2003.
13. H. S. Savci et al., MICS transceivers: Regulatory standards and applications (medical implant communications service), *IEEE Southeast Conference*, Ft. Lauderdale, Florida, April 2005.
14. J. F. Bêche and T. Levi et al., Real-time embedded signal processing for MEA-based neurobiological recording systems, *Proceedings of the MEA Meeting 2008*, Reutlingen, Germany July 8–11, 2008.
15. R. Escolá et al., Wavelet-based scale-dependent detection of neurological action potentials, *Proceedings of the 29th Annual International Conference of the IEEE EMBS*, Lyon, France, August 23–26, 2007.
16. M. S. Lewicki, A review of methods for spike sorting: The detection and classification of neural action potentials, *Computation in Neural Systems*, 4, R53–R78, 1998.
17. I. Obeid and P. Wolf, Evaluation of spike-detection algorithms for a brain–machine interface application, *IEEE Transactions on Biomedical Engineering*, 51, 905–911, 2004.
18. Z. Nenadic and J. W. Burdick, Spike detection using the continuous wavelet transform, *IEEE Transactions Biomedical Engineering*, 52(1), 74–87, 2005.
19. A. Zviagintsev, Y. Perelman and R. Ginosar, Algorithms and architectures for low power spike detection and alignment, *Journal of Neural Engineering*, 3, 35–42, 2006.
20. C.-C. Peng et al., Neural cache: A low-power online digital spike-sorting architecture, *Proceedings of the 30th Annual International IEEE EMBS Conference*, Vancouver, British Columbia, Canada, August 20–24, 2008.
21. J. F. Bêche et al., Real-time adaptive discrimination threshold estimation for embedded neural signals detection, *Proceedings of the fourth International IEEE EBMS Conference on Neural Engineering*, Antalya, Turkey, April 29–May 2, 2009.
22. K. Lee, Samsung semiconductor, *Conference on 3D Architectures for Semiconductor Integration and Packaging*, San Francisco, October 2006.
23. N. Magen et al., Interconnect-power dissipation in a microprocessor, *Proceedings of the 2004 International Workshop on System Level Interconnect Prediction*, Paris, France, pp. 7–13, 2004.
24. B. Yvert, CNRS, University of Bordeaux.

7 Technological Evolution of Wireless Neurochemical Sensing with Fast-Scan Cyclic Voltammetry

Dan P. Covey, Kevin E. Bennet, Charles D. Blaha, Pedram Mohseni, Kendall H. Lee, and Paul A. Garris

CONTENTS

7.1 INTRODUCTION

The brain has been called one of the last frontiers in all of biology. As such, a better understanding of how this complex organ functions will monumentally advance the life sciences as well as greatly impact medicine by improving the diagnosis and treatment of neuropathologies. Measuring the electrical and chemical activities of neurons, a cell type highly specialized for rapid, long-distance communication and information integration [1], has proven to be a complementary and effective strategy for investigating brain function, especially in the context of behavior. New technologies and refinement of existing ones are expected to play an important role in sustaining the success of this approach in the future.

While several methods have been developed for monitoring neural activity, this chapter focuses on electrochemistry for the *in situ* monitoring of neurotransmitters, the chemicals that bridge the extracellular cleft at the synapse between two neurons for signaling. Emphasis will be placed here on fast-scan cyclic voltammetry (FSCV), which like other modern electrochemical techniques, such as amperometry and high-speed chronoamperometry, supports real-time measurements of electroactive neurotransmitters [2]. However, FSCV affords superior chemical resolution by providing a unique signature of the detected species in the form of a voltammogram. Thus, the defining analytical characteristic of FSCV is the ability to interrogate the activity of a single neuron type by virtue of identifying the released neurotransmitter. Indeed, FSCV has recently achieved the key measurement milestone of selectively monitoring the neurotransmitter dopamine with subsecond temporal resolution (100 ms) at a brain-implanted, micron-sized probe during goal-directed behavior [3].

Technological innovation has driven the continued evolution of FSCV, and replacing the historical hardwired link between the chemical measurement and recording equipment with wireless communication is a logical, but critical, next step [4]. We describe here two new directions toward implementing this important engineering goal. The first direction developed small, battery-powered, board-level systems incorporating Bluetooth® telemetry. One device, called the wireless instantaneous neurotransmitter concentration system (WINCS), was designed specifically to be applied during human neurosurgical procedures such as deep brain stimulation (DBS) [5]. The second direction developed integrated circuits using very-large-scale integration (VLSI) techniques in standard complementary-metal-oxide-semiconductor (CMOS) technology. The long-term goal is to reduce size and power requirements sufficiently to support implantable devices for investigating brain–behavior relationships in untethered laboratory animals and, ultimately, "smart" neuroprostheses for clinical uses.

7.2 MONITORING NEURAL ACTIVITY

Neurons communicate via bioelectric and chemical signals [1]. As illustrated in Figure 7.1, communication along the length of one neuron's axon is achieved by conduction of the axon potential, a relatively large bioelectric signal originating from a transient (millisecond) change in membrane potential mediated by the flux of ions, typically Na^+ and K^+, through protein channels. The influx of Ca^{2+} at the axon terminal elicits the release of neurotransmitters from their vesicular package into the extracellular gap between two neurons separated by the synaptic cleft. These chemical messengers are released from the presynaptic neuron in response to the action potential, diffuse across the cleft, and bind to specific protein receptors on the postsynaptic neuron, where the chemical signal is transduced back into a bioelectric signal. Released neurotransmitters are typically taken up again into the presynaptic neuron to terminate synaptic signaling. Fast conduction velocities of the action potential (upwards of several meters per second) and the minimal delay for the neurotransmitter to diffuse across the short, ~25-nm distance of the cleft (milliseconds or less) ensure rapid, long-distance neuronal communication.

Monitoring bioelectric and chemical signals provides a quantitative and reliable index of neural activity for assessing brain function. Perhaps the most widespread measurement modality for this purpose is electrophysiology, which monitors bioelectric signals. Several configurations are commonly used, including patch clamp [6], intracellular recording with a sharp microelectrode [7], and

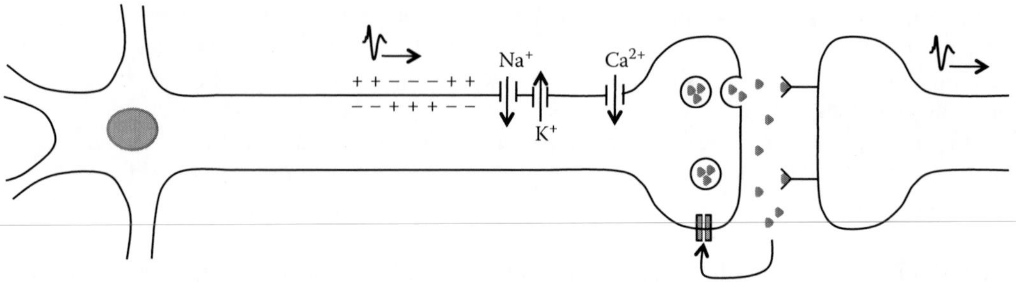

FIGURE 7.1 Neural signaling.

extracellular recording with saline-filled glass or metal microelectrodes [8]. In awake, behaving animals, the current state-of-the-art approach is a chronically implanted multiwire array electrode for high-density, simultaneous recording of extracellular action potentials or "units" across multiple experimental sessions [9]. Turnkey ensemble recording systems are now commercially available with hardwired (e.g., Plexon Inc.) and wireless (Triangle Biosystems Inc.) connections to the subject under investigation.

Although new optical methods are being developed [10], neurotransmitters have traditionally been measured by using microdialysis and voltammetry. In microdialysis, an analyte is physically removed from the brain extracellular fluid for an *ex vivo* determination [11]. Sophisticated analytical tools such as capillary electrophoresis, laser-induced fluorescence, and mass spectrometry have been coupled to this sampling technique, and these provide it with exquisite sensitivity and selectivity. However, large probe size (~200 μm) and slow sampling rates (minutes) are a limiting factor. Because neurotransmitters are directly monitored at an implanted microsensor using electrochemistry, voltammetry exhibits superior temporal and spatial resolution [12]. Previously criticized aspects of voltammetry are poor selectivity due to the plethora of easily oxidized species in the brain extracellular fluid, and poor sensitivity. As described in Section 7.3, recent advances in electrochemistry for neurochemical sensing have addressed these criticisms, and now this approach has become the technique of choice for many *in vivo* monitoring applications.

7.3 FAST-SCAN CYCLIC VOLTAMMETRY

7.3.1 Voltammetric Techniques

The general principle of voltammetry is that a voltage is applied to the microsensor and the resulting current is measured [13]. Faradaic current, due to analyte oxidation (i.e., loss of electrons) and/or reduction (i.e., gain of electrons), quantifies analyte concentration. Voltammetric techniques differ in how potential is applied. Older methods for *in vivo* neurochemical monitoring, such as differential pulse voltammetry, scanned potential slowly, which limited temporal resolution to the minute domain. In contrast, modern voltammetric techniques such as amperometry, high-speed chronoamperometry, and FSCV sample with subsecond temporal resolution. When coupled to a carbon–fiber microelectrode (CFM), the present microsensor of choice for *in vivo* voltammetry, these techniques also afford micron spatial resolution. The cylindrical CFM shown in Figure 7.2 was fabricated by aspirating a single carbon fiber ($r = 2.5$ μm) into a glass microcapillary tube and pulling to a taper. The active sensing surface is that portion of the carbon fiber extending from the glass insulation (~100 μm).

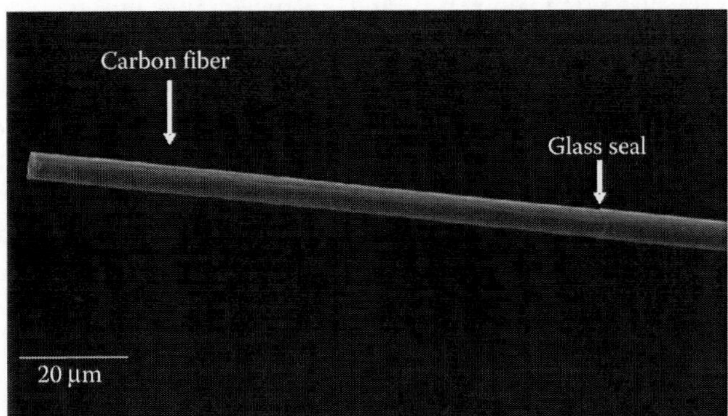

FIGURE 7.2 Scanning electron microscopic image of a CFM. (Reprinted from M. Roham, P. A. Garris, and P. Mohseni, *Proc. SPIE Symp. Nanoscience + Engineering*, 7035, 170350O-1–70350O-11, 2008. With permission.)

The simplest of the modern voltammetric techniques is amperometry, which applies a constant potential to the CFM. Although limited in chemical resolution, amperometric measurements can essentially be collected as fast as data acquisition permits, rendering this technique suitable for characterizing single-vesicle release from isolated cells with microsecond temporal resolution [15]. A voltage step is repetitively applied during high-speed chronamperometry, and faradaic current is typically monitored toward the end of the pulse after the charging current has subsided. Some chemical resolution is obtained by calculating the ratio of oxidative (positive step) and reductive (negative step) currents [16]. As described in more detail below, potential is linearly scanned in FSCV, which uniquely permits the determination of a voltammogram. It is this chemical signature that identifies the detected analyte and affords FSCV with its high degree of chemical resolution.

Voltammetric techniques are suitable for monitoring electroactive substances and several neurotransmitters important for normal brain function and associated with human neuropathologies. Dopamine, norepinephrine, serotonin, adenosine, and nitric oxide fall into this category [12,13]. Nonelectroactive neurotransmitters can also be measured electrochemically in real time using a biosensor approach [17]. For this strategy, a "biological recognition element" interacts with an analyte to produce an electroactive by-product. In the case of glutamate and gamma-aminobutyric acid, the two most prevalent neurotransmitters in the mammalian brain, an analyte-selective oxidase generates hydrogen peroxide that is detected electrochemically with amperometry [18]. Thus, voltammetric and biosensor approaches collectively have the capability of measuring a broad range of neurotransmitters.

7.3.2 Principles of FSCV

FSCV is the focus of the present chapter, because it exhibits the best chemical resolution of the real-time voltammetric techniques and it is therefore the most logical choice for incorporating into wireless devices supporting the monitoring of electroactive neurotransmitters. That said, a device that performs FSCV will also be able to support amperometry (and thus biosensors), high-speed chronoamperometry, and other forms of voltammetry with relatively straightforward changes in, for example, applied voltage, gain, and data acquisition and analysis.

The general scheme of FSCV is that, at regular intervals, the potential of the CFM is linearly and rapidly scanned from a resting or bias voltage to a peak voltage and back. The resulting applied waveform is thus triangular, and only during this voltage sweep is the analyte measured and are data acquired. The CFM is fixed at the bias potential in between scans. FSCV varies somewhat depending upon the application, but typical parameters for dopamine measurements in the awake rat are a bias potential (versus an Ag/AgCl reference electrode) of −0.4 V, a peak potential of +1.3 V, a scan rate of 400 V/s, and a scan interval of 100 ms. The negative bias potential advantageously promotes the adsorption of positively charged dopamine and preconcentrates this analyte in the time between scans. Because one concentration measurement is generated per scan, this interval means that the analyte is measured at a frequency of 10 Hz. The scan interval, and thus sampling frequency, is effectively determined by the duration of the scan. As a rule of thumb, the scan interval should be 10 times the scan duration to permit the relaxation of diffusion gradients produced during the scan.

As shown in Figure 7.3, a large background current is recorded at the CFM during the application of an individual voltage scan. This current is due to two phenomena: (1) charging the double-layer capacitance at the electrode–solution interface and (2) redox reactions of surface-bound chemical groups. The large background current, which cannot be avoided due to the high scan rate, masks the considerably smaller faradaic current due to the analyte, in this case, dopamine. Fortunately, the background current is stable, at least on short timescales (tens of seconds), and can be subtracted to reveal the faradaic current for the oxidation of dopamine to a quinone during the forward sweep and the reduction of the electroformed quinone back to dopamine during the reverse sweep. These time-dependent changes in the current relate to the applied voltage, with the peak potential for dopamine oxidization at ~+ 0.6 V and the one for quinone reduction at ~− 0.2 V. A plot of the measured

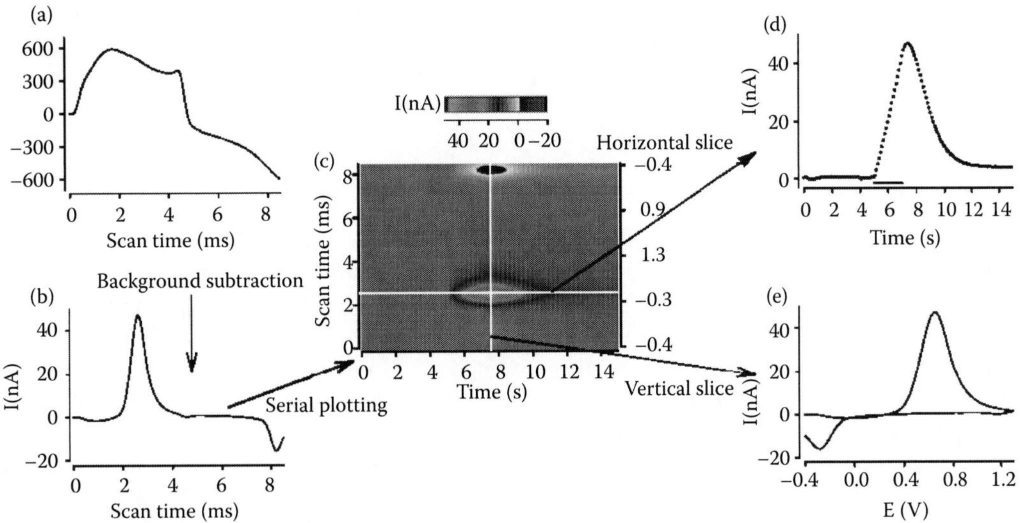

FIGURE 7.3 FSCV. (a) Background current recorded at the CFM. (b) Background-subtracted current for dopamine recorded at CFM. (c) Three-dimensional color plot serially plotting individual background-subtracted voltammograms, with time as the *x*-axis, applied voltage as the *y*-axis, and measured current as the *z*-axis. (d) Current measured at the peak oxidative potential for dopamine and plotted versus time. (e) Individual background-subtracted voltammogram for dopamine.

current versus the applied potential is called a voltammogram, and it is this chemical signature that is used to identify an analyte.

Individual voltammograms are plotted serially in time to reveal all of the electrochemical information collected during the measurement epoch using a three-dimensional color plot, with time as the *x*-axis, applied voltage as the *y*-axis, and measured current as the *z*-axis. The brown background color reflects zero current generated by the background subtraction procedure. This FSCV recording was collected in a urethane-anesthetized rat at a CFM implanted in the striatum, a densely dopamine-innervated region of the forebrain associated with motor control and Parkinson's disease [19]. Dopamine levels in the extracellular fluid were increased by means of electrical stimulation of the medial forebrain bundle, through which the dopaminergic neurons innervating the striatum ascend from their origins in the substantia nigra of the midbrain [20]. A 60 Hz, 2-s train, consisting of 4 ms, 300 μA biphasic pulses, was applied to an implanted bipolar stimulating electrode at 5 s.

The colors emerging from the brown background and coincident with stimulus application represent electrically evoked dopamine. The purple-green feature at ~+ 0.6 V is dopamine oxidation and the yellow-black feature at ~− 0.2 V is quinone reduction. Two accessory plots are constructed from the color profile and they provide better resolution of specific electrochemical information. The dynamic changes in dopamine are revealed by plotting current, measured along the horizontal line across the peak oxidation potential for dopamine, versus time and converting to concentration using postcalibration of the CFM with a flow injection analysis [21]. For this microsensor characterization technique, the CFM is placed in a flowing stream and exposed to a bolus injection of the analyte. In the first accessory plot, the increase in dopamine concentration during the pulse train is due to action potential-dependent neurotransmitter release, while the decrease after the stimulation is due to neuronal uptake.

For the second accessory plot, an individual background-subtracted voltammogram, representing the changes in electrochemistry between two time points, is constructed by plotting current, measured along the vertical line of the color profile, versus applied voltage. This folded or cyclic voltammogram shows the two characteristic peaks for dopamine occurring at +0.6 and −0.2 V for dopamine oxidation and quinone reduction, respectively. These two peaks also correspond to the color features in the three-dimensional plot (purple-green and black-yellow, respectively) showing all of the electrochemical information recorded during the measurement of the electrically evoked response. Of all the electroactive species identified in the brain, only norepinephrine has a similar voltammogram to that of dopamine [22].

7.3.3 Advances in FSCV

Since the introduction of FSCV at a CFM for *in vivo* neurochemical monitoring in 1984 [23], several innovations have advanced its utility for neurobiological applications. One prominent development was recording electrically evoked dopamine levels in ambulatory animals [24], which permitted investigating the role of dopamine in intracranial self-stimulation at the individual lever press level [25]. In this classic behavioral paradigm that has been used to study the brain reward system, animals learn to press a lever in order to obtain reinforcing electrical stimulation applied to an implanted electrode [26].

A state-of-the-art system for recording dopamine with FSCV at a CFM in an awake animal is described in Figure 7.4. Detailed later in this chapter, one long-term goal for instrumentation development is to replace this hardwired system with a wireless one. A photograph of the hardware attached to the animal is shown in Figure 7.4a. During preparatory surgery, a stimulating electrode is implanted in the medial forebrain bundle and cemented to the skull. A reference electrode positioned in the cortex and a hub centered over a skull burr hole above the striatum are also affixed to the skull. During recording, a micromanipulator housing a fresh CFM is attached to the hub for acute lowering of the microsensor in the awake animal. The micromanipulator is detachable; thus, it can be withdrawn and calibrated immediately after the experiment. Also affixed to the animal before measurements begin are a stimulating electrode cable and the board-level headstage housing the electronics for FSCV. The headstage is then connected to the CFM and reference electrode via jumper wires.

Figure 7.4b shows a schematic diagram of the measurement system for FSCV at a CFM in the awake rat. At the headstage level, a low-noise, high-bandwidth operational amplifier is configured as a current-to-voltage transducer (transimpedance amplifier), with the feedback resistor determining gain. The animal is maintained at ground through the reference electrode, and the voltage scan is applied directly to the CFM. A differential amplifier subsequently subtracts the applied triangle waveform from the measured signal (not shown). The animal is hardwired to recording and stimulating equipment via a commutator, which maintains electrical connections through a swivel while permitting 360° movement. Electrochemistry, electrical stimulation, and data acquisition are

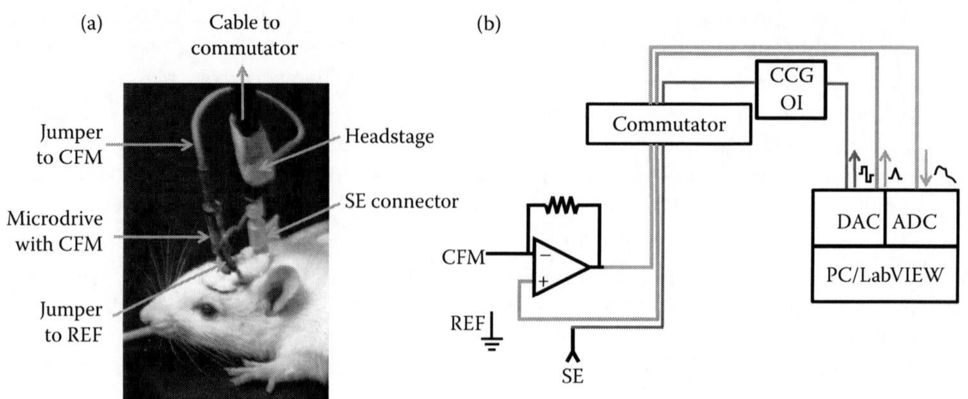

FIGURE 7.4 Headmounted hardware for FSCV in freely moving rats. (a) Photograph of hardware attached to the rat. (b) Schematic diagram of instrumental setup. Abbreviations: REF, reference electrode; SE, stimulating electrode; CCG, constant-current generator; OI, optical isolator

controlled using software written in LabVIEW® and National Instrument® PCI boards (Austin, TX, USA) running on a desktop PC. Measured signals are digitized by an analog-to-digital converter (ADC). The triangle waveform and stimulus pulses are generated by software and a digital-to-analog converter (DAC). Electrical stimulation is applied as a constant current and is optically isolated. Filtering and data analysis are performed offline by using LabVIEW software.

Further progress was made in recording dopamine with FSCV in awake animals through improvements in CFM sensitivity and chemical resolution. For example, the CFM can be rendered more sensitive to dopamine by extending the scanning potential from the traditional range of −0.4–1.0 V to either −0.4–1.3 V or even −0.6–1.4 V [27]. Extended scanning increases sensitivity by overoxidizing the carbon surface, which increases dopamine adsorption in the time between scans. This improvement in sensitivity has enabled the recording of dopamine transients, which are small, naturally occurring signals elicited by rewards and sensory cues predictive of these rewards [28]. Drugs of abuse are thought to activate dopamine transients and cause overlearning of cues predictive of drug availability [29]. Figure 7.5 shows the recording of dopamine transients in an awake rat administered the psychostimulant amphetamine. These phasic-type release events appear as small peaks in the trace (above) and color plot (below), and their voltammogram is consistent with dopamine (inset).

The analysis of dopamine transients has been improved by two mathematical procedures. In the first procedure, an automated algorithm was developed that "marches" through the voltammetric record and, using a moving background, calculates a background-subtracted cyclic voltammogram for each scan [30]. These voltammograms are then statistically compared using correlation to the voltammogram originating from electrically evoked dopamine, which is used as a standard reference signal. In Figure 7.5, electrically evoked dopamine is the larger signal in both the trace and the color plot. Also note how well the voltammograms for the evoked dopamine and the transient signal overlap (inset). In the second procedure, principal component regression is used to obtain a statistically verifiable dopamine trace [31], which is then amenable to analysis using peak-fitting algorithms [32]. This chemometrics approach is required for some applications, because the trace collected at the peak oxidation potential for dopamine may contain contributions from interferents whose voltammogram overlaps dopamine. Another advantage of principal component regression is that it can resolve slow changes in baseline dopamine levels.

The CFM is not only well suited for electrochemical measurements, but it is also an excellent, low-noise sensor for extracellular electrophysiology. This feature, combined with the intermittent nature of FSCV sampling, enables both electrochemistry and unit activity to be collected quasi-simultaneously at the same probe. This so-called time-share voltammetry and electrophysiology is described in Figure 7.6. In the time between scans, the CFM is switched from the current-to-voltage circuit for FSCV to a voltage-follower circuit for extracellular electrophysiology using a relay. Data for FSCV and electrophysiology are then collected and analyzed separately. The power of this approach is that dopamine and its effects on the postsynaptic neuron, in this case inhibition, can be monitored in the same locus. The typical sampling strategy is to decrease scan frequency from 10 to 5 Hz. Accounting for the additional time needed for circuit relaxation between switching, about 180 ms of each 200 ms recording epoch is available for electrophysiological measurements. More extended scan parameters, −0.6–1.4 V, are also used to offset the loss of sensitivity arising from the potential of the CFM floating between scans.

Another recent advance is the development of microelectrode arrays (MEAs) for electrochemical detection. MEAs have been microfabricated using platinum as the recording site on a ceramic [33] or silicon [34] substrate and pyrolyzed photoresist film, which exhibits a similar electrochemistry as a carbon fiber, on a silicon substrate [35]. In addition to increasing the number of recording sites interrogating brain chemistry, MEAs have the advantage of more reproducible fabrication compared to the hand-made CFM. Expanding recording channels up to 16 [36] has also exceeded the capabilities of conventional headstages, a problem that can be readily solved by integrated circuits as described later in this chapter.

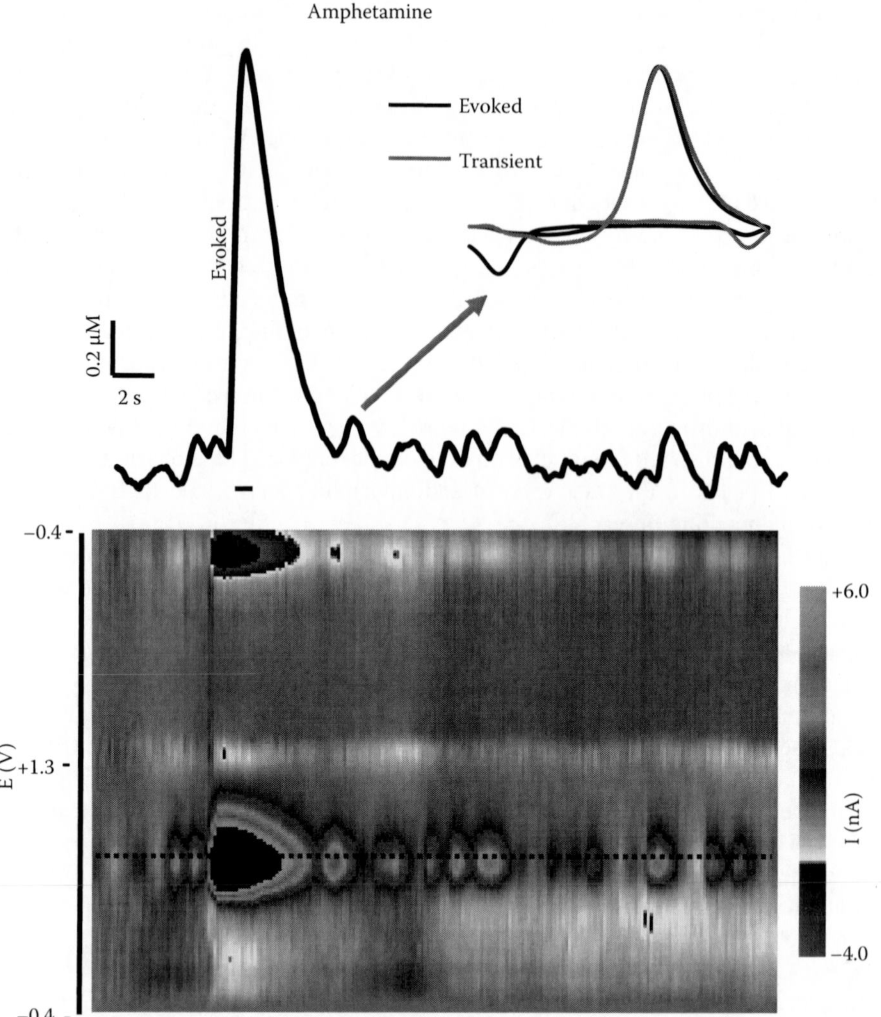

FIGURE 7.5 Dopamine recording in an awake rat following amphetamine administration. Electrically evoked dopamine is the larger signal in both the trace and the color plot, with much smaller transient release events occurring thereafter. The maximal current amplitude of background-subtracted cyclic voltammograms shown in the inset was normalized to 1.

7.4 BOARD-LEVEL SYSTEMS FOR WIRELESS NEUROCHEMICAL SENSING

7.4.1 Why Wireless?

A compelling justification can be put forth to replace the hardwired connection between recording and stimulating equipment by a wireless link. For example, physical restraint of the animal via the traditional tethering approach is a concern for altering behavior and also limits the use of important experimental paradigms involving enriched environments, social interaction, and long-term recording. Micromotion of cables during ambulation is also a significant noise source that seriously degrades measurement quality. Indeed, the intense stereotypy induced by psychostimulants, such as amphetamine, methamphetamine, and cocaine, may produce such robust movement artifacts that recordings are rendered unusable. While wireless systems for electrophysiology have been around for decades [4], incorporating telemetry into voltammetry has lagged behind considerably. Moreover,

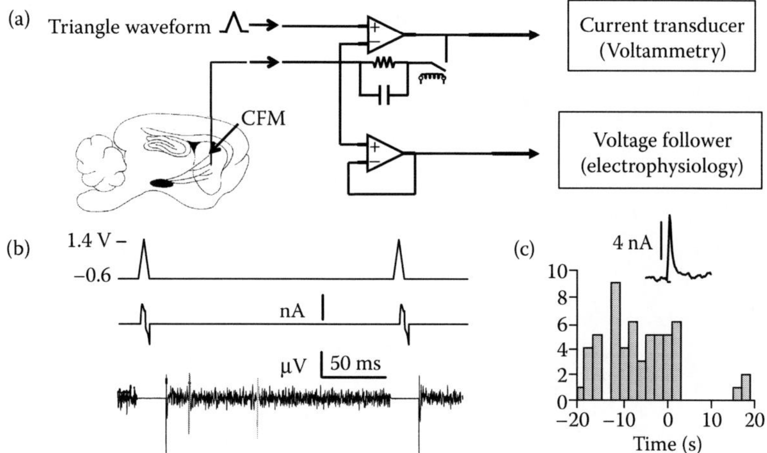

FIGURE 7.6 Time-share voltammetry and electrophysiology. (a) A simplified circuit diagram for switching between FSCV and electrophysiology. (b) Triangle voltage scans are applied to the CFM every 200 ms (top panel). During this time, electrochemical data are collected (middle panel), while electrophysiology is recorded in the time between scans (bottom panel). (c) Using the same probe to quasi-simultaneously monitor the effects of electrically evoked dopamine on the postsynaptic activity of a target neuron.

while board-level wireless devices supporting slow-scan voltammetry [37], chronoamperometry [38], and amperometry [39] have moved beyond development to application in awake animals, arriving at this same stage for wireless FSCV has presented unique challenges as discussed below.

7.4.2 Real-Time Animal Telemetry

We have developed a board-level wireless system called real-time animal telemetry (RAT) to support single-channel neurochemical monitoring with FSCV at a CFM and constant-current electrical stimulation at a bipolar electrode [4,40]. As shown in Figure 7.7, the RAT remote unit attached to the subject has four components: a Bluetooth transceiver (ROK 101008/21, Ericsson, Stockholm, Sweden), the main PC board, the electrical stimulation circuit, and battery. RAT communicates bidirectionally with the home-base station, a PC outfitted with an identical Bluetooth transceiver. This wireless module is accessed via a high-speed serial interface (460 kbps; 232PCI1A, B&B Electronics, Ottawa, IL, USA) and software written in LabVIEW.

Populated with surface mount components, the main board houses the front-end analog circuitry for FSCV and the microprocessor, and is connected to the brain-implanted CFM and reference electrode (Ag/AgCl). The feedback resistor of the current-to-voltage transducer circuit can be swapped to change gain. The analog stimulus generator was constructed on breadboard with conventional electronic devices, uses a separate and independent power supply, and applies constant-current and optically isolated pulses to a brain-implanted electrode with an impedance of ~5 kΩ. All four modules are folded together ($4 \times 2 \times 1.5$ cm^3; 17 g) and attached to the awake rat using a backpack. Since the stimulus device is passive, it can be detached from the main board in order to reduce the size of the remote unit for neurochemical recording only.

The microprocessor (C8051F007DK, Silicon Laboratories, Austin, TX, USA) performs several key functions of RAT, including control of FSCV, electrical stimulation, and data acquisition and transmission. It is also critical for device miniaturization by replacing large components of the hardwired system described above (Figure 7.4) for performing FSCV in an awake animal, such as the headstage and potentiostat, optical isolator/constant current generators, and computer PCI boards with ADC and DAC, and digital input/output (I/O), with a single chip without lost performance. For example, RAT collects FSCV at 100 kS/s with 12-bit resolution and applies

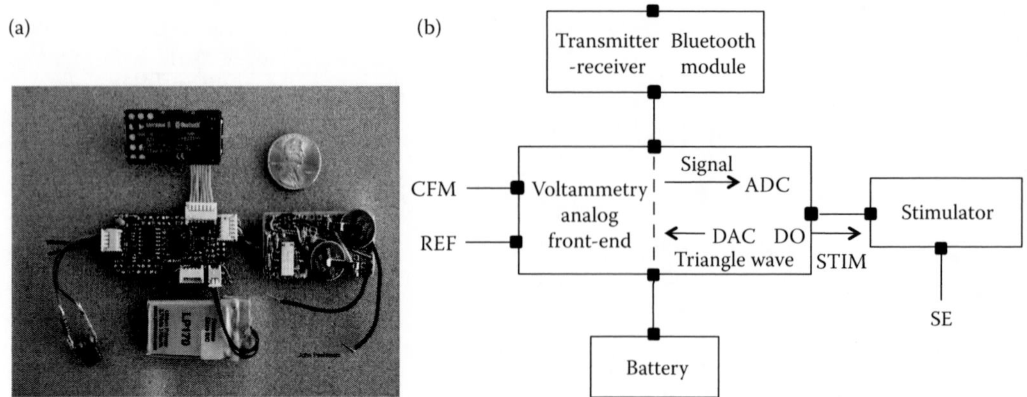

FIGURE 7.7 RAT. (a) Photograph of RAT hardware and (b) block diagram of RAT. (Modified from P. A. Garris et al. *Electrochemical Methods for Neuroscience*. A. C. Michael and L. M. Borland, Eds. Boca Raton, FL: CRC Press, pp. 233–259, 2007.)

constant-current, optically isolated biphasic stimulus pulses similar to the hardwired system. At the microprocessor level, ADC digitizes the CFM signal, DAC generates the triangle waveform and bias potential for FSCV, digital I/O communicates with the serial I/O of the Bluetooth module and sends positive and negative pulses to the stimulus generator, and software stored in FLASH memory controls all functions and timing.

The FSCV analog circuit of RAT is quite similar to that of the hardwired system. RAT amplifiers are configured such that the reference electrode is held at circuit common, while the potential of the CFM is scanned. This voltage scan is subtracted from the measured signal before digitization. Finally, the FSCV circuit is also operated in two-electrode mode (i.e., a working and a reference electrode). This mode is sufficient, because the small currents recorded at the CFM during FSCV do not require the use of an auxiliary electrode and, instead, can readily be passed through the reference electrode.

Bluetooth (802.15) was selected to provide the wireless link for RAT on the basis of several considerations, including commercial availability, signal fidelity and reliability, small size, low price, and low power requirements, relative to other digital telemetry options operating in the 2.4 GHz band such as Wi-FI (802.11 g) [41]. In general, digital telemetry was deemed necessary for this application in order to provide the requisite high-resolution acquisition of the voltammogram and to reduce susceptibility to transmission artifacts. The 2.4 GHz band also supports the high data rates required for FSCV. Although it is slower (1 versus 54 Mbps) and is transmitting shorter distances (9 versus 90 m) than Wi-Fi, Bluetooth, which uses frequency hopping spectrum spread modulation, is better suited for busy 2.4 GHz environments and is more resistant to multipath interference. High signal fidelity and reliability is achieved with this spread spectrum technology by jumping between 79 bands, 1 MHz each, according to a pseudorandom noise code at a rate of up to 3200 hops/s.

RAT has undergone extensive testing at the bench level: *in vitro* using flow injection analysis, and *in vivo* in the anesthetized rat for measuring dopamine levels in the striatum electrically evoked by stimulation of the medial forebrain bundle [4,40]. Overall, RAT performed similarly to a conventional hardwired system for FSCV, thereby establishing the first wireless measurement of FSCV at a CFM. The *coup de grace* demonstration of RAT's utility was the monitoring of dopamine in the awake, freely behaving rat. It should be noted that a design similar to RAT, but configured as a head-mounted device with provision for two-channel recording (but without electrical stimulation), has now been developed by Pinnacle Technology, Inc. (http://www.pinnaclet.com).

Importantly, RAT was less susceptible to ambient electrical noise than the conventional hardwired system [4,40]. This phenomenon was most likely due to digitization of the analog signal close to the measurement at the CFM (i.e., at the level of the animal) and the data transmission fidelity provided by Bluetooth digital telemetry. A desirable consequence of this attribute is the potential for performing experiments outside of the Faraday cage, which is normally essential for neurochemical monitoring with FSCV and other microelectrode measurements. For this reason and combined with its small size, we have also proposed RAT as a portable microsensor measurement system for real-time neurochemical monitoring applications [4]. Indeed, one such application was monitoring dopamine in the rat striatum during a model of transient focal ischemia. The portable and small RAT was an asset, because combining all of the surgical and monitoring equipment for the stroke experiment with a conventional hardwired system for FSCV inside a Faraday cage was not feasible.

7.4.3 Wireless Instantaneous Neurotransmitter Concentration System

RAT was used as a device template to develop another board-level, discrete system called WINCS, shown in Figure 7.8. In contrast to RAT, which was directed toward laboratory animals and basic neuroscience, the ultimate target of WINCS is the human during functional neurosurgical procedures and clinical research. WINCS is topical because currently there is no FDA-approved device for intraoperative neurochemical monitoring at an implanted microsensor in humans. Several important criteria were considered in developing WINCS. Foremost were patient safety, signal fidelity, and convenient integration into existing neurosurgical setups. These considerations are critical, because a sophisticated measurement approach is being added to already complex and highly invasive neurosurgical techniques, and these additions must not compromise patient outcome.

A small, wireless and battery-powered patient module unit akin to RAT was selected as the design strategy for WINCS. Such a device is readily attached to the stereotactic frame or another location in close proximity to the patient during the neurosurgical procedure and wirelessly transmits data to a remotely located base station, and so would not contribute to crowding in the busy space surrounding the patient. The susceptibility of electrochemical measurements to ambient noise inherent in the operating room is minimized by signal digitization near the site of measurement and Bluetooth telemetry. Safety issues related to line-powered devices are also eliminated by using a small battery. Of course, the patient module requires provisions for sterilization to reduce the risk for infection during surgery.

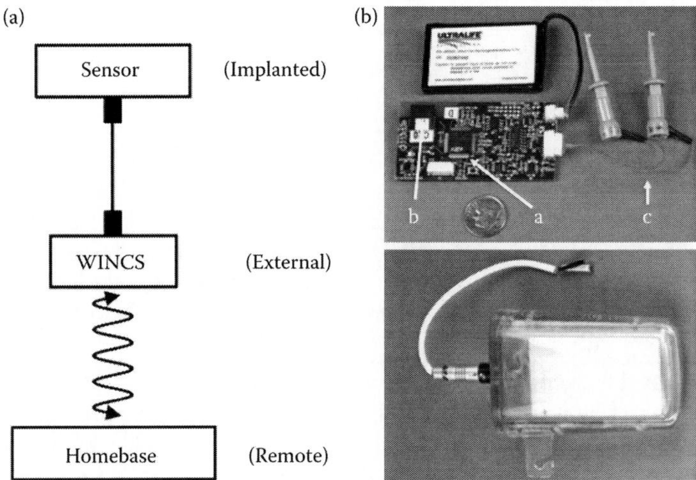

FIGURE 7.8 WINCS. (a) Operation of WINCS. (b) Photograph of WINCS circuit board with attached Ultralife® battery (a, microprocessor; b, Bluetooth transceiver; c, electrode leads). (c) WINCS encased in a hermetically sealed polycarbonate sheath for sterilization. (Reprinted from J. M. Bledsoe et al., *J. Neurosurg.*, 111(4), 712–723, 2009. With permission. Copyright 2009 Wolters Kluwer Health, Inc.)

WINCS was developed in compliance with FDA-recognized consensus standards for medical electrical device safety. Several improvements to the RAT design were implemented, including (1) a newer microprocessor with greater ADC bit resolution, more internal memory, and faster clock speed; (2) wirelessly programmable waveform parameters (scan bias, range, and rate) and offset; (3) a higher precision voltage reference for the microprocessor; (4) a more advanced Bluetooth module; (5) low-power mode to preserve battery life when idle; (6) battery voltage sensing and low-power alert; and (7) a longer lasting battery. The WINCS module circuitry and battery are packaged for use in a hermetically sealed, sterilizable polymer enclosure, with externally accessible connections. The home station is also now a PC laptop, which enhances portability, and front-end software, termed WincsWare, supports near real-time data display of the background current, cyclic voltammogram, current versus time curve at user-defined potential, and color plot of time, voltage, and current.

Like RAT, WINCS has been extensively tested at the bench-top level, *in vitro* with flow-injection analysis, and *in vivo* in the anesthetized rat, with great success [42–45]. RAT electrochemical measurements of dopamine have been extended with WINCS to include serotonin, norepineprhine, adenosine, ascorbic acid and pH with FSCV at a CFM and glutamate and adenosine with amperometric biosensors. WINCS has also been integrated into a large-animal model of functional neurosurgery, the domestic pig, to study the neurochemical mechanisms of DBS action [46]. DBS, a functional neurosurgical approach whereby neurological symptoms are treated by applying high-frequency pulse trains to a target-implanted stimulating electrode, has demonstrated efficacy in treating motor disorders such as Parkinson's disease, essential tremor, and dystonia, and is being increasingly applied to neuropsychiatric diseases such as intractable obsessive compulsive disorder [5]. The pig model incorporated key elements of the human DBS surgical procedure, including MR imaging, MR-compatible stereotaxic frame, neurosurgical planning software, electrophysiological verification of the target, and an Alpha Omega microdrive (Nazareth, Israel) connected to a Leksell Stereotactic System (Stockholm, Sweden). WINCS for intraoperative neurochemical monitoring in the human is now approved for DBS and epilepsy patients by the Institutional Review Board at Mayo Clinic Rochester (Rochester, MN, USA). Its establishment for this purpose is now under way at Mayo Clinic Rochester under the supervision of the neurosurgeon Dr. Kendall H. Lee.

7.5 VLSI-CMOS TECHNOLOGY FOR WIRELESS NEUROCHEMICAL SENSING

7.5.1 Why VLSI-CMOS Technology?

Although advances in the manufacture of discrete electrical components such as surface-mount devices have remarkably facilitated the implementation of board-level neurochemical recording systems with commercial off-the-shelf components, the majority still have prohibitively large dimensions, weight, or high power consumption, making them impractical for ultra-small-scale and low-power applications. Such limitations preclude applications in smaller, but neurobiologically relevant, animals such as hamsters, mice, and birds and even invertebrates including *Aplysia*, an important model organism for the study of learning and memory. Development of implantable devices for basic neuroscience research and ultimately "smart" neuroprostheses for treating human neuropathologies are also severely hampered.

As we discuss in this section, significant reductions in overall dimensions, total weight, and power consumption can be achieved using VLSI-CMOS technology. System integration will also increase the signal-to-noise ratio, while decreasing overall dimensions and weight by minimizing the number of external components necessary for system operation. More recording channels can be added as well, without prohibitively increasing the form factor, and when coupled with low-power design techniques, will afford using advanced batteries with smaller size and extended lifetime as power supplies. This will in turn reduce the overall device size and weight even further. The resulting small form factor should be suitable for long-term implantation.

7.5.2 Evolution of Integrated Circuits for FSCV

Low-noise, low-power microsystems for neurochemical sensing applications can be implemented with VLSI-CMOS technology. For example, integrated circuits have been developed for multichannel electrical stimulation, electrophysiology, and chemical recording using amperometry and chronoamperometry [47–49]. An inductively powered, 16-channel wireless device for amperometric recording has also been described [50]. We have focused our attention on developing the first-of-their-kind wireless integrated circuits supporting applications with FSCV.

Figure 7.9 shows the evolution of the three FSCV integrated circuits that we have developed to date. All were fabricated with the AMI 0.5 μm standard CMOS process, used RF-FSK wireless transmission operating at a frequency near 433 MHz, and shared common overall system architecture as described in more detail below. Functionality was added with each subsequent device. The first chip (2.2×2.2 mm^2) supported a single channel of either amperometry or FSCV, but required an external waveform generator to create the triangular waveform of FSCV [51]. The second chip (2.7×2.9 mm^2) expanded the number of recording channels to 16 and added an FSCV waveform generator [52]. Moreover, each channel could be independently configured for single-unit extracellular electrophysiology or FSCV. This chip, in particular, demonstrates the utility of VLSI-CMOS technology to add more recording channels and additional functionality without prohibitively increasing the form factor. Finally, while the third chip (1.8×2.8 mm^2) supported only four channels, each could be independently configured for one of three measurement modalities: FSCV, single-unit extracellular electrophysiology, or time-share voltammetry and electrophysiology [53]. Additionally, this chip housed an FSCV waveform generator and a constant-current electrical stimulator for neuroactivation.

System architecture for the third chip is shown in Figure 7.10. For neurochemical recording, a delta–sigma (ΔΣ) modulator converts the analog current measured at the CFM into a high-data-rate serial bit stream for subsequent data encoding and wireless transmission to the RF receiver at the base-station PC. The ΔΣ modulator, which provides a large dynamic range and high resolution for sampling low-frequency current signals, is functionally equivalent to the ADC of RAT and WINCS. Also similar to RAT and WINCS, the electrochemical circuit operates in the two-electrode mode. Voltage signals collected during neuroelectrical recording are first converted into current by a voltage-to-current circuit and then fed into the ΔΣ modulator. For time-share voltammetry and electrophysiology, a timing generator switches a channel between neurochemical and neuroelectrical recording modalities. Timing signals from the clock generator also control waveform and stimulus

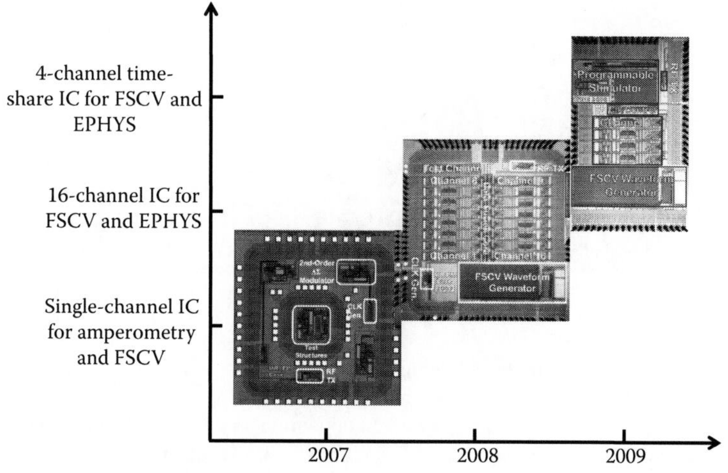

FIGURE 7.9 Evolution of FSCV integrated circuits.

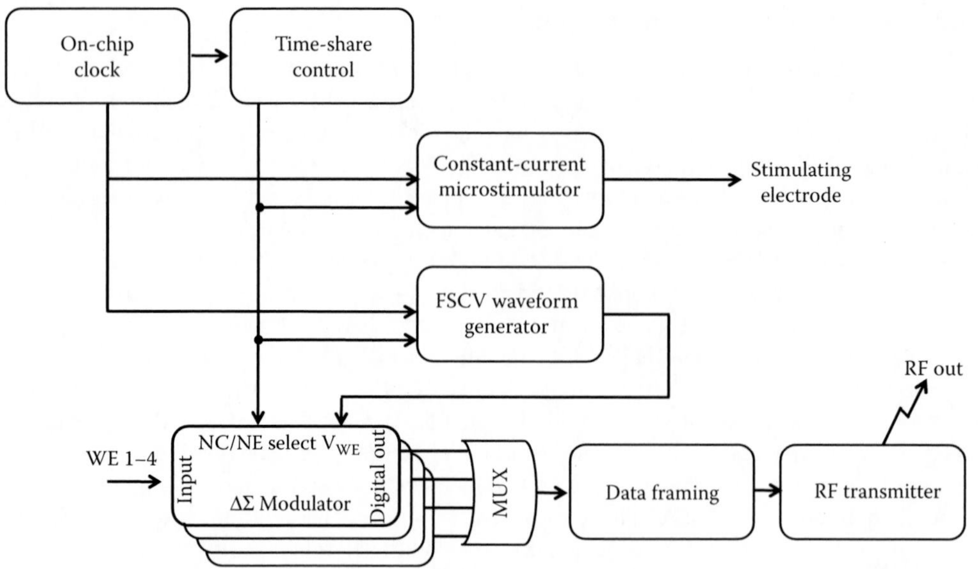

FIGURE 7.10 Simplified system architecture for an integrated circuit capable of voltammetry, electrophysiology, and time-share voltammetry and electrophysiology.

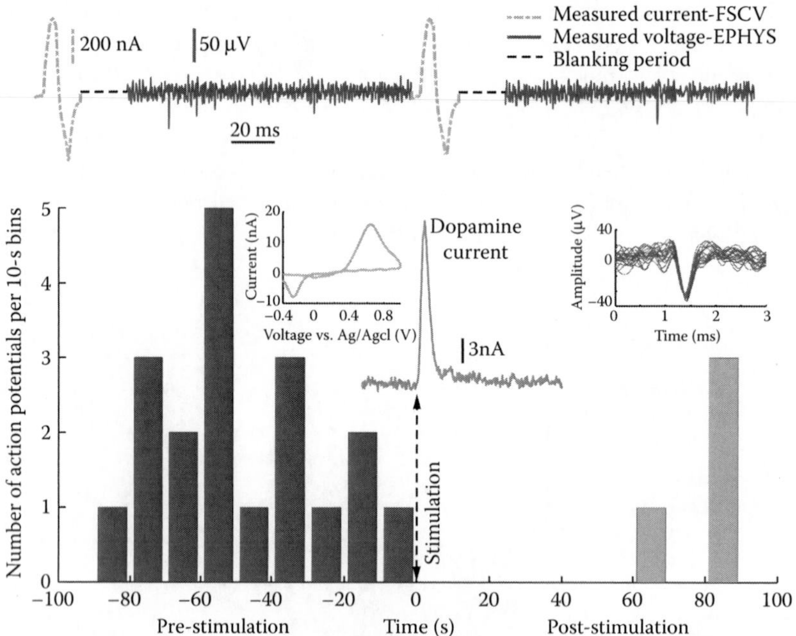

FIGURE 7.11 Time-share voltammetry and electrophysiology recorded by an integrated circuit in an anesthetized rat. The top panel shows alternate FSCV and electrophysiological recordings at the same CFM. The bottom panel displays the effects of electrically evoked dopamine on postsynaptic neuronal activity, plotted as the number of spikes per 10-s bin. Dopamine was identified by its characteristic cyclic voltammogram (inset, light gray), and single units were identified with offline analysis (inset, dark gray). (Reprinted from M. Roham et al., *IEEE J. Solid-State Circuits*, 44, 3645–3658, 2009. With permission. Copyright 2009 IEEE.)

generators. Biphasic electrical pulses are generated by a monolithic constant-current microstimulator incorporating stimulus waveform memory and a DAC. Similar to hardwired systems, pulses are applied in the time between waveform scans to minimize stimulus artifact.

The testing strategy was also similar to that for RAT and WINCS and consisted of bench-top engineering evaluation, *in vitro* flow injection analysis, and measurements of electrically evoked dopamine levels in the anesthetized rat. Single-unit extracellular electrophysiological recordings were additionally assessed *in vivo*. Overall, all three integrated circuits compared favorably to a conventional hardwired FSCV system. Figure 7.11 describes the evaluation of the third chip for the measurement modality of time-share voltammetry and electrophysiology in the anesthetized rat. The combined measurement clearly shows dopamine, evoked by electrical stimulation of the medial forebrain bundle at time zero, inhibiting spontaneously active units in the striatum in a manner consistent with the postsynaptic action of this neurotransmitter [54].

7.6 FUTURE DIRECTIONS

As is, WINCS is sufficiently advanced developmentally to be ready for broad applications, ranging from basic neuroscience research in laboratory animals to clinical research in humans. Like RAT, WINCS can also function as a portable microsensor measurement system and be conveniently incorporated into most preexisting experimental setups. Continued development of WINCS will enhance functionalities, including multiple channel recording, additional measurement modalities such as single-unit extracellular electrophysiology and time-share voltammetry and electrophysiology, and provision for electrical stimulation. While the downside is its relatively large size, which

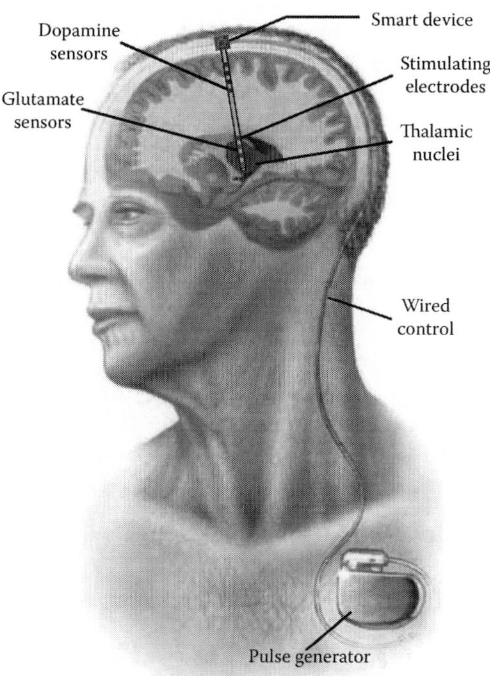

FIGURE 7.12 Neuroprosthesis concept: wireless, closed-loop system for neurorecording and neurostimulating. (Reprinted from K. H. Lee et al., *Neuromodulation*, 12, 85–103, 2009. With permission. Copyright 2008 Wiley-Blackwell.)

limits its use in small laboratory animals to anesthetized preparations, the future potential for neurochemical measurements in humans during neurosurgical procedures is clearly exciting.

Several future directions should be considered for continuing integrated circuit development. Basic neuroscience research in laboratory animals would benefit from a turnkey, fully implanted system, by which the subject is neurochemically interrogated in real time during behavioral paradigms without the requirement for handling to attach headstages and batteries, or insert microsensors. Chronically implantable CFMs are now available that retain sensitivity and response time to capture sensory cue-evoked dopamine transients with high fidelity [55]. These microsensors could be coupled with a rechargeable battery-powered implantable microsystem with functionalities similar to our time-share chip. A charging station using inductive powering could also be developed that functions in the home cage or be implemented prior to experiments. Additional chip development could also be directed toward "smart" devices that not only sense neurochemicals, but also use these signals as feedback in order to control neural activity at a desired level via electrical stimulation or drug injection [5]. As conceptualized in Figure 7.12, such neuroprostheses could one day be used for treating debilitating neuropathologies such as Parkinson's disease, dystonia, essential tremor, epilepsy, and obsessive–compulsive disorder. Supported by NSF (DBI-0754733 and -0754615) and NIH (DA-025809).

REFERENCES

1. L. R. Squire, D. Berg, F. Bloom, S. du Lac, and Ghosh, *Fundamental Neuroscience*, 3rd edn. New York, NY: Academic Press, 2008, p. 1256.
2. S. G. Sandberg and P. A. Garris, Neurochemistry of addiction: Monitoring essential neurotransmitters of addiction, in *Advances in the Neuroscience of Addiction*. C. M. Kuhn and G. F. Koob, Eds. Boca Raton, FL: CRC Press, 2010, pp. 101–136.
3. P. E. Phillips, G. D. Stuber, M. L. Heien, R. M. Wightman, and R. M. Carelli, Subsecond dopamine release promotes cocaine seeking, *Nature*, 422(6932), 614–618, 2003.
4. P. A. Garris, P. G. Greco, S. G. Sandberg, G. Howes, S. Pongmayteegul, B. A. Heidenreich, J. M. Casto et al., *In vivo* voltammetry with telemetry, in *Electrochemical Methods for Neuroscience*. A. C. Michael and L. M. Borland, Eds. Boca Raton, FL: CRC Press, pp. 233–259, 2007.
5. K. H. Lee, C. D. Blaha, P. A. Garris, P. Mohseni, A. Horne, K. E. Bennet, F. Agnesi et al., Evolution of deep brain stimulation: Human electrometer and smart devices supporting the next generation of therapy, *Neuromodulation*, 12, 85–103, 2009.
6. N. B. Standen and P. R. Stanfield, Patch clamp methods for single channel and whole cell recording, in *Monitoring Neuronal Activity: The Practical Approach*. J. Stamford, Ed. Oxford: Oxford University Press, pp. 59–84, 1992.
7. E. M. Silinksy, Intracellular recording methods for neurons, in *Monitoring Neuronal Activity: The Practical Approach*. J. Stamford, Ed. Oxford: Oxford University Press, pp. 29–58, 1992.
8. J. Millar, Extracellular single and multiple unit recording with microelectrodes, in *Monitoring Neuronal Activity: The Practical Approach*. J. Stamford, Ed. Oxford: Oxford University Press, pp. 1–28, 1992.
9. M. A. Nicolelis, D. Dimitrov, J. M. Carmena, R. Crist, G. Lehew, J. D. Kralik, and S. P. Wise, Chronic, multisite, multielectrode recordings in macaque monkeys, *Proc. Natl. Acad. Sci. USA*, 100(19), 11041–11046, 2003.
10. Q. T. Nguyen, L. F. Schroeder, M. Mank, A. Muller, P. Taylor, O. Griesbeck, and D. Kleinfeld, An *in vivo* biosensor for neurotransmitter release and *in situ* receptor activity, *Nat. Neurosci.*, 13(1), 127–132, 2010.
11. C. J. Watson, B. J. Venton, and R. T. Kennedy, *In vivo* measurements of neurotransmitters by microdialysis sampling, *Anal. Chem.*, 78(5), 1391–1399, 2006.
12. D. L. Robinson, A. Hermans, A. T. Seipel, and R. M. Wightman, Monitoring rapid chemical communication in the brain, *Chem. Rev.*, 108(7), 2554–2584, 2008.
13. L. M. Borland and A. C. Michael, An introduction to electrochemical methods in neuroscience, in *Electrochemical Methods for Neuroscience*. A. C. Michael and L. M. Borland, Eds. Boca Raton, FL: CRC Press, pp. 1–15, 2007.
14. M. Roham, P. A. Garris, and P. Mohseni, Wireless integrated microsystems for monitoring brain chemical and electrical activity, *Proc. SPIE Symp. Nanoscience + Engineering*, 7035, 170350O-1–70350O-11, 2008.

15. R. H. Chow, L. von Ruden, and E. Neher, Delay in vesicle fusion revealed by electrochemical monitoring of single secretory events in adrenal chromaffin cells, *Nature*, 356(6364), 60–63, 1992.
16. J. M. Gulley, G. A. Larson, and N. R. Zahniser, *Using High-Speed Chronoamperometry with Local Dopamine Application to Assess Dopamine Transporter Function*. Boca Raton, FL: CRC Press, pp. 83–102, 2007.
17. G. S. Wilson and R. Gifford, Biosensors for real-time *in vivo* measurements, *Biosens. Bioelectron.*, 20,(12), 2388–2403, 2005.
18. K. N. Hascup, E. C. Rutherford, J. E. Quintero, B. K. Day, J. R. Nickell, F. Pomerleau, P. Huettl, J. J. Burmeister, and G. A. Gerhardt, Second-by-second measures of L-glutamate and other neurotransmitters using enzyme-based microelectrode arrays, in *Electrochemical Methods for Neuroscience*. A. C. Michael and L. M. Borland, Eds. Boca Raton, FL: CRC Press, pp. 407–450, 2007.
19. C. W. Olanow and W. G. Tatton, Etiology and pathogenesis of Parkinson's disease, *Annu. Rev. Neurosci.*, 22, 123–144, 1999.
20. A. Bjorklund and O. Lindvall, Dopamine-containing systems in the CNS, in *Handbook of Chemical Neuroanatomy*. A. Bjorklund and T. Hokfelt, Eds. New York, NY: Elsevier, pp. 55–122, 1984.
21. E. W. Kristensen, R. M. Wilson, and R. M. Wightman, Dispersion in flow injection analysis measured with microvoltammetric electrodes, *Anal. Chem.*, 58, 986–988, 1986.
22. J. E. Baur, E. W. Kristensen, L. J. May, D. J. Wiedemann, and R. M. Wightman, Fast-scan voltammetry of biogenic amines, *Anal. Chem.*, 60(13), 1268–1272, 1988.
23. J. A. Stamford, Z. L. Kruk, J. Millar, and R. M. Wightman, Striatal dopamine uptake in the rat: *In vivo* analysis by fast cyclic voltammetry, *Neurosci. Lett.*, 51(1), 133–138, 1984.
24. P. A. Garris, J. R. Christensen, G. V. Rebec, and R. M. Wightman, Real-time measurement of electrically evoked extracellular dopamine in the striatum of freely moving rats, *J. Neurochem.*, 68(1), 152–161, 1997.
25. P. A. Garris, M. Kilpatrick, M. A. Bunin, D. Michael, Q. D. Walker, and R. M. Wightman, Dissociation of dopamine release in the nucleus accumbens from intracranial self-stimulation, *Nature*, 398(6722), 67–69, 1999.
26. R. A. Wise and P. P. Rompre, Brain dopamine and reward, *Annu. Rev. Psychol.*, 40, 191–225, 1989.
27. M. L. Heien, P. E. Phillips, G. D. Stuber, A. T. Seipel, and R. M. Wightman, Overoxidation of carbon-fiber microelectrodes enhances dopamine adsorption and increases sensitivity, *Analyst*, 128(12), 1413–1419, 2003.
28. R. M. Carelli and R. M. Wightman, Functional microcircuitry in the accumbens underlying drug addiction: Insights from real-time signaling during behavior, *Curr. Opin. Neurobiol.*, 14(6), 763–768, 2004.
29. S. E. Hyman, Addiction: A disease of learning and memory, *Am. J. Psychiatry*, 162(8), 1414–1422, 2005.
30. D. L. Robinson, M. L. Heien, and R. M. Wightman, Frequency of dopamine concentration transients increases in dorsal and ventral striatum of male rats during introduction of conspecifics, *J. Neurosci.*, 22(23), 10477–10486, 2002.
31. M. L. Heien, M. A. Johnson, and R. M. Wightman, Resolving neurotransmitters detected by fast-scan cyclic voltammetry, *Anal. Chem.*, 76(19), 5697–5704, 2004.
32. M. L. Heien, A. S. Khan, J. L. Ariansen, J. F. Cheer, P. E. Phillips, K. M. Wassum, and R. M. Wightman, Real-time measurement of dopamine fluctuations after cocaine in the brain of behaving rats, *Proc. Natl. Acad. Sci. USA*, 102(29), 10023–10028, 2005.
33. J. J. Burmeister, K. Moxon, and G. A. Gerhardt, Ceramic-based multisite microelectrodes for electrochemical recordings, *Anal. Chem.*, 72(1), 187–192, 2000.
34. M. D. Johnson, R. K. Franklin, M. D. Gibson, R. B. Brown, and D. R. Kipke, Implantable microelectrode arrays for simultaneous electrophysiological and neurochemical recordings, *J. Neurosci. Methods*, 174(1), 62–70, 2008.
35. M. K. Zachek, P. Takmakov, B. Moody, R. M. Wightman, and G. S. McCarty, Simultaneous decoupled detection of dopamine and oxygen using pyrolyzed carbon microarrays and fast-scan cyclic voltammetry, *Anal. Chem.*, 81(15), 6258–6265, 2009.
36. M. K. Zachek, J. Park, P. Takmakov, R. M. Wightman, and G. S. McCarty, Microfabricated FSCV-compatible microelectrode array for real-time monitoring of heterogeneous dopamine release, *Analyst*, 135(7), 1556–1563, 2010.
37. M. G. De Simoni, A. De Luigi, L. Imeri, and S. Algeri, Miniaturized optoelectronic system for telemetry of *in vivo* voltammetric signals, *J. Neurosci. Methods*, 33(2–3), 233–240, 1990.
38. M. Kagohashi, T. Nakazato, K. Yoshimi, S. Moizumi, N. Hattori, and S. Kitazawa, Wireless voltammetry recording in unanesthetised behaving rats, *Neurosci. Res.*, 60(1), 120–127, 2008.

39. G. Bazzu, G. G. Puggioni, S. Dedola, G. Calia, G. Rocchitta, R. Migheli, M. S. Desole, J. P. Lowry, R. D. O'Neill, and P. A. Serra, Real-time monitoring of brain tissue oxygen using a miniaturized biotelemetric device implanted in freely moving rats, *Anal. Chem.*, 81(6), 2235–2241, 2009.
40. P. A. Garris, R. Ensman, J. Poehlman, A. Alexander, P. E. Langley, S. G. Sandberg, P. G. Greco, R. M. Wightman, and G. V. Rebec, Wireless transmission of fast-scan cyclic voltammetry at a carbon-fiber microelectrode: Proof of principle, *J. Neurosci. Methods*, 140(1–2), 103–115, 2004.
41. C. J. Weisman, *The Essential Guide to RF and Wireless*. Upper Saddle River, Englewood Cliffs, NJ: Prentice-Hall, 2002, pp. 1–311.
42. J. M. Bledsoe, C. J. Kimble, D. P. Covey, C. D. Blaha, F. Agnesi, P. Mohseni, S. Whitlock et al., Development of the wireless instantaneous neurotransmitter concentration system for intraoperative neurochemical monitoring using fast-scan cyclic voltammetry, *J. Neurosurg.*, 111(4), 712–723, 2009.
43. C. J. Kimble, D. M. Johnson, B. A. Winter, S. V. Whitlock, K. R. Kressin, A. E. Horne, J. C. Robinson et al., Wireless instantaneous neurotransmitter concentration sensing system (WINCS) for intraoperative neurochemical monitoring, *Conf. Proc. IEEE Eng. Med. Biol. Soc.*, 1, 4856–4859, 2009.
44. F. Agnesi, S. J. Tye, J. M. Bledsoe, C. J. Griessenauer, C. J. Kimble, G. C. Sieck, K. E. Bennet, P. A. Garris, C. D. Blaha, and K. H. Lee, Wireless instantaneous neurotransmitter concentration system-based amperometric detection of dopamine, adenosine, and glutamate for intraoperative neurochemical monitoring, *J. Neurosurg.*, 111(4), 701–711, 2009.
45. C. J. Griessenauer, S. Y. Chang, S. J. Tye, C. J. Kimble, K. E. Bennet, P. A. Garris, and K. H. Lee, Wireless instantaneous neurotransmitter concentration system: Electrochemical monitoring of serotonin using fast-scan cyclic voltammetry—A proof-of-principle study, *J. Neurosurg.*, 113(3), 656–665, 2010.
46. Y. M. Shon, K. H. Lee, S. J. Goerss, I. Y. Kim, C. Kimble, J. J. Van Gompel, K. Bennet, C. D. Blaha, and S. Y. Chang, High frequency stimulation of the subthalamic nucleus evokes striatal dopamine release in a large animal model of human DBS neurosurgery, *Neurosci. Lett.*, 475(3), 136–140, 2010.
47. R. H. Olsson, III, D. L. Buhl, A. M. Sirota, G. Buzsaki, and K. D. Wise, Band-tunable and multiplexed integrated circuits for simultaneous recording and stimulation with microelectrode arrays, *IEEE Trans. Biomed. Eng.*, 52(7), 1303–1311, 2005.
48. K. Murari, M. Stanacevic, G. Cauwenberghs, and N. V. Thakor, Integrated potentiostat for neurotransmitter sensing. A high sensitivity, wide range VLSI design and chip, *IEEE Eng. Med. Biol. Mag.*, 24(6), 23–29, 2005.
49. R. R. Harrison, P. T. Watkins, R. J. Kier, R. O. Lovejoy, D. J. Black, B. Greger, and F. Solzbacher, A low-power integrated circuit for a wireless 100-electrode neural recording system, *IEEE J. Solid-State Circuits*, 42, 123–133, 2007.
50. K. Murari, C. M. Sauer, M. Stanacevic, G. Cauwenberghs, and N. Thakor, Wireless multichannel integrated potentiostat for distributed neurotransmitter sensing, *Proc. IEEE Eng. Med. Biology 27th Ann. Conf.*, 2005.
51. M. Roham, D. P. Daberkow, E. S. Ramsson, D. P. Covey, S. Pakdeeronachit, P. A. Garris, and P. Mohseni, A wireless IC for wide-range neurochemical monitoring using amperometry and fast-scan cyclic voltammetry, *IEEE Trans. Biomed. Circuits Syst*, 2, 3–9, 2008.
52. M. Roham, C. D. Blaha, P. A. Garris, K. H. Lee, and P. Mohseni, A configurable IC for wireless real-time *in vivo* monitoring of chemical and electrical neural activity, *Conf. Proc. IEEE Eng. Med. Biol. Soc.*, 1, 4222–4225, 2009.
53. M. Roham, D. P. Covey, D. P. Daberkow, E. S. Ramsson, C. D. Howard, B. A. Heidenreich, P. A. Garris, and P. Mohseni, A wireless IC for time-share chemical and electrical neural recording, *IEEE J. Solid-State Circuits*, 44, 3645–3658, 2009.
54. D. J. Surmeier, J. Ding, M. Day, Z. Wang, and W. Shen, D1 and D2 dopamine-receptor modulation of striatal glutamatergic signaling in striatal medium spiny neurons, *Trends Neurosci.*, 30(5), 228–235, May 2007.
55. J. J. Clark, S. G. Sandberg, M. J. Wanat, J. O. Gan, E. A. Horne, A. S. Hart, C. A. Akers et al., Chronic microsensors for longitudinal, subsecond dopamine detection in behaving animals, *Nat. Methods*, 7, 126–129, 2009.

8 Giga-Ohm High-Impedance FET Input Amplifiers for Dry Electrode Biosensor Circuits and Systems

Gaetano Gargiulo, Paolo Bifulco, Rafael A. Calvo, Maria Romano, Mariano Ruffo, Richard Shephard, Mario Cesarelli, Craig Jin, Alistair McEwan, and André van Schaik

CONTENTS

8.1 INTRODUCTION

Recently with rising health costs and an aging population, there is an increased demand for comfortable monitoring and sensing of biosignals in order to enable and encourage the transition of healthcare services into everyday living including the home, workplace, and during exercise. Sensors can be situated in objects that people interact with daily, such as within a computer, chair, bed, toilet, car, telephone, or any portable personal electronic device.

Moreover, the relatively recent wide availability of highly integrated, inexpensive microelectronics with embedded software, open-access wireless protocols, and high-power-density batteries has led many research groups to develop wearable, wireless biosignal sensor-based systems that are worn on the body and integrated into clothing, capable of interaction with other devices that are nowadays commonly in our possession such as a mobile phone, laptop, personal digital assistant (PDA), or Ipods.

As this wireless biomedical long-term monitoring moves toward personal monitoring, it demands very high input impedance systems capable of extending the reading of biosignal during daily activities offering a kind of "stress-free," convenient connection, with no need for skin preparation. In particular, we highlight the development and broad applications of our own circuits for wearable biopotential sensor systems enabled by the use of an field effect transistor (FET)-based amplifier circuit with sufficiently high impedance to allow the use of passive dry electrodes, which overcome the significant barrier of gel-based contacts.

First, we review the recent state of the art in noninvasive biosensor circuits and systems. Then we present the highlights of our own research on long-term monitoring, in particular for the brain computer interface (BCI), which aims to provide a new communication channel to the human brain that is independent of standard pathways such as muscles and nerves. This innovative and exciting research field is in need of a reliable and easy to use long-term recording system for brain signals (electroencephalogram (EEG)). We then discuss sensor impedance measurements and future directions in this exciting and highly active field and we conclude by presenting our own ideas and research plans for future works.

8.2 HIGH-IMPEDANCE BIOPOTENTIAL RECORDING SYSTEM DEVELOPMENT

8.2.1 BIOAMPLIFIER

Bioamplifiers used in skin contact recordings of biopotentials must have a suitable input impedance in order to overcome the contact impedance and its unpredictable shifts to obtain a repeatable biological measurement of biopotentials using skin contact electrodes [1–3]. It is vital that a biopotential recording system exhibits several important properties such as high noise immunity, suitable frequency bandwidth, and high common-mode rejection ratio (CMMR). Biopotentials are always measured as the voltage difference between two points [2] and so maximal CMMR will improve the immunity from large common-mode noise (e.g., magnetically induced currents from electrical power lines) [4].

In summary, the basic requirements of a biopotential recording system are

- The physiological process to be monitored should not be influenced in any way.
- The measured signal should not be distorted.
- The best possible separation of signal and interferences should be provided.
- The subject should be protected from any hazard (e.g., of electrical shock).
- The recording system itself should be protected against damages that might result from high input voltages as they occur during the application of defibrillators or electrosurgical instrumentation.

Typically, the biopotentials are recorded using a minimum of three electrodes. One is the reference and the other two record different biopotentials. The input signal to the amplifier consists of five components: (1) the desired biopotential, (2) undesired biopotentials, (3) external interference signals and their harmonics (e.g., power lines), (4) interference signals generated by the tissue/electrode interface, and (5) instrumentation noise [2,4].

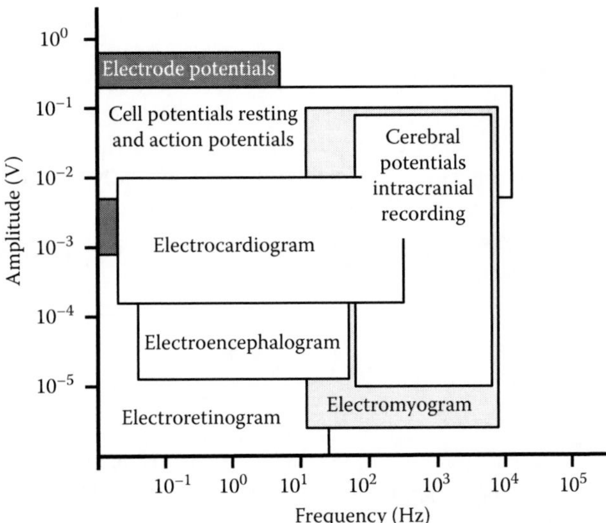

FIGURE 8.1 Amplitudes and spectral ranges of some important biosignals. (Adapted from J. D. Bronzino (Ed.), *The Biomedical Engineering Handbook*, second edition, Vol. 1. CRC Press, 2000.)

Owing to the very high number of different biopotentials and different diagnostic requirements needed, we start by highlighting the frequency/amplitude characteristics of the major biopotentials. We then delve into the history and details of existing bioamplifiers and the development of a new system. It is possible to infer from the chart depicted in Figure 8.1 that the various biopotentials completely cover the area from 10^{-6} V to almost 1 V and from dc to 10 kHz. This range is impossible to cover with any single fixed range device. Thus, the recording system should be designed for a particular application and with a multistage strategy, where a first stage (often referred to as a preamplifier) offers the correct interface to the measuring electrodes. This is usually followed by several stages of filtering/amplification to fulfill the application requirements. This situation is summarized in Figure 8.1, where three electrodes connect the patient to a preamplifier stage. After removing dc and low-frequency interferences, the signal is passed through an isolation stage which provides electrical safety to the patient, prevents ground loops, and reduces the influence of interference signals. The resulting signal is finally fed through a low-pass filter to remove unwanted higher frequencies [2].

The preamplifier stage is the crucial element of a biopotential measurement system; its main tasks are twofold: first, to sense the microvolt-level voltage between two measuring electrodes while rejecting the common-mode signal; second, by minimizing the dc effect of electrode polarization overpotentials. These unwanted signals are typically three to four orders of magnitude greater than the biopotential of interest demanding a CMRR of greater than 60 dB. Crucial for maintaining the performance of the preamplifier in practice is the input impedance, which should be as high as possible. Typical specifications include an input impedance of greater than 100 mega-ohms. Such a differential amplifier cannot be realized using a standard single operational amplifier (op-amp) design since this does not provide the necessary combination of high input impedance, CMRR, and gain over the required frequency range [2,4].

The typical solution is to implement an instrumentation amplifier using a differential amplifier configuration of three op-amps as is depicted in Figure 8.3. In this configuration, the rightmost amplifier, along with the resistors labeled R_2 and R_3, form a differential amplifier circuit, with a gain of R_3/R_2 and differential input resistance $2R_2$. The two amplifiers on the left are buffers to increase input impedance. With R_{gain} removed (open circuited), they are simple unity gain buffers; the circuit will work in that state, with gain simply equal to R_3/R_2. The buffer gain could be increased by putting resistors between the buffer inverting inputs and ground to shunt away some of the negative feedback; however, the single resistor R_{gain} between the two inverting inputs is a much more elegant method: it increases the differential-mode gain of the buffer pair while leaving the common-mode gain equal to one. This increases the CMRR of the circuit and also enables the buffers to handle much larger common-mode signals without clipping as would be the case if they were separate and had the same gain. Another benefit of the method is that it boosts the gain using a single resistor rather than a pair, thus avoiding a resistor-matching problem (although the two R_1s need to be matched, they may be smaller and have a closer matching for the same cost) and very conveniently allowing the gain of the circuit to be changed by changing the value of a single resistor. In this condition, the gain of the amplifier is expressed by [5]

$$\frac{V_{out}}{V_2 - V_1} = \frac{R_3}{R_2}\left(1 + \frac{2R_1}{R_{gain}}\right) \tag{8.1}$$

Ideally and theoretically, the common-mode gain of an instrumentation amplifier is zero in the circuit shown in Figure 8.3. In practice, there is significant common-mode gain caused by mismatch in the values of the equally numbered resistors, mismatch between the common-mode gains of the two input op-amps and mismatch between any stray impedances in the input paths. Therefore, it is not convenient to assemble such an amplifier with discrete components. Single-chip fabrication is far more successful with optimized matching of the input amplifier and resistors achieving CMRR values greater than 100 dB [2,4–5].

In order to give an idea of how a common-mode noise signal may enter the useful signal pathway, a case of ECG recording affected by power line and generic magnetic field interference is presented below [4].

An important practical source of noise that is not evident in Figure 8.2 is the power line coupling to the circuit and leads connecting the electrodes. This induced noise current can be measured between the patient's ground connection and the circuit grounding and has been observed to change with proximity to noise sources such as power lines. Therefore this noise signal will influence the quality of the measurement in an unpredictable way depending on the environment. Furthermore, a similar current may be induced directly from the power line to the subject. An additional induced noise source originates from a magnetic field generated by the subject itself. This magnetic field passes through an imaginary surface between leads, electrodes, and the circuit connections and induces currents in the patient leads. Any movement here will cause this noise source to be unpredictable and a common solution is to twist the electrode lead pairs. The twisted leads have been shown to be very successful in rejecting magnetically induced electric fields with perhaps the best

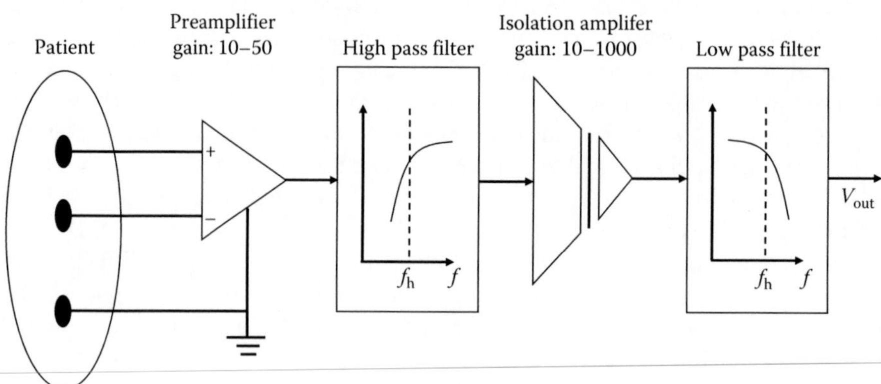

FIGURE 8.2 Schematic design of the main stages of a biopotential amplifier. (Adapted from J. D. Bronzino (Ed.), *The Biomedical Engineering Handbook*, second edition, Vol. 1. CRC Press, 2000.)

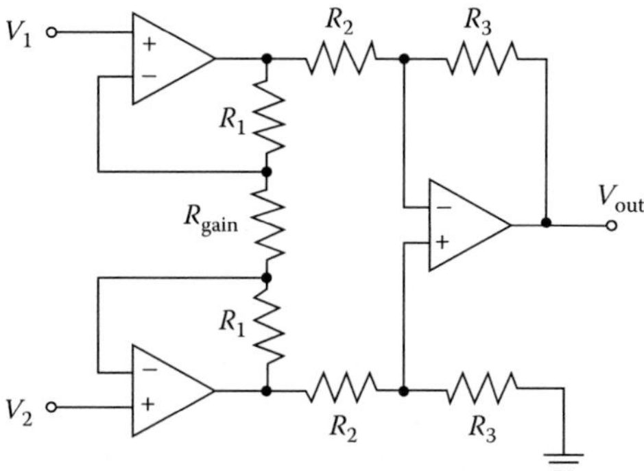

FIGURE 8.3 Classical differential amplifier implementation of an instrumentation amplifier using three op-amps.

example the enabling of recording of biopotentials inside the high-intensity magnetic field of an MRI device.

The last consideration on the schematic depicted in Figure 8.3 is about its input impedance. Without entering into too much detail, it is possible to say that such an impedance is as high as possible because at each input terminal, the signal source is directly connected to the input of an op-amp. These op-amps are specifically designed to offer the highest possible input impedance, with currently commercially available amplifiers offering input impedance of giga-ohms or greater.

Another crucial point in the implementation of the complete biopotential recording system is the subject protection. In Figure 8.2 it is represented by isolation amplifiers that are also useful for breaking ground current loops and eliminating source ground connections. However, in a biopotential recording system, the main purpose of the isolation amplifier is to protect the patient by eliminating the hazard of electric shock resulting from interactions among the patient, the amplifier, and other electric devices in the patient's environment, specifically defibrillators and electrosurgical equipment. Isolation amplifiers are realized in three different technologies: transformer isolation, capacitor isolation, and optical isolation. An isolation barrier provides a very high galvanic separation of the input side (i.e., the patient and the preamplifier) from all expected equipment on the output side. Ideally, there will be no flow of electric current across the barrier [2,4]. But, in practice, devices have an isolation of thousands of volts, which protects the subject from any reasonable risk they may encounter. Furthermore, advanced complete biopotential amplifier designs are completely floating and coupled wirelessly with data analysis stages. Here we have not addressed the filter design; however, this is highly dependent on application and the frequency range of the biopotentials of interest. The filter stages do not usually present great difficulties compared to the other issues such as contact impedance and safety concerns and so we believe that the filter stages are not as crucial as the preamplifier and insulation stages. These analog stages are followed by digitization via analog-to-digital conversion. Once the signal has been digitized it is much more flexible and convenient to apply sharp digital filters.

8.2.2 Galvanic Subject Isolation

When a living subject becomes part of an electrical circuit, the biological effect of the current may affect their safety—death or severe injuries may occur. As a consequence, safety precautions for the use of biomedical instruments (bioamplifiers in particular) must be put in place. The presence of leads and electrodes means that all possible precautions should be taken to reduce the possibility of injury or death if a malfunction occurs.

Medical devices can cause injury because of the actions or inactions of their inventors, designers, manufacturers, shippers, inspectors, maintainers, or operators. For example, the manufacturer may fail to properly assemble or construct an otherwise efficaciously designed medical device, or the shipper who transports a properly manufactured device could damage it in transit [6].

These regulations are detailed in [2,4,6–9]. However, it is important to bring forward two of the most relevant safety concerns associated with bioamplifiers: (1) the microshock and (2) the electromagnetic field irradiation due to microwave transmission systems.

Given the recent advances in the design of bioinstrumentation, bioamplifier designers must take into account both microshock and electromagnetic field irradiation. Microshock may arise from a faulty power supply unit; it is a key source of danger because of the presence of leads and electrodes that are directly connected to the subject. Moreover, damage may arise from the presence of a continuous electromagnetic field caused by the choice of a wireless insulation stage, such as the one depicted in Figure 8.2. Because of their importance, more details of these two sources of danger are provided.

8.2.2.1 Micro- and Macroelectrical Shock

There are two forms of shock: micro- and macroshock. The obvious difference between the two is the magnitude of the current that passes in the subject's body. It is well known that electrical current has many different effects on the human body, and that the impact of the effect will depend on its magnitude and the path it takes. Only the effect of alternating current (AC) from power distribution lines is considered because it is the primary current source for common appliances (120–220 V AC current at 50–60 Hz). The impact of AC current on the body is summarized in Table 8.1.

However, microshock, which can be cause of ventricular fibrillation, may occur with a current threshold as low as 20 μA when there is a direct low-impedance pathway (i.e., leads and electrodes) across the human heart [2,4,7,10]. The 20 μA threshold value has been recently updated at 50 μA and is specifically for broken skin connections that cross the heart? I think we would better check these against the IEC 60601 latest guidelines—also give the figure for unbroken skin, which is more relevant for noninvasive biosensing.

Therefore, bioamplifier design must take into account this potential danger. For example, the leakage currents must be kept below the cited limit and lead breaking circuits may be used in case of current overflow [2,4,7,10].

8.2.2.2 Electromagnetic Risk

This kind of safety concern is relatively new and specific publications on this matter have appeared only recently. Concern may have arisen due to the increasing use of personal transmission systems, which operate within the microwave bandwidth and consequently expose the human body to continuous electromagnetic irradiation.

The long-term effect of such exposure has not been clarified; however, there are some standards and guidelines that are available for the insulation stage and/or the communication unit where

TABLE 8.1
Human Response to Electrical Contact

Response	Average Minimum AC Current Level
Sensation-tingling (first perception)	1 mA
Painful shock but no loss of muscle control	9 mA
(Cannot) Let go	14 mA for males (10 mA for females)
Painful muscle contraction/difficulty breathing	23 mA
Ventricular fibrillation	50 mA (hand-to-hand contact)
Myocardial sustained contraction	Greater than 1 A
Burns (thermal injury)	Greater than 1 A

wireless microwave transmitters are adopted to communicate with large mainframes. Further details are available online and in [11].

8.2.2.3 Common Insulation Techniques

A complete description of the insulation techniques and classifications for biomedical instrumentation has not been provided in this chapter. However, given the safety risks mentioned in the previous section, bioamplifier designers must take into account the safety risk in producing a successful design. A brief discussion of the most important insulation techniques is provided below.

The most common technique used to obtain the galvanic insulation of the subject is to insulate the power supply unit of the bioamplifier. For this purpose, there are several medical grade chips available that provide the designer with a method for avoiding problems if creepage distances are observed [9].

In order to successfully transmit the detected signal to further stages without compromising the galvanic insulation, in addition to the already mentioned wireless radio technique, optical or capacitive coupling can be used.

In optical coupling, a light beam intensity is modulated by the information signal. At the other end, a light-sensitive element decodes the information received and translates it again into an electrical signal. The same principle is applied in the case of a capacitive coupler. In both cases, chips are available and the creepage distance once again must be respected.

Leads can be protected from overcurrent by using special lead breaker units. They are often used in combination with a gas discharger and clamping circuit. This also protects the preamplifier stage from defibrillator discharges [9]. Protection against leakage current may be easily achieved by adding a calibrated impedance prior to the electrode connection.

8.2.3 Review of Already Developed High-Impedance Biopotential Recording Systems

Here we present the concept of biopotential recording systems in the context of its history of development. We start from the well-explained instrumentation amplifier (see Section 8.1 and in particular Figure 8.2). Studying the available literature, it is in fact possible to observe that over the last two decades many researchers have attempted to solve the major problems affecting biopotential measurement instruments by redesigning the structure of the amplifier, or introducing new concepts, circuits, and electrodes. In this section, a review of the most important milestones in biopotential circuit design and implementation is presented.

Before introducing the reader to new concepts in biopotential recording design, it is noteworthy to analyze what improvements can be made to it, for example, to extend the bandwidth of the preamplifier stage to as close as possible to the DC mean value (ideally rejecting just the DC), without altering the DC coupling with the body. This technique is known as DC rejection, namely, the DC is erased using a feedback technique (for further theoretical details of this technique, see [9]). In this chapter, it is interesting to briefly introduce the DC rejection solution presented in [12], which used a feedback based on an optical transduction of the DC mean value.

Figure 8.4 presents a schematic diagram of the bioamplifier as it was proposed in [12]. The bioamplifier design is based on the classical three op-amp instrumentation amplifier with the gain value set by a single resistor (whose value is 220 Ω in Figure 8.4). As one should note from the figure, in parallel with the gain resistor there is an optical controlled voltage generator (transistors 4N35). This voltage source may have the same effect as a capacitive cell (high-pass effect) placed at the gain resistor place, when its voltage is controlled by a block having the same transfer function. In the proposed circuit, the controller has been realized with an integrator, thus realizing the feedback block with a transfer function of $1/s$.

The same authors [12] later proposed to move the feedback from the input stage of the instrumentation amplifier directly at the input at the differential stage (the rightmost amplifier in Figure 8.3) with a full differential network [13]. Such approach is depicted in Figure 8.5 limited to the instrumentation

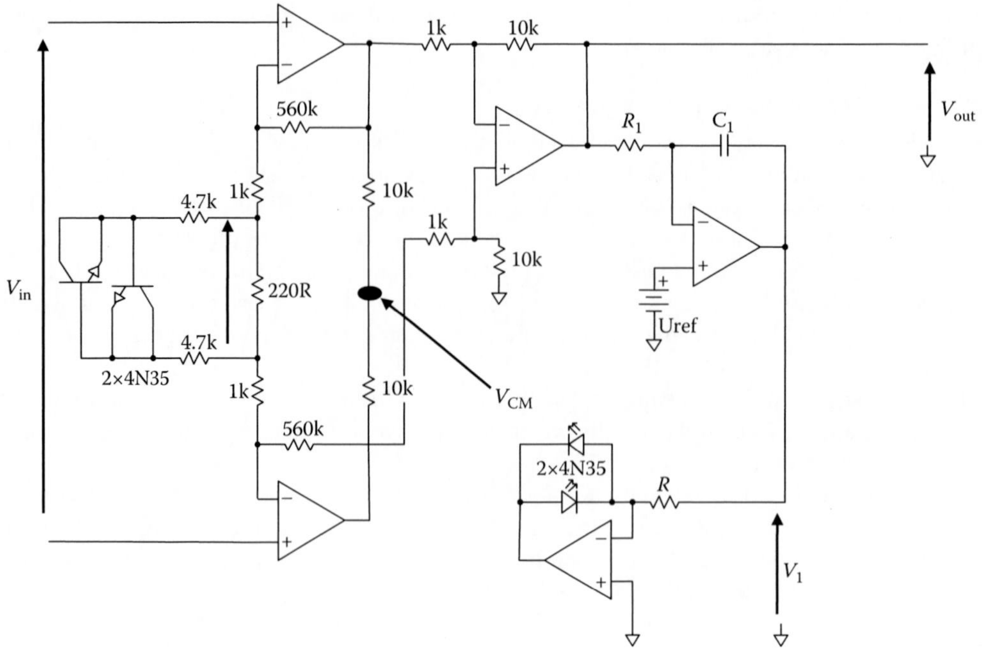

FIGURE 8.4 DC rejection bioamplifier as it is proposed in [12].

amplifier input stage and feedback network; in the figure, the transfer function in the larger block is obviously the one of an integrator circuit dimensioned to achieve the requested low-pass filtering. The other constant factors (1/α and 1/β) are the degrees of freedom that are to be balanced taking into account the remaining part of the instrumentation amplifier (not shown here); for further details see [13].

Another well-known methodology for realizing feedback that rejects the DC mean is referred to as the quasi-high-pass instrumentation amplifier [5]; this methodology is also well documented in several readily available instrumentation amplifier chips such as INA118 (by Burr Brown TI) [14]. Recalling the instrumentation amplifier schematic diagram as depicted in Figure 8.3, instead of applying the feedback at the input buffers, it may be applied at the ground terminal of the differential amplifier (the rightmost amplifier in Figure 8.3). Such an application to obtain high-pass behavior at 1.59 Hz is depicted in Figure 8.6 [14].

There is a well-described body of literature on improving the CMMR and reducing noise in biopotential recording systems. The first (and perhaps the most important) noise reduction technique was developed for electrocardiography several decades ago and it is referred to as right leg driver. In this circuit configuration the patient is not grounded, instead (in the exemplificative case

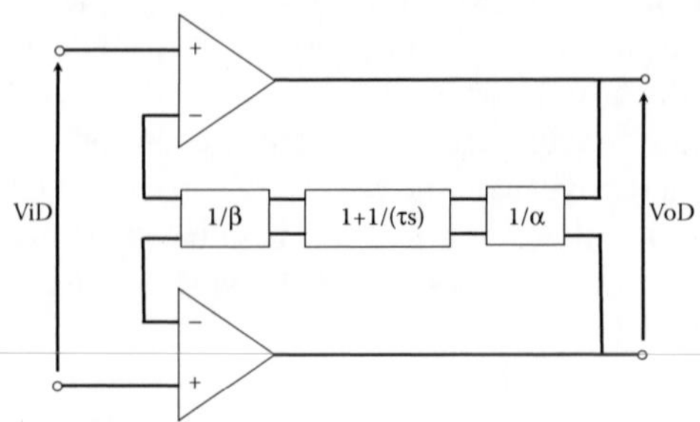

FIGURE 8.5 Fully differential DC mean feedback as proposed in [13].

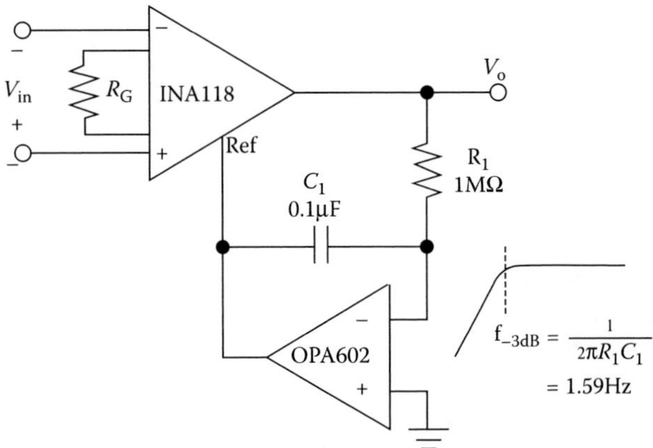

FIGURE 8.6 Quasi-high pass instrumentation amplifier. (Adapted from BurrBrown, INA 118 Precision low power Instrumentation Amplifier, *Technical data*, 2000.)

of the electrocardiogram (ECG)), the first two leads are used to record the ECG and the associated common-mode signal. This is inverted and fed back to the body via an additional fourth lead. This additional lead is not used for recording itself but improves the recording in the first two leads and the overall CMRR of the system [2,4,9,15].

A classical right leg driver (RLD) circuit and connection is depicted in Figure 8.7. As is clear from the figure, the common-mode voltage sensed by the resistors R_a and R_b is then inverted (with some amplification) and used to drive the entire body through the patient's right leg. In this way, the body common-mode voltage is driven to a lower value. Moreover, the body displacement current does not flow to the ground but flows through the driving amplifier, thus reducing the interferences captured by any ground loop [4]. This circuit also provides some electrical safety because it may increase the resistance between the body and the ground [4].

Over the last few years, the RLD circuit has evolved and may be present instead of a simple grounding in other bioamplifiers. Interesting to note is the modification to the RLD circuitry

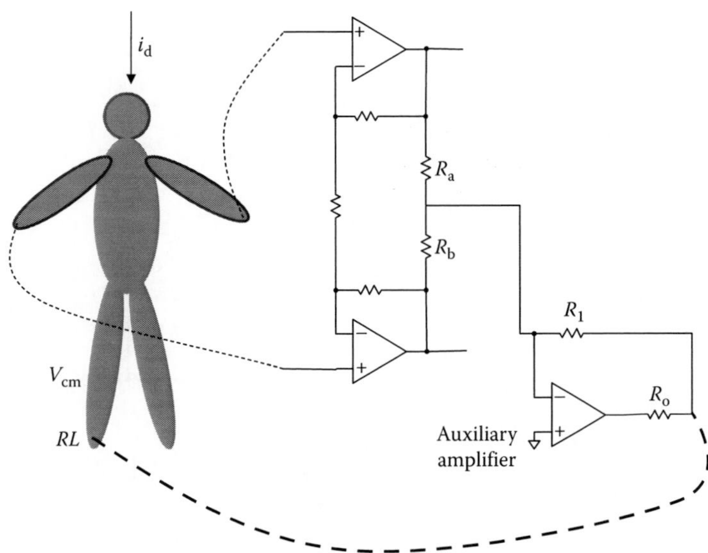

FIGURE 8.7 RLD for ECG application (Adapted from BurrBrown, INA 118 Precision low power Instrumentation Amplifier, *Technical data*, 2000.)

presented in [16] where a trans-conductance amplifier is used to drive the patient's body instead of a conventional voltage op-amp. This replacement results in some interesting features:

1. The amplifier's output is a current source; thus the circuit stability becomes independent of the impedances of the third electrode and the protection resistor [16].
2. The bandwidth of a typical trans-conductance amplifier is around a few mega-Hertz, so it does not contribute poles in the range of frequencies of interest [16].

There is another well-known technique for reducing the common-mode interference due to electromagnetic coupling of the body and the circuit with a large signal source (e.g., the power line). This technique, presented for the first time by Hewlett and Packard (HP) [17,18], is known as the bootstrapped common-mode circuitry. Namely, it does consist in driving the common terminal of the differential amplifier to the body voltage. The schematic diagram as it was presented by HP in 1978 is presented in Figure 8.8. In this diagram, the isolated common mode of the input amplifier is driven by the amplifier A3 to the body voltage, and the capacitor is added to block eventual voltage offset of this amplifier. Unlike the driven-right-leg circuit, the third electrode is not needed for driving the body potential [18]. More recent bootstrapped bioamplifier designs are available in the literature; for further design ideas, see [9,19].

However, many experimental results demonstrate that improving the design of the amplifier stage does not suffice for the requested noise immunity. In fact (as already mentioned in Section 8.1) noise may be captured as well at the leads and electrode level. To the best of our knowledge, the optimal way of reducing such noise capturing is to use shielded cable, the shortest possible cables and twisted leads [4].

A further action in the leads' noise immunization may be the use of the active guard ring [5]. This well-known technique has been used for years to protect the weak signals detected by sensors (in the biomedical case, electrodes) and to reduce the signal dispersion in shielded cables [5]. Ideally, shielding the cable carrying a weak signal would make the signal immune to any external electromagnetic noise interference. Unfortunately, the shielded cable may be regarded as a distributed capacitor; thus, any charge induced to the shield (one of the plates of the capacitor) may reflect on the core that carries the signal. While it seems to be an easy task to minimize this interference by driving the shield to the ground value, this action may increase the signal dispersion to the ground

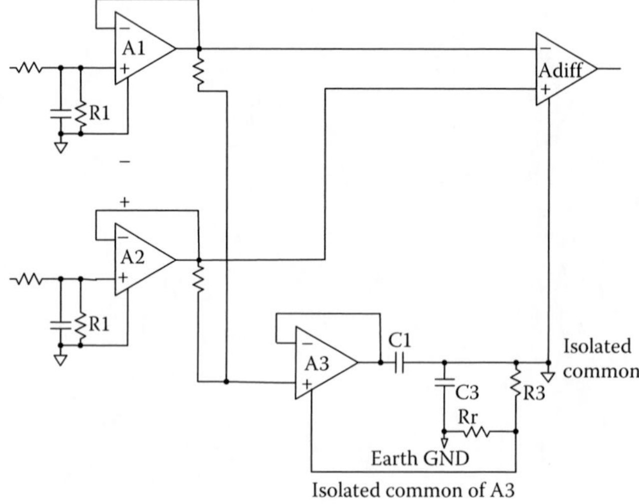

FIGURE 8.8 Bootstrapped common-mode circuitry as presented for the first time by Hewlett and Packard (HP). (Adapted from A. Miller, Coupling circuit with driven guard, US Patent 4191195, 1978; B. B. Winter and J. G. Webster, *IEEE Transaction of Biomedical Engineering,* BME-30, 58–62, 1983.)

because the resulting impedance through the ground is comparable with the input impedance of the amplifier. In order to minimize this effect, the shield should be driven with a signal as close as possible to the one present in the core. This concept is at the basis of the active guard circuitry [16] that is often used in biomedical applications by driving the shield to a potential close to the electrodes. This potential is derived from the bioamplifier itself. An example of the active guard joint with RLD for ECG applications can be found in the INA118 (by Burr Brown) application notes [14].

The recommendation that the leads be kept as short as possible has been taken literally by some researchers who have started investigating the possibility of building the front end directly at the electrode. This solution is often referred as an "active electrode" and has a number of advantages and some major drawbacks that still impede such technology. Historically, the necessity of buffering the signal at the electrode level was presented as a solution for paste-less or dry electrodes.

The general schematic diagram of an active electrode is depicted in Figure 8.9. As can be seen from the schematic diagram, it is essentially a voltage follower encapsulated in a guarded ring with a carefully calibrated biasing circuit. The voltage follower is used because of its very high input impedance (usually the same offered by the amplifier in use), and the guard ring, recalling the definition of the active guard explained above, is obtained from the amplifier output itself (ideally it is a replica of the input). The feedback and the biasing circuitry are to be designed in accordance with the amplifier in use; further details can be found in [9,20–26]. Without entering into too much detail, it is worth clarifying that some of the so-called active electrodes are also referred to as contactless [21,26]. The word "contactless" really means that the biopotential is detected remotely [21] or acts as a capacitively coupled rather than resistively coupled interface [9]. These can be made very sensitive as the impedance is very high and small potentials can be recorded. However, they are more sensitive to movement artifacts, first, due to the capacitive coupling, which will couple with anything in the environment including the subject, and second, due to the fact that these electrodes must be larger and heavier than simpler electrodes, leading to more movement. A block schematic of such system as presented in [26] is depicted in Figure 8.10.

Whichever is the case, the resulting circuit may be regarded as a real charge amplifier. In other words, if the buffer offers enough input impedance, the small biocurrent circulating in the skin electrode interface will be able to induce capacitively a charge flow at the conductive plate coupled with the amplifier. Thus, with the appropriate feedback, such a charge flow, which is a replica of the biocurrent circulating at the skin/electrode interface, is translated into a useful voltage signal that can be sensed by further stages of amplification (see Figure 8.11).

Despite the obvious advantages offered by the so-called active electrodes (such as the claimed signal-to-noise ratio improvement and the dry electrode capability), there are some drawbacks that impede such kinds of design to take off and overcome the so-called wet electrodes (traditional systems using gel).

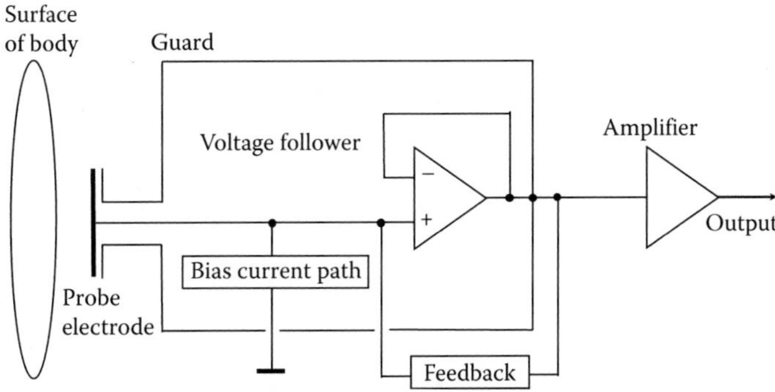

FIGURE 8.9 Active electrode general schematic. (Adapted from C. J. Harland et al., *Measurement Science and Technology Journal*, 13, 163–169, 2002.)

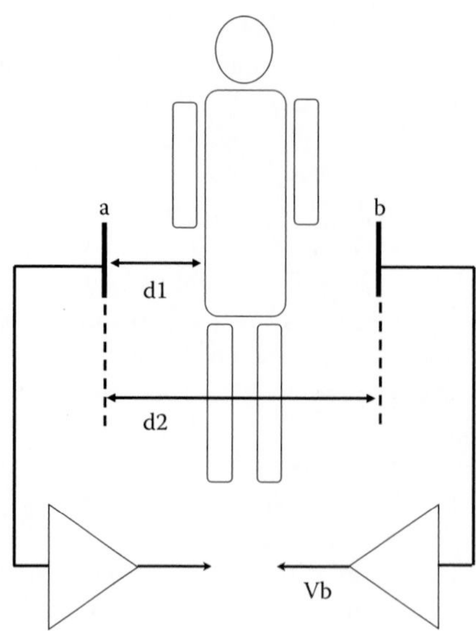

FIGURE 8.10 Remote biopotential recording as proposed in [21].

First, one should observe that active electrodes do not replace the bioamplifier; most of them are in fact designed (they have a unitary gain) to work in combination with them, presenting the disadvantage of a more complicated lead system. Because the active electrode circuit needs to be powered, each lead must carry signal and power supply, so it is not often possible to connect directly the active electrodes to the existing system in use (lack of power socket) and an alternative power source must be arranged.

Moreover, such electrodes present the disadvantage of cost. Often they are not disposable (because of the presence of the circuit) and they have to be cleaned and sterilized for use on the next patient. Again, the presence of a circuit inside may pose cleaning and sterilization problems. Furthermore, a significantly heavy printed circuit board (PCB) must be mounted close to the electrode, introducing additional mechanical strain on the contact [25]. Other active electrode implementations use as the electrode plate a micromachined metal plate that is designed and constructed

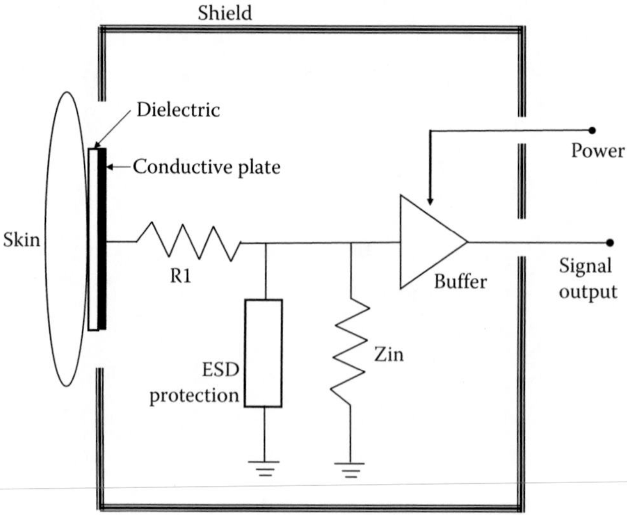

FIGURE 8.11 Insulated contact-less active electrode. (Adapted from D. Prutchi and M. Norris, *Design and Development of Medical Electronic Instrumentation*. John Wiley & Sons, Inc. Publication, 2005.)

with the same care of a microchip [24]. Finally, the majority of them are not directly serviceable, because for safety and sterilization reasons they have to be sealed.

8.2.4 Amplifier Front-End Basic Design

In this section, the development of a very high input impedance bioamplifier and its set of passive dry electrodes is discussed. As clarified in the text later, the proposed electrodes are designed to be passive and dry and in some cases insulated. However, they can also accommodate "wet" applications.

For the front-end design, particularly for the preamplification stage, a single chip is chosen. The chip is INA116 [27] (by Burr Brown TI). It is an instrumentation amplifier and the advantages of the use of a single instrumentation amplifier have been clarified in Section 8.1.

Even though this chip has been around for several years, it still has the highest input impedance available (10^{15} Ω). It has a maximum input bias current of 3 fA and an input current noise of 0.1 fA/√Hz. Furthermore, this IC also offers integrated active guard shielding, which is used to shield the electrodes. Moreover, it features built-in electrostatic discharge and overvoltage protection [27].

Figure 8.12 shows the first prototyped implementation of the front end. The INA116 is designed to work with a 9 V dual-power supply, but due to the very low bandwidth and the small amplitude of the biological signals we intend to measure, we were able to use it with a single-ended voltage supply as low as 2 V.

In this initial design, the total gain was configured to be ~700 V/V using the component values in Table 8.2. The total gain is given by the gain of the preamplification stage multiplied by the gain of the second stage. Because of the presence of artifacts and unpredictable skin/electrode contact impedance variation, which may generate large signals capable of bringing into saturation the preamplification stage, its gain is kept very low, ~6 V/V (in accordance with the INA116 specifications when a resistor of 10 kΩ is used [27]).

This circuit is preferably operated from a single battery. Thus, a virtual signal ground is derived from the battery using a compensated voltage divider (R_5/R_6). The virtual ground is also buffered to provide a driven ground connection via a coupling impedance R_{couple}. R_{couple} (placed before any electrode connection) is needed for protecting the subject from potentially large currents in the case of device malfunctions. Malfunctions and their effect on the body have been discussed in Section 8.2.3.

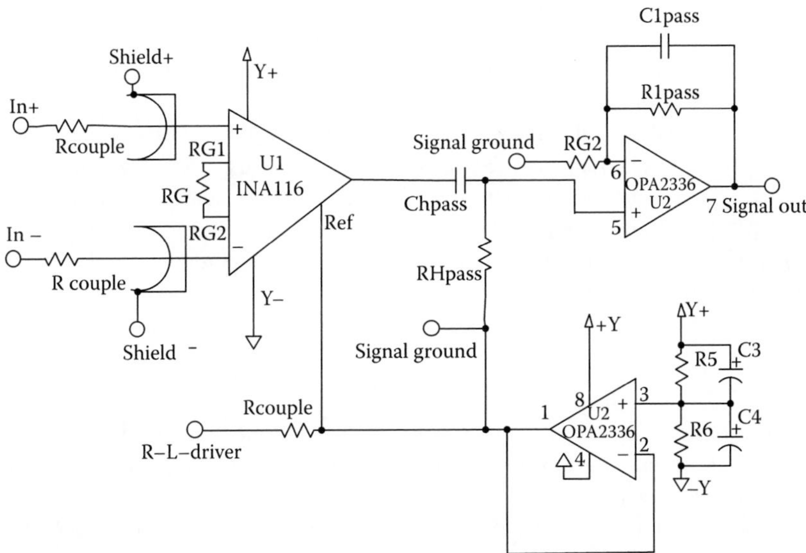

FIGURE 8.12 Front-end schematic. (Courtesy of HEARD Systems Pty Ltd, Sydney, Australia.)

TABLE 8.2
Component Specification

R_{Hpass}	390 kΩ	C_{Hpass}	1 μF
R_{Lpass}	1 MΩ	C_{Lpass}	3.3 nF
R_5/R_6	170, 102 kΩ	C3, C4	1 μF
RG	10 kΩ	RG2	7.5 kΩ
R_{couple}	100 kΩ	Cb2, Cb4, Cb6	100 nF
Cb1, Cb3, Cb5	10 μF		

However, to avoid introducing an imbalance at the input of the amplifier, care must be taken in matching the coupling impedance between each of the electrodes, including the driven ground. Such an imbalance may result in the degradation of the circuit's total CMMR.

The analog front end contains a low-pass filter and a high-pass filter to limit the bandwidth of the recorded signal. The cutoff frequency for the high-pass filter is tunable from near DC up to 5 Hz by changing the value of C_{Hpass} while R_{Hpass} is kept fixed at 390 kΩ. The cutoff frequency of the low-pass filter is regulated by tuning C_{Lpass} while keeping R_{Lpass} fixed at 1 MΩ.

The choice of fixing the circuit's bandwidth tuning capacitors instead of resistors may appear strange at first. However, it makes sense because as inferred by the schematic depicted in Figure 8.12, variance of the value of the resistor labeled R_{Lpass} to tune the low-pass frequency cutoff may badly affect the chosen gain. This implies that fine calibration of the resistor labeled R_{G2} should be an additional consideration. Given the large bandwidth span of biomedical signals (almost two decades, see the introduction to Chapter 3), the R_{Lpass} resistor value span could give very low corresponding values for the resistor RG2. Additionally, using commercially available component values, resistor/capacitors pairs are chosen in such a way that always the corner frequency is below (greater than) the standard used frequencies in the case of the low (high) pass filtering cell. Fine-tuning of the filter may always be achieved in postprocessing by using proper high-order filters.

Using commercially available precision components, for this prototype, we chose to implement a bandwidth of 0.38–44 Hz (±5%) suitable for most ECG as well as EEG applications [28]. It is possible to extend the circuit bandwidth up to ~1000 Hz (using commercially available capacitors of 15 nF) and down to ~0.04 Hz (using commercially available capacitors of 10 μF).

However, given that our aim was to monitor day-to-day activities and athletes, we chose to not extend the bandwidth. It is known that a value as low as 0.04 Hz for the high pass frequency would make the use of the monitoring device impractical because of the long recovery time associated with an amplifier saturation due to large body movements.

Moreover, extending the bandwidth up to 100 Hz or more would require an increase of the sample rate and the amount of EMG signal capturing will increase, especially in athlete monitoring.

The second stage of amplification and the driven ground are implemented using a low-power, precision op-amp (OPA2336 from Burr-Brown [29]). The second stage of amplification together with the band-pass filtering provides sufficient gain and high-frequency suppression to directly feed the analogue to digital converter (ADC).

8.2.5 Electrodes

Because of the number of issues raised by the use of conventional gel-based electrodes ("wet electrodes") and the skin preparations used for biomedical signal recording, there is an urgent need to find solutions to those issues.

A possible solution could be the use of the so-called "passive dry electrodes" [28,30–33]. These are distinct from active dry electrodes that require local active electronics, power supply over cables, additional manufacturing, and hermetic enclosures. Passive dry electrodes have no local active electronics, so it is possible to integrate them into garments or clothes, resulting in fewer restrictions for daily life activities.

Conductive rubber has several attributes useful for use in dry electrodes. Electrodes made from conductive rubber are durable, washable, and re-usable. The carbon and silicon materials, commonly used in conductive rubber, are biocompatible, and they provide a smoother and more uniform contact surface with the skin. They can be thin, flexible, and easily applied to a variety of substrates [34,35]. However, they have a much higher impedance than conventional wet electrodes [36].

Alternatively, textile electrodes, which can be embedded in clothes, can also be used as dry electrodes. These offer a high degree of patient autonomy and freedom of movement and are suitable for long-term monitoring. Textile electrodes are typically made of synthetic materials that endure abrasion very well. They do not irritate the skin, and are lightweight and washable. A major drawback is the high contact impedance of these electrodes, typically 1–5 $M\Omega/cm^2$, compared to the 10 $k\Omega/cm^2$ impedance for the disposable Ag/AgCl electrodes [37].

In fact, the high electrode impedance is a common issue with all types of dry electrodes. Therefore, to use these electrodes they must be connected to instrumentation amplifiers with extremely high input impedances [9].

The passive dry electrodes are made from commercially available 1.5 mm thick silicone conductive rubber shaped as discs of 8 mm diameter. Figure 8.13 provides a diagram of a dry electrode assembly. The active side of the electrode is capacitive coupled through a layer of insulating silicon rubber with a metal shield wired to the active guard shield.

The impedance of the realized electrodes at 100 Hz is greater than 20 MΩ with a parasitic capacitance not greater than 2 pF. Laboratory tests demonstrate that even a tolerance of 20% for the electrode's impedance is acceptable and does not influence the quality of the measurement, even in a multichannel montage.

To avoid any accidental contact with the electrode's shield or with the optional grounded cable sleeve, a final layer of insulation rubber (not shown in Figure 8.13) is poured to cover them [28,30]. The quality of the measurement is not influenced by the contact impedance imbalance between electrodes. In fact, it is possible to mix the electrodes—some dry and some wet—in our system.

In some applications (e.g., installation of the electrodes inside a standard EEG cap), the conductive layer is realized with thick conductive rubber in order to improve the hair penetration of the electrode. The electrode and the carrier act like a hair brush, thus improving the percentage of the electrode area in contact with the skin.

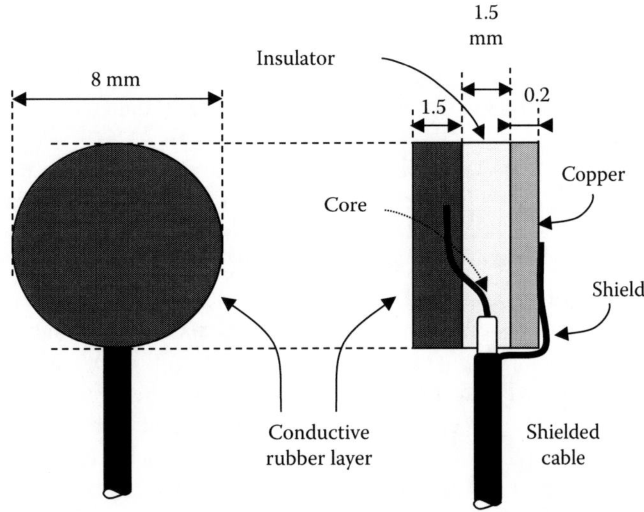

FIGURE 8.13 Passive dry electrode schematic.

8.2.6 Prototype Bench Tests

First, the amplifier has been tested using a patient simulator (Philips Fluke Medsim 300B) to ensure its biosignal compatibility (gain and bandwidth). The input impedance measurement was attempted on a Teflon-based PCB; however, none of the commercially available instruments are capable of reaching values as high as $10^{15}/2$ (Ω/pF), so a value denoting the open circuit (infinite) was reported.

CMMR was evaluated using the recommended testing circuits mentioned in [5,38]. Results were always within the typical range of 80–90 (dB) as specified by the producer [27].

Safety of the prototype was evaluated using a safety analyzer approved for these tests (Metron Q80A). In all the tests that could be conducted on a floating, battery-powered instrument, the current dispersion to the grounded case was always below 2 μA (the threshold for approved devices is set to 50 μA).

The internally generated noise was evaluated as the input electrodes were shortened [5]. Data were recorded using a sample rate of 2 kHz with shielded leads 1 m in length (as this is the length most likely to be used) terminated with electrodes as depicted in Figure 8.13. The two electrodes were kept in contact with each other using a nonmetallic clamp. The measured total input referred noise in the frequency band from 0.1 to 100 Hz was 0.660 μV_{rms} [33].

8.2.7 Multichannel Connection

As mentioned, biosignals, in accordance with the applications (e.g., ECG and EEG), are supposed to be measured either bipolarly or unipolarly. Often unipolar signals are referred to a single recording site (common reference) and all possible combinations of bipolar signals are then built offline by simple time-domain signal subtraction.

While a bipolar multichannel connection does not pose any circuital problem, a unipolar connection may pose problems that are to be taken into account. In some cases (e.g., the Wilson central terminal), the common point is derived by interconnecting the reference channels with a high value resistor. This solution may decrease the input impedance offered to the reference electrode when this is connected to the subject's body. When all the channels are equal, the input impedance offered to the reference electrode may be approximated with the relationship:

$$Z_{common} = \frac{Z_{in}^{-}}{n} \tag{8.2}$$

where Z_{in}^{-} indicates the input impedance offered by the inverting input of each channel and n is the total number of channels.

It should be clear from the previous discussion that the input impedance for dry electrode systems should be as high as possible in order to deal with the problems of (a) random contact impedance and (b) even worse, the random contact impedance imbalance between channels. The latter is even more critical for a passive dry electrode system that has to rely completely on the input impedance value of the amplifier to work properly.

To solve this problem without disrupting the input impedance of the proposed system, a special input circuitry has been developed.

Figure 8.14 presents (limited to the preamplifier sections) the interconnection between two channels with a single common reference. Namely, the guard terminal from the inverting input of the preamplifier is used to spread the signal to the next channel. In this circuit, the contact impedance offered to the reference electrode connected to the body is as high as possible and eventual impedance imbalance between channels is not greater than the normal components (INA116) tolerance.

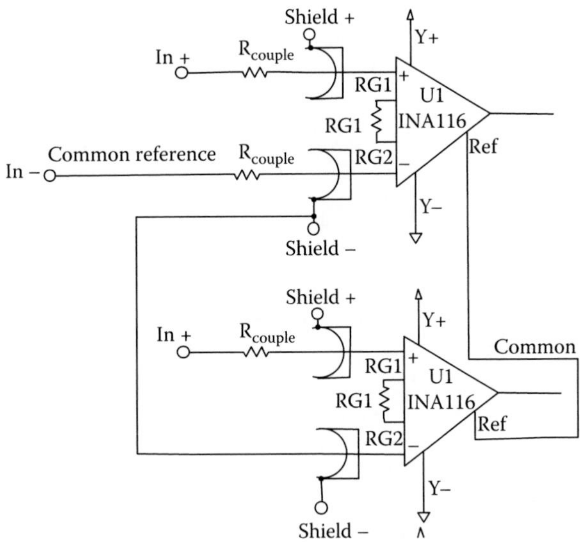

FIGURE 8.14 Multichannel wiring. (Courtesy of HEARD Systems Pty Ltd, Sydney, Australia.)

8.2.8 Analog Front-End Improvements

As mentioned in Section 1.3, it is possible to improve CMMR and electromagnetic noise capturing immunity by using the well-known technique of voltage bootstrapping.

The circuit schematic diagram depicted in Figure 8.12 has been improved by adding an improved bootstrapping technique. Thanks to the features offered by the preamplifier chip (INA116), the input circuitry can be simplified and the amplifiers A1 and A2 in Figure 8.8 are not needed. In fact the INA116 has the replica of the input voltage at the guard terminals readily available [27]. So the sum of the replicas can be used directly to drive the INA116 grounding terminal.

This solution has been used to draw the circuit schematic diagram shown in Figure 8.15 [32]. As can be seen from the picture, the signals from the shielding outputs are summed (using as weights an impedance R_{couple}) and then used to drive the reference terminal of the entire circuit including the virtual ground terminal.

Using the component values as reported in Table 8.2, there is no change of the input referred noise; however, laboratory comparison experiments showed that the circuit depicted in Figure 8.15 is more robust in terms of noise, and it can work in hostile environments such as on a farm for agricultural applications. We have found that it can be used with highly noncompliant subjects such as large farm animals.

An additional third connection to the patient (see Figure 8.15) may be obtained from the summing point. This optional connection should be connected to a neutral point on the subject's body (e.g., the nose tip in EEG recordings). In this configuration it can be said that a point on the body is used as the summing point of the general body common voltage itself and the common voltage as sensed at each electrode. When the resulting voltage is used to drive the amplifier common point, it erases the common body voltage from the output signal.

Because in this way the reference value for the preamplifier may change with the common-mode signal, it follows that the output dynamic excursion may be reduced at the expense of these improvements, and in fact, if the summed voltage rises too high, it will bring the driven common point close to one rail, and the output waveform may be deformed (i.e., clipping at the closest rail). Moreover, when adopting this technique care should be taken in choosing the R_{couple} impedance values to ensure that a current greater than 50 μA cannot flow through the subject [4].

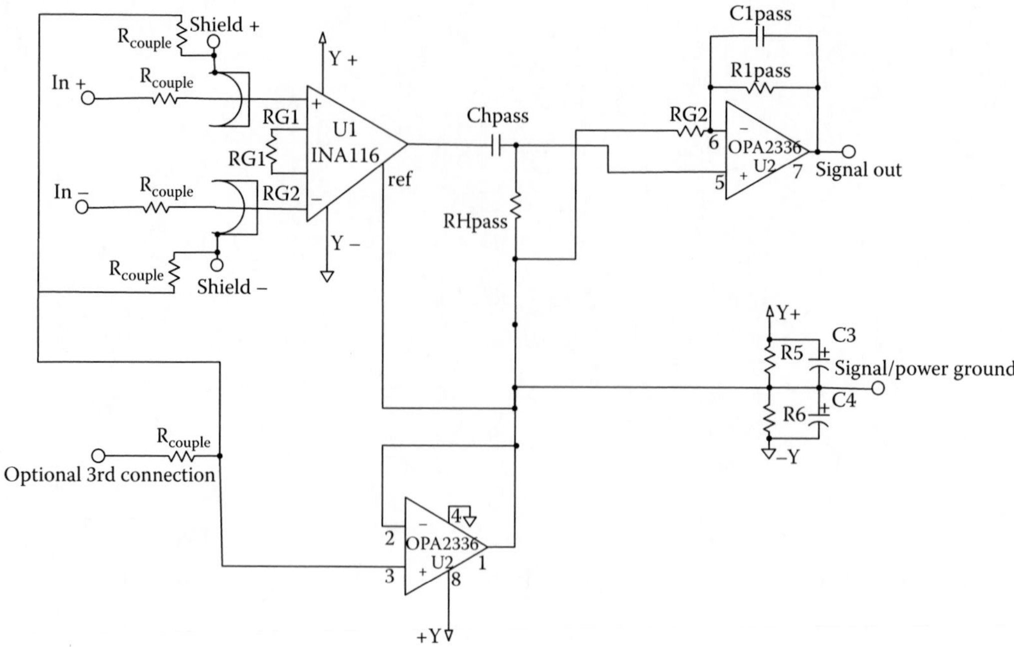

FIGURE 8.15 FVEP recording solid line: dry electrode; dashed line reference system. (Adapted from G. Gargiulo et al., *Clinical Neurophysiology,* 121(5), 686–693, 2010.)

8.2.9 Signal Shielding and Patient Insulation

For data transmission and patient insulation we use the BluesenseAD Bluetooth transceiver (by CorScience), which fulfills the EN 60601-1-2 medical electrical equipment standard [39]. It has an integrated 12-bit ADC and is designed to accept input signals up to 3.6V_{pp}. We chose to operate our analog front end with a 4.8 V supply and a limiting circuit has been added to the input of the ADC to protect the circuit. Figure 8.16 shows the BlueSenseAD schematic diagram including the necessary voltage regulators at 3.3 V for the digital circuitry and 3.6 V for the analog power. The

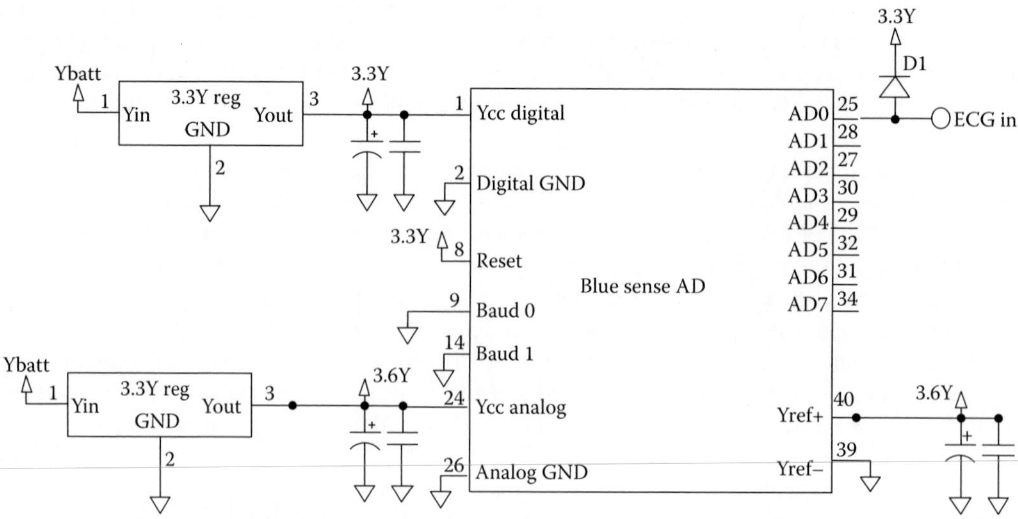

FIGURE 8.16 Schematic drawing of the BlueSenseAD connections [33].

BlueSenseAD can operate in standard mode or in SNIFF mode. In the standard mode, the trans-receiver consumes up to 160 mW, while in SNIFF mode, the power consumption drops to <30 mW. In SNIFF mode, the maximum data rate is only 10 kbs, limiting the maximum sample rate to 500 Hz, which is enough for most of our applications [40].

8.2.10 ECG Validation

For standard ECG measurements, electrodes are usually attached to the patient's skin after full skin preparation, which includes cleaning, shaving, mechanical abrasion to remove dead skin, and moisturizing. Moreover, a layer of electrically conductive gel is applied in between the skin and the electrodes to reduce the contact impedance [41].

However, the electrolytic gel in wet electrodes dehydrates over time, which reduces the quality of the recorded signals; this is the major problem that can affect long-term recording of ECG signals, for example, Holter recording. In addition, the gel might leak, particularly when monitoring an athlete during training or where the performance causes sweating, which could short circuit the recording sites. Short circuit between recording sites is even a bigger problem for monitoring athletes who are immersed in water.

Securing the wet electrodes in place is also complicated, since the electrodes cannot be glued directly to the skin due to the presence of the gel. The use of dry or insulating electrodes avoids these problems [42].

In order to confirm the ECG recording capability of the new system, it was first tested with a suitable signal simulator (Philips Fluke Medsim 300B). This kind of simulator is designed to ensure that both the ECG and the patient monitor are in working order. It is capable of simulating ECG signal on all the 12 leads simultaneously with standard-level outputs (up to 5 mV_{pp}).

The new system was then tested on a volunteer subject in parallel with a standard medical approved device. The reference device was g.Bsamp, which is used in the biomedical engineering department at "Federico II," the University of Naples. Parameters including signal bandwidth, and the gain of the new system were adjusted as much as possible to match the reference machine.

Figure 8.17 shows a direct comparison between signals recorded in parallel (Lead I) from the signal simulator using the new system (bold black line) and a commercial biopotential amplifier (g.Bsamp, dashed gray line). The reference signal (thin black line) is generated by the simulator. The g.Bsamp exhibits a second-order high-pass filter response close to DC, whereas our amplifier has a first-order high-pass filter response (see Section 1.4 for details). Point-to-point correlation between

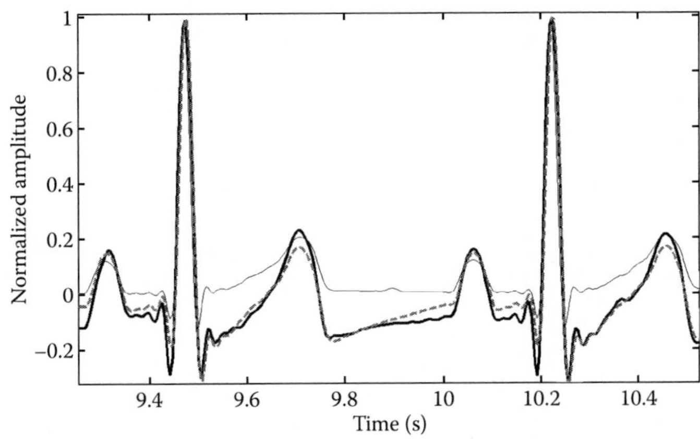

FIGURE 8.17 Direct ECG signal recording comparison: thin line reference signal, dashed grey g.Bsamp, bold our amplifier.

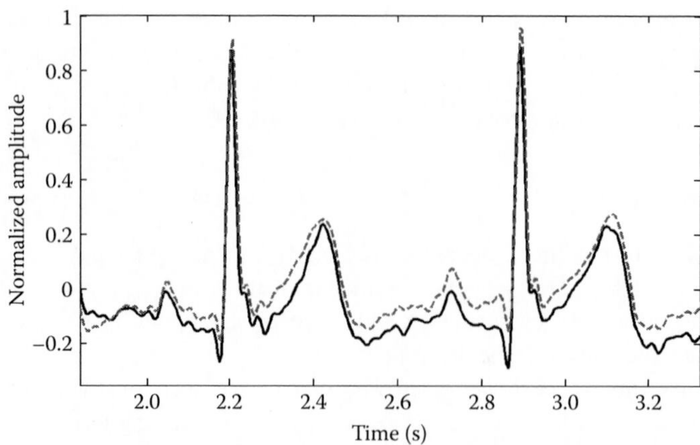

FIGURE 8.18 Direct ECG comparison lead I, bold line new system, dashed grey line g.Bsamp.

each of the signals is at least 0.94. Correlation between the recordings made with our amplifier and those made with g.Bsamp is larger than 0.96 [30,33].

The ECG capability of the new system was then completed by performing a parallel recording (using for both system standard Ag/AgCl electrodes) from a volunteer; an excerpt of such data is depicted in Figure 8.18, and the point-to-point correlation index was greater than 0.96 [33].

8.2.10.1 Passive Dry Electrodes versus Wet Electrodes

Recall that the system is completed by its passive dry electrodes as introduced in Section 1.5. The dry electrodes shown in Figure 8.13 are placed on the chest of a volunteer at the side of the ribs, held with an elastic band (approximating Lead I). They are located as close as possible to Holter long-lasting Ag/AgCl electrodes as used with the g.Bsamp system. No skin preparation was used for the dry electrodes, but preparation was necessary for the wet ones.

Visual inspection of the data (depicted in Figure 8.19) shows no evident differences between the signals confirmed by analytical analysis. Point-to-point correlation between the two recordings was scoring always larger than 0.96. Data recorded after the electrodes were left in place on the subject

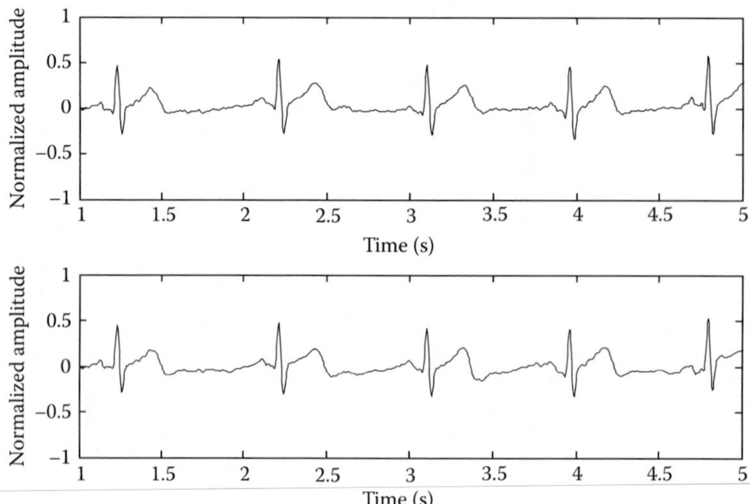

FIGURE 8.19 Direct comparison of ECG signals recorded from freshly installed electrodes (top) proposed system, (bottom) g.Bsamp using Holter Ag/AgCl electrodes.

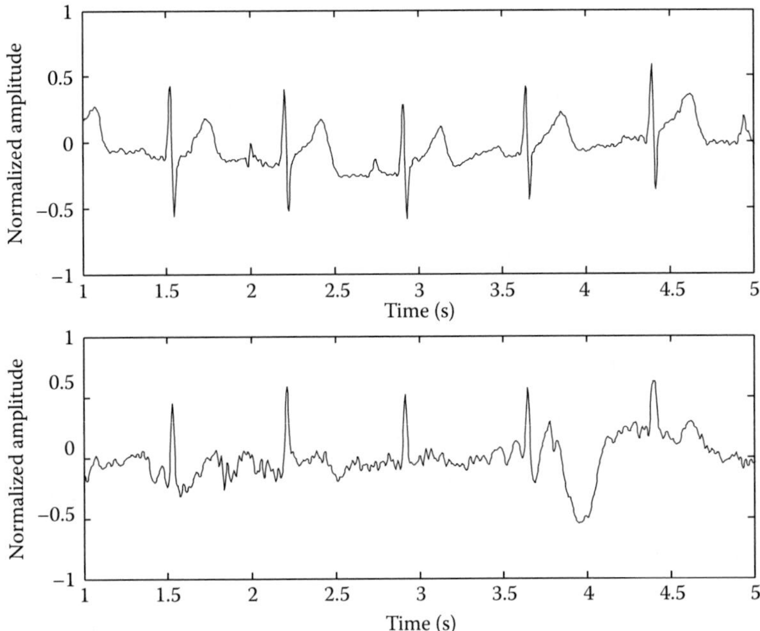

FIGURE 8.20 Direct comparison of ECG signals recorded after 48 hours (top) proposed system, (bottom) g.Bsamp using Holter Ag/AgCl electrodes.

for 48 h showed evident differences between the signals with an evident information loss for the system using the wet electrodes (see Figure 8.20).

8.2.11 EEG Validation

This section presents the EEG validation of the biomedical signal recording system described above as presented in [28,43]. As discussed, the standard procedure for the use of the so-called wet electrodes when performing EEG recordings involves substantial preparation and the application of conductive gels and glues [44].

Such preparation typically consists of head measurement, accurate electrode placement, and skin preparation which may involve an abrasive paste or soap [44]. Single electrodes are often kept in position using collodion. This method of electrode placement allows reliable, stable, and repeatable EEG recordings. It is a recommended practice to maintain the electrode contact impedance below 5 kΩ and any impedance imbalance to within 1 kΩ.

Long-term EEG recordings pose their own unique set of challenges that include the desiccation of the conductive gel or paste. The drying decreases the signal-to-noise ratio and increases the contact impedance, and when added with sweat and gel leakage, electrical short circuits between adjacent sites can result.

The use of dry electrodes may be a possible solution for stable long-term EEG recordings, and they are easier to use. There are a number of advantages that our dry electrode system offers. First, it does not require conductive gel or paste between the skin and the electrode surface to record a signal. Furthermore, it does not require any skin/scalp preparation. We have also developed a simple methodology to apply our flexible, dry, and flat electrode to the scalp without the need to shave hair.

It is thought that an advantage of the wet electrodes system is the application of a conductive gel that allows contact of the electrode with the scalp without the need to remove scalp hair. However, the same feat is accomplished with our dry electrode system without the use of a conductive gel.

Of course, shaving may provide some improvements of performance, but none of the subjects in our experiments were shaved [43].

8.2.11.1 EEG Recording Capability of the New Hardware

Evaluation of EEG systems can be difficult, since many parameters are involved, and EEGs cannot be reproduced in different recording sessions. The evaluation of new EEG recording systems is normally conducted by making a comparison with a reference system using two methods. In one method, referred to as the parallel method, electrodes for the test and reference EEG systems are placed at neighboring locations on the scalp and the signals are examined simultaneously in the time and frequency domains [45]. In another method, referred to as the serial method, the comparison between the reference and test systems is made serially by first connecting the reference system to a subject who performs a particular task and then repeating this measurement with the test system [46].

In order to demonstrate the EEG capability of the new hardware, our approach combined both techniques in three experiments. We used the parallel method to record simultaneously EEG signals for a reactive alpha rhythm. In addition, we used the serial method in a third experiment to record EEG signals from the same position on the scalp, in different trials during a reproducible task associated with flash visual-evoked potentials (FVEPs).

Prior to each comparison experiment, both systems were examined using a signal generator to determine hardware features such as filter cutoff frequencies and gain. An exact match of these hardware features was neither expected nor possible due to the presence of various hardware notch filters and varying filter responses (see Table 8.3). In addition, we note that an experienced electroencephalographer examined the recorded EEG signals for the three presented experiments; thus we can say that the EEG signals recorded from all the subjects, from both the test and reference EEG systems, demonstrated normal brain activity in awake subjects [43].

TABLE 8.3
Specifications of the Different Equipment Used

	New System	RPAH	g.BSamp GT201
HW bandwidth	0.05/0.5–40/150 (Hz) selectable	0.5–35 (Hz)	0.01–1000 Hz selectable
Filter order	Single	Single	Multiple
HW gain	6,000–60,000 (V/V)	Software regulated	160,000 (V/V)
HW input impedance	$>10^{15}$ Ω/2 pF	Not known	$>10^{11}$ Ω
Electrode ohmic resistance DC	~100 Ω	~0.4 Ω	~0.4 Ω
Recommended electrode–body contact impedance	Any, tested up to 10^9 Ω	<5 kΩ	<5 kΩ
Voltage supply	3.3 V up to 6 V	Not known	12 V
Maximum current absorption	6 mA + 36 mA (Radio) measured	Not known	1 A rated not including AD module
Power consumption	<250 mW full power <50 mW using SNIFF radio feature	Not known	9.6 W rated not including AD module
Weights	<400 g including battery	n/a	2 kg excluding battery and AD system
Input referred noise	<2 μV_{pp} DC ÷ 10 Hz	n/a	< 0.30 μV_{pp} DC ÷ 10 Hz
Special features	Active guarded shielded leads and electrodes	50 Hz, 60 Hz hardware notch filters	50 Hz, 60 Hz selectable hardware notch filter

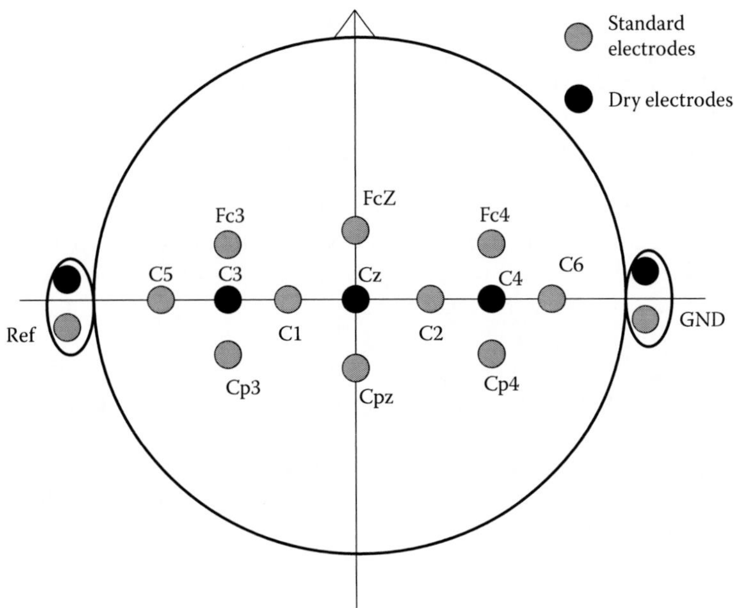

FIGURE 8.21 Experimental EEG montage (Adapted from G. Gargiulo et al., *Clinical Neurophysiology*, 121(5), 686–693, 2010.)

We first used the parallel method to record EEG signals. The test EEG system was configured with dry electrodes placed in the standard positions C3, C4, and Cz. The reference system (Compumedics®, Abbotsford, Victoria used at Royal Prince Alfred Hospital, Sydney, NSW) recorded simultaneously from standard locations Fc3, Fc4, Fcz, C1, C2, C5, C6, PC3, PC4, and PCz is depicted in Figure 8.21. The reference EEG system used standard golden brass cup electrodes with conductive gel (wet electrode) held in position using collodion. Each dry electrode was surrounded by four wet electrodes. These experiments were performed on eight healthy volunteers (seven male and one female, age range between 25 and 45 years old) [43].

In this first part of the evaluation experiment, we evaluated the alpha rhythm [47]. This is because the alpha rhythm is easily recognizable as one of the strongest brain signals in the EEG and it was also the very first signal correlated with real brain activity [41].

The EEG signals recorded with both systems were band-pass filtered (bandwidth 0.5–35 Hz; 50th-order finite impulsive response (FIR)) and an additional 50th-order infinite impulsive response (IIR) notch filter at 50 Hz was applied for the first two comparison experiments; see Table 8.3 for further details.

The serial comparison experiment involved recording a visual-evoked response. The visual-evoked potential is a transient response elicited by specific visual stimuli. It is used in combination with continuous EEG recordings to document the integrity of neural pathways and does not require a motor response. An example of such elicited responses is the FVEP. Despite the fact that FVEPs are very variable, they are often used in general medical practice to assess the eyes to cortex pathway integrity [48,49]. In this experiment, we compare the test EEG system configured with dry electrodes with a reference system referred to as the g.BSamp system which used standard brass golden cup electrodes. The g.BSamp system is in use at the biomedical lab at the University of Naples. Once again, as previously mentioned, both systems were first tested using a signal generator. Also, as previously mentioned, the EEG signals recorded with both systems were filtered using a software band-pass filter, 0.05 –100 Hz (50th-order FIR) and an additional 50th-order IIR notch filter at 50 Hz was applied.

The experiment was conducted following standard FVEP recommendations [50]. We recorded FVEP from three subjects. All subjects were male, healthy, and without any known visual or mental impairments. They had normal visual acuity and did not require refractive glasses and their age ranged from 24 to 30 years.

For this experiment electrodes were placed at standard position Oz. An additional ground electrode was placed on the right ear lobe. The recording positions were marked on the head using an eyeliner pencil and our dry electrodes were secured in position using an elastic band to avoid entangling the hair.

The subjects were asked to sit in an armchair for 30 min in a dimly lit room to allow light adaptation. After this period, a flash of light in front of the subject would produce the necessary stimuli as previously described [50]. The stimuli were randomly presented by the operator with an average interval of 2 s. Signals from the flash trigger and a light detector were recorded simultaneously with the EEG signal. The starting time for each trial was defined as 1 ms after the flash trigger. Consecutive trials showing an intertrial interval less than 1.1 s were rejected, as well as trials with an EEG peak signal amplitude greater than 50 μV_{pp}, since these trials would in all probability have been caused by eye blinks.

To compare the VEP waveforms between the two systems, signal averaging was performed for an identical number of trials with a minimum of 32 trials per system for each subject. We evaluated FVEP from the standard lead: Oz was referred to the left ear. The reference and test EEG systems were compared serially with a 30-min break in between the recording sessions. For the reference EEG system, the marked recording positions were prepared by the operator using a standard EEG preparation paste, that is, the wet electrodes were gelled, and secured in position using a bandage glued with collodion. The contact impedance was kept below 5 kΩ. Signal evaluation was performed with regard to looking for a peak in the evoked average potential at a standard time lag and amplitude for the P100 component [49,51].

While preparing the subject for the first experiment, the preparation time per electrode was recorded and averaged for all of the subjects. Based on our measurements, the average setup time for the reference system using standard wet electrodes is within the range of 2–3 min/electrode and includes: spot preparation using specialized abrasive paste, adding gel to the electrodes, electrode placement, sticking the electrode with bandage, and checking the contact impedance (and eventual electrode replacement in case the impedance is too large). The average setup time per dry electrode is about 10 s, which is mostly taken up by the time it takes the collodion to dry. Figure 8.22 shows a photograph of the electrode montage. In this figure, the dry electrodes are indicated by the arrows and it is possible to observe that they are directly in contact with the scalp through a thin film of collodion, while the wet electrodes are covered by white bandages (which are soaked in collodion).

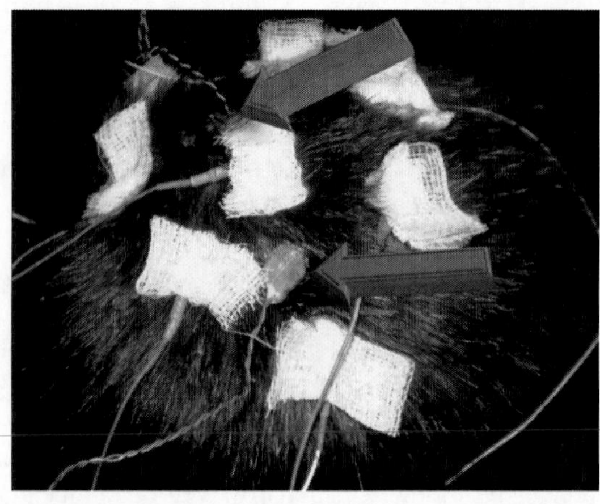

FIGURE 8.22 Photography of the experimental montage.

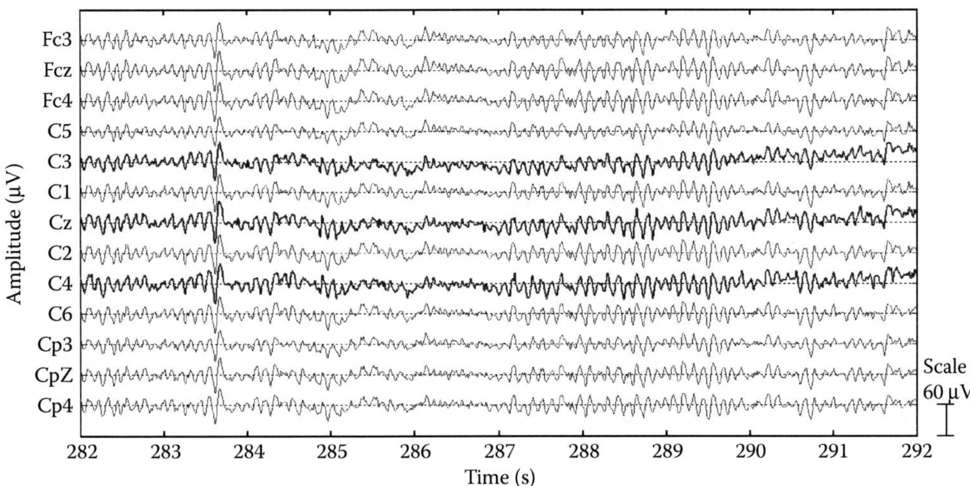

FIGURE 8.23 Alpha wave replacement, dry electrodes are in bold. (Adapted from G. Gargiulo et al., *Clinical Neurophysiology*, 121(5), 686–693, 2010.)

Recordings of the alpha rhythm were made using both the new EEG system and the reference EEG system. Visual inspection was used to ensure qualitative match between the two systems, before continuing with analytical comparisons. Figure 8.23 shows a recording in the time domain (10 s) of the signals recorded at the RPA hospital from one subject using the electrode montage depicted in Figure 8.21. In Figure 8.23 dry electrode signals are represented in bold. The phenomenon is more apparent in the frequency domain as shown in Figure 8.24. Observe the difference in the spectrum around 9 Hz between the eyes open (top panel) and eyes closed (bottom panel) cases as recorded by a dry electrode (solid line) and a standard wet electrode (dashed line) recorded in standard positions C4 and Cp4, respectively. Visually, both the dry and wet electrodes yield similar results and the data shown are representative of the recordings across the eight subjects. As the test and reference EEG signals were recorded on different computers, the signals were time-aligned by selecting the time alignment that maximizes the cross-correlation of the two signals. Analytical comparisons, after appropriate time alignment of the signals, showed that the average correlation coefficient between the dry electrode signal and the average of the four surrounding standard electrode signals was 0.82 (across all the subjects) [43].

When the correlation analysis was performed processing only the clean signals, the best correlation between the dry electrodes and the average of the surrounding electrodes was 0.94 with an average of 0.83.

The results obtained in the two field experiments, conducted to compare the new system with various different reference EEG systems, indicated that the alpha rhythm signals were highly correlated with signals recorded in parallel with a clinically approved system. The FVEP patterns (see Figure 8.25) had differences smaller that 10% in the amplitude of the P100 feature, which is considered as a marginal difference in clinical applications.

Thus, it is possible to affirm that passive dry electrodes may offer advantages for EEG monitoring (e.g., ease of application, stability, and reliability). Generally, the time required to apply collodion to the dry electrodes (10 s/electrode) is much less than the time required to prepare wet electrodes, while the time that the dry electrodes remain viable once attached is longer than that for wet electrodes. In summary, this new EEG system moves the state of the art closer toward one of the holy grail for the EEG recording system, namely (1) easy to use, requiring little time to install and remove; (2) portable, so people can use it at home and during daily activities; and (3) wireless, so in applications such as BCI and neurofeedback the data can be processed remotely by a more powerful computer.

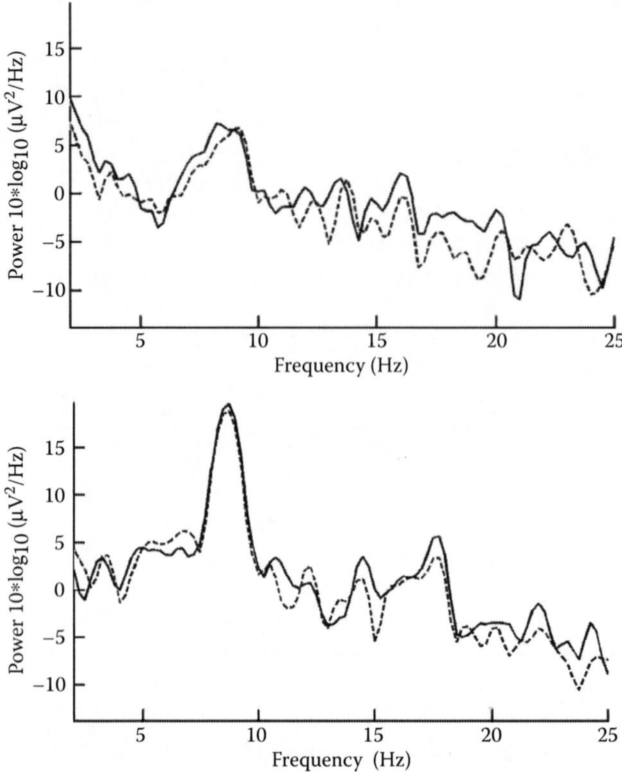

FIGURE 8.24 Power spectral density showing alpha wave replacement eyes open (top), closed (bottom) [43].

8.2.12 Application to Veterinary Science

The system performs well, and the combination of passive dry electrodes and the use of an ultrahigh input impedance front end suggests that the system could be successfully employed in veterinary science. The capability of obtaining recordings without performing skin preparations on noncompliant patients would be a considerable advantage. The next section discusses the applications being developed by HEARD System Pty Ltd.

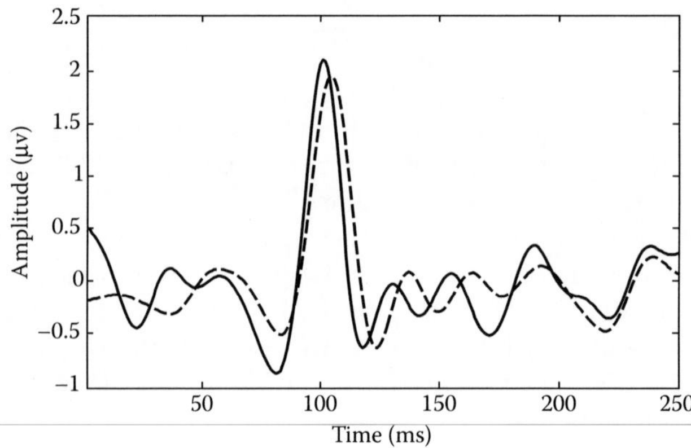

FIGURE 8.25 FVEP recording solid line: dry electrode; dashed line reference system. (Adapted from G. Gargiulo et al., *Clinical Neurophysiology,*121(5), 686–693, 2010.)

8.2.12.1 Early Pregnancy Detection in Large Farm Animal (Courtesy of HEARD Systems)

Pregnancy diagnosis is one of the most frequently performed diagnostic procedures undertaken on cattle [52–56]. Timely testing of individual cows for pregnancy supports optimal management of individual animals and the maximization of farm profit for both the dairy and beef production systems [57,58]. The current recommendations from the major beef and dairy industry research and development organizations in Australia are for each mated female to be pregnancy tested at least once per year [57,58].

The two most frequently used methods for pregnancy diagnosis of cattle are manual palpation of the reproductive tract (per rectum) and transrectal ultrasonography of the reproductive tract [53]. Alternative sample-based methods are under development. At present, no commercially viable test is available. These require the collection of either a milk or (invasive) blood sample, do not operate "cow side" or in real-time, can be of varying accuracy, and are usually not economical on a per test basis [59–61].

Furthermore, it is possible to say that both manual and assay-based tests in their current forms have limitations concerning practical use. The necessity to use highly skilled contractors to undertake either manual or ultrasound-based pregnancy testing effectively limits usage. Most testing using these methods is applied at the herd level—little testing of individual animals is performed and generally this cannot be conducted on demand. As a result, many animals are not tested at the optimal time for accurate diagnosis or for tailored management decisions to be made. In many countries and regions of the world, there is also a shortage of contractors to provide these services [62]. Rectal palpation is strenuous physical work for the operator. Increasing herd sizes are increasing the risk of fatigue-related and repetitive strain injuries among veterinarians and contractors providing whole-herd pregnancy testing services [63,64]. The high cost of ultrasound equipment and the extensive training required to achieve a suitable level of competence are a barrier to entry for new contractors. In many countries and jurisdictions, invasive pregnancy testing remains an act of veterinary science and nonveterinarians are unable to operate. Thus, a system based upon the noninvasive detection of the fetal heartbeat may allow the development of a real-time, noninvasive, and rapid pregnancy diagnostic system for cattle.

Such a system is currently under development by HEARD Systems. Field trials have captured fetal signals from cows from the 6th week of pregnancy onwards. The novel device developed by HEARD Systems is applied to the flank of the animal to detect physiological signals related to the pregnancy such as fetal ECG and fetal heart sounds.

The concept is well proven and an excerpt from a combined recording of fetal and maternal ECG is depicted in Figure 8.26. An excerpt from a fetal ECG (multileads recording) recorded with dry electrodes is depicted in Figure 8.27.

8.3 CONCLUSION

Giga-ohm input impedance FET amplifiers enable the recording of biopotentials in a range of important applications: ECG in athlete monitoring, EEG in long-term recordings such as the BCI, and fetal ECG detection in noncompliant subjects such as cattle. Important considerations must be made when designing the leads, electrodes, and printed circuit boards to maintain noise immunity, input impedance, and high CMRR. Safety is an important consideration where the increasing availability of wireless and low-power instrumentation enables ideal isolation from high-voltage supplies but at the same time introduces a further concern due to the RF radiation. The availability of optimized instrumentation amplifiers such as INA116 allows dry recordings without the need for active electrodes that are associated with increased costs and mechanical instability. These amplifiers also conveniently allow single referenced setups to avoid the use of common-mode feedback—difficult to provide with dry electrodes in the past due to increased contact impedance. The contact impedance has

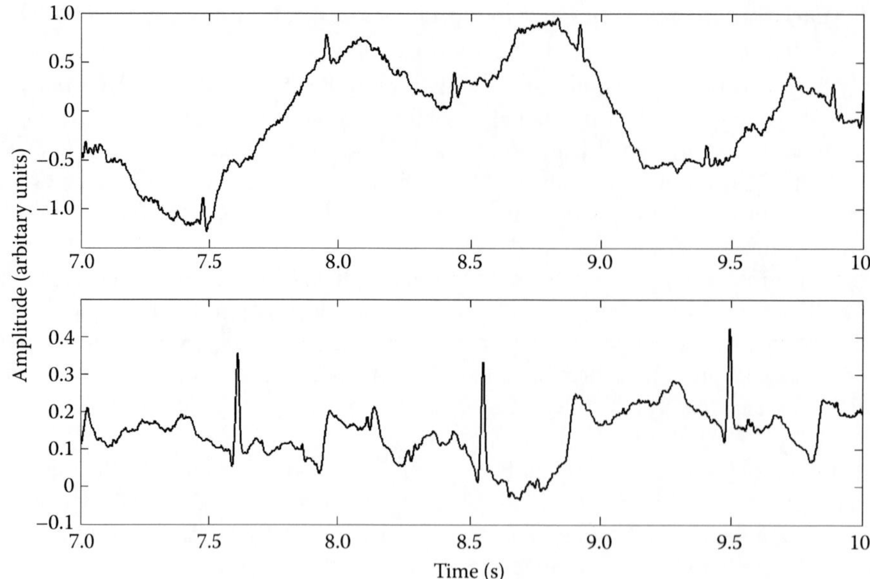

FIGURE 8.26 Combined recording of fetal (top) and maternal (bottom) ECG from a 16-week pregnant cow. (Courtesy of HEARD system.)

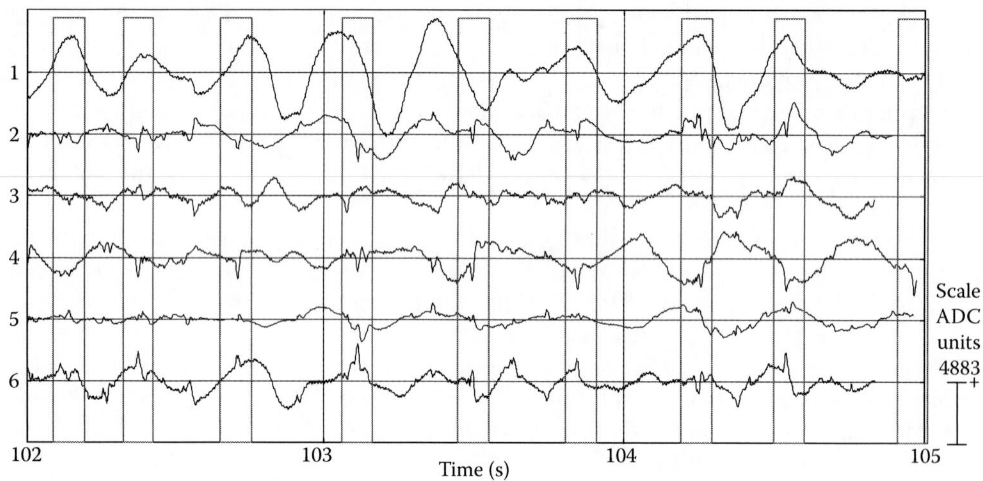

FIGURE 8.27 Fetal ECG recorded from a 18–20-week pregnant cow using dry electrodes. (Courtesy of HEARD Systems Pty Ltd, Sydney, Australia.)

been a concern in the past for dry electrode recordings; however, the high input impedance of the bioamplifier can now overcome this limitation. For safety it is also important to preserve contact impedance as it occurs as part of the body's natural protection against electric currents.

REFERENCES

1. J. D. Enderle, *Bioinstrumentation*, Vol. 6. Morgan & Claypool, San Rafael, CA, 2006.
2. J. D. Bronzino (Ed.), *The Biomedical Engineering Handbook*, second edition, Vol. 1. CRC Press, Boca Raton, FL, 2000.

3. J. G. Webster (Ed.), *Encyclopedia of Medical Devices and Instrumentation*, Vol. 1. John Wiley & Sons, Inc. Publication, New York, NY, 2006.
4. J. G. Webster (Ed.), *Medical Instrumentation Application and Design.* John Willey, New York, FL, 1998.
5. P. Horowitz and W. Hill, *The Art of Electronics.* Cambridge, New York, NY, 2002.
6. J. G. Webster (Ed.), *Encyclopedia of Medical Devices and Instrumentation*, Vol. 6. John Wiley & Sons, Inc. Publication, New York, NY, 2006.
7. M. Akay (Ed.), *Wiley Encyclopedia of Biomedical Engineering.* John Wiley & Sons, Inc. Publication, New York, NY, 2006.
8. J. Moore and G. Zouridakis (Eds), *Biomedical Technology and Devices Handbook.* CRC Press, Boca Raton, FL, 2004.
9. D. Prutchi and M. Norris, *Design and Development of Medical Electronic Instrumentation.* John Wiley & Sons, Inc. Publication, Hoboken, NJ, 2005.
10. J. Moore and G. Zouridakis (Eds), *Biomedical Technology and Devices Handbook.* CRC Press, Boca Raton, FL, 2004.
11. COMAR, IEEE Committee on Man and Radiation. (2000, Human Exposure to Radio Frequency and Microwave Radiation from Portable and Mobile Telephones and Other Wireless Communication Devices. Available at: http://ewh.ieee.org/soc/embs/comar/index.html
12. E. M. Spinelli and M. A. Mayosky, AC coupled three op-amp biopotential amplifier with active DC suppression, *IEEE Transaction on Biomedical Engineering*, 47, 1616–1619, 2000.
13. E. M. Spinelli et al., A novel fully differential biopotential amplifier with DC suppression, *IEEE Transactions on Biomedical Engineering*, 51(8), 1444–1448, 2004.
14. BurrBrown, INA 118 Precision low power Instrumentation Amplifier, *Technical data*, 2000.
15. J. G. Webster (Ed,), *Encyclopedia of Medical Devices and Instrumentation*, Vol. 3. John Wiley & Sons, Inc. Publication, New York, NY, 2006.
16. N. H. M. ı. Enrique Mario Spinelli, and Miguel Angel Mayosky, A trans-conductance driven-right-leg circuit, *IEEE Transactions on Biomedical Engineering*, 46, 1466–1470, 1999.
17. A. Miller, Coupling circuit with driven guard, US Patent 4191195, 1978.
18. B. B. Winter and J. G. Webster, Reduction of interference due to common mode voltage in biopotential amplifiers, *IEEE Transaction of Biomedical Engineering*, BME-30, 58–62, 1983.
19. D. P. Dobrev et al., Bootstrapped two-electrode biosignal amplifier, *Medical and Biological Engineering and Computing*, 46, 613–619, 2008.
20. C. J. Harland et al., Electric potential probes—new directions in the remote sensing of the human body, *Measurement Science and Technology Journal*, 13, 163–169, 2002.
21. C. J. Harland et al., Remote detection of human electroencephalograms using ultrahigh input impedance electric potential sensors, *Applied Physics Letters*, 81(17), 3284–3286, 2002.
22. E. R. Valverde et al., Effect of the electrode impedance in improved buffer amplifier for bioelectric recordings, *Journal of Medical Engineering and Technology*, 5, 2004.
23. M. J. Burke and D. T. Gleeson, A micropower dry-electrode ECG preamplifier, *IEEE Transaction on Biomedical Engineering*, 47(2), 155–162, 2000.
24. E. S. Valchinov and N. E. Pallikarakis, An active electrode for biopotential recording from small localized bio-sources. *Biomedical Engineering Online*, 3(25), 2004.
25. R. J. Prance et al., An ultra-low-noise electrical-potential probe for human-body scanning, *Measurement Science and Technology Journal*, 11, 291–297, 2000.
26. W. J. Smith and J. R. LaCourse, Non-contact biopotential measurement from the human body using a low-impedance charge amplifier, Bioengineering Conference, 2004. *Proceedings of the IEEE 30th Annual Northeast,* 31–32, 2004.
27. BurrBrown, INA116. *Technical Data*, 2008.
28. G. Gargiulo et al., A mobile EEG system with dry electrodes, in *IEEE BIOCAS*, Baltimore, USA, 2008.
29. BurrBrown, OPA336-2336-4336. *Technical Data*, 2008.
30. G. Gargiulo et al., Mobile biomedical sensing with dry electrodes, in *ISSNIP*, Sydney (NSW), 2008.
31. G. Gargiulo et al., Non-invasive electronic biosensor circuits and systems, in *Intelligent and Biosensors*, V. S. Somerset, Ed., IN-TECH, Rijeka, Croatia, 2010.
32. G. Gargiulo, A system for sensing electrophysiological signals, International Patent, 2009.
33. G. Gargiulo et al., An ultra-high input impedance ECG amplifier for long-term monitoring of athletes, *Medical Devices: Evidence and Research*, 3(3), 1–9, 2010.
34. S. Chang et al., Rubber electrode for wearable health monitoring, in *2005 IEEE Engineering in Medicine and Biology 27th Annual Conference*, Shanghai, China, 2005.

35. J. Muhlsteff and O. Such, Dry electrodes for monitoring of vital signs in functional textiles, in *26th Annual International Conference of the IEEE Engineering in Medicine and Biology Society (EMBC)*, San Francisco, CA, 2004, pp. 2212–2215.
36. A. Baba and M. J. Burke, Measurement of the electrical properties of ungelled ECG electrodes, *International Journal of Biology and Biomedical Engineering*, 2, 89–97, 2008.
37. M. Catrysse et al., Fabric sensors for measurement of physiological parameters, in *IEEE The 12th International Conference on Solid State Sensors, Actuators and Microsystems*, Boston, USA, 2003.
38. A. S. Sedra and K. C. Smith, *Microelectronic Circuits*, fifth edition. Oxford University Press, New York, NY, 2004.
39. P. Bifulco et al., Bluetooth portable device for continuous ECG and patient motion monitoring during daily life, in *MEDICON*, Ljubljana, Slovenia 2007.
40. CORSCIENCE, Blusense AD Data Sheet V 1.2, 2006.
41. J. G. Webster, *Medical Instrumentation Application and Design*. John Wiley, New York, NY, 1998.
42. A. Searle and L. Kirkup, A direct comparison of wet, dry and insulating bioelectric recording electrodes, *Physiological Measurement*, 21, 271–283, 2000.
43. G. Gargiulo et al., A new EEG recording system for passive dry electrodes, *Clinical Neurophysiology*, 121(5), 686–693, 2010.
44. M. Teplan, Fundamentals of EEG measurement, *Measurement Science Review*, 2, 1–11, 2002.
45. H. Iguchi et al., Wearable electroencephalograph system with preamplified electrodes, *Medical and Biological Engineering and Computing*, 32, 459–461, 1994.
46. F. Popescu et al., Single trial classification of motor imagination using 6 dry EEG electrodes, *PLoS One*, 2, e637, 2007.
47. P. V. Mohanan and K. Rathinam, Biocompatibility studies on silicone rubber, *14th Conference of the Biomedical Engineering Society of India,* pp. 4/12, 1995.
48. R.-C. Wu et al., Applications of event-related-potential-based brain computer interface to intelligent transportation systems, in *IEEE International Conference on Networking, Sensing and Control*, Taipei, Taiwan, 813–818, 2004.
49. P.-L. Lee et al., Visual evoked potential actuated brain computer interface: A brain-actuated cursor system, *Electronics Letters*, 41, 2005.
50. J. V. Odom et al., Visual evoked potentials standard (2004), *Documenta Ophthalmologica*, 108, 115–123, 2004.
51. K. Takei et al., Analysis of the components of electrically evoked response using a monopolar recording technique, *Investigative Ophthalmology and Visual Science*, 34, 1923–1929, 1993.
52. N. C. Friggens et al., Improved detection of reproductive status in dairy cows using milk progesterone measurements, *Reproduction in Domestic Animals*, 43, 113–121, 2008.
53. J. E. Romano et al., Early pregnancy diagnosis by transrectal ultrasonography in dairy cattle, *Theriogenology*, 66, 1034–1041, 2006.
54. S. McDougall et al., Pregnancy loss in dairy cattle in the Waikato region of New Zealand, *New Zealand Veterinary Journal*, 53, 279–287, 2005.
55. P. M. Fricke and G. C. Lamb, Potential applications and pitfalls of reproductive ultrasonography in bovine practice, *The Veterinary Clinics of North America—Food Animal Practice*, 21(2), 419–436, 2005.
56. O. Szenci et al., Comparison of ultrasonography, bovine pregnancy-specific protein B, and bovine pregnancy-associated glycoprotein 1 tests for pregnancy detection in dairy cows, *Theriogenology*, 50, 77–88, 1998.
57. Meat & Livestock Australia, *More Beef from Pastures: The Producer's Manual. More Beef from Pastures.* Sydney: Meat & Livestock Australia, 2004.
58. Dairy Australia, *The InCalf Book for Dairy Farmers*. Melbourne: Dairy Australia, 2003.
59. B. Kornmatitsuk et al., Measurement of faecal progesterone metabolites and its application for early screening of open cows post-insemination, *Reproduction in Domestic Animals*, 42, 238–242, 2007.
60. D. Cavestany and C. S. Galina, Evaluation of an artificial insemination programme in a seasonal breeding dairy system through milk progesterone, *Reproduction in Domestic Animals*, 36, 79–84, 2001.
61. D. Cavestany and C. S. Galina, Factors affecting the reproductive efficiency of artificial insemination programmes in a seasonal breeding pasture-based dairy system with the aid of milk progesterone, *Reproduction in Domestic Animals*, 36, 85–89, 2001.
62. P. T. Frawley, *Review of Rural Veterinary Services: Report/Reviewer: Peter T. Frawley*. Canberra: Department of Agriculture, Fisheries & Forestry Australia, Commonwealth Department of Education, Science and Training, 2003.
63. J. Landercasper et al., Trauma and the veterinarian, *Journal of Trauma*, 28, 1255–1259, 1988.
64. H. M. Busch, Jr. et al., Blunt bovine and equine trauma, *Journal of Trauma*, 26, 559–60, 1986.

9 Retinal Prostheses
Current Approaches, Challenges, and Outlook

Luke Theogarajan, John Wyatt, and Joseph Rizzo, III

CONTENTS

9.1 BACKGROUND AND MOTIVATION

9.1.1 WHY, WHERE, AND HOW?

Vision is arguably the most important sense that we possess and diseases that cause an impairment of this sense result in a debilitating condition. Additionally age-related causes of blindness, such as age-related macular degeneration (AMD), are exacerbated by the increase in average lifespan, especially in developed countries. It is imperative then that a means of restoring a useful level of vision to these patients who have become blind be pursued.

Three main questions naturally arise and must be addressed at the outset. (1) What are the diseases that will be amenable to restoration by an engineering approach? (2) Where is the ideal placement of this device? (3) What are the strategies that one could use to restore vision?

The retina is often referred to as an approachable part of the brain [1] and is composed of exquisite neural circuitry that performs an amazing level of processing. Hence, the greatest chance of building a successful retinal prosthesis is to start with diseases that leave much of the retinal architecture intact. There are two such diseases that affect only the sensory transduction layer, the photoreceptor layer, of the retina. The first is AMD and the second is retinitis pigmentosa; both these diseases result in a loss of photoreceptors (see Figure 9.1).

The answer to the second question needs careful consideration of the pros and cons of placing the device in a specific location. There are three logical placements of the device: (1) the retina, which can be further divided into the epiretinal and the subretinal, the epiretinal referring to the side that faces the vitreous and the subretinal to the side that is adjacent to the choroid; (2) the visual cortex; and (3) the optic nerve.

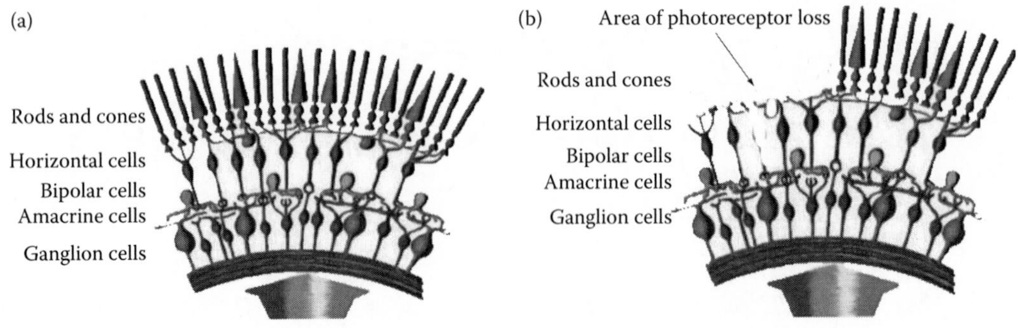

FIGURE 9.1 Schematic representation of retinal degeneration. (a) Normal retina and (b) degenerated retina.

If the device were placed in the retina and if we are able to harness much of the processing capability of the remaining intact neural tissue, it offers the most seamless and natural method. This is mainly due to the fact that it does not bypass the natural flow of information. However, it also places the most stringent demands on the prosthesis. The retina is an extremely delicate tissue with the consistency of wet tissue paper; placing a device here is a daunting surgical challenge. As to epiretinal versus subretinal, the epiretinal approach is easier from a surgical point of view but the mechanical anchoring of the implant to the epiretinal surface is difficult [2]. A schematic representation of the epiretinal approach is shown in Figure 9.2. This can be alleviated by placing the device subretinally [3], see Figure 9.3, although the surgery becomes more difficult.

Cortical implants (see Figure 9.4), offer another means of restoring visual function by placing a device that interfaces directly with the brain. This is advantageous since it does not require an intact optic nerve and hence has a wider range of diseases that can be treated. However, the columnar organization of the visual cortex [4], and the fact that much of the preprocessing that occurs in the retina and the lateral geniculate nucleus is bypassed, makes the conversion of the visual image into a meaningful cortical stimulus rather difficult.

The optic nerve [5] is another possible location; this has the advantage of easy surgical access but the bundle organization makes the spatiotemporal mapping onto the optic nerve rather challenging. Although it is partially the present author's bias, placing the prosthesis in the retina seems to be the best choice. Furthermore, since mechanical anchoring seems to be more difficult than the surgical task, subretinal implantation is preferred to epiretinal implantation.

9.1.2 Electrical Stimulation

The key to action potential generation is the control of the membrane potential. A very simple and intuitive model can be developed [6] and more sophisticated models are available; see [7,8,9,10]. Ideally, a voltage would be placed across the membrane; unfortunately, one cannot do this without causing damage to the cell. Hence, a noninvasive method needs to be adopted. Considering the electrical model of the membrane patch in Figure 9.5, it would be natural to think that applying an extracellular potential would couple it intracellularly via the resistances in the membrane. However, these resistances are ion specific and are not electrically accessible since the rearrangement of ions due to an applied potential is not ion specific. Furthermore, these ions will predominantly be composed of sodium and chlorine ions since they are the dominant species extracellularly and the channels at rest are highly impermeable to these ions. So, from an electrical perspective, the ion channels can be neglected and the access is primarily via the membrane capacitance. This rules out the direct modulation of the intracellular potential via an extracellular applied voltage.

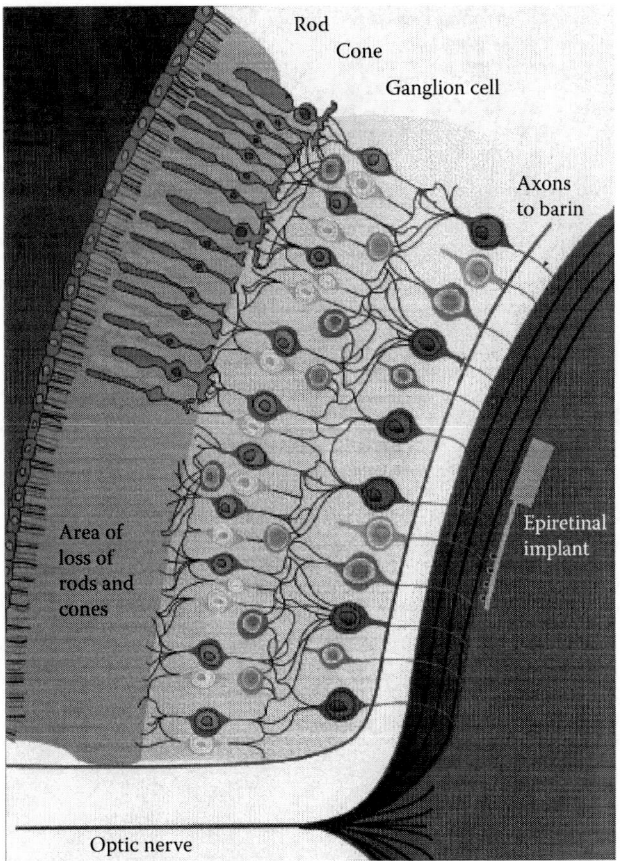

FIGURE 9.2 Epiretinal placement of a retinal prosthesis. (From J. F. Rizzo and J. L. Wyatt, *Neuroscientist*, 3(4), 251–262, 1997. With permission.)

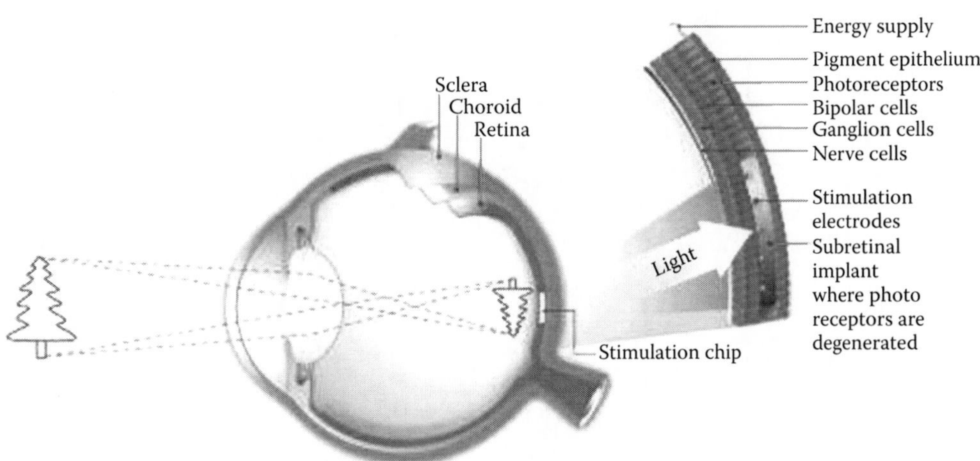

FIGURE 9.3 Subretinal approach for a retinal prosthesis. (From http://www.eye-chip.com)

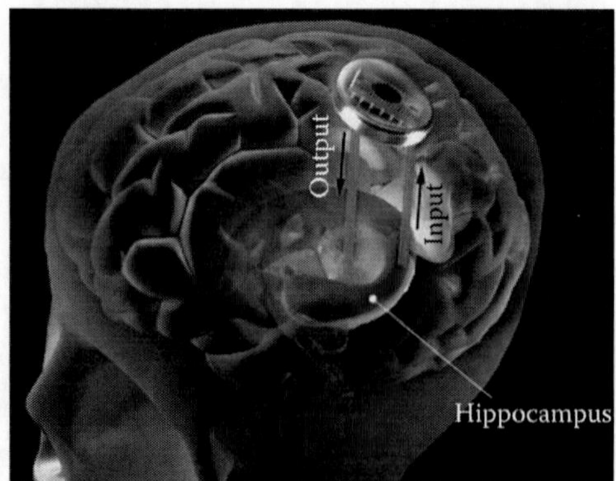

FIGURE 9.4 Schematic representation of a cortical prosthesis. (From http://met.usc.edu/research/projects/bio-implantation/cortical.jpg)

An alternative is to inject current in the vicinity of the neural membrane, as shown in Figure 9.6. Some of this current will charge the membrane, with current flowing out of the membrane depolarizing the membrane and current flowing into the membrane hyperpolarizing it. Hence for a patch that depolarizes there will be another patch nearby that will hyperpolarize due to the change in the current direction [11]. For electrical stimulation to be highly effective the electrode must be fairly close to the neuron. The other problem is that the low resistivity of the surrounding electrolyte compared to the neural membrane will also shunt much of the current away from the nerve if the electrode is not very close.

9.2 ELECTRONIC VISUAL PROSTHESIS

As explained in the preceding sections, the goal of an artificial retinal prosthesis is to stimulate the remaining healthy layers of retinal neurons using brief biphasic pulses of current. These current pulses produce a sensation of vision in the brain that is termed a phosphene. We hope that over time the patient will be able to integrate these phosphenes into useful vision. A key step toward this goal

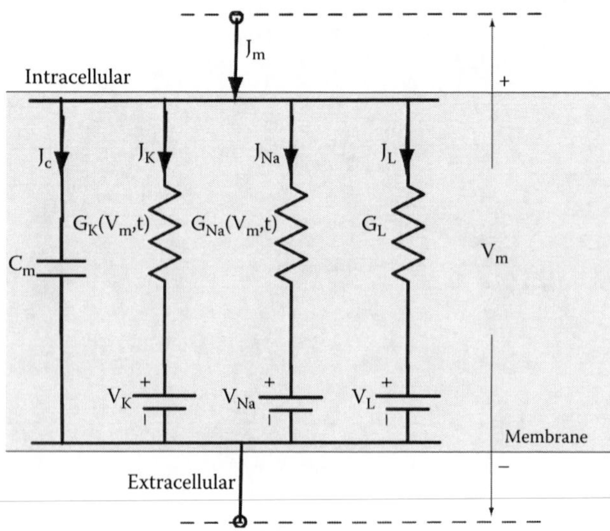

FIGURE 9.5 Electrical model of a patch of the neural membrane. The values of the voltages are equal to the resting Nernst potential for that ion.

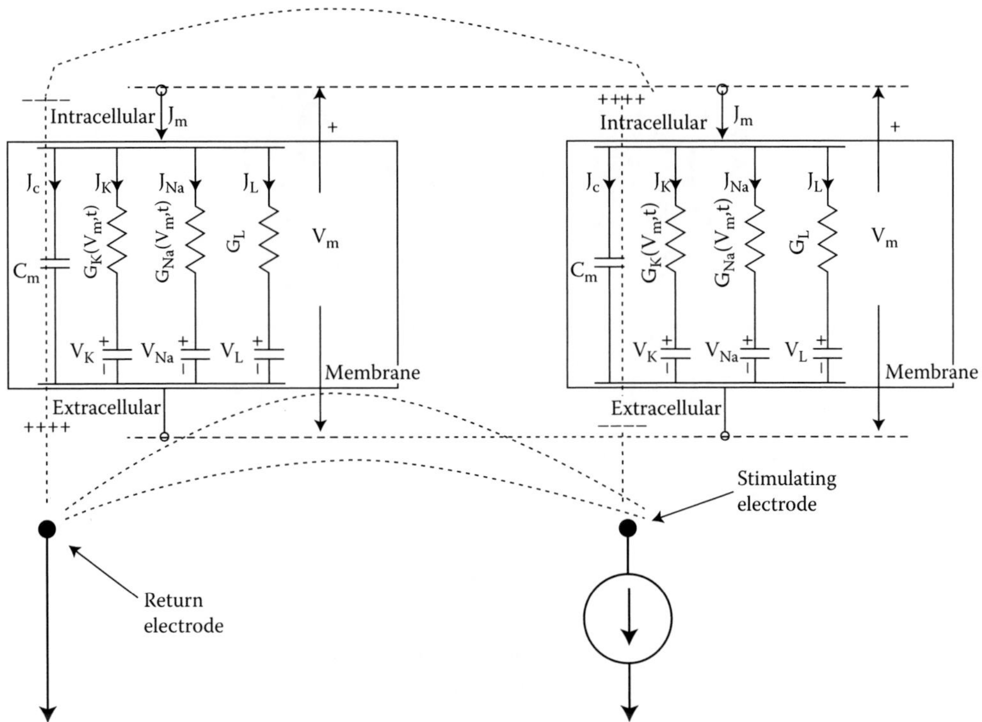

FIGURE 9.6 Electrical stimulation of neurons by injecting a current in the vicinity of the neuron. A fraction of the current will flow through the membrane capacitance charging the membrane; see text for details.

is the development of a chronic implant. Our design philosophy is based on the following requirements: (1) the implant must be powered via an external source (i.e., no batteries); (2) an ability to communicate wirelessly with the implant via external commands; (3) allowing for parameter tuning, that is, current amplitude, duration, and interpulse timing. The first and second constraints were met by using an inductively coupled power and data link. The third was enabled by implementing a flexible stimulator chip architecture as discussed in Section 9.3.1.

Our physical implant design is based on a minimally invasive *ab externo* approach, which is schematically shown in Figure 9.7. In this approach, only the electrode array is placed in the subretinal space (underneath the retina), while the secondary coils and stimulator chip are placed outside on the eyeball. This technique minimizes the number of components that are placed in these retinal spaces, which provides the following key advantages: (1) minimizes the risk of infection due to the implant; (2) increases the amount of power that can be safely transmitted to the secondary coil; and (3) larger physical space in which the implant resides, which allows for larger secondary coils.

9.3 STIMULATOR CHIP

9.3.1 Architectural Overview

The basic architecture of the stimulator chip is shown in Figure 9.8. The chip is powered via an inductive link; the power signal is rectified and filtered using off-chip diodes and capacitors with the nominal supply voltage being ±2.5 V. The data are received through a separate coil placed concentric to the power coil. The digital data are transmitted using an amplitude shift keyed (ASK) waveform. The carrier frequencies of the power and data are 125 kHz and 13.56 MHz, respectively. The front-end decouples the power and data signals, demodulates, and restores the data signal to digital levels. The symbol is encoded as a pulse-width-modulated signal, a 50–50% duty cycle encodes a 0,

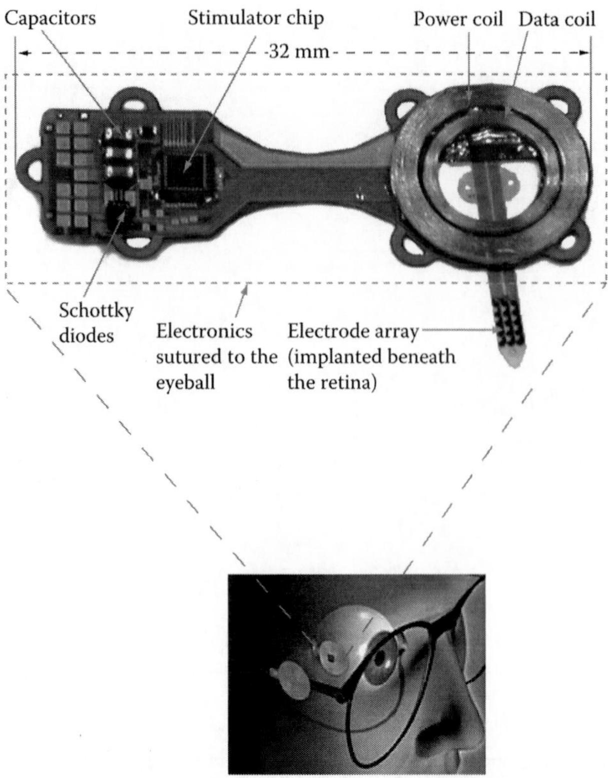

FIGURE 9.7 Schematic representation of the minimally invasive *ab externo* approach. The transmitter coils are placed outside on a pair of eyeglasses and the receiver coils and the stimulator chip are placed on the eyeball. The electrode array is placed in the subretinal space through a scleral flap.

while a 30–70% duty cycle encodes a 1. The data and clock are recovered by the delay locked loop and fed to a control logic block. The signals from the control block control the current driver array, which outputs biphasic current pulses to the electrode array. Complete circuit details of the chip have been previously published by the chapter authors [12].

9.3.2 Power Supply Considerations

Unlike other implant designs, the power supply of this chip is lower. This is not a concern in this design since this chip drives an electrode array made of iridium oxide, which unlike platinum has intrinsically higher charge capacities [13] ($\cong$ 10×). An electrode in an electrolyte can be modeled as a resistance in series with a capacitor to first order [14], assuming that the charge transfer resistance is large, which is true in this case. The large charge capacity of iridium oxide translates into a large capacitor; in our electrodes the series resistance is 2.04 kΩ and the capacitance is 1.13 μF (see Figure 9.10). It should be noted that the series resistance seems to double to $\cong$4 kΩ in animal experiments conducted by others in our group (S. K. Kelly, personal communication, 2007). Experiments on human volunteers that have been previously performed in our group [15] have determined the current levels that are needed to elicit the sensation of perception for a given pulse duration (see Table 9.1). Using a conservative swing of 2.1 V that allows the current source devices to remain in saturation, one can calculate the maximum allowed current for a given duration using a series RC electrode model, with an R of 4.09 kΩ and a C of 1.13 μF. Using such a calculation it can be seen from Table 9.1 that the chip can either meet or exceed the needed current levels for a human implant. Furthermore, a recent chronic study in three patients [16] used 1-ms pulse durations exclusively and the thresholds, for a majority of the electrodes, were below the 420 μA driving capability of this

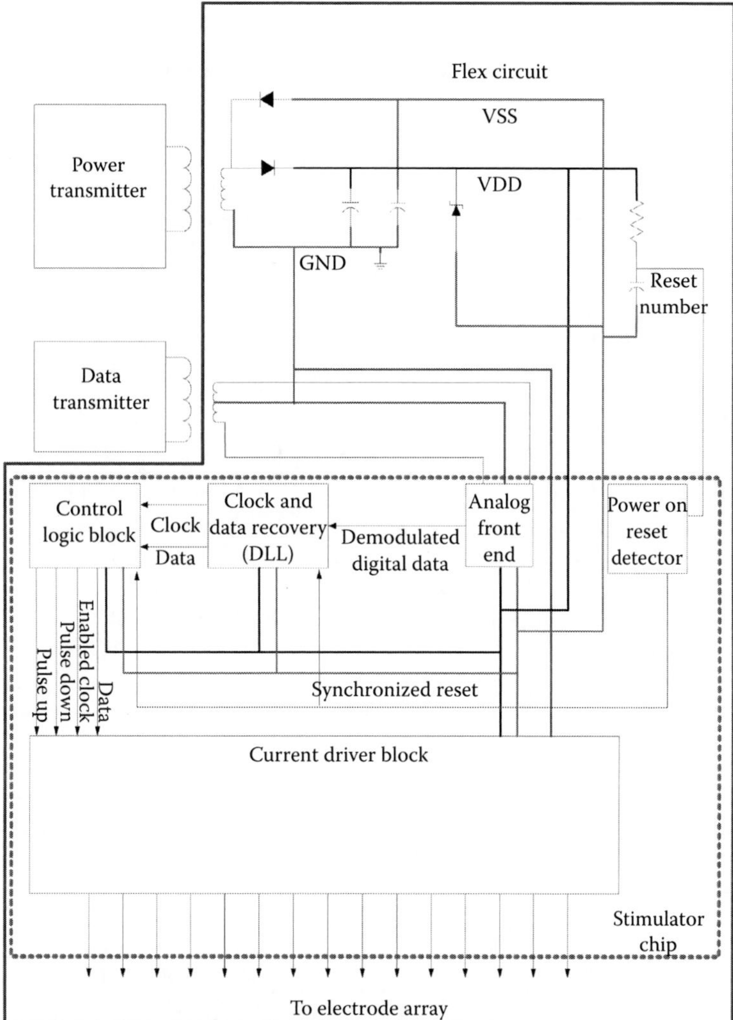

FIGURE 9.8 Architectural overview of the current retinal implant. The blocks that correspond to the stimulator chip are outlined by a dotted line. The chip receives data and power through two separate inductive links, demodulates the signal, recovers the data and the clock, and outputs biphasic current pulses upon receiving the appropriate commands.

chip (see Table 9.1). From a pragmatic standpoint, if an electronic retinal implant is to become a reality, employing current levels greater than 100–200 μA is impractical for an implant with a large number of electrodes. Under these constraints, it seems that the practical choice is the use of larger pulse durations, lower currents, iridium oxide electrodes, and lower power supplies.

9.3.3 Full Chip Experimental Results

The microphotograph of the chip is shown in Figure 9.9. The first step was to evaluate whether the implantable retinal stimulator chip would function as designed when powered wirelessly while driving a 400-μm diameter iridium oxide electrode immersed in saline. The results of this experiment are shown in Figure 9.10; the separation between the primary and secondary coils is 15 mm. The data from the register were additionally recorded to ensure data integrity. The full metrics of the chip are listed in Table 9.2. Another metric of interest is the power consumption as a function of data

TABLE 9.1
Comparison of the Chip Current Delivering Capability versus Requirement of Human Implant

Human Perceptual Threshold		Chip Capability	
Current Amplitude	**Pulse Duration**	**Max. Current at Given Duration**[c]	**Useful for Human Implant**
		Acute Experiment[a]	
1.6–1.5 mA	250 μs	480 μA	No
800–350 μA	1 ms	420 μA	Yes[d]
200–100 μA	4 ms	270 μA	Yes
150–100 μA	16 ms	120–90 μA[e]	Yes
		Chronic Experiment[b]	
24–720 μA	1 ms	420 μA	Yes[f]

[a] Data taken from Rizzo et al. [15]; this was an acute experiment on blind human volunteers. The electrode used was an iridium oxide electrode 400 μm in diameter. The upper and lower limits are from two different patients, respectively.

[b] Chronic implant data from Mahadevappa et al. [16].

[c] The maximum current possible was calculated using a simplified RC electrode model with a 4.09-kΩ resistor and a 1.13-μF capacitor with a maximum allowed swing of 2.1 V, the equation being $I = V_{swing}/(R_{elec} + t_{pulse}/C_{elec})$.

[d] The current meets the lower limit of the threshold requirement but not the upper limit.

[e] Calculation yields 120 μA for 15 ms and 90 μA for 20 ms; the total charge delivered exceeds the requirement for the lower limit of the threshold.

[f] The thresholds reported in [16] were for three different subjects for an implant with 16 platinum electrodes; only four electrodes in patient 1 and patient 2 had thresholds exceeding 420 μA.

Source: Adapted from M. Mahadevappa et al., *IEEE Transactions on Neural Systems and Rehabilitation Engineering*. 13(2), 201–206, 2005; J. F. Rizzo et al., *Investigative Ophthalmology & Visual Science*, 5355–5361, 2003.

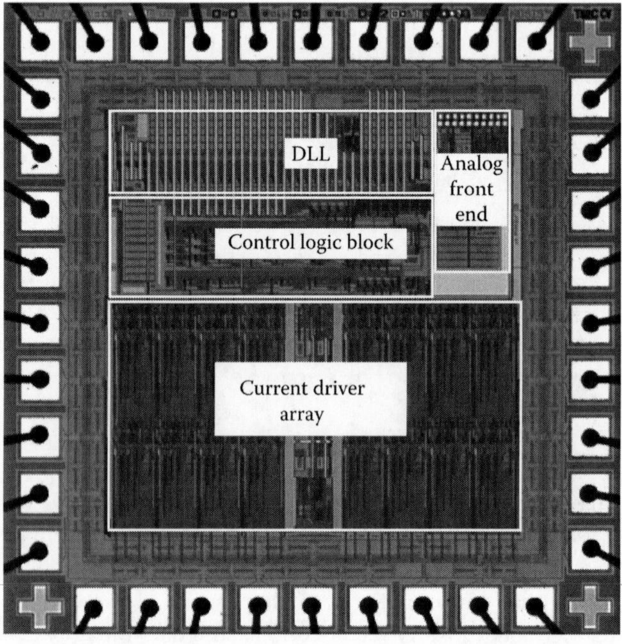

FIGURE 9.9 Microphotograph of the stimulator chip.

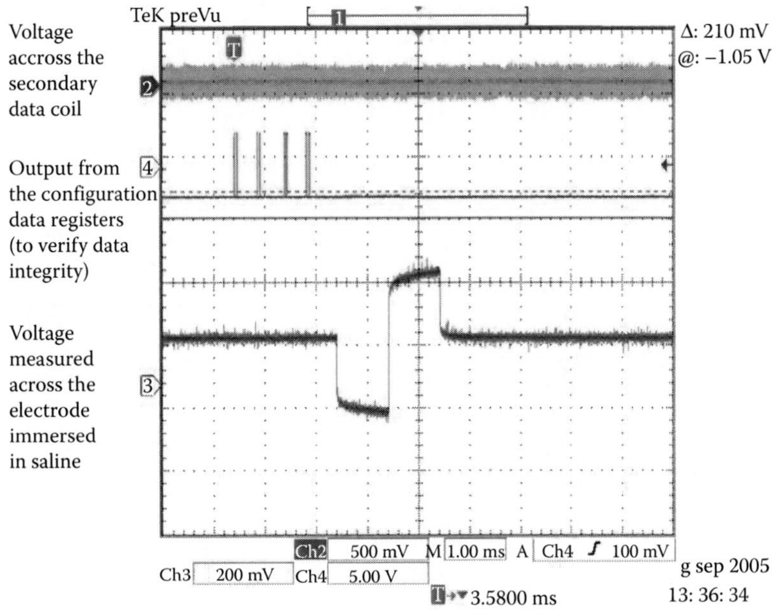

FIGURE 9.10 Output of the wirelessly driven and powered stimulator chip driving an electrode immersed in saline. The separation between the primary and secondary coils is 15 mm.

frequency and the experimental results are shown in Figure 9.11. It can be seen that the increase in power is an order of magnitude smaller than the increase in the data rate, demonstrating the scalability of this architecture.

We have recently implanted our retinal prosthesis in a Yucatan minipig [17] and the results from the animal experiments are shown in Figure 9.12. The basic implant function was tested by measuring the stimulus artifact by commanding up-down current pulses from the implant via wireless commands.

9.4 CHALLENGES

Although we have successfully demonstrated the design, fabrication and implantation of a preliminary visual prosthesis, much remains to be done. The first major challenge that stands out is the

TABLE 9.2
Full Chip Metrics

Technology	AMI 0.5 μm
Die size	2.3 mm × 2.3 mm
Carrier frequency[a]	5–9 MHz
Number of current generators[b]	15
Number of electrodes	15
Data rate	25–714 kb/s
Current amplitude resolution	5 bits
Timing resolution	1.4–4 μs (data rate dependent)
Power consumption	Min.–1.2 mW at 25 kb/s Max.–3.2 mW at 714 kb/s
Maximum frame rate with 1 ms up and down pulses	440 frames/s

[a] This limit is imposed by the data coil characteristics and not by the chip.

[b] It is actually implemented as 16 drivers with two driving a single electrode to enable large currents to study electrode integrity.

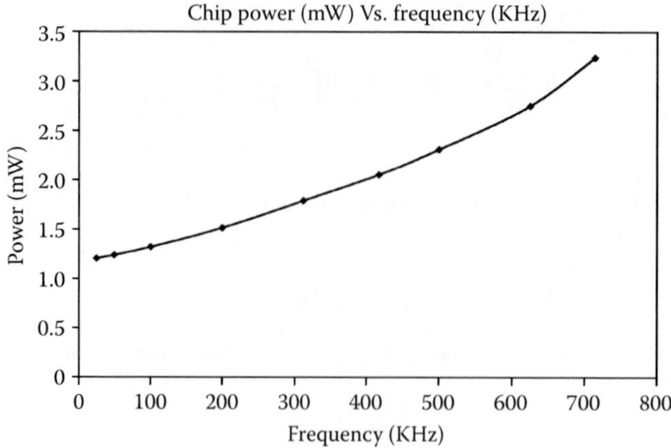

FIGURE 9.11 Power consumed by the chip (excluding the current sources) at different data rates. As the data rate increases by a factor of 28, the chip power increases by a factor of 2.7.

number of electrodes in the current implant. For investigative purposes we had designed a 15-channel implant. However, for a successful human implant we envision that we would need at least 100 electrodes or more. A reasonable estimate that compromises between high visual acuity and power would probably be around 1000 electrodes. From earlier human studies by our group and others [15], the work [16] suggests a current level of at least 200 μA and pulse widths of 4 ms. We need a minimum supply voltage of 5 V, provided that the electrodes are large (≅ 400 μm in diameter), to meet the required compliance voltage. This gives us 500 W/electrode since we swing symmetrically around ground. This implies that we need 500 mW for a 1000 electrode array, which is of course impossible to achieve while maintaining cell viability due to the amount of heat dissipation. Of course, things are not quite this much bleak, since all electrodes are not switching at the same time. If we assume that we limit the array to a 0.3 activity factor we still need 150 mW; this still exceeds the safety limit, which is around 10–50 mW [18]. The use of a switched supply design using capacitor banks can mitigate some of the power losses [19] and thereby lower the power required.

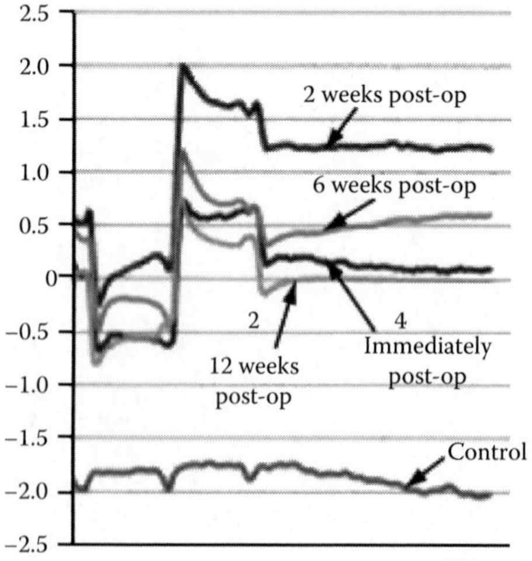

FIGURE 9.12 Stimulus artifacts recorded from an implanted Yucatan minipig while the implant was powered wirelessly and commanded wirelessly to output biphasic current pulses.

An alternative way of approaching the problem is to design better electrode architectures that can be placed closer to the retinal tissue and thereby lowering the current required for stimulation. An encouraging note is that routinely in the laboratory we use 1–10 A to stimulate retina *in vitro* [20] where the stimulating electrode is placed very close to the cell. Another approach for enhancing proximity is to induce neurons to grow toward the electrode by using drug-eluting electrodes [21]. The next major challenge is biocompatibility of the retinal implant. Although polymer coatings such as paralyene, polyimide, and polysiloxanes are currently being used in neural prosthesis [22], they degrade over time. Metal encapsulation such as titanium packaging is another possibility although this may make the implant bulky and surgically hard to handle. Apart from general biocompatibility, there is also the issue of tissue encapsulation of the electrodes, which increases the access resistance of the electrodes. The use of special coatings near the vicinity of the electrode array may overcome this [22].

From a VLSI design and test standpoint, many improvements can be made. Currently, many transmission schemes have been investigated, such as ASK, FSK, and DPSK [12,23,24], each of them having its own advantages. As electrode counts increase, the data rate increases and advanced low-power, high-data-rate transmission schemes need to be investigated. However, the bigger obstacle is efficient power transmission, which is severely impeded by the low coupling between primary and secondary coil. One approach might be to use a rechargeable battery in order to wireless recharge it [25], although battery lifetime becomes an obstacle. Instead of using a fixed current level that is imposed from the outside, it may be better to use a closed-loop feedback system where the output of the neuron is coupled to the stimulator and the current necessary to elicit a neural response is determined by this loop. The overall viability of the implant must be continuously monitored to ensure safety and efficacy of the implant. One important parameter that needs to be regularly monitored is the impedance of the electrode.

We have only addressed, albeit briefly, the challenges from a design standpoint. There remain numerous challenges in the areas of behavioral studies, brain plasticity, and patient training that need to be addressed and are outside the scope of this work.

9.5 CONCLUSION

We have recently designed, fabricated, and implanted a visual prosthesis. Animal studies show that the implant remains viable postoperation. There exist numerous challenges in moving the implant from the bench to the bedside, and a concerted effort from scientists in different disciplines to come together is required. We hope that in the future we will eventually take the important step as we are able to perform human studies to understand the efficacy of a chronic retinal implant.

ACKNOWLEDGMENTS

The authors thank the Catalyst Foundation for funding this project and MOSIS for their generosity in fabricating the chips, especially Cesar Pina and Wes Hansford. The help provided by Greg Swider, Bill Drohan, Mariana Markova, Milan Raj, Doug Shire, and Shawn Kelly in the fabrication and experimental measurements is gratefully acknowledged.

REFERENCES

1. J. E. Dowling, *The Retina: An Approachable Part of the Brain*, Belknap Press, Cambridge, MA, 1987.
2. J. F. Rizzo and J. L. Wyatt, Prospects for a visual prosthesis. *Neuroscientist*, 3(4), 251–262, 1997.
3. E. Zrenner, Will retinal implants restore vision? *Science*, 295(8), 1022–1025, 2002.
4. R. J. Jensen, J. F. Rizzo III, O. R. Ziv, A. Grumet, and J. Wyatt, Ferrier lecture: Functional architecture of macaque monkey visual cortex, *Proceedings of the Royal Society of London. Series B, Biological Sciences*, 198(1130), 1–59, 1977.

5. C. Veraart, C. Raftopoulos, J. T. Mortimer, J. Delbeke, D. Pins, G. Michaux, A. Vanlierde, S. Parrini, and M-C. Wanet-Defalque, Visual sensations produced by optic nerve stimulation using an implanted self-sizing spiral cuff electrode, *Brain Research*, 813, 181–186, 1998.
6. D. R. McNeal, Analysis of a model of a model for excitation of mylineated nerve. *IEEE Transactions on Biomedical Engineering*, 23, 329–337, 1976.
7. N. W. Eduardo, W. M. Grill, and D. Durand, Modeling the effects of electric fields on nerve fibers: Determination of excitation thresholds, *IEEE Transactions on Biomedical Engineering*, 39(12), 1244–1254, 1992.
8. F. Rattay, The basic mechanism for the electrical stimulation of the nervous system, *Neuroscience*, 89(2), 335–346, 1999.
9. F. Rattay, S. Resatz, P. Lutter, K. Minassian, B. Jilge, and M. R. Dimitrijevic, Mechanisms of electrical stimulation with neural prostheses, *Neuromodulation*, 6(1), 42–56, 2003.
10. M. A. Schiefer and W. M. Grill, Sites of neuronal excitation by epiretinal electrical stimulation, *IEEE Transactions on Neural Systems and Rehabilitation Engineering*, 14(1), 5–13, 2006.
11. J. B. Ranck, Which elements are excited in electrical stimulation of mammalian central nervous system: A review, *Brain Research*, 98, 417–440, 1975.
12. L. Theogarajan, J. Wyatt, J. Rizzo, B. Drohan, M. Markova, S. Kelly, G. Swider et al., Minimally invasive retinal prosthesis, *ISSCC 2006 Digest of Technical Papers*, 99–108, 2006.
13. J. D. Weiland, D. J. Anderson, and M. S. Humayun, *In vitro* electrical properties for iridium oxide versus titanium nitride stimulating electrodes, *IEEE Transactions on Biomedical Engineering* 49(12), 1574–1579, 2002.
14. A. J. Bard and L. R. Faulkner, *Electrochemical Methods: Fundamentals and Applications*, 2nd Edition. Wiley, New York, NY, 2000.
15. J. F. Rizzo, J. Wyatt, J. Loewenstein, S. Kelly, and D. Shire, Methods and perceptual thresholds for short-term electrical stimulation of human retina with microelectrode arrays, *Investigative Ophthalmology & Visual Science*, 44(12), 5355–5361, 2003.
16. M. Mahadevappa, J. D. Weiland, D. Yanai, I. Fine, R. J. Greenberg, and M. S. Humayun, Perceptual thresholds and electrode impedance in three retinal prosthesis subjects, *IEEE Transactions on Neural Systems and Rehabilitation Engineering*, 13(2), 201–206, 2005.
17. S. K. Kelly, J. Chen, P. Doyle, M. D. Gingerich, S. F. Cogan, W. A. Drohan, O. Mendoza et al., Development and implantation of a minimally invasive wireless subretinal neurostimulator, *IEEE Transactions on Biomedical Engineering*, 56(10), 2502–2511, 2009.
18. R. R. Harrison, The design of integrated circuits to observe brain activity, *Proceedings of IEEE*, 96(7), 1203–1216, 2008.
19. J. Wyatt and S. K. Kelly, A power-efficient voltage-based neural tissue stimulator with energy recovery, *International Solid State Circuits Conference,* 1, 228–524, 2004.
20. R. J. Jensen, J. F. Rizzo III, O. R. Ziv, A. Grumet, and J. Wyatt, Thresholds for activation of rabbit retinal ganglion cells with an ultrafine, extracellular microelectrode, *Investigative Ophthalmology & Visual Science*, 44(8), 3533–3543, 2003.
21. J. O. Winter, S. F. Cogan, and J. F. Rizzo III, Neurotrophin-eluting hydrogel coatings for neural stimulating electrodes, *Journal of Biomedical Materials Research Part B: Applied Biomaterials*, 81B(2), 551–563, 2007.
22. C. Scholz, Perspectives on materials aspects for retinal prostheses, *Journal of Bioactive and Compatible Polymers*, 22(5), 539–568, 2007.
23. K. Najafi and M. Ghovanloo. A wireless implantable multichannel microstimulating system-on-a-chip with modular architecture, *IEEE Transactions on Neural Systems and Rehabilitation Engineering*, 15(3), 449–457, 2007.
24. M. R. Yuce, W. Liu, and M. Zhou, A non-coherent dpsk data receiver with interference cancellation for dual-band transcutaneous telemetries, *IEEE Journal of Solid-State Circuits*, 43(9), 2003–2012, 2008.
25. P. Li and R. Bashirullah, A wireless power interface for rechargeable battery operated medical implants, *IEEE Transactions on Circuits and Systems II: Express Briefs*, 54(10), 912–916, 2007.

10 A Biomorphic Active Cochlear Model *In Silico*

Bo Wen and Kwabena Boahen

CONTENTS

10.1 EMULATING THE COCHLEA IN VERY-LARGE-SCALE-INTEGRATED CIRCUITS

10.1.1 The Biological Cochlea

The human auditory system exhibits extraordinary ability for sensing sound, distinguishing frequencies, and maintaining satisfactory performance in natural and adverse acoustic environments. Its front end, the cochlea, converts sound-induced fluid pressure fluctuations into neuronal spikes in the auditory nerve (AN), decomposing the mixture of frequencies, amplifying low-level sound, compressing high-level sound, and producing interference between different frequencies. For decades, engineers have made efforts to build a hearing machine or computer that can emulate the function and efficiency of the cochlea and the human auditory system. However, no engineered device to date is capable of performing as well as its biological counterpart.

Neuromorphic engineers have taken an unconventional approach in which they reverse engineer the human brain, with the goal to morph or capture both the organization and the function of the nervous system. For about two decades, neuromorphic systems have modeled sensory systems, including the retina [1–4] and the cochlea [5–7], cortical functions, mainly including visual cortex [8,9], developmental processes based on axon guidance [10], and memory and learning [11,12]. While artificial retinomorphic chips have meticulously copied the detailed neuronal biophysics and complex synaptic organizations in the retina, the silicon cochleae have benefited relatively less from morphing the biology because the cochlear amplifier mechanism that accounts for the cochlea's characteristic behavior remains a mystery [13].

Advances in physiological measurements and mathematical modeling in the last few decades have revealed the cochlear mechanics to some extent, although much is yet to be uncovered. In the mammalian cochlea, the nonuniform basilar membrane (BM) vibrates in response to fluid pressure, providing broad frequency tuning that is then enhanced and reshaped by the hypothesized cochlear amplifier. Bridging the gap between the dead cochlea's response and that of living cochleae, the postulated cochlear amplifier refers to the selective amplification process occurring within the cochlear partition (CP) that enhances cochlear behavior: Exquisite sensitivity, remarkable frequency selectivity, and nonlinearities. In short, the BM preliminarily detects and filters sound signals and the cochlear amplifier selectively amplifies the BM's responses, resulting in nonlinear active cochlear behavior.

Since the discovery of the electromotility of outer hair cells (OHCs) in the mammalian cochlea [14,15], cochlear modeling, as a powerful supplementary tool for physiological studies, has been focusing on exploring the detailed manner in which OHCs' motile forces enhance the BM's vibration. The OHC forces can be transmitted, somehow through the complex organizations of the organ of Corti, onto the BM to affect its motion. Enormous modeling efforts have been made to incorporate the OHC motility in cochlear models, with differing hypotheses to account for the cochlear amplifier [16–18]. Responses to sound in most active cochlear models were either unrealistic [19] or missing important characteristic cochlear behaviors, for instance nonlinearity [16,17]. We recently proposed a novel cochlear amplifier mechanism, in which the cochlear microanatomy is considered critical in transmitting OHC forces onto the BM [20,21]. Simply by employing active coupling between neighboring BM segments, this cochlear model reproduced characteristic cochlear responses, which motivated us to build a nonlinear active silicon cochlea based on our proposed cochlear amplifier mechanism.

10.1.2 Why Build Silicon Cochleae?

Silicon cochleae emulate cochlear processing of sound stimuli in very-large-scale-integrated (VLSI) circuits, attempting to match the biological cochlea's sound sensitivity, frequency selectivity, and dynamic range. The effort to build artificial cochleae in silicon has been largely motivated by their potential applications in hearing aids, cochlear implants, and other portable devices that demand real-time, low-power signal processing for speech recognition; these requirements favor subthreshold analog VLSI designs [22]. Furthermore, analog VLSI is amenable to cochlea-like distributed processing due to its compact computational elements, large numbers of which can be integrated in a small area of silicon. However, digital outputs are easier to interface with higher-level processing, whether performed by other neuromorphic chips or implemented in computer software. Thus, a mixed-mode approach, where the cochlea's analog outputs are converted to digital pulses (a function performed by the AN), is most attractive.

Silicon cochleae take the form of a bank of low-pass or band-pass filters, with exponentially decreasing resonant frequencies, connected in cascade or in parallel. Cascaded filter banks, introduced in the first silicon cochlea [5], rely on gain accumulation, with each filter's gain being small. Their major drawbacks are excessive delay and noise accumulation [23], and poor fault tolerance. Parallel filter banks require each filter to generate the desired gain and tuning by itself, falling short of the biological cochlea's frequency tuning and cutoff slopes [24]. A variation of the parallel architecture introduced by Watts [6] passively couples the filters together through a resistive grid that models the cochlear fluid. Although this coupled architecture emulates the cochlea more faithfully, its gain is diminished by destructive interactions [7].

Our silicon cochlea aims to overcome existing architectures' shortcomings by mimicking the cochlea's micromechanics, in particular the intricate anatomical arrangement of OHCs and other structural cells in the organ of Corti. Although how exactly OHC motile forces, discovered in mammalian cochlea over two decades ago [15], boost the BM's vibration remains a mystery, cochlear microanatomy provides clues. Based on these clues, we previously proposed a novel mechanism for the cochlear amplifier—active bidirectional coupling (ABC) [20]. Here, we report a mixed-signal VLSI chip that implements ABC, the first cochlear chip that employs active behavior (i.e., negative damping [25–28], instead of passive behavior, that is, undamping [27,29]).

By counteracting the passively coupled architecture's destructive interference, ABC promises frequency tuning comparable to human performance. The psychophysically measured auditory filter width, or critical band, is about 1/3 to 1/6 octave [30]. This bandwidth suggests a Q_{10}—center frequency divided by width 10 dB below the peak—of between 3 and 6 at the BM. In fact, Q_{10} values measured from cat AN fibers increase from 1 to above 6 from 200 to 20k Hz [31]. In comparison, the highest Q_{10} reported for the cascade and parallel architectures are 0.92 [5] and 0.42 [24], respectively. In the former, the individual filter Q must be limited to manage noise accumulation [32]; in the latter, individual filters had to achieve the desired performance on their own. By avoiding these constraints, the passively coupled architecture achieved a best-case Q_{10} of 2.34—the highest to date—despite a 25 dB gain-drop due to destructive interference [7]. Our software simulations suggested that ABC could counteract this destructive interference [20], thereby achieving performance comparable to humans. However, this proved challenging in silicon: We discovered that reflections were caused by abrupt changes in BM properties (due to transistor mismatch).

10.1.3 Digital or Analog VLSI?

While our software simulations demonstrated ABC's promise as a cochlear amplifier [20,21], implementing it in digital or analog VLSI presents challenges. According to our simulations, a large gain (over 60 dB) is achieved when negative damping (i.e., active amplification) occurs over many BM segments (about 60). This requirement necessitates a large number of segments per octave (about 45) if sharp tuning ($Q_{10} > 5$) is desired as well. The upshot is about 450 segments are needed to span the audio-frequency range (20–20k Hz or 10 octaves), presenting challenges for both digital and analog implementations.

As to digital VLSI, although the bit-serial technique offers implementation efficiency, it is hard-pressed to fit several hundreds of segments on a chip. This approach yielded 71 second-order sections in a 40 mm^2 1.2 µm-CMOS ASIC [33] and 88 sections in a Xilinx Virtex XCV1000 FPGA [34]. Extrapolating these numbers yields 409 sections in a 10 mm^2 0.25 µm-CMOS ASIC and 334 sections in a Xilinx Virtex II XC2V8000, but this does not include the fluid model nor does it include ABC. Adding this functionality, which requires two multiply-accumulate operations for ABC and about 10 for the fluid (per section), will double the complexity of the system, and halve the number of sections.

As to analog VLSI, fitting several hundred segments on a single chip is possible if small transistors and capacitors are used, but these are prone to mismatch and noise. However, given that the biological cochlea itself is built out of imprecise components, we conjectured that ABC will be robust to mismatch and noise in silicon devices. For instance, noise in transistors used to model the fluid in the silicon cochlea parallels Brownian motion of water molecules impinging on the BM. Our motivation for implementing ABC in analog VLSI was to explore this conjecture—if indeed ABC inherited its biological counterpart's robustness. To this end, we integrated hundreds of BM segments in a single chip, passively and actively coupled by transistors mimicking the cochlear fluid and

ABC, respectively. In addition, the chip includes silicon neurons that convert analog signals, representing BM velocity, into digital pulse streams, representing AN fibers' spike trains.

10.2 MODELING THE NONLINEAR ACTIVE COCHLEA

10.2.1 Cochlear Mechanics and the Cochlear Amplifier

The cochlea actively amplifies acoustic signals as it performs spectral analysis. Incoming sound moves the oval window (stapes) at the cochlea's base, which in turn sets the cochlear fluid in motion (Figure 10.1). The fluid interacts with the BM, the cochlea's main vibrating organ, forming a traveling wave that propagates toward the cochlea's apex. From the base to the apex, BM transverse fibers increase in width and decrease in thickness, resulting in an exponential decrease in stiffness, which gives rise to broad frequency tuning of the cochlea, the passive cochlear behavior.

The cochlea exhibits exquisite sound sensitivity, fine frequency discrimination, and nonlinearity. These characteristic active behaviors have been attributed to the cochlea amplifier, with OHCs widely thought to be its key element, making an essential contribution to active cochlear responses. Physiological experiments have revealed that OHCs contract or elongate when electrically or acoustically stimulated (electromotility) [15]. Their contraction or extension can enhance sensitivity by amplifying BM vibration, and can enhance frequency discrimination as well if the amplification is

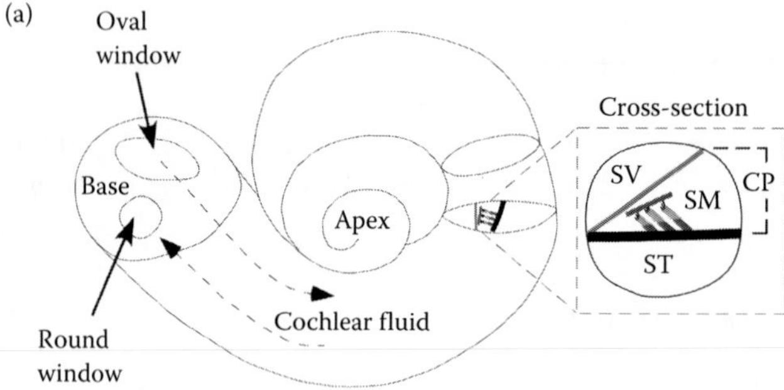

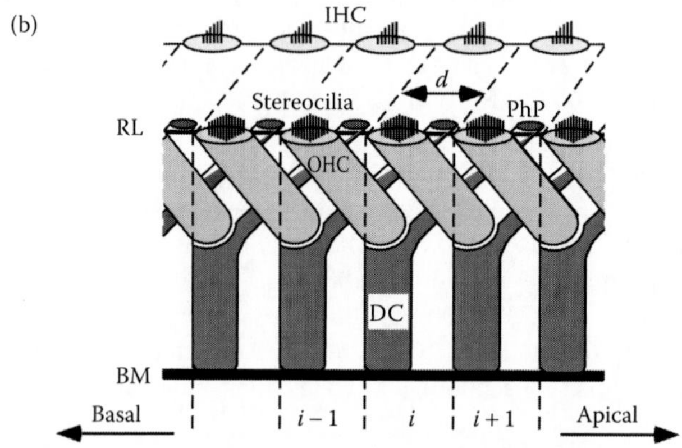

FIGURE 10.1 The cochlea. (a) Cutaway showing cochlear ducts, comprising (inset) the scala vestibuli (SV), scala media (SM), and scala tympani (ST). The cochlear partition (CP) separates the two perilymphatic scalae. (Adapted from C. A. Mead, *Analog VLSI and Neural Systems*. Reading, MA: Addison-Wesley, 1989.) (b) Longitudinal view of the CP. Outer hair cells (OHCs) tilt toward the base while Deiters' cells' (DC) phalangeal processes (PhP) tilt toward the apex; their bases rest on the basilar membrane (BM) and their tips form the reticular lamina (RL). *d* is the tilt distance. (Adapted from W. E. Brownell et al., *Science*, 227, 194–196, 1985; C. D. Geisler, *From Sound to Synapse: Physiology of the Mammalian Ear*. New York, NY: Oxford University Press, 1998.)

applied to a restricted region. However, how exactly OHC forces enhance BM vibration in a frequency-selective fashion remains elusive due to the difficulties in accessing and exploring the functional roles of different components in the CP [13,19].

OHCs have a unique cortical structure in their lateral surface [38], which is believed to be responsible for their ability to change their cell body length—at acoustic frequencies—when acoustically or electrically stimulated. Basically, the OHC's lateral surface consists of three layers: the plasma membrane, the helical circumferential filaments, and the lateral cisternae, from outside to inside [38]. It is widely held that the plasma membrane's array of large bound particles plays an important role in OHC motility [39]. The idea is that these membrane-bound particles undergo conformational changes when the transmembrane voltage changes. Upon depolarization, the particle's effective diameter decreases, their packing density increases, and the OHC's surface area shrinks. In contrast, hyperpolarization expands the OHC's surface area. The change in surface area translates into a change in cell body length.

Although the speed limit of OHC electromotility has not yet been determined, deformation of OHCs can be considered to be "rapid" [19]. Therefore, it is reasonable to assume that OHC forces can follow acoustic frequencies on a cycle-by-cycle basis. Thus, we assumed that OHC forces are exerted onto the BM instantaneously and are not filtered. For exploring the cochlear amplifier mechanism, we also assumed that the cochlear microanatomy, that is, the complex organization and unique architecture of the CP, especially of the organ of Corti, plays a critical role in transmitting OHC electromotile forces onto the BM, thus affecting the BM's motion.

10.2.2 Cochlear Microanatomy and the ABC Mechanism

Our hypothesized cochlear amplifier mechanism incorporates the cochlear microanatomy, particularly the bidirectional transmission of OHC forces, a mechanism we named *active bidirectional coupling* (ABC) [20]. We posited that the triangular mechanical unit formed by an OHC, a phalangeal process (PhP) extended from the Deiters' cell (DC) on which the OHC sits, and a portion of the reticular lamina (RL), between the tips of the OHC and the PhP, plays an active role in enhancing the BM's vibration [20] (Figure 10.1).

Bidirectional coupling comprises both forward coupling due to the OHC's basal tilt and backward coupling due to the PhP's apical tilt. Forward coupling, proposed in [16,40], posits that the OHC's basal tilt transmits OHC forces to an adjacent downstream BM segment. Backward coupling, the novel component of ABC, posits that the PhP's apical tilt transmits OHC forces to an adjacent upstream BM segment. Thus, these forward and backward OHC forces couple together the otherwise weakly coupled BM transverse fibers. In contrast, either tilt alone—OHC or PhP—realizes unidirectional coupling due to forward or backward forces.

Bidirectional force transmission can be modeled when the cochlea is segmented along its longitudinal axis (Figure 10.1b). Each segment includes one DC, one PhP tip, and one OHC tip, both attached to the RL. When an OHC's tip lies in segment $i-1$, its end lies in the immediately apical segment i. Meanwhile, the DC in segment i extends a PhP that angles toward the apex of the cochlea, with its tip inserted just behind the tip of the OHC in segment $i+1$. Note that this arrangement of the cells is a simplified description of the anatomy; the PhP's tip may extend three to four segments apically, depending on the species [36,37].

As is widely accepted, segment i's BM fiber's upward or downward motion deflects the stereocilia in that segment, due to shear between the RL and the TM as the fiber pivots at the arches of Corti (see [21] for details). The resulting depolarization contracts or hyperpolarization expands the OHC whose stereocilia tip is in segment i, which pulls up or pushes down segment $i+1$'s BM fibers due to the OHC's basal tilt. Meanwhile, this OHC also moves the RL down or up, which causes segment i-1's BM fibers to be pushed down or pulled up by the apical tilt of the PhP whose tip lies next to the stereocilia in segment i. We made the distances over which the forward and backward forces act (tilt distance d) equal to the width of a BM segment for simulation efficiency.

10.2.3 Mathematical ABC Cochlear Model: Formulation and Simulation

A cochlea model that includes ABC can be formulated as follows. Both the cochlea's length (BM) and height (cochlear ducts) are discretized into a number of segments, with the original aspect ratio of the cochlea maintained. In the following expressions, x represents the distance from the stapes along the CP, with $x = 0$ at the base (or the stapes) and $x = L$ (uncoiled cochlear duct length) at the apex; y represents the vertical distance from the BM, with $y = 0$ at the BM and $y = \pm h$ (cochlear duct height) at the top/bottom wall.

The BM's up–down motion is driven by the fluid pressure difference P_d between the two fluid ducts (the scala vestibule (SV) and the scala tympani (ST)), as described by

$$P_d(x) + F_{OHC}(x) = S(x)\delta(x) + \beta(x)\dot{\delta}(x) + M(x)\ddot{\delta}(x), \tag{10.1}$$

where $S(x)$ is the stiffness, $\beta(x)$ is the damping ($\beta(x) = \zeta\sqrt{S(x)M(x)}$ where ζ is the damping ratio), and $M(x)$ is the mass, per unit area, of the BM; δ is the BM's downward displacement. The fluid velocity (components V_x and V_y) is obtained by assuming incompressibility, which yields $\nabla^2\phi(x, y, t) = 0$, where $\partial\phi/\partial x = -V_x$ and $\partial\phi/\partial y = -V_y$ define the velocity potential $\phi(x, y, t)$ (∇^2 is the Laplacian operator). Then the pressure difference is calculated by applying Newton's second law, which yields $P_d = \rho\partial(\phi_{SV}(x, y, t) - \phi_{ST}(x, y, t))/\partial t = 2\rho\dot{\phi}$, where $\phi(x, y, t)$ is evaluated at the BM ($y = 0$); ρ is the fluid density.

The $F_{OHC}(x)$ term, combining both forward and backward OHC forces, is described by

$$F_{OHC}(x) = \alpha S(x)\{\gamma T(\delta(x - d)) - T(\delta(x + d))\}, \tag{10.2}$$

where α represents OHC motility, expressed as a fraction of BM stiffness, and γ is the ratio of forward to backward coupling, representing relative strength of OHC forces exerted on the BM segment directly through a DC on which the OHC sits (first term), and indirectly via a PhP attached to the RL (second term). $\delta(x - d)$ and $\delta(x + d)$ are the displacement of adjacent upstream and downstream BM segments, respectively; d denotes the tilt distance, the horizontal displacement between the source and the recipient of the OHC force, assumed to be equal for the forward and backward cases. The function T models saturation of OHC forces, a nonlinearity evident in physiological measurements [19].

To visualize the traveling wave behavior, we obtained the velocity potential in the fluid and the BM displacement in both a passive and an active cochlear model* (Figure 10.2). In the passive case, the BM displacement amplitude is only about 23 dB and the Q_{10} is 0.6, while the active response reaches 85 dB and Q_{10} is 5.4. The wavelength decreases as the wave travels; near its peak (short-wave region), the wave becomes more localized in the vertical direction. In particular, the wave extends from the BM for about 77 μm deep into the fluids, which is comparable to its longitudinal wavelength.

In our model, the forward-to-backward ratio, γ, describes the contribution of feedforward and feedbackward OHC forces to the BM's motion. In order to demonstrate the effect of adding feedforward and/or feedbackward OHC forces to a passive model (without OHC motility), we explored three force-transmission configurations: bidirectional (both OHC and PhP tilts), feedforward (only

* The model parameters used for simulation are as follows. Cochlear duct height $h = 1.0$ mm and length $L = 25.0$ mm; fluid density $\rho = 1.0^*10^{-3}$ g/mm^3; BM mass per unit area $M(x) = 3.0^*10^{-5}$ g/mm^2; stiffness per unit area $S(x) = 5.0^*10^6\, e^{-0.4x}$ g/(mm^2 s^2); and damping ratio $\zeta = 0.2$. Tilt distance $d = 71.0^*10^{-3}$ mm; OHC motility factor $\alpha = 0.0$–0.2; and forward-to-backward ratio $\gamma = 0.3$. For the simulation of the linear ABC model, the cochlea was discretized into 350 segments longitudinally and 13 segments vertically, while for that of the nonlinear ABC model (Section 10. 2.5), 150 longitudinal and six vertical segments were used to save computation time.

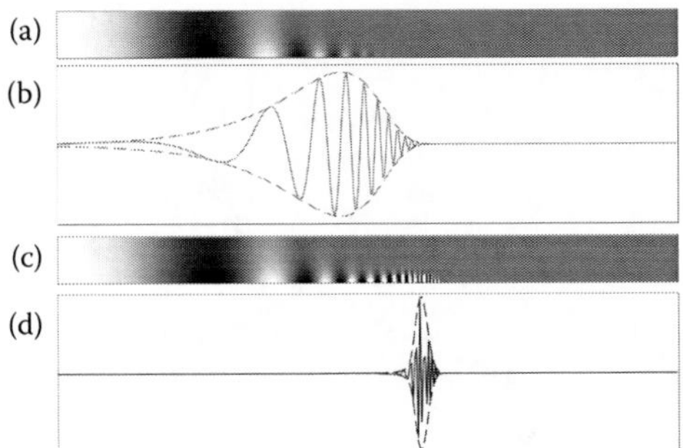

FIGURE 10.2 Snapshots of the traveling wave in the passive and active cochlear models. The input is a 2-kHz pure tone. The passive case ($\alpha = 0$): (a,b). The active case ($\alpha = 0.15$): (c,d). Traveling wave in the fluid: (a,c). Traveling wave along the BM: (b,d). Note that the plots for the passive and active cases are on different scales: The peak amplitude is 23 dB in the passive case and 86 dB in the active case—1265 times greater.

OHC tilt), and feedbackward (PhP tilt with upright OHCs). (Note that upright OHCs produce negligible change in BM stiffness as the force constant is small.) Of the three configurations, only the feedforward case was investigated previously (the so-called feedforward models) [16,18,40]. The same parameter values were used for all these simulations when applicable; the OHC motility factor α was 0.15 and the ratio between feedforward and feedbackward coupling γ was 0.3 (in the case when feedbackward OHC forces were present).

Peak amplitude, phase accumulation, and Q_{10} were obtained by evaluating the model response quantitatively. Figure 10.3a shows the amplitude and phase of the BM displacement, normalized by the stapes displacement, when driven by a 2 kHz tone for the three different configurations as well as the passive case. Quantitative results are listed in Table 10.1. The BM response is least amplified (peak < 20 dB) and most broadly tuned (Q_{10} is as small as 0.6) in the passive case, where the cochlear amplifier mechanism—ABC—is absent; feedforward forces alone increase the amplification (peak reaches around 54 dB) and sharpen the tuning (Q_{10} is about 2.6) to a limited extent; feedbackward forces alone increase the amplification a little more (peak reaches about 57 dB) and sharpen the tuning to a much larger extent (Q_{10} is 7.0); the BM displacement is the largest (peak is above 80 dB) and most realistically tuned (Q_{10} is 6.1) when both feedforward and feedbackward forces are included.

Regarding the phase, the four cases show different phase accumulations at the peak (Figure 10.3b). The passive and feedbackward cases result in the smallest phase lag; the bidirectional case has moderate phase lag at the peak; while the feedforward case has the largest phase lag ($-25.6\ \pi$ rads). Thus, feedforward OHC forces alone result in too much phase shift; feedbackward OHC forces alone give rise to too sharp tuning with a not-large-enough peak; while feedforward and feedbackward OHC forces combined (i.e., ABC) produce the most realistic responses, in terms of peak amplitude, phase, and frequency tuning of the BM responses, compared to physiological measurements [13].

10.2.4 Negative Damping and Spatial Filtering

Impedance quantifies resistance to motion. While mechanical impedance is defined as the ratio of the driving force to the velocity it imparts, the effective acoustic impedance of the BM is calculated as the pressure difference acting on a BM segment divided by the velocity of that segment. For a passive BM (without OHC forces exerted on it), the real part of the acoustic impedance is the BM damping and the imaginary part is the difference of BM mass and stiffness. In contrast, for an active BM (with OHC forces exerted on it), the real part and the imaginary part of the impedance will be altered due to the additional OHC forces. Thus, exploring the BM's acoustic impedance reveals how OHC forces contribute to its vibration, which eventually leads to large amplification and sharp tuning.

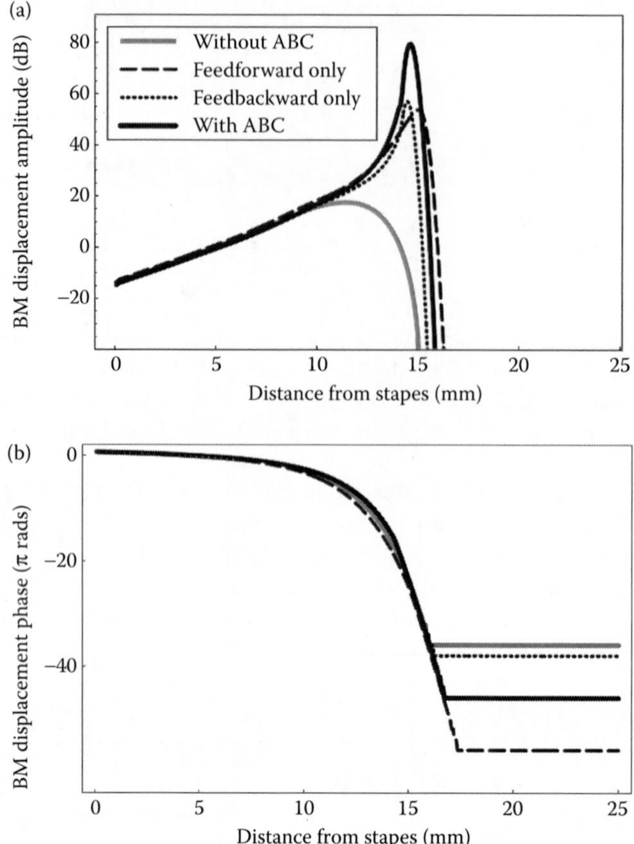

FIGURE 10.3 Comparison between unidirectional and bidirectional coupling. BM displacement responses to a 2-kHz pure tone, normalized by the stapes displacement: (a) Amplitude and (b) phase. Four cases were simulated for comparison: Without ABC, feedforward only, feedbackward only, and with ABC. (ABC: Active bidirectional coupling.)

Transmitting OHC forces bidirectionally gives rise to negative damping in a circumscribed region basal to the characteristic place. Abstract and functional cochlear models have long predicted that reduced or negative damping is required to replicate cochlear sensitivity and selectivity [15,41–43]. The real and imaginary components of the BM impedance, normalized by the critical damping (i.e., mass and stiffness component at resonance, $\sqrt{S(x)M(x)}$, are obtained for a 2-kHz pure tone (Figure 10.4). The impedance's reactive component is almost the same in the passive and active cases (Figure 10.4b), indicating that BM stiffness and mass are not altered by OHC motility.

TABLE 10.1
Bidirectional versus Unidirectional Coupling: Simulation Results

Model	Peak Gain (dB)	Peak Phase (π rads)	Q_{10}	Peak Position (mm)
Without ABC	17.6	−5.1	0.6	11.4
Feedforward only	53.9	−25.6	2.6	15.1
Feedbackward only	57.1	−17.4	7.0	14.5
With ABC	79.5	−19.2	6.1	14.6

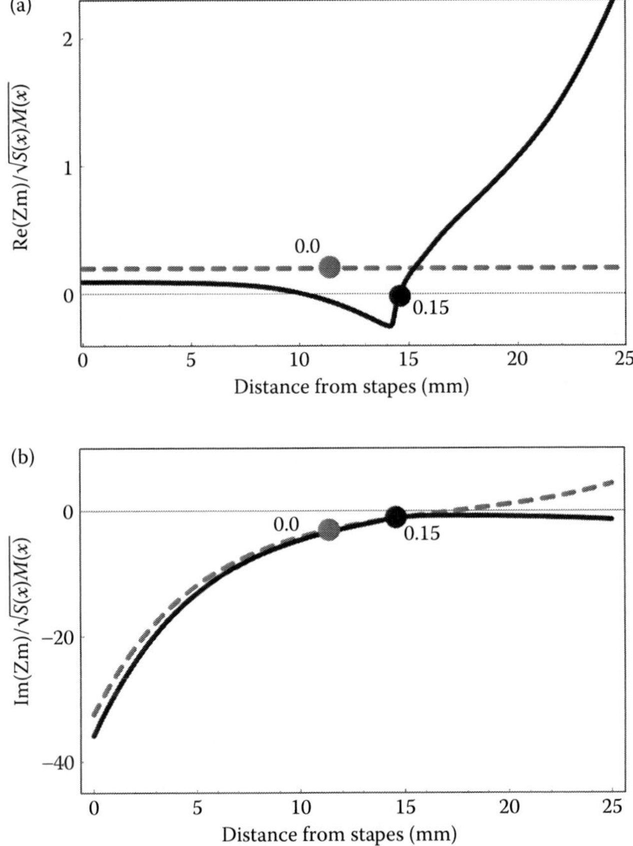

FIGURE 10.4 The BM's effective impedance. The BM's impedance is normalized by the critical damping, $\sqrt{S(x)M(x)}$, at a 2-kHz pure-tone input. (a) Resistive component or the damping ratio. (b) Reactive component. Gray curve: The passive case ($\alpha = 0.0$). Black curve: The active case ($\alpha = 0.15$). The dots mark where the peaks occur. As expected, the damping ratio in the passive case is a constant (i.e., 0.2). In contrast, in the active case in which ABC is included, the damping ratio becomes negative right before the peak while it is affected only slightly near the base.

The impedance's resistive component, which when normalized equals the damping ratio, is no longer constant in the active case (Figure 10.4a), implying that ABC actually modifies the damping. It decreases from 0.2 to a value closer to zero, becomes negative right before the characteristic place, and then rises abruptly to a positive value after the characteristic place. As a result, the BM vibration is large around the characteristic place and then cuts off sharply.

Active coupling's frequency selectivity arises from its wavelength dependence (Figure 10.5). Where the wave is long (small phase differences between adjacent BM segments), the coupling forces are in phase with BM displacement (except for a sign flip for the backward force). This renders them ineffective in amplifying BM's motion—they even cancel each other to a certain extent. Where the wave is short (the phase difference approaches ~90°), the coupling forces are in phase with BM velocity. This is the optimal timing to amplify BM motion—corresponding to negative damping. Our simulation results validated this reasoning: For a 2-kHz pure-tone input, negative damping is maximal when the wave is 278 μm long, which is approximately four times the tilt distance (71 μm).

In summary, ABC generates characteristic cochlear responses (see [20] for details of mathematical model simulation), amplifying the traveling wave locally in a frequency-selective fashion. The peak in BM velocity is higher and sharper in the active case (i.e., with ABC) than in the passive case

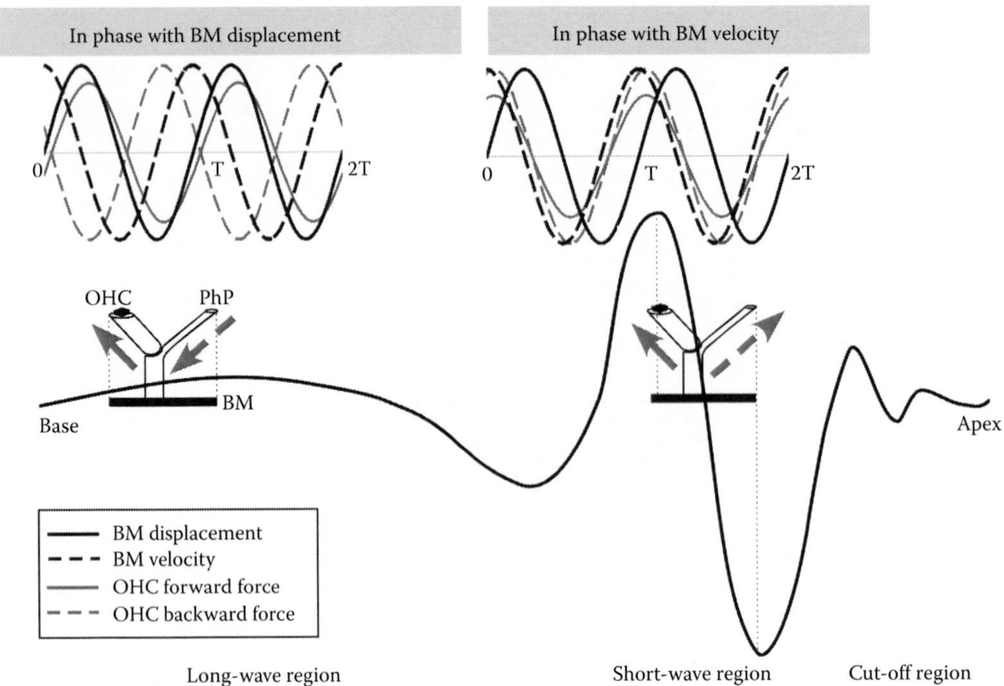

FIGURE 10.5 How negative damping arises. When the wave (continuous line) is long, forces transmitted by the OHC and the PhP are in phase or counter phase with the BM displacement, resulting in a (slight) decrease or increase in stiffness. When the wave is short, these forces are ±90° out of phase with the BM displacement (i.e., in phase with the BM velocity), giving rise to negative damping.

(i.e., without ABC), similar to the difference between a live and a dead cochlea. This frequency-selective amplification arises because ABC produces negative damping when the wavelength of the cochlear traveling wave matches the tilt distance.

10.2.5 Compressive Growth and Automatic Gain Control

The cochlea processes sounds nonlinearly, mainly evident in the compressive growth of its response amplitude with increasing input intensity [13]. Nonlinear cochlear behavior can be obtained in the ABC cochlear model by incorporating saturation of OHC forces, which is assumed to be the origin of the cochlear nonlinearity [13]. The assumption that the OHC forces saturate is supported by physiological observations: the OHC's receptor potential saturates with the acoustic pressure and the change in an OHC's cell body length saturates with the receptor potential [16,19].

In the nonlinear active model, we investigated the compressive growth of BM responses with increasing input levels. For simplicity, our present model assumes that OHC forces saturate with a symmetric profile for both contraction and expansion. That is, the function T in Equation 10.2 takes the form of a hyperbolic tangent (tanh), which is applied to both the feedforward and feedbackward OHC forces. We stimulated the model with a 5-kHz pure tone at various intensities in 20 dB steps and obtained BM velocity responses (Figure 10.6). Clearly seen from Figure 10.6a, the BM amplitude response grows but becomes more broadly tuned as the input level increases, resulting in compressive growth. Specifically, when the input level is at 0 and 20 dB sound pressure level (SPL), the BM velocity amplitude exhibits sharp tuning (Q_{10} = 4.2 and 5.3, respectively); when the input level is at 100 dB SPL, the BM velocity amplitude shows broad tuning (Q_{10} = 1.6), resembling the passive cochlea's response. As a result, the input dynamic range of 100 dB is compressed in the nonlinear active cochlear model, yielding a compression of ~50 dB, which is comparable to physiological data

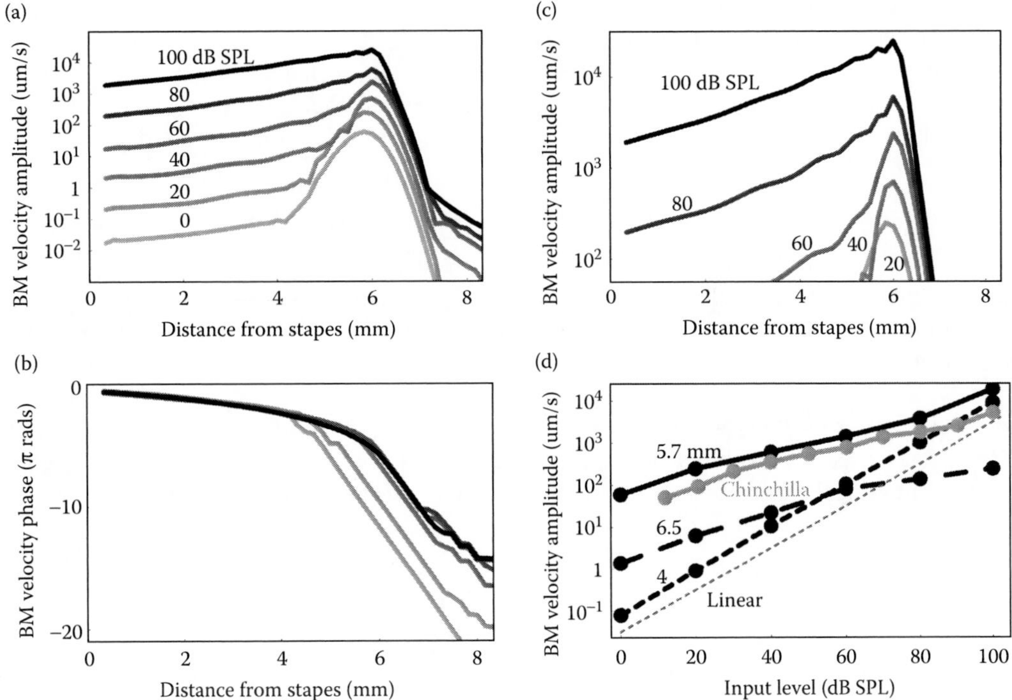

FIGURE 10.6 Cochlear nonlinearity—Compressive growth in the ABC model. BM velocity responses in the ABC model are obtained at various input levels. (a) BM velocity amplitude grows in a compressive manner, exhibiting sharp tuning at low input levels while showing broad tuning (passive behavior) at high levels. Only part of the cochlea (0–8 mm) is shown. (b) BM velocity phase responses, which are almost independent of input levels. (c) Partial plots highlight the small localized cochlear region that is stimulated by low-level sound, compared to much broader activity at high sound levels. (d) BM velocity amplitude versus input level at three different cochlear locations: 4 mm, 5.7 mm (where the BM velocity peaks at 0 dB SPL), and 6.5 mm. The BM shows linearly increasing responses basal to the peak but nonlinear (saturating) responses (i.e., compression at high input levels) at and apical to the peak.

[44]. Consistent with physiological data, the phase of BM displacement does not show significant variation with the input level (Figure 10.6b).

This peak-specific high-level compression is further evident when the BM input–output (I/O) function is plotted at three different cochlear positions (i.e., BM velocity amplitude response versus input level; Figure 10.6d). At the peak (5.7 mm from the base, the characteristic place at the lowest input level in the simulation), the I/O function showed lower slopes at low, medium, and high sound levels (0.62, 0.40, and 0.70, respectively, on a log–log plot). This compressive growth around the peak is comparable with physiological measurements obtained from the chinchilla's cochlea (Figure 10.6d; chinchilla data are from [44]). At a cochlear position slightly apical to the peak (6.5 mm), the I/O function is also compressive, with a slope of 0.48 at high input levels. In contrast, in the region basal to the peak (4 mm), the I/O function is linear. Therefore, compressive growth only occurs around the peak, where saturation of OHC forces takes effect. This saturation is readily implemented in a cochlear chip, realizing automatic gain control.

10.3 BUILDING AN ABC ANALOG VLSI COCHLEA

We set out to build an analog VLSI cochlear model based on the ABC cochlear amplifier mechanism, mainly motivated by the following considerations. On the one hand, the ABC cochlear amplifier mechanism is able to simulate the major characteristic cochlear responses, including large amplification, sharp frequency tuning, and automatic gain control. And more importantly, it takes a form that is simple enough to be implemented in an analog VLSI chip at a reasonable cost. Doing so provides us the opportunity to validate the robustness of ABC, a biology-inspired cochlear amplifier mechanism, by employing a large number of imprecise components, much like the biological cochlea itself.

10.3.1 Design of an ABC Silicon Cochlea: Circuit Synthesis and Analysis

Based on the mathematical ABC cochlear model, we design a two-dimensional (2D) nonlinear active cochlear circuit in analog VLSI, taking advantage of the 2D nature of silicon chips. We start by synthesizing a passive model, and then extend it to a nonlinear active one by including ABC with saturation.

10.3.1.1 Passive Cochlear Circuit

The model consists of two fundamental parts: the cochlear fluid and the BM. First, we design the fluid circuit using the discrete version of Laplace's equation (in one dimension for simplicity):

$$\frac{1}{\Delta x}\left(\frac{\phi_{n+1}-\phi_n}{\Delta x}-\frac{\phi_n-\phi_{n-1}}{\Delta x}\right)=0.$$

where $\phi_n = \phi\ (n\Delta x)$. The velocity potential may be represented in one of two ways: If node n's voltage represents ϕ_n (voltage mode), resistors connect adjacent nodes. If node n's voltage represents $\log(\phi_n)$ (log-domain), subthreshold metal–oxide–semiconductor (MOS) transistors (diffusors) connect adjacent nodes [45,46]. The latter is simpler to implement (see Figure 10.10): We used nMOS transistors for the diffusors and pMOS transistors to take the antilog, yielding a current I_ϕ that is proportional to ϕ_n^κ, a good approximation if the pMOS transistors' κ(subthreshold slope-coefficient) is close to one.

Second, we design a BM segment, and thus the BM. If I_ϕ represents $2\rho\phi$ (the velocity potential scaled by the fluid density) and I_{mem} represents $\dot{\delta}$ (BM velocity), the BM boundary condition (Equation 10.1) can be expressed as

$$\dot{I}_{\text{j}} = S(x)\int I_{\text{mem}}\text{d}t + \beta(x)I_{\text{mem}} + M(x)\dot{I}_{\text{mem}}.$$

(The F_{OHC} term is dealt with later.) Taking the first time-derivative and working in the s-domain ($s = \text{j}\omega$) yields

$$I_\phi s^2 = S(x)I_{\text{mem}} + \beta(x)I_{\text{mem}}s + M(x)I_{\text{mem}}s^2 \tag{10.3}$$

We synthesized this second-order system from two low-pass filters (LPFs), using a custom *Mathematica* program to find a decomposition that provides economy and accommodates ABC readily:

$$\begin{aligned}
\tau_1 I_s s + I_s &= -I_\phi + I_o,\\
\tau_2 I_o s + I_o &= I_\phi - bI_s,\\
I_{\text{mem}} &= I_\phi + I_s - I_o.
\end{aligned} \tag{10.4}$$

The LPFs' outputs are I_s and I_o (also known as state variables); their time-constants are τ_1 and τ_2, respectively; b is a gain factor.

The BM's velocity matches the fluid's and thus we must ensure that

$$I_{\text{mem}} = -\frac{I_\phi(x,\Delta y) - I_\phi(x,0)}{2\rho\Delta y}$$

(Recall that, by definition, $V_y = -\ \partial\phi/\partial y$.) The right-hand side is proportional to the current in the diffusor that connects these two nodes. Therefore, we can satisfy this constraint simply by connecting the BM circuits' current output (I_{mem}) to the fluid circuit—and setting the diffusors' gate voltage (V_{fld}; see Figure 10.10) appropriately (i.e., $\rho \propto e^{-\kappa V_{\text{dd}}/u_T}$, where κ is the nMOS transistors' subthreshold slope coefficient, and u_T is the thermal voltage 25.6 mV at room temperature).

Given Equation 10.4, I_ϕ, I_s, and I_o can be expressed in terms of the output current I_{mem}:

$$\begin{aligned} I_\phi &= \frac{(b+1)+(\tau_1+\tau_2)s+(\tau_1\tau_2)s^2}{\tau_1\tau_2 s^2} I_{\text{mem}}, \\ I_s &= -\frac{1}{\tau_1 s} I_{\text{mem}}, \\ I_o &= \frac{(b+1)+\tau_1 s}{\tau_1\tau_2 s^2} I_{\text{mem}}. \end{aligned} \tag{10.5}$$

By comparing the expression for I_ϕ with the design target (Equation 10.3), we obtain the circuit counterparts:

$$S(x) = \frac{b+1}{\tau_1\tau_2}, \quad \beta(x) = \frac{\tau_1+\tau_2}{\tau_1\tau_2} \quad \text{and} \quad M(x) = 1, \tag{10.6}$$

where the mass M is normalized. These analogies require that the time-constants (τ_1 and τ_2) increase exponentially to simulate the exponentially decreasing BM stiffness (and damping). b allows us to achieve a larger quality factor (a measure of frequency selectivity) for a given choice of τ_1 and τ_2 (limited by capacitor size C: $\tau = Cu_T/\kappa I_\tau$, where I_τ is the current level). That is

$$Q = \frac{\sqrt{S(x)M(x)}}{\beta(x)} = \frac{\sqrt{b+1}}{\sqrt{\tau_1/\tau_2} + \sqrt{\tau_2/\tau_1}}.$$

These circuit–biology relationships help determine the parameter values used in circuit simulation and chip operation.

10.3.1.2 Active Cochlear Circuit

We synthesized an active BM segment by following the same procedure we used for the passive one, but with the F_{OHC} term included. The design target equation becomes

$$I_\phi s^2 = S(x)I_{\text{mem}} + \beta(x)I_{\text{mem}}s + M(x)I_{\text{mem}}s^2 - \alpha S(x)\left\{\gamma T\left(I_{\text{mem}}(x-d)/s\right)s - T(I_{\text{mem}}(x+d)/s)s\right\}.$$

We find I_{mem}/s (i.e., the time-integral) by observing that the state variable I_s in the passive design (Equation 10.5) is related to I_{mem} by $I_s = -I_{\text{mem}}/(\tau_1\ s)$.

Thus,

$$I_{\text{mem}}(x-d)/s = -\tau_{1f}I_{sf}, \quad I_{\text{mem}}(x+d)/s = -\tau_{1b}I_{sb},$$

where I_{sf} and I_{sb} represent the output currents, and τ_{1f} and τ_{1b} the time-constants, of the first LPF in the upstream and downstream BM segment, respectively. We replace τ_{1f} and τ_{1b} by τ_1—the receiving segment's time-constant—a good approximation due to the small change in τ between neighboring segments. Therefore, the design target becomes

$$I_{in}s^2 = S(x)I_{mem} + \beta(x)I_{mem}s + M(x)I_{mem}s^2 - r_{ff}S_0(x)T(-I_{sf})s + r_{fb}S_0(x)T(-I_{sb}),$$

where $S_0(x) = S(x)\ \tau_1 = (b+1)/\tau_2$ (see Equation 10.6—τ_1 was factored out by rescaling T); $r_{ff} = \alpha\gamma$ and $r_{fb} = \alpha$ denote the forward and backward OHC force factors, respectively.

We synthesized the circuit following a procedure similar to that used in the passive design. Only the second equation changed:

$$\tau_2 I_o s + I_o = I_\phi - bI_s - a_{ff}T(-I_{sf}) + a_{fb}T(-I_{sb}), \tag{10.7}$$

where $a_{ff} = r_{ff}(b+1)$ and $a_{fb} = r_{fb}(b+1)$. Note that, to include ABC, we need to only add two currents to the input of the second LPF in each BM segment circuit; these currents are from its adjacent neighbors. Specifically, I_{sf} and I_{sb} are the output currents (I_s) of the first LPF in the upstream (basal) and downstream (apical) BM segments, respectively.

10.3.1.3 Circuit Building Block: Log-Domain Class AB LPF

Based on our synthesized design, we implement a Class AB log-domain circuit for the BM segment. We employ the log-domain filtering technique [47] to realize current-mode operation. In addition, we adopt Class AB operation to increase dynamic range, reduce the effect of mismatch, and lower power consumption [4,48,49]. This differential signaling is inspired by the biological cochlea—the BM's displacement is driven by the pressure difference across it. We present the transistor-level schematics in this section as well as a silicon neuron that converts the segment's output current into a pulse stream.

Taking a bottom-up approach, we start by designing a Class AB LPF, a building block for the BM circuit. An LPF is described by

$$\tau I_{out}s + I_{out} = I_\phi,$$

where I_ϕ is the input current, I_{out} is the output current, and τ sets the time-constant. Its differential counterpart is

$$\tau\left(I_{out}^+ - I_{out}^-\right)s + \left(I_{out}^+ - I_{out}^-\right) = I_\phi^+ - I_\phi^-,$$

where each signal is expressed as the difference between its positive (+) and negative (–) components. The common-mode constraint is

$$\tau I_{out}^+ I_{out}^- s + I_{out}^+ I_{out}^- = I_q^2,$$

where I_q sets the geometric mean of the output current's components.

Combining the common-mode constraint with the differential design equation yields the positive path's nodal equation (the negative path has superscripts + and – swapped) [4]:

$$C\dot{V}_{out}^+ = I_\tau\left(\left(I_\phi^+ - I_\phi^-\right) + \left(I_q^2/I_{out}^+ - I_{out}^+\right)\right)\Big/\left(I_{out}^+ + I_{out}^-\right),$$

This nodal equation suggests the half-LPF circuit shown in Figure 10.7a. V^+_{out}, the voltage on the positive capacitor (C^+), gates a pMOS transistor to produce the corresponding current signal, I^+_{out} (V^-_{out} and I^-_{out} are similarly related). The bias V_q sets the quiescent current I_q while V_τ determines the current I_τ, which is related to the time-constant by $\tau = Cu_T/\kappa I_\tau$. Two of these subcircuits, connected in push–pull, form a complete LPF (Figure 10.7b). Specifically, when the input I^+_ϕ charges C^+, it also discharges C^-; similarly, I^-_ϕ charges C^- and discharges C^+.

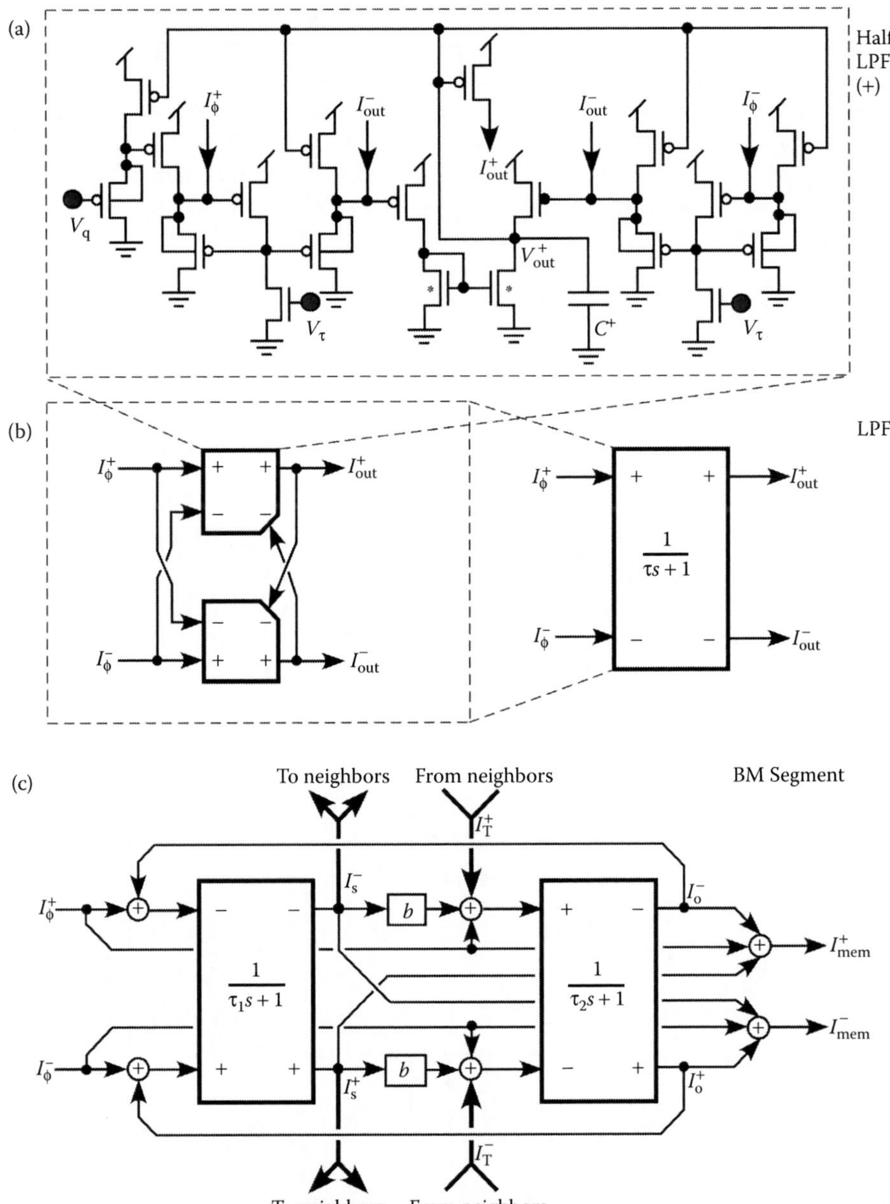

FIGURE 10.7 LPF and BM-segment circuits. (a) Half-LPF circuit (* denotes a complex current mirror). (b) Complete LPF circuit formed by two half-LPF circuits. (c) BM-segment circuit. It consists of two LPFs and is connected to its neighbors, sending current I_S and receiving current I_T (the last two terms in Equation 10.7, corresponding to ABC). In (b) and (c), current splitting implies current copying.

10.3.1.4 BM Circuit

The BM-segment circuit (Figure 10.7c) is implemented using two LPFs interacting in accordance with the synthesized design equations. I_{mem} is the sum of three signals, I_{ϕ}, I_s, and I_o (Equation 10.4). The positive and negative components of I_s, I_s^+, and I_s^-, are the differential output currents of the first LPF (with time-constant τ_1), corresponding to I_{out}^+ and I_{out}^- in the LPF symbol (see Figure 10.7b), respectively. Similarly, I_o^+ and I_o^- are the output currents of the second LPF (with time-constant τ_2). Summing (+) is implemented by exploiting Kirchhoff's current law; scaling (*b*) is implemented by biasing a pMOS transistor's source–voltage (see [21] for transistor-level circuit figures).

ABC is implemented by exchanging currents between neighboring BM segments (Figure 10.8). Each BM sends out I_s and receives I_T, a saturated and scaled version of its neighbor's I_s (Equation 10.7). The saturation is accomplished by a current-limiting transistor, which yields $I_T = T(I_s) = I_s I_{sat}/(I_s + I_{sat})$ [50], where I_{sat} is set by a bias voltage V_T. We used a subtract circuit (see [51] for a transistor-level circuit) to take the difference first because saturation is applied to the differential signal, not to its positive and negative components. The scaling corresponds to the gain factors a_{ff} and a_{fb} in Equation 10.7, implemented by biasing a pMOS transistor's source-voltage (V_{ff} and V_{fb} in Figure 10.7b, respectively).

10.3.1.5 Spiral Ganglion Cell Circuit

In the biological cochlea, the BM's velocity, sensed by inner hair cells (IHCs), is encoded by spiral ganglion cells (SGCs). Behaving like pulse-frequency modulators, SGCs convey information about sound stimuli—including frequency, level, and timing—over the AN (axons of SGCs). Their spikes are evoked by neurotransmitters released from IHCs, each of which drives 10–30 SGCs, increasing from the apex to the base [52]. In our silicon cochlea, this fanout is 6.

The IHC circuit has three functional components (Figure 10.9a): A current mirror takes the difference between I_{mem}'s positive and negative components. A current splitter half-wave rectifies the difference. And a Class A log-domain LPF filters the half-wave-rectified currents. The bias voltages (V_{gain} and V_{sat}) can be varied to yield distinct rate–level relations (i.e., sound level to spike rate).

Augmenting its static rate-level relation, an SGC's dynamic properties enhance the encoding of a sound stimulus' temporal features: It fires at a higher rate at stimulus onset, due to the

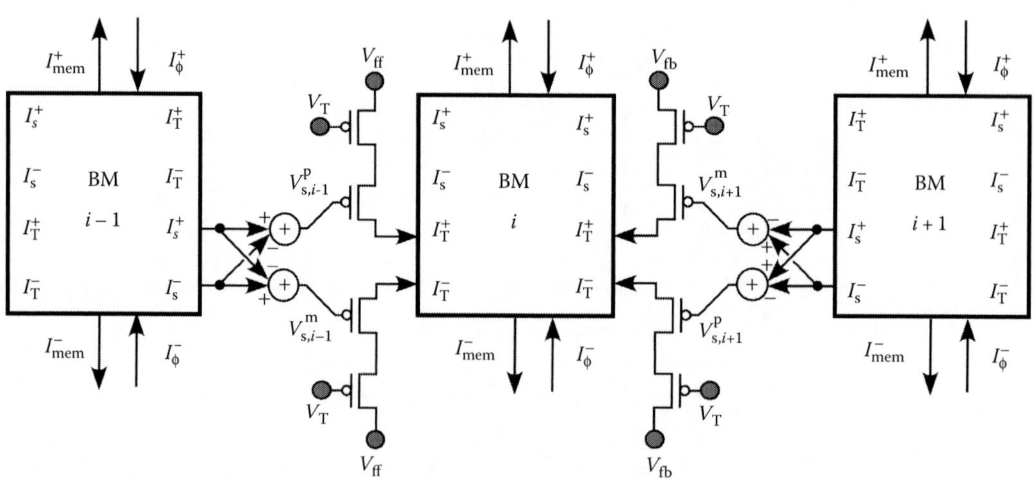

FIGURE 10.8 Active-coupling circuitry. BM Segment i receives a scaled and saturated version of Segment $i-1$ and $i+1$'s I_s outputs. The circuitry that couples Segment i to Segments $i-1$ and $i+1$ is omitted for clarity. V_{ff} and V_{fb} set the gain of feedforward and feedbackward coupling, respectively; V_T sets their saturation levels.

presence of a Ca-concentration-dependent K-current [53]. And from cycle to cycle, it is more likely to fire when the sinusoid is rising most rapidly (phase locking [54]), due to the presence of a low-threshold K-current [55,56]. In addition to these two K-currents, the SGC circuit models a Na-current that generates an all-or-none spike and a high-threshold K-current that resets the membrane [57] (Figure 10.9b).

An address-event encoder transmits the SGC circuits' spikes off-chip [58–60]. To communicate with the address-event encoder, the SGC makes a request when it spikes and clears this signal when acknowledged (Req and Ack in Figure 10.9b). The spike is encoded as a unique address (specifying the row and the column). The receiver chip decodes this address and delivers the spike to the target neuron.

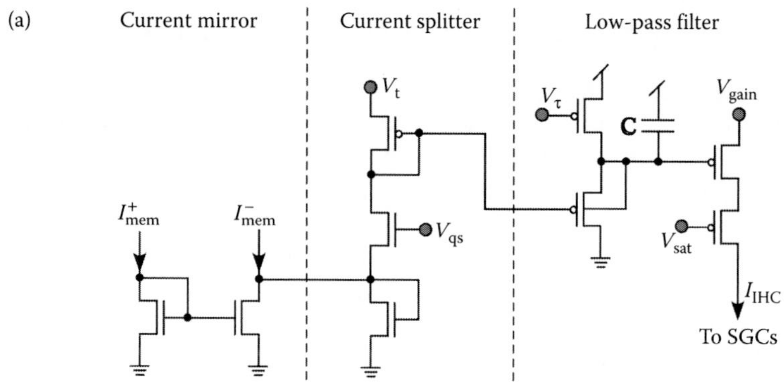

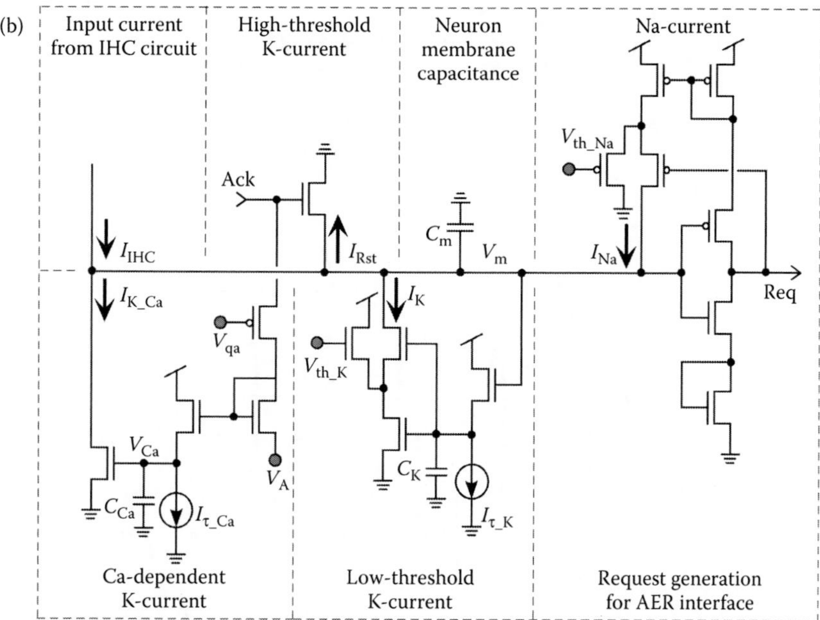

FIGURE 10.9 IHC and SGC circuits. (a) The IHC circuit converts differential currents, representing the BM velocity, into a low-pass filtered, half-wave rectified current that drives the SGC circuits. V_{qs} sets the quiescent level; V_t sets the current splitter's gain; V_τ sets the LPF's time-constant; V_{gain} sets the synaptic efficacy, and V_{sat} sets the maximum amplitude. (b) The SGC circuit models three membrane-voltage-dependent currents (I_{Na}, I_{Rst}, and I_K) and one Ca-concentration-dependent current (I_{K_Ca}). These currents turn on when V_m exceeds certain levels (set by V_{th_Na} and V_{th_K}) or when a spike occurs (activates Req, which activates Ack). I_{τ_K} sets I_K's time-constant; V_{qa} and I_{τ_Ca} set the Ca-concentration's increment (per spike) and time-constant, respectively.

10.3.2 Cochlear Chip Architecture

We fabricated a version of this design with 360 BM-segment circuits, two 4680-element (360 × 13) fluid grids, and 2160 (360 × 6) SGC circuits (Figure 10.10). The number of BM segments was chosen to satisfy the requirements of our software simulation—the chip has approximately 55 segments per octave (assuming a 200–20k Hz range or 6.6 octaves). The fluid-element grids' height (13) was chosen to match the biological cochlea's aspect ratio, a factor important in controlling the traveling wave's behavior [6]. The number of SGC circuits per BM segment (6) was chosen to ensure that the stimulus evokes multiple spikes per cycle—an octave-wide response will produce up to 33,000 spikes/s (assuming a maximum spike-frequency of 100 Hz). A die photograph of the chip is shown in Figure 10.11.

10.4 RESPONSES OF THE ABC SILICON COCHLEA TO SOUND

We measured the silicon cochlea's BM responses to pure tones and AN responses to complex sounds. To supply sinusoidal current as input, we applied the logarithm of a half-wave rectified sinusoid to the top and bottom fluid grids; these two voltage signals were 180° out-of-phase. Scaled to match the pMOS transistors' subthreshold slope-coefficient ($\kappa = 0.58$, measured), the half-wave

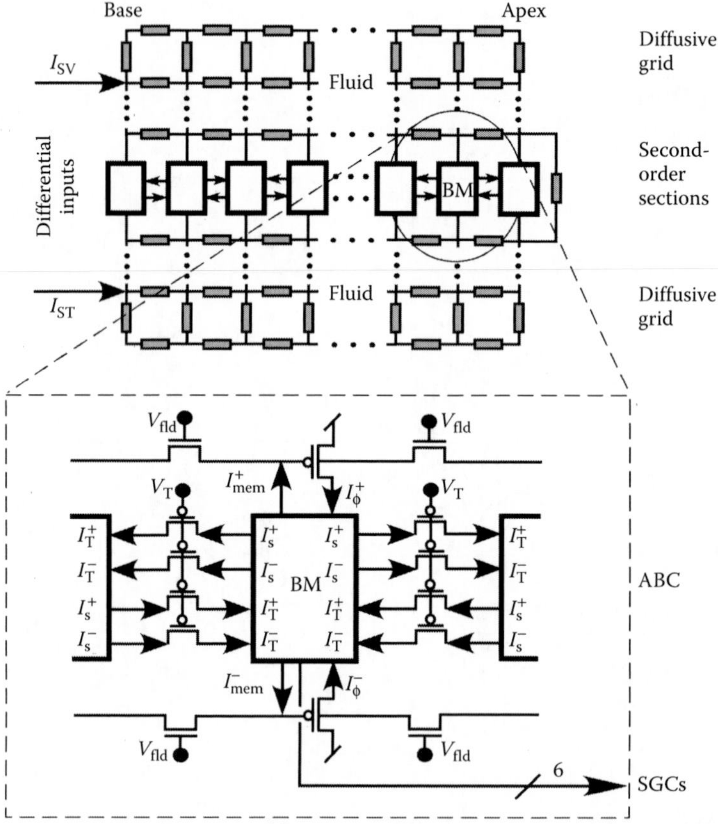

FIGURE 10.10 Active-coupling architecture. Differential audio signals are applied at the base of two diffusive-element grids (representing the top and bottom fluids, respectively; V_{fld} determines the fluids' density), connected at the apex by a single diffusive element (representing the helicotrema). Second-order sections (representing the BM segments) embedded between the grids' send/receive currents to/from their immediate neighbors (V_T as in Figure 10.8), realizing ABC. Their output currents (I_{mem}, representing BM velocity) each drive six pulse-frequency-modulation circuits (representing the SGCs).

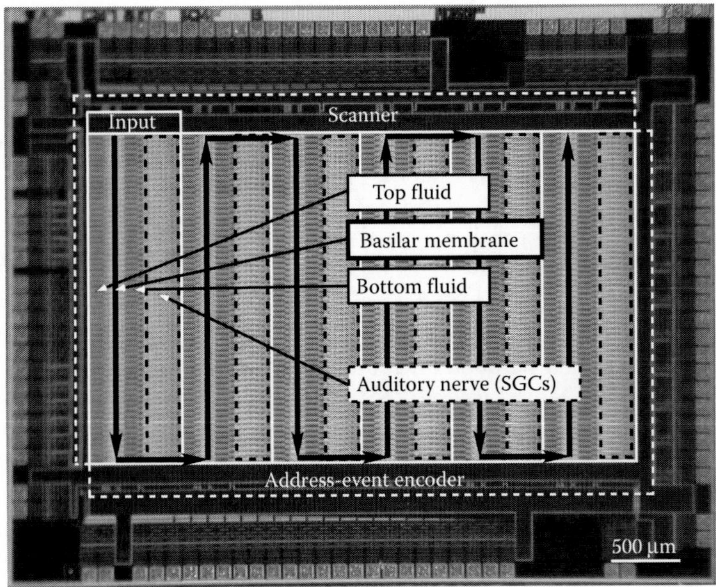

FIGURE 10.11 A die photograph of the chip. Fabricated in a 5 M 1P 0.25-μm CMOS process, the ABC cochlea, with six 60-segment columns snaking to yield a desirable aspect ratio, occupies 10.9 mm^2. The input, BM, top/bottom fluid, AN (axon of SGCs), scanner, and address-event encoder circuits are labeled.

rectified voltage signals' peak amplitude varied from 0.12 to 0.36 V, dropping from a baseline of 2.26 V ($V_{dd} = 2.4$ V), in 0.04 V steps. These values correspond to input current amplitudes of 0–48 dB, increasing in 8 dB steps, with 24 dB corresponding to a medium sound level. We set up the cochlea chip's time-constant-setting voltages ($V_{\tau2}$ and $V_{\tau2}$) by tuning the base and the apex to approximately 20 kHz and slightly below 200 Hz, respectively. Linear interpolation (implemented with two polysilicon lines spanning the silicon cochlea's length) gave rise to exponentially decreasing time-constant currents. The saturation level of ABC currents was set to its maximum level ($V_T < 1.7$ V, putting the pMOS transistor above-threshold) unless otherwise stated.

10.4.1 Frequency and Longitudinal Responses

We measured frequency responses as well as longitudinal responses. To obtain frequency responses, we swept the input frequency and measured BM current outputs (from both positive and negative paths) at a particular segment (with segment numbers increasing from the base to the apex, starting from 1). To obtain longitudinal responses, we kept the input frequency fixed and measured current outputs at consecutive segments along the cochlea's length. Selecting a particular segment or sweeping through consecutive ones is realized with a built-in scanner (modified from [61] to accommodate snaking). AN responses, on the other hand, were measured in parallel by capturing (time-stamped) address-events over a USB link.

Here we present frequency responses measured from linearly spaced BM segments and longitudinal responses to octave-spaced pure tones, both at an input level of 24 dB. We also present frequency responses obtained at various input intensities (0–48 dB), demonstrating automatic gain control. We then demonstrate the role of ABC by disabling it. Finally, we present the chip's real-time responses to a chirp-click sound sequence.

Frequency responses reveal the tuning of individual BM segments (Figure 10.12) (segments beyond 240 were not considered because they did not respond robustly, probably due to the large discontinuity we observed at each U-turn (segments 60, 120, 180, etc.)), presumably caused by doping-level deviations at the array's edges (dummy cells were not deployed). Despite some irregularities in response shape and peak height (due to transistor mismatch), the chip's responses captured the characteristics of the biological responses, at least qualitatively. Frequency responses are peaked and the cutoff slope is steep (more so in some segments than in others), with peak or characteristic frequencies (CFs) ranging from 13.8 kHz to 218 Hz for these six BM segments (40-segment spacing). Phase accumulates gradually at first, then more rapidly near the peak (marked by dots in Figure 10.12b), and plateaus after the peak. The large accumulation indicates a traveling wave; the plateau indicates its extinction.

Longitudinal responses give a snapshot of the entire BM, thereby providing a direct measurement of the traveling wave, to whose wavelength ABC is sensitive. They also show how the wave's amplitude builds up as it travels from the base to the apex, providing evidence that ABC acts in a distributed fashion. The chip's longitudinal responses show large variations from segment to segment (due to mismatch), which we filtered with a 10-segment moving average in order to estimate the response characteristics (Figure 10.13a).

We measured longitudinal responses to four pure tones, with octave spacing (Figure 10.13b). A 4-kHz tone elicits a peak response at Segment 85 (characteristic place), while a 500-Hz tone travels further and peaks at Segment 178. The characteristic places for the two intermediate frequencies

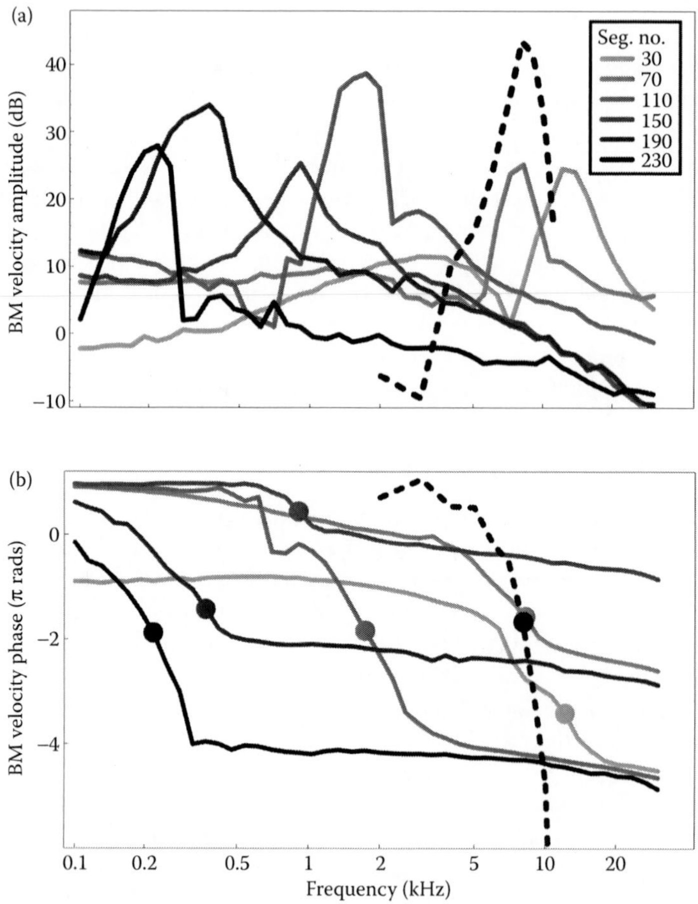

FIGURE 10.12 Measured frequency responses. Velocity frequency responses of six BM segments, spaced 40 segments apart, from 30 to 230 (24-dB input level): (a) Amplitude and (b) phase (dots mark the CFs). Biological data are provided for comparison (dashed line: chinchilla measurement at medium sound level. (From M. A. Ruggero et al., *J. Acoust. Soc. Am.*, 101, 2151–2163, 1997. With permission.)

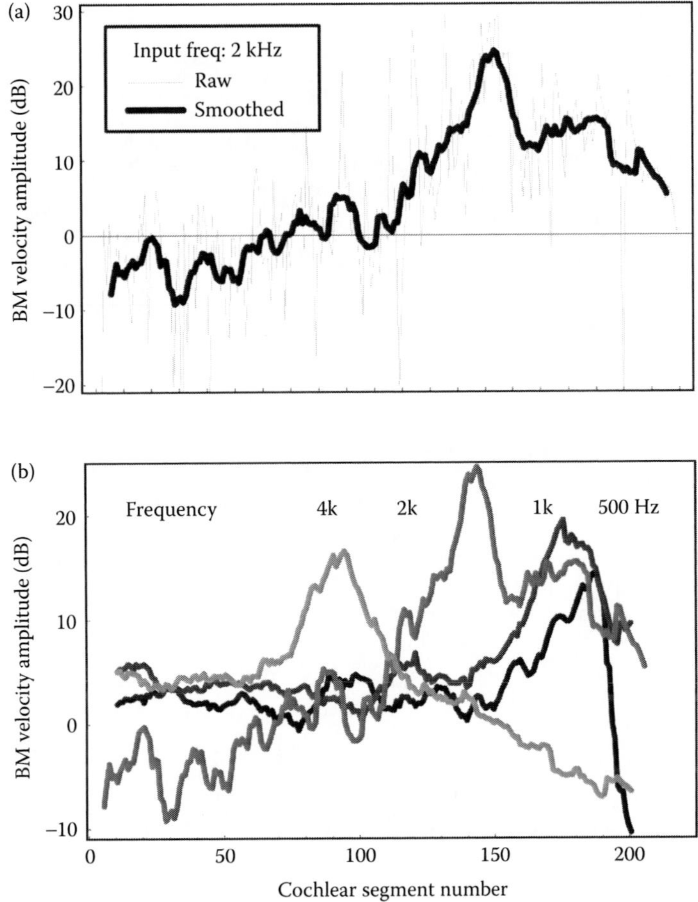

FIGURE 10.13 Measured longitudinal responses. (a) Raw and smoothed longitudinal BM velocity responses (2-kHz pure-tone input at 24 dB). A 10-segment moving average removes the large segment-to-segment variations. (b) Smoothed longitudinal responses to four octave-space frequencies. As frequency increases (from 500 to 4k Hz), the BM response peaks closer to the silicon cochlea's base.

(1 and 2 kHz) are Segments 166 and 139, respectively. Tip-to-tail ratios range from 12 to 32 dB; Q_{10} values range from 0.9 to 1.2; and cutoff slopes range from −16 to −70 dB/octave.*

10.4.2 Nonlinear Responses

I/O functions reveal the silicon cochlea's nonlinear behavior. We increased the input amplitude exponentially by increasing the voltage applied linearly, calculating the corresponding amplitude (in dB) based on the chip's subthreshold slope-coefficient (measured experimentally). The amplitude range applied was constrained on the high side by strong inversion (leaving the subthreshold region) and on the low side by the noise floor. We set $V_T = 1.9$ V to saturate active coupling at the upper end of this range, thereby producing compression.

BM responses show compressive growth, first at the CF and then at nearby frequencies (Figure 10.14). As a result, BM responses become more broadly tuned with increasing input amplitude; Q_{10} drops from 1.8 to 1.1. There is a corresponding decrease in cutoff slope, which drops from −44 to −13 dB/octave. Unlike biology, where there is a basal shift (to lower frequency) [13], the CF hardly changes,

* The number of segments spanned by an octave was calculated from the CF range of the first 240 segments.

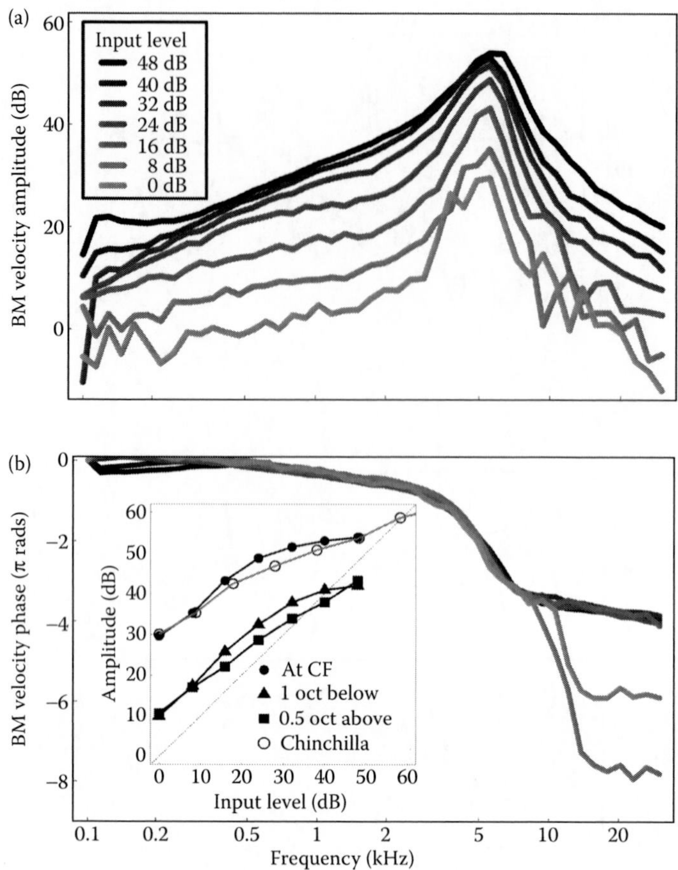

FIGURE 10.14 Nonlinear compression. BM-velocity frequency responses for different input amplitudes (BM Segment 100; CF: 5.6 kHz). (a) Amplitude. Equally-spaced responses indicate linear behavior. (b) Phase. Inset: I/O functions, measured at CF, an octave below, and half an octave above. Biological measurement is provided for comparison (open circles: chinchilla measurement from (M. A. Ruggero et al., *J. Acoust. Soc. Am.*, 101, 2151–2163, 1997), shifted to align the lowest input level tested with that of the chip). Dotted line: Identity ($y = x$). (From B. Wen and K. A. Boahen, *IEEE Trans. Biomed. Circuits Syst.*, 3, 444–455, 2009. With permission.)

probably due to insufficiently high input levels. The phase of BM responses does not change significantly; the case in biology as well. The larger phase plateaus (exactly 2π apart) at low input amplitudes (0 and 8 dB) are due to noisy responses in the cutoff region.

Compression does not occur symmetrically around the peak: It sets in at lower intensities for frequencies below the CF (see Figure 10.14, inset). Whereas at the CF (5.6 kHz) compression sets in when input amplitude exceeds 24 dB, one octave below (2.8 kHz) it happens at 32 dB, and half an octave above (7.9 kHz) it happens at 48 dB (the largest amplitude applied). This result suggests that upstream segments (higher CFs) contribute to automatic gain control, more so than downstream segments (lower CFs).

The chip's CF behavior agrees qualitatively with the chinchilla measurements (see Figure 10.14, inset), except that at high intensities, which the chip input did not reach, the chinchilla's I/O function became linear again, resembling a passive cochlea. Above or below the CF, the chip's I/O functions are less linear (more compressive) than the chinchilla's (data not shown), presumably because the chip's tuning is broader such that compression at high sound levels occurs with a larger spread.

To find the lowest detectable input amplitude, we measured the SNR at the output (defined as signal-squared over noise-squared) for various input amplitudes and extrapolated to 0 dB (see [21] for details). Output SNR increased from 2.8 to 19 dB as input amplitude increased from 0 to 48 dB. We fitted the SNR's initial increase and asymptotic behavior using a Michaelis–Menten function and obtained an output SNR of 1 (i.e., 0 dB) at an input amplitude of −4 dB by extrapolating the fit, which indicated a 52 dB input dynamic range.

10.4.3 Effect of ABC

Varying the coupling's saturation level (through V_T) demonstrates ABC's role. In all responses presented so far, except for Section 10.4.2, the saturation level was high enough to avoid saturation. It gets progressively lower as V_T (which gates pMOS transistors) increases, producing saturation at lower and lower input levels. Coupling is negligible for $V_T = 2.2$ V, which corresponds to a passive cochlea.

We obtained a series of frequency responses from Segment 100 with different saturation levels (Figure 10.15a). Decreasing saturation levels resulted in smaller response amplitudes. Amplitude decreased monotonically from 33.3 to 15.1 dB (arbitrary scale) at the CF, an 18 dB drop. Because decreases were more prominent in this region, responses became more broadly tuned; Q_{10} decreased

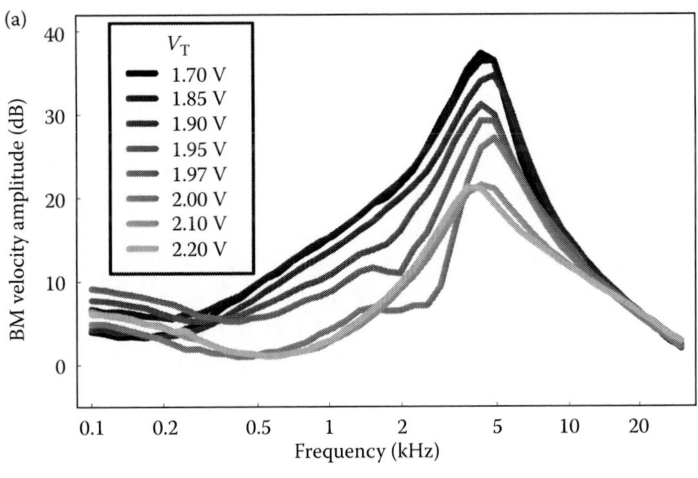

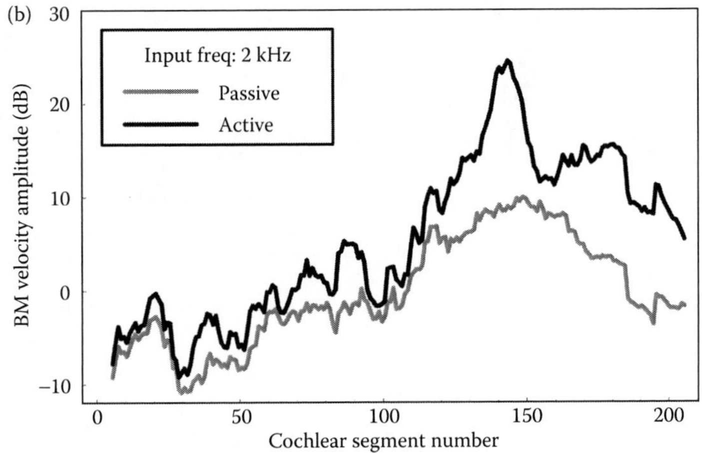

FIGURE 10.15 Effect of active coupling. (a) BM amplitude frequency responses for various coupling saturation levels (Segment 100; 16-dB input level). The saturation level decreases as V_T increases. (b) Longitudinal responses with (active; black) and without (passive; gray) coupling (2-kHz pure-tone input at 24 dB).

monotonically from 1.14 to 0.45. We also measured longitudinal responses to a 2-kHz tone with ($V_T = 0.26$ V) and without ($V_T = 2.35$ V) coupling (Figure 10.15b). Peak amplitude was 14.6 dB larger with coupling; the cutoff slope was 35 dB/octave steeper; Q_{10} increased from 0.39 to 1.16. These increases are comparable to those seen in Segment 100's frequency response (increases of 18.2 dB, 22.0 dB/octave, and 0.69, respectively).

In summary, ABC implemented in the analog VLSI chip increases gain and sharpens tuning, achieving responses that are qualitatively comparable to physiological measurements. Indeed, the cases with and without ABC resemble live (active) and dead (passive) cochlea, respectively; thus ABC captures the role of OHC electromotility—at least qualitatively.

10.4.4 Responses of the Silicon AN to Chirp-Click Sound

We visualized the silicon AN's response by constructing a cochleagram (Figure 10.16). This raster plot displays spike trains of all SGCs in Segments 1–240, a total of 1440 (240 × 6) outputs (SGCs from Segments 241–360 were omitted for the same reason stated earlier). Segment number runs from the top (base) to the bottom (apex)—high to low frequency—while time runs from left to right.

The silicon AN responds to the chirp-click sequence with a wave of spike activity followed by a flash (Figure 10.16). The wave propagates from the base to the apex in response to the chirp's decreasing frequency. It becomes more sharply defined after the first 60 segments (i.e., 360 SGCs), indicating the extent to which frequency selectivity arises cooperatively. The flash lights up all outputs simultaneously in response to the click's broad frequency content, except for the apex, where it is masked by the chirp's close proximity in time (contiguity). This masking is due to SGC spike-rate adaptation, which emphasizes sound onsets. A few highly excitable SGCs (e.g., Channels 223 and 480) respond throughout most of the stimulus; this behavior is due to transistor mismatch.

In summary, the silicon AN encodes a sound's frequency, intensity, and timing. It uses a place code for frequency: only neurons at a certain location fire. It uses a rate code for intensity: these neurons spike at higher rates. And it uses a real-time code for timing: spike rates change in real time, with sound onset emphasized by SGC spike-rate adaptation. The chip's specifications are summarized in Table 10.2 (mean ± standard deviation is quoted for $n = 12$ measurements).

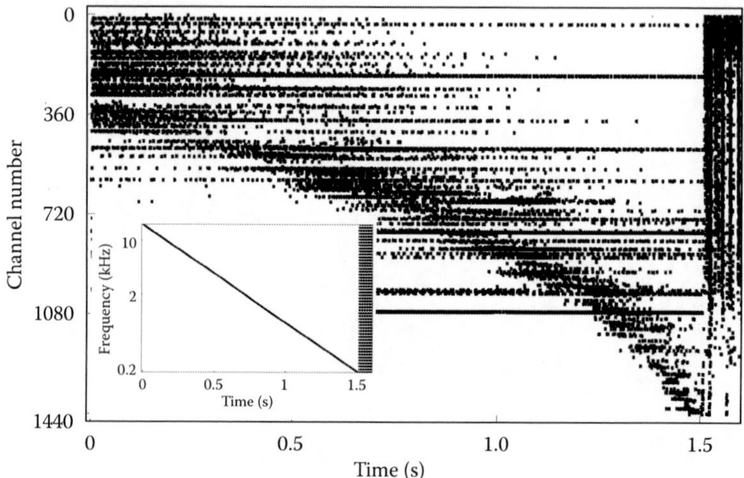

FIGURE 10.16 Chirp-click cochleagram. The chirp invokes a wave that propagates from the base (top) toward the apex (bottom). The click invokes a flash that lights up all but the lowest-frequency outputs. Inset: Chirp-click sound. On a logarithmic scale, the 1.5-s chirp's frequency decreases linearly and the 0.1-s click's 50 discrete frequencies are equally spaced; both span 16 kHz to 200 Hz.

TABLE 10.2
Silicon Cochlea Specifications

Specification	Values
Fabrication process	5M 1P 0.25 μm CMOS
Chip die dimensions	3.76 × 2.91 mm²
Transistors	115,000
Cochlear segments	360
SGC spike outputs	2160
Frequency range	200–20k Hz
Input dynamic range	52 dB
Signal-to-noise ratio	11.9 ± 4.0 dB
Tip-to-tail ratio	26.9 ± 11.7 dB
Phase at peak	−1.38 ± 1.31 π rads
Q_{10}	1.16 ± 0.92
Cutoff slope	−19.6 ± 17.5 dB/octave
Compression at peak	24 dB
Supply voltage	$AV_{dd} = 2.4$ V; $DV_{dd} = 2.5$ V
Total power	51.8 mW (35.9 mW for the analog core)

10.4.5 Impact of Transistor Mismatch on Chip Responses

The chip measurements presented here demonstrate that ABC overcomes the major shortcomings of previous silicon cochlea architectures, summarized in Table 10.3. In the cascade architecture, noise increased a hundredfold (asymptoting after 30 segments) [32]. With ABC, noise does not accumulate, as demonstrated by our SNR measurements (see [51] for details). In the passively coupled architecture, gain decreased by 25 dB [7]. With ABC, this destructive interference is overcome, as demonstrated by our gain and tuning measurements (Figure 10.15). However, ABC's gain-increase was limited to 18 dB by mismatch-induced traveling-wave reflections. We confirmed that these reflections can reduce gain and broaden tuning by performing simulations with mismatch included.

The dominant source of transistor mismatch is threshold-voltage variation, which has been shown to be Gaussian distributed, with variance inversely proportional to the transistor's channel area [64]. When transistors operate in weak-inversion for low-power consumption, their currents are log-normally distributed. For instance, in a 0.35-μm CMOS process, the currents' coefficient of variation (standard deviation over mean), or CV, is 9.2% and 22% for 11.4 × 11.4 λ and 4.6 × 4.6 λ ($\lambda = 0.18$ μm) nMOS transistors, respectively [65]. Given the transistor sizes in our circuits (see [51] for details), we used log-normally distributed parameter values with CVs ranging up to 25% in our simulations (see [51] for details).

We quantified the mismatch's effect on active amplification (tip-to-tail ratio) and tuning sharpness (Q_{10}), extracted from smoothed BM velocity responses. With OHC motility factor $\alpha = 0.15$,

TABLE 10.3
Silicon Cochlea Architectures

Architecture	Major Issues
Cascade [5,29,62]	Noise and delay accumulate; poor fault tolerance
Passive coupling [6,7,63]	Destructive interference occurs due to large phase changes at resonance
Active coupling (this work)	Reflections occur when device mismatch causes abrupt changes

these metrics dropped from 85 ± 4 (mean ± standard deviation) to 41 ± 7 dB and from 5.2 ± 0.6 to 1.1 ± 0.8, respectively, as CV increased from 5% to 25%, becoming similar to the passive case ($\alpha = 0$), albeit with substantially larger variance. This loss of sensitivity and selectivity could be counteracted by increasing α. For CV = 25%, increasing α from 0.15 to 0.25 increased peak gain from 41 ± 7 to 70 ± 13 dB and Q_{10} from 1.1 ± 0.8 to 3.6 ± 1.5, with variance increasing dramatically in both cases. For comparison, with $\alpha = 0.15$, these metrics were 89 dB and 5.6, respectively, in the absence of mismatch.

These simulation results suggest that mismatch accounts for shortfalls in the chip's overall performance as well as variability among its segments. For the value of α the chip used (0.14—estimated from bias voltages that determine a_{ff}, a_{fb}, and b), the simulations reproduce the range of values we measured for the tip-to-tail ratio and Q_{10} with a parameter-CV of slightly above 20% (see [51] for details), twice the 10% current-CV of the chip's (mostly) 10 × 10 λ transistors.* We could not confirm the predicted performance improvement with values of α greater than 0.14 because they produced instability in the chip.

These simulation results also suggest that ABC has the potential to exceed the best performance achieved by silicon cochleae to date. Sarpeshkar et al.'s hybrid parallel–cascade architecture achieved a tip-to-tail ratio of 77 dB [32]. In contrast, Fragniere's passively coupled architecture achieved a Q_{10} of 2.34 [7]. In comparison, our simulations predict that, with the practical OHC motility factor of 0.14, ABC can achieve a tip-to-tail ratio of 85 ± 4 dB and a Q_{10} of 5.2 ± 0.6 if parameter-CV is reduced to 10%. This requires decreasing the current-CV from 10% to 5% by increasing transistor sizes from 10 × 10 to 20 × 20 λ. These larger transistors would only increase the chip's size from 10.9 to 14.3 mm^2, since the BM segments currently occupy only 10.3% of its area (excluding the capacitors). However, this promised performance remains to be proven in silicon.

10.5 CONCLUSIONS AND FUTURE WORK

We presented a nonlinear active cochlear model based on a novel cochlear amplifier mechanism, ABC. ABC offers a plausible way in which OHC electromotile forces are transmitted to the BM through the unique microanatomy and the architecture formed by several types of cells within the organ of Corti. Specifically, ABC postulates that both the basal tilt of OHCs and the apical tilt of PhPs play a critical role in delivering OHC forces onto the BM, thus affecting its vibration. We showed, through mathematical simulations, that the ABC cochlear model is able to reproduce the characteristic cochlear responses, including large amplification and sharp frequency tuning at low sound levels, and compressive growth of response gain and broadened frequency tuning at mid-to-high sound levels. We further explored the way in which ABC enhances the BM motion in a frequency-selective fashion and found that ABC generates negative damping before the characteristic place over a restricted cochlear region. Thus, ABC amplifies the cochlear traveling wave only in the short-wave region, increasing the response gain as well as sharpening the frequency tuning at the peak.

We then presented a bioinspired mixed-signal VLSI implementation of an active cochlear model that utilizes the cochlear amplifier mechanism, ABC. *In silico*, ABC produces large amplification and sharp tuning to soft sound and nonlinear compression and broad tuning to loud sound. Rather than detecting signal amplitude and implementing an AQC loop, ABC simply mimics OHC-force saturation, which acts instantaneously; and ABC senses the wavelength, which adds frequency selectivity. It successfully combats destructive interference in the coupled architecture.

ABC was vulnerable to reflections that occur when BM properties change abruptly due to device mismatch. However, reducing mismatch by increasing transistor area will decrease the number of

* Note that this doubling could be produced by cascading two current mirrors. That this is less than the actual number of mirroring operations in a BM segment is explained by the averaging that occurs when several segments' outputs are actively and passively coupled together to yield the measured response.

BM segments per octave, which will broaden frequency tuning. Alternatively, as mismatch perturbs BM properties at the finest spatial scale, it could be counteracted by increasing the wavelength, something the three-to-five-OHC tilt observed in the organ of Corti [39,66] would achieve. The caveat is that lengthening the wavelength will also broaden tuning. Further study is required in order to determine which approach offers the most favorable trade-off.

REFERENCES

1. C. A. Mead and M. A. Mahowald, A silicon model of early visual processing, *J. Neural Networks*, 1, 91–97, 1988.
2. K. A. Boahen, A retinomorphic vision system, *IEEE Micro*., 16, 30–39, 1996.
3. K. A. Boahen, The retinomorphic approach: Pixel-parallel adaptive amplification, filtering, and quantization, *J. Analog Integr. Circuits Signal Process.*, 13, 53–68, 1997.
4. K. Zaghloul and K. A. Boahen, An on-off log-domain circuit that recreates adaptive filtering in the retina, *IEEE Trans. Circuits Syst. I. Reg. Papers*, 52, 99–107, 2005.
5. R. F. Lyon and C. A. Mead, An analog electronic cochlea, *IEEE Trans. Acoust. Speech Signal Process.*, 36, 1119–1134, 1988.
6. L. Watts, *Cochlear Mechanics: Analysis and Analog VLSI*, PhD dissertation, California Institute of Technology, Pasadena, CA, 1993.
7. E. Fragnière, A 100-channel analog CMOS auditory filter bank for speech recognition, in *Proc. IEEE Int. Solid-State Circuits Conf. Dig. Tech. Papers*, San Francisco, CA, 2005, pp. 140–141.
8. P. Merolla and K. A. Boahen, A recurrent model of orientation maps with simple and complex cells, in *Advances in Neural Information Processing Systems*, Vol. 16, S. Thrun and L. Saul, Eds. Cambridge, MA: MIT Press, 2004, pp. 995–1002.
9. T. Y. W. Choi, P. A. Merolla, J. V. Arthur, K. A. Boahen, and B. E. Shi, Neuromorphic implementation of orientation hypercolumns, *IEEE Trans. Circuits Syst. I: Reg. Papers*, 52, 1049–1060, 2005.
10. B. Taba and K. A. Boahen, Topographic map formation by silicon growth cones, in *Advances in Neural Information Processing Systems*, Vol. 14, S. Becker, S. Thrun, and K. Obermayer, Eds. Cambridge, MA: MIT Press, 2002, pp. 1139–1146.
11. J. V. Arthur and K. A. Boahen, Recurrently connected silicon neurons with active dendrites for one-shot learning, in *Proc. IEEE Int. Joint Conf. Neural Networks*, Budapest, Hungary, 2004, pp. 1699–1704.
12. J. V. Arthur and K. A. Boahen, Learning in silicon: Timing is everything, in *Advances in Neural Information Processing Systems*, Vol. 17, B. Sholkopf and Y. Weiss, Eds. Cambridge, MA: MIT Press, 2006, pp. 75–82.
13. L. Robles and M. A. Ruggero, Mechanics of the mammalian cochlea, *Physiol. Rev.*, 81, 1305–1352, 2001.
14. W. E. Brownell, Observation on a motile response in isolated hair cells, in *Mechanism of Hearing*, W. R. Webster and L. M. Aiken, Eds. Melbourne, Australia: Monash University Press, 1983, pp. 5–10.
15. W. E. Brownell, C. R. Bader, D. Bertrand, and Y. Deribaupierre, Evoked mechanical responses of isolated cochlear outer hair cells, *Science*, 227, 194–196, 1985.
16. C. D. Geisler and C. Sang, A cochlear model using feed-forward outer-hair-cell forces, *Hear. Res.*, 86, 132–146, 1995.
17. T. Fukazawa, How can the cochlea amplifier be realized by the outer hair cells which have nothing to push against? *Hear. Res.*, 172, 53–61, 2002.
18. K. Lim and C. R. Steele, A three-dimensional nonlinear active cochlear model analyzed by the WKB-numeric method, *Hear. Res.*, 170, 190–205, 2002.
19. C. D. Geisler, *From Sound to Synapse: Physiology of the Mammalian Ear*. New York, NY: Oxford University Press, 1998.
20. B. Wen and K. A. Boahen, A linear cochlear model with active bi-directional coupling, in *Proc. 25th Annu. Int. Conf. IEEE Eng. Med. Biol. Soc.*, Cancun, Mexico, 2003, pp. 2013–2016.
21. B. Wen, *Modeling the Nonlinear Active Cochlea: Mathematics and Analog VLSI*, Philadelphia, PA: University of Pennsylvania, 2006.
22. J.-J. Sit and R. Sarpeshkar, A cochlear-implant processor for encoding music and lowering stimulation power, *IEEE Pervasive Comput.*, 1, 40–48, 2008.
23. R. Sarpeshkar, R. F. Lyon, and C. Mead, A low-power wide-dynamic-range analog VLSI cochlea, *J. Analog Integr. Circuits Signal Process.*, 16, 245–274, 1998.

24. R. Sarpeshkar, C. Salthouse, J.-J. Sit, M. W. Baker, S. M. Zhak, T. K.-T. Lu, L. Turicchia, and S. Balster, An ultra-low-power programmable analog bionic ear processor, *IEEE Trans. Biomed. Eng.*, 52, 711–727, 2005.
25. B. Wen and K. A. Boahen, Active bidirectional coupling in a cochlear chip, in *Advances in Neural Information Processing Systems*, Vol. 18, Y. Weiss, B. Scholköpf, and J. Platt, Eds. Cambridge, MA: MIT Press, 2006, pp. 1497–1504.
26. S. Martignoli, J.-J. van der Vyver, A. Kern, Y. Uwate, and R. Stoop, Analog electronic cochlea with mammalian hearing characteristics, *Appl. Phys. Lett.*, 91, 064108, 2007.
27. T. J. Hamilton, C. Jin, A. van Schaik, and J. Tapson, An active 2-D silicon cochlea, *IEEE Trans. Biomed. Circuits Syst.*, 2, 30–43, 2008.
28. T. J. Hamilton, C. Jin, J. Tapson, and A. van Schaik, A 2D cochlea with Hopf oscillators, in *Proc. IEEE Biomed. Circuits Syst. Conf.*, Montreal, Canada, 2007, pp. 91–94.
29. R. Sarpeshkar, R. F. Lyon, and C. Mead, An analog VLSI cochlea with new transconductance amplifiers and nonlinear gain control, in *Proc. IEEE Int. Symp. Circuits and Systems*, Atlanta, GA, 1996, pp. 292–295.
30. B. C. J. Moore, *An Introduction to the Psychology of Hearing*. New York, NY: Elsevier Academic Press, 2004.
31. W. S. Rhode and P. H. Smith, Characteristics of tone-pip response patterns in relationship to spontaneous rate in cat auditory-nerve fibers, *Hear. Res.*, 18, 159–168, 1985.
32. R. Sarpeshkar, R. F. Lyon, and C. Mead, A low-power wide-dynamic-range analog VLSI cochlea, in *Neuromorphic Systems Engineering-Neural Networks in Silicon*, T. S. Lande, Ed. Boston: Kluwer Academic Publishers, 1998, pp. 49–103.
33. C. D. Summerfield and R. F. Lyon, ASIC implementation of the Lyon cochlea model, in *Proc. IEEE Int. Conf. Acoust. Speech and Signal Process.*, San Francisco, CA, 1992, pp. 673–676.
34. M. P. Leong, C. T. Jin, and P. H. W. Leong, An FPGA-based electronic cochlea, *EURASIP J Appl. Signal Process.*, 7, 629–638, 2003.
35. C. A. Mead, *Analog VLSI and Neural Systems*. Reading, MA: Addison-Wesley, 1989.
36. Y. Raphael, M. Lenoir, R. Wroblewski, and R. Pujol, The sensory epithelium and its innervation in the mole rat cochlea, *J. Comp. Neurol.*, 314, 367–382, 1991.
37. I. J. Russell and K. E. Nilsen, The location of the cochlear amplifier: Spatial representation of a single tone on the guinea pig basilar membrane, *Proc. Nat. Acad. Sci. USA*, 94, 2660–2664, 1997.
38. P. Dallos, The active cochlea, *J. Neurosci.*, 12, 4575–4585, 1992.
39. F. Kalinec and B. Kachar, Structure of the electromechanical transduction mechanism in mammalian outer hair cells, in *Active Hearing*, A. A. Flock, D. Ottoson, and M. Ulfendahl, Eds. Kidlington: Pergamon, 1995, pp. 181–193.
40. C. R. Steele, G. Baker, J. Tolomeo, and D. Zetes, Electro-mechanical models of the outer hair cell, in *Proc. Int. Symp. Biophysics of Hair Cell Sensory Systems*, H. Duifhuis, J. W. Horst, P. van Dijk, and S. M. van Netten, Eds. Singapore: World Scientific, 1993.
41. G. Zweig, Finding the impedance of the organ of Corti, *J. Acoust. Soc. Am.*, 89, 1229–1254, 1991.
42. S. T. Neely, A model of cochlear mechanics with outer hair cell motility, *J. Acoust. Soc. Am.*, 94, 137–146, 1993.
43. P. Kolston, The importance of phase data and model dimensionality to cochlear mechanics, *Hear. Res.*, 145, 25–36, 2000.
44. M. A. Ruggero, N. C. Rich, S. S. Narayan, and L. Robles, Basilar membrane responses to tones at the base of the chinchilla cochlea, *J. Acoust. Soc. Am.*, 101, 2151–2163, 1997.
45. K. A. Boahen and A. G. Andreou, A contrast sensitive silicon retina with reciprocal synapses, in *Advances in Neural Information Processing Systems*, Vol. 4, J. E. Moody and R. P. Lippmann, Eds. San Mateo, CA: Morgan Kaufmann, 1992, pp. 764–772.
46. A. G. Andreou and K. A. Boahen, Translinear circuits in subthreshold MOS, *J. Analog Integr. Circuits Signal Process.*, 9, 141–166, 1996.
47. D. R. Frey, Log-domain filtering: An approach to current-mode filtering, *IEE Proc. G Circuits Devices Syst.*, 140, 406–416, 1993.
48. T. Y. W. Choi, B. E. Shi, and K. A. Boahen, An on-off orientation selective address event representation image transceiver chip, *IEEE Trans. Circuits Syst. I: Reg. Papers*, 51, 342–353, 2004.
49. W. K. Chen, *The VLSI Handbook*. Boca Raton, FL: CRC Press, 2000.
50. T. Delbrück, "Bump" circuits for computing similarity and dissimilarity of analog voltages, in *Proc. Int. Joint Conf. Neural Networks*, Seattle, Washington, 1991, pp. I-475–479.

51. B. Wen and K. A. Boahen, A silicon cochlea with active coupling, *IEEE Trans. Biomed. Circuits Syst.*, 3, 444–455, 2009.
52. M. C. Liberman, L. W. Dodds, and S. Pierce, Afferent and efferent innervation of the cat cochlea: Quantitative analysis with light and electron microscopy, *J. Comp. Neurol.*, 301, 443–460, 1990.
53. C. L. Adamson, M. A. Reid, Z. L. Mo, J. Browne-English, and R. L. Davis, Firing features and potassium channel content of murine spiral ganglion neurons vary with cochlear location, *J Comp Neurol*, 447, 331–350, 2002.
54. J. H. Wittig and K. A. Boahen, Silicon neurons that phase-lock, in *Proc. IEEE Int. Symp. Circuits and Systems*, 2006, pp. 4535–4538.
55. J. Santos-Sacchi, Voltage-dependent ionic conductances of Type-I spiral ganglion-cells from the guinea-pig inner-ear, *J. Neurosci.*, 13, 3599–3611, 1993.
56. E. J. Moore, D. B. Hall, and T. Narahashi, Sodium and potassium currents of type I spiral ganglion cells from rat, *Acta Oto-Laryngol.*, 116, 552–560, 1996.
57. K. Yamaguchi and H. Ohmori, Voltage-gated and chemically gated ionic channels in the cultured cochlear ganglion neurone of the chick, *J. Physiol.*, 420, 185–206, 1990.
58. J. Lazzaro, M. Wawrzynek, M. Mahowald, M. Sivilotti, and D. Gillespie, Silicon auditory processors as computer peripherals, *IEEE Trans. Neural Networks*, 4, 523–528, 1993.
59. K. A. Boahen, A burst-mode word-serial address-event channel-I: Transmitter design, *IEEE Trans. Circuits Syst. Reg. Papers*, 51, 1269–1280, 2004.
60. V. Chan, S.-C. Liu, and A. van Schaik, AER EAR: A matched silicon cochlea pair with address event representation interface, *IEEE Trans. Circuits Syst. I.*, 54, 48–59, 2007.
61. C. A. Mead and T. Delbrück, Scanners for visualizing activity of analog VLSI circuitry, *J. Analog Integr. Circuits Signal Process.*, 1, 93–106, 1991.
62. A. van Schaik, E. Fragnière, and E. A. Vittoz, Improved silicon cochlea using compatible lateral bipolar transistors, in *Advances in Neural Information Processing Systems*, Vol. 8, D. S. Touretky, M. C. Mozer, and M. E. Hasselmo, Eds. Cambridge, MA: MIT Press, 1996, pp. 671–677.
63. A. van Schaik and E. Fragnière, Pseudo-voltage-domain implementation of a design of two-dimensional silicon cochlea, in *Proc. IEEE Int. Symp. Circuits Syst.*, 2001, pp. 185–188.
64. P. R. Kinget, Device mismatch and tradeoffs in the design of analog circuits, *IEEE J. Solid-State Circuits*, 40, 1212–1224, 2005.
65. B. Linares-Barranco, T. Serrano-Gotarredona, R. Serrano-Gotarredona, and G. Vicente-Sanchez, On mismatch properties of MOS and resistors calibrated ladder structures, in *Proc. IEEE Int. Symp. Circuits Syst*, Vancouver, Canada, 2004, pp. 377–380.
66. Y. Raphael and R. A. Altschuler, Reorganization of cytoskeletal and junctional proteins during cochlear hair cell degeneration, *Cell Motility Cytoskeleton*, 18, 215–227, 1991.

11 Micropower Adaptive VLSI Systems for Acoustic Source Localization and Separation

Milutin Stanaćević and Gert Cauwenberghs

CONTENTS

11.1 INTRODUCTION

Blind separation of real-world acoustic sources is generally considered a hard and unsolved problem, with mixed degree of success in practical realizations. Closely linked to acoustic source separation is the problem of source localization, or bearing angle estimation. Wave propagation of sound complicates the task of separating multiple coexisting sources using independent component analysis (ICA) [1], which conventionally assumes instantaneous mixture observations. In contrast, convolutive ICA techniques explicitly assume convolutive or delayed mixtures in the source observations. Convolutive ICA techniques [2–4] are usually much more involved and require a large number of parameters and long adaptation time horizons for proper convergence. Inspiration from biology suggests that for very small aperture (spacing between acoustic sensors, i.e., tympanal membranes), small differences (gradients) in sound pressure level are more effective in resolving source direction than actual (microsecond scale) time differences. The remarkable auditory localization capability of certain insects at a small (1%) fraction of the wavelength of the source owes itself to highly sensitive differential processing of sound pressure through intertympanal mechanical coupling [5] or interaural coupled neural circuits [6].

In this chapter, we present an approach, gradient flow, that avoids the problem of separating delayed mixtures in the case of arrays of very small aperture, that is, of dimensions significantly smaller than the shortest wavelength in the sources. The delayed signals observed on the array are expended in series of terms that only contain the instantaneous signals and their time derivatives. By taking spatial derivatives of these delayed signals, we are able to isolate terms of various orders in the temporal derivatives, all indirectly contributing observations of linearly independent instantaneous mixtures of the source signals [7]. This formulation is equivalent to that of standard ICA. The mixing coefficients obtained from ICA yield the angles of the incoming waves. Therefore this method can be seen as a combination of the wave sensing idea and ICA, performing at once blind separation and localization of traveling waves. We present a mixed-signal very-large-scale integration (VLSI) adaptive microsystem implementing gradient flow interfaced with a miniature microphone array that performs real-time acoustic source separation and localization at microwatts of power, for use in intelligent hearing aids and acoustic surveillance.

11.2 MICROPOWER ACOUSTIC LOCALIZER

In this section, we present the gradient flow principle of sensing the acoustic field and demonstrate how the problem of estimating time delays simplifies to the least-squares problem in the case of acoustic localization of a single source.

11.2.1 Gradient Flow Principle

A spherical traveling wave emitted by a point source $\mathcal{S}$ propagates through space and is observed by a sensor at location $\mathbf{r}_s$ in space, with respect to the source position, as

$$\mathcal{S}(\mathbf{r}_s,t) = A(\mathbf{r}_s)\mathcal{S}(t+\tau(\mathbf{r}_S)), \tag{11.1}$$

where $\tau(\mathbf{r}_s)$ represents time traversed along the path from the source to the sensor, and $A(\mathbf{r}_s)$ accounts for the dependence of amplitude on distance from the source, as shown in Figure 11.1. The propagation model (Equation 11.1) can be applied to an electromagnetic wave as well as to an acoustic wave. The points in space lying on the surface of a sphere, with the center at the source, have a common phase and belong to the same wavefront. In the far-field condition, when the distance $|\mathbf{r}_s|$ from the source is large, the wavefront becomes a flat plane of constant phase, resulting in a plane wave.

Let us assume that a signal is observed on the sensor array. The distribution of sensors could be continuous or discrete. We define $t_0 = \tau(\mathbf{r}_0)$ as the time traveled from the source to the center of the array that coincides with the "center of mass" of the sensor distribution and located at position $\mathbf{r}_0$ relative to the source. The signal observed at the center is denoted as

$$S(t) = \mathcal{S}(\mathbf{r}_0,t) = A(\mathbf{r}_0)\mathcal{S}(t+t_0). \tag{11.2}$$

Let the coordinate system $\mathbf{r}$ have the origin in the center of the array. We define $\tau(r)$ as the time lag between the wavefront at point $\mathbf{r}$ and the wavefront at the center of the array, that is, the

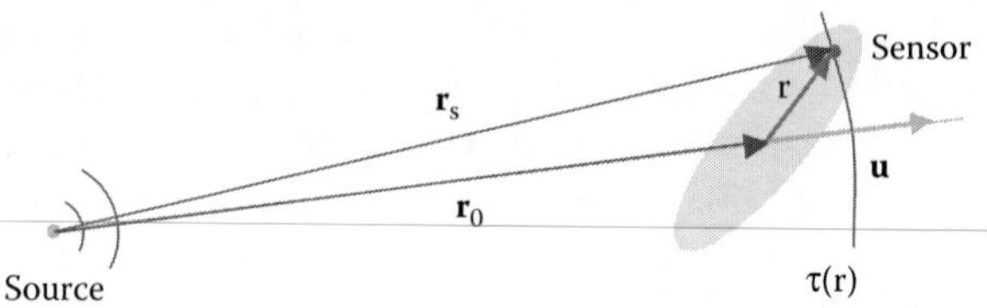

FIGURE 11.1 A traveling wave, emitted by the point source, is received at the sensor at location $\mathbf{r}_s$.

propagation time $\tau(\mathbf{r})$ is referenced to the center of the array. The signal measured at the sensor at location $\mathbf{r}$ is

$$\begin{aligned} \mathcal{S}(\mathbf{r},t) &= A(\mathbf{r}_s)\mathcal{S}((t+t_0)+(\tau(\mathbf{r}_s)-t_0)) \\ &= A(\mathbf{r}_s)\mathcal{S}(t+t_0)+\tau(\mathbf{r})). \end{aligned} \tag{11.3}$$

For miniature sensor arrays, in the far-field approximation, the distance from the source is much larger than the dimensions of the sensor array and the amplitude of the signal $A(\mathbf{r}_s)$ at the sensor will be approximately equal to the amplitude of signal $A(\mathbf{r}_0)$ at the center of the array. The measured signal at the sensor is then a delayed version of the signal observed at the center of the array

$$\mathcal{S}(\mathbf{r},t) = s(t+\tau(\mathbf{r})). \tag{11.4}$$

The wavefront delay $\tau(\mathbf{r})$ is approximately linear in the projection of $\mathbf{r}$ on the unit vector $\mathbf{u}$ pointing toward the source,

$$\tau(\mathbf{r}) \approx \frac{1}{c}\mathbf{r}\cdot\mathbf{u}, \tag{11.5}$$

where c is the speed of (acoustic or electromagnetic) wave propagation.

The signal observed at the sensor at location $\mathbf{r}$ can be expanded about the center of the array in the power series expansion,

$$x_{\mathbf{r}}(t) = s(t+\tau(\mathbf{r})) = s(t)+\tau(\mathbf{r})\dot{s}(t)+\tfrac{1}{2}\tau(\mathbf{r})^2\ddot{s}(t)+\cdots. \tag{11.6}$$

The relative size of terms in the series expansion, or the scale on which the signals are sampled, depends on the frequency content of the source signal and the size of the array. The Fourier transform of Equation 11.6 in time corresponds to a frequency-domain transfer function with series approximation

$$\exp(+j\omega\tau(\mathbf{r})) = 1+j\omega\tau(\mathbf{r})-\tfrac{1}{2}(\omega\tau(\mathbf{r}))^2+\cdots. \tag{11.7}$$

The series (Equation 11.7) converges uniformly for all ω, but the number of terms needed increases rapidly with $|\omega\tau(\mathbf{r})|$. On the other hand, for the purposes of time delay estimation from physical observations of individual terms in the series, the ratio of consecutive terms in the series cannot be too small. A trade-off between approximation and resolution power is thus obtained when

$$\varepsilon \le |\omega\tau(\mathbf{r})| \le \alpha, \tag{11.8}$$

where ε is sufficiently above the observation noise floor, and α is not too large. In the far-field approximation,

$$\omega\tau(\mathbf{r}) = -\mathbf{k}\cdot\mathbf{r}, \tag{11.9}$$

where $\mathbf{k}$ is the wave vector,

$$\mathbf{k} = -\frac{\omega}{c}\mathbf{u} = -\frac{2\pi}{\lambda}\mathbf{u}, \tag{11.10}$$

and condition (11.8) translates to

$$\varepsilon\lambda_{\max} \leq |\mathbf{r}| \leq \alpha\lambda_{\min}, \tag{11.11}$$

where $\lambda_{\min} = c/f_{\max}$ is the shortest wavelength present in the spectrum of the traveling wave and $\lambda_{\max} = c/f_{\min}$ is the largest. In other words, we consider array dimensions not much larger than the smallest wavelength, but not too small compared with the largest wavelength. Note that α in the upper limit depends on the number of terms in the expansion.

In the special case of a two-dimensional (2D) array of sensors, the position vector $\mathbf{r}$ can be decomposed in the direction of the position coordinates p and q as $\mathbf{r} = p\mathbf{r}_1 + q\mathbf{r}_2$, where $\mathbf{r}_1$ and $\mathbf{r}_2$ are orthogonal unit vectors in the sensor plane. In a similar fashion, the time delay of source signal observed at the sensor at location $\mathbf{r}$ can also be decomposed as

$$\tau_{pq} = p\tau_1 + q\tau_2, \tag{11.12}$$

where τ_1 and τ_2 are the intertime differences (ITDs) of the source between adjacent sensors on the grid along the p and q place coordinates, respectively,

$$\begin{aligned} \tau_1 &= \frac{1}{c}\mathbf{r}_1 \cdot \mathbf{u}, \\ \tau_2 &= \frac{1}{c}\mathbf{r}_2 \cdot \mathbf{u}, \end{aligned} \tag{11.13}$$

as illustrated in Figure 11.2a. Under the assumption (Equation 11.11), we can concentrate on the first two terms in the series expansion (11.6) and the signal observed at the sensor at location $\mathbf{r}$, with spatial coordinates p and q, becomes

$$x_{pq}(t) \approx s(t) + (p\tau_1 + q\tau_2)\dot{s}(t) + n_{pq}(t). \tag{11.14}$$

We can now define gradient flow representation through spatial gradient decomposition, which relates the spatial and temporal gradients. We take spatial derivatives of various orders i and j along the position coordinates p and q, around the origin $p = q = 0$, and apply the series expansion model from Equation 11.14 to obtain

$$\begin{aligned} \xi_{ij}(t) &\equiv \left.\frac{\partial^{i+j}}{\partial^i p \partial^j q} x_{pq}(t)\right|_{p=q=0} \\ &= (\tau_1)^i (\tau_2)^j \frac{\mathrm{d}^{i+j}}{\mathrm{d}^{i+j} t} s(t) + \nu_{ij}(t), \end{aligned} \tag{11.15}$$

where ν_{ij} are the corresponding spatial derivatives of the sensor noise n_{pq} around the center. For the first-order case $k = 1$, Equation 11.15 becomes

$$\begin{aligned} \xi_{00}(t) &= s(t) + \nu_{00}(t), \\ \xi_{10}(t) &= \tau_1 \dot{s}(t) + \nu_{10}(t), \\ \xi_{01}(t) &= \tau_2 \dot{s}(t) + \nu_{01}(t). \end{aligned} \tag{11.16}$$

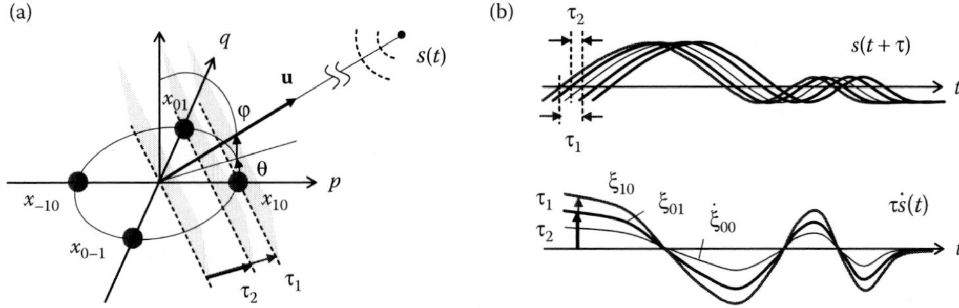

FIGURE 11.2 Gradient flow principle. (a) Sensor geometry and source direction coordinates Time-delayed observations of a wave signal $s(t)$ at four closely spaced sensor locations. (b) Top: Time-delayed observations of a wave signal $s(t)$ at four closely spaced sensor locations. Bottom: Gradient flow converts delays into relative amplitudes of the temporal derivative of the signal as observed in the spatial gradients of the wave signals over the array.

The first-order spatial gradients are linearly scaled versions of the time derivative of the source signal measured at the center of the array. Time delays linearly enter the spatial gradient equations and are isolated in the p and q directions. By taking the time derivative of ξ_{00}, we obtain three independent observations of the time derivative of the source signal and the problem of estimating time delays translates to the standard least-square problem in the unknown delays.

In practice, spatial derivatives (Equation 11.17) are approximated by discrete sampling on the grid $x_{pq}(t)$. Finding the proper sampling coefficients on a grid to approximate derivatives is a well-studied problem in digital signal processing [8]. For dense sensor arrays, an alternative is to approximate the derivatives using moments over the sensor distribution, giving estimates that are more robust to noise. Distributed sensors that acquire spatial gradients directly are also implementable in MEMS technology [9]. Estimates of ξ_{00}, ξ_{10}, and ξ_{01} (precise up to terms at least of third order) are obtained with just four sensors x_{pq} in the configuration shown in Figure 11.2a:

$$\begin{aligned}\xi_{00} &\approx \tfrac{1}{4}(x_{-1,0} + x_{1,0} + x_{0,-1} + x_{0,1})\\ \xi_{10} &\approx \tfrac{1}{2}(x_{1,0} - x_{-1,0})\\ \xi_{01} &\approx \tfrac{1}{2}(x_{0,1} - x_{0,-1})\end{aligned} \tag{11.17}$$

In Figure 11.2b, the sensor observations and spatial gradient signals are illustrated. From least-squares estimates of the time delays, we can directly obtain estimates of azimuth angle θ and elevation angle ϕ.

11.2.2 Mixed-Signal VLSI Implementation

Gradient flow principle is implemented in ultrapower mixed-signal VLSI application specific integrated circuit (ASIC) for 3D localization of a broadband acoustic source. The system block diagram implementing gradient flow for bearing estimation is shown in Figure 11.3. By adopting a mixed-signal architecture in the implementation, we combine the advantages of both approaches: an analog data path directly interfaces with inputs without the need for data conversion; and digital adaptation offers the desired outputs as digital values, performing "smart" analog-to-digital conversion. Estimation of the gradients is implemented using sampled-data switched-capacitor (SC) circuits. The advantage of this realization is application of correlated-double sampling (CDS) that significantly reduces common-mode offsets and 1/*f* noise [10], the dominant noise source at low frequencies. The spatial gradients are computed in the fully differential mode, to provide increased clock and supply

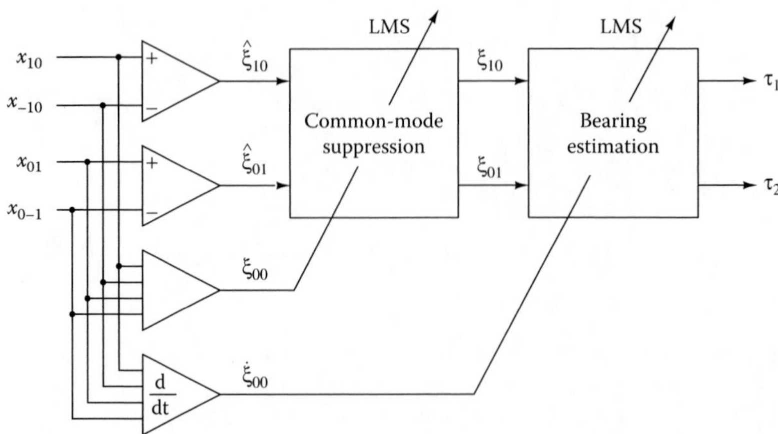

FIGURE 11.3 System block diagram.

feedthrough rejection. A cascoded nMOS inverter implements a simple high-gain amplifier in all of the SC circuits, supporting high density of integration and high energetic efficiency.

11.2.2.1 Gradient Computation

Spatial gradients are approximated by evaluating finite differences over the four sensors on the planar grid shown in Figure 11.2a [11]. Accurate bearing estimation assumes accurate sensing of the gradients. One significant advantage of gradient flow localization is that it relaxes requirements on sampling rate, governed by signal bandwidth (sub-kHz for acoustic surveillance) as opposed to the desired resolution of ITD estimation (microseconds). However, it is crucial to ensure that the signals be properly bandlimited, and that all signal components including spatial and temporal gradients be synchronously sampled.

The common-mode component is decomposed in differential form $\xi_{00}[n] = \xi_{00}^{+}[n] - \xi_{00}^{-}[n]$ with

$$\begin{aligned}\xi_{00}^{+}[n] &= \frac{1}{8}\left(x_{10}\left[n-\frac{1}{2}\right] + x_{-10}\left[n-\frac{1}{2}\right] + x_{01}\left[n-\frac{1}{2}\right] + x_{0-1}\left[n-\frac{1}{2}\right]\right),\\ \xi_{00}^{-}[n] &= -\frac{1}{8}(x_{10}[n] + x_{-10}[n] + x_{01}[n] + x_{0-1}[n]).\end{aligned} \tag{11.18}$$

The timing of common-mode acquisition is illustrated in Figure 11.4a. The contribution ξ_{00}^{+} to ξ_{00} represents the estimate of the average signal at time instance $nT - T/2$, while the contribution ξ_{00}^{-} represents the inverted estimate at time instance nT. The difference between both contributions hence produces an unbiased estimate of ξ_{00} centered at time $nT - T/4$ (as the average of the estimates at times $nT - T/2$ and nT).

SC realization of the common-mode estimation is given in Figure 11.4b. In the sampling phase ϕ_1, input signals are sampled on the capacitors C_1 in the branch computing ξ_{00}^{+}, while the zero-level reference voltage V_{ref} (set to $V_{dd}/2$) is sampled in the branch computing ξ_{00}^{-}. The feedback capacitors C_2 are precharged to zero-level reference voltage and the inverters are reset. In the computation phase ϕ_2, the common-mode output signal is established by feedback of C_2 with the order of switches in the input stage reversed, connecting sampling capacitors C_1 to zero-level reference in the positive branch and to the input voltages in the negative branch. The clocks ϕ_1 and ϕ_2 are nonoverlapping, and ϕ_{1e} replicates ϕ_1 with its falling edge slightly preceding the falling edge of ϕ_1. All the switches are complementary transmission gate field-effect transistors (FETs), except the switches controlled by ϕ_{1e}, which are *n*-channel FETs. The estimate ξ_{00} is used for suppressing the leakage of the common-mode component in the spatial gradient signals through least-mean-square (LMS) adaptation.

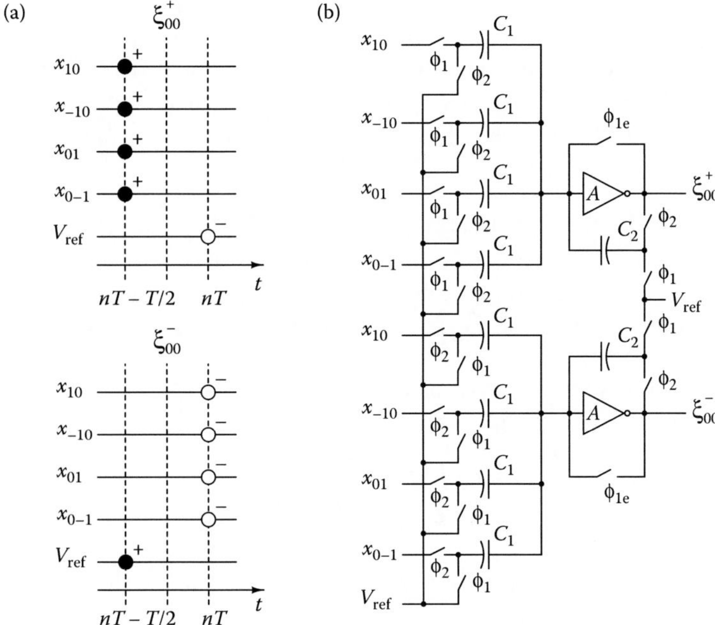

FIGURE 11.4 (a) Estimation of the spatial common-mode signal ξ_{00}. (b) SC realization.

Temporal derivative $\dot{\xi}_{00}$ is estimated independently. The estimate $\dot{\xi}_{00}$, centered at the same time instance $nT - T/4$, is computed differentially in a manner similar to ξ_{00}

$$
\begin{aligned}
\dot{\xi}_{00}^{+}[n] &= 0,\\
\dot{\xi}_{00}^{-}[n] &= -\frac{1}{8}(x_{10}[n] + x_{-10}[n] + x_{01}[n] + x_{0-1}[n])\\
&\quad + x_{10}\left[n-\frac{1}{2}\right] + x_{-10}\left[n-\frac{1}{2}\right]\\
&\quad + x_{01}\left[n-\frac{1}{2}\right] + x_{0-1}\left[n-\frac{1}{2}\right].
\end{aligned}
\tag{11.19}
$$

$\dot{\xi}_{00}$ is obtained as the difference of common-mode signals at time instances $nT - T/2$ and nT and approximately equals the time derivative of the common-mode signal at $nT - T/4$ scaled by $T/2$.

The small aperture of the sensor array poses a design challenge in resolving small signal spatial gradients amidst a large common-mode signal pedestal. Differential low-noise amplification eliminates the common-mode component and boosts differential sensitivity. The first-order spatial gradient in the p direction ξ_{10}, also centered at time $nT - T/4$, is computed as the average of ξ_{10} estimates at time instances $nT - T/2$ and nT. For amenable implementation, the contributions to ξ_{10}^{+} and ξ_{10}^{-} are distributed in the following manner:

$$
\begin{aligned}
\xi_{10}^{+}[n] &= \frac{1}{4}\left(x_{10}\left[n-\frac{1}{2}\right] - x_{-10}[n]\right),\\
\xi_{10}^{-}[n] &= \frac{1}{4}\left(x_{-10}\left[n-\frac{1}{2}\right] - x_{10}[n]\right),
\end{aligned}
\tag{11.20}
$$

as illustrated in Figure 11.5a. The SC realization shown in Figure 11.5b includes provisions for common-mode suppression, described in Section 11.2.2.2. In the sampling phase ϕ_1, input signal x_{10} is sampled on capacitor C_1 in the branch computing ξ_{10}^{+}, while in the branch computing ξ_{10}^{-} signal x_{-10} is sampled. In the computation phase ϕ_2, spatial gradient signal is computed by exchanging the inputs selected to the sampling capacitors. The first-order spatial gradient in the q direction, ξ_{01}, is computed in an identical fashion.

11.2.2.2 Common-Mode Suppression

Mismatch across the sensor array introduces errors in estimation of the spatial gradients, which translates to errors in bearing estimates. To mitigate this effect, common-mode correction of the gain mismatch errors in the sensors is applied to the estimated spatial gradients, prior to bearing estimation.

Common-mode offsets can be represented to first order as

$$\begin{aligned}\hat{\xi}_{10} &\approx \xi_{10} + \varepsilon_1 \xi_{00} \\ &\approx \sum_{\ell} \tau_1^{\ell} \dot{s}^{\ell}(t) + \varepsilon_1 \sum_{\ell} s^{\ell}(t)\end{aligned} \tag{11.21}$$

From second-order statistics, the correlation between any signal and its time-derivative is zero:

$$E[\dot{s}(t)s(t)] = 0, \tag{11.22}$$

which implies that the correlation between common-mode and gradient variable is also zero:

$$\begin{aligned}E[\xi_{00}\xi_{10}] &= 0, \\ E[\xi_{00}\xi_{01}] &= 0.\end{aligned} \tag{11.23}$$

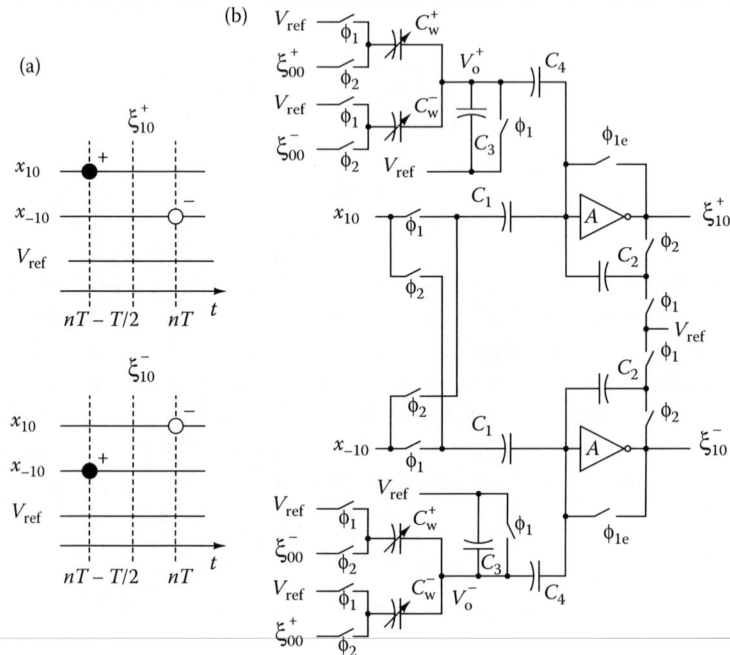

FIGURE 11.5 (a) Estimation of first-order spatial gradient along the p direction, ξ_{10}. (b) SC differential realization.

The spatial gradient with eliminated systematic common-mode error can then be estimated using adaptive least-squares calibration with the value of ε_1 ideally equal to

$$\varepsilon_1 = -\frac{E\left[\xi_{00}\hat{\xi}_{10}\right]}{E\left[\xi_{00}^2\right]}. \tag{11.24}$$

To efficiently implement the correction factor ε_1 in the digital domain, a sign–sign least-mean-square (SS-LMS) adaptation rule is used [12]. ε_1 is stored as the digital value in a 12-bit counter and it is represented in two's complement. The update is performed by incrementing or decrementing the counter based on the polarities of spatial gradient and common-mode signals

$$\begin{aligned} \varepsilon_1^+[n+1] &= \varepsilon_1^+[n] \\ &\quad + \operatorname{sgn}\left(\xi_{10}^+[n]-\xi_{10}^-[n]\right)\operatorname{sgn}\left(\xi_{00}^+[n]-\xi_{00}^-[n]\right] \\ \varepsilon_1^-[n+1] &= 2^{12}-1-\varepsilon_1^+[n+1]. \end{aligned} \tag{11.25}$$

The eight most significant bits (MSBs) are presented to multiplying D/A capacitor arrays to construct the LMS error signal and the correction term $\varepsilon_1\xi_{00}$. Capacitive coupling of the D/A arrays to nodes V_0^+ and V_0^- in Figure 11.5b establishes the corrected gradient estimate

$$\begin{aligned} \xi_{10}^+[n] &= \hat{\xi}_{10}^+[n]-\left(\varepsilon_1^+\xi_{00}^+[n]+\varepsilon_1^-\xi_{00}^-[n]\right), \\ \xi_{10}^-[n] &= \hat{\xi}_{10}^-[n]-\left(\varepsilon_1^-\xi_{00}^+[n]+\varepsilon_1^+\xi_{00}^-[n]\right). \end{aligned} \tag{11.26}$$

In phase ϕ_1, both capacitor arrays are precharged to zero-level reference voltage V_{ref}. In phase ϕ_2, a fraction of the capacitance corresponding to ε_1^+ (the number of unit capacitors is equal to the 8-bit representation) couples ξ_{00}^+ to the branch ξ_{10}^+, while the complement (the remainder of the capacitor array) couples ξ_{00}^- to ξ_{10}^+. To implement the complement ε_1^- in branch ξ_{10}^-, the connections to ξ_{00}^+ and ξ_{00}^- in the capacitor array are exactly reversed. The additional four bits of the stored ε_1 value provide a digital buffer integrating LMS contributions that offers flexibility in the choice of the learning rate, regulated by the frequency of updating.

The capacitor array is implemented as an array of 15 columns each containing 16 unit capacitors, controlled by the four MSBs presented in thermometer code, and a column of 15 identical unit capacitors controlled by the next four less significant bits in thermometer code. To reduce the size of the array, bottom plate sampling was not implemented. The bottom plate common for all unit capacitors is connected to the amplifier's virtual ground node.

The range of common-mode error correction is designed to compensate for at most 5% of common-mode leakage in the spatial gradient estimates. Since the minimum size of a capacitor array is constrained by the size of a unit capacitor, a T-cell is used to attenuate the output swing of the multiplying D/A capacitor array. While the T-cell leads to nonlinearity in the transfer characteristic, it does not affect the monotonicity of the D/A which is sufficient for LMS convergence. Stray sensitivity in the T-cell does not influence the differential linearity.

11.2.2.3 Bearing Estimation

Estimation of bearing ITDs is implemented with digital SS-LMS differential online adaptation, using architecture similar to common-mode error correction. Bearing estimates are represented as 12-bit values in two's complement

$$\begin{aligned} \tau_1^+[n+1] &= \tau_1^+[n] \\ &\quad + \operatorname{sgn}(e_{10}^+[n]-e_{10}^-[n])\operatorname{sgn}(\xi_{10}^+[n]-\xi_{10}^-[n]] \\ \tau_1^-[n+1] &= 2^{12}-1-\tau_1^+[n+1], \end{aligned} \tag{11.27}$$

where the eight MSBs are used for computation of LMS error signal

$$\begin{aligned} e_{10}^{+}[n] &= \xi_{10}^{+}[n] - (\tau_1^{+}\dot{\xi}_{00}^{+}[n] + \tau_1^{-}\dot{\xi}_{00}^{-}[n]), \\ e_{10}^{-}[n] &= \xi_{10}^{-}[n] - (\tau_1^{-}\dot{\xi}_{00}^{+}[n] + \tau_1^{+}\dot{\xi}_{00}^{-}[n]). \end{aligned} \tag{11.28}$$

The SS-LMS adaptation stage and multiplying D/A capacitor array are identical to the ones described in Section 11.2.2.2.

The minimum observable ITD delay relative to the sampling interval T equals $T/640$, and the maximum observable ITD delay equals $2/5T$. The number of update iterations (Equation 11.27) to convergence depends on the signal and by virtue of the SS-LMS rule does not exceed 2^{12} update cycles, determined by the register length.

11.2.3 Localization Performance

The VLSI acoustic localizer measures 3 mm × 3 mm in 0.5 μm CMOS technology. Figure 11.6 shows the micrograph of the chip, highlighting the functional blocks. The digital ITD estimates τ_1 and τ_2, obtained directly from the bearing registers (Equation 11.27) at convergence, are output in bit-serial format using a separate clock. The chip also outputs the gradient signals ξ_{10}, ξ_{01}, and $\dot{\xi}_{00}$, for use in separation and localization of multiple (up to three) acoustic sources, as described in Section 11.2.3.1. The ability to resolve delays that are a small fraction (0.4%) of the sampling interval is characteristic of gradient flow, and allows to reduce the power. At the 2 kHz clock (suitable for acoustic surveillance applications), the power consumption was measured to be 30 μW from the analog (3 V) supply, and 1.8 μW from the digital supply, for a total of 32 μW. At the 16 kHz clock (for hearing aid and audio-range multimedia applications), measured power increased to 54 μW. About 30% of these figures account for the power consumed by the sample-and-hold output buffers, not used in localization but used for observing the gradient signals.

To evaluate localization performance in the audio range of designed ASIC, the experimental setup with one directional source was used. We considered two scenarios in our tests: localization

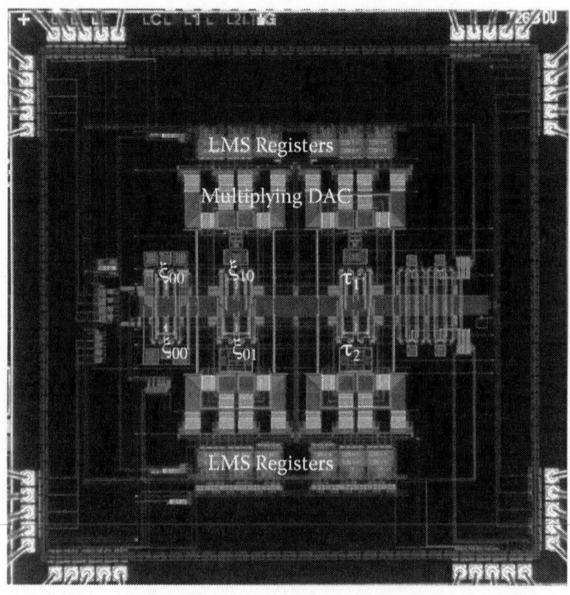

FIGURE 11.6 Micrograph of a 3 × 3 mm chip in 0.5 μm CMOS technology.

of ground-based vehicles, such as jeeps and tanks, in open-field environment and localization of speakers in a room environment.

11.2.3.1 Ground-Based Vehicles Localization

For experiments assessing the performance of localization of ground-based vehicles, the acoustic localizer chip was integrated and placed in the bottom, squared chamber of acoustic surveillance unit (ASU) enclosure, designed and implemented by Signal Systems Corporation (SSC) [13]. Measuring 16 cm in diameter, the ASU also contained four Knowles SiSonic MEMS microphones of the topology shown in Figure 11.2a and signal conditioning circuitry. The conditioning circuitry contained an amplification stage with a gain of 1084 and frequency characteristic of a first-order bandpass filter. The low cutoff frequency of a bandpass filter was set at 10.6 Hz and the high cutoff frequency was set at 473 Hz. The larger 16 cm aperture is desirable for the frequency range of interest with vehicles emitting motor noise in the 100–300 Hz range. To accommodate this range the sampling clock frequency of the chip was set to 2 kHz. The ASU, including the gradient flow localization chip, was powered with a chain of three AA batteries without a voltage regulator.

The bearing accuracy was obtained in experiments with high signal-to-noise ratio (SNR) conditions and control of the frequency content and amplitude of the sounds. Two different sound sources, broadband bandlimited (20–300 Hz) Gaussian signal and narrowband signal, were presented through a subwoofer under the same conditions. The distance between the loudspeaker and the microphone array was approximately 18 m. The SNR was around 25–30 dB. For this experimental setup and the broadband acoustic source, the calculated Cramer–Rao bound was around 1°. For each bearing angle the sound source was played for 10 s, and at the end of each 1-s wide window, the bearing estimate was reported by the acoustic localizer ASIC. The accuracy of the ASIC for different ranges of bearing angles is summarized in Table 11.1.

After assessing the localization performance with synthesized sounds in controlled experiments, tests were conducted in the open field with the chip tracking different types of ground-based vehicles, plus some occasional airborne traffic.

Ground-based vehicles were driven around a 662 × 108 m oval-shaped track at different speeds, and tracked with three ASUs positioned at points S_1, S_2, and S_3 approximately 90 m apart as illustrated in Figure 11.7. The tests were performed with relatively loud ambient background noise. The range at which the localizer was able to track the vehicles depended on the type of vehicle and varied from 350 to 600 m, limited by test conditions.

The standard Unattended Ground Sensor (UGS) processing was implemented by SSC in a real-time microprocessor and used as a metric to compare to the gradient flow chip bearings [13]. The standard UGS bearings were calculated using a delay and sum beamformer, beam interpolation, narrowband tone detection, and harmonic association. The gradient flow chip had compatible performance to that of the standard UGS processing, but at a few orders of magnitude lower power consumption. The average bias error and bearing standard deviation for both systems are shown in Table 11.2.

As an example of tracking performance, tracking of one vehicle moving clockwise around the oval is illustrated in Figure 11.7. The bearing ITD estimates were recorded at 1-s time intervals and converted to azimuth and elevation angles. Only the azimuth angles θ are shown for ground vehicles, since the ASU microphone arrays were oriented horizontally. Estimates of true bearing angles

TABLE 11.1
Accuracy of the ASIC as the Mean of Standard Deviation in Degrees

Range	[−90, +90]	[−95, −85]	[−50, −40]
Mean STD BBN	1.06	0.92	0.98
Mean STD NB	1.18	0.93	1.11

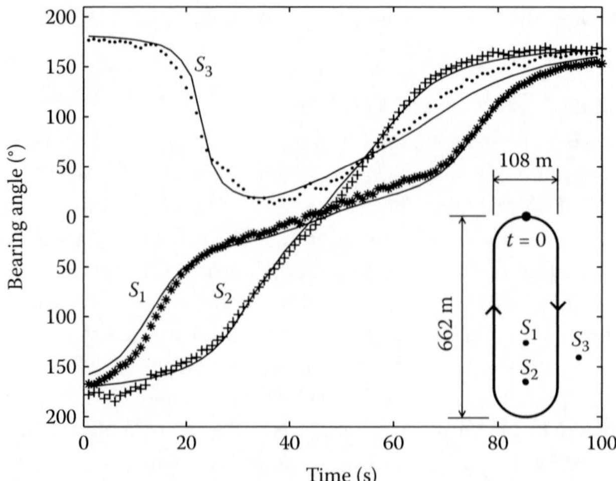

FIGURE 11.7 Experimental tracking of a ground vehicle using three acoustic localization sensor nodes positioned in the field as shown in the inset. Solid lines indicate ground truth estimates from GPS measurement.

θ from GPS tracking of the vehicles, accounting for the approximate geometry of the track and ASUs and correcting for delays in acoustic wave propagation, are also depicted as "ground truth" in Figure 11.7. In tests with multiple vehicles moving together or in opposite directions, the localizer chip tracked the loudest (received) target. An F/A-18 fighter jet flying overhead at ~3000 m was also successfully tracked by the localizer chip, accounting for elevation besides azimuth.

11.2.3.2 Speaker Localization

The planar array of four omnidirectional hearing aid miniature microphones (Knowles IM-3268), shown in the inset of Figure 11.8a, was used for speaker localization experiments. Opposing pairs of microphones in the array are oriented identically, rather than symmetrically, to minimize differences in microphone response due to mismatch in directionality pattern. The common-mode suppression (Section 11.2.2.2) compensates for up to 5% in gain mismatch between microphones. Phase mismatch is unaccounted for, except for linear phase errors (pure delay differences), which introduce offset in ITD estimation that can be digitally subtracted (not implemented).

A single acoustic source was presented through a loudspeaker positioned at 1 m distance from the array in a mild reverberant room. For precise control of angle θ in the experiments, the platform containing the array and the chip was rotated, using a stepper motor, around the axis through the center of the array perpendicular to the plane.

The system sampling frequency of the chip was set to 16 kHz. A broadband bandlimited (100–1000 Hz) Gaussian signal was presented. The corresponding SNR was around 35 dB. Expressions for the Cramer–Rao lower bound on variance of the bearing angle estimate predict an achievable angular resolution of around 1° under these conditions and a 1-s observation interval. For each setting of the bearing angle, 10 samples of ITD estimates were recorded from the chip at 1 s intervals.

TABLE 11.2
Bearing Accuracies of ASU in Ground Vehicle Tracking

Bearing Estimation Type	Average Bias Error (deg)	Bearing Standard Deviation (deg)
Standard UGS	5.45	2.69
Gradient flow	6.13	1.49

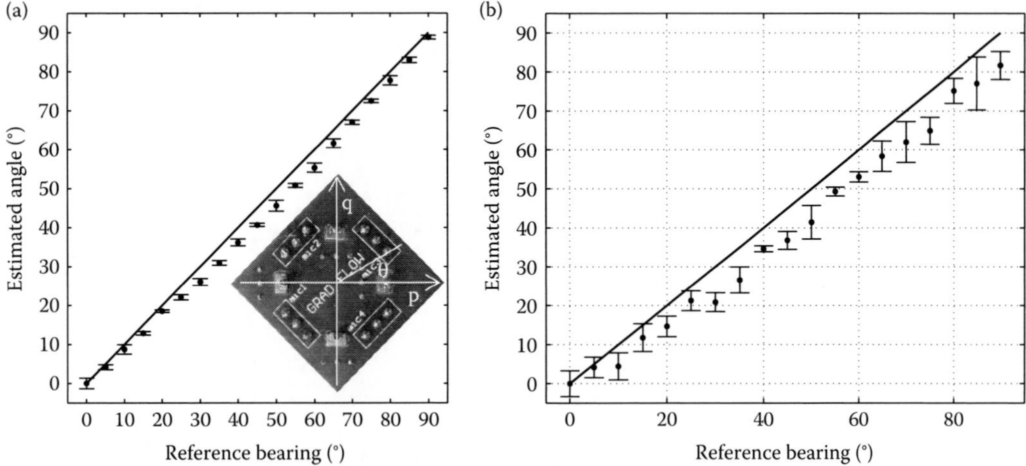

FIGURE 11.8 Localization results in a room environment with (a) a bandlimited (100–1000 Hz) Gaussian source and (b) a speech signal source.

The platform was rotated in increments of 5° until it reached 90° from the initial position. The absolute angle θ between the speaker and the microphone array ranged from around 70° to –20°. The mean and variance of estimated bearing angles normalized from the initial position are shown in Figure 11.8a. The same experiment was repeated for speech signal and the results are shown in Figure 11.8b.

11.3 GRADIENT FLOW ICA

A single source localization by estimation of direction cosines τ_1 and τ_2 from Equation 11.16 has been known for years in monopulse radar. The novelty of the proposed method lies in the application of spatial gradient sensing to a more complex environment with multiple signal sources present. When multiple sources are present, the signal observed at the sensor at the location **r** is a mixture of time-delayed source signals. In the far-field approximation (Equation 11.5), each source signal s^ℓ contributing to $x_{pq}(t)$ is advanced in time by τ_{pq}^ℓ

$$x_{pq}(t) = \sum_{\ell}^{\mathcal{L}} s^\ell\left(t + \tau_{pq}^\ell\right) + n_{pq}(t), \tag{11.29}$$

where $\mathcal{L}$ represents the number of sources in the environment and $\tau_{pq}^\ell(\mathbf{r})$ is the waveform delay for source s^ℓ. Knowledge of τ_{pq}^ℓ uniquely determines the direction vector $\mathbf{u}^\ell$ along which source s^ℓ impinges the array, in reference to the sensor plane. We now extend spatial gradient sensing to the case of multiple sources $s^\ell(t)$ that can be jointly separated and localized using essentially the same principle:

$$\begin{aligned} \xi_{00}(t) &= \sum_{\ell} s^\ell(t) + \nu_{00}(t), \\ \xi_{10}(t) &= \sum_{\ell} \tau_1^\ell \dot{s}^\ell(t) + \nu_{10}(t), \\ \xi_{01}(t) &= \sum_{\ell} \tau_2^\ell \dot{s}^\ell(t) + \nu_{01}(t), \end{aligned} \tag{11.30}$$

where ν_{00}, ν_{10}, and ν_{01} represent common-mode and spatial derivative components of additive noise in the sensor observations. Taking the time derivative of ξ_{00}, we thus obtain from the sensors a linear instantaneous mixture of the time-differentiated source signals,

$$\begin{bmatrix} \dot{\xi}_{00} \\ \xi_{10} \\ \xi_{01} \end{bmatrix} \approx \begin{bmatrix} 1 & \cdots & 1 \\ \tau_1^1 & \cdots & \tau_1^L \\ \tau_2^1 & \cdots & \tau_2^L \end{bmatrix} \begin{bmatrix} \dot{s}^1 \\ \vdots \\ \dot{s}^L \end{bmatrix} + \begin{bmatrix} \dot{\nu}_{00} \\ \nu_{10} \\ \nu_{01} \end{bmatrix}, \tag{11.31}$$

an equation in the standard form

$$\mathbf{x} = \mathbf{A}\mathbf{s} + \mathbf{n}, \tag{11.32}$$

where $\mathbf{x}$ is given and the mixing matrix $\mathbf{A}$ and sources $\mathbf{s}$ are unknown. Ignoring the noise term $\mathbf{n}$, this problem setting is standard in ICA, and three independent sources can be identified from the three gradient observations. Various formulations of ICA exist to arrive at estimates of the unknown $\mathbf{s}$ and $\mathbf{A}$ from observations $\mathbf{x}$. ICA algorithms typically specify some sort of statistical independence assumption on the sources $\mathbf{s}$ either in distribution over amplitude [2] or over time [14].

11.3.1 ICA Processor Architecture

Gradient flow and ICA combine to yield both separation and localization of multiple independent signal sources. Implementation of ICA in mixed-signal VLSI that interfaces with the gradient flow processor described in Section 11.2.2 presents a mixed-signal VLSI system for separation and localization of traveling wave sources. The mixed-signal VLSI implementation of the ICA processor uses a combination of analog and digital VLSI technology to maximize flexibility in programming and configuring adaptation rules at minimal power dissipation. An analog data path directly interfaces with inputs without the need for data conversion and provides analog output signals; and digital adaptation offers flexibility in selection of learning rules and digital values of mixing coefficients that correspond to directional angles of the source signals. As in the implementation of the gradient flow processor, the mixed-signal ICA architecture is implemented using fully differential SC sampled-data circuits.

A general mixed-signal parallel architecture that can be configured for implementation of various ICA update rules is shown in Figure 11.9 [15]. The input signals are the observed signals linearly mixed as in Equation 11.32. In the gradient flow framework, the input signals are temporal and spatial gradient observations ξ_{10}, ξ_{01}, and $\dot{\xi}_{00}$. To obtain estimates $\mathbf{y} = \hat{\mathbf{s}}$ of the sources $\mathbf{s}$, a linear transformation with matrix $\mathbf{W}$ is applied to the gradient signals $\mathbf{x}$, $\mathbf{y} = \mathbf{W}\mathbf{x}$. Each cell representing an adaptive coefficient in the unmixing matrix in the implemented architecture contains a counter, a decoder, and D/A capacitor arrays for discrete updates.

Efficient implementation in parallel architecture requires a simple form of the update rule, which avoids excessive matrix multiplications and inversions. A variety of ICA update algorithms can be cast in a common, unifying framework of outer-product rules [15]. In the proposed implementation of the update rule, diagonal terms are fixed $w_{ii} \equiv 1$, and off-diagonal terms adapt according to

$$\Delta w_{ij} = -\mu f(y_i) g(y_i), \quad i \neq j, \tag{11.33}$$

where f and g are odd-symmetric functions. The implemented update rule (Equation 11.33) (for $f(y) \equiv \tanh(y)$ and $g(y) \equiv y$) can be seen as a nonholonomic (zero-diagonal) version of the gradient of *InfoMax* [2] multiplied by $\mathbf{W}^T$, rather than the natural gradient multiplication factor $\mathbf{W}^T\mathbf{W}$. To obtain

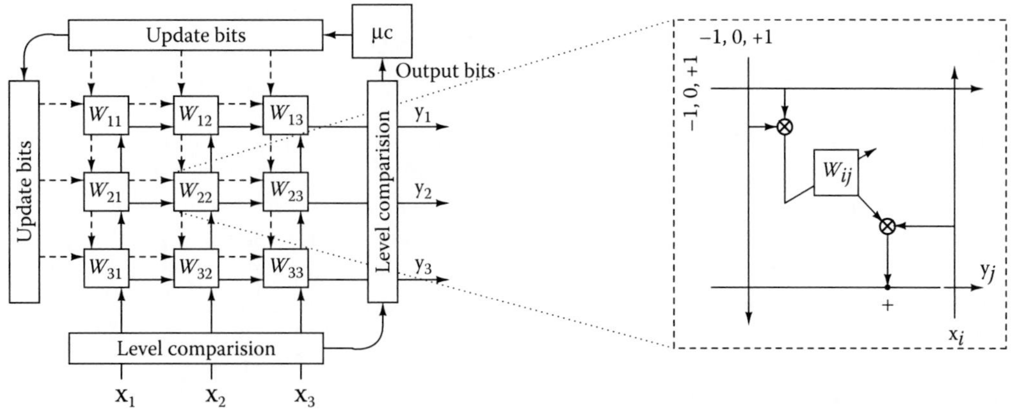

FIGURE 11.9 Reconfigurable mixed-signal ICA architecture implementing general outer-product forms of ICA update rules.

the full natural gradient in outer-product form, it is necessary to include a back-propagation path in the network architecture, and thus additional silicon resources, to implement the vector contribution $\mathbf{W}^T y$ in the update rule [15]. Interestingly, however, in the special case of a 2-input, 2-output network, the update rule (Equation 11.33) is equivalent to natural gradient ICA in nonholonomic form [16], without the need for the backward signal path in the architecture.

Scalar functions $f(y)$ and $g(y)$ appearing in learning rule (Equation 11.33) can be implemented as discrete approximations through level comparisons. The functions proposed in (Equation 11.33) are cumulative distribution functions of source signal for f and linearity for g. As an example, for the problem of separating speech signals, the following function approximations represent the optimal choice. Since speech signals are approximately Laplacian distributed, the nonlinear scalar function $f(y)$ is approximated by sign(y) and implemented using single-bit quantization. Conversely, a linear function $g(y) \equiv y$ in the learning rule is approximated by a three-level staircase function (–1,0, +1) using 2-bit quantization. The quantization of the f and g terms in the update rule (Equation 11.33) simplifies the implementation to that of discrete counting operations.

The functional block diagram of a 3 × 3 outer-product incremental ICA architecture, shown in Figure 11.9, supports a quantized form of the general update rule (Equation 11.33). Coefficients in the unmixing matrix **W** are stored digitally in each cell of the architecture. The update is performed locally by once or repeatedly incrementing, decrementing, or holding the current value of the counter based on the learning rule served by the external microcontroller. A microcontroller provides flexibility in the implementation of different learning rules. The eight MSBs of the 14-bit counter holding and updating the coefficients are presented to a multiplying D/A capacitor array to linearly unmix the separated signal. The remaining six bits in the coefficient registers provide flexibility in programming the update rate to tailor convergence.

11.3.1.1 Vector Matrix Multiplication

The block diagram of the ICA prototype indicates that its main functionality is a vector (3 × 1)-matrix(3 × 3) multiplication Wx. The output signal is decomposed in differential form as

$$
\begin{aligned}
y_i^+ &= -\sum_{j=1}^{3} (W_{ij}^+ x_j^- + W_{ij}^- x_j^+), \\
y_i^- &= -\sum_{j=1}^{3} (W_{ij}^+ x_j^+ + W_{ij}^- x_j^-).
\end{aligned} \tag{11.34}
$$

The input vector is analog signal, while the matrix elements have adaptive digital values. The multiplication is performed through multiplying D/A capacitor arrays and the output of each of these DACs represents the product $W_{ij}x_j$. The implementation of the multiplying capacitor arrays is identical to that discussed in Section 11.2.2.2.

Figure 11.10 shows the SC circuit for computing one output component in the architecture that is obtained through a linear sum of the weighted input contributions. Each output signal y_i is computed by accumulating outputs from all the DAC cells in the ith row. In the precharging phase ϕ_1, all the unit capacitors in the array are precharged to the zero-level reference voltage V_{ref} (set to $V_{dd}/2$), as well as the feedback capacitor C_2. The inverters are reset. In the computation phase ϕ_2, the input signals are sampled on unit capacitors and the accumulation is performed on C_2 by switch-cap amplifier, yielding the valid output signals during ϕ_2 phase.

11.3.1.2 Update Rule Implementation

To efficiently implement ICA learning rule (Equation 11.33), the functions f and g are approximated as discrete, and adaptation is performed through discrete updates. The weights, coefficients of the unmixing matrix W, are represented as 14-bit values in two's complement and are stored in a counter. The update is performed by incrementing, decrementing, or holding the current value of the counter

$$\begin{aligned} W_{ij}^{+}[n+1] &= W_{ij}^{+}[n] - \text{sgn}(y_i[n])\ \text{quant}(y_j[n]), \\ W_{ij}^{-}[n+1] &= 2^{14} - 1 - W_{ij}^{+}[n+1], \end{aligned} \tag{11.35}$$

where quant(y) is a three-level staircase function (–1,0, +1), which is coded using 2-bits, sgn and mag. Different learning rules could be implemented through multiple updates. The eight most significant bits in the binary representation of the weights are presented to multiplying D/A capacitor array in thermometer code to construct the output signals.

The discrete values of the functions $f(y)$ and $g(y)$ are obtained through level comparisons. The implementation of a comparator that is able to compare signals with variable levels is shown in Figure 11.10. While the output signals are valid, y_i^+ is sampled in phase ϕ_1^c on capacitor C_3. The sign of the comparison of y_i with variable level threshold V_{th} is computed in the evaluate phase ϕ_1^c, through capacitive coupling into the amplifier input node. The change in voltage V_th in phase ϕ_1^c will lead to multiple-level comparison in a single clock cycle. The clocks ϕ_1^c and ϕ_2^c are nonoverlapping

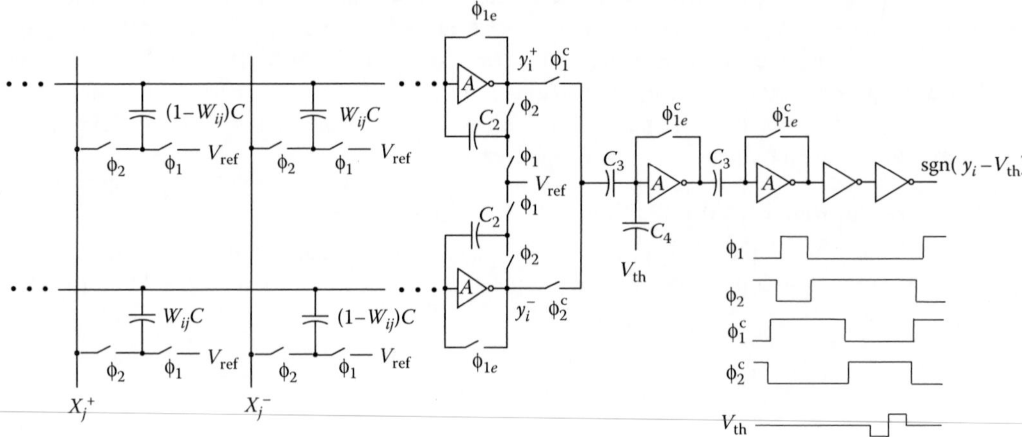

FIGURE 11.10 Correlated CDS SC fully differential circuits implementing linearly weighted summing in the mixed-signal ICA architecture.

and their relative timing with respect to clocks ϕ_1 and ϕ_2 is shown in the inset of Figure 11.10, as well as the changes in threshold voltage V_{th} for three-level comparison.

11.3.2 Real-World Speech Separation and Localization Experiments

A prototype 3 × 3 mixed-signal ICA processor was designed, fabricated, and tested. The architecture is integrated on a single 3 mm × 3 mm chip fabricated in 0.5 μm 3M2P CMOS technology. The differential analog input channels directly interface with gradient output signals from a previously developed gradient flow processor for acoustic localization, to extend its functionality to joint separation and localization of up to three acoustic sources. Figure 11.11 shows the micrograph of the chip, highlighting the functional blocks. The measured power consumption of the chip was 70 μW at 2 kHz sampling rate and 180 μW at 16 kHz sampling rate at 3 V supply. The external microcontroller can be taken out of loop by fixing a specific learning rule leading to a completely autonomous system. The integration of the gradient flow computation and the ICA processor on a single substrate would lead to system-on-chip solution for blind localization and separation. The digital estimates of coefficients W_{ij} in the unmixing matrix are obtained directly from the counters at convergence and are output at 4 bits at a time. The chip also outputs the estimated source signals $y_i(t)$. The output signals are presented in complementary analog format through sample-and-hold buffers.

To demonstrate source separation and localization in a real environment [17], two mixed-signal VLSI ASICs, the gradient flow and the ICA processor, were interfaced with four omnidirectional miniature microphones (Knowles FG-3629). Microphones are arranged in a circular array with a radius of 0.5 cm. The sensitivity of microphones is –53 dB and the typical noise level is at 27 dB. At the front end, the microphone signals were passed through a second-order bandpass filter with the low-frequency cutoff set at 130 Hz and the high-frequency cutoff set at 4.3 kHz. The signals were also amplified by a factor of 20.

The experimental setup is shown in Figure 11.12. The speech signals were presented through loudspeakers positioned at 1.5 m distance from the array. The system sampling frequency of both chips was set to 16 kHz. A male and a female speaker from the TIMIT database were chosen as sound sources. To provide the ground truth data and full characterization of the systems, speech segments were presented individually through either loudspeaker at different time instances. The data were recorded for both speakers, archived, and presented to the gradient flow chip. Localization

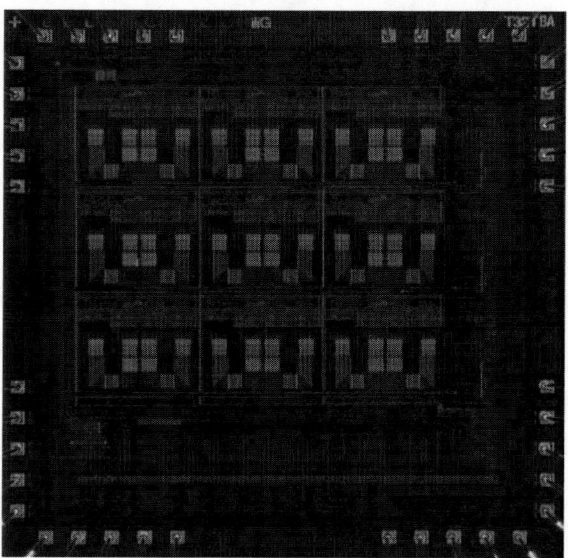

FIGURE 11.11 Micrograph of a 3 × 3 mm chip in 0.5 μm CMOS technology.

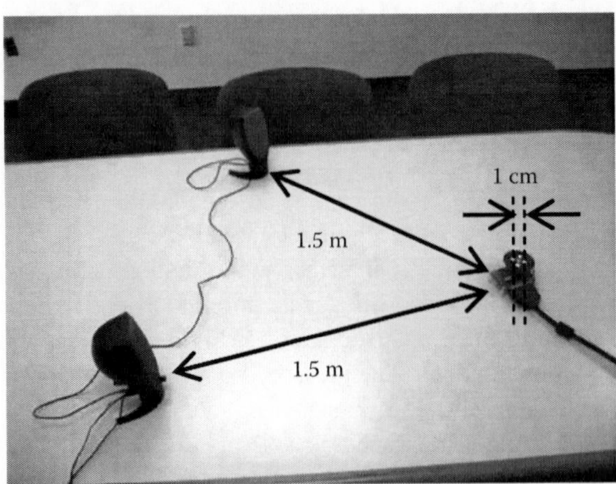

FIGURE 11.12 Experimental setup for the separation of two acoustic sources in a conference room environment.

results obtained by gradient flow chip through LMS adaptation are reported in Table 11.3. The two recorded data sets were then added, and presented to the gradient flow ASIC. The gradient signals obtained from the chip were then presented to the ICA processor, configured to implement the outer-product update algorithm in Equation 11.33. The quantization level in three-level approximation of the function g was set to 100 mV amplitude change in voltage V_{th}. The observed convergence time was around 2 s. From the recorded 14-bit digital weights, the angles of incidence of the sources relative to the array were derived. These estimated angles are reported in Table 11.3. As seen, the angles obtained through LMS bearing estimation under individual source presentation are very close to the angles produced by ICA under joint presentation of both sources. The original sources and the recorded source signal estimates, along with recorded common-mode signal and first-order spatial gradients, are shown in Figure 11.13.

11.4 CONCLUSIONS

The task of blind source localization and separation can greatly benefit from the exciting opportunities presented by advances in MEMS microarrays and miniaturization of integrated systems at the sensor array interfaces. The gradient flow technique, based on wavefront sensing and ICA, presents a unique approach for the task of acoustic source separation using miniature microphone arrays. The instantaneous static formulation of gradient flow is convenient, and avoids the need for non-static (convolutive) ICA to separate delayed mixtures of traveling wave sources (in free space). Although the application of static ICA is limited by reverberation, the perceptual quality of the separated outputs owes itself to the elimination of the direct path in the residuals. Gradient flow also satisfies the requirements for implementation in a real-time low-power system. The miniature size of the microphone array enclosure (1 cm diameter) and micropower consumption of the VLSI hardware (250 μW) are key advantages of the approach, with applications to hearing aids, conferencing, multimedia, and surveillance.

TABLE 11.3
Localization Performance

	Male Speaker	Female Speaker
Single-source LMS localization	–31.11	40.95
Dual-source ICA localization	–30.35	43.55

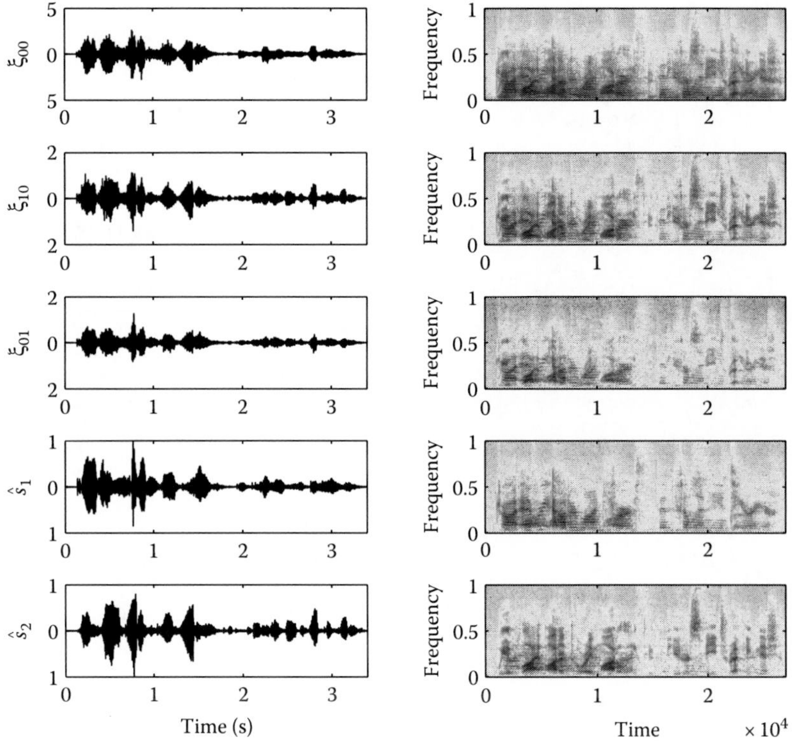

FIGURE 11.13 Time waveforms and spectrograms of the presented sources s_1 and s_2, observed common-mode and gradient signals ξ_{00}, ξ_{10} and ξ_{01} by the gradient flow chip, and recovered sources $\hat{s}_1$ and $\hat{s}_2$ by the ICA chip.

REFERENCES

1. A. Cichocki and S. Amari, *Adaptive Blind Signal and Image Processing: Learning Algorithms and Applications*, New York, NY: John Wiley, 2002.
2. A. Bell and T. Sejnowski, An information maximization approach to blind separation and blind deconvolution, *Neural Computation*, 7, 1129–1159, 1995.
3. K. Torkkola, Blind separation of delayed sources based on information maximization, *Proc. IEEE Int. Conf. Acoustics, Speech and Signal Processing* (*ICASSP'96*), Atlanta, GA, 1996.
4. R. Lambert and A. Bell, Blind separation of multiple speakers in a multipath environment, *Proc. IEEE Int. Conf. Acoustics, Speech and Signal Processing* (*ICASSP'97*), Münich, 1997.
5. D. Robert, R. N. Miles, and R. R. Hoy, Tympanal hearing in the sarcophagid parasitoid fly *Emblemasoma* sp.: The biomechanics of directional hearing, *Journal of Experimental Biology*, 202, 1865–1876, 1999.
6. R. Reeve and B. Webb, New neural circuits for robot phonotaxis, *Philosophical Transactions of the Royal Society A*, 361, 2245–2266, 2002.
7. M. Stanacevic, G. Cauwenberghs, and G. Zweig, Gradient flow adaptive beamforming and signal separation in a miniature microphone array, *Proc. IEEE Int. Conf. Acoustics Speech and Signal Processing* (*ICASSP'2002*), 4, 4016–4019, Orlando, FL, 13–17, 2002.
8. L. R. Rabiner and R.W. Schafer, On the behavior of minimax relative error FIR digital differentiators, *Bell System Technical Journal*, 53, 333–361, 1974.
9. A. G. Andreou, D. H. Goldberg, E. Culurciello, M. Stanacevic, and G. Cauwenberghs, Heterogeneous integration of biomimetic acoustic microsystems, *Proc. IEEE Int. Symp. Circuits and Systems* (*ISCAS'2001*), Sydney, Australia, May 6–9, 2001.
10. C. C. Enz and G.C. Temes, Circuit techniques for reducing the effects of Op-Amp imperfections: autozeroing, correlated double sampling, and chopper stabilization, *IEEE Proceedings*, 84(11), 1584–1614, 1996.

11. M. Stanacevic and G. Cauwenberghs, Micropower gradient flow VLSI acoustic localizer, *IEEE Transactions on Circuits and Systems I: Regular Papers*, 52(10), 2148–2157, 2005.
12. L. Der and B. Razavi, A 2-GHz CMOS image-reject receiver with LMS calibration, *IEEE Journal of Solid-State Circuits*, 38(2), 167–175, 2003.
13. L. Riddle et al., VLSI acoustic surveillance unit, *Proc. GOMAC*, 12–13, 2004.
14. L. Molgedey and G. Schuster, Separation of a mixture of independent signals using time delayed correlations, *Physical Review Letters*, 72(23), 3634–3637, 1994.
15. A. Celik, M. Stanacevic, and G. Cauwenberghs, Mixed-signal real-time adaptive blind source separation, *Proc. IEEE Int. Symp. Circuits and Systems* (*ISCAS'2004*), 5, 760–763, Vancouver, Canada, May 23–26, 2004.
16. M. Cohen and G. Cauwenberghs, Blind separation of linear convolutive mixtures through parallel stochastic optimization, *Proc. IEEE Int. Symp. Circuits and Systems* (*ISCAS'98*), Monterey CA, 3, 17–20, 1998.
17. A. Celik, M. Stanacevic, and G. Cauwenberghs, Gradient flow independent component analysis in micropower VLSI, *Adv. Neural Information Processing Systems* (*NIPS'2005*), Cambridge: MIT Press, Vol. 18, 2005.

12 Remote Frequency Calibration of Passive Wireless Microsystems

Nima Soltani and Fei Yuan

CONTENTS

12.1 INTRODUCTION

In wireless communication systems, a mobile station must be able to both receive data from a base station and transmit packets of data back to the base station over wireless channels. In active mobile stations, such as cellular phones, large energy storage devices, that is, batteries, allow for the filtering and amplification of incoming signals as small as a few microvolts of amplitude and peak transmission output power as large as a few watts. In passive mobile stations, such as radio-frequency-identification (RFID) tags, however, the only source of energy available to the systems is the power of the radio-frequency (RF) waves from the base station. Due to the unavailability of large storage capacitors in these passive systems and the fast communication requirement of these systems, it is impractical to store energy for later usage [1]. Therefore, the design constraints of practical passive mobile wireless systems are (1) the total change of energy over each transaction is zero or negative (inward flow) and (2) all the power entering the system shall exit shortly afterwards.

One immediate consequence of these two constraints is that the power of the output signal from the transponder is directly sourced from the power of the input signal it receives. Because a portion of the input power will be dissipated by the transponder in the form of heat once it enters the system, the maximum output power that can only be delivered by the transponder is to immediately reflect the incoming signal before it enters the system. This method is known as backscattering and is a widely used method of data communication from a passive transponder to its reader. Figure 12.1 provides a graphical view of the transponder-to-reader link using both direct transmission and

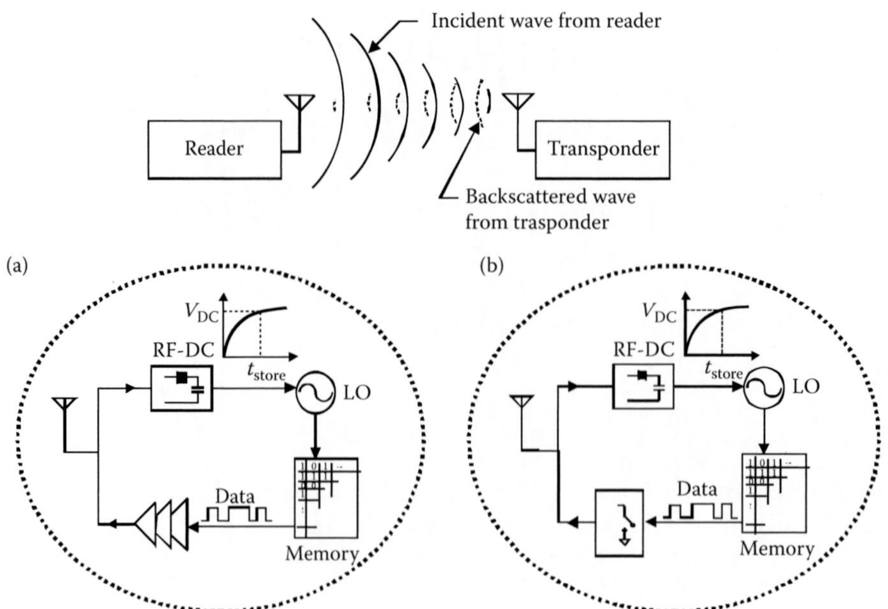

FIGURE 12.1 Block diagram of reader–transponder links. (a) Direct transmission. (b) Backscattering.

backscattering. It can be seen from the figure that in backscattering, the unmodulated sinusoidal wave emitted by the reader is reflected from the transponder antenna in the form of a modulated sinusoidal wave. The transponder modulates the reflected sinusoidal wave by varying the antenna load in accordance with the baseband signal. The baseband signal and the operation of a passive transponder are typically controlled by an on-chip local oscillator. The oscillator provides the clock signal that is used to serialize the data fetched from the memory of the transponder. In addition, it controls the operation of the modulator where the serialized data are converted to a digital waveform. The waveform is then used to modulate the load of the antenna to complete the backscattering communications with the reader. If sensors are present, the oscillator also controls the operation of the sensors. Clearly, the local oscillator determines the data rate or equivalently the bandwidth of the backscattered signal. This point is illustrated in Figure 12.2a where the amplitude of the backscattered signal is in the same range as that of the incoming carrier at the transponder.

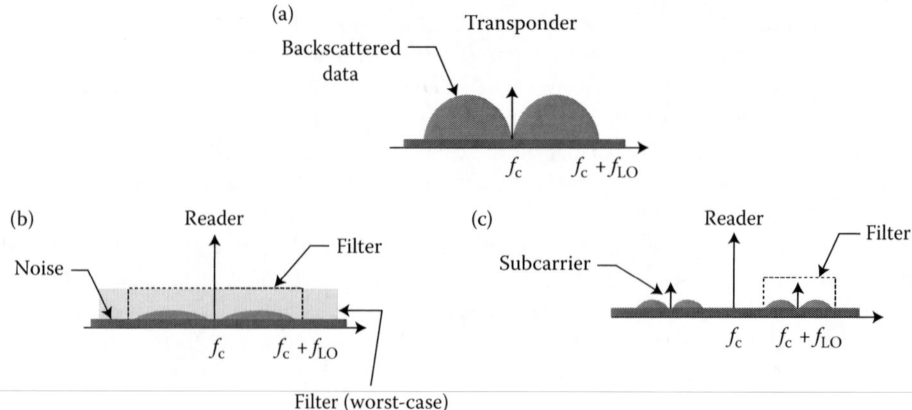

FIGURE 12.2 Power spectrum of signals (a) at the transponder, (b) at the reader without a subcarrier, and (c) at the reader with a subcarrier.

When the backscattered signal reaches the reader, it will be severely attenuated. In Figure 12.2b, the backscattered signal manifests itself in the form of an extremely attenuated signal at the reader. The amplitude of the backscattered signal could be attenuated by five orders of magnitude when reaching the reader [1]. Filtering and retrieving such a weak signal at the reader end is extremely challenging. It imposes stringent constraints on the sensitivity and dynamic range of the reader. The channel select filter of the reader must be designed in such a way that the pass band of the filter is centered at the frequency of the backscattered signal. To achieve this, the reader must have the prior knowledge of the spectrum of the backscattered signal with a high degree of fidelity. Figure 12.2c shows another approach of backscattering where the data to be transmitted to the reader are first premodulated by a signal of an intermediate frequency. The modulated signal is then used to modulate the antenna load for backscattering. This scheme is known as *backscatter modulation with subcarriers*. Because the location of the poles and zeros of the retrieving filter is preciously set by the frequency of the local oscillator of the transponder, a prior knowledge of the spectrum of the backscattered signal is also essential.

Passive wireless microsystems such as RFID tags, smart dusts, and temperature sensors for environmental monitoring are usually fabricated using low-cost complementary metal-oxide-semiconductor (CMOS) technologies. These low-cost processes typically have a large degree of process variation. As a result, the oscillation frequency of the local oscillator of these systems is intrinsically bound to have a high degree of uncertainty. For example, the frequency of a relaxation oscillator designed in a typical 0.18 μm CMOS technology will have an approximately ±30% error. Supply voltage fluctuation and temperature variation will further contribute to the uncertainty of the frequency of the local oscillator. It is evident that the oscillation frequency of the local oscillator of a transponder must be calibrated prior to each backscattering data transaction with the reader [1].

12.2 REMOTE FREQUENCY CALIBRATION SCHEMES

Owing to the unavailability of crystal oscillators and other precision reference components in a passive wireless transponder, the timing reference required for calibrating the frequency of the local oscillator of the transponder must be provided by the reader. Based on how the timing reference is recovered from the signal transmitted by the reader, the mechanisms for remote frequency calibration of passive wireless microsystems can be loosely categorized into the following two groups: *carrier-based frequency calibration* and *envelope-based frequency calibration*. In what follows, we will investigate them in detail.

12.2.1 Carrier-Based Frequency Calibration

The unmodulated carrier sent by a reader to a transponder provides the operation power of the transponder. This signal can also be used as a timing reference to calibrate the frequency of the local oscillator of the transponder. Since the local oscillator is used to control the operation of the baseband blocks of the transponder, its oscillation frequency is typically much smaller as compared with the frequency of the carrier. The frequency of the carrier must therefore be scaled down. This is typically done using frequency dividers, as shown graphically in Figure 12.3, where a low-frequency clock is generated from an unmodulated high-frequency carrier using a chain of D-flipflops. The first stage of the frequency divider must operate at the carrier frequency and therefore consumes most of the power, often exceeding the total power budget of passive transponders. An alternative is to use more power-efficient injection-locked frequency dividers [2]. Since the division ratio of injection-locked frequency dividers is typically low, these frequency dividers are typically used in the first stage of the frequency divider chain where the power consumption is the highest. The rest of the divider-by-2 blocks are implemented using conventional digital blocks [3]. The main drawback of carrier-based frequency calibration is its high power consumption, mainly due to the high operation frequency.

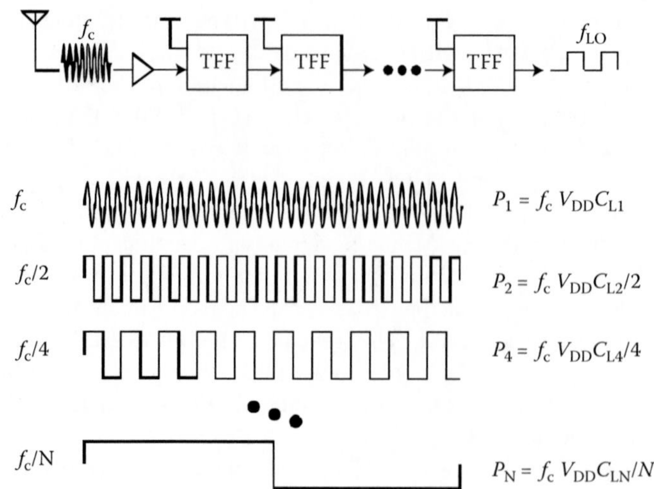

FIGURE 12.3 Timing reference recovery from the carrier using multiple frequency dividers.

12.2.2 Envelope-Based Frequency Calibration

A timing reference can be sent by the carrier in the form of an amplitude-modulated signal (envelope). The modulated timing reference can be a periodic signal with a reference frequency or a long pulse with a reference duration, as shown in Figure 12.4. The amplitude of the envelope containing the reference frequency changes periodically. Since in a passive transponder the envelope signal is also used to power the transponder, the envelope containing a reference frequency will cause frequent power interruptions to the transponder. For this reason, the calibration scheme using a long reference timing pulse is generally preferred.

12.2.3 Calibration Using Timing Reference Pulses (Digital Timing Feedback Loop)

Calibration using timing reference pulses employs a digital timing feedback loop to adjust the frequency of the local oscillator in N iterations where N is the number of pulses used in calibration [4,5]. The block diagram of the digital timing feedback loop is shown in Figure 12.6. It is similar to a digital phase-locked loop. The timing pulse is logic-1 for t_{ref} during which the oscillator clocks the M-bit counter. The calibrated frequency of the oscillator is M/t_{ref}. The frequency of the local oscillator is controlled by a successive approximation register (SAR), governed by an N-bit control word. After one timing pulse, if the counter overflow bit is ON, the most significant bit of the SAR is set to 1. Otherwise it is set to 0. This procedure continues until all the SAR bits are set to either 1 or 0. At this point, the frequency of the local oscillator is calibrated with the maximum error of $100\%/2^N$. As shown in Figure 12.5, calibrating an oscillator to a reference frequency of $1/T$ and the maximum error of $100\%/2^N$ will take exactly $N \times 2^M \times T$. For instance, using an 8-bit counter, calibrating the

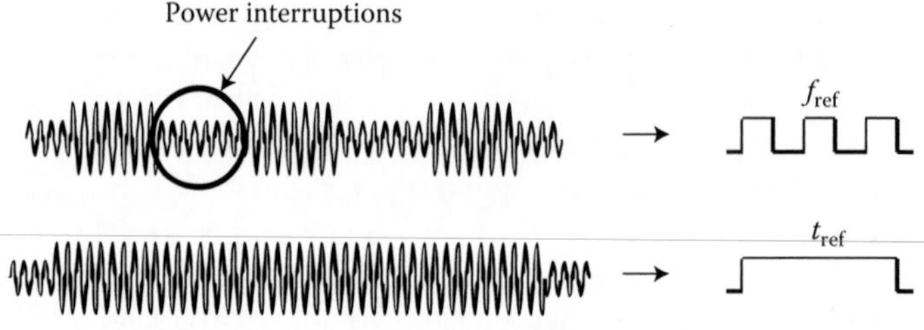

FIGURE 12.4 Top: Modulated reference frequency signal. Bottom: Reference time signal.

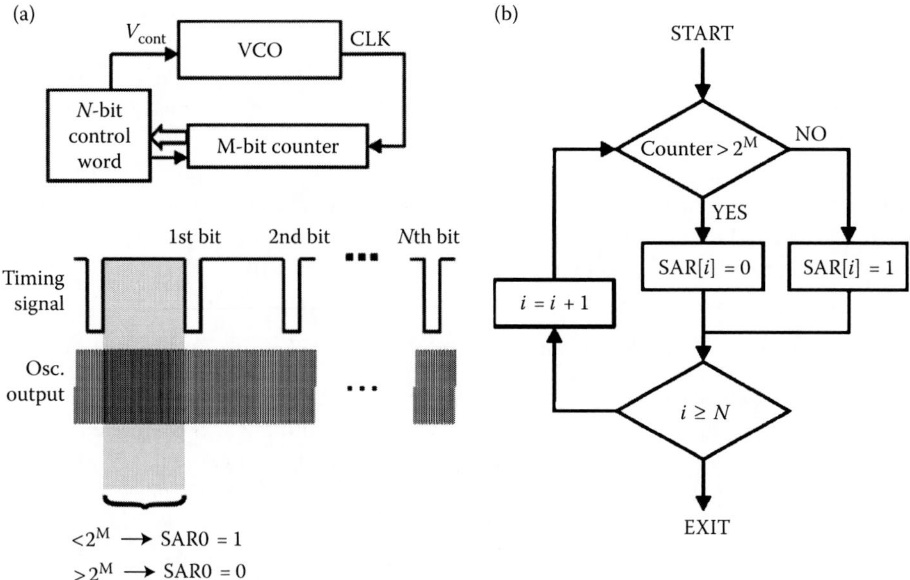

FIGURE 12.5 (a) Frequency calibration using a digital timing feedback loop. (b) Flow diagram of digital calibration using a digital timing feedback loop.

frequency of the local oscillator to a 1 MHz reference frequency with an error less than 4% will take about 4 ms using this method. The major drawback of using a digital timing feedback loop is the long calibration time required for achieving a small calibration error. One possible way of reducing the calibration time is to use a shorter timing reference pulse (smaller *M*'s), but this will mean more frequent dips in the amplitude modulation (AM) envelope and subsequently more interruptions in delivery of power to the transponder.

12.3 INJECTION LOCKING

When two oscillators with different but close frequencies are weakly coupled, they synchronize each other such that in the steady state they both oscillate at the same frequency. First observed by

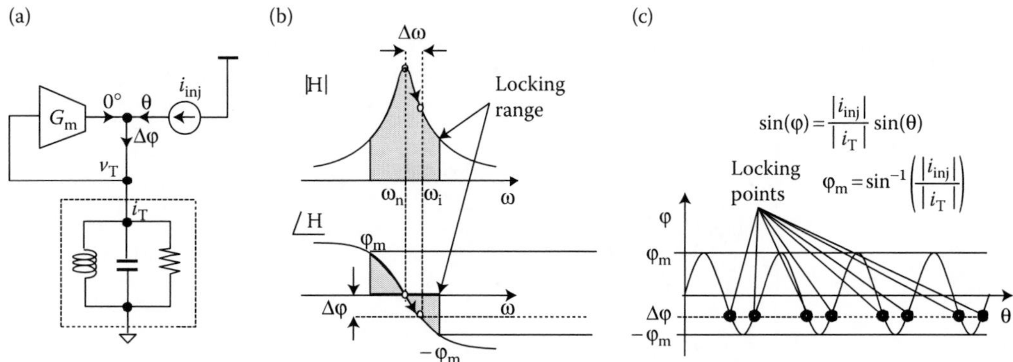

FIGURE 12.6 (a) Oscillator under injection. The phase contributed by injection signal i_{inj} causes the tank frequency to shift by $\Delta\omega$, which will in turn change the phase of the tank again. If within the locking range, this loop will become stable when $\omega_n + \Delta\omega = \omega_i$. (b) Phase and amplitude in injection-locking. The loop is stable ($\omega_{ss} = \omega_i$) when the frequency of the injected signal is within the locking range of the oscillator. (c) Effect of injection on the phase and frequency of the oscillator under injection.

Christiaan Huygens, the inventor of pendulum clock, this phenomenon is known as injection locking. A detailed study of the injection-locked oscillator is available in [6]. Since injection locking can synchronize the frequency of an oscillator to that of its injection-locking signal of small amplitude, it has been widely used as a power-efficient means for clock recovery and phase locking in RF and mixed-mode circuits.

The principle of injection locking is demonstrated in Figure 12.6 where the behavior of an LC tank oscillator under injection is used as an example. The extra phase (θ) contributed by the injected current (i_{inj}) causes the tank frequency to shift from the resonant point toward the injection frequency. If injection is strong enough, the loop in Figure 12.7a will stabilize at $\omega_T = \omega_i$.

12.3.1 Frequency Calibration Using Injection Locking

Injection locking can be used to calibrate the frequency of the local oscillator of a passive wireless transponder with the calibrating reference signal of small amplitude sent by the reader. Since the modulated reference frequency signal needs only be of small amplitude, the injection signal can be carried by the carrier and the transmission of an AM injection signal will not cause a significant power interruption to the transponder, as shown in Figure 12.8.

Figure 12.8 illustrates graphically how the frequency of the local oscillator can be adjusted to the reference frequency by injecting the reference signal into the oscillator. The injection-locked frequency calibration system, shown in Figure 12.8, suffers from the following drawbacks. (1) The initial free-running frequency of the oscillator has to be close enough to the reference frequency. In other words, the reference frequency has to be within the locking range of the oscillator. Otherwise, the frequency of the local oscillator will only be disturbed by the injection, a phenomenon known as injection pulling. (2) In the absence of the injection signal, the frequency of the local oscillator will revert to its oscillation frequency without injection. In other words, the frequency of the local oscillator will only be held to that of the reference signal when the reference signal is present.

12.3.2 Frequency Calibration Using Injection Locking with Integrating Feedback

By accumulating the difference between the frequency of the local oscillator and that of the reference signal and adding it to the control voltage of the local oscillator, the two drawbacks of the frequency calibration system of Figure 12.8 can be eliminated [7]. Figure 12.9 illustrates how the integrating feedback is added to the control of an injection-locked oscillator to force the oscillator to lock to the injection signal.

By adding the integrating feedback to the injection-locked local oscillator, the correcting effect of the injection is translated to the control voltage of the oscillator, and the frequency of the oscillator

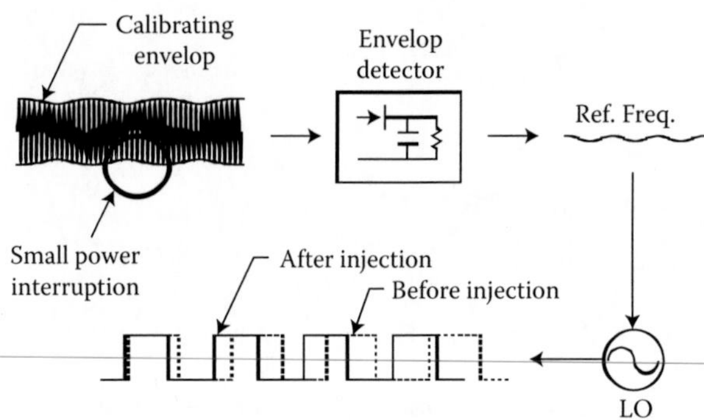

FIGURE 12.7 Frequency adjustment using injection-locking.

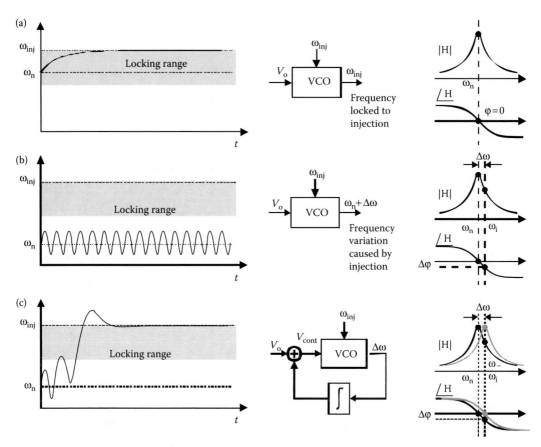

FIGURE 12.8 Variations of frequency when the injection-locked oscillator is within the locking range of the injection signal (a), when it is outside the locking range (b), and when it is outside the locking range with integrating feedback added to the system (c).

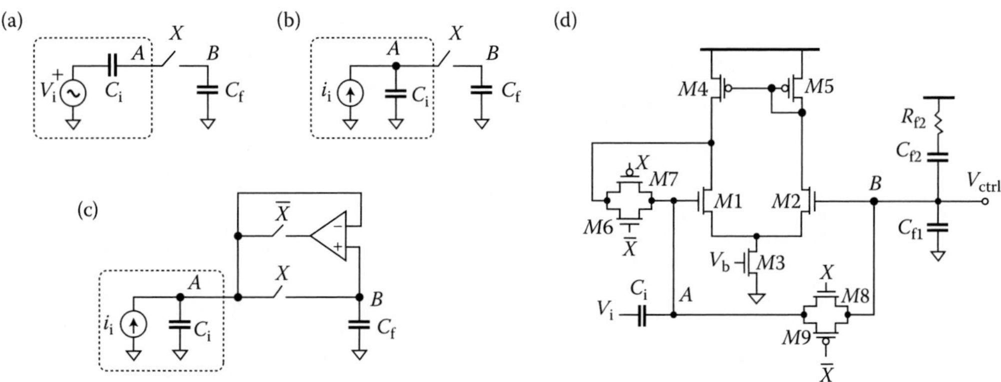

FIGURE 12.9 (a) Construction of integrating feedback from injection signal (v_i, i_i) and oscillator square-wave output (X). (a) Integrating voltage-mode injection signal, v_i. (b) Norton equivalent circuit. (c) Integrating feedback with a unity-gain buffer to preserve the DC component of the capacitor C_i when $X = 0$. (d) Schematic diagram of integrating feedback.

is adjusted. Since the control voltage of the oscillator is adjusted, after the injection-locking signal is removed, the frequency of the local oscillator will be held at the calibrated value. The integrating feedback can be constructed by mixing the oscillator output and the injection signals and integrating the resulting value. The circuit to perform this operation is shown in Figure 12.9 where TG switches are used to mix the two signals and a metal–insulator–metal (MIM) capacitor is used for performing integration. Also, according to the simulation and measurement results given in Figure 12.10, integrating feedback increases the locking range by approximately 13 times, ensuring that the local oscillator can be locked to the injection signal.

Figures 12.11 and 12.12 show the control voltage and frequency of the injection-locked local oscillator with integrating feedback. It is seen that the control voltage is adjusted by the integrating feedback even after injection-locking occurs to produce the permanent calibration of the frequency of the oscillator.

12.4 LOCAL OSCILLATOR

The local oscillator of a passive transponder typically oscillates at a few megahertz with its power consumption below 1 mW. Due to the constraints of extremely low power consumption and relatively low oscillation frequencies, these oscillators are usually implemented as either current-starved ring oscillators or relaxation oscillators. LC tank oscillators are not suitable for these applications due to the need for impractically larger passive inductors in order to oscillate at baseband frequencies.

12.4.1 Current-Starved Ring Oscillators

By limiting the current supplied to a ring oscillator, the power consumption and oscillation frequency of the oscillator can be reduced significantly. Figure 12.13 shows the block diagram of a current-starving ring oscillator. Current-starving ring oscillators can be designed to have power consumption below 1 μW. The major problem with ring oscillators is their high sensitivity to process,

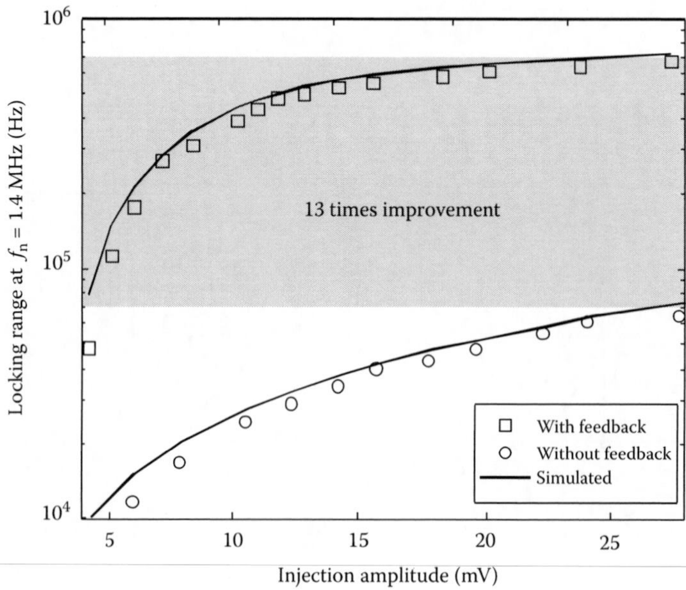

FIGURE 12.10 Simulated and measured locking range of the injection-locked local oscillator with and without integrating feedback.

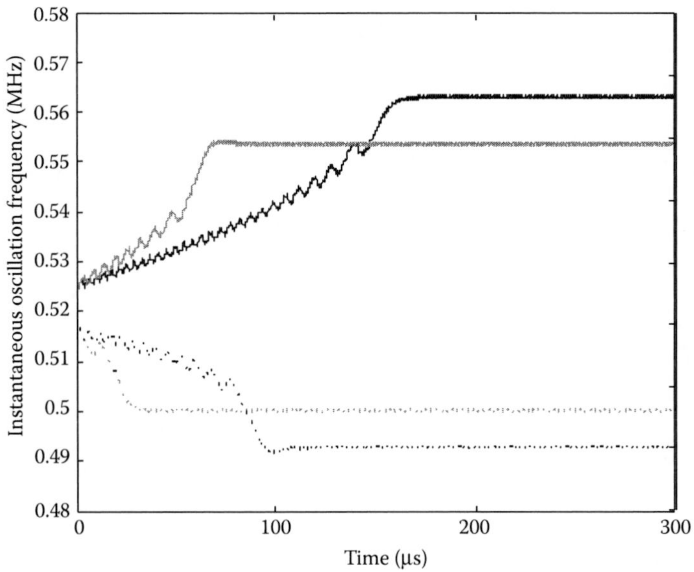

FIGURE 12.11 Simulated control voltage of the injection-locked local oscillator with integrating feedback. (Copyright © IEEE.)

supply voltage, and temperature (PVT) variations. This is because the oscillation frequency of these oscillators is controlled by active components. The oscillation frequency of current-starving oscillators is even more sensitive to process variation than that of conventional ring oscillators. As shown in Figure 12.13, the current-starving configuration dwells longer in the subthreshold region than do the conventional ring oscillators. The subthreshold current of a transistor is much more process-sensitive than the triode and saturation currents [8].

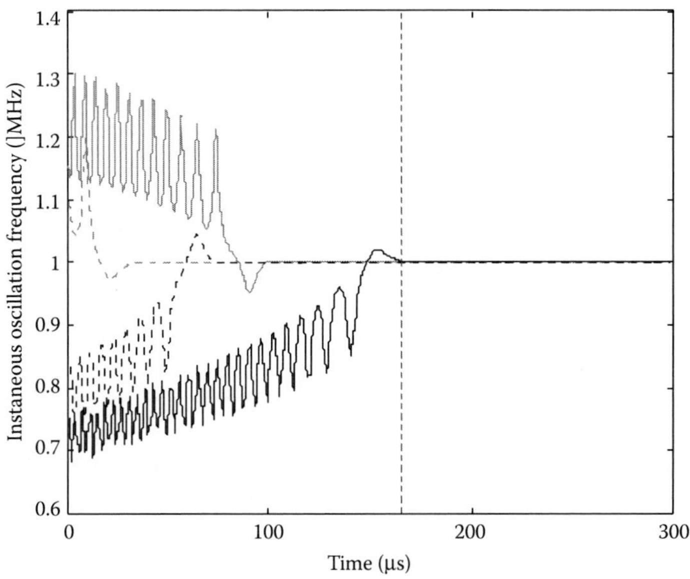

FIGURE 12.12 Simulated frequency of the injection-locked local oscillator with integrating feedback. (Copyright © IEEE.)

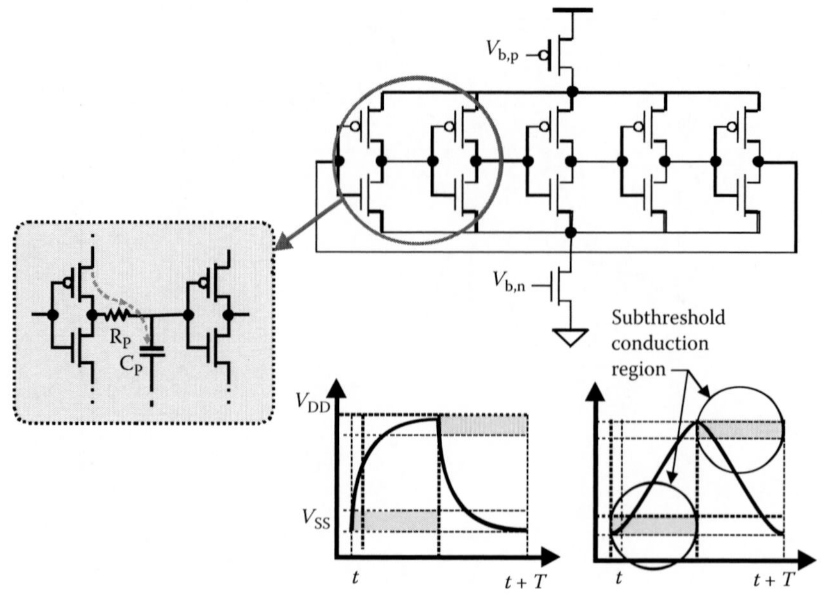

FIGURE 12.13 Block diagram and operation of the current-starving ring oscillator.

12.4.2 Relaxation Oscillators

The block diagram of a conventional relaxation oscillator is shown in Figure 12.14. The charge pump charges and discharges the timing capacitor. Once the voltage of the timing capacitor exceeds the thresholds, the state of the output of the comparator will change subsequently the direction of the current of the charge pump. The oscillation frequency of the relaxation oscillator is determined by the current of the charge pump, the capacitance of the timing capacitor, and the hysteresis width of the comparator.

$$f_{osc} = \frac{I_{CP}}{C \times \Delta V_{TH}}, \tag{12.1}$$

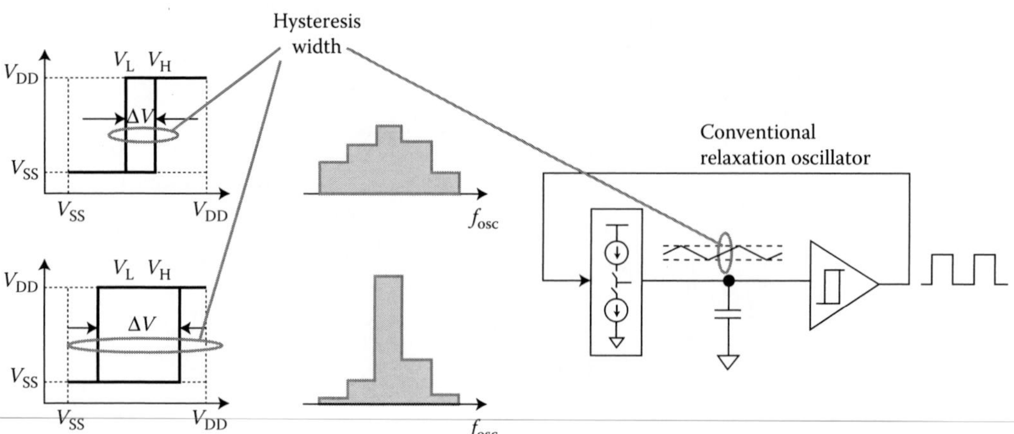

FIGURE 12.14 Block diagram of the conventional relaxation oscillator and the relationship between hysteresis width and frequency variation (dispersion of the frequency histogram).

$$\left|\frac{df_{osc}}{f_{osc}}\right| = \left|\frac{\partial I_{CP}}{I_{CP}}\right| + \left|\frac{\partial C}{C}\right| + \frac{\left|\partial V_{TH}^{+}\right| + \left|\partial V_{TH}^{-}\right|}{\left|\Delta V_{TH}\right|} \tag{12.2}$$

where ΔV_{TH} is the hysteresis width of the comparator and I_{CP} is the current of the charge pump. Since I_{CP} is typically supplied by transistors biased in saturation, its value is less sensitive to process variation as compared with the current of transistors in the subthreshold. Also, the timing capacitor is typically implemented as a MIM capacitor whose value has a much lower uncertainty as compared with the capacitances of transistors, which determine the oscillation frequency of ring oscillators. As a result, relaxation oscillators are less sensitive to PVT as compared with current-starving ring oscillators.

From Equation 12.2, we can verify that the sensitivity of the frequency of relaxation oscillators to process variations can be further reduced by increasing the hysteresis width of the comparator [9]. As shown in Figure 12.14, the frequency of the relaxation oscillator with a large hysteresis has a much lower frequency variation as compared with the frequency of the relaxation oscillator with a small hysteresis. The hysteresis width of CMOS Schmitt triggers is limited by the headroom voltage $V_{DD} - (V_{T,N} + |V_{T,P}|)$. Due to the low supply voltage of passive transponders, this headroom voltage is quite small, usually in the range of 100–200 mV. Employing conventional CMOS Schmitt triggers will therefore cause the oscillation frequency of the oscillator to be more sensitive to process variation due to a limited hysteresis width caused by the low supply voltage of passive transponders. This is why most current designs avoid using standard CMOS Schmitt triggers. Instead, the hysteresis required for oscillation is created by using an set-reset (SR)-latch, two timing capacitors, and two comparators without hysteresis [10,11]. In this chapter, we introduce a new relaxation oscillator that provides rail-to-rail hysteresis using only one timing capacitor and one comparator.

12.4.3 Relaxation Oscillator with Current Pulse Generator

The block diagram of the relaxation oscillator is shown in Figure 12.15a. The hysteresis required for oscillation is created by the current pulse generator, a schematic diagram of which is shown in Figure 12.15b. Each time the voltage of the timing capacitor reaches the threshold level ($V_{DD}/2$), the comparator output makes a transition. If the transition is a rising edge, the current pulse generator produces a positive current pulse of short width. This current pulse charges the timing capacitor to V_{DD}. If the transition is a falling edge, the current pulse generator will generate a negative current pulse of narrow width that will discharge the timing capacitor. The waveforms of the voltage of the timing capacitor and the output of the current pulse generator are shown in Figure 12.15c. Since the oscillation is controlled by charging and discharging the timing capacitor only, this relaxation oscillator is particularly suitable for injection locking as we can easily control the frequency of the oscillator by injecting a control current to the timing capacitor.

12.5 SUMMARY

Design techniques for remote frequency calibration of passive wireless microsystems have been reviewed. An injection-locking remote frequency calibration method that allows a passive wireless microsystem to adjust the oscillation frequency of its local oscillator to a desired frequency has been presented. A new relaxation oscillator with a current pulse generator and a single MIM capacitor to generate the effective hysteresis needed for oscillation with a low supply voltage has also been proposed. Integrating feedback has been employed to increase the lock range and withhold the oscillation frequency of the oscillator when the injection signal is removed. The locking range of the proposed injection-locked-phase-locked loop is approximately 13 times that of the corresponding injection-locked oscillator without integrating feedback. When the injection signal is removed, the frequency of the oscillator with the integrating feedback drifts at a rate of 5 Hz/ms. This drift is

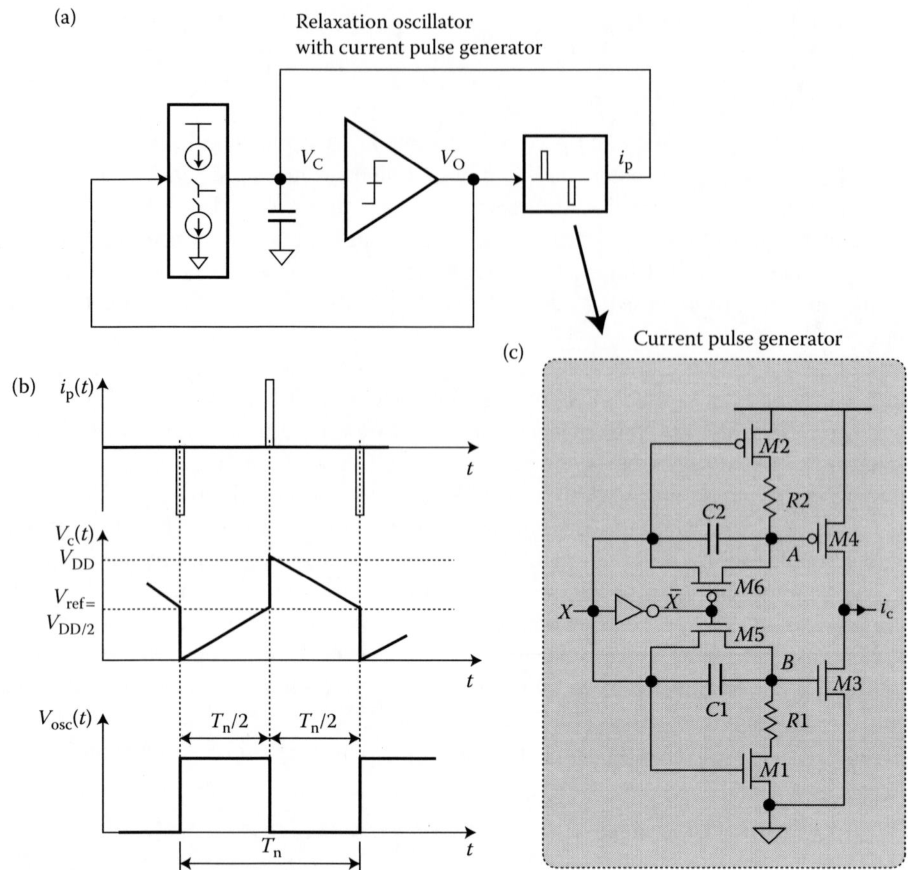

FIGURE 12.15 (a) Block diagram of the relaxation oscillator with a current pulse generator. (b) Waveforms of the relaxation oscillator. (c) Simplified schematic diagram of the current pulse generator. (Copyright © IET.)

negligible as backscattering from transponders to their base station typically takes only a few milliseconds to complete. For the same argument, the effect of temperature variation on the frequency of the oscillator during backscattering can also be neglected.

REFERENCES

1. K. Finkenzeller, *RFID Handbook—Radio-frequency Identifications Fundamentals and Applications*, 2nd edn, Wiley, New York, 2003.
2. F. Kocer and M. Flynn, A new transponder architecture with on-chip ADC for long-range telemetry applications, *IEEE J. Solid-State Circuits*, 41, 5, 1142–1148, 2006.
3. L. Leung and H. Luong, A 7 μW clock generator in 0.18 μm CMOS for passive UHF RFID EPC G2 tags, *Proc. European Solid-State Circuits Conf.*, Muenchen, Germany, pp. 412–415, 2007.
4. N. Tran, B. Lee, and J. Lee, Development of long-range UHF-band RFID tag chip using Schottky diodes in standard CMOS technology, *Proc. IEEE Radio Frequency Integrated Circuits Symp.*, Grapevine, Texas, pp. 281–284, September 2007.
5. N. Panitantum, K. Mayaram, and T. Fiez, A 900- MHz low-power transmitter with fast frequency calibration for wireless sensor networks, *IEEE Custom Integrated Circuits Conf.*, San Jose, CA, pp. 595–598, September 2008.
6. B. Razavi, A study of injection locking and pulling in oscillators, *IEEE J. Solid-State Circuits*, 40, 11, 2193–2202, 2005.

7. N. Soltani and F. Yuan, Non-harmonic injection-locked phase-locked loops with applications in remote frequency calibration of passive wireless transponders, *IEEE Trans. Circuits and Systems I*, 57(12), 2381–2393, 2010
8. B. Razavi, *Fundamentals of Microelectronics*. Wiley, NJ, 2006.
9. F. Yuan and N. Soltani, A low-voltage low VDD sensitivity relaxation oscillator for passive wireless microsystems, *IET Electronics Letters*, 45(21), 1057–1058, 2009.
10. R. Barnett and J. Liu, A 0.8 V 1.52 MHz MSVC relaxation oscillator with inverted mirror feedback reference for UHF RFID, *Proc. IEEE Conf. Custom Integrated Circuits*, San Jose, CA, pp. 769–772, September 2006.
11. Y. Tokunaga, S. Sakiyama, A. Matsumoto, and S. Dosho, An on-chip CMOS relaxation oscillator with power averaging feedback using a reference proportional to supply voltage, *IEEE Int. Solid-State Circuits Conf.*, San Francisco, CA, pp. 404–405, 405a, February 2009.

Part II

Photonics and Imaging

13 Terahertz Imaging and Spectroscopy

State-of-the-Art and Future Trends

Daryoosh Saeedkia

CONTENTS

13.1 INTRODUCTION

Terahertz science and technology has entered an unprecedented revolutionary era with ever-growing applications in biology and medicine, monitoring and spectroscopy in pharmaceutical industry and science, medical imaging, material spectroscopy and sensing, security, and high-data-rate communications. Recent innovations offering both powerful and reliable terahertz sources together with high-performance terahertz spectroscopy and imaging systems have exposed remarkable new opportunities in science and technology. Although major gains in performance and functionality are still anticipated, present commercially available terahertz devices and systems have already made the terahertz spectrum accessible to many scientists and technologists in diverse areas, ranging from biology and medicine to chemical, pharmaceutical, and environmental sciences to revisit their scientific problems under the light of terahertz waves. In this chapter, the recent advances in terahertz devices and systems for imaging, spectroscopy, and sensing applications will be reviewed and the future outlook of the terahertz technology at the device and system level will be presented.

13.2 TERAHERTZ SOURCE TECHNOLOGIES

13.2.1 Electron Beam Sources

Gyrotrons [1], free electron lasers (FELs) [2], and backward wave oscillators (BWOs) [3] are electron beam sources that generate relatively high power terahertz signals. These devices work based on the interaction of a high-energy electron beam with a strong magnetic field inside resonant cavities or waveguides, which results in an energy transfer between the electron beam and an electromagnetic wave. Gyrotrons with 1 MW power at 140 GHz have been successfully developed [4]. An FEL is a gyrotron with very high operating frequencies and wider frequency tuning range [5]. BWOs can be electrically tuned over a bandwidth of more than 50% of their operation frequencies, and can generate up to 50 mW of power at 300 GHz going down to a few mW at 1 THz [6]. Complete systems are heavy and large, and need a high bias voltage and usually a water cooling system [7]. Microfabrication and microassembly technologies are promising approaches to reduce the size of these devices and to make them more suitable for terahertz applications [8].

13.2.2 Solid-State Sources

Solid-state sources include resonant tunneling diodes (RTDs) [9], Gunn or transferred electron devices [10,11], and transit time devices such as impact avalanche transit time diodes and tunnel injection transit time (TUNNETT) diodes. Gunn devices generating 0.2–5 μW power in the 400–560 GHz frequency range are now feasible [12]. TUNNETT diodes with operation frequency as high as 355 GHz with 140 μW output power have been reported [13].

13.2.3 Frequency Multipliers

In a terahertz frequency multiplier, the frequency of a driver source is multiplied in a nonlinear device in order to generate higher-order harmonic frequencies. Planar Schottky varactor diodes are commonly used in frequency multipliers, taking advantage of GaAs substrateless technology to reduce substrate loss. The drive sources can be BWOs or solid-state sources such as Gunn and IMPATT oscillators, with relatively high output power in the range of 50–150 GHz. Microwave frequency synthesizers in combination with high-gain power amplifiers fabricated by the monolithic microwave-integrated circuit technology can generate high output power above 100 GHz [14]. The most efficient terahertz frequency multipliers are realized by series chains of frequency doublers and frequency triplers [15]. Signals up to 2 THz are achievable from frequency multipliers [16,17]. However, using a hybrid system consisting of a BWO and a chain of frequency multipliers, it is possible to generate THz signals with frequencies higher than 2.5 THz [18].

13.2.4 Terahertz Semiconductor Lasers

The most promising terahertz semiconductor lasers are quantum cascade lasers [19,20]. A quantum cascade laser is a unipolar laser, in which the conduction band or the valence band is divided into a few subbands. The carrier transition occurs between these discrete energy levels within the same band. The discrete energy levels are created in a semiconductor heterostructure containing several coupled quantum wells. Quantum cascade lasers with around 10 mW output power at 2 THz have been demonstrated. An operation temperature as high as 93 K has been reported for a terahertz quantum cascade laser at 3.2 THz [21].

13.2.5 Optically Pumped Far-Infrared Gas Lasers

These THz sources consist of a pump laser radiating into a cavity filled with a gas that lases at the terahertz frequency range [22,23]. The lasing frequency is dictated by the filling gas. Power levels of 1–20 mW are common for 20–100 W laser pump power.

13.2.6 Terahertz Optoelectronic Sources

Terahertz photoconductive antennas (photomixers) are widely used to generate terahertz broadband pulses and terahertz narrowband continuous-wave (cw) signals [24,25]. In terahertz photomixers, two cw laser beams, with their frequency difference in the THz range, combined either inside an optical fiber or properly overlapped in space, are mixed in a photo-absorbing medium and generate a beat frequency signal [26,27]. Terahertz signals with a frequency linewidth as low as a few KiloHertz can be generated by photomixers. The frequency of the terahertz signal can be tuned by tuning the wavelengths of the lasers. The output power in conventional photomixers falls from ≈2 μW at 1 THz to below 0.1 μW at 3 THz [28–30].

Broadband terahertz pulses can be generated by exciting a photoconductive antenna by a femto-second short-pulse laser [31]. Using a typical femto-second laser with 100 fs optical pulse duration and a few 100 mW average power, terahertz pulses with their frequency content extended up to around 5 THz and an average power of a few microwatts can be achieved [32,33]. Broadband terahertz pulses can also be generated in electrooptic crystals excited by femto-second short-pulse lasers [34].

Terahertz signals can be generated via parametric interaction of near-infrared photons and optical vibration modes inside an optical crystal [35]. Using this technique, the generation of a quasi-cw terahertz signal with the pulse duration of 3.6 ns, an average power of 9 nW, and a frequency tuning range of 0.7–2.4 THz has been reported [36].

Terahertz signals can also be generated through difference frequency mixing in nonlinear crystals [35]. Mixing a dual-wavelength Yb-fiber laser with the pulse duration of 1 ns in a $ZnGeP_2$ crystal, 2 mW average terahertz power was generated at 2.45 THz [37].

Figure 13.1 compares some of the terahertz sources in terms of their output powers and operation frequencies [35].

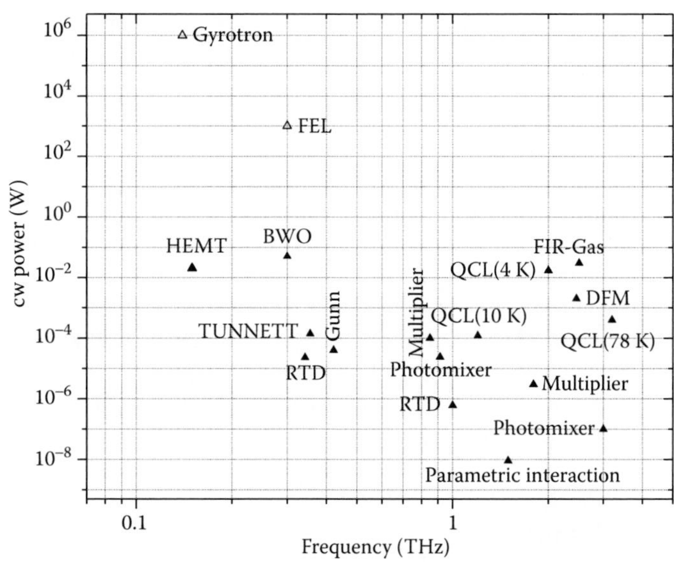

FIGURE 13.1 Comparison of some of the terahertz sources in terms of their output power and operation frequency. (FEL: free-electron laser; BWO: backward wave oscillator; RTD: resonant tunneling diode; TUNNETT: tunnel injection transit time diode; PI: parametric interaction in nonlinear crystals; DFM: difference frequency mixing in nonlinear crystals; FIR-Gas: far-infrared gas laser; QCL: quantum cascade laser; HEMT: high-electron mobility transistor.) (Courtesy of D. Saeedkia and S. Safavi-Naeini, *IEEE/OSA J. Lightwave Technol.*, 26(15), 2409–2423, 2008.)

13.3 TERAHERTZ DETECTOR TECHNOLOGIES

13.3.1 Homodyne Detectors

In homodyne (or direct) detection techniques, the incident terahertz wave on a detector is converted into a measurable electrical signal. Thermal detectors form a large class of the homodyne detectors. The incident terahertz signal on a thermal detector is absorbed by a material whose physical properties such as volume, electric conductivity, and dielectric properties change with temperature. Thermal detectors are square law devices, in which their output signals are proportional to the square of the incident field. The phase information of the incident signal is not directly measured by thermal detectors. Most of the thermal detectors have relaxed intrinsic frequency limitation due to their purely thermal sensing principle, and they are usually slow response devices. The figure of merit for thermal detectors is their noise equivalent power (NEP; in W $Hz^{-1/2}$), defined as the input signal power required to deliver an output signal-to-noise ratio equal to unity in 1 Hz bandwidth, or the noise equivalent temperature difference (NETD or NEΔT; in K), which is defined as the equivalent temperature difference on the object that results in a signal-to-noise ratio of unity at the detector output. Golay cells, pyroelectric detectors, thermoelectric detectors or thermopiles, and bolometers are among the most widely used thermal detectors.

In Golay cells, the incident power is absorbed by a thin absorber membrane that heats up a sealed volume of gas. The change in gas volume can be measured either by a sensitive microphone or by changing the angle of a mirror in an optical amplifier. Their typical responsivity at 1 THz with 10 Hz modulation frequency is around 10^5 V/W with the NEP of around 10^{-10} $WHz^{-1/2}$.

In pyroelectric detectors, the incident signal changes the dielectric constant of a material inside a voltage-biased capacitor and consequently generates a measurable current proportional to the rate of change in the dielectric constant of the absorbing material. Pyroelectric detectors are mostly used as the infrared detectors with a typical NEP of 5×10^{-10} $WHz^{-1/2}$ at 1 MHz modulation frequency and $\lambda = 10$ μm wavelength range. Their sensitivity drops at far-infrared and terahertz frequencies.

Bolometers form a large class of thermal detectors [38,39]. In a bolometer, a resistance thermometer is thermally attached to an absorber material and measures the temperature change of the absorber due to the incident radiation. The absorber material has a large absorptivity and a low heat capacity, and can be made of a normal metal, a doped semiconductor, or a superconductor film. The NEPs for room temperature bolometers with normal metal absorbers are in the range of 5×10^{-10} $WHz^{-1/2}$ with the responsivity of 100 V/W and 1 μs response time. For liquid nitrogen-cooled bolometers the NEP can be as low as 2.5×10^{-12} $WHz^{-1/2}$ with the responsivity of 4000 V/W and 200 ns response time. The most sensitive bolometers are liquid-helium-cooled bolometers with their NEP in the range of 1×10^{-18} $WHz^{-1/2}$ with the responsivity of 10^9 V/W and 1 μs response time.

Another class of room temperature homodyne terahertz detectors is demonstrated based on plasma wave oscillation in field effect transistors [40] with typical NEP around 1×10^{-10} $WHz^{-1/2}$ and the responsivity of 200 V/W [41–43]. The resonance absorption frequency can be tuned over a wide range by tuning the gate voltage. Devices compatible with standard complementary metal-oxide- semiconductor (CMOS) technology have been demonstrated and are promising candidates for low-cost terahertz array detector technologies [41].

13.3.2 Heterodyne Detectors

In a heterodyne detection scheme [44,45], the input terahertz signal is multiplied by a signal from a local oscillator in a nonlinear mixer device such as a Schottky mixer, a hot electron bolometer (HEB) mixer, or a superconductor–insulator–superconductor (SIS) mixer, and the resulting intermediate frequency (IF) signal containing both amplitude and phase information of the input terahertz signal is amplified, filtered, and processed in the back-end IF electronic stages [46]. The figure of merit for heterodyne detectors is their noise temperature (NT; in K). The Schottky mixers can operate at room temperature with 10^4 K noise temperature at 1.5 THz and need relatively high local oscillator power in the range of 1–10 mW. HEB mixers operating at the liquid nitrogen temperature can work at frequencies up to 3 THz, where the SIS mixers fail to operate, and need very low local oscillator power in the range of 10 nW. The SIS mixers with 1 μW local oscillator power working at the liquid helium temperature exhibit the highest sensitivity among the heterodyne mixers with the noise temperature on the order of 400 K at 1 THz.

13.3.3 Optoelectronic Detectors

Optoelectronic techniques exhibit alternative solutions for extracting both amplitude and phase information of a terahertz signal incident on an optically gated terahertz photoconductive antenna [31] or a nonlinear electrooptic crystal [34]. The gating laser beam can come from a short-pulse laser or from a pair of cw lasers with their frequency difference being equal to the frequency of the incident cw terahertz signal [47]. In the photoconductive antenna detection scheme, the amplitude of the generated photocurrent on the receiver antenna is proportional to the amplitude of the incident terahertz electric field.

In the case of the electrooptic detection scheme, the incident terahertz wave copropagates with the gating laser beam inside an electrooptic crystal and induces a change in the polarization state of the linearly polarized laser beam. The change in the polarization state of the gating laser beam is proportional to the amplitude of the terahertz electric field, which can be detected as a voltage at the output of a pair of balanced photodiode detectors. In both the photoconductive antenna and electrooptic detection schemes, the phase information of the received terahertz signal can be extracted by controlling the arrival time of the gating laser beam with respect to the arriving time of the incident terahertz signal.

13.4 TERAHERTZ IMAGING

Over the last few years, many terahertz imaging techniques and instruments have been developed for a variety of different applications ranging from proof of principle studies to the system development for real-world applications [48]. Terahertz waves penetrate into many materials and compositions and exhibit relatively high resolution images, a unique property of terahertz waves that makes them attractive for nondestructive and noninvasive imaging with potential applications in security, pharmaceutical industry, medical imaging, monitoring and quality control in food industries, and electronic circuit inspection. In recent years, the main focus of the terahertz imaging technology development activities has been on the system development for stand-off detection of hidden objects and concealed threats, and on the compact and portable system development for cancer detection and for tablet analysis and quality control of pharmaceutical products.

In a contrast (gray scale) imaging system, the detection technique is either direct (homodyne) detection with amplitude image construction capability or heterodyne detection with the possibility of constructing both amplitude and phase images. These systems are either passive imagers not needing illuminating sources or active imagers usually equipped with cw terahertz sources to illuminate the target. Most of the demonstrated imaging systems for stand-off hidden object detection applications have been contrast-imaging systems [49–53].

Another series of terahertz imaging systems use cw tunable terahertz sources or broadband terahertz pulse sources to construct two-dimensional (2D) and 3D images with the possibility of extracting spectroscopic information of the images [54–61]. These systems are particularly attractive for explosive and illicit drug detection applications as well as for pharmaceutical product monitoring and classification and counterfeit drug-sensing applications [62–65].

An active terahertz imaging system has been recently demonstrated for stand-off imaging applications, containing two optically pumped far-infrared gas lasers with 100 mW output power at 1.56 THz, one used as the illumination source and the other as the local oscillator for the heterodyne Schottky diode receiver [50]. The illuminating terahertz beam is scanned over the object using a commercial scanning mirror system. Both the amplitude and phase of the received signal were measured using a lock-in amplifier system. The system is designed for a 2.5-m stand-off scan with a capacity for imaging a 0.5 m × 0.5 m scene with 1.5 cm resolution with an image rate of 2 frames/s.

The U.S. Defense Advanced Research Projects Agency has initiated two programs toward the development of active imaging systems for stand-off imaging applications at 340 and 670 GHz. The first program called Submillimeter Wave Imaging Focal Plane Technology started in 2006, aimed at the development of an imaging system at 340 GHz, using InP HEMT sources with 50 mW output power and an array of 1 × 128 pixel heterodyne receiver. The second program is called Terahertz Imaging Focal-Plane Technology, aimed at the development of sources and detectors at 670 GHz frequency with more than 10 mW output power for the sources and NEP less than 10^{-12} $WHz^{-1/2}$ for the detectors.

13.4.1 Passive Terahertz Imaging

In the passive imaging approach, the target is not illuminated by a terahertz source, and the natural radiation from the target and/or the reflected/scattered ambient radiation off the target is detected by sensitive detectors [49,51,66]. The image contrast in passive imaging comes from the difference in emissivity of different objects in the scene. Both homodyne (direct) and heterodyne detectors can be used in terahertz passive imaging systems. Since the receiving signal is too small in a passive imaging scheme, the direct detectors have to be supersensitive with an NEP in the range of 10^{-14} $WHz^{-1/2}$ or an NETD less than 1 K. Cryogenically cooled detectors are needed in order to address these sensitivity requirements. Using a low-noise amplifier (LNA) before the detector module can increase the input signal level to the point that room temperature direct detectors with NEPs in the range of 10^{-12} $WHz^{-1/2}$ are suitable for passive imaging applications [67–69]. However, adding the LNA modules to the system increases the complexity and cost of the system and limits the operation frequencies to mostly below 300 GHz. The heterodyne detectors exhibit larger signal-to-noise ratios and can also operate at room temperature, but the system becomes complex and expensive.

The passive imaging systems have been mostly used in the stand-off detection and people screening applications. The fact that the target is not illuminated by a terahertz radiation makes the passive imaging less invasive and more suitable for ethics and public safety involving types of applications. ThruVision offers a commercially available terahertz passive imaging system targeted toward people screening applications at airports, border checkpoints, entrances to public buildings, shopping malls, sporting events, and police deployments. The system can monitor targets indoor and outdoor at distances up to 25 m.

13.4.2 Active Terahertz Imaging

In the active imaging approach, the target is illuminated by a terahertz source and the transmitted signal through the target or the reflected/scattered signal off the target is detected by a terahertz detector [48,50,52,53,55,59]. The image contrast in active imaging comes from the difference in reflectivity or transparency of the object. Different types of terahertz sources and detectors have been used for terahertz active imaging, and several commercially available systems have been developed to address various applications ranging from security and mail inspection [70] to tablet coating analysis [63], integrated circuit inspection [71,72], and artwork analysis [73,74]. Compared to the passive imaging modality, in terahertz active imaging systems the signal-to-noise ratio is much higher and less-expensive room temperature detectors can be used to achieve video-rate imaging performance. Most of the commercially available active imaging systems for stand-off detection and people screening applications work at frequencies below 300 GHz. A higher image resolution can be achieved by moving into the higher frequencies, or for the same image resolution, the overall size of the system can be reduced by working at higher frequencies. The major difficulties with

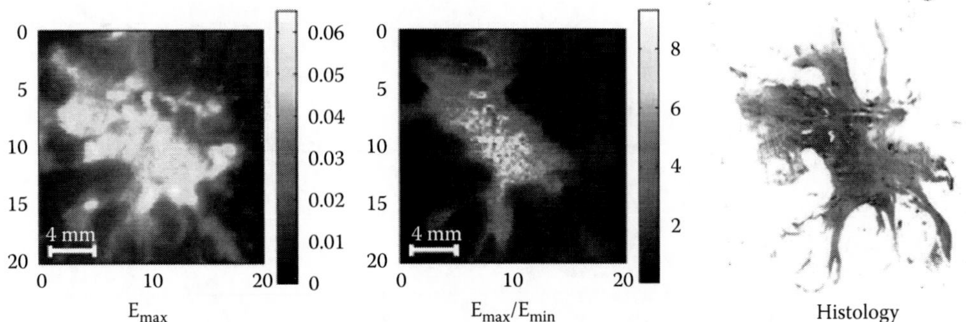

FIGURE 13.2 Terahertz pulsed spectroscopy of freshly excised human breast cancer. (From C. Ashworth et al., *Opt. Express*, 17(15), 12444–12454, 2009. With permission.)

performing active imaging at frequencies above 300 GHz are the higher absorption and scattering losses and the smaller reflectivity of materials, higher atmospheric attenuation (with a few open windows around 340 GHz, 420 GHz, 650 GHz, 850 GHz, and 1.5 THz), and less available terahertz power from existing terahertz source technologies.

Active imaging systems have also been developed for medical imaging and particularly for cancer detection applications. The majority of the demonstrated systems use optoelectronic techniques for terahertz pulsed and cw signal generation and detection with the capability of operating in both transmission and reflection modes [58,75–78].

Figure 13.2 shows the images of freshly excised human breast tissues taken by a terahertz pulse imaging system [76]. The cancerous regions are well correlated with the tumor shown in the histology image. The tissue samples were collected from 20 patients containing healthy tissues and cancerous tissues. Samples were compressed between two quartz windows and were scanned across the terahertz beam in a transmission-mode measurement scheme. The complex refractive indices of the samples were determined and it was shown that the samples containing cancer had a higher refractive index and absorption coefficient in the range of 0.15–2.0 THz.

13.4.3 Terahertz Near-Field Imaging

In a diffraction-limited imaging scenario, where the source of illumination and the detector are both far from the target, the highest achievable resolution is in the range of half of the wavelength of illuminating signal. At the frequency of 1 THz, for example, this translates into an image resolution around 150 μm. One way of increasing the resolution is to bring the source and/or the detector close to the target and perform a near-field imaging [79–81]. Another approach for achieving a resolution beyond the diffraction limit is to employ a subwavelength size aperture between the target and the terahertz source [82–84]. In the case of optoelectronic detection schemes, the subwavelength spatial resolution can also be achieved by limiting the active imaging area to the beam size of a focused laser beam [85,86]. Increasing the spatial resolution beyond the diffraction limit by means of a subwavelength aperture usually comes with the price of reducing the signal-to-noise ratio of the imaging system. Figure 13.3 shows an image of a nanoscale transistor using the terahertz near-field nanoscopy technique at 2.54 THz (λ = 118 mm) based on terahertz scattering at atomic force microscope tips [87]. Using this technique, features as small as 40 nm (λ/3000) can be resolved.

13.4.4 Single Pixel and Array Detectors: Real-Time Terahertz Imaging

The dominant imaging technique in the existing terahertz imaging systems is based on single-point detection configuration, where the transmitted terahertz signal through the target or the reflected/

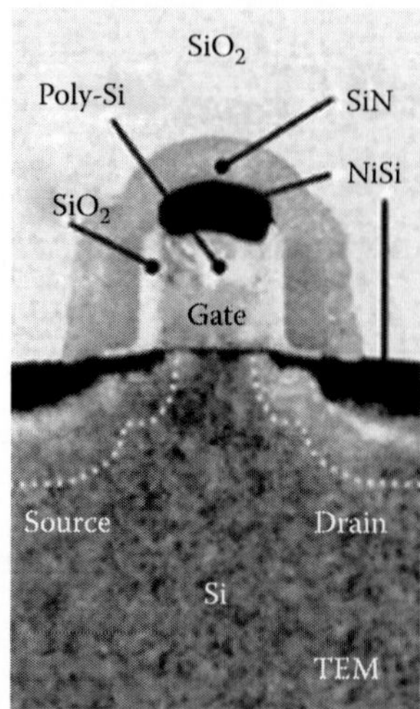

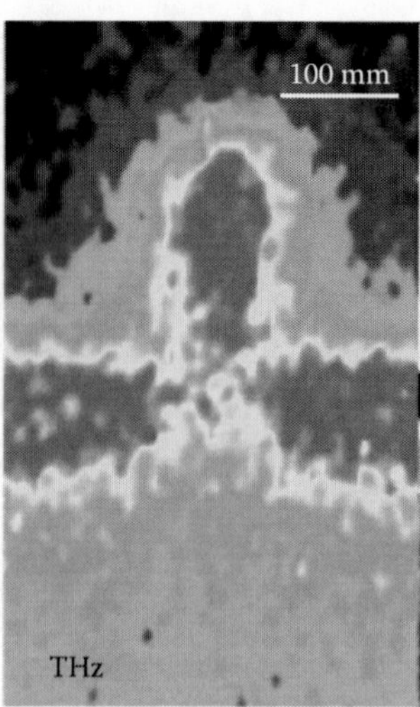

FIGURE 13.3 Image of nanoscale transistors using THz near-field nanoscopy technique at 2.54 THz (λ = 118 mm). 40 nm (λ/3000) features are resolved. (From A. J. Huber et al., *Nano Lett.*, 8(11), 3766–3770, 2008. With permission.)

scattered terahertz signal off the target is detected by a single-pixel detector unit. To acquire a 2D image of a target, the incident terahertz signal is scanned across the target and/or the target is raster scanned across the incident terahertz beam, and the transmitted and/or reflected/scattered terahertz signal for each pixel is individually detected by the single-pixel detector unit. Using this technique, the image acquisition time substantially increases when a large cross section of an object needs to be imaged, making it impractical for many real-world applications, where high-resolution real-time or quasi-real-time imaging is required. Single-pixel detection schemes in combination with compressed sensing techniques have been investigated to demonstrate fast 2D terahertz imaging [88–90].

To reduce the image acquisition time, array detectors have been developed and their applications in real-time imaging have been investigated [51,66,67,69,91–94]. A focal-plane array detector based on low-cost CMOS technology has been developed and its application in terahertz imaging at 0.65 THz has been demonstrated [95,96].

For the systems using high-power terahertz sources, real-time imaging has been demonstrated using commercially available room temperature pyroelectric [97] and microbolometer [98–100] cameras.

Real-time 2D terahertz imaging has also been demonstrated using a commercial charge-coupled device (CCD) camera in a terahertz imaging system containing an electrooptic crystal and a readout laser beam [101–106]. In this system, the polarization state of the readout laser beam is modulated by the electric field of a copropagating terahertz beam and then converted into an intensity modulation using an arrangement of optical polarizers. The intensity modulation on the readout laser beam carries the image information and is displayed by the CCD camera.

13.5 TERAHERTZ SPECTROSCOPY AND SENSING

Many organic and inorganic materials and compositions have distinct fingerprints in the terahertz spectrum, a unique property of terahertz waves making them attractive for material spectroscopy and sensing applications [107–109]. Terahertz spectroscopy and sensing techniques have been shown to be useful for polymorph recognition [110] and active ingredient fingerprinting and quantification [111] in pharmaceutical science and industry, resonance absorption [112,113] and refractive index contrast [114–116] sensing of biomolecules [54,117,118], cancer cell detection [76], and explosives [119] and biohazards [70] detection and identification.

Wideband terahertz pulse sources or widely tunable cw terahertz sources are needed to acquire spectroscopic information over a wide range of terahertz frequencies. Among the existing terahertz source and detector technologies, terahertz optoelectronic sources and detectors such as photoconductive antennas in pulsed and cw modes and electrooptic crystals are dominantly used for terahertz spectroscopy and sensing applications [107,110,111,114,116,118]. Terahertz parametric sources have also been used for drugs of abuse detection and mail inspection applications [64,70].

Figure 13.4 shows the absorption features of D-tartaric acid over a range of terahertz frequencies measured in a terahertz time-domain system. The D-tartaric acid powder was mixed with polyethylene powder and the mixture was exposed to the terahertz wave in a terahertz time-domain system. The terahertz path was purged with dry nitrogen to remove the water vapor. Compared to the reference spectrum, the pronounced absorption fingerprint of the D-tartaric acid around 1.08 THz is believed to be due to the intermolecular bond vibrations of the crystal structure of the material. Unlike infrared spectroscopy, which mainly records the intramolecular vibrations of molecules, terahertz spectroscopy reveals the spectroscopic features of the intermolecular bond vibrations, which are directly related to the molecular conformations and the crystalline structure of the material.

Figure 13.5 shows the terahertz absorption features of two different polymorphs of carbamazepine (CBZ), namely form I and form III [110]. Difference in the crystalline structures of the two forms of CBZ results in a distinct difference in their absorption fingerprints in the terahertz spectrum.

Integrated terahertz sensor modules where the generation, guidance, interaction with samples, and detection of the terahertz wave all take place on a single chip have been studied and demonstrated by several groups [120–126]. An integrated terahertz biochip contains a terahertz source, a sensor transducer, and a detector element integrated on a single substrate [122,125]. The laser excitation on the source and the detector sites can be pulsed or cw laser beams. In the edge-coupled guided wave optical excitation scheme, the laser beam is guided inside an integrated optical waveguide structure [127] and is absorbed by an overlying ultrafast photoabsorbing layer for terahertz generation and detection purposes [124,125]. Terahertz biochip sensors have been used to differentiate between single-strand DNA (ss-DNA) and double-strand DNA (ds-DNA) molecules. The operation principle in demonstrated terahertz biochip sensors is based on the change in resonance

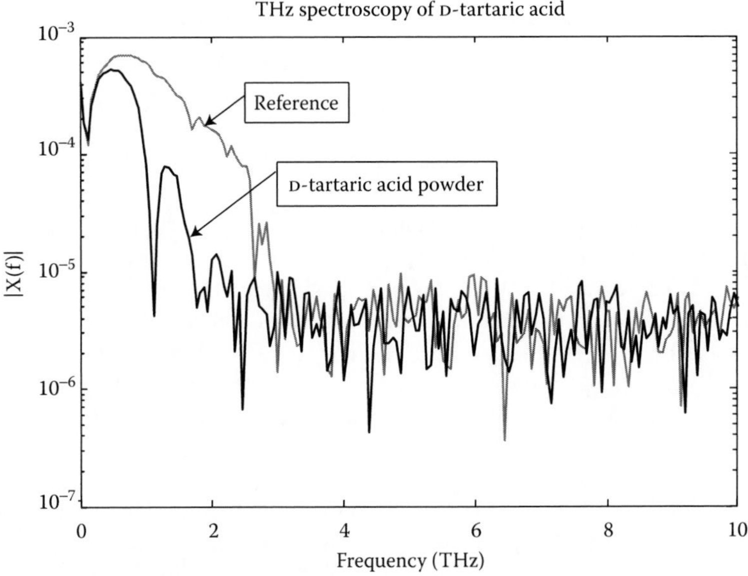

FIGURE 13.4 Absorption features of D-tartaric acid over a range of terahertz spectra measured in a terahertz time-domain system.

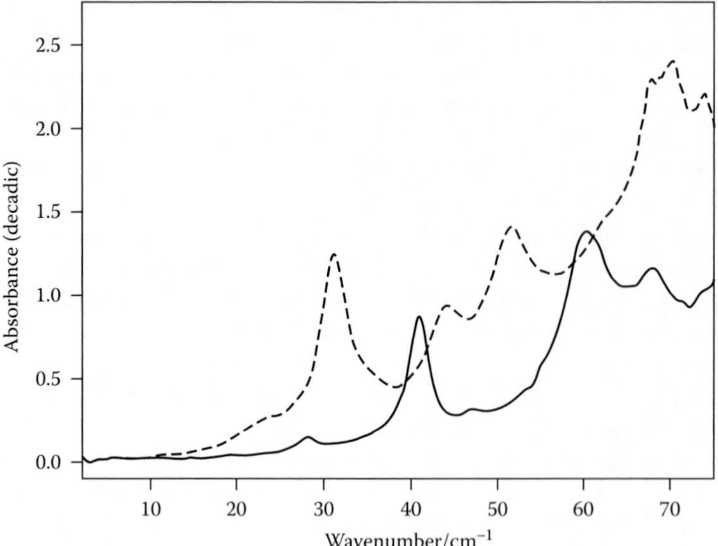

FIGURE 13.5 Absorption spectra of CBZ form III (solid line) and CBZ form I (dashed line) mixed with polyethylene powder. (From J. Strachan et al., *Chem. Phys. Lett.*, 390(1–3), 20–24, 2004. With permission.)

frequency and/or quality factor of the terahertz resonator due to the presence of biosamples with different refractive indices and the attenuation coefficients. This can be attributed to the change in the effective refractive index of the resonator's surrounding medium after adding the biomolecule samples. A significant advantage of using resonators as transducers in a biosensing system is that the volume of the sample required for reliable detection is reduced dramatically (more than three orders of magnitudes) compared to the free-space spectroscopy approach [126], which results in a much higher analytic sensitivity.

13.6 CONCLUDING REMARKS AND FUTURE TRENDS

Terahertz imaging technology is moving toward the development of low-cost, high-resolution, and real-time 2D and 3D imaging systems with the possibility of extracting spectroscopic information from the recorded signals. For security applications, both passive and active imaging systems will continue to emerge. Developing passive imaging systems with highly sensitive room temperature detectors not needing the LNA stages before the sensor modules can make passive imagers the dominant technology for people screening applications. Low-cost, compact, ruggedized and low-weight, and portable active terahertz imaging systems utilizing high-power and tunable terahertz sources and sensitive 2D array detectors can open up a large market for terahertz spectroscopy and imaging technologies in medical imaging and many other industries. Developing fiber-coupled terahertz optoelectronic spectrometer and imager systems working in the telecom wavelength range and developing 2D terahertz cameras compatible with low-cost CMOS technology combined with image enhancement software/hardware techniques are among the most promising paths toward these goals.

Subwavelength terahertz sensing and imaging techniques using novel device and system concepts can play an important role in introducing the terahertz technology as a unique solution to various industrial problems. Near-field imaging and sensing techniques and field enhancement techniques over subwavelength regions using surface plasmon, photonic band gap, and metamaterial structures are among the most promising approaches for achieving resolutions beyond the diffraction limit.

REFERENCES

1. K. Flech, B. G. Danly, H. R. Jory, K. E. Kreischer, W. Lawson, B. Levush, and R. J. Temkin, Characteristics and applications of fast wave gyrodevices, *Proc. IEEE*, 87(5), 752–781, 1999.
2. S. Krishnagopal and V. Kumar, Free-electron lasers, *Radiat. Phys. Chem.*, 70(4,5), 559–569, 2004.
3. R. Kompfner and N. T. Williams, Backward-wave tubes, *Proc. IRE*,41, 1602–1610, 1953.
4. G. Dammertz *et al.*, Development of a 140-GHz 1-MW continuous wave gyrotron for the W7-X stellarator, *IEEE Trans. Plasma Sci.*, 30(3), 808–818, 2002.
5. L. Granatstein, R. K. Parker, and C. M. Armstrong, Vacuume electronics at the dawn of the twenty-first century, *Proc. IEEE*, 87(5), 702–716, 1999.
6. L. P. Schmidt, S. Biber, G. Rehm, and K. Huber, THz measurement technologies and applications, in *Proc. 14th Int. Conf. Microwaves, Radar and Wireless Communications*, Gdansk, Poland, 2, pp. 581–587, 2002.
7. R. L. Ives, D. Marsden, M. Caplan, C. Kory, J. Neilson, and S. Schwartzkopf, Advanced terahertz backward wave oscillators, in *Proc. 4th IEEE Int. Conf. Vacuum Electronics*, Seoul, Korea, pp. 20–21, May 2003.
8. R. L. Ives, Microfabrication of high-frequency vacuum electron devices, *IEEE Trans. Plasma Sci.*, 32(3), 1277–1291, 2004.
9. E. R. Brown and C. D. Parker, Resonant tunnel diodes as submillimetre-wave sources, *Philos. Trans. R. Soc. London*, 354, 2365–2381, 1996.
10. H. Eisele and R. Kamoua, Submillimeter-wave InP Gunn devices, *IEEE Trans. Microw. Theory Tech.*, 52(10), 2371–2378, 2004.
11. L. Wandinger, mm-wave InP Gunn devices: Status and trends, *Microw. J.*, 24(3), 71–78, 1981.
12. H. Eisele, M. Naftaly, and R. Kamoua, Generation of submillimeter wave radiation with GaAs TUNNETT diodes and InP Gunn devices in a second or higher harmonic mode, *Int. J. Infrared Millim. Waves*, 26(1), 1–14, 2005.
13. H. Eisele, InP Gunn devices for 400–425 GHz, *Electron. Lett.*, 42(6), 358–359, 2006.
14. L. A. Samoska, T. C. Gaier, A. Peralta, S. Weibreb, J. Bruston, I. Mehdi, Y. Chen et al., MMIC power amplifiers as local oscillator drivers for FIRST, in *Proc. SPIE Conf.*, Munich, Germany, 4013, 275–284, 2000.
15. P. H. Siegel, Terahertz technology, *IEEE Trans. Microw. Theory Tech*, 50(3), 910–928, 2002.
16. J. Ward, E. Schlecht, G. Chattopadhyay, A. Maestrini, J. Gill, F. Maiwald, H. Javadi, and I. Mehdi, Capability of THz sources based on Schottky diode frequency multiplier chains, in *Proc. IEEE Microwave Theory and Techniques Soc. Int. Microwave Symp. Dig.*, Fort Worth, Texas, 3, 1587–1590, 2004.
17. V. Krozer, G. Loata, J. G. de la Fuente, and P. Sanz, Limitations in THz power generation with Schottky diode varactor frequency multipliers, in *Proc. IEEE 10th Int. Conf. Terahertz Electronics*, Cambridge, pp. 109–112, September 2002.
18. C. P. Endres, H. S. P. Muller, S. Brunken, D. G. Paveliev, T. F. Giesen, S. Schlemmer, and F. Lewen, High resolution rotation-inversion spectroscopy on doubly deuterated ammonia, ND_2H, up to 2.6 THz, *J. Mol. Struct.*, 795(1), 242–255, 2006.
19. J. Faist, F. Capasso, D. L. Sivco, C. Sirtori, A. L. Hutchinson, and A. Y. Cho, Quantum cascade laser, *Science*, 264(5158), 553–556, 1994.
20. F. Capasso *et al.*, Quantum cascade lasers: Ultrahigh-speed operation, optical wireless communication, narrow linewidth, and far-infrared emission, *IEEE J. Quantum Electron.*, 38(6), 511–532, 2002.
21. S. Kumar, B. S. Williams, S. Kohen, Q. Hu, and J. L. Reno, Continuous-wave operation of terahertz quantum-cascade lasers above liquid-nitrogen temperature, *Appl. Phys. Lett.*, 84(14), 2494–2496, 2004.
22. T. Y. Chang and T. J. Bridges, Laser action at 452, 496, and 541 μm in optically pumped CH_3F, *Opt. Commun.*, 1, 423–426, 1970.
23. M. Inguscio, G. Moruzzi, K. M. Evenson, and D. A. Jennings, A review of frequency measurements of optically pumped lasers from 0.1 to 8 THz, *J. Appl. Phys.*, 60(12), R161–R192, 1986.
24. E. R. Brown, THz generation by photomixing in ultrafast photoconductors, *Terahertz Sensing Technology*, Vol. 1: *Electronic Devices and Advanced Systems Technology*. Eds. D. L. Woolard, W. R. Loerop, and M. S. Shur. Singapore: World Scientific, 2003, pp. 147–195.
25. D. Saeedkia and S. Safavi-Naeini, A comprehensive model for photomixing in ultrafast photoconductors, *IEEE Photon. Technol. Lett.*, 18(13), 1457–1459, 2006.
26. D. Saeedkia, S. Safavi-Naeini, and R. R. Mansour, The interaction of laser and photoconductor in a continuous-wave terahertz photomixer, *IEEE J. Quantum Electron.*, 41(9), 1188–1196, 2005.
27. D. Saeedkia, R. R. Mansour, and S. Safavi-Naeini, Modeling and analysis of high-temperature superconductor terahertz photomixers, *IEEE Trans. Appl. Supercond.*, 15(3), 3847–3855, 2005.

28. J. E. Bjarnason, T. L. J. Chan, A. W. M. Lee, E. R. Brown, D. C. Driscoll, M. Hanson, A. C. Gossard, and R. E. Muller, ErAs:GaAs photomixer with two-decade tunability and 12 μW peak output power, *Appl. Phys. Lett.*, 85(18), 3983–3985, 2004.
29. P. Kordos, M. Marso, and M. Mikulics, Performance optimization of GaAs-based photomixers as sources of THz radiation, *Appl. Phys. A*, 87, 563–567, 2007.
30. E. A. Michael, Travelling-wave photonic mixers for increased continuous-wave power beyond 1 THz, *Semicond. Sci. Technol.*, 20(7), S164–S177, 2005.
31. R. A. Cheville, Terahertz time-domain spectroscopy with photoconductive antennas, *Terahertz Spectroscopy Principles and Applications*. Ed. S. L. Dexheimer. Boca Raton, FL: CRC Press, pp. 1–39, 2008.
32. D. Saeedkia, M. R. Esmaili-Rad, and M. Nagel, Photoconductive aperture antenna arrays for generation and detection of terahertz radiation, in *Proc. 34th Int. Conf. Infrared, Millimeter, and Terahertz Waves*, Busan, Korea, 2009.
33. D. Saeedkia, Resonantly enhanced terahertz power spectrum in terahertz photoconductive antennas, in *Proc. 34th Int. Conf. Infrared, Millimeter, and Terahertz Waves*, Busan, Korea, 2009.
34. I. Wilke and S. Sengupta, Nonlinear optical techniques for terahertz pulse generation and detection—optical rectification and electrooptic sampling, *Terahertz Spectroscopy Principles and Applications*. Ed. S. L. Dexheimer. Boca Raton, FL: CRC Press, pp. 41–72, 2008.
35. D. Saeedkia and S. Safavi-Naeini, Terahertz photonics: Optoelectronic techniques for generation and detection of terahertz waves, *IEEE/OSA J. Lightwave Technol.*, 26, 15, 2409–2423, 2008.
36. K. Kawase, J. Shikata, and H. Ito, Terahertz wave parametric source, *J. Phys. D, Appl. Phys.*, 34, R1–R14, 2001.
37. D. Creeden, J. C. McCarthy, P. A. Ketteridge, T. Southward, P. G. Schunemann, J. J. Komiak, W. Dove, and E. P. Chicklis, Compact fiber-pumped terahertz source based on difference frequency mixing in ZGP, *IEEE J. Sel. Top. Quantum Electron.*, 13(3), 732–737, 2007.
38. P. L. Richards, Bolometers for infrared and millimetre waves, *J. Appl. Phys.*, 76(1), 1–24, 1994.
39. A. J., Kreisler and A. Gaugue, Recent progress in high-temperature superconductor bolometric detectors: From the mid-infrared to the far-infrared (THz) range, *Supercond. Sci. Technol.*, 13, 1235–1245, 2000.
40. M. Shur and V. Ryzhii, Plasma wave electronics, terahertz sensing technology, Vol. 1: *Electronic Devices and Advanced Systems Technology*. Eds. D. L. Woolard, W. R. Loerop, and M. S. Shur. Singapore: World Scientific, pp. 225–250, 2003.
41. R. Tauk, F. Teppe, S. Boubanga, D. Coquillat, W. Knap, Y. M. Meziani, C. Gallon et al., Plasma wave detection of terahertz radiation by silicon field effects transistors: Responsivity and noise equivalent power, *Appl. Phys. Lett.*, 89, 253511-1–3, 2006.
42. A. Lisauskas, W. von Spiegel, S. Boubanga-Tombet, A. El Fatimy, D. Coquillat, F. Teppe, N. Dyakonova, W. Knap, and H.G. Roskos, Terahertz imaging with GaAs field-effect transistors, *Elect. Lett.*, 44(6), 408–409, 2008.
43. A. El Fatimy, J. C. Delagnes, A. Younus, E. Nguema, F. Teppe, W. Knap, E. Abraham, and P. Mounaix, Plasma wave field effect transistor as a resonant detector for 1 terahertz imaging applications, *Opt. Commun.*, 282, 15, 3055–3058, 2009.
44. H.-W. Hubers, Terahertz heterodyne receivers, *IEEE J. Sel. Top. Quantum Electron.*, 14, 2, 378–391, 2008.
45. P. H. Siegel and R. J. Dengler, Terahertz heterodyne imaging part I: Introduction and techniques, *Int. J. Infrared Millim. Waves*, 27(4), 465–480, 2006.
46. P. H. Siegel, THz technology: An overview, terahertz sensing technology, Vol. 1: *Electronic Devices and Advanced Systems Technology*. Eds. D. L. Woolard, W. R. Loerop, and M. S. Shur. Singapore: World Scientific, pp. 1–44, 2003.
47. S. Verghese, K. A. McIntosh, S. Calawa, W. F. Dinatale, E. K. Duerr, and K. A. Molvar, Generation and detection of coherent terahertz waves using two photomixers, *Appl. Phys. Lett.*, 73(26), 3824–3826, 1998.
48. S. P. Mickan and X.-C. Zhang, T-ray sensing and imaging, terahertz sensing technology, Vol. 1: *Electronic Devices and Advanced Systems Technology*. Eds. D. L. Woolard, W. R. Loerop, and M. S. Shur. Singapore: World Scientific, pp. 251–326, 2003.
49. D. T. Petkie, C. Casto, F. C. De Lucia, S. R. Murrill, B. Redman, R. L. Espinola, C. C. Franck et al., Active and passive imaging in the THz spectral region: Phenomenology, dynamic range, modes, and illumination, *J. Opt. Soc. Am. B*, 25(9), 1523–1531, 2008.
50. T. M. Goyette, J. C. Dickinson, K. J. Linden, W. R. Neal, C. S. Joseph, W. J. Gorveatt, J. Waldman, R. Giles, and W. E. Nixon, 1.56 Terahertz 2-frames per second standoff imaging, *Proc. SPIE*, 6893, 68930J, 2008.

51. A. Luukanen1, P. Helistö, P. Lappalainen, M. Leivo, A. Rautiainen, H. Toivanen, H. Seppä, Z. Taylor, C. R. Dietlein, and E. N. Grossman, Stand-off passive THz imaging at 8-meter stand-off distance: Results from a 64-channel real-time imager, *Proc. SPIE*, 7309, 73090F, 2009.
52. K. B. Cooper, R. J. Dengler, N. Llombart, T. Bryllert, G. Chattopadhyay, E. Schlecht, J. Gill et al. Penetrating 3D imaging at 4 and 25 meter range using a submillimeter-wave radar, *IEEE Trans. Microw. Theory Tech.*, 56, 2771–2778, 2008.
53. W. von Spiegel, C. am Weg, R. Henneberger, R. Zimmermann, T. Loeffler, and H. G. Roskos, Active THz-imaging system with improved frame rate, *Proc. SPIE*, 7311, 73110O, 2009.
54. J.-H. Son, Terahertz electromagnetic interactions with biolocical matter and their applications, *J. Appl. Phys.*, 105(10), 102033, 2009.
55. M. Hangyo, M. Tani, T. Nagashima, H. Kitahara, and H. Sumikura, Spectroscopy and imaging by laser excited terahertz waves, *Plasma Fusion Res.*, 2, S1020, 2007.
56. I. S. Gregory, H. Page, and L. Spencer, *Continuous-wave Terahertz Photomixer System for Real-World Applications, Ser. Terahertz Frequency Detection and Identification of Materials and Objects: NATO Science for Peace and Security Series-B: Physics and Biophysics.* New York, NY: Springer, pp. 167–184, 2007.
57. K. Shibuya, M. Tani, M. Hangyo, O. Morikawa, and H. Kan, Compact and inexpensive continuous-wave subterahertz imaging system with a fiber-coupled multimode laser diode, *Appl. Phys. Lett.*, 90(16), 161127, 2007.
58. T. Löffler, K. J. Siebert, H. Quast, N. Hasegawa, G. Loata, R. Wipf, T. Hahn, M. Thomson, R. Leonhardt, and H. G. Roskos, All-optoelectronic continuous-wave terahertz systems, *R. Soc. London Trans. Ser. A*, 362(1815), 263–281, 2004.
59. Q. Song, Y. Zhao, A. Redo-Sanchez, C. Zhang, and X. Liu, Fast continuous terahertz wave imaging system for security, *Opt. Commun.*, 282(10), 2019–2022, 2009.
60. B. M. Fischer, H. Helm, and P. Uhd Jepsen, Chemical recognition with broadband THz spectroscopy, *Proc. IEEE*, 95(8), 1592–1604, 2007.
61. K. Kawase, Terahertz imaging for drug detection and large-scale integrated circuit inspection, *Opt. Photon. News*, 15(10), 34–39, 2004.
62. P. F. Taday, Recent work on imaging using time-domain based interferometry: Applications to the pharmaceutical industry, in *Proc. 32th Int. Conf. Infrared, Millimeter, and Terahertz Waves*, Cardiff, pp. 644–646, 2009.
63. Y.-C. Shen and P. F. Taday, Development and application of terahertz pulsed imaging for nondestructive inspection of pharmaceutical tablet, *IEEE J. Sel. Topl Quantum Electron.*, 14(2), 407–415, 2008.
64. K. Kawase, A. Dobroiu, M. Yamashita, Y. Sasaki, and C. Otani, *Terahertz Rays to Detect Drugs of Abuse, Ser. Terahertz Frequency Detection and Identification of Materials and Objects: NATO Science for Peace and Security Series-B: Physics and Biophysics.* New York, NY: Springer, pp. 241–250, 2007.
65. J. A. Zeitler and L. F. Gladden, *In-vitro* tomography and non-destructive imaging at depth of pharmaceutical solid dosage forms, *Eur. J. Pharm. Biopharm.*, 71(1), 2–22, 2009.
66. T. May, G. Zieger, S. Anders, V. Zakosarenko, H.-G. Meyer, M. Schubert, M. Starkloff, M. Rößler, G. Thorwirth, and U. Krause, Safe VISITOR: VISible, Infrared and Terahertz Object Recognition for security screening application, *Proc. SPIE*, 7309, 73090E, 2009.
67. J. A. Cox, R. Higashi, F. Nusseibeh, K. Newstrom-Peitso, C. Zins, R. Osiander, J. Lehtonen, and E. Dodson, Uncooled MEMS-based detector arrays for THz imaging applications, *Proc. SPIE*, 7311, 73110R, 2009.
68. J. J. Lynch, J. N. Schulman, and H, P. Moyer, Low noise direct detection sensors for millimeter wave imaging, in *Technical Digest IEEE Compound Semiconductor Integrated Circuit Symposium*, San Antonio, TX, pp. 215–218, 2006.
69. D. Wikner and E. Grossman, Demonstration of a passive, low noise, millimeter-wave detector array for imaging, *Proc. SPIE*, 7309, 730909, 2009.
70. H. Hoshina, Y. Sasaki, A. Hayashi, C. Otani, and K. Kawase, Non-invasive mail inspection system with terahertz radiation, *Proc. SPIE*, 7311, 731103, 2009.
71. M. Yamashita, C. Otani, K. Kawase, K. Nikawa, and M. Tonouchi, Noncontact inspection technique for electrical failures in semiconductor devices using a laser terahertz emission microscope, *Appl. Phys. Lett.*, 93(4), 041117, 2008.
72. M. Yamashita, C. Otani, K. Kawase, T. Matsumoto, K. Nikawa, S. Kim, H. Murakami, and M. Tonouchi, Backside observation of large-scale integrated circuits with multilayered interconnections using laser terahertz emission microscope, *Appl. Phys. Lett.*, 94(190), 191104, 2009.

73. R.M. Groves, B. Pradarutti, E. Kouloumpi, W. Osten, and G. Notni, 2D and 3D non-destructive evaluation of a wooden panel painting using shearography and terahertz imaging, *NDT & E International*, 42(6), 543–549, 2009.
74. K. Fukunaga, I. Hosako, I. N. Duling III, and M. Picollo Terahertz imaging systems: A non-invasive technique for the analysis of paintings, *Proc. SPIE*, 7391, 73910D, 2009.
75. E. Pickwell-MacPherson and V. P. Wallace, Terahertz pulsed imaging—A potential medical imaging modality?, *Photodiagnosis and Photodynamic Therapy*, 6(2), 128–134, 2009.
76. P. C. Ashworth, E. Pickwell-MacPherson, E. Provenzano, S. E. Pinder, A. D. Purushotham, M. Pepper, and V. P. Wallace, Terahertz pulsed spectroscopy of freshly excised human breast cancer, *Opt. Express*, 17(15), 12444–12454, 2009.
77. A. J. Fitzgerald, V. P. Wallace, M. Jimenez-Linan, L. Bobrow, R. J. Pye, A. D. Purushotham, and D. D. Arnone, Terahertz pulsed imaging of human breast tumors, *Radiology*, 239(20), 533–540, 2006.
78. S. J. Oh, J. Kang, I. Maeng, J.-S. Suh, Y.-M. Huh, S. Haam, and J.-H. Son, Nanoparticle-enabled terahertz imaging for cancer diagnosis, *Opt. Express*, 17(50), 3469–3475, 2009.
79. M. Wächter, M. Nagel, and H. Kurz, Tapered photoconductive terahertz field probe tip with subwavelength spatial resolution, *Appl. Phys. Lett.*, 95(4), 041112, 2009.
80. V. Astley, H. Zhan, R. Mendis, and D. M. Mittleman, A study of background signals in terahertz apertureless near-field microscopy and their use for scattering-probe imaging, *J. Appl. Phys.*, 105(11), 113117, 2009.
81. M. Awad, M. Nagel, and H. Kurz, Tapered Sommerfeld wire terahertz near-field imaging, *Appl. Phys. Lett.*, 94(5), 051107, 2009.
82. C.-M. Chiu, H.-W. Chen, Y.-R. Huang, Y.-J. Hwang, W.-J. Lee, H.-Y. Huang, and C.-K. Sun, All-terahertz fiber-scanning near-field microscopy, *Opt. Lett.*, 34(7), 1084–1086, 2009.
83. B. Gompf and M. Dressel, THz-micro-spectroscopy, *IEEE J. Sel. Top. Quantum Electron.*, 14(2), 470–475, 2008.
84. J. F. Federici and H. Grebel, Characteristics of nano-scale composites at THz and IR spectral regions. Terahertz sensing technology, Vol. 1: *Electronic Devices and Advanced Systems Technology*. Eds. D. L. Woolard, W. R. Loerop, and M. S. Shur. Singapore: World Scientific, pp. 67–91, 2003.
85. J. R. Knab, A. J. L. Adam, M. Nagel, E. Shaner, M. A. Seo, D. S. Kim, and P. C. M. Planken, Terahertz near-field vectorial imaging of subwavelength apertures and aperture arrays, *Opt. Express*, 17(17), 15072–15086, 2009.
86. A. Bitzer and M. Walther, Terahertz near-field imaging of metallic subwavelength holes and hole arrays, *Appl. Phys. Lett.*, 92(23), 231101, 2008.
87. A. J. Huber, F. Keilmann, J. Wittborn, J. Aizpurua, and R. Hillenbrand, Terahertz near-field nanoscopy of mobile carriers in single semiconductor nanodevices, *Nano Lett.*, 8(11), 3766–3770, 2008.
88. W. L. Chan, K. Charan, D. Takhar, K. F. Kelly, R. G. Baraniuk, and D. M. Mittleman, A single-pixel terahertz imaging system based on compressed sensing, *Appl. Phys. Lett.*, 93(12), 121105, 2008.
89. W. L. Chan, M. L. Moravec, R. G. Baraniuk, and D. M. Mittleman, Terahertz imaging with compressed sensing and phase retrieval, *Opt. Lett.*, 33(9), 974–976, 2008.
90. A. Heidari and D. Saeedkia, A 2D camera design with a single-pixel detector, in *Proc. 34th Int. Conf. Infrared, Millimeter, and Terahertz Waves*, Busan, Korea, September 2009.
91. M. A. Dem'yanenko, D. G. Esaev, B. A. Knyazev, G. N. Kulipanov, and N. A. Vinokurov, Imaging with a 90 frames/s microbolometer focal plane array and high-power terahertz free electron laser, *Appl. Phys. Lett.*, 92(13), 131116, 2008.
92. T. Pope, M. Doucet, F. Dupont, L. Marchese, B. Tremblay, G. Baldenberger, S. Verreault, and F. Lamontagne, Uncooled detector, optics, and camera development for THz imaging, *Proc. SPIE*, 7311, 7311oL, 2009.
93. D. R. Denison, M. E. Knotts, M. E. McConney, and V. V. Tsukruk, Experimental characterization of mm-wave detection by a micro-array of Golay cells, *Proc. SPIE*, 7309, 73090J, 2009.
94. D. Grbovic and G. Karunasiri, Fabrication of bi-material MEMS detector arrays for THz imaging, *Proc. SPIE*, 7311, 731108, 2009.
95. E. Öjefors, U. R. Pfeiffer, A. Lisauskas, and H. G. Roskos, A 0.65 THz focal-plane array in a quarter-micron CMOS process technology, *IEEE J. Solid-State Circuits*, 44(7), 1968–1976, 2009.
96. U. R. Pfeiffer, E. Ojefors, A. Lisaukas, D. Glaab, and H. G. Roskos, A CMOS focal-plane array for heterodyne terahertz imaging, in *Proc. IEEE Radio Frequency Integrated Circuits Symposium*, Boston, MA, pp. 433–436, 2009.
97. S. Ruan, J. Yang, and M. Zhang, Real-time terahertz imaging using a 1.63 THz optically-pumped terahertz laser and a pyroelectric camera, *Proc. SPIE*, 7126, 71261U, 2009.

98. B. N. Behnken, G. Karunasiri, D. R. Chamberlin, P. R. Robrish, and J. Faist, Real-time imaging using a 2.8 THz quantum cascade laser and uncooled infrared microbolometer camera, *Opt. Lett.*, 33(5), 440–442, 2008.
99. J.-P. Caumes, B. Chassagne, D. Coquillat, F. Teppe, and W. Knap, Focal-plane micro-bolometer arrays for 0.5 THz spatial room-temperature imaging, *Elect. Lett.*, 45(1), 34–35, 2009.
100. Q. Hu, Terahertz quantum cascade lasers and video-rate THz imaging, in *Proc. 32th Int. Conf. Infrared, Millimeter, and Terahertz Waves*, Cardiff, 24–25 September 2007.
101. Q. Wu, T. D. Hewitt, and X.-C. Zhang, Two-dimensional electro-optic imaging of THz beams, *Appl. Phys. Lett*, 69(8), 1026–1028, 1996.
102. Z. Jiang, X. G. Xu, and X.-C. Zhang, Improvement of terahertz imaging with a dynamic subtraction technique, *Appl. Opt.*, 39(17), 2982–2987, 2000.
103. A. Nahata, J. T. Yardley, and T. F. Heinz, Two-dimensional imaging of continuous-wave terahertz radiation using electro-optic detection, *Appl. Phys. Lett.*, 81(6), 963–965, 2002.
104. M. Usami, M. Yamashita, K. Fukushima, C. Otani, and K. Kawase, Terahertz wideband spectroscopic imaging based on two-dimensional electro-optic sampling technique, *Appl. Phys. Lett.*, 86(14), 141109, 2005.
105. H. Kitahara, M. Tani, and M. Hangyo, Two-dimensional electro-optic sampling of terahertz radiation using high-speed complementary metal-oxide semiconductor camera combined with arrayed polarizer, *Appl. Phys. Lett.*, 94(9), 091119, 2009.
106. L. Zhang, H. Zhong, Y. Zhang, N. Karpowicz, C. Zhang, Y. Zhao, and X.-C. Zhang, Terahertz wave focal-plane multiwavelength phase imaging, *J. Opt. Soc. Am. A*, 26(5), 1187–1190, 2009.
107. H.-B. Liu and X.-C. Zhang, Terahertz spectroscopy for explosive, pharmaceutical, and biological sensing applications, *Ser. Terahertz Frequency Detection and Identification of Materials and Objects: NATO Science for Peace and Security Series-B: Physics and Biophysics*. New York, NY: Springer, 2007, pp. 251–323.
108. E. J. Heilweil and D. F. Plusquellic, Terahertz spectroscopy of biomolecules, *Terahertz Spectroscopy Principles and Applications*. Ed. S. L. Dexheimer. Boca Raton, FL: CRC Press, 2008, pp. 269–297.
109. J. A. Zeitler, T. Rades, and P. F. Taday, Pharmaceutical and security applications of terahertz spectroscopy, *Terahertz Spectroscopy Principles and Applications*. Ed. S. L. Dexheimer. Boca Raton, FL: CRC Press, 2008, pp. 299–323.
110. C. J. Strachan, T. Rades, D. A. Newnham, K. C. Gordon, M. Pepper, and P. F. Taday, Using terahertz pulsed spectroscopy to study crystallinity of pharmaceutical materials, *Chem. Phys. Lett.*, 390(1–3), 20–24, 2004.
111. P. F. Taday, Applications of terahertz spectroscopy to pharmaceutical sciences, *Philos. Trans. R. Soc. Lond. A*, 362(1815), 351–364, 2004.
112. T. Globus, D. Woodlard, M. Bykhovskaia, B. Gelmont, L. Werbos, and A. Samuels, THz-frequency spectroscopic sensing of DNA and related biological materials, *Terahertz Sensing Technology*, Vol. 2: *Emerging Scientific Applications and Novel Device Concepts*. Eds. D. L. Woolard, W. R. Loerop, and M. S. Shur. Singapore: World Scientific, 1–34, 2003.
113. J.-I. Nishizawa, T. Sasaki, and T. Tanno, Coherent terahertz-wave generation from semiconductors and its applications in biological sciences, *J. Phys. Chem. Solids*, 69(2,3), 693–701, 2008.
114. M. Nagel, M. Forst, and H. Kurz, THz biosensing devices: Fundamentals and technology, *J. Phys.: Condens. Matter*, 18(18), S601–S618, 2006.
115. A. G. Markelz, Terahertz dielectric sensitivity to biomolecular structure and function, *IEEE J. Sel. Top. Quantum Electron.*, 14(1), 180–190, 2008.
116. T. L. J. Chan, J. E. Bjarnason, A. W. M. Lee, M. A. Celis, and E. R. Brown, Attenuation contrast between biomolecular and inorganic materials at terahertz frequencies, *Appl. Phys. Lett.*, 85(13), 2523–2525, 2004.
117. D. F. Plusquellic, K. Siegrist, E. J. Heilweil, and O. Esenturk, Applications of terahertz spectroscopy in biosystems, *Chem. Phys. Chem.*, 8(17), 2412–2431, 2007.
118. E. R. Brown, J. Bjarnason, T. L. J. Chan, D. C. Driscoll, M. Hanson, and A. C. Gossard, Room temperature, THz photomixing sweep oscillator and its application to spectroscopic transmission through organic materials, *Rev. Sci. Instrum.*, 75(12), 5333–5342, 2004.
119. C. Konek, J. Wilkinson, O. Esenturk, E. Heilweil, and M. Kemp, Terahertz spectroscopy of explosives and simulants—RDX, PETN, sugar and L-tartaric acid, *Proc. SPIE*, 7311, 73110K, 2009.
120. N. Zamdmer, Q. Hu, K. A. McIntosh, S. Verghese, and A. Forster, Onchip frequency-domain submillimeter-wave transceiver, *Appl. Phys. Lett.*, 75(24), 3877–3879, 1999.
121. T.-I. Jeona and D. Grischkowsky, Direct optoelectronic generation and detection of sub-ps-electrical pulses on sub-mm-coaxial transmission lines, *Appl. Phys. Lett.*, 85(25), 6092–6094, 2004.

122. M. Nagel, F. Richter, P. Haring-Bolivar, and H. Kurz, A functionalized THz sensor for marker-free DNA analysis, *Philos. Trans. R. Soc. London*, 48, 3625–3636, 2003.
123. J.-Y. Lu, L.-J. Chen, T.-F. Kao, H.-H. Chang, H.-W. Chen, A.-S. Liu, Y.-C. Chen et al. Terahertz microchip for illicit drug detection, *IEEE Photon. Technol. Lett.*, 18(21), 2254–2256, 2006.
124. H. Page, S. Malik, M. Evans, I. Gregory, I. Farrer, and D. Ritchie, Waveguide coupled terahertz photoconductive antennas: Toward integrated photonic terahertz devices, *Appl. Phys. Lett.*, 92(16), 163502, 2008.
125. M. Neshat, D. Saeedkia, R. Sabry, and S. Safavi-Naeini, An integrated continuous-wave terahertz biosensor, *Proc. SPIE*, 6549, 65409E, May 2007.
126. P. H. Bolivar, M. Nagel, F. Richter, M. Brucherseifer, H. Kurz, A. Bosserhoff, and R. Büttner, Label-free THz sensing of genetic sequences: Towards THz biochips, *Philos. Trans. R. Soc. London*, 362, 323–335, 2003.
127. D. Saeedkia and S. Safavi-Naeini, Modeling and analysis of a multilayer dielectric slab waveguide with applications in edge-coupled terahertz photomixer sources, *IEEE/OSA J. Lightwave Technol.*, 25(1), 432–439, 2007.

14 Terahertz Technology Based on Nanoelectronic Devices

Yukio Kawano

CONTENTS

14.1 INTRODUCTION

Since the establishment of the Maxwell equation and the discovery of the electromagnetic wave, researchers have been devoting themselves to the development of a number of technologies based on the electromagnetic wave, bringing about a lot of changes in human life. High-frequency electronics technology has provided the radio, television, cellular phone, and so on. From optics and photonics, optical communication, the LED lamp, the endoscope, and so on have resulted.

The terahertz (THz, 10^{12} Hz) frequency region is located in between the microwave region and the visible light region (Figure 14.1). This region was studied by merely a small number of researchers in limited fields, such as chemical spectroscopy, astronomy, and solid-state physics. However, THz technology is nowadays in strong demand in a large variety of fields, ranging from basic science such as biochemical spectroscopy, astronomy, and materials science to practical science such as environmental science, medicine, agriculture, and security [1,2]. Why does the THz wave attract so much interest? The advantageous properties of the THz wave are that it can be transmitted through objects

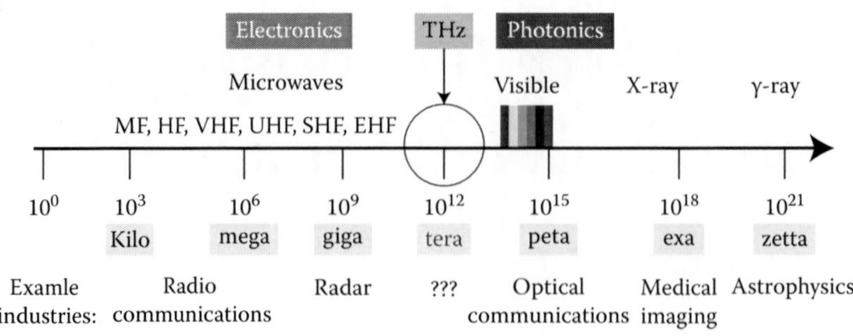

FIGURE 14.1 Chart of the electromagnetic wave spectrum. (Adapted from THz Science & Technology Network (http://thznetwork.net/).)

opaque to visible light and that the corresponding photon energy, 1–100 meV, is in the important energy spectrum for various materials and biomolecules. These features allow various applications of imaging and spectroscopy in this frequency band. Figure 14.2 displays several examples of applications of the THz waves. In the THz measurements shown in Figure 14.2, one illuminates the THz waves onto the object and maps intensity distributions of reflected or transmitted THz waves. In some situations, by simultaneously measuring frequency spectra, one is able to identify the contents and to characterize their physical/chemical properties. The technique can therefore be used for nondestructive inspection, which is based on the fact that the THz wave is much safer and does not cause much damage, compared to x-ray. In addition to industrial and medical applications, THz technology is also of much importance in basic sciences. For example, in astronomy, materials science, and biochemistry, the detection of very weak THz radiation from interstellar matter in space, electrons in

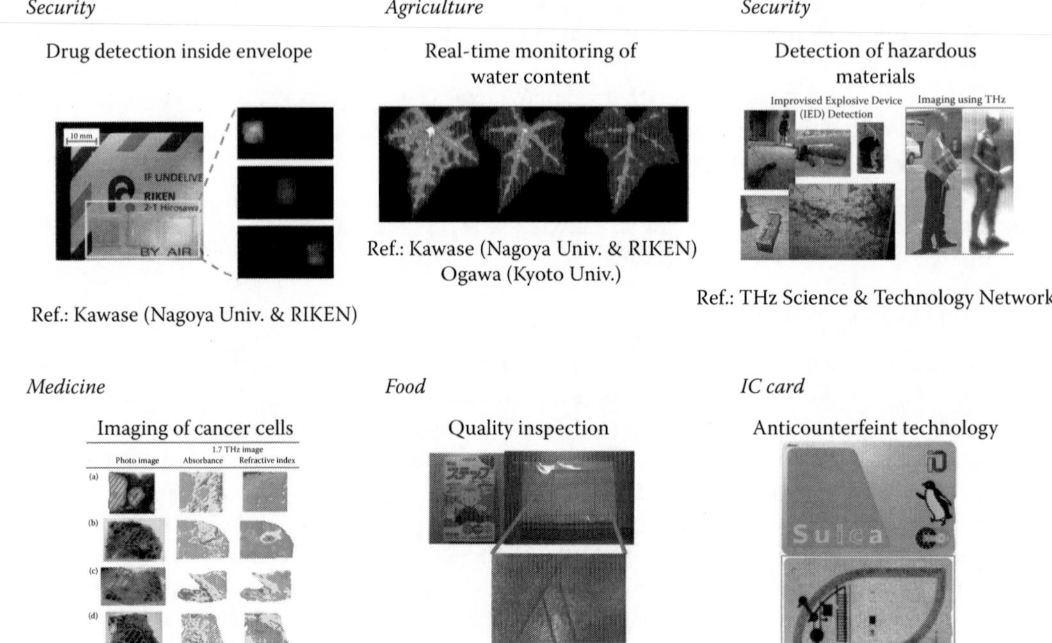

FIGURE 14.2 Various applications of THz imaging and spectroscopy.

materials, and biomolecules is expected to unlock the mysteries underlying the creation of the universe, quantum effect in materials and life activity, respectively.

In the THz region, however, even basic components such as the detector and the source have not been fully established, compared to the technically mature, other frequency regions. This is because the frequency of the THz wave is too high to be handled with conventional high-frequency semiconductor technology. In addition, the photon energy of the THz wave is much lower than the band gap energy of semiconductors. For the above reasons, the THz wave is not easy to be handled from either the side of electronics or the side of optics/photonics. In imaging technology, the THz wave also has the problem of low spatial resolution, which results from the much longer wavelengths of THz waves compared to those of visible light.

The applications of nanoscale materials and devices, however, are opening up new opportunities to overcome such difficulties. Nanostructured devices based on the superconductor, semiconductor, and carbon nanotube (CNT) have enabled significant improvements in detection sensitivity and spatial resolution. In this chapter, a new THz sensing and imaging technology based on such nanoelectronic devices is described. Moreover, the applications of cutting-edge THz measurements in materials research, which have provided new insights into the electronic properties of the materials, are shown.

14.2 THz DETECTOR

14.2.1 Overview

THz detectors can be generally classified into three types: bolometric (thermal) detection, wave detection, and quantum detection. In addition, they are also used as photoconductive antennas, electrooptic devices, and frequency mixers for heterodyne detection. In this section, an overview of various THz detectors is presented and their advantages and disadvantages are discussed briefly.

14.2.1.1 Bolometric (Thermal) Detection

This type of detector utilizes the temperature rise via THz absorption. As the crystal temperature of the detector decreases, the detection sensitivity is improved, but the detection speed becomes low (a typical time constant is of the order of milliseconds below 4 K). The detected signal is mostly resistance change arising from the rise in crystal temperature because of THz absorption. There is another type of readout mechanism: measuring gas pressure via thermal expansion (the Golay cell detector). Since all the detectors based on bolometric detection respond to electromagnetic waves in a wide-frequency region, one needs a frequency cutoff filter. The work [3] has recently reported a nanoscaled superconductor bolometer with the capacity for a single THz-photon detection.

14.2.1.2 Wave Detection

This detector senses the THz electromagnetic wave as a high-frequency "wave." A representative device is a Schottky-barrier diode detector. The advantages of this detector are high-speed detection (a time constant of approximately nanoseconds) and room-temperature operation. This detector is often used in sub-THz regions, because the sensitivity becomes low with increasing the frequency of the incident THz wave.

14.2.1.3 Quantum Detection

In contrast to wave detection, this type of detector senses photons of the THz electromagnetic wave. Solid-state devices based on materials such as superconductors and semiconductors usually have energy-level spacing corresponding to the THz photon energy (1–100 meV): for example, the energy gap of a superconductor, the impurity level of a semiconductor and the energy-level spacing due to quantum electron confinement of the semiconductor quantum structure. It follows that excess carriers are generated in the devices when these devices absorb the THz waves. One can detect the

THz wave by recording electric signals produced by the carriers. THz detectors based on a nanoscale island connected to electrodes, such as superconductor junctions [4] and semiconductor quantum dots (QDs) [5,6], have been presented earlier and have been demonstrated to exhibit ultrahigh sensitivity including single-photon detection. However, the operation of superconductor and semiconductor detectors needs a very low-temperature environment (<0.3 K). This situation forces one to use a dilution refrigerator or a ^{3}He refrigerator, restricting the range of practical uses.

14.2.1.4 Others

THz time-domain spectroscopy (TDS) is nowadays widely employed in THz research fields. As detectors, photoconductive antennas and electrooptic devices are used. This measurement allows real-time observation of the oscillatory electric field of THz waves, providing information about both the amplitude and phase of the THz electric field. Although these detectors work at room temperature, their operation requires an expensive femto-second pulse laser.

Further, a frequency mixer using a superconductor is known in which a beat signal corresponding to the frequency difference with a local oscillator is measured. This type of detector is often used in the fields of astronomy and environmental science.

14.2.2 CNT-Based THz Detector

CNT is expected to be applicable as a building block for future nanoelectronics, nanophotonics, and nanomechanics owing to its unique one-dimensional (1D) structure [7]. From the viewpoint of application to THz detectors, the CNT also has been regarded as a promising candidate. In fact, near-infrared sensors using the CNT transistor have been successfully developed [8,9]. In the THz region, although there are several reports [10,11], much higher performance has not been achieved to date, compared to other existing detectors.

In the following section, the recent development of CNT-based THz detectors are introduced [12,13]. We have created a highly sensitive and frequency-tunable THz-photon detector using the CNT and GaAs/AlGaAs transistors. This detector has two detection mechanisms: photon-assisted tunneling (PAT) [12] and current-peak shift [13]. For the latter, THz irradiation causes peak shift of CNT currents relative to gate voltage, leading to the realization of ultrahigh-sensitivity THz-photon detection.

14.2.2.1 PAT in CNT

In 1963, Tien and Gordon proposed a theory on the interaction of a nanoscale island with an electromagnetic wave [14]. The essence of their discussion is that new energy bands, the so-called photon sidebands, are formed by the ac electric potential of the electromagnetic wave at intervals of nhf (n is the integer number, h the Planck constant, and f the frequency of the electromagnetic wave).

A QD structure connected to the source, the drain, and gate electrodes is a promising device for examining their model, because the QD with the electrodes works like a single-electron transistor (SET). By sweeping either the gate voltage or the source–drain voltage and measuring the resulting source–drain current, spectroscopic information about energy states in the QD can be directly obtained. The photon sidebands in the QD can be thus observed as the generation of new current signals via an inelastic electron tunnel when electrons exchange photons. This phenomenon is known as PAT (Figure 14.3a). With microwave irradiation of superconductor tunneling devices [14–16] and semiconductor QDs [17,18], the PAT has been successfully observed.

Compared to conventional QDs based on superconductors and semiconductors, a QD using a CNT has the following unique properties: its characteristic energy or charging energy and energy level spacing due to quantum electron confinement typically reach ~10 meV, corresponding to a THz frequency (~2.4 THz). This energy range is by a factor of 10 larger than the energy range of conventional QDs. These advantageous properties potentially lead to device applications of CNT-QDs in the THz region. In this context, we have studied the THz response of the CNT-QDs [12].

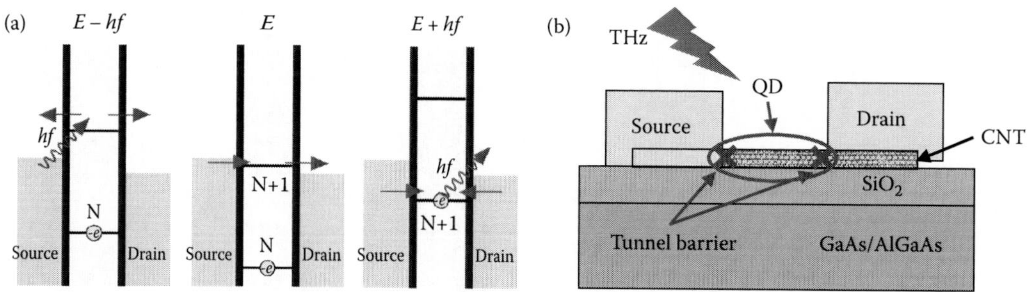

FIGURE 14.3 (a) Schematic diagram of electron tunneling processes in a QD under the electromagnetic wave irradiation. Middle panel: when the Fermi level in the source lead aligns with a level in the QD, a source–drain current is passed via elastic tunneling. Left and right panels: when electrons interact with photons, a new current flows via inelastic tunneling, that is, PAT. (b) Sketch of a CNT-QD. (Adapted from Y. Kawano et al., *J. Appl. Phys*, 103, 034307, 2008.)

Figure 14.3b schematically represents the CNT-QD structure. The CNT-QD was fabricated as follows: first, CNTs were dispersed on a semiconductor (GaAs/AlGaAs) wafer, whose surface was covered with a SiO_2 film of ~100 nm thickness. We mapped the topography of the device surface with an atomic force microscope, and specified locations of single-wall CNTs with a diameter of ~1 nm. Based on the images obtained, source and drain electrodes with an interval of ~600 nm and side-gate electrodes were patterned with electron-beam lithography. In this device, electrons are confined to a very small area of 1×600 nm^2, forming a QD. Metallic CNTs were used.

The CNT device was mounted in a ^{4}He cryostat at a temperature of 1.5 K, and the device was irradiated with a THz wave through an optical window made from a mylar sheet. As a THz illumination source, a THz gas laser pumped by a CO_2-gas laser was used.

Figure 14.4 shows the data about the effect of THz irradiation on the CNT-QD. Differently from the black curve for the data without THz irradiation, new satellite current peaks are generated for the illumination of the THz wave. It is also seen that its position relative to gate voltage shifts in the positive direction with increasing frequency, f, of the THz wave. The inset of Figure 14.4 displays the energy spacing, $\kappa\Delta V_G$, between the original peak and the satellite peaks as a function of the photon energy, hf, of the THz wave. From the measurement of the differential conductance dI_{SD}/dV_{SD} as a function of source–drain voltage V_{SD} and gate voltage V_G (Coulomb-diamond measurement), we derived the conversion factor, $\kappa = 0.18$, which is defined as the conversion ratio of V_G into energy. The data clearly show good agreement between $\kappa\Delta V_G$ and hf, providing evidence for the THz-PAT in the CNT-QD. It is thus demonstrated that the CNT-QD works as a THz detector with frequency tunability by the application of the gate voltage.

It should be noted that the satellite current is only observed on the positive V_G side with respect to the original peak. The occurrence of the satellite current corresponds to the electron tunneling from the QD to the drain lead (the right-side panel of Figure 14.3a). The side of V_G on which the satellite current is clearly seen depends on the sample properties. This is possibly due to tunnel barrier asymmetry between the source and drain electrodes.

The theory by Tine and Gordon says that the tunneling rate into the photon sidebands should follow the Bessel functions of the illuminated power [14]. In order to examine this feature, we measured the THz intensity dependence of the THz-PAT in the CNT-QD. In the measurements, we inserted THz attenuating filters between the THz laser and the sample. The result is displayed in Figure 14.5. The general tendency is as expected, but we could not get a perfect fit to the Bessel functions. We speculate that since the single QD was used, the tunneling processes via the electrodes would make it difficult to analyze the result accurately with this model. We plan to study the THz intensity dependence in more detail by using a double-coupled CNT-QD, in which the PAT occurs as a consequence of electron transitions between two well-defined discrete levels. In this device, we anticipate that frequency selectivity would be improved compared to the single CNT-QD.

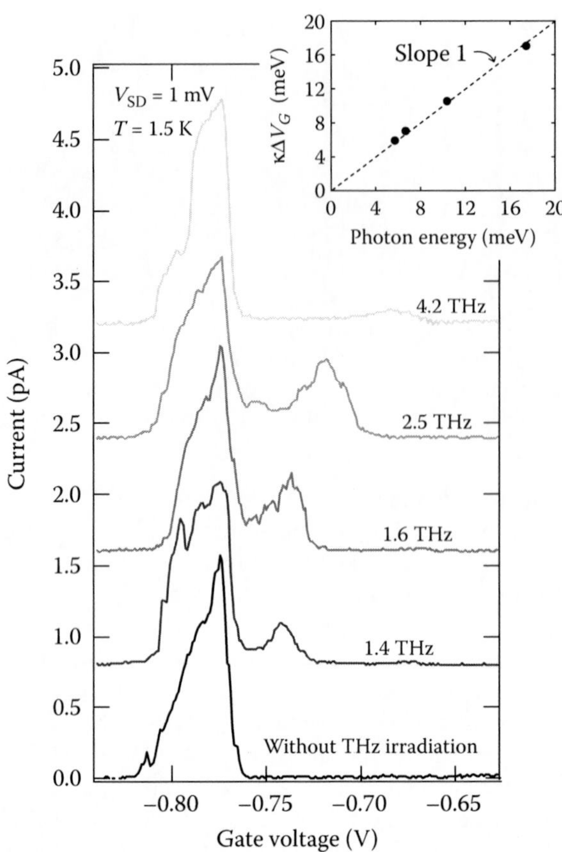

FIGURE 14.4 Source–drain current I_{SD} versus gate voltage V_G for the frequency of the THz wave, $f = 1.4$, 1.6, 2.4, and 4.2 THz. The experimental curves for the THz irradiation are offset by multiples of 0.8 pA for clarity. The inset shows the energy spacing, $\kappa\Delta V_G$, between the original peaks and the satellite peaks as a function of the photon energy, *hf*, of the THz wave. The dashed line in the inset is a guide to the eyes, corresponding to $\kappa\Delta V_G = hf$. (Adapted from Y. Kawano et al., *J. Appl. Phys*, 103, 034307, 2008.)

14.2.2.2 THz-Photon Detection with a CNT/2DEG Hybrid Device

In the CNT THz detector described in the previous section, although frequency-selective THz detection has been achieved, the detection sensitivity is not high. This is because in this detection mechanism, one-photon absorption generates only one electron even if a quantum efficiency of 100% is achieved. This limits the detection sensitivity. In order to resolve this problem, we have created a newly designed device [13]: a CNT-SET is integrated with a GaAs/AlGaAs heterostructure chip (Figure 14.6a). The hybrid structure is divided into two separate roles of THz absorption (two-dimensional electron gas (2DEG)) and signal readout (CNT-SET). The basic idea of THz detection with this device is that the CNT-SET senses electrical polarization induced by THz-excited electron–hole pairs in the 2DEG. Since the SET works as an ultrasensitive electrometer, the CNT/2DEG device is expected to exhibit ultimate sensitivity photon detection.

Figure 14.6b shows the transport properties of the CNT without THz irradiation: the data about I_{SD} versus V_G at $V_{SD} = 1.5$ meV. This result shows the oscillatory behavior of I_{SD}, indicating that the fabricated CNT device properly functions as an SET.

Figure 14.7 displays the THz response of the 2DEG/CNT device and the dependence on the magnetic field, *B*, applied perpendicular to the 2DEG plane. The experimental setup for the THz measurements shown here is similar to that for the THz-PAT in the previous section. The laser

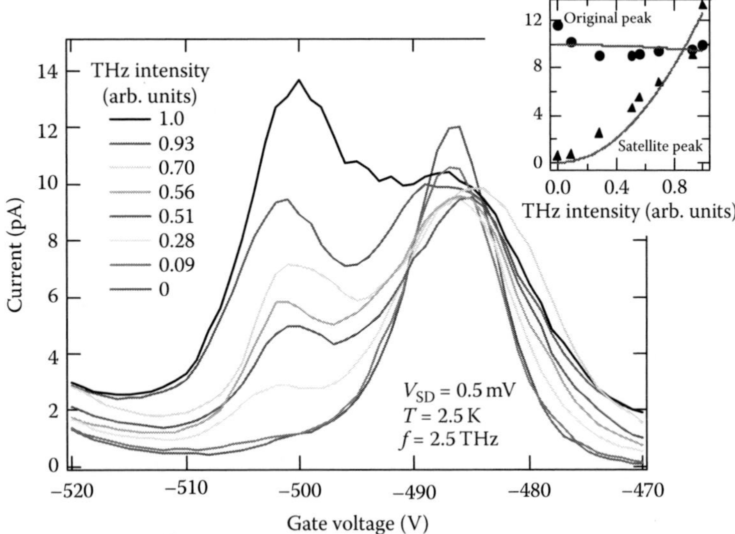

FIGURE 14.5 THz intensity dependence of I_{SD} versus V_G. The inset shows the THz intensity dependence of the amplitudes of a satellite peak and the one of an original peak. The solid lines in the inset are fitted curves based on the square of the *n*th order Bessel functions. (Adapted from Y. Kawano et al., *J. Appl. Phys*, 103, 034307, 2008.)

intensity was reduced with a set of THz attenuating filters and the intensity of the THz radiation applied to the sample is estimated to be 0.75 nW/mm^2.

The results of Figure 14.7 show that the THz irradiation caused a shift in the current peak position in the direction of positive V_G. The data for the irradiation at 1.6 THz reveals that the shift was monotonically enhanced with increasing B up to 3.95 T, then decreased when B was further raised beyond $B = 3.95$ T. On the other hand, in the case of the 2.5-THz irradiation, the B value for the maximum of the peak shift changed to 6.13 T.

The physical meaning underlying the features seen in Figure 14.7 is as follows: in the presence of magnetic field, the energy state of the 2DEG forms Landau level. When the 2DEG is illuminated with a THz wave whose photon energy hf is equal to Landau-level separation eB/m^*, the 2DEG absorbs well the THz wave (cyclotron resonance). Here, e is the elementary charge, and m^* is the cyclotron effective mass for the crystal used. The experimental data ($B = 3.95$ T for $f = 1.6$ THz and $B = 6.13$ T for $f = 2.5$ THz) show that the f value is proportional to the B value for the maximum of the peak shift, which is characteristic of the cyclotron resonance. In addition, from these data, the associated m^* value is derived to be $0.067m_0$, where m_0 is the free electron mass. This value is in

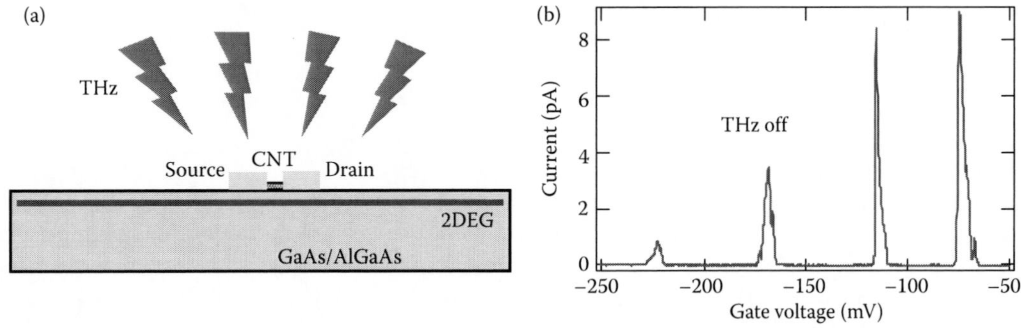

FIGURE 14.6 (a) THz detector using the CNT/2DEG hybrid device. (b) Source–drain current I_{SD} as a function of gate voltage V_G of the CNT-SET when the THz is off.

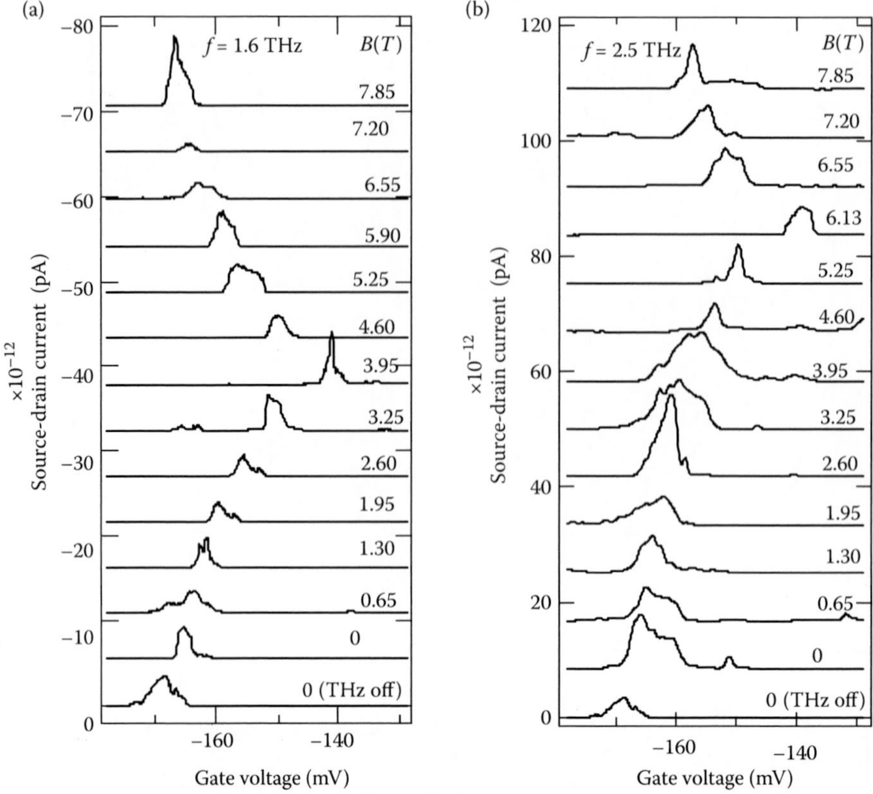

FIGURE 14.7 Magnetic field dependence of source–drain current I_{SD} versus gate voltage V_G of the CNT under THz irradiation. The magnetic field B was applied to the detector perpendicular to the 2DEG plane, and the B values in units of Tesla (T) are given on the right-hand side of the figures. The data with THz irradiation are offset for clarity. (Adapted from Y. Kawano, T. Uchida, and K. Ishibashi, *Appl. Phys. Lett*, 95, 083123, 2009.)

good agreement with the cyclotron effective mass for a GaAs-based 2DEG [19]. These facts indicate that the current peak shift of the CNT-SET originates from the THz absorption by the 2DEG.

The author explains the microscopic carrier dynamics associated with the THz detection. It is well known that a 2DEG has a random potential with a typical period of 20–100 nm [20]. It follows that the THz-excited electrons and holes drift in the opposite directions through the local electric field gradient due to the random potential [21]. As a result, they are spatially separated from each other. Such a separation of electron–hole pairs generates electrical polarization in the 2DEG. This situation is equivalent to the application of an effective gate voltage to the CNT-SET, resulting in the current peak shift.

We then measured the temporal trace of the THz signal (the I_{SD} change associated with the current peak shift) as the THz irradiation was cycled on and off. Here we used cyclotron radiation [22] from another 2DEG in a different GaAs/AlGaAs chip. The intensity of this THz source can be continuously changed by altering the current to the 2DEG of the THz source. We reduced its intensity to an extremely low level, on the order of 0.1 fW. We mounted, face to face, the sample and the 2DEG-based THz source in the same superconducting magnet so that the 2DEGs of the sample and the source were both in cyclotron resonance condition. Figure 14.8 displays time response of I_{SD} for an on/off sequence of the THz irradiation at $V_G = -169$ mV, $V_{SD} = 1.5$ mV, $B = 3.95$ T, and $f = 1.6$ THz. This result shows that the CNT-SET current was stable when the THz is off, whereas it repeatedly switched during the THz irradiation. This behavior means that the CNT-SET senses temporal processes of excitation and recombination of THz-excited carriers in the 2DEG.

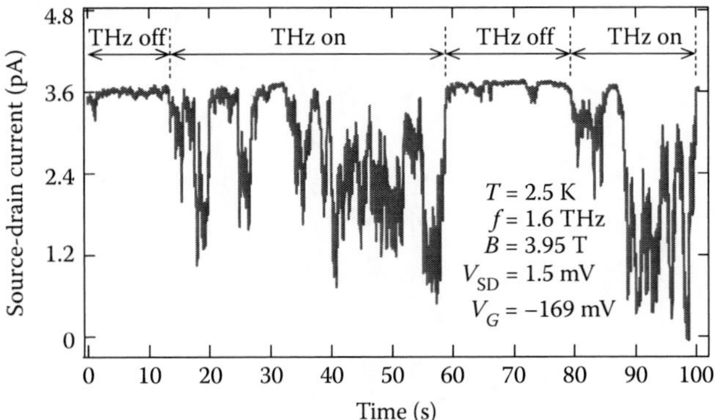

FIGURE 14.8 Time trace of the THz-detected signal (the CNT-SET current I_{SD}) as the THz irradiation is cycled on and off. In this measurement, THz cyclotron radiation emitted from another 2DEG was used with a very low intensity of ~0.1 fW. (Adapted from Y. Kawano, T. Uchida, and K. Ishibashi, *Appl. Phys. Lett*, 95, 083123, 2009.)

The author notes that the CNT-2DEG distance is 120 nm, the relative dielectric constant of GaAs is 13, and the separation length of excited electron–hole pairs is 20–100 nm [20,21]. Based on these values, the potential change caused by the polarization of a single electron–hole pair is estimated to be 0.4–10 meV. This value is comparable to the width of the current peak of the CNT-SET (~3 meV). This shows that single carrier charging via single THz-photon absorption in a 2DEG can generate an observable current peak shift and the resulting current switching. The data of Figure 14.8 thus demonstrate that the CNT/2DEG device is capable of detecting a few THz photons.

The power of 0.1 fW at 1.6 THz is equivalent to about 10^5 photons/s. This means that the detector does not sense all incident THz photons, which is due to the much smaller detection area as compared to the wavelength of the incident THz wave. The author expects that this problem would be resolved by fabricating a device having appropriate antenna-shaped electrodes for the CNT-SET.

The present detector can work at 6–7 K. This performance eliminates the use of a dilution or ^{3}He refrigerator with a low cooling capacity and complex systems. The device can therefore be used in a standard ^{4}He refrigerator or a compact cryo-free mechanical refrigerator with a much higher cooling capacity and much greater ease of use. This advantageous property makes it possible to extend the usable range of ultrasensitive THz measurements.

14.3 THz IMAGING

Enhancing the spatial resolution of THz imaging is one of the central issues in THz technology. Nevertheless, this is a formidable task, because the basic components necessary for obtaining high resolution, such as high-transmission wave lines and highly sensitive detectors, have not been well established as compared to other frequency regions.

There are, generally, two methods for realizing high resolution in optical imaging: the solid immersion lens and the near-field imaging technique. The applications of these techniques to THz imaging are explained below.

14.3.1 Solid Immersion Lens

In a standard optical imaging system such as the use of a lens, the spatial resolution of an optical image is proportional to the wavelength of light. The solid immersion lens utilizes the fact that the wavelength in a material with a high dielectric constant is reduced compared to that in vacuum. Therefore, a lens with a large refractive index leads to high resolution.

Figure 14.9 depicts an example of THz imaging based on the solid immersion lens [23]. A hyper-hemispherical lens made of Si is in contact with the back surface of a sample. The sample is a 2DEG

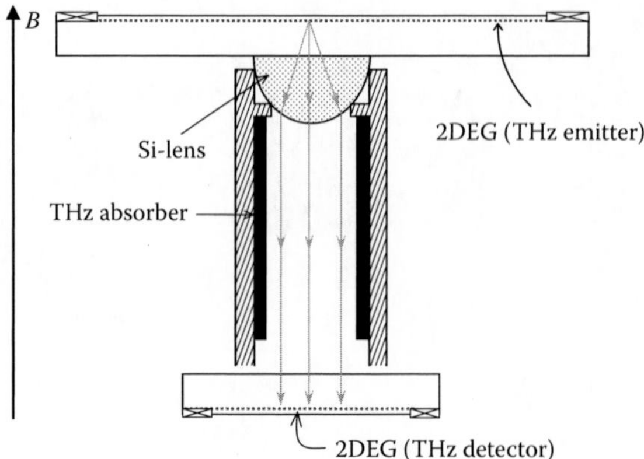

FIGURE 14.9 THz microscope based on a solid immersion lens.

in GaAs/AlGaAs heterostructure. A THz emission from the 2DEG is radiated as a consequence of inter-Landau-level transitions of electrons under magnetic field, that is, cyclotron emission (CE) [22]. The focal point of the lens is designed to be on the 2DEG layer of the sample. The CE from the focal point is collimated via the lens and is guided through a metallic light pipe to a THz detector. Off-axis light is filtered by a black polyethylene pipe. The sample is scanned relative to the lens by the use of an X–Y translation stage, while the optical system including the detector is stationary. The relatively large refractive index of GaAs and Si ($n \sim 3.4$) allows a resolution much higher than that obtained with a remote lens system.

The work [23] reported that for the solid immersion lens system, the resolution is about 50 μm at 130 μm, the wavelength of CE in vacuum. This value is improved by a factor of 6, compared to the resolution (300 μm) for the remote Si lens.

14.3.2 Near-Field Imaging

Although the solid immersion lens system enables relatively high resolution, the resolution is still determined by the diffraction limit. A powerful technique for overcoming the diffraction limit is near-field imaging [24]. When an electromagnetic wave is illuminated onto an aperture smaller than a wavelength, a localized evanescent field (near-field) is generated just behind the aperture. The size of the evanescent field is just determined by the aperture size and not the wavelength. By illuminating and/or detecting the evanescent field, it is possible to get a resolution beyond the diffraction limit.

Conventional systems for near-field imaging have an aperture type and an aperture-less (scattering) type. In the visible and near-infrared regions, either a tapered, metal-coated optical fiber (aperture type) [25] or a metal tip (aperture-less type) [26] is used. In the microwave region, either a sharpened waveguide (aperture type) [27] or a coaxial cable (aperture-less type) [28] is used. Since the intensity of the evanescent field is very weak, the realization of near-field imaging needs a highly sensitive detection scheme, such as high transmission wave lines and highly sensitive detectors.

14.3.2.1 Near-Field Imaging in the THz Region

Several methods for near-field imaging in the THz region have been presented. In the aperture type, a metal hole was used to obtain a resolution better than $\lambda/4$ [29]. This method, however, has the drawback of low wave transmission through the small aperture, which requires detecting very weak waves. Moreover, the spatial resolution is not so high. As the aperture-less type, a sharpened antenna [30], a metal tip [31], and a cantilever [32] were reported. Although the aperture-less technique allows high spatial resolution, it has the problem of separation from a far-field component of an incident wave, which generates a large background signal. For this reason, in most instances the

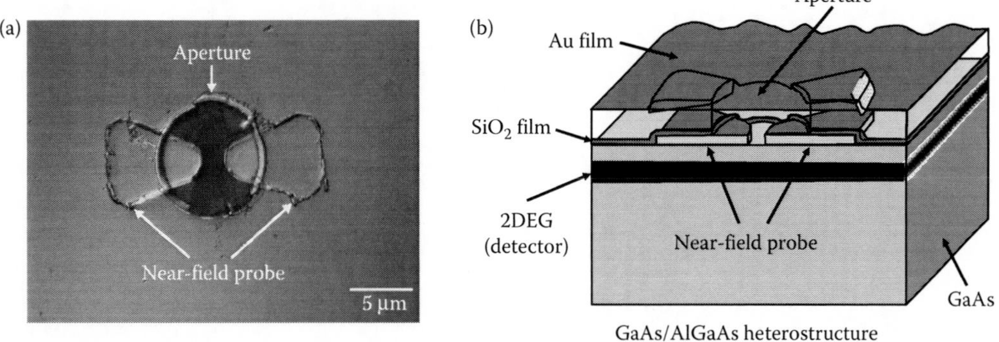

FIGURE 14.10 (a) Photograph of the near-field THz imaging device and (b) its schematic view.

probe position is modulated and synchronously detected signal is measured. However, this scheme makes the whole system and its operation complicated.

At the present stage, near-field THz imaging has not been fully established, and several other techniques are proposed and attempted. This is still an ongoing issue.

14.3.2.2 Near-Field THz Imaging on One Chip

Here, the author explains a unique type of near-field THz imaging—on-chip THz imaging with an integrated semiconductor device [33,34]. The problems of other techniques were low efficiency of near-field detection and complicated systems. The new integrated device enables near-field THz imaging in a much simpler manner. As shown in Figure 14.10, an aperture with 8 μm diameter and a planar probe were deposited on the surface of a GaAs/AlGaAs heterostructure chip. The aperture and the probe are insulated by a 50-nm thick SiO_2 layer. The GaAs chip has an electron mobility of 18 m^2/Vs and a sheet electron density of 4.4×10^{15} m^{-2} at 77 K. The two ohmic contacts were extended to the side surfaces of the chip, to each of which an electrical wire was attached. A 2DEG, located 60 nm below the chip surface, works as a THz detector. In this device structure, all the components, namely an aperture, a probe, and a detector, are integrated on one GaAs/AlGaAs chip. This scheme eliminates any optical and mechanical alignments between each component, leading to an easy-to-use and robust system.

An advantage of this device structure is that the presence of the planar probe changes the distribution of the evanescent field, enhancing the coupling of the evanescent field to the 2DEG detector. This is expected to lead to an increase in detection sensitivity. Moreover, the 2DEG detector is not affected by the far-field wave owing to the close vicinity to the aperture and the probe, allowing the detection of the evanescent field alone.

Figure 14.11 shows calculations of THz electric field distributions near the aperture using a finite-element method. Compared are the device of the aperture alone and that of the aperture plus

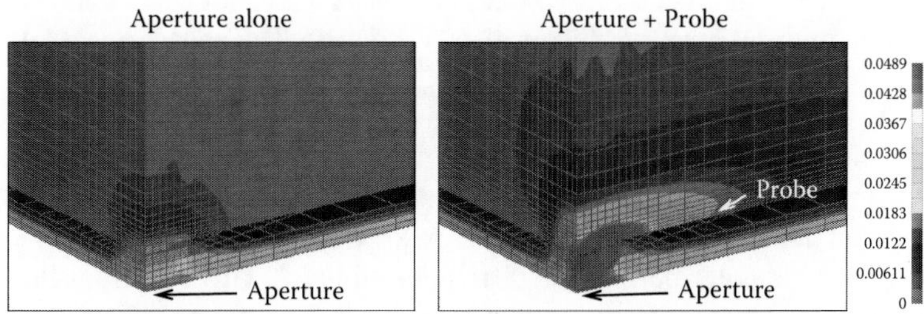

FIGURE 14.11 Calculations of THz electric field distributions in the vicinity of the aperture for the device with the aperture and probe (left) and for the device with the aperture alone (right).

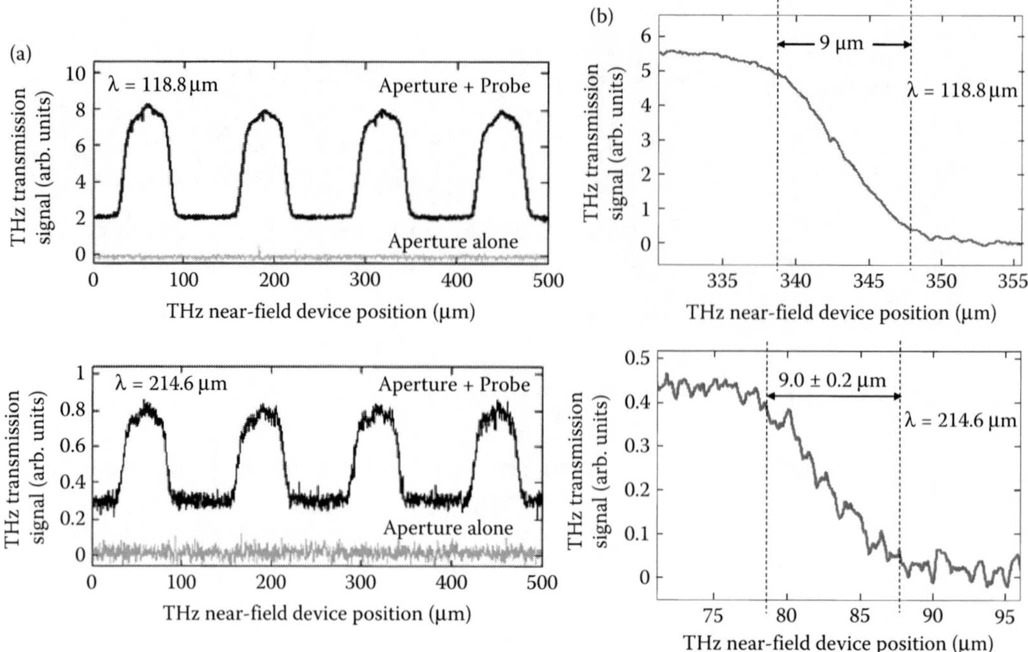

FIGURE 14.12 (a) THz transmission signal versus the position of the near-field THz detector. (b) Decay curves of the signals in (a).

the probe, where the aperture diameters are the same. For the case of the aperture alone, the electric field is localized close to the aperture. This explains why the conventional aperture-based technique suffers from low transmission through the aperture. On the other hand, when the probe is present just behind the aperture, the electric field extends into the interior region of the GaAs substrate. This result indicates that the presence of the probe changes the distribution profile of the evanescent field, enhancing the coupling between the evanescent field and the 2DEG detector.

In order to confirm experimentally the above calculations, we measured the THz transmission distribution by scanning the device across a sample. In the measurements, the THz gas laser pumped by the CO_2-gas laser was used as a THz source. The THz radiation was chopped at 16 Hz and the amplitude modulation of the detected signal (the voltage change of the 2DEG) was measured with a lock-in amplifier. The THz near-field device relative to the sample was scanned with a translation stage based on a piezoelectric stick–slip motion. The sample is made up of a THz transparent substrate, the surface of which is covered at regular intervals by THz opaque Au films. The widths of THz opaque and transparent regions across the scan direction are 80 and 50 μm, respectively. Two types of near-field THz devices were used: the aperture plus the probe and the aperture alone. As displayed in Figure 14.12a, in the former case, a clear signal is visible, whereas in the latter case, no signal is observed. This feature does not depend on the wavelength of the incident THz wave. The enhancement ratio of the signal amplitude, on comparison of the two devices, was found to be 41 for $\lambda = 118.8$ μm and 67 for $\lambda = 214.6$ μm. These results clearly demonstrate that the distribution of the THz evanescent field is largely enhanced due to the presence of the probe, leading to an improvement of detection sensitivity.

The decay curves of Figure 14.12b show that the near-field THz device has a spatial resolution of 9 μm. The important points of the data are that the resolution does not depend on the wavelength of the THz wave and that it is far beyond the diffraction limit $\lambda/2$ (107.3 μm) for the wavelength of $\lambda = 214.6$ μm. These features are characteristic of the near-field effect. The present device, hence, properly functions as a near-field THz imaging detector. Using this device, a high-resolution image of THz CE distribution in another 2DEG has been obtained [35].

In general, when one improves the spatial resolution, one encounters the problem that it is necessary to largely enhance detection sensitivity. This is because the intensity of the wave to be detected is strongly reduced as the sensing area becomes small. This situation imposes one to produce a scheme of highly sensitive detection in a tiny region. The author expects that one promising approach for tackling this problem in the THz region will be to use the CNT/2DEG THz detector [13], described in the previous section. Compared to the 2DEG detector, the CNT/2DEG detector exhibits much higher sensitivity in a much smaller sensing area of submicrometer. When this detector is integrated with an aperture and a probe as shown in Figure 14.10, the device would enable THz imaging with ultrahigh sensitivity and a sub-micron resolution.

14.4 THz APPLICATION

14.4.1 Applications to Materials Research

The photon energy and the period of the THz wave with 1 THz are about 4 meV and 1 ps, respectively. In these energy and time regions, there are many important materials and their physical properties, such as energy gap of superconductor, impurity level of semiconductor, phonon energy, and Landau-level separation. THz spectroscopy and imaging can be thus exploited as a powerful tool for investigating and characterizing various materials.

There are a number of THz applications to materials research. The work [36] reported the mapping of supercurrent distributions in a high-temperature superconductor by means of the THz imaging technique. The THz-TDS is a very powerful tool for investigating electron dynamics in materials. This technique provides two kinds of information: real-time dynamics and frequency spectra. With this method, a great deal of important information was successfully derived and the related electronic properties were clarified. For example, by using this method, earlier works reported THz conductivity in an MgB_2 superconductor [37], Bloch oscillation in a semiconductor superlattice [38], ballistic electron motion in a CNT [39], and the dynamics of the spin-density-wave gap in a quasi-1D organic conductor [40].

14.4.2 Applications to Semiconductors

14.4.2.1 Imaging Energy Dissipation in 2DEG

When the 2DEG is subjected to a perpendicular magnetic field, it exhibits dramatic properties known as the quantum Hall effect (QHE) [41,42]. In the QHE regime, the longitudinal resistance vanishes and the Hall resistance is precisely quantized. The basis of the QHE is the formation of Landau level, which originates from the quantization of electron cyclotron motion. Studying the electron distribution of an excited Landau level (the distribution of energy relaxation of excited electrons) is one of the critical issues regarding the QHE. The reason is as follows: earlier works reported that the electron relaxation from excited Landau level involves a slow physical process, the typical time scale being as long as 10–100 ns [43]. Moreover, the equilibrium length of the excited electrons L_E was shown to reach a macroscopic value of ~0.1 mm [44,45]. This leads us to expect that the spatial distribution of the excited electrons will be strikingly different from that of the ground-state electrons and will drastically depend on sample dimensions, in relation to L_E. However, this issue has not been satisfactorily clarified.

Several imaging techniques have been applied to obtain information about dissipation distributions in the QHE systems. By using the fountain-pressure effect of superfluid liquid helium, Klaß et al. demonstrated that in the QHE state, dissipation takes place almost totally at the diagonally opposite electron entry and exit corners of the sample (hot spots) [46]. A similar conclusion has been derived from the experiments of Russell et al., which applied the local bolometry technique [47]. Unfortunately, since these earlier experiments probe the lattice temperature related to Joule heating, they do not exclusively observe the distribution within the 2DEG, that is, the effective temperature of the excited electrons. Thus, until now no experimental techniques were available for imaging only the dissipation distribution in the 2DEG.

In contrast, since CE is radiated with the transition of electrons from higher Landau levels to lower Landau levels, mapping the CE intensity with the THz microscope provides a direct probe of the excited electrons. In the following section, investigations on the spatial properties of 2DEGs using THz-CE imaging are discussed.

14.4.2.2 Separate Imaging of Ground and Excited Levels

In order to enable separate imaging of the ground-state electrons and the excited-state electrons, we have developed a combined system of an electrometer with a THz microscope [48]. In the electrometer technique, we are able to map voltage distributions [49,50]. Hence, comparing the two kinds of mapped data (voltage and CE) allows us to distinguish between the contributions of the ground-state and excited-state electrons to the generation of the voltage.

Figure 14.13 depicts the setup of the combined imaging system. An electrometer (small Hall bar) and a hyperhemisphere Si lens are in contact with the front and back surfaces of the sample, respectively. A THz detector is mounted at the bottom of the system. The electrometer, the sample, and the THz detector were fabricated on GaAs/AlGaAs heterostructure wafers having the 2DEGs, 0.1 μm beneath the crystal surfaces. In imaging experiments, the sample alone was moved with an X–Y stage, while the electrometer and the optical system were spatially fixed. The whole system was directly immersed in liquid ^{4}He and was subjected to a perpendicular magnetic field B.

The detection mechanism of the electrometer is as follows: as shown in Figure 14.14, the distance between the two 2DEG layers is very short and consequently they are capacitively coupled. It follows that when a current I_S is passed through the sample, excess charges ΔQ are induced into the 2DEGs, according to $CV(x,y) = \Delta Q$. Here, $V(x,y)$ is a local voltage in the sample right below the electrometer, and C is the capacitance between the two 2DEG layers. The generation of ΔQ leads to the change, ΔR_E, in the longitudinal resistance of the electrometer. By translating the electrometer over the sample surface and measuring $\Delta R_E \times I_E$, we are able to image 2D distributions of $V(x,y)$ in the sample (I_E is the bias current for the electrometer). The electrometer was processed into a Hall bar geometry from a GaAs/AlGaAs heterostructure with an electron mobility $\mu_H = 18$ m^2/Vs and a sheet electron density $n_s = 2.2 \times 10^{15}$ m^{-2} at 4.2 K. The device has a 2DEG channel with a length

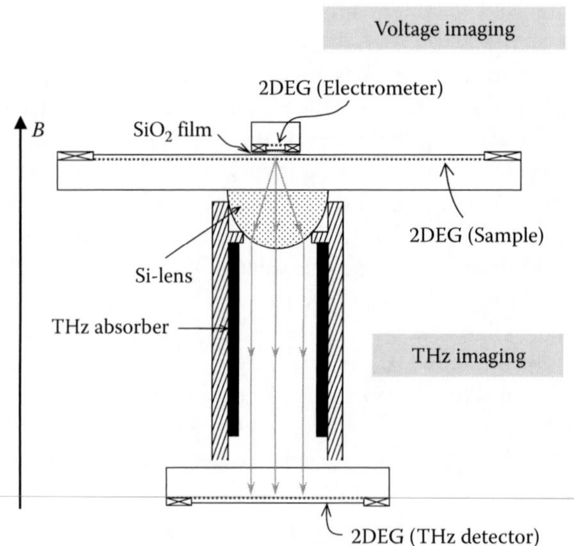

FIGURE 14.13 Combined imaging system of the electrometer and the THz microscope.

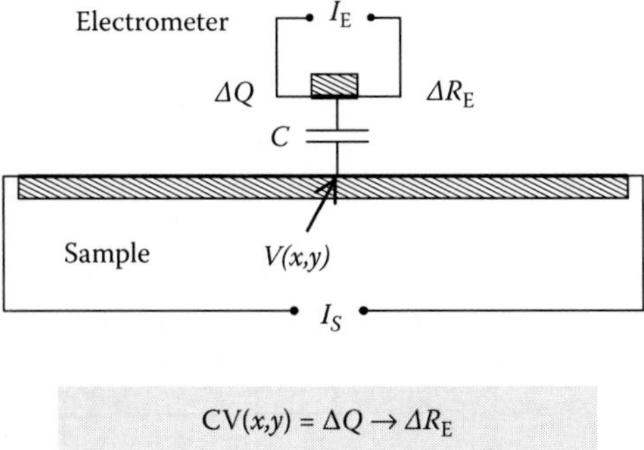

FIGURE 14.14 Equivalent circuit of the scanning electrometer system and the detection mechanism.

$L = 200$ μm and a width $W = 1.5$ μm, and the two voltage probes with the interval of 2.3 μm. Spatial resolution of this system is about 2 μm, which is determined by the sensing 2DEG area of the electrometer.

The sample studied has a Hall bar geometry with $L = 2.8$ mm and $W = 1$ mm, which is fabricated from a GaAs/AlGaAs heterostructure with $\mu_H = 53$ m²/Vs and $n_s = 2.4\times 10^{15}$ m^{-2} at 4.2 K. In imaging measurements, the voltage $V(x,y)$ and the CE intensity $V_{CE}(x,y)$ were simultaneously obtained with two lock-in amplifiers, where a 30-Hz rectangular-wave current alternating between zero and a given finite value I_S was passed through the sample. All measurements were carried out at 4.2 K.

Figure 14.15 displays images of the longitudinal voltage Vxx and V_{CE} at three current levels, $I = 20$, 70, and 140 μA, and at $B = 5.75$ T (the Landau level filling factor, 1.74, of the sample). We obtained the Vxx(x,y) data by differentiating $V(x,y)$ over a distance of 50 μm in the direction of the length of the sample: $V\text{xx}(x,y) = V(x + \Delta x,y) - V(x,y)$ with $\Delta x = 50$ μm. The 20-μA data show that Vxx is seen over the whole 2DEG area, whereas CE occurs only in the two diagonally opposite corners. This directly indicates that the observed Vxx (except at the two spots) arises from scattering of the ground-state electrons. It is known that the CE at the two spots takes place via tunneling injection of nonequilibrium

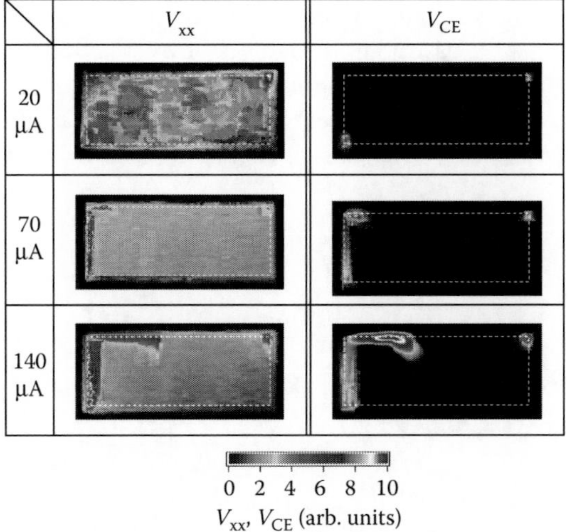

FIGURE 14.15 Distribution images of the longitudinal voltage Vxx (left) and the CE intensity V_{CE} (right) at three current levels, $I = 20$, 70, and 140 μA. The white broken lines denote the 2DEG boundaries of the sample. In the Vxx (V_{CE}), for clarity, the signals at $I = 20$ and 70 μA are magnified, respectively, by factors of 15 (18) and 9 (3) compared to that at $I = 140$ μA. (Adapted from Y. Kawano and T. Okamoto, *Phys. Rev.*, B 70, 081308(R), 2004.)

electrons from the source contact and inter-Landau-level tunneling of electrons near the drain contact [22]. The *V*xx data at $I = 70$ and 140 μA show that an additional *V*xx is generated around the source contact and, with increasing current, the area covered by the additional *V*xx expands toward the interior 2DEG region. Comparing with the V_{CE} data reveals that a strong CE is radiated in a similar region, indicating that the *V*xx observed on the source-contact side mostly originates from the scattering of the excited electrons. *V*xx is also visible over the whole 2DEG region, whereas CE remains absent (except in the two diagonally opposite corners). This situation is similar to that observed at $I = 20$ μA, showing again that the *V*xx associated with the ground-state electrons is generated over the entire 2DEG area. We confirmed that the pattern of these features systematically changes upon reversing *B* and *I*, and that they are also observed for other Landau level filling factors and for other samples fabricated from different wafers. This indicates that they are due an intrinsic nature of the 2DEG and are not due to inhomogeneity of the electron density.

Let me explain the origin of the difference in distributions between the ground-state electrons and the excited electrons. A summary of the experimental findings is schematically shown in Figure 14.16; the scattering distribution of the ground-state electrons spreads over the entire 2DEG region, whereas that of the excited electrons is localized in the two corners and around the source contact. The result indicates large differences in the scattering processes and in their characteristic lengths. The scattering length of excited electrons was shown to be a very long scale of 10–300 μm [44,45]. On the other hand, although there is no clear experimental information about the ground-state electrons, one can consider that the scattering rate will be much higher because the scattering does not require much energy. The main scattering mechanism of the ground-state electrons is possibly impurity scattering, originating from ionized donors in the AlGaAs layer. The characteristic scattering length of the ground-state electrons can be regarded as period of the ionized impurity potential 0.05–0.3 μm, which is much shorter than L_E. This explains the contrasting situation regarding spatial distributions of ground- and excited-state electrons. The electron transport process is discussed in more detail below.

14.4.2.3 Macroscopic Channel-Size Effect of THz Image

The experimental data given above showed that the macroscopically long value of L_E results in an asymmetric distribution of the excited electrons. From this fact, the following interesting phenomenon is expected: the spatial distribution of the excited electrons will drastically depend on sample dimensions, in relation to L_E. We have addressed this issue by studying the channel-size dependence of the CE distribution by the use of THz imaging [51].

The experimental setup of the THz microscope is similar to that shown in Figure 14.9. Three samples with different widths of $W = 1.2$, 0.3, and 0.02 mm (length $L = 4$ mm) were investigated, all

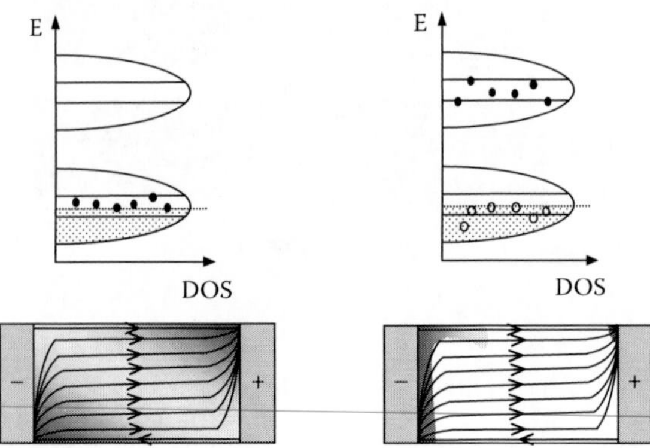

FIGURE 14.16 Sketch of scattering distributions of the ground-state electrons (left) and of the excited-state electrons (right).

of which were fabricated from the same GaAs/AlGaAs heterostructure crystal with $\mu_H = 62\ m^2/Vs$ and $n_s = 2.4 \times 10^{15}\ m^{-2}$ at 4.2 K. In CE measurements, the detected signal was recorded with a lock-in amplifier, where 20-Hz rectangular wave currents alternating between zero and a given finite value I were transmitted through the sample. All the measurements were carried out at 4.2 K.

Figure 14.17 shows a comparison of the CE images for the three samples. In the widest sample ($W = 1.2$ mm), CE takes place mostly in the two diagonally opposite corners and in a localized region near the source contact. In the data for $W = 0.3$ mm, CE expands into the more interior 2DEG region. Furthermore, when $W = 0.02$ mm, CE takes place over the entire region of the interior 2DEG channel. We confirmed that the pattern of these features systematically changed upon reversing B and I and that they were also observed for other samples fabricated from different GaAs/AlGaAs wafers.

The significant change with W observed shows the validity of the above expectation: the spatial distribution of the excited electrons is considerably influenced by the very long length scale of L_E. This means that the electrons travel the macroscopic distance L_E to lead to an appreciable generation of CE. On the basis of this, the transport process of the excited electrons are explained below.

In the QHE devices, it is known that a high electric field is concentrated in the two diagonally opposite corners, which are also the electron entry and exit corners [52]. It follows that as the current increases, electron excitation into higher Landau level starts in the vicinity of the two current contacts. On the source-contact side, CE begins to take place in the electron entry corner S_E (Figure 14.18). At $W \gg L_E$, although the electric field decreases away from S_E, the excitation process can continue toward the opposite corner (S_O) over the distance L_E. As the applied electric field becomes higher, such as 0.4 and 1.5 A/m in the sample with $W = 1.2$ mm, the area where such excitation occurs further expands through S_O toward the interior region of the 2DEG channel. A similar excitation process takes place along the boundary of the drain contact. In this region, on the other hand, electrons travel from the opposite corner (D_O) to the electron exit corner (D_E), which is opposite to that on the side of the source contact. As a result, although electron excitation starts around D_O, CE does not appreciably occur there and CE mostly occurs at D_E.

In contrast, when W is smaller than L_E, CE is not generated in the vicinity of the source contact. This is because in such narrow devices, electron excitation can take place only as the electrons

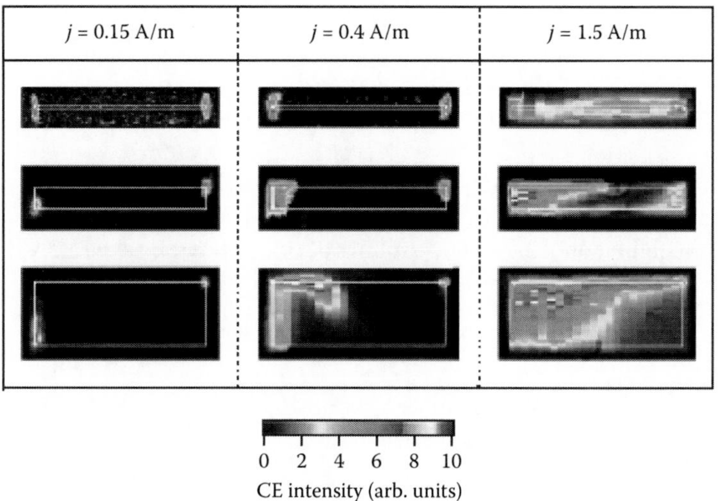

FIGURE 14.17 CE images at three current densities $j = 0.15$, 0.4, and 1.5 A/m and for the three samples with different channel widths $W = 20$, 300, and 1200 μm. The white solid lines denote the 2DEG boundaries of the samples. For clarity, the signals are magnified by factors of 1300 (20, 0.15), 360 (20, 0.4), 23 (20, 1.5), 70 (300, 0.15), 18 (300, 0.4), 3 (300, 1.5), 14 (1200, 0.15), and 5 (1200, 0.4), respectively, compared to that for (1200, 1.5), where (A, B) represents (W in μm, j in A/m). (Adapted from Y. Kawano and T. Okamoto, *Phys. Rev. Lett.*, 95, 166801, 2005.)

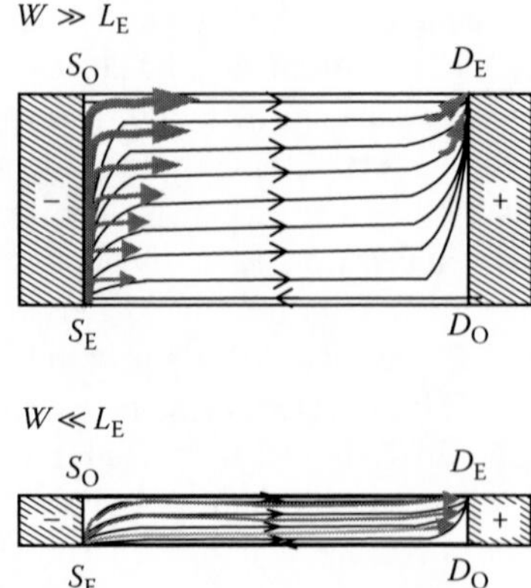

FIGURE 14.18 Schematic view of trajectories (thick lines) of excited electrons in the QHE device for a wide Hall bar with $W >> L_E$ (upper panel) and a narrow Hall bar with $W << L_E$ (lower panel).

traverse the Hall bar along the length direction of the 2DEG channel. The CE thus occurs over the whole region of the interior 2DEG channel, which is in strong contrast to the CE distribution for the devices with $W \gg L_E$.

14.5 CONCLUSION AND OUTLOOK

This chapter presents novel THz sensing and imaging devices based on nanoelectronic materials and devices: 2D semiconductors and CNTs. These detectors enable THz wave sensing with high sensitivity and high spatial resolution. The applications of THz measurements to materials research are discussed. The experimental data have successfully revealed the spatial properties of electrons in the 2DEG, which were not revealed by conventional transport measurements.

The next key devices for future THz technology will be the THz camera, THz video, and THz communication. Once these devices are realized in portable size, THz technology would widely spread into our daily life. For reaching this goal, achieving higher detection sensitivity and higher power generation will become increasingly important. The development should require further breakthroughs in materials, device structure, operation principle, and so on. The author anticipates that nanotechnology would still be one of the keys for enhancing the performance of THz technology.

Regarding the next target, the author plans to create a THz-photon counting video, which is a strongly desired device in many fields. When many CNT-based THz-photon detectors [13] are integrated in a 2D configuration [53,54], the resulting device will work as a THz video for real-time, high-resolution THz imaging.

REFERENCES

1. B. Ferguson and X.-C. Zhang, Materials for terahertz science and technology, *Nat. Mater.*, 1, 26, 2002.
2. M. Tonouchi, Cutting-edge terahertz technology, *Nat. Photon.*, 1, 97, 2007.
3. J. Wei, D. Olaya, B. S. Karasik, S. V. Pereverzev, A. V. Sergeev, and M. E. Gershenson, Ultrasensitive hot-electron nanobolometers for terahertz astrophysics, *Nat. Nanotechnol.*, 3, 496, 2008.
4. S. Ariyoshi, C. Otani, A. Dobroiu, H. Matsuo, H. Sato, T. Taino, K. Kawase, and H. Shimizu, Terahertz imaging with a direct detector based on superconducting tunnel junctions, *Appl. Phys. Lett.*, 88, 203503, 2006.
5. S. Komiyama, O. Astafiev, V. Antonov, H. Hirai, and T. Kutsuwa, A single-photon detector in the far-infrared range, *Nature*, 403, 405, 2000.
6. P. Kleinschmidt, S. Giblin, A. Tzalenchuk, H. Hashiba, V. Antonov, and S. Komiyama, Sensitive detector for a passive terahertz imager, *J. Appl. Phys*, 99, 114504, 2006.

7. R. Saito, G.. Dresselhaus, and M. S. Dresselhaus, *Physical Properties of Carbon Nanotubes*, Imperial College Press: London, 1998.
8. P. W. Barone, S. Baik, D. A. Heller, and M. S. Strano, Near-infrared optical sensors based on single-walled carbon nanotubes, *Nat. Mater.*, 4, 86, 2005.
9. M. E. Itkis, F. Borondics, A. Yu, and R. C. Haddon, Bolometric infrared photoresponse of suspended single-walled carbon nanotube films, *Science*, 312, 413, 2006.
10. T. Fuse, Y. Kawano, M. Suzuki, Y. Aoyagi, and K. Ishibashi, Coulomb peak shifts under terahertz-wave irradiation in carbon nanotube single-electron transistors, *Appl. Phys. Lett.*, 90, 013119, 2007.
11. K. Fu, R. Zannoni, C. Chan, S. H. Adams, J. Nicholson, E. Polizzi and K. S. Yngvesson, Terahertz detection in single wall carbon nanotubes, *Appl. Phys. Lett*, 92, 033105, 2008.
12. Y. Kawano, T. Fuse, S. Toyokawa, T. Uchida, and K. Ishibashi, Terahertz photon-assisted tunneling in carbon nanotube quantum dots, *J. Appl. Phys*, 103, 034307, 2008.
13. Y. Kawano, T. Uchida, and K. Ishibashi, Terahertz sensing with a carbon nanotube/two-dimensional electron gas hybrid transistor, *Appl. Phys. Lett*, 95, 083123, 2009.
14. P. K. Tien and J. P. Gordon, Multiphoton process observed in the interaction of microwave fields with the tunneling between superconductor films, *Phys. Rev*, 129, 647, 1963.
15. J. M. Hergenrother, M. T. Tuominena, J. G. Lua, D. C. Ralpha, and M. Tinkham, Charge transport and photon-assisted tunneling in the NSN single-electron transistor, *Physica*, B 203, 327, 1994.
16. B. Leone, J. R. Gao, T. M. Klapwijk, B. D. Jackson, W. M. Laauwen, and G. de Lange, Electron heating by photon-assisted tunneling in niobium terahertz mixers with integrated niobium titanium nitride striplines, *Appl. Phys. Lett*, 78, 1616, 2001.
17. T. H. Oosterkamp, L. P. Kouwenhoven, A. E. A. Koolen, N. C. van der Vaart, and C. J. P. M. Harmans, Photon sidebands of the ground state and first excited state of a quantum dot, *Phys. Rev. Lett*, 78, 1536, 1997.
18. T. H. Oosterkamp, T. Fujisawa, W. G. van der Wiel, K. Ishibashi, R. V. Hijman, S. Tarucha, and L. P. Kouwenhoven, Microwave spectroscopy of a quantum-dot molecule, *Nature*, 395, 873, 1998.
19. F. Thiele, U. Merkt, J. P. Kotthaus, G. Lommer, F. Malcher, U. Rossler, and G. Weimann, Cyclotron masses in *n*-GaAs/Ga_{1-}xAlxAs heterojunctions, *Solid State Commun.*, 62, 841, 1987.
20. S. H. Tessmer, P. I. Glicofridis, R. C. Ashoori, L. S. Levitov, and M. R. Melloch, Subsurface charge accumulation imaging of a quantum Hall liquid, *Nature*, 392, 51, 1998.
21. Y. Kawano, Y. Hisanaga, H. Takenouchi, and S. Komiyama, Highly sensitive and tunable detection of far-infrared radiation by quantum Hall devices, *J. Appl. Phys.*, 89, 4037, 2001.
22. Y. Kawano, Y. Hisanaga, and S. Komiyama, Cyclotron emission from quantized Hall devices: Injection of nonequilibrium electrons from contacts, *Phys. Rev*, B 59, 12537 1999.
23. Y. Kawano and S. Komiyama, Spatial distribution of non-equilibrium electrons in quantum Hall devices: Imaging via cyclotron emission, *Phys. Rev*, B 68, 085328, 2003.
24. M. Ohtsu, ed. *Near-Field Nano/Atom Optics and Technology*, Springer-Verlag, Berlin, 1998.
25. T. Saiki, S. Mononobe, M. Ohtsu, N. Saito and J. Kusano, Tailoring a high-transmission fiber probe for photon scanning tunneling microscope, *Appl. Phys. Lett*, 68, 2612, 1996.
26. F. Zenhausern, Y. Martin, and H. K. Wickramasinghe, Scanning interferometric apertureless microscopy: Optical imaging at 10 Angstrom resolution, *Science*, 269, 1083, 1995.
27. W. C. Symons III, K. W. Whites, and R. A. Lodder, Theoretical and experimental characterization of a near-field scanning microwave microscope (NSMM), *IEEE Trans. Microwave Theory Tech*, 51, 91, 2003.
28. M. Tabib-Azar and Y. Wang, Design and fabrication of scanning near-field microwave probes compatible with atomic force microscopy to image embedded nanostructures, *IEEE Trans. Microwave Theory Tech*, 52, 971, 2004.
29. S. Hunsche, M. Koch, I. Brener, and M. C. Nuss, THz near-field imaging, *Opt. Commun.*, 150, 22, 1998.
30. N. C. J. van der Valk and P. C. M. Planken, Electro-optic detection of subwavelength terahertz spot sizes in the near field of a metal tip, *Appl. Phys. Lett.*, 81, 1558, 2002.
31. H. T. Chen, R. Kersting, and G. C. Cho, Terahertz imaging with nanometer resolution, *Appl. Phys. Lett.*, 83, 3009, 2003.
32. A. J. Huber, F. Keilmann, J. Wittborn, J. Aizpurua, and R. Hillenbrand, Terahertz near-field nanoscopy of mobile carriers in single semiconductor nanodevices, *Nano Lett.*, 8, 3766, 2008.
33. Y. Kawano and K. Ishibashi, An on-chip near-field terahertz probe and detector, *Nat. Photon.*, 2, 618–621, 2008.
34. Y. Kawano, Terahertz Detectors: Quantum dots enable integrated terahertz imager, *Laser Focus World*, 45(7), 45–47, 50, 2009.

35. Y. Kawano and K. Ishibashi, On-chip near-field terahertz detection based on a two-dimensional electron gas, *Physica E*, 42, 1188, 2010.
36. S. Shikii, T. Kondo, M. Yamashita, M. Tonouchi, M. Hangyo, M. Tani, and K. Sakai, Observation of supercurrent distribution in $YBa_2Cu_3O_{7-\delta}$ thin films using THz radiation excited with femtosecond laser pulses, *Appl. Phys. Lett.*, 74, 1317, 1999.
37. R. A. Kaindl, M. A. Carnahan, J. Orenstein, D. S. Chemla, H. M. Christen, H.-Y. Zhai, M. Paranthaman and D. H. Lowndes, Far-infrared optical conductivity gap in superconducting MgB_2 films, *Phys. Rev. Lett.*, 88, 027003, 2001.
38. N. Sekine and K. Hirakawa, Dispersive terahertz gain of non-classical oscillator: Bloch oscillation in semiconductor superlattices, *Phys. Rev. Lett.*, 94, 057408, 2005.
39. Z. Zhong, N. M. Gabor, J. E. Sharping, A. L. Gaeta, and P. L. McEuen, Terahertz time-domain measurement of ballistic electron resonance in a single-walled carbon nanotube, *Nat. Nanotechnol.*, 3, 201, 2008.
40. S. Watanabe, R. Kondo, S. Kagoshima, and R. Shimano, Observation of ultrafast photoinduced closing and recovery of the spin-density-wave gap in $(TMTSF)_2PF_6$, *Phys. Rev.*, B 80, 220408(R), 2009.
41. K. von Klitzing, G. Dorda, and M. Pepper, New method for high-accuracy determination of the fine-structure constant based on quantized Hall resistance, *Phys. Rev. Lett.*, 45, 494, 1980.
42. D. C. Tsui, H. L. Stormer, and A. C. Gossard, Two-dimensional magnetotransport in the extreme quantum limit *Phys. Rev. Lett.*, 48, 1559, 1982.
43. B. R. A. Neves, N. Mori, P. H. Beton, L. Eaves, J. Wang, and M. Henini, Landau-level populations and slow energy relaxation of a two-dimensional electron gas probed by tunneling spectroscopy, *Phys. Rev.*, B 52, 4666, 1995.
44. S. Komiyama, Y. Kawaguchi, T. Osada, and Y. Shiraki, Evidence of nonlocal breakdown of the integer quantum Hall effect, *Phys. Rev. Lett.*, 77, 558, 1996.
45. I. I. Kaya, G. Nachtwei, K. von Klitzing, and K. Eberl, Spatially resolved monitoring of the evolution of the breakdown of the quantum Hall effect: Direct observation of inter-Landau-level tunneling, *Europhys. Lett.*, 46, 62, 1999.
46. U. Klaβ, W. Dietsche, K. von Klitzing, and K. Ploog, Imaging of the dissipation in quantum-Hall-effect experiments, *Z. Phys.*, B 82, 351, 1991.
47. P. A. Russell, F. F. Ouali, N. P. Hewett, and L. J. Challis, Power dissipation in the quantum Hall regime, *Surf. Sci.*, 229, 54, 1990.
48. Y. Kawano and T. Okamoto, Imaging of intra- and inter-Landau-level scattering in quantum Hall systems, *Phys. Rev.*, B 70, 081308(R), 2004.
49. Y. Kawano and T. Okamoto, Scanning electrometer using the capacitive coupling in quantum Hall effect devices, *Appl. Phys. Lett.*, 84, 1111, 2004.
50. Y. Kawano and T. Okamoto, Noise-voltage mapping by a quantum-Hall electrometer, *Appl. Phys. Lett.*, 87, 252108, 2005.
51. Y. Kawano and T. Okamoto, Macroscopic channel-size effect of nonequilibrium electron distributions in quantum Hall conductors, *Phys. Rev. Lett.*, 95, 166801, 2005.
52. J. Wakabayashi and S. Kawaji, Hall effect in silicon MOS inversion layers under strong magnetic fields, *J. Phys. Soc. Jpn.*, 44, 1839, 1978.
53. N. R. Franklin, Q. Wang, T. W. Tombler, A. Javey, M. Shim, and H. Dai, Integration of suspended carbon nanotube arrays into electronic devices and electromechanical systems, *Appl. Phys. Lett.*, 81, 913, 2002.
54. H. Tabata, M. Shimizu, and K. Ishibashi, Fabrication of single electron transistors using transfer-printed aligned single walled carbon nanotubes array, *Appl. Phys. Lett.*, 95, 113107, 2009.

15 Design and Assessment Principles of Semiconductor Flat-Panel Detector-Based X-Ray Micro-CT Systems for Small-Animal Imaging

Alejandro Sisniega, J. J. Vaquero, and M. Desco

CONTENTS

15.1 INTRODUCTION

In recent years, the number of animal models of human disease has increased and their use is now widespread. The need to study biological processes and morphological features in small-animal models—and to do so noninvasively so that the process can be tracked over time—has stimulated the development of high-resolution biomedical imaging devices. Nowadays, drug development relies heavily on the use of small-animal models and molecular imaging techniques, such as positron emission tomography (PET) or single-photon emission computed tomography (SPECT) to provide the required functional information that characterizes the behavior of the drug. However, the results obtained are sometimes difficult to interpret due to the lack of a reliable anatomical localization of tracer uptake. In order to avoid this problem, registration of PET and SPECT images with accurate anatomical images [1] has proven to be an appropriate choice in new multimodality systems.

Among the different anatomical imaging techniques, x-ray microcomputed tomography (micro-CT) is the preferred complement to preclinical functional imaging modalities, due to its high-resolution capabilities and the possibility of integration with other imaging systems.

As well as complementing the information obtained using molecular imaging techniques, micro-CT in itself is a valuable tool in small-animal imaging and is commonly used in research fields associated with the morphology of the sample (e.g., bone studies) [2–6].

In the development of x-ray micro-CT systems, most approaches make use of detectors based on x-ray image intensifiers and charge-coupled devices (CCDs) to which a scintillator screen is connected either directly or using light guides (e.g., fiber optic plates) [7–9]. Recent developments in semiconductor detectors have made it possible to use new, compact devices—flat-panel detectors—for x-ray detection. These flat-panel devices can be categorized into two different groups according to the process carried out to convert the x-ray photons (primary quanta) to electric charges that are gathered and converted into a digital signal. The first approach makes use of photoconductors that directly convert the incident x-ray radiation into electric charges as secondary quanta. Devices that conform to this approach are called direct conversion flat-panel detectors. The second approach is based on scintillation screens that stop incident x-ray photons, thus producing optical photons as secondary quanta. These optical photons are then stopped by a photodiode array that provides the electric charges required by the device readout electronics. The detectors that implement this scheme are known as indirect conversion flat-panel detectors.

Direct conversion detectors based on amorphous selenium (a-Se), indirect conversion detectors based on amorphous silicon (a-Si) coupled to scintillation screens, and indirect conversion detectors based on CCDs connected to scintillation screens using fiber tapers are compared in [10]. The authors conclude that the final reconstructed CT image quality cannot be predicted from differences in the quantum efficiency of the detectors studied, due to stability issues.

In the past 10 years, different micro-CT systems based on microfocus x-ray tubes and semiconductor-based flat-panel detectors arranged in cone-beam geometry have been developed, and their suitability has been proved [11,12]. Flat-panel-based cone-beam configurations present advantages over other configurations (e.g., pencil or fan-beam geometries) used in clinical or preclinical applications. These advantages include reduction in acquisition time, large axial field of view (FOV) with no geometrical distortions, optimization of radiated dose per time and data acquired, and a more compact, space-saving design. Additionally, indirect conversion semiconductor flat panels are particularly interesting for small-animal imaging due to their high-resolution capability, especially when the microcolumnar scintillation screen is directly grown on the semiconductor detector. Current advances in semiconductor technology point to improved features in the future [13,14].

The main topics to be addressed during the design of micro-CT systems are reviewed below, with special emphasis on x-ray detector features and management. The performance of the system is also analyzed. This review is based on a state-of-the-art x-ray micro-CT [15] used as an add-on for small-animal PET systems [16,17]. The micro-CT system was designed to achieve an FOV that is appropriate for small rodents, a spatial resolution better than 50 μm, and a minimal radiated dose.

The tomography system includes a flat-panel detector (complementary metal-oxide semiconductor (CMOS) technology with a columnar cesium iodide scintillator plate) with a 50-μm pixel size, and a micro-focus x-ray source with a nominal focal spot of 35 μm. Both elements are placed in a rotating gantry according to the cone-beam geometry. The magnification factor of 1.6 was obtained by applying the design specification for final resolution, FOV size, and mechanical constraints defined by the system size and radiation shields.

The performance of the flat-panel detector was evaluated to validate its suitability for the micro-CT scanner. In order to validate its use for preclinical *in vivo* imaging as an add-on system for PET/SPECT tomographs or as a standalone unit, the overall performance of the system was evaluated in terms of spatial resolution, image contrast, exposure dose, and image acquisition and reconstruction time.

15.2 SMALL-ANIMAL MICRO-CT DESIGN CONSIDERATIONS

Small-animal micro-CT imaging systems are usually designed to provide complementary information for molecular imaging systems. The main design issues are image quality and the radiation delivered to the study animal.

Early implementations of x-ray micro-CT systems were aimed at nondestructive testing for industrial applications or at the *in vitro* study of biological tissues [18]. The main design goal for these systems was to achieve high image quality (resolution and contrast), regardless of the radiation dose delivered. They were not designed to facilitate the use of equipment for *in vivo* imaging, such as anesthesia equipment or vital sign monitoring devices. Thus, the mechanical setup was such that the x-ray source and the detector were fixed while the sample was rotated between these devices. This made system calibration easier and ensured long-term stability.

In vitro micro-CT scanners can achieve very high spatial resolution values (~5 μm) using micro-focus x-ray sources and area detectors such as CCDs or flat-panel detectors. However, to obtain an appropriate signal-to-noise ratio (SNR), it is necessary to perform long acquisitions at high radiation doses. Furthermore, the desired resolution in the reconstructed volume is commonly obtained in practice by using high magnification values (>3), which require the detector to be situated at some distance from the sample; therefore, such mechanical arrangements are only feasible if the x-ray source and the detector are assembled on a horizontal flat surface. A typical configuration for an x-ray *in vitro* system is depicted in Figure 15.1.

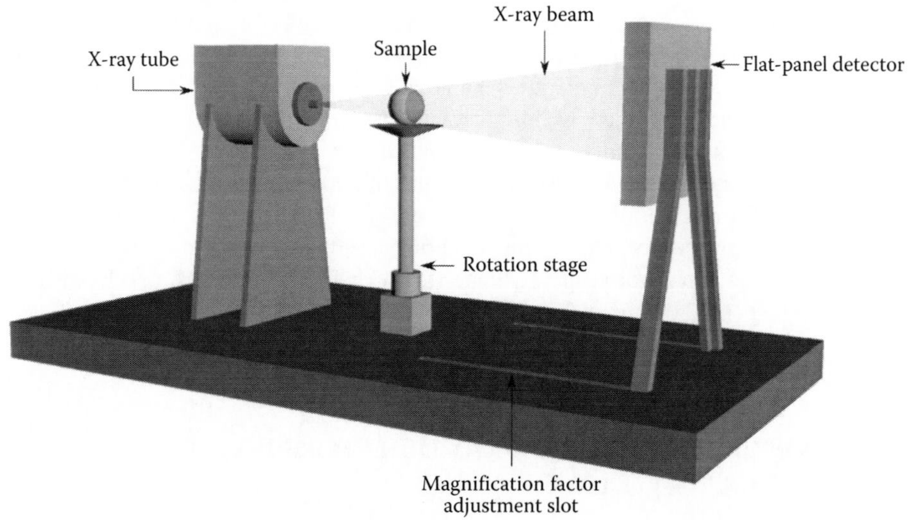

FIGURE 15.1 Typical configuration of an *in vitro* micro-CT scanner. The magnification factor can be adjusted by varying the distance between the sample and the flat-panel detector.

Small-animal micro-CT scanners also offer a reasonably high spatial resolution with sufficient image quality, although they require acquisition time and radiation dose to be as low as possible. These two additional constraints reveal the need for a new approach to the implementation of the system. Therefore, a compromise must be sought between image quality, spatial resolution, acquisition time, and dose delivered. Furthermore, during the acquisition process, the animal must be kept steady while the gantry holding the x-ray source and detector rotates around it. This is an important requirement, since it is necessary to minimize the disturbance to the animal and to avoid inconsistent projection data derived from any organ displacement that may occur if the animal is moving. Anesthesia equipment and monitoring devices (heartbeat, breathing rate) must be correctly placed, as monitoring becomes somewhat challenging if the animal is rotating.

The constraints imposed by *in vivo* requirements demand a more sophisticated and careful design if the system is to be compact. This requirement is even more important when space is scarce. In this setting, the mechanical features of the x-ray source and detector become more important, since these devices should be placed on a rotating gantry to keep the subject in a fixed position. In order to avoid instability during rotation, the weight and size of the devices should be as low as possible, and mechanical elements are necessary to counterbalance the system. Although some scanners make use of slip rings, this is not the most common solution, as they are expensive and rotation speed is not the most constraining factor. Therefore, the signal and power cables must be placed in such a way that they do not disturb the image acquisition process. This usually involves an extension of cable lengths, thus increasing signal losses and deteriorating the SNR in the acquired data.

Sensor specifications are also an important issue. Fast and sensitive detectors are extremely desirable for small animal micro-CT, given that acquisition time and dose delivered are paramount.

Since the acquired x-ray micro-CT projection data must be highly stable along the acquisition path, it is necessary to use highly stable x-ray sources and detectors. If the detector is not stable, it becomes necessary to acquire several correction datasets during a single acquisition process, thus increasing the total acquisition time.

Different approaches can be adopted in the selection of the detector. Nowadays, CCDs connected optically to a scintillation screen are the most widely used detectors in small-animal micro-CT systems. These detectors show good spatial resolution (usually depending on the coupling between scintillator and sensor) and the fastest image rate. However, these devices are usually too bulky to integrate in a moving gantry. Another drawback is that the sensor can be seriously damaged by x-ray radiation [19] and must be carefully shielded, thus increasing the size and weight of the system.

Modern designs make use of the so-called flat-panel x-ray detectors (semiconductor-based light detector matrices coupled to scintillator screens [20] or direct conversion semiconductor detectors), due to their high resolution (equal to or better than that achieved by CCDs) and image quality, combined with a compact design and low weight that simplifies integration in the rotating gantry. Their main drawback is that most of them are slower than CCDs.

Some experimental developments [21–24] make use of photon-counting detectors based on cadmium telluride (CdTe) or cadmium zinc telluride sensors. These devices are able to classify the incoming photons according to their energy, enabling accurate correction of energy-related artifacts, such as beam hardening or scatter. Much effort is being made in the development of x-ray photon-counting detectors for micro-CT systems, but these are still at an early stage. The quality and image rate of the data acquired by state-of-the-art devices are not sufficient to allow them to be used in commercial preclinical imaging systems.

15.3 OVERVIEW OF FLAT-PANEL X-RAY DETECTORS FOR CONE-BEAM MICRO-CT

Flat-panel digital detectors are one of the most widely used x-ray detection devices for small-animal imaging. Several comprehensive reviews of flat-panel x-ray detector technology [20,25–27] address topics not included in the present work and could prove useful for the interested reader. This section

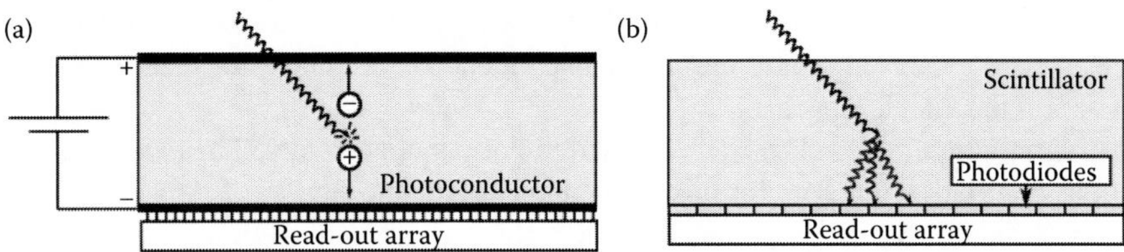

FIGURE 15.2 Scheme of direct (a) and indirect (b) detection approaches used in x-ray flat-panel detectors.

presents a brief overview of the state-of-the-art technology of the aforementioned detectors, focusing on their suitability for small-animal cone-beam micro-CT.

Flat-panel detectors can be classed as direct conversion and indirect conversion devices (Figure 15.2). Below, the features of flat-panel detectors are presented according to this classification. A comparative study of direct and indirect conversion flat-panel detectors can be found in [28].

Since x-ray detectors can be simply modeled using cascaded devices [29–32], for the sake of clarity the following explanation divides signal generation into two different stages, namely, x-ray conversion and data readout. Information on the position, where the x-ray photon is detected, and on its deposited energy, is generated at the beginning of the first stage where the x-ray photons (primary quanta) are stopped. Subsequent steps do not add new information to form the image. Thus, it is important to have a low noise level and adequate amplification in the stages following x-ray capture to ensure that no information is lost after the x-ray photons are detected. The stage with the poorest quanta detection capability, the quantum sink, limits system performance in terms of SNR. Since the information lost in the quantum sink cannot be recovered, a well-designed detector should have its quantum sink at the very first stage of image formation, namely, when x-ray photons are stopped [20].

15.3.1 Indirect Conversion Flat-Panel Detectors

15.3.1.1 X-Ray Conversion Stage

Indirect conversion flat-panel detectors detect individual x-ray photons by generating optical photons as secondary quanta. A subsequent step is needed to convert the optical photons into electric charges on each pixel. Integrated over a period of time; this charge is then amplified and digitized.

The outer layer of the detector is made of a scintillation material, which provides a variable number of optical photons per x-ray photon stopped, depending on the energy involved in the interaction.

The scintillation materials used in x-ray flat-panel detectors are usually inorganic compounds such as cesium iodide or gadolinium oxysulfide. Scintillation in such materials is based on energy transfer to the molecules of the scintillator, depending on the energy states determined by the crystal lattice of the material. In insulator or semiconductor materials, electrons remain in a discrete number of energy bands. The two main energy bands are the valence band and the conduction band. Electrons with an energy state that places them in the valence band are bound to the crystal lattice and, therefore, fixed. However, those electrons with sufficient energy to reach the conduction band can move across the crystal. The band between the conduction and valence bands is the forbidden band, where no electrons can be found in a pure crystal.

If a photon with sufficient energy reaches an electron in the valence band, it can increase its energy so as to reach the conduction band, thus leaving a hole in the valence band. The excited electron returns to the valence band by emitting a photon of energy equal to the difference between the energy levels. This energy is usually too high and the emitted photon energy does not correspond to the visible light range.

In order to increase the number of visible light photons emitted, dopants are added to the crystal [33]. These materials create defects in the crystal lattice, where the normal energy band structure is modified, thus creating energy levels within the forbidden band. Excited electrons can fall first into one of these energy levels and later into the stable valence band, and emit photons with an energy that falls within the visible range.

Several scintillation materials have been used in flat-panel detectors. The most desirable characteristics of a scintillation material for this application are the possibility of implementing large-area screens, the production of a high number of optical photons per x-ray photon detected, high sensitivity to the energy spectrum of the x-ray beam, and a high degree of correlation between the direction of propagation of the incident x-ray photon and that of the optical photons generated. It is also important that the energy spectrum of the photons emitted by the scintillation material fits the reception spectrum of the photodiodes used in the second detection stage.

Currently, the two scintillation materials most commonly used in flat-panel detectors are terbium-doped gadolinium oxysulfide (Gd_2O_2S:Tb) and thallium-doped cesium iodide (CsI:Tl).

Gd_2O_2S:Tb has traditionally been used to detect x-rays and can be manufactured easily and cost-effectively using well-known technology [20]. It comes in the form of a powder [34] composed of microscopic particles with a density of 7.3 g/cm^3. The particles are bound together by an acrylic binder to form a homogeneous paste that is usually applied as a coat on a glass or plastic support. A reflector can be added to increase light collection in the detector.

Gd_2O_2S:Tb has one of the highest figures of merit (defined as the best balance between high light production, fast response, and appropriate energy spectra) among powder scintillators: it is highly efficient and has a very low afterglow and an appropriate energy emission spectrum, centered at 540 nm. However, achievable spatial resolution is limited by the lateral scattering of the photons generated. Thicker scintillation screens offer a longer path for the optical photons, thus increasing scattering and worsening spatial resolution, while thinner screens stop a low fraction of the received x-ray photons, thus decreasing detector sensitivity. Therefore, a compromise must be reached between x-ray stopping power and achievable spatial resolution.

Microstructured scintillation screens based on CsI:Tl were developed to meet the main imaging needs of x-ray systems, namely, the increase in x-ray stopping power while maintaining good spatial resolution.

The manufacturing process of this type of scintillation screen is based on the deposition by thermal evaporation of long thin needle-shaped structures on a glass or plastic support or directly on top of the semiconductor light detectors. Each of the needle-shaped structures behaves as a light pipe, confining optical photons inside it and thus avoiding most of the lateral scattering present in nonstructured screens (Figure 15.3). This light confinement makes it possible to increase the thickness of the scintillation screen (up to 1–2 mm), while maintaining good spatial resolution. Furthermore, light production, needle stability and shape, and resolution of the scintillator screen are highly dependent on manufacturing conditions [35], namely, thallium concentration, pressure, temperature, and postprocessing.

The scintillator needle layer can be deposited directly on the semiconductor detector surface without degrading the properties of the photodetector elements in the array, thus achieving optimal spatial resolution and high x-ray detection efficiency, as optical coupling agents are not necessary to glue the scintillator screen over the semiconductor surface. Besides the aforementioned advantages

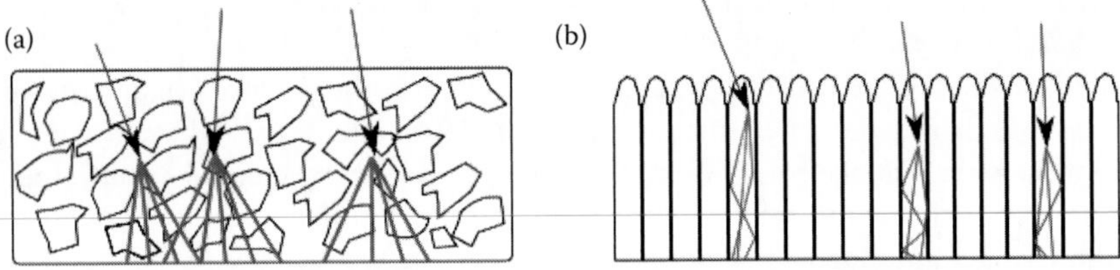

FIGURE 15.3 Simplified light transport in a granular nonstructured scintillator screen (a) and in a microcolumnar-structured scintillator screen (b).

of this kind of scintillator, the light production per photon stopped of CsI:Tl is among the highest known, and the peak of the emitted spectrum is at 550 nm, a value that matches the spectral response of most semiconductor photodetectors currently used in the development of x-ray flat-panel detectors [36,37]. Due to its advantages over other scintillation materials, CsI:Tl is becoming the preferred material for the x-ray photon conversion stage in flat-panel detectors. However, it does have certain drawbacks, the most important being its relatively slow response time, as compared to that of Gd_2O_2S:Tb.

15.3.1.2 Secondary Quanta Detection and Read-Out

Secondary quanta conversion and data read-out in indirect flat-panel x-ray detectors has traditionally been implemented as a pixel array based on hydrogenated amorphous silicon (aSi:H) and thin-film transistor (TFT) technology. Each pixel consists of a reverse-biased photodiode and a TFT that acts as a switch. During exposure, charges are accumulated in the photodiode. After exposure, a gate pulse is generated for each row of pixels, thus switching the TFT of the given row of pixels to release the accumulated charges through the data line. The released charges are amplified and converted into a voltage using an array of charge-integrating amplifiers, with one amplifier per pixel in the row. The voltage signals from the row of pixels are then multiplexed and digitized.

The technology described has mainly been used for digital radiography detectors; however, devices using this technology show a long signal decay time and a poor fill factor due to the wide electrode width and switch size [36]. These drawbacks impair the development of sensors with an appropriate frame rate and small pixel size, thus hampering the use of this technology for micro-CT image acquisition.

A newer technology for the read-out of indirect x-ray flat-panel detectors consists of sensors based on CMOS technology. CMOS image sensors are composed of a matrix of identical pixels that have a photodiode and a MOS switch transistor [37], two scan circuits which address the different rows and columns of the sensor matrix, and an output amplifier.

The image formation process for the simplest CMOS image sensor, based on passive pixel elements, is quite similar to that of the pixel array based on aSi:H and TFT technology. First, the photodiodes are reverse biased. The incoming photons cause a decrease in the voltage of the photodiode, which is measured at the end of the imaging process. The drop in voltage gives an estimation of the number of photons that have reached the given pixel. After the pixel reading, the photodiode is reset.

Current CMOS sensors use more sophisticated pixel designs, where every pixel has an active element that acts as an individual amplifier, thus reducing the noise level of the final image. Improvements in active pixel design have led to the development of the pinned photodiode pixel that is in use for most current CMOS image sensors. In this kind of sensor, two measurements are taken and subtracted for each image pixel (correlated double sampling, CDS). The first contains information about the number of photons reaching the pixel, while the second gives an estimation of the photodiode offset voltage. This kind of design allows a further reduction in the noise level and dark current of the detector. A sketch of a CMOS sensor with active pixels and CDS circuits is shown in Figure 15.4.

15.3.2 Direct Conversion Flat-Panel Detectors

15.3.2.1 X-Ray Conversion Stage

The detection of x-ray photons to generate secondary quanta in a direct conversion flat-panel detector consists of a layer of photoconductor material. Unlike indirect conversion detectors, the secondary quanta generated are already electric charges, thus avoiding the need for an intermediate stage to convert the secondary quanta into electric charges.

The process by which electric charges are generated from stopped x-ray photons is the same for all photoconductor materials. Stopped x-rays with sufficient energy generate an electron–hole pair that drifts through the photoconductor material under the action of an externally applied electrical

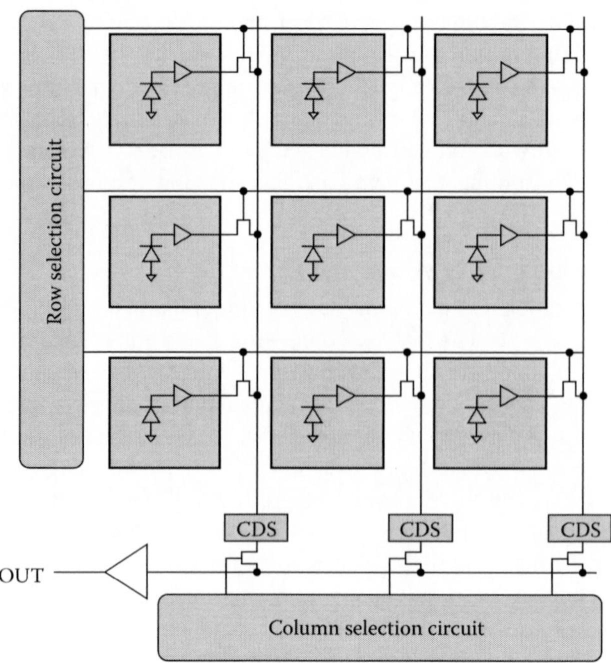

FIGURE 15.4 Sketch of a typical CMOS image sensor with active pixels and CDS.

field. Each portion of the photoconductor layer that defines a pixel has a capacitor which accumulates the charge generated by the stopped x-rays inside the current pixel. This accumulated charge is later measured and converted to form a pixel of the final image.

The photoconductor materials used to detect x-ray photons should be as efficient as possible in the conversion of x-ray photons to electric charges. Conversion efficiency depends on several factors associated with the photoconductor material, its manufacturing process, and the operating conditions. The main factors affecting sensor efficiency are x-ray stopping power, the number of electric charges generated from the absorbed radiation, and the number of electric charges that reach the end of the photoconductor layer and can be collected by the capacitive elements [20,26].

X-ray stopping power (i.e., the number of x-ray photons stopped) is highly associated with the density of the photoconductor material, its atomic number, and the energy of the incident photons. Materials with a high density and atomic number have a larger absorption coefficient and stop more x-ray photons. Thus, photoconductor materials for x-ray flat-panel detectors should be dense and made of elements with a high atomic number.

The number of electric charges generated from the stopped radiation depends on the energy necessary to create an electron–hole pair in the photoconductor material, that is, the ionization energy. Low ionization energy is highly desirable when attempting to generate a high number of electric charges from the incident radiation. The charge generated [26] is given by expression (15.1)

$$Q = \frac{eE}{W_{\pm}} \tag{15.1}$$

where Q stands for the generated electric charge, e is the charge of the electron, E is the energy of the incoming radiation, and $W_{\pm}$ is the ionization energy of the photoconductor. The ionization energy depends on the energy band gap (E_g) of the material used and, in some cases, it can be modified by means of an electric field. One of the materials that allow its $W_{\pm}$ value to be modified by applying an electric field is a-Se, the material most widely used in the development of x-ray direct flat-panel detectors.

The fraction of the generated charge that reaches the sensor surface and can be gathered by the capacitive elements is determined by the drift mobility of the electrons and holes generated inside the photoconductor, and the mean time that electrons and holes can drift without being trapped. Taking into account the applied electric field, it is possible to define the *Schubweg*, which is the mean distance traveled by a charge carrier before being trapped [38] and is given by (15.2)

$$S = \mu\tau F \tag{15.2}$$

where μ stands for the drift mobility of the charge carriers, τ is the mean time before being trapped, and F is the applied electric field.

As mentioned above, the most commonly used photoconductor for the development of direct x-ray flat-panel detectors is a-Se, despite the fact that pure a-Se has some undesirable properties, namely, the material is thermally unstable and crystallizes after a variable period depending on ambient conditions. In order to prevent crystallization and stabilize the material, some additives—usually small amounts of arsenic and a halogen (e.g., chloride)—are mixed with the original a-Se. The doped material, known as "stabilized a-Se," is more stable, thus enabling its deposition as flat screens. However, doping with a-Se can worsen the performance of the photoconductor screen. The most important drawback is the decrease in carrier mobility, which, in turn, increases the number of trapped carriers. The increase in the number of trapped carriers causes image lag and a decrease in sensor sensitivity that hamper the use of this kind of detector for the acquisition of micro-CT images. Both these effects are caused by the delayed freeing of carriers trapped during previous x-ray exposures. The image correction procedures applied to the acquired projections (see below) assume that every projection image is acquired under approximately the same conditions (dark current and x-ray conversion efficiency). Image lag prevents the fulfillment of these requirements, thus leading to inconsistent datasets when image correction is performed using a correction dataset acquired before the actual acquisition process. This problem can be solved by using several correction datasets acquired during the CT image acquisition, albeit at the cost of increasing acquisition time and dose delivered.

Recent developments point to CdTe (and CdZnTe) as a photoconductor material for stopping x-ray radiation. However, in most cases, development is at an early stage and there are few manufactured devices (mainly for dental and industrial radiography).

Early studies on the properties of these photoconductor materials conclude that the sensitivity of a sensor based on CdTe or CdZnTe can be up to four times higher than that achieved using a-Se–based sensors [39], but they also show a strong afterglow effect [40] and poor spatial resolution [39].

Recent developments show a reduction in the afterglow and better resolution while maintaining the predicted enhancement in sensitivity. There is also a high correlation between the design of the contacts deposited over each of the material surfaces and the amount of dark current present in the detector that degrades the performance of the device, especially the achievable energy resolution [41,42]. Depending on the design of the contact plates, there are two main detector types: Ohmic detectors and Schottky detectors [41,43]. Ohmic detectors have two contacts made of platinum, while in Schottky detectors one of the contacts is made of titanium and indium, thus forming a Schottky contact that reduces the injection of holes for the same voltage bias, thus reducing the dark current of the device. The main drawback of Schottky contacts is the so-called polarization effect, which consists of a very slow increase in the number of holes trapped near the positive electron [44]. This trapping effect leads to a decrease in sensitivity and in the charge collected per detected photon [45]. There are several ways to overcome this phenomenon, the simplest and most common being to reset the bias voltage when the effect is noticeable (about 60 min after the bias voltage is applied, for modern devices) [41,42].

15.3.2.2 Signal Read-Out

In detectors based on a-Se screens, the electric charges generated within the photoconductor are gathered by capacitive elements connected to TFTs that act as switches. The reading process is almost identical to the one used for indirect x-ray flat-panel detectors based on a-Si:H and TFT technology. Each row of pixels is addressed using a pulse that activates the TFTs of the desired pixel row, and the signal accumulated at each pixel in the row is read and converted into a voltage. This voltage is multiplexed with the rest of the voltages coming from the different pixels in the row and the values are digitized, thus forming the image. The process is performed for every row of pixels in the sensor.

For CdTe and CdZnTe detectors, the read-out matrix is generally implemented using a CMOS or TFT application-specific integrated circuit (ASIC), although in this case, the photoconductor cannot be directly deposited over the ASIC; therefore, the ASIC is built separately and at a later stage, and the crystal is placed on top of the read-out circuit. Both are connected by flip-chip bonding using a conductive resin.

15.4 DESIGN OF AN X-RAY MICRO-CT SYSTEM

15.4.1 Components of a Small-Animal Micro-CT System

The main components of a micro-CT system based on flat-panel detectors are the x-ray detector and the microfocus x-ray source. The constraints imposed by the application determine the type of flat-panel detector chosen by the designer.

In small-animal micro-CT systems, it is important to use a detector with an appropriate image resolution to obtain the high-quality images necessary for preclinical applications. The maximum pixel size and minimum resolution of the detector depend on the geometrical configuration of the system (see below). High sensitivity and low noise level are also highly desirable features when attempting to minimize the radiation delivered.

The output of the x-ray tube must be stable enough to ensure a constant radiation level during the acquisition process. Its focal spot size must be sufficiently small so as not to degrade system resolution. The maximum admissible size for the focal spot is determined by the detector pixel size and the geometrical configuration of the system. Furthermore, highly stable motorized devices are used in the design of small-animal micro-CT systems to place the animal within the FOV and to perform the rotational movement of the x-ray source–detector assembly around the sample. Finally, control components (e.g., computer, motion control drivers, shutter) and shield elements must be incorporated to ensure simple and safe operation.

This section summarizes the main elements of a commercial state-of-the-art *in vivo* micro-CT system, the Argus PET/CT (Sedecal, Madrid, Spain).

15.4.1.1 System Components

A complete description of the different components included in the design of the micro-CT system used as an example in this section can be found in [15].

The scanner design includes a computer that controls the microfocus x-ray tube and the CMOS flat-panel detector, both of which are assembled in a common rotating gantry. A linear motion stage is used to displace the sample along the FOV, thus enabling the tomograph to perform whole body scans (Figure 15.5). The assembly is enclosed in a radiation-shielded cabinet with openings for animal positioning, anesthesia gas lines, and physiological monitoring cables.

The computer synchronizes the gantry motions with the image integration in the detector. The data acquired from each angular position are captured by a digital frame grabber. Raw data are processed simultaneously with the acquisition, thus saving processing time during the subsequent reconstruction stage and taking advantage of the full potential offered by the system computer.

15.4.1.1.1 Flat-Panel Detectors

The x-ray flat-panel detector used in the Argus PET/CT is the C7940DK-02 model (Figure 15.6) from Hamamatsu Photonics K.K. (Hamamatsu City, Japan). A complete description and an

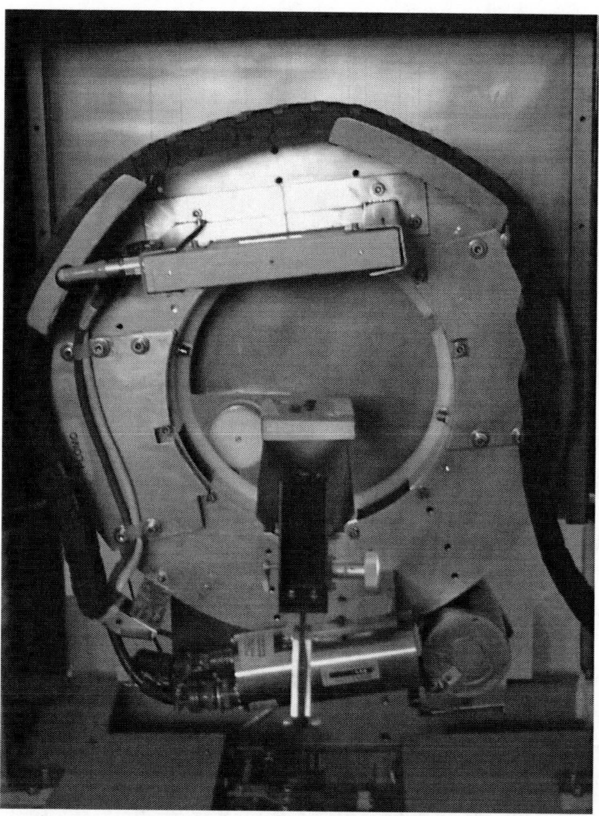

FIGURE 15.5 Small-animal CT prototype showing its components attached to the rotating gantry: micro-focus cone-beam x-ray tube (bottom), object bed (center), and CMOS digital imaging sensor (top). The radiation shielding cabinet is not shown.

evaluation of some of the performance parameters can be found in [36]. This is an indirect flat-panel detector based on a CsI:Tl scintillator screen and a high-fill-factor CMOS image sensor to detect the optical photons. The features of the flat-panel detector as reported by the manufacturer are summarized in Table 15.1.

The scintillator layer of the flat-panel detector consists of a matrix of 150- μm–long needle-like CsI:Tl crystal structures directly deposited over the CMOS photodiode matrix surface (Figure 15.6). A photodiode matrix with active pixel elements connected to CMOS transistor switches enables detection and read-out of the visible photons generated on the scintillation screen. The photodiode

TABLE 15.1
Features of an X-Ray Flat-Panel Detector

Pixel size	50, 100, 200 μm (Binning 1, 2, 4)
Photodiode area	120 × 120 mm
Number of pixels (total/active)	2400 × 2400/2240 × 2344
Frame rate	2, 4, 9 frames/s (Binning 1, 2, 4)
Noise (rms)	1100 electrons
Saturation charge	2.2 M electrons
Dynamic range	2000
Sensitivity (at 80 kV)	25 LSB/mR

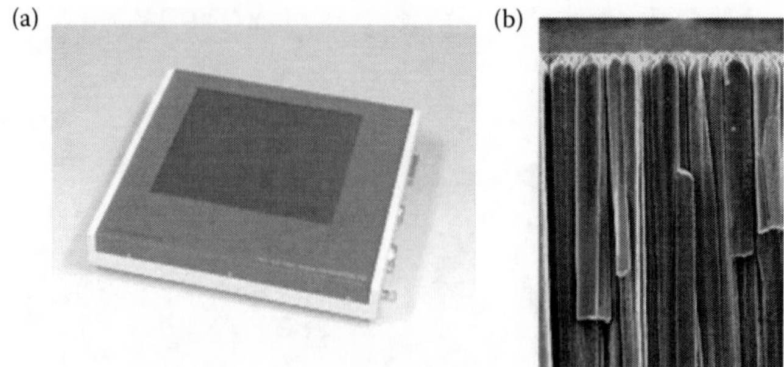

FIGURE 15.6 Hamamatsu C7940DK-02 x-ray flat-panel detector (a) and details of the needle-like CsI:Tl crystal structures on the scintillator layer (b). (Images courtesy of Hamamatsu Photonics K.K.)

CMOS matrix has 2 × 2 and 4 × 4 binning capabilities and a high fill-factor (79%). The on-chip signal amplification channels have a low noise level, and an offset suppression circuit based on CDS is assigned to each of these channels. This design achieves a high degree of image uniformity and a low noise level. However, correction tasks must be performed after acquisition of an image in order to obtain the best achievable quality. In addition to the noise-reduction stages, every pixel in the matrix implements an overflow drain function to avoid possible blooming.

15.4.1.1.2 X-Ray Source

The scanner uses the XTG5011 Apogee microfocus x-ray source (Oxford Instruments, Scotts Valley, CA). This tube has a stationary tungsten anode, a 127- μm-thick beryllium window, and a Gaussian-like focal spot measuring 46.5 μm × 49.1 μm, according to the manufacturer's measurements. The tube also has a maximum anode power of 75 W, limited to 50 W by the high voltage power supply (50 kV for an anode current of 1 mA).

The working settings for this component (i.e., anode current and voltage) are managed by the control computer through an I2C interface. In order to reduce the radiated dose during scans and the presence of artifacts arising from the polychromatic properties of the generated x-ray beam (e.g., beam hardening), two different elements have been added to the source output window:

- A tungsten shutter to block the x-ray beam during the intervals in which the detector is not integrating a valid image, that is, when the gantry is moving. This shutter has a maximum operating frequency of 10 Hz and a minimum opening time of 20 ms. The nominal beam extinction ratio increases to 10^4 for a maximum beam energy of 30 keV, as stated by the manufacturer. Practical measurements of the beam extinction fraction for the particular settings of the current system (40 keV, 200 μA) reveal a ratio of 1:4 × 10^3; therefore, exposure to radiation could be considered negligible when the shutter is closed.
- An aluminum filter (thickness ranging from 0.1 to 2 mm) to filter the low-energy region of the emission spectrum, thus improving beam mono-chromaticity and reducing superficial dose and image artifacts.

Minimal beam collimation is performed using a lead collimator, since most of the x-ray cone beams are used for imaging.

15.4.1.1.3 Mechanical Subsystem

The x-ray source, with its associated elements, and the flat-panel detector are placed on a circular aluminum plate fixed to a rotational motion stage. The projection dataset to be reconstructed is acquired by rotating the whole set 180° or 360° around the subject. The gantry stage is driven by a controller and a stepper motor. The main features of the rotational stage are shown in Table 15.2.

TABLE 15.2
Rotation Stage Features

Axis diameter	78 mm
Resolution	0.001°
Accuracy	0.010°
Repeatability	0.002°
Maximum centered load	1800 N
Maximum inertia	3 kg m^2
Maximum speed	20°/s

The system is provided with a linear motion stage to place the sample into the x-ray beam during the acquisition process. The sample is placed on a carbon-fiber bed with the appropriate dimensions for small animals (rats and mice). The carbon-fiber structure is attached to the linear motion stage using a metallic holder, which incorporates controls to adjust the height and lateral shift of the animal bed.

The whole mechanical system is controlled by the control computer, which interfaces with the stepper motors using motor controller circuits. These are enclosed in an electronic box containing the auxiliary electronic systems for the interlock that prevents accidental radiation leakages due to incorrect operation of the radiation-shielded cabinet elements.

15.4.2 Geometrical Configuration

Small-animal micro-CT systems based on cone-beam geometry should accomplish two basic design criteria: the resolution of the reconstructed data has to be high enough to image anatomical structures with the appropriate level of detail (~100 μm), and the transaxial FOV has to be large enough for small laboratory rodents (about 75 mm in diameter). The distances from the source to the object (D_{so}) and from the object to the detector (D_{od}) determine the size of the FOV and the magnification factor, according to the following expressions [1,46,47]:

$$\mathrm{FOV} = \frac{T_d}{M} \tag{15.3}$$

$$M = \frac{D_{so} + D_{od}}{D_{so}} \tag{15.4}$$

where T_d is the size of the flat-panel detector active area and M is the magnification factor. The useful FOV is defined as the length of the rotation axis intersected by the effective cone beam (Figure 15.7); the "effective" section of the cone beam is that which intersects the active area of the detector.

In order to assess the suitability of the design parameters, the theoretical system resolution can be estimated as the convolution of the effects of the finite focal spot size in the source (ρ_f) and the intrinsic resolution of the detector (ρ_d) [47].

The component of system resolution due to the detector (θ_d) can be calculated at the center of the FOV using the following expression:

$$\theta_d = \frac{\rho_d}{M} \tag{15.5}$$

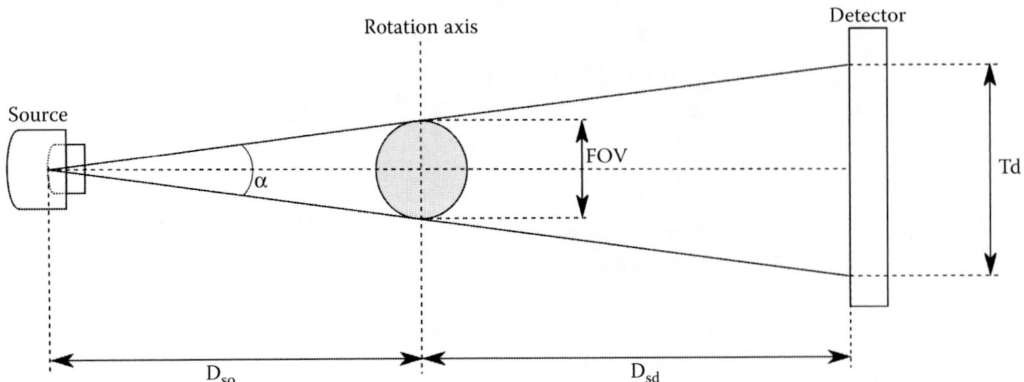

FIGURE 15.7 Geometry of the micro-CT system. T_d refers to the usable size of the x-ray CMOS detector.

If ρ_f is the focal spot size of the source, then θ_f at the center of the FOV is

$$\theta_f = \rho_f \frac{M-1}{M} \tag{15.6}$$

Assuming a Gaussian distribution for θ_f and θ_d, the resulting resolution for the reconstructed images can be estimated theoretically according to the formula

$$\theta = \sqrt{\theta_d^2 + \theta_f^2} \tag{15.7}$$

System resolution could be degraded by other factors associated with the tomographic reconstruction process and by submillimetric mechanical misalignments. Correct alignment between the source and the detector is critical to achieve the theoretical resolution value and avoid the presence of artifacts in the reconstructed image [48]. There are several suitable methods of experimentally estimating the differences between the geometrical parameters of the real system and those of the original design [49–52]. These methods are usually based on the acquisition of a phantom with a known geometry whose projection trajectories are fitted to the theoretical trajectories (derived from the ideal geometrical arrangement) to calculate the deviation between the real and theoretical configuration parameters.

The geometrical parameters of the micro-CT subsystem of the Argus PET/CT (D_{so} = 219.8 mm and D_{od} = 131.9 mm, α = 19.4°, T_d = 120 mm) were selected to meet the design constraints, namely, resolution, FOV size, and available space. The adopted solution leads to a magnification factor (M) of 1.6 and to a theoretical resolution of 12 cycles/mm (measured as the modulation transfer function [MTF] 10%), or about 40 μm in the spatial domain.

In this system, the geometrical deviation from the original design is measured by means of an analytical procedure based on the assessment of the elliptical trajectories shown by two ball bearings placed in a soft material, such as foam, as described in [51]. Using this method it is possible to estimate the values of two of the three tilt angles of the detector, the position of the real center for the image (i.e., the projection pixel for the central and orthogonal ray), and the actual distance between the x-ray source and the flat-panel detector. The remaining angle, although not as critical as the previous two [51,53,54], should first be reduced as much as possible to be able to assume that its value is close to zero. The correct alignment in the direction of this angle is mechanically assessed. The estimated angular deviations are mechanically corrected. The offset of the central ray position is corrected online during the acquisition process.

15.4.3 Data Acquisition

Several acquisition schemes make it possible to obtain the projection data for the different angular positions. There are two main trends for the acquisition of micro-CT data. Some devices use a continuous rotation acquisition protocol, where a moving gantry performs a continuous motion while projection data are acquired. This approach has the advantage of faster acquisition times when a fast detector is used, although the effect of image lag and mechanical imperfections are more conspicuous. An alternative is the acquisition of a stack of frames for each angular projection, with the gantry steady during the acquisition (step-and-shoot). While the gantry rotates, no image is acquired and the radiation beam is blocked to minimize the effect of image lag.

The step-and-shoot approach used in the Argus PET/CT system is implemented by means of an event-driven finite-state machine with two possible states to take advantage of the maximum detector transfer rate [55] and to reduce acquisition time and delivered dose. The first state (step) is used to move the gantry to the next angular position and, if needed, to save data from RAM memory to a disk. The second (shoot) performs two tasks:

1. Launching the acquisition of either a single frame or a frame sequence in the current angular position.
2. Processing the dataset acquired in the previous gantry position.

The transition between states is triggered in synchrony with the detector integration period (T_{vc}), as shown in Figure 15.8.

The processing tasks necessary to generate a projection image are performed online during the shoot state. The correction procedures are explained in the following section.

Quality of the projection images can be improved by acquiring and averaging several frames per angular position. In this case, the finite-state machine remains in shoot state for a time equal to T_{VC}*N, where N is the desired number of frames, until the last frame of the current projection

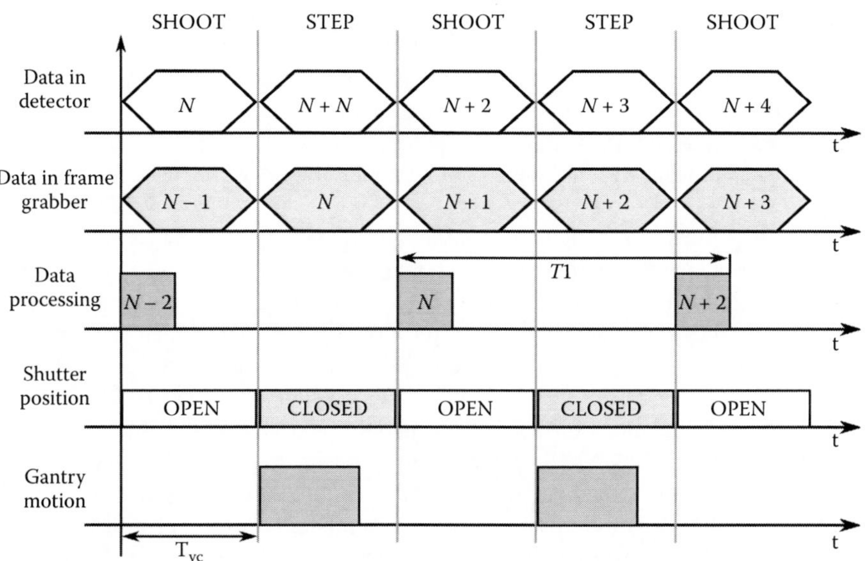

FIGURE 15.8 High-speed acquisition protocol. T_{vc} stands for the integration period in the detector and $T1$ represents the time elapsed between triggering of an image acquisition and storage of already processed images in RAM before they can be saved to disk. The state transitions are shown in the last row of the chronogram and the gray rectangle indicates the time spent by the acquisition software to process the dataset acquired in the previous gantry position.

arrives. Therefore, in the multiframe case there are several "state 1" periods between two "state 2" periods. Additional prereconstruction processing, such as filtering, can be performed during "state 1" intervals, when the CPU is idling.

If the sample is too large to fit inside a single axial FOV, the whole volume can be acquired by performing rotations combined with axial shifts of the bed. From the parameters of the detector and the requirements of the given acquisition, it is possible to calculate the time taken by the acquisition process. This effective acquisition time (excluding warm-up and sample positioning) is given (in seconds) by the following expression:

$$T_{\text{acq}} = \left(\frac{1}{FR}\right) \cdot (Av_{\text{img}} + N_{\text{loss}}) \cdot N_{\text{p}} \cdot N_{\text{FOV}} \tag{15.8}$$

where

- FR is the frame rate from the detector in images per second.
- Av_{img} is the number of averaged frames per projection image.
- N_{loss} is the number of frames lost due to the motion of the rotating stage per each angular projection (one in the current implementation).
- N_{p} is the number of angular views acquired over the defined gantry rotation span.
- *N*FOV is the number of axial bed positions.

These parameters can be balanced to configure different acquisition protocols: for example, one option could be a high-speed, low-resolution, and low-dose scan, or alternatively a slower, high-resolution, and high-dose scan. In each case, the exposure time is controlled by synchronizing the gantry rotation and shutter with the master timing from the frame grabber.

15.4.3.1 Online Correction of Raw Data

Most of the corrections to be applied to the projections can be performed online during the acquisition process, thus reducing processing time for tomographic image reconstruction.

First, despite the offset subtraction performed by the CDS circuit, every pixel has a slight offset level that must be canceled to obtain optimal image quality. In order to estimate this offset level, it is necessary to acquire an image with no x-ray radiation reaching the detector (dark current image) at the same temperature and with the same binning configuration as that used for tomographic data acquisition.

After offset correction, the spatial variation of pixel sensitivity must be reduced. Pixel response can be equalized by acquiring an image with a homogeneous radiation field and no object between the x-ray source and the detector (flood-field image). Again, the acquisition setting must match the one planned for the subsequent tomographic acquisition. In order to calculate the equalized image, the offset corrected image is divided by the flood-field image, thus providing a flat sensitivity profile across the image pixels.

Once the image is equalized, a further correction must be performed to obtain a projection dataset free of artifacts. Due to the CMOS manufacturing process, some lines, columns, or single pixels of the pixel matrix (usually called "dead elements") do not show an appropriate response to the incoming radiation, thus giving a minimum or maximum signal value regardless of the radiation intensity. The correction is performed by linear interpolation of the value given by the adjacent elements of the detector.

Finally, the attenuation image is generated by calculating the logarithm of the corrected projection image [56].

The different correction steps, as well as their effect on the image, are shown in Figure 15.9.

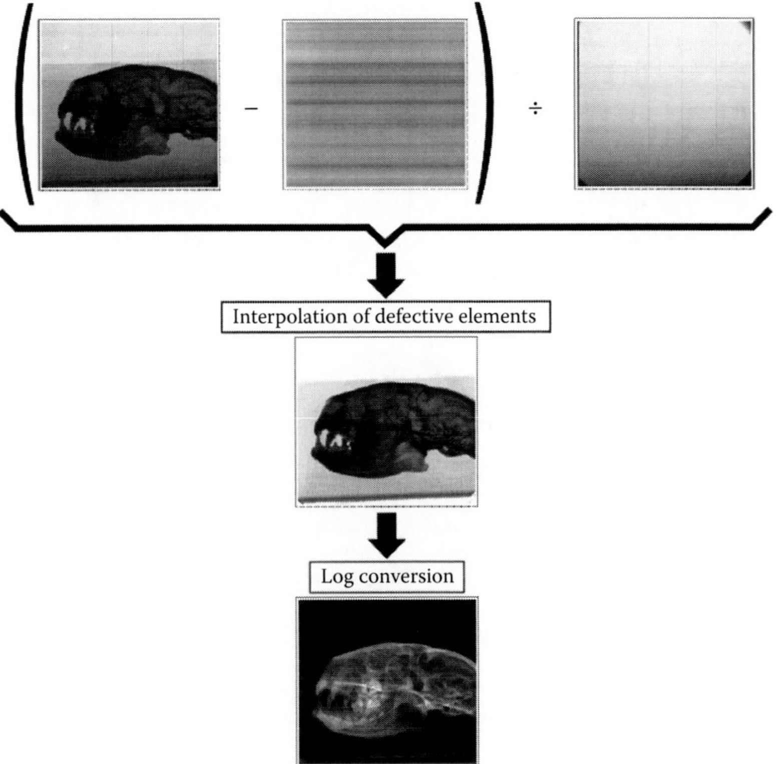

FIGURE 15.9 Raw image correction stages.

15.4.4 Tomographic Image Reconstruction

Data obtained by cone-beam micro-CT systems with a circular orbit do not fulfill Tuy's condition, which is required to guarantee consistency in an analytical reconstruction [57]. Therefore, to obtain the reconstructed volume, it is necessary to use approximated algorithms derived from filtered backprojection (FBP)—such as the one proposed by Feldkamp, Davis, and Kress, known as FDK, first described in [58]—or iterative approaches. Approximated algorithms reconstruct the image by performing a modified FBP that minimizes the effects of the inconsistency of acquired data. Iterative and statistical algorithms, on the other hand, are intrinsically able to deal with data inconsistency. Iterative algebraic algorithms, such as the algebraic reconstruction technique [59], model the reconstruction problem as a set of algebraic equations and solve the inverse problem to obtain the attenuation value for each voxel in the reconstructed volume. One special category of iterative reconstruction methods includes those based on a statistical treatment of acquired data. These techniques treat the reconstruction as a statistical estimation problem and model the noise properties of the acquired data, achieving the best results when the original data are very noisy (e.g., at low radiation doses).

Statistical methods are now the preferred reconstruction strategy in other biomedical imaging techniques such as PET or SPECT. However, these methods present a much larger computational burden than the analytical algorithms; therefore, FDK-based methods are the preferred reconstruction technique for cone-beam micro-CT [9].

In order to provide consistent attenuation values for different materials, regardless of the scanner settings used in the experiment, the resulting volumetric data are usually represented in Hounsfield units (HU), which relate the attenuation of the different materials with that of water and are not affected by the spectral properties of the x-ray beam [18]. The conversion into HU requires a previous calibration step for different spectral configurations using several materials with a known HU value.

In the Argus PET/CT, reconstruction is performed by means of a modified FDK algorithm with a Ram–Lak filter. The algorithm is adapted to the specific geometry of the scanner, and includes beam hardening correction and HU calibration, using a phantom with seven different known materials (air, water, PMMA, Nylon, Delrin, PTFE, and aluminum). The calibration parameters are obtained for four standard settings of the x-ray beam. The reconstruction software, together with the real-time preprocessing during acquisition, achieves reasonable reconstruction times on standard personal computers (100 seconds to reconstruct a 512^3 voxels volume using a 2.80-GHz dual-core CPU with 8 GB of RAM).

15.5 EVALUATION OF MICRO-CT SYSTEMS

An evaluation of small-animal micro-CT performance enables us to determine the quality of the projection images and reconstructed data and to estimate the dose received by the sample.

The following sections present different techniques to evaluate the performance of small-animal micro-CT systems, based on the results obtained for the Argus PET/CT. A complete description of these results can be found in [15].

15.5.1 X-Ray Flat-Panel Detectors

The features that give flat-panel detectors a greater impact on the quality of the final images are temporal stability, gain linearity, noise level, and resolution. Temporal instability increases artifacts introduced by the detector, and gain linearity affects the accuracy of tomographic image quantification and introduces ring artifacts. The noise level of the projection data is translated into noise in the reconstructed images, and the intrinsic resolution of the detector limits the final resolution that the system can achieve, as shown in Equations 15.5 through 15.7. Detective quantum efficiency for this type of detector has been evaluated in [12,60].

A possible protocol for the measurement of the different parameters and the results obtained for the C7940DK-02 is provided below.

15.5.1.1 Detector Stability

One way to estimate the temporal stability of the detector involves acquisition of a set of flood-field images over a given period of time for a fixed x-ray source setting. Between consecutive acquisitions, the x-ray beam must be stopped to allow for scintillation decay to remove any potential afterglow contamination on the next measurement. The stability of the device can be assessed by plotting the mean pixel value as a function of time.

In order to illustrate this procedure using the CA7940DK-02 system, 360 consecutive flood-field images were acquired at 30 kV and 0.4 μA with no object between the source and the detector. Exposures were separated by 10-s intervals.

Measurements show a peak-to-valley ratio during the experiment lower than 0.05% of the mean pixel value. This result indicates that the flat-panel detector is stable enough and the reconstructed images will not be affected by this parameter.

15.5.1.2 Detector Gain Linearity

The linearity of the detector response with the radiation received can be measured by plotting the mean pixel value as a function of the anode current. Since radiation intensity is directly proportional to the anode current [61], a linear trend is expected for the mean pixel value. For the test carried out on the C7940DK-02 system, the x-ray beam peak energy was set at 40 kV, with anode current ranging from 200 to 500 μA. A 1-mm-thick aluminum filter was placed in front of the x-ray source to reproduce a setup commonly used for CT acquisition. The images were acquired with a homogeneous radiation field and no object between the x-ray source and detector. The result of the test shows an excellent degree of linearity ($R^2 > 0.99$) over the dynamic range of the detector.

15.5.1.3 Detector Noise Level

The noise level in the acquired projection data has a considerable impact on the final achievable quality. It can be measured by the SNR of a set of flood-field images as a function of the anode current.

The SNR was measured as a function of anode current for the C7940DK-02. As in the previous measurement, peak x-ray beam energy was set at 40 kV, with anode current ranging from 200 to 500 μA and a 1-mm-thick aluminum filter. The trend observed was as expected.

15.5.1.4 Detector Spatial Resolution

The resolution of x-ray imaging detectors is usually expressed in terms of the presampled MTF. This describes the signal transfer characteristics as a function of spatial frequency taking into account all the detection stages except for sampling. If the sampling stage is included in the calculation, the detector spatial response may become undersampled, leading to aliasing errors in the estimated MTF.

Among the different methods proposed to estimate the presampled MTF, those based on imaging a slanted slit or a slanted edge are the most widely used due to their relatively easy implementation and accurate results.

The following sections present a brief description of the procedure proposed in [62,63], which implements a variation of the slanted-edge method. A comprehensive review of the different versions of the slanted-edge approach can be found in [64]. The selected algorithm is based on the analysis of the edge response function (ERF), which is obtained by imaging a phantom consisting of an x-ray-opaque object with a polished edge. The phantom is placed directly over the detector surface at a shallow angle (1.5°–3°) with respect to the pixel matrix. The edge position is estimated with subpixel accuracy in the image area by using linear interpolation. This position is then fitted to a straight line by linear regression.

The slope of this line is used to determine the number of rows (N_{av}) necessary for a 1-pixel lateral shift of the edge position in the original image (Figure 15.10).

The algorithm generates an oversampled ERF using the pixel value at the edge position for N_{av} consecutive rows. As depicted in Figure 15.10, the value of the pixel in the first row (triangular mark) corresponds to the first data point of the ERF. Then, the pixel value of the second row (square mark) yields the second data point, and so on. Finally, the pixel value of the N_{av}th row (fifth row in Figure 15.10) is the last data point of the ERF.

The detector area is split up into groups of N_{av} rows, and oversampled ERFs are estimated for each of the groups according to the process explained. These calculated ERFs are then aligned by linear regression and averaged to reduce noise.

The line spread function (LSF) is estimated as the 3-point derivative of the average ERF. Finally, an estimation of the MTF is obtained as the Fourier transform of the LSF. The calculated estimation

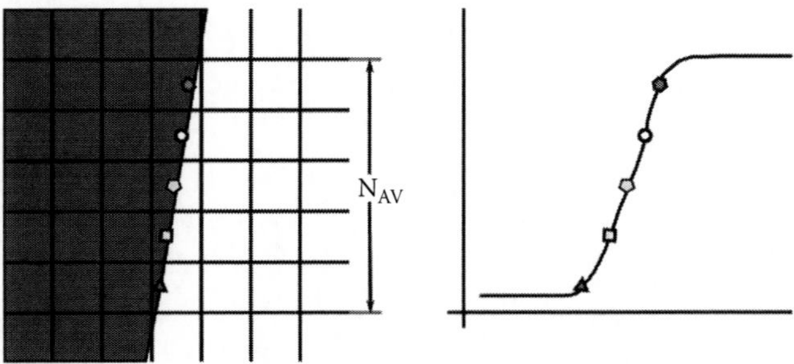

FIGURE 15.10 Estimation of the oversampled ERF from the slanted-edge images.

is corrected for the sinc function introduced by the derivative operation, and the frequency axis is corrected for the slant angle. The result is an accurate estimation of the presampled MTF.

Another interesting parameter is the effective MTF of the system that reflects the combined effect of the detector and the finite focal spot size of the source. This can be obtained by imaging the same phantom at nominal system magnification [46] and estimating the actual resolution of the projection data of a sample placed at the center of rotation of the micro-CT system. Figure 15.11 plots the presampled MTF obtained for the flat-panel detector of the C7940DK-02. The spatial frequency where the MTF falls to 10% of the zero-frequency value (MTF10%) was 8.1 lpmm, a figure compatible with the manufacturer's specifications. MTF10% measured at the nominal system magnification was 11.85 cycles/mm, almost 1.6 times the intrinsic resolution, as expected due to the magnification factor used.

15.5.2 Quality Evaluation of Reconstructed Images

The quality of the reconstructed images determines their utility in preclinical studies. However, in longitudinal *in vivo* studies it is necessary to reach a trade-off between image quality and accumulated radiation dose, as several CT scans are usually acquired during the experiment.

The parameters that determine the quality of the final images in preclinical applications are the noise in the reconstructed image, the contrast-to-noise ratio (CNR), spatial resolution, and HU accuracy.

Various strategies are available to measure each of the aforementioned parameters. The methods presented in [15] were used to assess the Argus PET/CT, as described below.

Noise in reconstructed images was evaluated on a homogeneous water phantom by measuring the standard deviation of the signal in HU as a function of radiated dose. The phantom was acquired six times at 25 kV and 0.6 μA at different doses (different number of averaged images for each angular position).

The measured noise level decreased proportionally to the square root of the dose, as expected, according to theoretical noise models for CT images [65]. A good soft tissue contrast is achieved for a noise level below 50 HU, which corresponded to a radiated dose of 75 mGy in our system. The curve of noise level as a function of dose can be found in Figure 15.12.

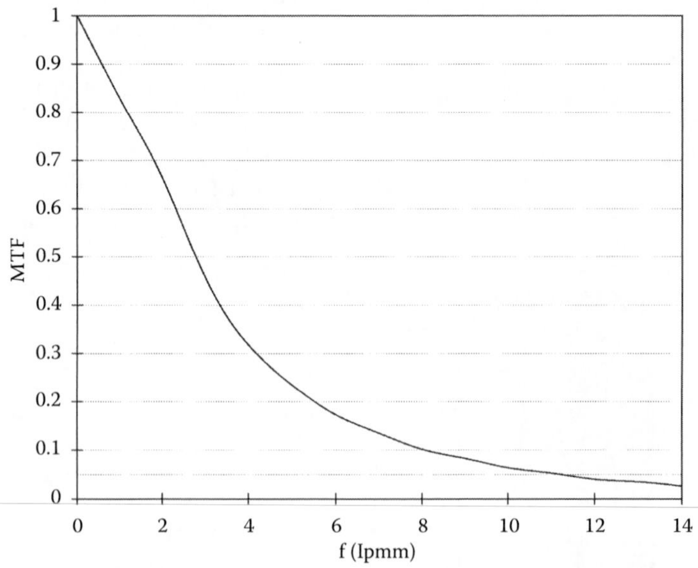

FIGURE 15.11 Presampled modulation transfer function measured with a slanted-edge method.

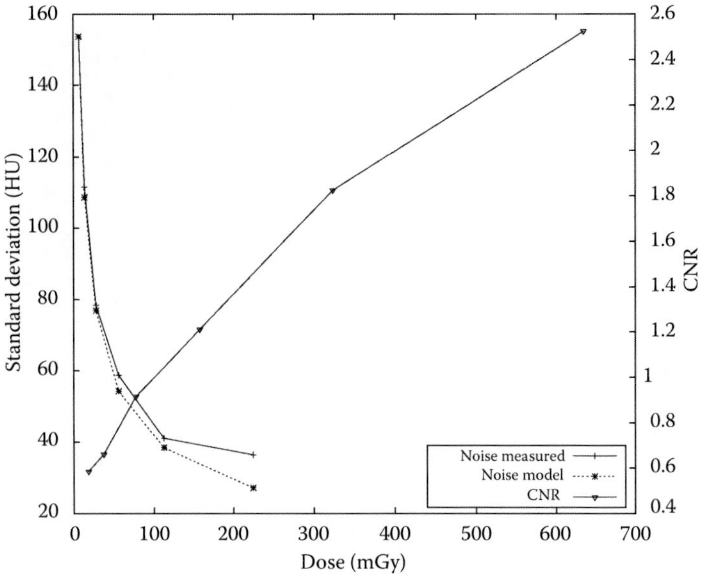

FIGURE 15.12 Noise level (standard deviation) in HUs measured and estimated using the Gaussian model and measured CNR as a function of radiated dose.

Image CNR was measured as a function of radiated dose using a contrast phantom consisting of a nylon cylinder (1.15 g/cm^3) immersed in a water container. CNR is defined as

$$\mathrm{CNR} = \frac{|\mu_n - \mu_w|}{\sqrt{\sigma_n^2 + \sigma_w^2}} \tag{15.9}$$

where μ and σ represent, respectively, the mean and standard deviation of the pixel values in the reconstructed images corresponding to water (μ_w, σ_w) and nylon (μ_n, σ_n), obtained from regions of interest created by gray-level thresholding.

Figure 15.12 shows a plot of the CNR versus the radiated dose. CNR increases almost proportionally to the square root of the dose. The CNR obtained for a dose of 75 mGy is 0.98.

The system resolution was measured following the standard test method E1695–95 [66], which is based on the examination of the CT image of a uniform disk of polycarbonate (1.18 gr/cm^3) (Figure 15.13). The resolution value is derived from an analysis of the edge of the disk; in other words, the ERF is obtained and the LSF and MTF are calculated. The cutoff point where the MTF decreases below 10% of its maximum value is given as the standard resolution measurement.

In the Argus PET/CT, the MTF at 10% was 11.3 cycles/mm, or 44 μm in the spatial domain (Figure 15.13). The difference between the actual resolution obtained from the reconstructed images and the resolution measured in projection data is due to the reconstruction process and possible submillimetric misalignments [51].

The accuracy of the HU values has been assessed with the calibration phantom previously described. The phantom was previously imaged using a properly calibrated clinical CT scanner (Toshiba Aquillion 16) for two x-ray peak energy settings. The values obtained for each of the materials on the phantom were averaged over the whole area covered by them.

The same values were obtained from a third acquisition of the phantom with the small-animal micro-CT system.

Finally, the values obtained by both scanners were compared, assuming those measured by the clinical system as the gold standard.

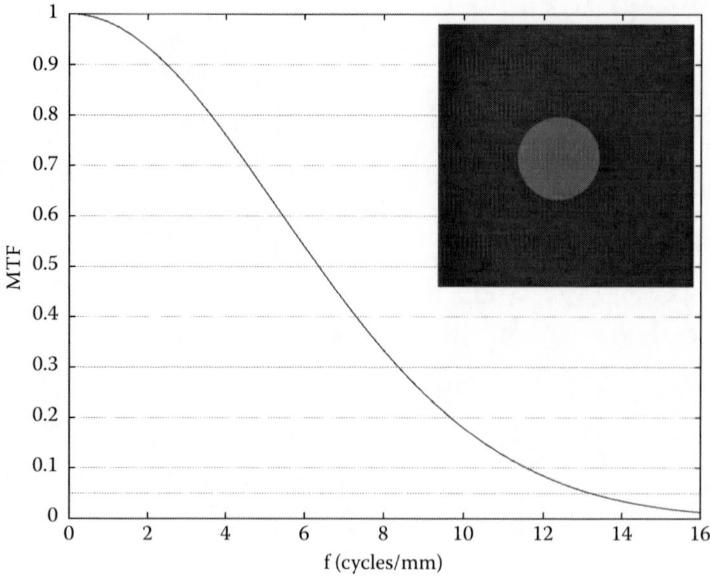

FIGURE 15.13 Modulation transfer function after tomographic reconstruction calculated using the standard protocol E1695–95. In the upper right corner of the plot a transaxial image of the polycarbonate disk used is shown.

The results of the cross-validation of the HU conversion are shown in Table 15.3. The data obtained by the micro-CT agree to a large extent with those provided by the clinical scanner, thus proving the accuracy of the HU conversion. A strong deviation for very dense materials such as metals, due to the low peak energy of the spectra generated by the micro-focus x-ray source, can be observed.

15.5.3 Radiation Dose

Another important consideration in the design of *in vivo* micro-CT systems is the dose delivered to the animal. Therefore, it is necessary to provide software and hardware tools to allow the user to select the best settings for each application. Of particular importance is the resolution setting, because, if the image resolution is doubled for a given x-ray setting, voxel noise increases four times and the dose has to increase 16 times to maintain the same SNR [67]. For this reason, special care must be taken with x-ray settings for ultrahigh-resolution protocols.

TABLE 15.3
HUs Evaluation Results

Material	Toshiba Aquillion 16 (Peak Energy 120 kV)	Toshiba Aquillion 16 (Peak Energy 135 kV)	Micro-CT (Peak Energy 45 kV)
Air	−1005	−1002	−998
Water	−4	−1	1
PMMA	124	118	120
Nylon	242	290	224
Delrin	567	626	640
PTFE	885	960	937
Aluminum	4100	4070	4892

TABLE 15.4
X-Ray Settings and Radiation Dose for Acquisition Protocols

Voltage (kV)	Current (μA)	Time	Resolution (μm)	Radiation Dose (mGy)
25	600	6′00″	200	33.73
40	750	6′30″	100	165.2

The measurement of absorbed dose may provide a more reliable assessment of *in vivo* biological effects than that offered by the incident radiation measurements. In the example system, thermoluminescent dosimeters (STI, TLD-100) were introduced into representative organs in euthanized rats that had undergone standard acquisition protocols.

The dose values obtained show the potential damage to the animal for different acquisition settings.

Table 15.4 shows the results and acquisition settings for two standard protocols. The first, which is intended to provide anatomical information for PET-CT studies, does not provide high spatial resolution, as PET image resolution is usually worse than 1 mm. The second protocol represents a high-resolution setting for bone tissue, which needs higher voltage and current. The radiation doses obtained (Table 15.4) were, respectively, 0.5% and 2% of the LD50/30 (~7.3 Gy) for small rodents [67,68]. Typical results reported in the literature of delivered dose to the animal in micro-CT scans are about 100–300 mGy [69,70].

15.5.4 Small-Animal Studies

To illustrate the performance of micro-CT scanners in small-animal *in vivo* imaging and the kind of information that they can provide to the user, two examples of datasets acquired on real experiments are shown in this section. Figure 15.14 depicts a coronal view of a tomographic reconstruction of a mouse study where anatomical x-ray images and functional PET data were used. The image shows a high contrast in the abdominal area, allowing the segmentation of the different organs and muscles from the surrounding adipose tissue. No contrast agent was used in this protocol.

Figure 15.15 is a volumetric render of the same tomographic dataset. Note the high level of detail obtained in the bony structures.

15.6 CONCLUSIONS

The design of *in vivo* micro-CT scanners for small-animal imaging must address a number of requirements that differ widely from those of other applications, such as *in vitro* micro-CT scanners

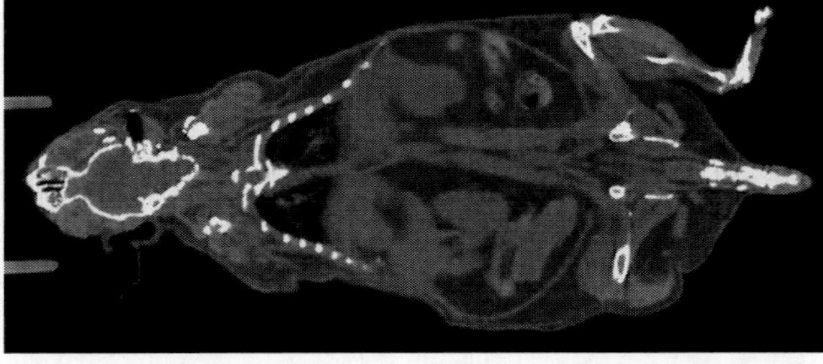

FIGURE 15.14 Coronal slice of a large mouse whole body study. The volume was acquired in two FOV positions with a 125-μm pixel size, 360 angular projections, 8 images averaged per projection, 40-kV peak x-ray beam energy, and a 200-μA x-ray source anode current.

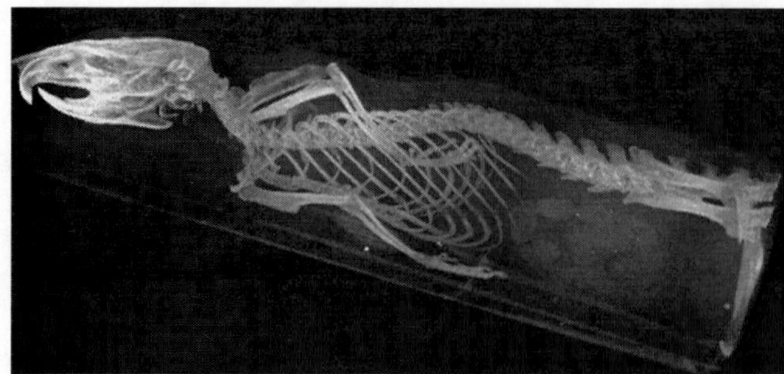

FIGURE 15.15 Volume render of a rat study, 3 beds and pixel size of 0.125 mm. The acquisition parameters were 40 kV, 200 μA, 360 angular projections, 0.125 mm pixel size, and eight images averaged per projection.

or regular clinical CT scanners. The impact of the detector device on the quality of the final image and on the mechanical constraints of the system makes it necessary to select the most appropriate detector from the different commercially available options.

The general overview presented in this chapter should prevent designers with the basic aspects of the development of *in vivo* micro-CT systems. The example used was the Argus PET/CT. A complete assessment of its performance was provided with emphasis on the detector component.

The size of commercial CMOS flat-panel detectors makes them a suitable choice for small-animal imaging, since they are more compact than CCDs, the most widely used small-animal imaging system.

State-of-the-art CMOS flat-panel detectors offer good results in terms of noise, contrast, and resolution, thus making it possible to optimize image quality in terms of dose radiated.

When using low-power x-ray sources, one way to improve the SNR and, therefore, contrast of images in soft tissue, is to optimize exposure time. In this context, optimization of the acquisition protocol allows the designer to better exploit the features of the detector, thus improving system performance with regard to per-animal screening time.

The resolution of the reconstructed data should be in the tens-of-micrometer range in most multimodality preclinical experiments. This high-resolution value is achieved, thanks to the magnification effect inherent to the cone-beam geometry and to the detector and x-ray tube features. High-resolution *in vivo* imaging may show slight quality degradation due to movements such as breathing or heartbeat. Gating the projection acquisition or performing retrospective gating over multiple exposures per projection [71] can help to recover this resolution loss at the cost of increased radiation dose and acquisition time. In addition, high-resolution imaging requires precise characterization of the system alignment; mechanical misalignments that could not be corrected have to be taken into account during the image reconstruction process, and this may prevent the use of symmetries, thus increasing reconstruction time considerably.

Equations 15.5 through 15.7 describe how the detector and source components affect the final resolution and show that the limiting factor in regular *in vivo* micro-CT systems is the intrinsic resolution of the detector, since the size of the finite focal spot has a negligible impact due to the magnification factor used in systems based on microfocus x-ray tubes.

REFERENCES

1. M. J. Paulus, S. S. Gleason, S. J. Kennel, P. R. Hunsicker, and D. K. Johnson, High resolution x-ray computed tomography: An emerging tool for small animal cancer research, *Neoplasia*, 2, 62–70, 2000.
2. H. Ebina, J. Hatakeyama, M. Onodera, T. Honma, S. Kamakura, H. Shimauchi, and Y. Sasano, Micro-CT analysis of alveolar bone healing using a rat experimental model of critical-size defects, *Oral Diseases*, 15, 273–280, 2009.

3. N. M. Harrison, P. F. McDonnell, D. C. O'Mahoney, O. D. Kennedy, F. J. O'Brien, and P. E. McHugh, Heterogeneous linear elastic trabecular bone modelling using micro-CT attenuation data and experimentally measured heterogeneous tissue properties, *Journal of Biomechanics*, 41, 2589–2596, 2008.
4. J. U. Umoh, A. V. Sampaio, I. Welch, V. Pitelka, H. A. Goldberg, T. M. Underhill, and D. W. Holdsworth, *In vivo* micro-CT analysis of bone remodeling in a rat calvarial defect model, *Physics in Medicine and Biology*, 54, 2147–2161, 2009.
5. T. Engelhorn, I. Y. Eyupoglu, M. A. Schwarz, M. Karolczak, H. Bruenner, T. Struffert, W. Kalender, and A. Doerfler, *In vivo* micro-CT imaging of rat brain glioma: A comparison with 3 T MRI and histology, *Neuroscience Letters*, 458, 28–31, 2009.
6. H. Parameswaran, E. Bartolak-Suki, H. Hamakawa, A. Majumdar, P. G. Allen, and B. Suki, Three-dimensional measurement of alveolar airspace volumes in normal and emphysematous lungs using micro-CT, *Journal of Applied Physiology*, 107, 583–592, 2009.
7. S. C. Thacker, V. V. Nagarkar, and H. J. Liang, Characterization of a novel microCT detector for small animal computed tomogaphy (CT), *Medical Imaging 2007: Physics of Medical Imaging, Pts 1–3*, 6510, U1511–U1522, 2007.
8. V. V. Nagarkar, S. V. Tipnis, I. Shestakova, V. Gaysinskiy, B. Singh, M. J. Paulus, and G. Entine, A high-speed functional microCT detector for small animal studies, *IEEE Transactions on Nuclear Science*, 53, 2500–2505, 2006.
9. C. T. Badea, M. Drangova, D. W. Holdsworth, and G. A. Johnson, *In vivo* small-animal imaging using micro-CT and digital subtraction angiography, *Physics in Medicine and Biology*, 53, R319–R350, 2008.
10. A. L. Goertzen, V. Nagarkar, R. A. Street, M. J. Paulus, J. M. Boone, and S. R. Cherry, A comparison of x-ray detectors for mouse CT imaging, *Physics in Medicine and Biology*, 49, 5251–5265, 2004.
11. D. A. Jaffray and J. H. Siewerdsen, Cone-beam computed tomography with a flat-panel imager: Initial performance characterization, *Medical Physics*, 27, 1311–1323, 2000.
12. H. K. Kim, S. C. Lee, M. H. Cho, S. Y. Lee, and G. Cho, Use of a flat-panel detector for microtomography: A feasibility study for small-animal imaging, *IEEE Transactions on Nuclear Science*, 52, 193–198, 2005.
13. I. Fujieda, G. Cho, J. Drewery, T. Gee, T. Jing, S. N. Kaplan, V. Perezmendez, D. Wildermuth, and R. A. Street, X-ray and charged-particle detection with Csi(Tl) layer coupled to a-Si-H photodiode layers, *IEEE Transactions on Nuclear Science*, 38, 255–262, 1991.
14. E. Miyata, M. Miki, N. Tawa, D. Kamiyama, and K. Miyaguchi, Development of new x-ray imaging device sensitive to 0.1–100 keV, *Nuclear Instruments and Methods in Physics Research Section A—Accelerators Spectrometers Detectors and Associated Equipment*, 525, 122–125, 2004.
15. J. J. Vaquero, S. Redondo, E. Lage, M. Abella, A. Sisniega, G. Tapias, M. L. S. Montenegro, and M. Desco, Assessment of a new high-performance small-animal x-ray tomograph, *IEEE Transactions on Nuclear Science*, 55, 898–905, 2008.
16. J. J. Vaquero, E. Lage, L. Ricon, M. Abella, E. Vicente, and M. Desco, rPET detectors design and data processing, *2005 IEEE Nuclear Science Symposium Conference Record*, 1–5, 2885–2889, 2005.
17. Y. C. Wang, J. Seidel, B. M. W. Tsui, J. J. Vaquero, and M. G. Pomper, Performance evaluation of the GE healthcare eXplore VISTA dual-ring small-animal PET scanner, *Journal of Nuclear Medicine*, 47, 1891–1900, 2006.
18. W. A. Kalender, *Computed Tomography: Fundamentals, System Technology, Image Quality, Applications* (2 edn), Erlangen, Publicis, 2005.
19. D. Okkalides, Contrast reduction in digital images due to x-ray induced damage to a TV camera's CCD image receptor, *Physics in Medicine and Biology*, 44, N63–N68, 1999.
20. H. K. Kim, I. A. Cunningham, Z. Yin, and G. Cho, On the development of digital radiography detectors: A review, *International Journal of Precision Engineering and Manufacturing*, 9, 86–100, 2008.
21. C. Frojdh, H. Graafsma, H. E. Nilsson, and C. Ponchut, Characterization of a pixellated CdTe detector with single-photon processing readout, *Nuclear Instruments and Methods in Physics Research Section A—Accelerators Spectrometers Detectors and Associated Equipment*, 563, 128–132, 2006.
22. K. Kowase and K. Ogawa, Photon counting x-ray CT system with a semiconductor detector, *IEEE Nuclear Science Symposium Conference Record*, 5, 3119–3123, 2006.
23. Y. Onishi, T. Nakashima, A. Koike, H. Morii, Y. Neo, H. Mimura, and T. Aoki, Material discriminated x-ray CT by using conventional microfocus x-ray tube and CdTe imager, *2007 IEEE Nuclear Science Symposium Conference Record*, 1–11, 1170–1174, 2007.
24. J. P. Schlomka, E. Roessl, R. Dorscheid, S. Dill, G. Martens, T. Istel, C. Baumer et al., Experimental feasibility of multi-energy photon-counting K-edge imaging in pre-clinical computed tomography, *Physics in Medicine and Biology*, 53, 4031–4047, 2008.

25. W. A. Kalender and Y. Kyriakou, Flat-detector computed tomography (FD-CT), *European Radiology*, 17, 2767–2779, 2007.
26. S. O. Kasap, M. Z. Kabir, and J. A. Rowlands, Recent advances in x-ray photoconductors for direct conversion x-ray image detectors, *Current Applied Physics*, 6, 288–292, 2006.
27. J. Yorkston, Recent developments in digital radiography detectors, *Nuclear Instruments and Methods in Physics Research Section A—Accelerators Spectrometers Detectors and Associated Equipment*, 580, 974–985, 2007.
28. T. Gomi, K. Koshida, T. Miyati, J. Miyagawa, and H. Hirano, An experimental comparison of flat-panel detector performance for direct and indirect systems (initial experiences and physical evaluation), *Journal of Digital Imaging*, 19, 362–370, 2006.
29. G. Hajdok, J. J. Battista, and I. A. Cunningham, Fundamental x-ray interaction limits in diagnostic imaging detectors: Spatial resolution, *Medical Physics*, 35, 3180–3193, 2008.
30. G. Hajdok, J. J. Battista, and I. A. Cunningham, Fundamental x-ray interaction limits in diagnostic imaging detectors: Frequency-dependent Swank noise, *Medical Physics*, 35, 3194–3204, 2008.
31. G. Hajdok, J. Yao, J. J. Battista, and I. A. Cunningham, Signal and noise transfer properties of photoelectric interactions in diagnostic x-ray imaging detectors, *Medical Physics*, 33, 3601–3620, 2006.
32. H. K. Kim, S. M. Yun, J. S. Ko, G. Cho, and T. Graeve, Cascade modeling of pixelated scintillator detectors for x-ray imaging, *IEEE Transactions on Nuclear Science*, 55, 1357–1366, 2008.
33. G. F. Knoll, *Radiation Detection and Measurement* (3 ed.), New York: John Wiley & Sons, 2000.
34. M. Nikl, Scintillation detectors for x-rays, *Measurement Science and Technology*, 17, R37–R54, 2006.
35. B. K. Cha, J. H. Shin, J. H. Bae, C. H. Lee, S. H. Chang, H. K. Kim, C. K. Kim, and G. Cho, Scintillation characteristics and imaging performance of CsI:Tl thin films for x-ray imaging applications, *Nuclear Instruments and Methods in Physics Research Section A—Accelerators Spectrometers Detectors and Associated Equipment*, 604, 224–228, 2009.
36. H. Mori, R. Kyuushima, K. Fujita, and M. Honda, High resolution and high sensitivity CMOS PANEL SENSORS for x-ray, *2001 IEEE Nuclear Science Symposium, Conference Records*, 1–4, 29–33, 2002.
37. A. Theuwissen, CMOS image sensors: State-of-the-art and future perspectives, *ESSDERC 2007: Proceedings of the 37th European Solid-State Device Research Conference,* 21–27, Munich, 2007.
38. J. A. Rowlands and J. Yorkston, Flat panel detectors for digital radiography, in *Handbook of Medical Imaging Vol. 1—Physics and Psychophysics,* J. Beutel, H. L. Kundel, and R. L. Van Metter, Eds., Bellingham, WA: SPIE Press, 223–328, 2000.
39. Y. Izumi, O. Teranuma, T. Sato, K. Uehara, H. Okada, S. Tokuda, and T. Sato, Development of flat-panel x-ray image sensors. *Sharp Technical Journal*, 80, 25–30, 2001. Available: http://sharp-world.com/corporate/info/rd/tj3/3-6.html
40. S. Ricq, F. Glasser, and M. Garcin, Study of CdTe and CdZnTe detectors for x-ray computed tomography, in *11th International Workshop on Room-Temperature Semiconductor X- and Gamma-Ray Detectors and Associated Electronics*, Vienna, Austria, pp. 534–543, 1999.
41. M. Funaki, Y. Ando, R. Jinnai, A. Tachinaba, and R. Ohno. Development of CdTe detectors in Acrorad. Available at : http://www.acrorad.jp/pdf/Development_of_CdTe_detectors.pdf.
42. M. Tamaki, Y. Mito, Y. Shuto, T. Kiyuna, M. Yamamoto, K. Sagae, T. Kina, T. Koizumi, and R. Ohno, Development of 4-sides buttable CdTe-ASIC hybrid module for x-ray flat panel detector, *IEEE Transactions on Nuclear Science*, 56, 1791–1794, 2009.
43. K. Kim, S. Cho, J. Suh, J. Won, J. Hong, and S. Kim, Schottky-type polycrystalline CdZnTe x-ray detectors, *Current Applied Physics*, 9, 306–310, 2009.
44. H. B. Serreze, G. Entine, R. O. Bell, and F. V. Wald, Advances in CdTe gamma-ray detectors, *IEEE Transactions on Nuclear Science*, 21, 404–407, 1974.
45. A. Cola and I. Farella, The polarization mechanism in CdTe Schottky detectors, *Applied Physics Letters*, 94, 102113, 2009.
46. S. Redondo, J. J. Vaquero, E. Lage, M. Abella, G. Tapias, A. Udias, and M. Desco, Assessment of a new CT system for small animals, in *IEEE Nuclear Science Symposiun and Medical Imaging Conference*, San Diego, 2006.
47. E. Van de Casteele, Model-based approach for beam hardening correction and resolution measurements in microtomography, Department Natuurkunde Antwerpen, University Antwerpen, Antwerpen, 2004.
48. I. Vidal-Migallón, M. Abella, A. Sisniega, J. J. Vaquero, and M. Desco, Simulation of mechanical misalignments in a cone-beam micro-CT system, in *2008 IEEE Nuclear Science Symposium and Medical Imaging Conference*, Dresden, Alemania, 2008.

49. Y. Kyriakou, R. M. Lapp, L. Hillebrand, D. Ertel, and W. A. Kalender, Simultaneous misalignment correction for approximate circular cone-beam computed tomography, *Physics in Medicine and Biology*, 53, 6267–6289, 2008.
50. C. Mennessier, R. Clackdoyle, and F. Noo, Direct determination of geometric alignment parameters for cone-beam scanners, *Physics in Medicine and Biology*, 54, 1633–1660, 2009.
51. F. Noo, R. Clackdoyle, C. Mennessier, T. A. White, and T. J. Roney, Analytic method based on identification of ellipse parameters for scanner calibration in cone-beam tomography, *Physics in Medicine and Biology*, 45, 3489–3508, 2000.
52. K. Yang, A. L. C. Kwan, D. F. Miller, and J. M. Boone, A geometric calibration method for cone beam CT systems, *Medical Physics*, 33, 1695–1706, 2006.
53. G. T. Gullberg, B. M. W. Tsui, C. R. Crawford, J. G. Ballard, and J. T. Hagius, Estimation of geometrical parameters and collimator evaluation for cone beam tomography, *Medical Physics*, 17, 264–272, 1990.
54. J. Y. Li, R. J. Jaszczak, H. L. Wang, K. L. Greer, and R. E. Coleman, Determination of both mechanical and electronic shifts in cone-beam SPECT, *Physics in Medicine and Biology*, 38, 743–754, 1993.
55. Hamamatsu Photonics K. K.—Solid state division, *X-ray flat panel sensor application manual,* rev. 4.3. Hamamatsu city: Hamamatsu Photonics K. K., 2008. Available: http://sales.hamamatsu.com/en/support/application-notes.php
56. E. Lage, J. J. Vaquero, S. Redondo, M. Abella, G. Tapias, A. Udias, and M. Desco, Design and development of a high performance micro-CT system for small-animal imaging, in *IEEE Nuclear Science Symposium and Medical Imaging Conference*, San Diego, 2006.
57. H. K. Tuy, An inversion-formula for cone-beam reconstruction, *SIAM Journal on Applied Mathematics*, 43, 546–552, 1983.
58. L. A. Feldkamp, L. C. Davis, and J. W. Kress, Practical cone-beam algorithm, *Journal of the Optical Society of America a-Optics Image Science and Vision*, 1, 612–619, 1984.
59. R. Gordon, R. Bender, and G. T. Herman, Algebraic reconstruction techniques (Art) for 3-dimensional electron microscopy and x-ray photography, *Journal of Theoretical Biology*, 29, 471–81, 1970.
60. U. Ewert, U. Zscherpel, and K. Bavendiek. (2007, 2009). Replacement of film radiography by digital techniques and enhancement of image quality. Available at: www.ndt.net/search/docs.php3?id=4516.
61. J. M. Boone, X-ray production, interaction and detection in diagnostic imaging, in *Handbook of Medical Imaging Vol. 1—Physics and Psychophysics,* J. Beutel, H. L. Kundel, and R. L. Van Metter, Eds., Bellingham, WA: SPIE Press, 1–78, 2000.
62. E. Buhr, S. Gunther-Kohfahl, and U. Neitzel, Simple method for modulation transfer function determination of digital imaging detectors from edge images, *Medical Imaging 2003: Physics of Medical Imaging, Pts 1 and 2*, 5030, 877–884, 2003.
63. E. Buhr, S. Gunther-Kohfahl, and U. Neitzel, Accuracy of a simple method for deriving the presampled modulation transfer function of a digital radiographic system from an edge image, *Medical Physics*, 30, 2323–2331, 2003.
64. E. Samei, E. Buhr, P. Granfors, D. Vandenbroucke, and X. H. Wang, Comparison of edge analysis techniques for the determination of the MTF of digital radiographic systems, *Physics in Medicine and Biology*, 50, 3613–3625, 2005.
65. H. H. Barrett, S. K. Gordon, and R. S. Hershel, Statistical limitations in transaxial tomography, *Computers in Biology and Medicine*, 6, 307–323, 1976.
66. ASTM Standard E1695-95, Standard test method for measurement of computed tomography (CT) system performance, West Conshohocken, PA: ASTM International, 2001.
67. N. L. Ford, M. M. Thornton, and D. W. Holdsworth, Fundamental image quality limits for microcomputed tomography in small animals, *Medical Physics*, 30, 2869–2877, 2003.
68. A. Obenaus and A. Smith, Radiation dose in rodent tissues during micro-CT imaging, *Journal of X-Ray Science and Technology*, 12, 241–249, 2004.
69. J. M. Boone, O. Velazquez, and S. R. Cherry, Small-animal x-ray dose from micro-CT, *Molecular Imaging*, 3, 149–158, 2004.
70. M. J. Paulus, S. S. Gleason, M. E. Easterly, and C. J. Foltz, A review of high resolution x-ray computed tomography and other imaging modalities for small animal research, *Lab Animal*, 30, 36–45, 2001.
71. C. Chavarrias, J. J. Vaquero, A. Sisniega, A. Rodriguez-Ruano, M. L. Soto-Montenegro, P. Garcia-Barreno, and M. Desco, Extraction of the respiratory signal from small-animal CT projections for a retrospective gating method, *Physics in Medicine and Biology*, 53, 4683–4695, 2008.

16 Portable High-Frequency Ultrasound Imaging System Design and Hardware Considerations

Insoo Kim, Hyunsoo Kim, Flavio Griggio, Richard L. Tutwiler, Thomas N. Jackson, Susan Trolier-McKinstry, and Kyusun Choi

CONTENTS

16.1 INTRODUCTION

Ultrasound techniques have wide use in various applications in numerous fields. The frequency range from 10 kHz to 1 MHz is widely used for sound navigation and ranging (SONAR), ultrasonic welding, therapeutic ultrasound, and humidifiers. A frequency range of 1–50 MHz is commonly used in diagnostic sonography and nondestructive testing to find flaws in materials. Micron-sized silicon surface detection utilizes a frequency range of 50–200 MHz [1], and surface acoustic wave (SAW) devices use frequencies ranging from 1 to 10 GHz.

Ultrasound techniques are also commonly used in diagnostic imaging and often supersede x-ray imaging in the medical sector [2]. The vast majority of medical ultrasound imaging occurs at frequencies between 1 and 50 MHz. For example, a diagnostic imaging that is designed to penetrate tissues to a depth of 5–20 cm uses frequencies between 1 and 10 MHz. Recently, studies for imaging smaller organs or surfaces, such as skin, the gastrointestinal tract, and intravascular blood vessels, have emerged that utilize ultrasound with frequencies over 20 MHz. However, there is still a need for better clinical ultrasound imaging for detecting skin, eye, and prostate cancers as well as many other diseases, *in vivo*. Imaging techniques with a resolution below 100 μm for these situations would minimize the need for biopsies [2].

Moreover, the medical community has recently expressed the desire for an ultrasound imaging system that would not only provide appropriate resolution, but also be portable [3]. For example, veterinarians would be well served by the development of a portable ultrasound imaging system for onsite diagnosis of pets and zoo and farm animals. The conventional system's size is due to the complex front-end electronics that consist of a discrete chip set for pulsers, preamplifiers, time gain controls (TGCs), analog/digital (A/D) converters, and memory devices. In addition, the conventional design of the transducer arrays requires high transmit-drive voltages on the order of 100 V.

During the past 20 years or so, many researchers have tried to produce miniaturized and integrated ultrasound imaging systems [4–10]. The reason is because integrating all electronic components into a single integrated circuit (IC) chip will afford a smaller system size, higher speed, and lower power consumption than building the system with discrete chipsets. The earliest ultrasound application-specific integrated circuit (ASIC) chips were reported by Black et al. and Hatfield et al. in 1994. The ASIC chips contained 16 channels of transmitters and current amplifiers with integrated transducers [4] and digital transmitters [5]. Since 2000, with the rapid development of mixed-signal IC design technology, closed-coupled ultrasound front-end electronics have emerged for high-frequency ultrasound imaging systems. Wygant et al. [6] developed a Capacitive Micromachined Ultrasound Transducer (CMUT) with closed-coupled electronics, which contain 16 receive–transmit channels. Johansson et al. [7] introduced a portable ultrasound system using a battery-operated voltage-boosting scheme. The Sonic Window, developed by Fuller et al. [8] in 2005, included one of the most integrated ultrasound front-end IC chip concepts to date. Developed for guiding needle and catheter insertion, biopsies, and other invasive procedures for which only a basic aid to diagnosis is necessary, the sonic window can also be used for C-mode ultrasound imaging.

Kim et al. [9] introduced a high-frequency system with a fully integrated, custom-designed ultrasound front-end IC chip that includes both transmit and receive electronics with A/D converters (ADCs) and high-capacity on-chip memory. The design has integrated electronics with thin-film transducers small enough to construct a portable, ultracompact, low-power consumption ultrasound imaging system. Unlike other works mentioned above, which still require a significantly higher drive voltage for the excitation of transducers, the transceiver chip interfaces with thin-film transducer arrays that operate below 5 V, so that the limitations of high-voltage excitation become moot.

This chapter focuses on introducing the architecture and design of a fully integrated ultrasound transceiver chip. Section 16.2 outlines the key points of ultrasound imaging fundamentals: ultrasound physics, the basics of B-mode ultrasound imaging, and beamforming architectures. Section 16.3 investigates the design consideration for the ultrasound transceiver chip in portable high-frequency ultrasound imaging systems. Section 16.4 presents the Penn State portable ultrasound imaging system. The design specifications and details of the circuit components on the transceiver chip are described. In addition, the characteristics of the transceiver chip and the measured signal acquisition results from the Penn State ultrasound imaging system along with the thin-film ultrasound transducer arrays are shown. Finally, the summary and conclusions are given in Section 16.5.

16.2 B-MODE ULTRASOUND IMAGING SYSTEM

16.2.1 Ultrasound Imaging Basics

An ultrasound wave is a longitudinal wave in which oscillations are in the same direction as propagation. In addition, the ultrasound wave is attenuated as it propagates through the medium. Several factors contribute to this attenuation. One of the most significant factors is the absorption of ultrasound energy by the medium and its conversion into heat. The ultrasound wave loses its acoustic energy continuously as it moves through the medium. Scattering and refraction also result in some loss of energy and contribute to overall attenuation.

Reflection is an important physical phenomenon of an ultrasound wave, and it is also a key characteristic used for ultrasound imaging. A reflection occurs at any boundary between two media having different densities and/or acoustic velocities. When an ultrasound wave encounters the boundary between two media, only a portion of the wave's acoustic energy will be transmitted, and the rest of the acoustic energy will be reflected. B-mode ultrasound imaging is based on the pulse–echo (backscattering) response of an ultrasound wave, and provides a two-dimensional (2D), cross-sectional reflection image of the scanned object [10]. The amplitude of the reflection signal is converted to the brightness information of the target object. Higher amplitude creates a brighter image, and weaker amplitude creates a dark image.

In the meantime, the ultrasound wave is attenuated as it propagates through the medium. Several factors contribute to this attenuation. One of the most significant factors is the absorption of ultrasound energy by the medium and its conversion into heat. The ultrasound wave loses its acoustic energy continuously as it moves through the medium. Scattering and refraction also result in some loss of energy and contribute to overall attenuation. A simple exponential loss of pressure amplitude expresses the attenuation of an ultrasound wave [11]:

$$p(z) = p_0 \, e^{-\alpha(f)\cdot z}, \tag{16.1}$$

where p_0 is the initial pressure amplitude and $\alpha(f)$ is the attenuation coefficient that is a function of frequency. This implies that the reflection signals from the medium that is closer to the observation point is stronger than the reflection signals from the medium that is far away from the observation point even if the media are the same. Therefore, the TGC is necessary in the ultrasound front-end electronics to compensate for signal attenuation as a function of depth.

Resolution is one of the most important properties to consider in designing an ultrasound imaging system. Resolution involves two factors in a B-scan: (1) resolution in the direction of the transducer motion, known as "lateral" or "transverse" resolution, and (2) resolution in the direction of acoustic pulse propagation, known as "axial" resolution.

Lateral resolution of an ultrasound imaging system (resolution in the direction of transducer motion) is the system's ability to discriminate between two closely adjacent structures placed at the same depth from the transducer surface. The ultrasound's beam width at a specific depth determines lateral resolution. The beam width varies as the wave propagates in and out of the focal region; therefore, the focusing property of the transducer is

$$\mathrm{LR} = f^{\#}\lambda = \frac{f}{a}\lambda, \tag{16.2}$$

where $f^{\#}$ is the f-number, a is the aperture of the transducer, f is the focal length, and λ is the wavelength. Practically, lateral resolution is proportional to 2λ [12].

Axial resolution of an ultrasound imaging system (resolution in the direction of ultrasound wave propagation) is the ability to discriminate between two closely placed structures lying along the length of the ultrasound wave. The important factor in determining axial resolution is the spatial pulse length (λ) and the number of pulses (N):

$$\mathrm{AR} = \frac{N\lambda}{2}. \tag{16.3}$$

From both Equations 16.2 and 16.3, notably, the wavelength, and consequently the frequency, directly determines the resolution of an ultrasound system. In general, a higher-frequency ultrasound wave is more desirable for higher resolution. However, arbitrarily increasing the ultrasound wave frequency to obtain finer resolution is not desirable because the attenuation rate of ultrasound waves increases as the frequency increases. Therefore, in determining frequency, a necessary consideration is the trade-off between the resolution and the penetration distance of the ultrasound wave. Having set the frequency of an ultrasound wave, the specification for the front-end electronics, such as input buffer bandwidth and A/D conversion speed, can be determined.

16.2.2 B-Mode Imaging System Hardware

A block diagram of a general B-mode ultrasound imaging system appears in Figure 16.1. The following subsections generically describe the processing blocks.

16.2.2.1 Control Host

This grouping includes microprocessors or a host computer and postprocessors. The computer or microprocessors control the entire hardware system to function in the desired modes and to provide a control interface to the front-end electronics. The postprocessor performs scan conversions (i.e., imaging formation), image processing, and display.

16.2.2.2 Transmit/Receive Switch

Generally, the transmit pulses use a very high voltage, typically up to 200 V, while the receiver electronics process uses lower voltage signals, in the 10^{-3} V range. Modern complementary

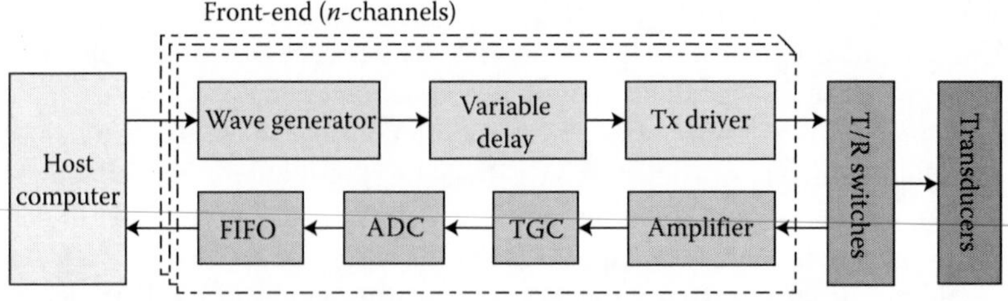

FIGURE 16.1 A block diagram of a general B-mode ultrasound imaging system.

metal-oxide-semiconductor (CMOS) technology uses a power supply below 5 V. Therefore, the receiver should be isolated from transmit pulses in order to protect inner circuits. The transmit/receive (T/R) switch connects transducers to the transmitter during transmit mode operation; conversely, the switch connects the transducer to the receiver during receive mode operation.

16.2.2.3 Amplifier

The amplifier is a key component in the ultrasound imaging system. It performs two functions. First, it receives the reflected signals from the transducers. This means that the dynamic range of the amplifier is crucial because attenuation of an ultrasound wave is sometimes over 100 dB. Impedance matching between the amplifier and transducers is also important for reception. A low-noise amplifier, which has both high dynamic range and good impedance-matching properties, is preferred for the preamplifier. Second, the preamplifier enhances the received signals, but careful preamplifier gain selection avoids amplified signal saturation.

16.2.2.4 Time-Gain Control

The TGC provides time-varying gain for the reflected ultrasound signal whose attenuation varies as a function of depth and the attenuation coefficient of the medium. From Equation 16.1, ultrasound waves attenuate on a logarithmic scale rather than a linear scale. This means that the TGC should express a variable linear gain range in the decibel scale. The TGC can be a variable gain amplifier (VGA).

16.2.2.5 ADC and Memory

As stated earlier, every receive channel needs one or more ADCs for digital beamforming (DBF). Conversion rates 3–5 times the highest center frequency are necessary in order to reduce beamforming quantization errors [13]. As conversion speed increases, memory devices may be needed to store the digitized data and to interface the ADC with the receive beamformer.

16.2.3 Beamforming

Modern ultrasound imaging systems often use multichannel transducer arrays to increase beam flexibility, spatial converge, and resolution. Ultrasound pulses from each channel should have a delay in order to form a wave front that converges on a specified focal point. The transmit beamformer generates delays for each channel to focus and steer the transmit beam, and the receive beamformer performs focusing and steering of the scattered radio-frequency (RF) signals to create the B-mode images. In certain systems, the transmitter consists of delay networks. A single cycle pulse excitation signal is ideal for B-mode imaging since it yields better axial resolution. Typical systems have the flexibility to generate multiple-gated bursts of sinusoidal excitation as well as coded excitation. The delay network focuses the amount of transmitted energy into the medium and has the capability for pulse and pulsed-wave Doppler transmit modes. The receive beamformer also generates delays for each channel in inverse order of transmit delays to align the amplified signals at the reference time. Then, the postprocessor adds the delay compensated signals and generates a large imaging signal for further image processing.

16.2.3.1 Analog Beamforming versus Digital Beamforming

Beamforming architectures are of two types: analog beamforming (ABF) and digital beamforming (DBF). ABF for ultrasound waves first appeared in the 1960s. Researchers developed DBF in the 1980s; however, not until the 1990s did DBF become feasible because that period made available fast, high-precision ADCs necessary for these systems. The recent development of very large-scale integration (VLSI) techniques enables designing real-time digital receive beamformers, and allows amplified signals from receive channels to be coherently added after digitization [14].

The main difference between ABF and DBF, as compared in Figure 16.2, is the method of achieving beamforming. In ABF, analog delay lines for each channel delay the transmit pulses; then

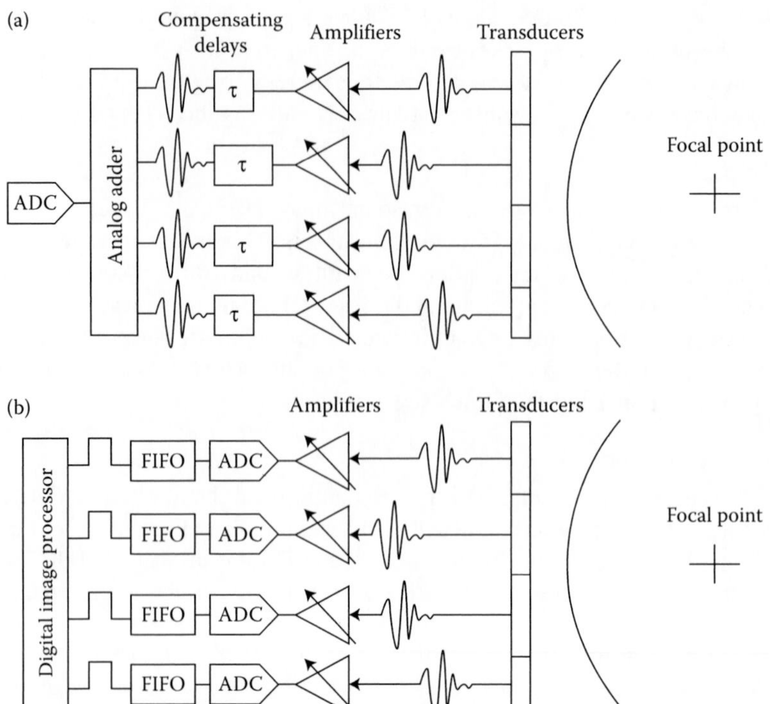

FIGURE 16.2 Simple block diagram of a typical DBF system. (a) The receive ABF system. (b) The receive DBF system.

the beam is formed. In receive mode, the amplified and delayed, reflected analog signal compensates for the transmit delays, which are subsequently accumulated to construct a large analog imaging signal. Then, an ADC digitizes the analog signal for further image processing.

Unlike the signals in an ABF system, the signals in a DBF system are sampled as close to the transducer elements as possible in receive mode, and then delayed and summed digitally. Thus, a DBF system needs an ADC for each channel. Since modern DBF systems use multichannels and arrays of transducers, DBF requires a large number of ADCs. This creates a considerable disadvantage for DBF systems since ADCs consume significant power.

However, DBF systems also have considerable advantages over ABF systems. First, DBF has better control over time delay quantization errors. Analog delay lines tend to be poorly matched between channels. In DBF, synchronization with a high-frequency clock source can greatly improve delay accuracy. Second, DBF provides a finer resolution of ultrasound images. Typical analog delay accuracy is on the order of 20 ns, which constrains lateral resolution [12], but digital delay accuracy in modern digital circuit technology is on the order of a few hundreds of picoseconds with a few gigahertz clock sources and phase-locked loops (PLLs) [15]. Finally, since the digitized data are much less susceptible to noise than analog signal, DBF systems, in stark contrast to ABF systems, can deliver clearer display images than ABF systems, which may have analog noise throughout its entire system.

16.3 CHALLENGES TO THE PORTABLE HIGH-FREQUENCY ULTRASOUND IMAGING SYSTEM

16.3.1 Low-Voltage High-Frequency Transducer

The majority of existing transducers for medical imaging still need a significantly higher drive voltage for excitation (above 60 V). High-voltage excitation pulses result in more complex system designs requiring protection T/R switches, digital controls, and charge-pump circuitry for the transmitter. Thus, the high-voltage system is apt to consume high power and, consequently, is not suitable for portable systems. In addition, the existing systems interface the transducer array elements with the RF front-end by coaxial cable networks. The cables are specifically 50 Ω impedance matched to the RF front-end interface. The existence of T/R switches between the cable network and front-end electronics makes impedance matching even more complex.

Therefore, low-voltage high-frequency ultrasound transducer arrays are crucial in portable high-frequency ultrasound imaging systems. The low-voltage transducers make the imaging system capable of integrating front-end electronics with transducers without charge-pump circuitry and RF coaxial cables. In addition, receiver protection devices are likely to be unnecessary because the transmit voltage is of the same magnitude as the CMOS logic voltage level. The integrated electronics also produces better signal integrity and noise immunity than conventional, analog, front-end electronics, which consist of discrete chipsets. Digital signal interfacing has wide acceptance for much higher signal-to-noise ratio (SNR) compliance than analog signal interfacing. In conventional systems, substantial efforts are necessary to control SNR in analog signal interfacing. However, in the integrated system, only chip-to-chip interfacing is necessary via digital signals because all analog signal processing occurs inside the chip and chips produce only digital outputs.

Studies on developing low-voltage high-frequency ultrasound transducers are in demand. First, the high-frequency $PbZr_{0.52}Ti_{0.48}O_3$ (PZT) thin-film ultrasound transducer arrays using microelectromechanical system technology were proposed in [16]. The PZT layers can be thin, and allow the reduction of the required voltages for exciting the transducer. The center frequency of the thin-film transducer is 30–70 MHz with a bandwidth of 60–100%. Because the piezoelectric layer is a thin film (<1 μm thickness), the transducer array utilizes CMOS-compatible, low-level (below 5 V) excitation voltages. This technology enables the thin-film ultrasound transducers to be placed in close proximity to the electronics.

In addition, a 20-element high-frequency ultrasound transducer array using the micromolding technique is introduced in [17]. The array used piezocomposite material and thin-film Cr–Au electrodes in a mask-based process, packaged in epoxy with external connectors. The center frequency of the transducer is about 35 MHz with a bandwidth of 74% at 6-dB points.

16.3.2 Hardware Specifications

Achieving the required design specification for a high-frequency ultrasound imaging system is challenging. The linear dynamic range for an analog amplifier has a limitation of 100 dB in practical systems. However, the required dynamic range of the preamplifiers is sometimes higher than 100 dB for an ultrasound imaging system [18]. An even more critical obstacle is the requirement for the ADC. While the earliest commercially available digital beamformers became available in the early 1980s, they did not begin to have a significant impact until the early 1990s. Much of this delay was due to the need for ADCs with a sufficiently large number of bits and sufficiently high sampling rates.

Figure 16.3 shows the ADC development trends, presented in the recent publications of two major international conferences: the International Solid State Circuits Conference (ISSCC) and the VLSI (Symposia on VLSI Technology and Circuits) [19]. The dynamic range and the bandwidth of the ADCs show an inversely proportional relationship, and the majority of the recent studies on ADCs focused on mid-resolution (50–70 dB, i.e., 8–12 bit) and mid-frequency (10–100 MHz) ranges. The requirements for high-resolution (~10 μm minimum feature size), high-frequency (30–150 MHz center frequency of the transducers) ultrasound imaging systems are 50–70 dB dynamic range and 75–400 MHz bandwidth (gray box in the figure). As seen in this figure, a state-of-the-art ADC is a fundamental requirement for the success of the development of portable high-frequency ultrasound imaging systems.

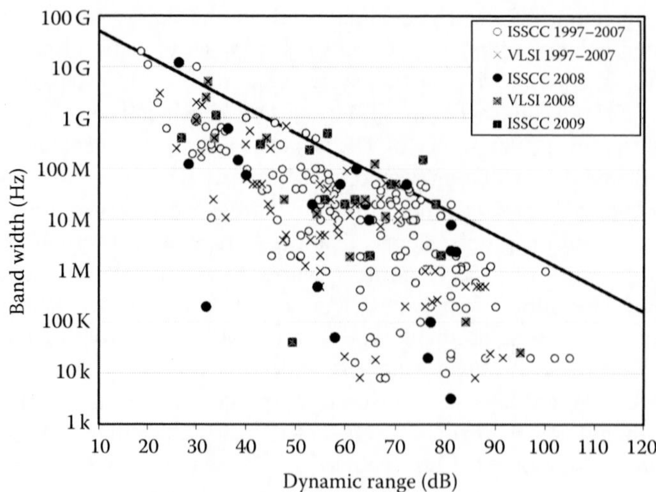

FIGURE 16.3 Dynamic range and bandwidth trends of recently published ADCs.

16.3.3 System Architecture

The novel design architecture is essential for achieving low power consumption while adapting DBF architecture. DBF architecture consumes considerable power because of the need for a dedicated ADC and memory blocks for the receive channel. The need for an ADC per receive channel in a typical DBF system is a substantial disadvantage because of high power consumption and large system size as compared to an ABF system that delays the received signals, sums them by analog circuitry, and then converts them to a digital signal by an ADC.

According to Murmann [20], the power dissipation of the recently published ADCs in ISSCC and VLSI is about 2×10^{-11} to 2×10^{-8} J at 50 dB dynamic range, as shown in Figure 16.4. For example, assuming the system has 256 receive channels (i.e., it needs 256 ADCs with DBF architecture), the power dissipation of the ADC is 5×10^{-10} J (the median value), and the sampling rate

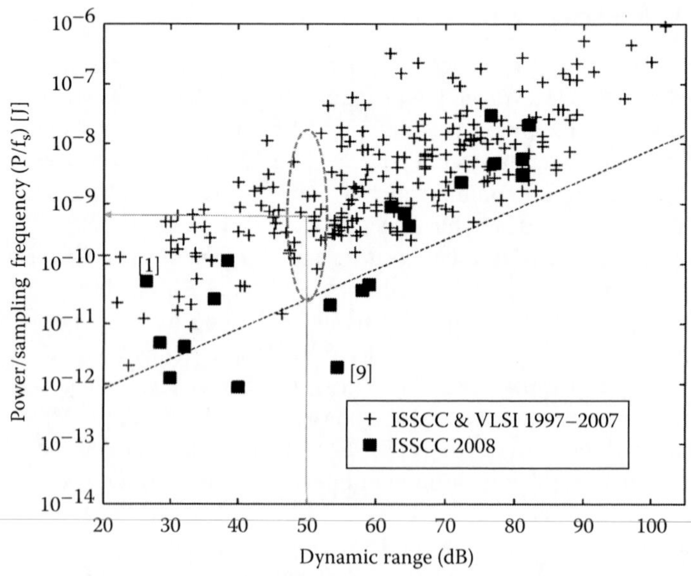

FIGURE 16.4 Power efficiency versus dynamic range in recently published ADCs.

is 250 MHz, the system consumes 32 W (= 5×10^{-10} J × 250 MHz × 256) only for 256 ADCs. This consumption is rarely practical or even possible considering power consumption limitations in a portable system. For example, the AD9271 chipset has a total of eight receive channels with dedicated ADCs per channel and consumes 1.5 W of maximum power. Thus, it needs 48 W of maximum power to build 256 receive channels using the AD9271 chips, which may not be suitable for portable devices.

16.3.3.1 Shared ADC Architecture

To overcome the problem stated above, the transceiver chip has only one ADC shared by the 16 receivers via a 16:1 analog multiplexer (aMUX) as proposed in [9]. Consequently, this configuration creates a DBF system but of the same order of size and power consumption as an ABF system. However, the prototype device operates 16 times slower than a conventional system because the shared ADC architecture performs 16 iterative operations accessing different channels to complete one scan. Another drawback is that the architecture requires extra digital controls.

An evaluation of the effectiveness of the shared ADC architecture, the performance of the shared ADC architecture, and the typical DBF architecture is presented as a comparison in Table 16.1. In this comparison, the number of channels in the typical DBF architecture varies from 1 to 16, while the number of channels in the shared ADC architecture remains at 16, and the number of shared channels varies from 4 to 16. The sizes of one receive and transmit channel, an ADC, and the 3-kbyte static random-access memory (SRAM) are assumed to be 0.175, 0.9, and 2.16 mm^2, respectively. These sizes are estimates based on the actual layout sizes of each component in the transceiver chip. The size of digital control circuitry, needed only for the shared ADC architecture, is expected to be 0.2 mm^2. In addition, the assumed power consumption of one receive and transmit channel, an ADC, 3-kbyte SRAM, and the digital controls are 2, 100, 130, and 8 mW, respectively. These data were also estimated from SPICE simulation results of each component with postlayout parameters. The time for 1-scanning is calculated based on the operational sequence and time for one complete scanning of the Penn State ultrasound imaging system described in Section 16.4.

Table 16.1 also indicates the trade-off relationship among operational speed for 1-scanning, chip size, and power consumption. Thus, to determine the optimal number of shared channels, the maximum time for 1-complete-scanning allowed for real-time imaging is a consideration. Having established the maximum time, the total number of channels can be determined considering the chip size and power consumption specifications. For example, if the maximum allowable time for 1-scanning is 800 μs, the 16 channels can be shared. Then, if the chip size is 25 mm^2 and power consumption is 1 W, the optimal number of total channels will be 64 (16 channels of each are shared).

TABLE 16.1
Performance Comparison among Shared ADC and Typical DBF Architectures

	Typical DBF Architecture: Number of Channels			Shared ADC Architecture: Number of Shared Channels[a]		
	1	**8**	**16**	**4**	**8**	**16**
Numbers of required ADC and SRAM	1	8	16	4	2	1
Chip size (mm^2)	3.24	25.9	51.8	15.2	9.1	6.1
Power consumption (mW)	240	1864	3720	960	500	270
Time for 1-scanning (μs)	50	50	50	200	400	800

[a] Total number of channels: 16.

16.4 PENN STATE PORTABLE HIGH-FREQUENCY ULTRASOUND IMAGING SYSTEM

16.4.1 Configuration of the Penn State Ultrasound Imaging System

Conventional front-end electronics consist of discrete chipsets for transmitters, preamplifiers, TGCs, ADCs, and memory devices, all mounted on several printed circuit boards (PCBs). Therefore, the systems are not only large and expensive, but also they have difficulty with high-speed operation. The Penn State ultrasound imaging system integrates the complete ultrasound front-end electronics onto a single IC chip with closed-coupled thin-film ultrasound transducers, and then constructs high-resolution ultrasound images. The system requires (1) a multichannel analog signal processing system including high-speed ADCs and a transmit beamformer integrated on a single transceiver chip and (2) auxiliary digital controls on a field programmable gate array (FPGA) chip with several discrete chipsets such as an RS232 chip, a D/A converter (DAC), and a 250-MHz crystal oscillator. These specifications enable the creation of an ultracompact, low-cost, high-speed, and high-resolution ultrasound imaging system.

The FPGA chip has been programmed to control the ultrasound transceiver chip, and helps the transceiver chip to communicate with the imaging host via an RS-232 chip. The main control interfaces with other circuitry such as mode set, memory, and the transceiver chip according to commands received from the user. The clock buffer receives a 250-MHz clock signal from an external clock oscillator and distributes it to other circuit blocks and to the transceiver chip. The mode set consists of 1-bit serial pipeline registers that store data preset by the user, for example, channel and the preamplifier gain selection information. The 48-kbyte internal memory's assignment is to store image information from the transceiver chip. The stored data, transferred to the host computer through the serial port in the FPGA chip and the RS-232 chip, allows subsequent image creation. The counter's design permits the generation of digital codes that increase as an exponential function of time. The digital codes produce a pseudoexponential analog signal for the VGA in the transceiver chip.

Figure 16.5 shows a block diagram of the transceiver chip. The receiver consists of a preamplifier and a TGC that compensates for signal attenuation as a function of depth. The TGC consists of an on-chip VGA and an external 10-bit 50-MHz DAC (AD9760, Analog Devices, Inc., MA). A time-varying control signal, applied to the VGA gain control input, ensures that the signal strength at the VGA output is constant over time (i.e., depth). An 8-bit ADC digitizes the compensated signals. The ADC output connects to a 3-kbyte on-chip SRAM, which is large enough to store all the scanned image data for a specified depth range. In this work, the transceiver chip has 16 transmit and receive channels. The number of channels can be increased. The transceiver chip has only one ADC and SRAM to reduce chip area and power consumption, but the system needs an aMUX and auxiliary

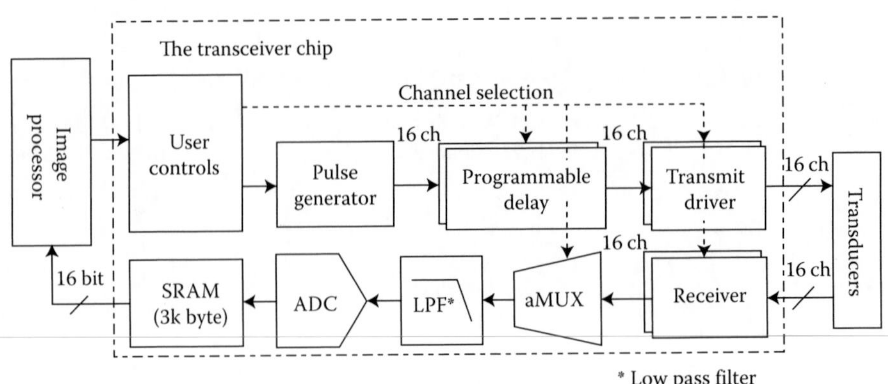

FIGURE 16.5 Simplified block diagram of the transceiver chip.

digital controls for channel selection. A 16:1 aMUX allows these two components to share 16 receive channels. Section 16.4.2 discusses the architectural advantage of the transceiver chip.

The transmit signal generator produces and sends a 50-MHz pulse to the thin-film ultrasound transducers through programmable delay chains to enable electronic beam focusing in the transmit mode. In a DBF system, focusing occurs by introducing delays to the transmit pulse on the elements so that emitted ultrasonic beams can be made constructively at the target of interest. Therefore, excitation pulses should be delivered to the transducer elements in an order that allows convergence of a composite wave front to a focal point. The variable delay chains in the figure determine the excitation order of the transducers.

16.4.2 Receiver

16.4.2.1 Required Specifications

The most important design specification of the system is the bandwidth of the receiver. The required bandwidth of the receiver is determined by the center frequency and bandwidth of the transducer. In this study, the target frequency of the transducers is 50 MHz with 100% bandwidth; thus, the input frequency range is 25–75 MHz [16]. Therefore, the receiver circuitry must be capable of a flat frequency response over the bandwidth of the transducer elements up to 75 MHz with a maximum gain of 20 dB.

In addition, the ratio between the ADC aperture and the maximum preamplifier input amplitude determines the gain of the preamplifier according to

$$\text{Gain}_{\text{preamp}} = 20 \cdot \log_{10}\left(\frac{\text{Max ADC Input}}{\text{Max Preamp Input}}\right) \pm (\text{Design Margin}). \tag{16.4}$$

In this design, the maximum input of the preamplifier is set to 0.3 V_{P-P}, and the ADC aperture is 1.5 V_{P-P}. Thus, the preamplifier gain is 14 dB ± (design margin). Since the thin-film transducers are currently under development, the design margin is set to ±6 dB. Therefore, the gain of the preamplifier can be changed over a range from 8 to 20 dB at the discretion of the user.

The dynamic range of the preamplifier is another important factor in the receive circuitry. The dynamic range of the receiver determines the minimum and maximum signal amplitudes that the system can process. Therefore, the attenuation rate and depth range of the target medium can determine the required dynamic range. Assuming that the attenuation rate in soft tissue is 0.5 dB/MHz/cm [21], the total attenuation is 45 dB at 50 MHz for a penetration depth of 9 mm (i.e., the total signal path of 18 mm considering signal reflection). Adding a minimum display resolution of 30 dB, image saturation allowance of 6 dB, and noise threshold of 6 dB [22] provides a dynamic range of 87 dB [23]. Therefore, the SNR of the ADC needs to be greater than 87 dB, which corresponds to 15-bit resolution, according to the relationship [22]

$$\text{SNR}_{\text{ideal}} = 6.02N + 1.76 \text{ (dB)}, \tag{16.5}$$

where N is the bit resolution of an ADC.

However, this dynamic range is too great for current high-speed ADCs. The use of a VGA reduces the dynamic range requirement. Since the main purpose of the VGA is to compensate for signal attenuation as a function of the depth of targets, the maximum gain of the VGA is bounded by the total signal attenuation, that is, 45 dB. The optimal gain range of the VGA is selectable according to the dynamic range of the ADC. For example, if the SNR of the ADC is 42 dB, 45 dB of variable gain range is the requirement. In this design, the target SNR of the ADC is 48 dB (i.e., 8 bit); thus, the required gain range of the VGA is 37 dB. Figure 16.6 illustrates the gain and dynamic range requirements.

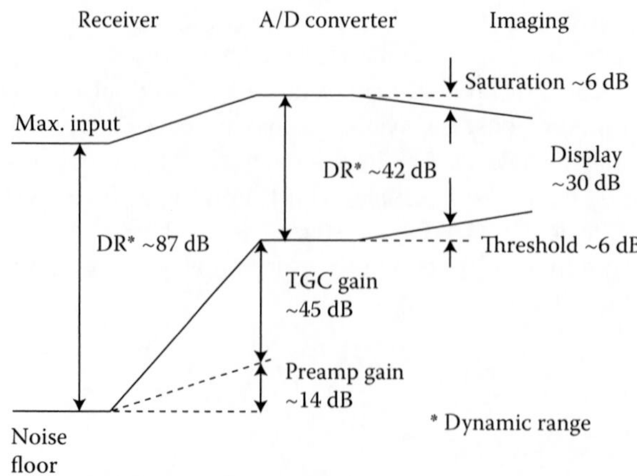

FIGURE 16.6 Transceiver chip gain and dynamic range requirements.

16.4.2.2 Circuit Design Details

The receive circuitry consists of two on-chip components (the preamp and the VGA) and several off-chip components. The counter included in the FPGA chip generates time-varying digital codes that convert to the pseudoexponential analog control signals through an external DAC. The VGA can produce a time-varying gain on a linear decibel scale with pseudoexponential control signals.

Figure 16.7 shows the simplified circuit schematic diagram of the preamplifier. The analog signals from the transducers connect to IN+ and the common ground of the transducer arrays connects to IN−. The resistance ratio of the transistors M1 and M2 and the resistors R1 and R2 determine the gain. The voltage gain of the amplifier is expressed as

$$A_V = -g_{m1,2} \cdot \left(r_{O1,2} \| r_{O3,4} \| R_{1,2}\right), \tag{16.6}$$

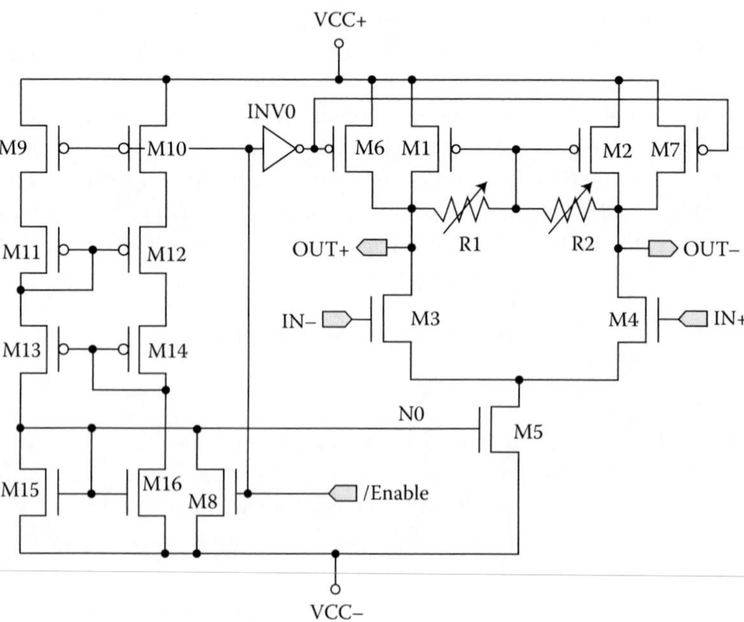

FIGURE 16.7 Preamplifier core circuit schematic.

where $g_{m1,2}$ is the transconductance of M1 and M2, $r_{O1,2}$ is the output resistances of transistors M1 and M2, and $r_{O3,4}$ is the output resistances of transistors M3 and M4. R1 and R2 in the design vary the resistance value from 4 to 20 kΩ so that the user can preset the gain.

The combination of transistors M6–M10 and the inverter INV0 forms the enable/disable switch. This internal switch eliminates external T/R switches (required in typical ultrasound transceivers) in the analog signal path. When "/Enable" is HIGH, transistor M8 turns OFF so that the voltage of the node N0 goes to ground, and transistors M6 and M7 turn ON so that OUT+ and OUT– are tied to VCC+ regardless of the amplifier's inputs. The speed of the switch is fast enough for the amplifier to be stable before signal acquisition starts. Transistors M9–M16 generate bias voltages, independent of the power supply voltages, for the amplifier.

Since an ultrasound wave attenuates its power traveling in tissue on a decibel scale, the gain of the VGA also needs to have the capability to be changed linearly in decibel [21]. Therefore, the gain of the VGA must be linear-in-dB over the linear control voltage range. To achieve this relationship, the proposed design adapts a Gilbert-type four-quadrant multiplier, whose output is equal to the product of the two inputs [24], and the generated pseudoexponential control voltages use external circuitry with an FPGA chip and a DAC. Figure 16.8 depicts the folded Gilbert cell, in which the bottom differential pair of the original Gilbert cell folds without degrading performance in order to reduce the number of cascode transistors. The derivation of the analytic relationship between input and output is the following [25]:

$$\begin{aligned} V_o &= (g_{m3,4} - g_{m5,6}) \cdot R_D \cdot (V_{in}^+ - V_{in}^-) \\ &= \sqrt{\frac{k_N (W/L)}{2I_{SS}}} \cdot g_{m1,2} (V_{cp} - V_{cn})(V_{in}^+ - V_{in}^-), \end{aligned} \tag{16.7}$$

where $g_{m1,2}$, $g_{m3,4}$, and $g_{m5,6}$ are the transconductances of transistors M1 and M2, M3 and M4, and M5 and M6, respectively; $k_N = \mu_N \cdot C_{OX}$ (μ_N is the electron mobility and C_{OX} is the gate capacitance of the NMOS transistor); W is the channel width of transistors M1–M4; and L is the channel length of transistors M1–M4. Transistors M9–M16 constitute a linear voltage converter.

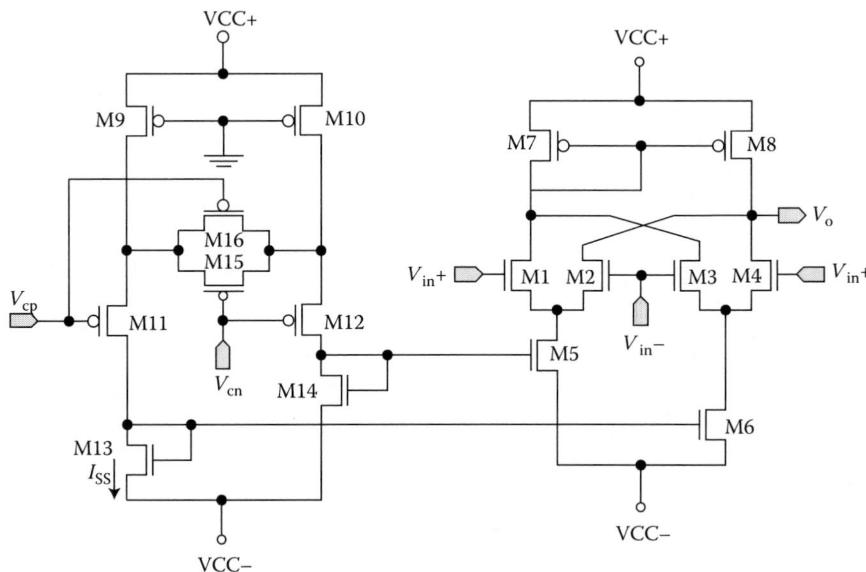

FIGURE 16.8 Folded Gilbert cell-based VGA circuit schematic.

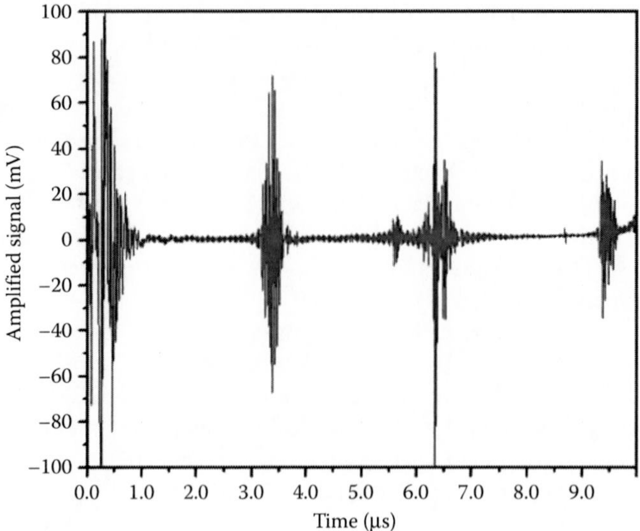

FIGURE 16.9 Amplified signals by the receiver with the VGA functioning. See Section 16.4.6 for details of the experimental setup for this testing.

Figure 16.9 presents the measured output of the receive circuitry including the preamplifier and the VGA. The preamplifier gain is set to 14 dB and the linear gain control range of the VGA is 23 dB with a control voltage of 0.1–1.0 V, which is generated using the FPGA chip (Spartan III, Xilinx, Inc.) and a 10-bit DAC (AD 9760, Analog Devices, Inc.). The results demonstrate the function of the receiver: the amplitudes of the second and third peaks are similar to that of the first peak due to the increasing gain over time.

16.4.3 A/D Converter

The sampling rate of the ADC can be determined by the Nyquist sampling theorem [26], which states that reconstruction of a continuous-time signal from its samples is possible if the sampling frequency is greater than twice the signal bandwidth. If the center frequency of the target transducer is 50 MHz with 100% bandwidth, the bandwidth of the reflected signals will be 25–75 MHz. Given the 20 MHz design margin of the antialiasing filter located between the VGA and the ADC, the signal bandwidth will be 5–95 MHz. Therefore, the required minimum sampling rate of the ADC is 190 MHz according to the Nyquist theorem.

A further important determination is the effective bit resolution. This consideration depends on the characteristics of the medium. In this design, the target medium is tissue in human organs, which requires at least a 50-dB image resolution [22]. Therefore, the required effective bit resolution of the ADC is set to 50 dB, that is, an 8-bit resolution.

16.4.3.1 TIQ-Based ADC

The design of a 190-MS/s ADC is a challenge in 0.35 μm CMOS technology. To achieve the ADC requirements, a threshold inverter quantization ADC (TIQ ADC), known for its fast conversion speed [27], has been designed. Although flash-type ADCs have several disadvantages in terms of higher power consumption, occupying a larger area than other types of ADCs, the shared ADC architecture described in Section 16.3 overcomes the drawbacks of the flash ADC. Since this architecture, reportedly, has the operation speed, gain, and DC offset variations of up to 18% due to process and temperature variations [27], a sampling rate of 250 MHz rather than the required sampling rate of 190 MHz is the target for the proposed design.

A TIQ comparator is one of the most important circuits in a flash ADC. It converts an analog input voltage into a digital logic output "1" or "0," depending on the reference voltage of the comparator. In a traditional flash ADC, a differential comparator, which needs a resistor–ladder circuit as an external voltage reference, is commonly used. On the other hand, the TIQ comparator, which consists of two cascaded CMOS inverters, does not need a resistor–ladder circuit because it uses the built-in voltage reference of the CMOS inverters [28].

As an example of TIQ ADC operation, Figure 16.10a shows the schematic of a 2-bit TIQ ADC comprising three TIQ comparators, three gain boosters, and an encoder (notably, an n-bit TIQ ADC consists of $2^n - 1$ comparators and gain boosters and an n-bit encoder). The TIQ comparator consists of two cascaded inverters; the first inverter sets the analog signal quantization according to its logic threshold and the second inverter increases the gain of the comparator. If the analog input is higher than the logic threshold, the digital output is logic "1"; otherwise, the digital output is logic "0."

A particular output voltage (V_{out}) that is the same as input voltage (V_{in}), that is, $V_{in} = V_{out}$, determines the logic threshold of the TIQ comparator. And the logic threshold changes depending on the width ratios of the PMOS and NMOS. If P1 is the largest PMOS and P5 is the smallest PMOS, and if N1 is the smallest NMOS and N5 is the largest NMOS, as shown in Figure 16.10a, the top comparator output corresponds to C_3, the middle comparator corresponds to C_2, and the bottom comparator output corresponds to C_1 as in Figure 16.10b. Clearly, the three different ratios of the PMOS and NMOS widths result in three different logic thresholds: The logic threshold value of the top comparator is the largest and the logic threshold of the bottom comparator is the smallest.

With fixed lengths for the PMOS and NMOS transistors, increasing or decreasing the width of the PMOS or NMOS, respectively, produces the desired values for the logic thresholds. Since the TIQ comparator is used in a flash ADC, a $2^n - 1$ set of TIQ comparators is necessary in order to design an n-bit flash ADC. Therefore, finding the exact $2^n - 1$ different logic thresholds as the reference voltages of the TIQ comparator in an input voltage range is necessary. For example, all 63 TIQ comparators for a 6-bit flash ADC have transistors of different sizes, so all the comparators have different logic threshold values.

16.4.3.2 Design Automation for the TIQ Comparator

The simple architecture of the TIQ ADC is an advantage; however, for a TIQ ADC, the TIQ comparators' design must be precisely sized to be different from one another. Achieving the required

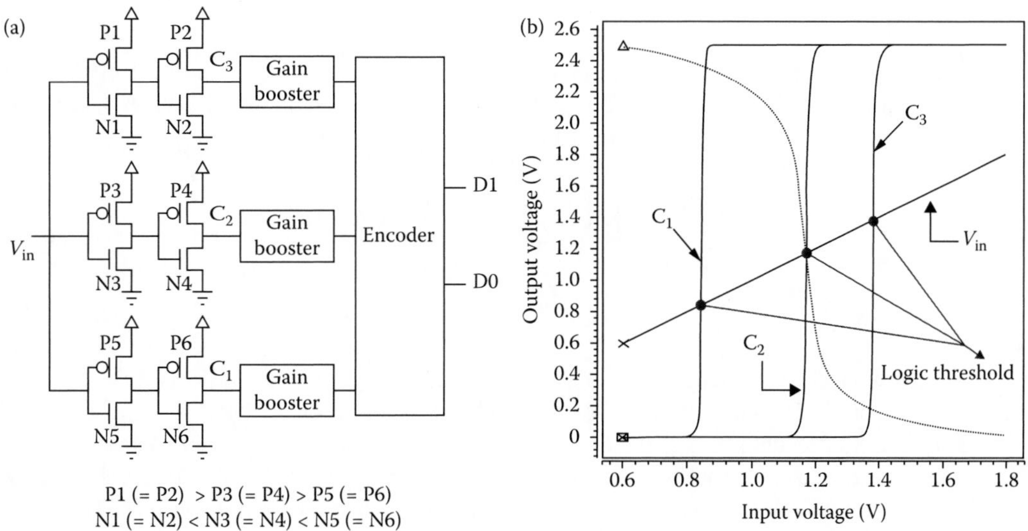

FIGURE 16.10 TIQ comparator design: (a) Example of 2-bit TIQ ADC and (b) VTC of a TIQ comparator.

dynamic range makes designing this feature a somewhat difficult task. Mitigating the difficulty is the use of a computer-aided design (CAD) tool, which automates TIQ comparator design and implementation. The systematic size variation (SSV) technique is the proposed method for easing, comparatively, the choice of needed logic thresholds from the many possible comparators [28]. The SSV technique chooses V_m from a reduced range of 3D plots. The diagonal line drawn in the 3D plots is the optimal line, which maintains a systematic increasing and/or decreasing order of transistor sizes. Keeping the transistor size in increasing and/or decreasing order significantly improves the linearity of the ADC in relationship to fabrication process variations. This method also significantly reduces the number of simulations needed for transistor size selection. The simulation is needed only along the diagonal-line region rather than on the full 3D surface.

Using the SSV could save this design time. However, it is still time consuming due to simulating all possible combinations of the PMOS and NMOS. For example, according to [29], about 4 h were necessary to find 6-bit TIQ comparators using the SSV technique, and five Sun-Blade 2000 machines performed 28,000 simulations to find 63 TIQ comparators. Notably, the total design time increases exponentially as the bit resolution of a TIQ ADC increases.

An improved TIQ comparator design methodology has been proposed in [29]. The proposed method introduces an analytical TIQ model to overcome the drawbacks of the SSV technique. The analytical model has advantages over the SSV technique in terms of simulation time as well as accuracy.

Since the logic threshold (V_m) is a voltage in which the output voltage is equal to the input voltage ($V_{out} = V_{in} = V_m$), the mathematical expression of V_m can be derived from drain current equations for both PMOS and NMOS devices. For simplicity, only a TIQ model using a Level 1 SPICE model has been derived here. More sophisticated models, such as BSIM3 (Berkeley Short-channel IGFET Model) or BSIM4 [30], may improve the model's accuracy. Also, the assumption is that the channel lengths of PMOS and NMOS devices are long enough; that is, velocity saturation does not occur. The drain currents of NMOS and PMOS, $I_{DS,NMOS}$, $I_{DS,NMOS}$, respectively, can be written as

$$I_{DS,NMOS} = \frac{k_N}{2}\left(\frac{W_N}{L_N}\right)(V_m - V_{THN})^2(1+\lambda_N V_{DS}), \tag{16.8}$$

$$I_{DS,PMOS} = \frac{k_P}{2}\left(\frac{W_P}{L_P}\right)(V_{DD} - V_m - |V_{THP}|)^2(1+\lambda_P V_{DS}), \tag{16.9}$$

where $k_N = \mu_N \cdot C_{OXN}$ (μ_N is the electron mobility and C_{OXN} is the gate capacitance of NMOS), and $k_P = \mu_P \cdot C_{OXP}$ (μ_P is the hole mobility and C_{OXP} is the gate capacitance of PMOS). When the channel lengths of both transistors are the same, the logic threshold, V_m, yields

$$V_m = \frac{V_{THN} + (V_{DD} - |V_{THP}|)\cdot \Lambda \cdot \sqrt{(k_P W_P / k_N W_N)}}{1+\sqrt{(k_P W_P / k_N W_N)}}, \tag{16.10}$$

where $\Lambda = \sqrt{2+\lambda_P V_{DD}/2+\lambda_N V_{DD}}$.

From Equation 16.10, the dependency of V_m on the width ratio of PMOS and NMOS (W_P/W_N) can be derived. Figure 16.11 shows a comparison of the V_m dependencies on the width ratios in analytical models and the SSV technique. A standard 0.35 μm CMOS technology is used for this graph, and the SSV technique generates a set of 63 TIQ comparators for a 6-bit TIQ ADC. The V_m curve from the BSIM3 model shows excellent accuracy with an average mismatch rate of less than 1%. The maximum error is about 5%, and the average error is less than 1%. Therefore, a set of width ratios, according to ideal V_m values, can be found using the TIQ model rather than the SSV technique.

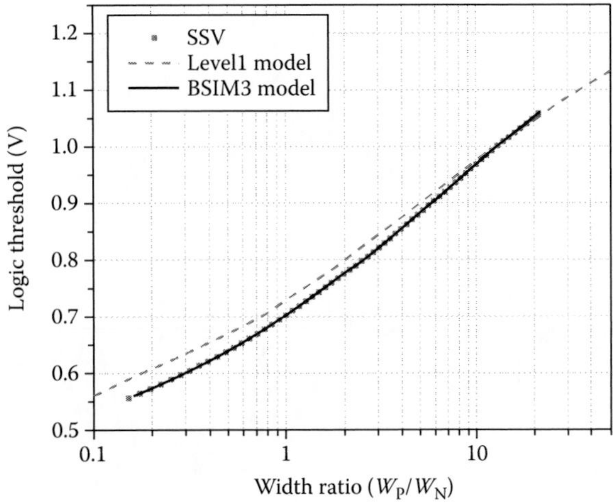

FIGURE 16.11 Accuracy comparison of various TIQ comparator models.

As an alternate form of Equation 16.10, a set of widths can be expressed as a function of V_m. This alternate set is

$$\left(\frac{W_P}{W_N}\right) = \frac{k_N\left(V_m - V_{THN}\right)^2\left(2+\lambda_N V_{DD}\right)}{k_P\left(V_{DD} - V_m - \left|V_{THP}\right|\right)^2\left(2+\lambda_P V_{DD}\right)}. \tag{16.11}$$

Equation 16.11 provides the width ratio for each ideal V_m. The width ratios of the TIQ comparators can be expressed as

$$\frac{W_P(i)}{W_N(i)} = R(i), \qquad (i = 1 - 2^n - 1), \tag{16.12}$$

where $W_P(i)$ is the ith PMOS width; $W_N(i)$ is the ith NMOS width, and $R(i) >$ is the ith width ratio for the n-bit TIQ comparator set.

However, the widths of NMOS and PMOS devices cannot be determined using only Equation 16.12 without another relationship between W_P and W_N. The relationship arises from the projection of the line on the x–y plane, as illustrated in Figure 16.12. The line expression, in general form, is

$$a \cdot W_P + b \cdot W_N = c, \tag{16.13}$$

where a, b, and c are constants. In the case of process variation, shifting the NMOS and PMOS at the same ratio is desirable. Thus, a and b can be set to 1. Therefore, Equation 16.13 can be denoted as

$$W_P(i) + W_N(i) = k. \tag{16.14}$$

From Equations 16.12 and 16.14, W_P(i) and $W_N(i)$ can be derived as

$$W_P(i) = \frac{k \cdot R(i)}{1 + R(i)} \tag{16.15}$$

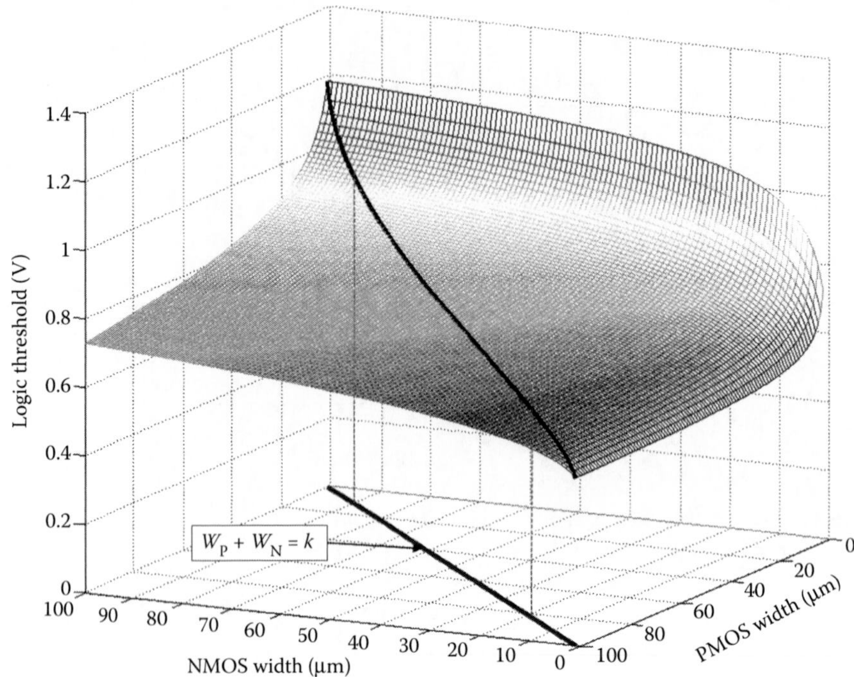

FIGURE 16.12 A 3D plot of the V_m and width size relationship of NMOS and PMOS of the TIQ comparator analytical model.

and

$$W_N(i) = \frac{k}{1+R(i)}. \tag{16.16}$$

The optimal transistor width derives from considering the relationship between transistor length and data conversion speed. In general, a longer transistor length in a TIQ comparator is desirable for achieving higher gain, that is, higher sensitivity, less noise, and less process variation sensitivity. However, a longer transistor yields a slower data comparison speed in the TIQ comparator. If the conversion target speed is 1 GSPS, a maximum transistor length of about 1 μm is allowed in a 0.18 μm standard CMOS technology [29]. Consequently, the optimal value of the transistor length in a TIQ comparator can be set to 1 μm for a 1-GSPS TIQ ADC.

16.4.4 Static Random-Access Memory

16.4.4.1 Required Specifications

The SRAM included in the design reduces the data transfer rates from the ADC to the imaging host processor. Since the sampling rate of the ADC is 250 MS/s and the bit resolution is 8 bits, the digitized image data transfer to the host at the data bandwidth of 2 GBPS. However, such high-speed data transfer is not only difficult to be achieved using less expensive circuit boards, but also generates substantial digital noise (jitters) that negatively affects the analog signal integrity of the receiver. On-chip memory devices overcome these problems. Therefore, a SRAM that can write data with a data bandwidth of 2 GBPS and that can read data with a lower data transfer rate of 250 Mbps became elements of the design for the CMOS transceiver chip.

Another key specification of the on-chip memory is capacity. The calculation of the memory capacity uses the relationship

$$\text{Capacity} = \frac{t_{\text{Travel}}}{t_{\text{sample}}} = \frac{D/c}{t_{\text{sample}}}, \tag{16.17}$$

where t_{Travel} is the total (i.e., two-way) travel time of the ultrasound wave in the medium; t_{sample} is the sampling interval of the ADC; D is the total distance that the ultrasound wave travels in the medium; and c is the speed of the ultrasound wave in the medium. Estimates indicate that a 3-kbyte buffer length is necessary for $t_{\text{sample}} = 4$ ns, $D = 18$ mm, and $c = 1500$ m/s.

16.4.4.2 SRAM Design Details

Figure 16.13 shows the functional block diagram of a 3-kbyte SRAM. This SRAM operates in two modes: data write mode and data read mode with auto precharge. Once the data write or data read operation begins, the operation continues until the all 3-kbyte cells are written to or read by the address counter, which automatically, incrementally sweeps all 3000 addresses.

The SRAM design adopts asymmetric operating speed between data write and data read. As described earlier, the data write speed is faster than 125 MHz; however, a 125-MHz data readout speed could be a disaster in some inexpensive applications. Thus, this design uses two different speed clocks for data write and date read. First, a 250-MHz clock is used for data conversion and storing. Next, a 50-MHz clock is for the input/output (I/O) system. Thus, the data readout uses the 50-MHz clock. The main I/O clock offers an inexpensive and easy way of transferring data.

The asymmetric operating speed between data write and data read occurs by a 2:1 multiplexer. During write operations, the SRAM shares the ADC clock, and the SRAM uses the main I/O clock during the readout operation. Figure 16.14 presents the SPICE simulation results of the SRAM clock transition. Until 700 ns, the SRAM writes the data in the memory cells in the two subbanks with a 250-MHz clock speed as shown in Figures 16.14b and c. Clearly, the subbanks operate one after the other as mentioned earlier. At 700 ns, the read command comes in, and the clock changes from 250 to 50 MHz. Thus, the read operation performs with the 50 MHz clock.

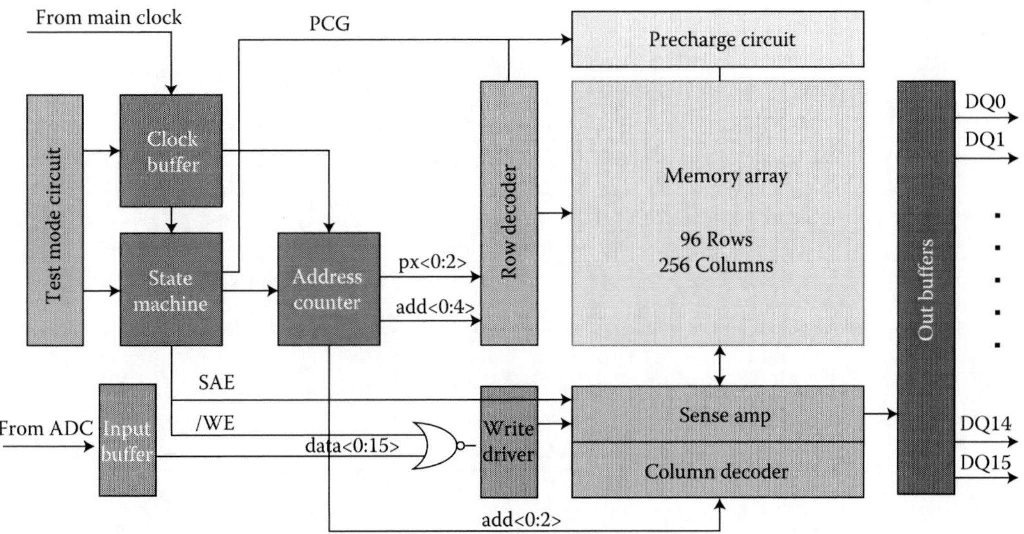

FIGURE 16.13 Functional block diagram of the 3-kbyte SRAM.

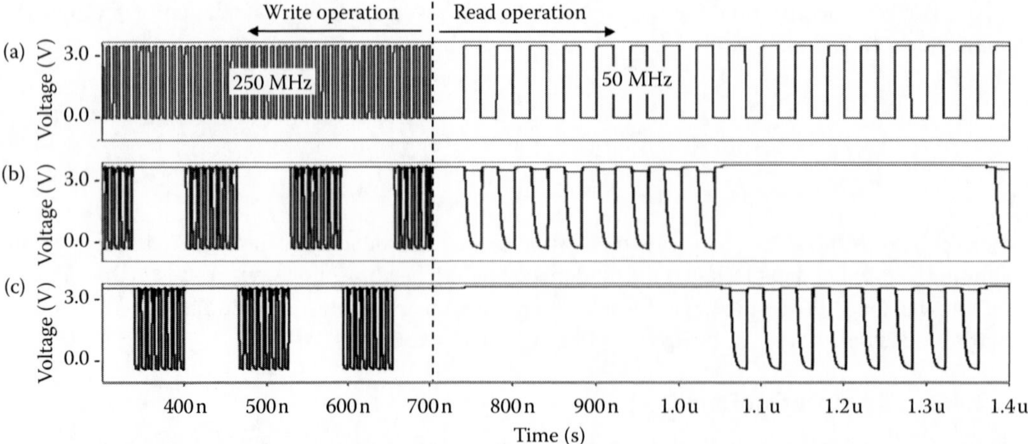

FIGURE 16.14 Simulation results of the SRAM clock modulation: (a) clock transition, (b) memory cell data in Bank 0, and (c) memory cell data in Bank 1.

Figure 16.15 presents the measured outputs of the SRAM, which transferred at a rate of 400 MBPS as described earlier. In this figure, only 6 bit outputs are presented because the ADC shows linear characteristics with 6 bits. 85 kHz of sawtooth wave was generated by a function generator and fed to the ADC. The analog signal was sampled at a speed of 250 MS/s, and then converted into digital signals. The SRAM stored the digital data at the same speed as the ADC's sampling rate. The test results prove the functionality of the SRAM and ADC.

16.4.5 Transmitter

The major function of the transmitter is to excite the transducer elements and to focus and/or steer the ultrasound beam. Focusing and steering the ultrasonic beam requires time delays to compensate

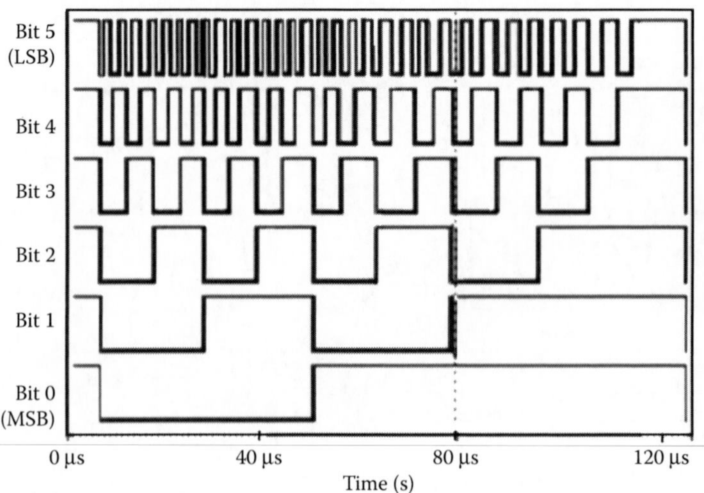

FIGURE 16.15 Measured outputs of the SRAM with the transfer rate of 400 MBPS.

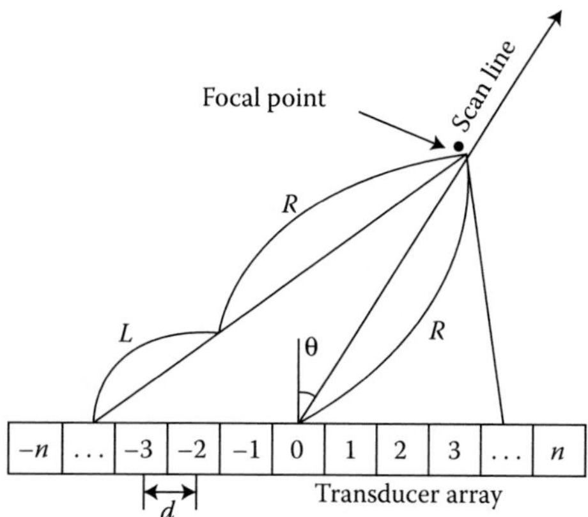

FIGURE 16.16 Dynamic focusing and steering delay.

for the acoustic signal path length differences from the transducer array to the target of interest. The expression for the focused signal $f(t)$ is

$$f(t) = \sum_{n=-N/2}^{n=N/2} X_n(t - \tau_n), \tag{16.18}$$

where N is the total number of transducer elements; X_n is the received reflected signal; and τ_n is the channel delay time for the nth transducer element [15]. The delay time, τ_n, derives from Figure 16.16. Assuming a signal, transmitted with the steering angle θ by exciting a transducer located at 0, a reflected signal propagates back from the focal point to the transducer array. When the distance from the focal point to the transducer center is R, the distance from the focal point to the nth transducer has the expression $L + R$, as shown in Figure 16.16. By denoting the space between adjacent channels, d, the channel delays are expressed as

$$\tau_n = \tau_n(R) = \frac{R}{c}\left[\sqrt{1 + \left(\frac{nd}{R}\right)^2 + 2\left(\frac{nd}{R}\right)\sin\theta} - 1\right], \tag{16.19}$$

where c is the average propagation speed of ultrasound in the medium [31].

The design of the programmable delays provides different delay times for each of the elements in a 16 × 1 array configuration. Implementing such a fine delay step in a CMOS technology is challenging in beamformer design. The most recently designed digital clock delay schemes use PLLs [15,31]. However, a 20-ps delay step would need at least a 10-GHz clock using these methods. This is not feasible in a 0.35-μm standard CMOS technology. Therefore, this work adopts an analog delay chain method. Figure 16.17 is a block diagram of the proposed delay chain. One of five delay buffers can be selected for coarse delay time setting with a 100-ps step. Then four different loading options can be added for the 20-ps fine delay step. Every channel on the chip has the channel delay setting circuit; therefore, a host computer can control delays between pulses by transmit beam focusing. Although required channel delays are 20–160 ps, the channel delays are programmable from 20 to 480 ps in order to compensate for the initial channel delay mismatch.

Figure 16.18 illustrates the transmit pulses generated by the transceiver chip. The transmit pulses can be delayed from 20 to 500 ps as described in Section 16.4.4. The delays by the programmable delay chain in the chip are measured with a high-precision digital oscilloscope (Agilent Infiniium 8000). Notably, the signals shown in this figure are calibrated to compensate for the initial channel

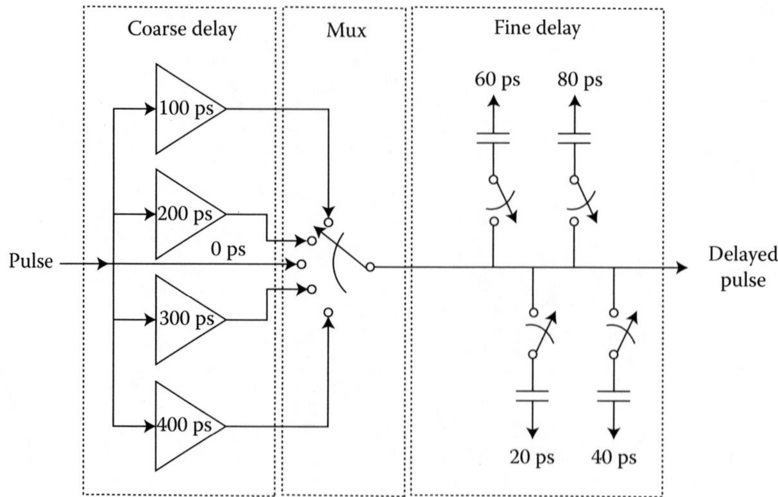

FIGURE 16.17 Circuit schematic of programmable delays for beam focusing.

delays due to signal line mismatches on the PCB. The frequency of the pulses can be varied from 1 to 100 MHz, where 5 MHz pulses are shown in this figure.

16.4.6 Experimental Results

16.4.6.1 Prototype Experimental Board

The transceiver chip was fabricated using a TSMC 0.35 μm, double-poly, four-metal process through MOSIS. The die size was 10 mm². Figure 16.19 shows the mounting of the transceiver chip and the thin-film transducers on the test board (a) and a microphotograph of the first-generation transceiver chip (b). The average power consumption in the receive mode, consisting of 16 receiver channels, ADC, and SRAM, operating simultaneously, is approximately 270 mW with a 3.3 V power supply. The shared ADC and SRAM architecture, which reduced the number of ADCs and SRAMs from 16 to 1, resulted in smaller chip area and lower power consumption. This size and power consumption is reasonable for a portable ultrasound imaging system using the transceiver chip; it can be decreased further if a state-of-the-art process technology, for example, a 90-nm or

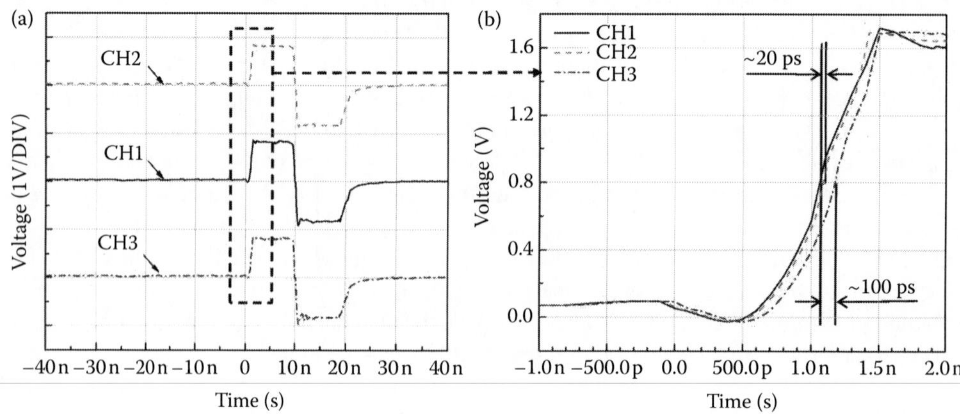

FIGURE 16.18 Measured delay of transmit channels: (a) transmit pulses with various channel delays (50 MHz) and (b) magnified view of the box in blank on (a).

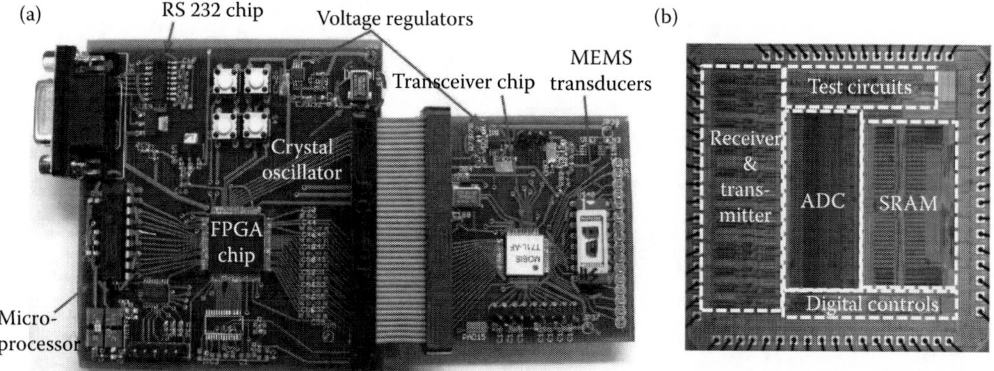

FIGURE 16.19 (a) Test board for the transceiver chip with the thin-film transducer array and (b) microphotograph of the CMOS transceiver chip.

0.13-μm CMOS process technology, is used. Table 16.2 summarizes the specifications for the transceiver chip.

16.4.6.2 Thin-Film Ultrasound Transducer Array

T-bar-shaped ultrasound PZT transducer arrays have been developed and documented in [16]. PZT layers can be thin, and allow reduction of the required voltages for exciting the transducer. Therefore, directly driving the transducers with low-voltage CMOS signals is possible. The thin-film transducers' fabrication employed a sol–gel and multilayer dry-etching process. Ti/Pt bottom electrodes were deposited on a silicon wafer on which a 300-nm thermal silicon dioxide film was preformed. The total of 0.5–0.6 μm PZT films was deposited using the sol–gel process over the bottom electrode; then, Pt top electrodes were formed. Finally, the T-bar shape transducer array structure was patterned by dry-etching. Figure 16.20 shows a scanning electron microscopy (SEM) image of the transducer array (a) and its frequency spectrum (b). The dimensions of a T-bar structure are 30 μm in width and 300 μm in length. Details of the thin-film transducers can be found in [16]. The target,

TABLE 16.2
CMOS Transceiver Chip Specifications Summary

Preamp	Gain (dB)	5–20
	Bandwidth (MHz)	>75
	Dynamic range (dB)	90
	Noise figure (dB)	10
VGA	Gain range (dB)	46
	Bandwidth (MHz)	250
	Noise figure (dB)	6–12
ADC	Resolution (bit)	6
	Conversion speed (MHz)	250
Memory	Capacity (byte)	3 K
	Data bandwidth (Mbps)	250
Transmitter	Pulse frequency (MHz)	1–100
	Delay step (ps)	20
Total chip	Noise figure (dB)	9.7–14.5
	Power consumption	270 mW
	Process technology	TSMC 0.35 μm
	Chip size	10 mm^2

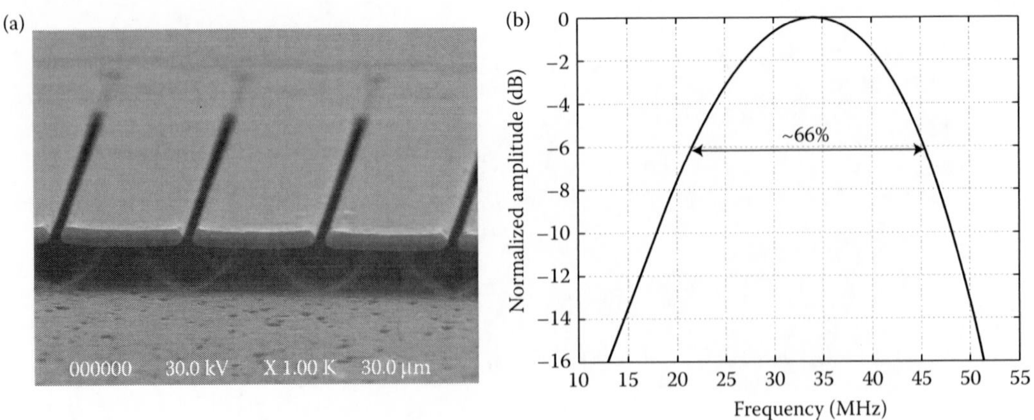

FIGURE 16.20 The SEM image of the thin-film transducer array (a) and its frequency spectrum (b).

center frequency of the thin-film transducer is 30–70 MHz, and that of the particular transducer array in these experiments is 35 MHz, with a bandwidth of 66% at 6-dB points. The capacitance of the 30-μm-wide transducer element is 145.1 pF, which indicates a dielectric constant of ~1000 at 1 kHz (as high as 1500) along with a low dielectric loss (<4%). Thus, the transducer appears to be a pure capacitance load for the preamplifier in the transceiver chip.

16.4.6.3 Pulse–Echo Experiments

The ultrasound signal acquisition experiments were conducted using the thin-film transducer with the transceiver chip. Figure 16.21 illustrates the pitch-catch-mode experimental setup. The stainless steel target object was located at a distance of about 3 mm away from the transducers in a water tank. A 50-MHz transmit pulse sent to the thin-film transducers from the transceiver chip via an external pulser allowed an increase of acoustic energy. The adjacent transducer in the same array received the reflected signals; then the transceiver chip amplified the received signals.

The gain of the preamplifier is set to 14 dB, and the gain of the VGA increased from 0 to 20 dB using varied control signals (0.15–1.0 V). Figure 16.22 shows the amplified and time-compensated ultrasound signals obtained from the VGA output using the thin-film transducer. The high-amplitude

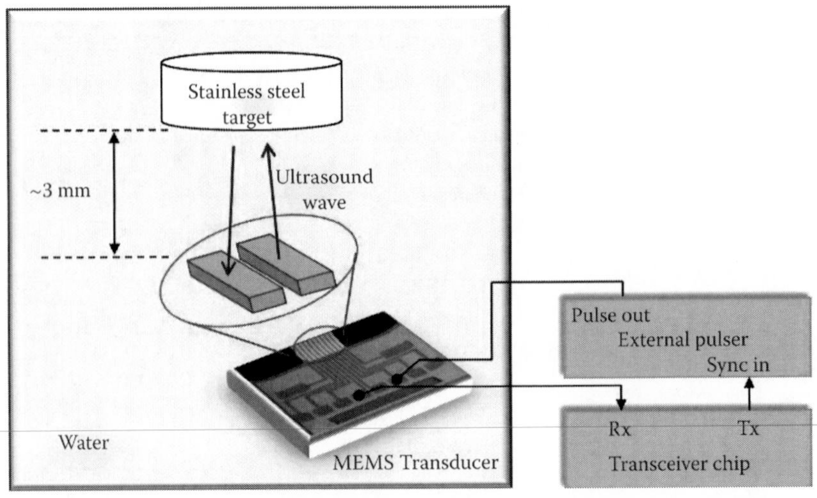

FIGURE 16.21 The pitch–catch-mode experimental setup.

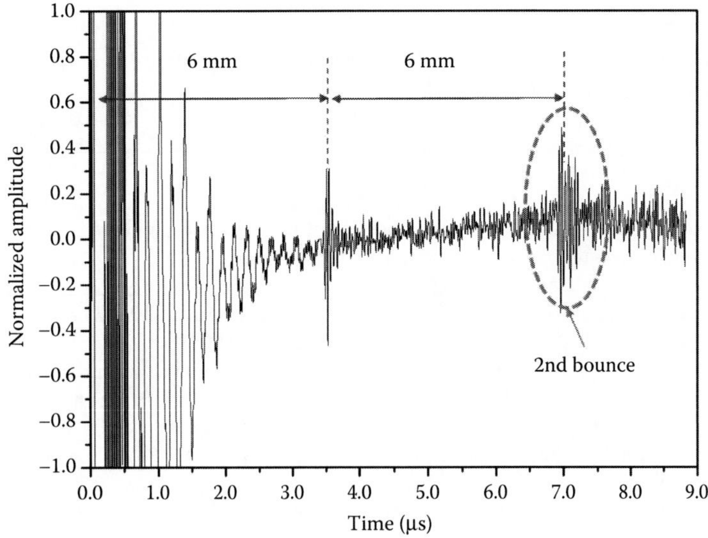

FIGURE 16.22 Thin-film transducer array pitch–catch-mode test results.

signal before 2.5 μs in this figure is from cross talk with a transmit pulse. The first peak of the detected ultrasound wave appeared around 3.5 μs, which is the first echo signal; the second peaks, around 7 μs, underwent multiple bounces. The second peaks, amplified by the VGA, compensated for the attenuation in the water. Notably, the amplitude of the second peaks is similar to that of the first peak due to the increasing gain over time.

16.5 CONCLUSION

This chapter explains the ultrasound imaging fundamentals and system considerations for developing a portable high-frequency ultrasound imaging system. The low-voltage transducer is crucial for developing a portable, ultracompact ultrasound imaging system because it enables the transducer to be placed with close-coupled ultrasound front-end electronics without using any expensive coaxial cables. Thus, reasonably, some cost reductions will accrue. Also, the fully integrated ultrasound transceiver chip with the shared ADC architecture is an effective solution for the portable imaging systems. It greatly decreases system size and power consumption, compared to conventional DBF ultrasound imaging systems currently marketed.

This chapter also introduces the Penn State portable ultrasound imaging system as an example of existing portable high-frequency ultrasound imaging systems. The Penn State ultrasound imaging system consists of a low-voltage-operated thin-film transducer array and a fully integrated custom-designed CMOS transceiver chip. A 16-channel ultrasound receiver is shared with an ADC and a 3-kbyte SRAM. The chip also makes it feasible for the transducers to be fabricated on the same package or board with the chip, and anticipates more cost and size reduction. Initial pulse–echo experiments using the imaging system were performed and the experimental results demonstrate the shared ADC architecture and the transceiver chip component designs.

REFERENCES

1. F. S. Foster, C. J. Pavlin, J. A. Harasiewicz, D. A. Christopher, and D. H. Turnbull, Advances in ultrasound biomicroscopy, *Ultrasound in Medicine and Biology*, 26(1), 1–27, 2000.
2. P. A. Payne, J. V. Hatfield, A. D. Armitage, Q.X. Chen, P. J. Hicks, and N. Scales, Integrated ultrasound transducers, *Proceedings of IEEE Ultrasonic Symposium*, 3, 1523–1526, 1994.

3. R. Reeder and C. Petersen, The AD9271—A revolutionary solution for portable ultrasound, *Analog Dialogue*, 41–07, July 2007. Available at: http://www.analog.com.
4. W. C. Black, Jr. and D. N. Stephens, CMOS chip for invasive ultrasound imaging, *IEEE Journal of Solid-State Circuits*, 29(11), 1994.
5. J. V. Hatfield, N. R. Scales, A. D. Armitage, P. J. Hicks, Q. X. Chen, and P. A. Payne, An integrated multi-element array transducer for ultrasound imaging, *Sensors and Actuators A: Physical,* 41(1–2), 167–173, 1994.
6. I. O. Wygant, D. T. Yeh, X. Zhuang, S. Vaithilingam, A. Nikoozadeh, O. Oralkan, A. Sanli Ergun, G. G. Yaralioglu, and B. T. Khuri-Yakub, Integrated ultrasound imaging systems based on capacitive micromachined ultrasonic transducer arrays, *2005 IEEE Sensors*, 2005.
7. J. Johansson, M. Gustafsson, and J. Delsing, Ultra-low power transmit/receive ASIC for battery operated ultrasound measurement systems, *Sensors and Actuators A: Physical*, 125, 317–328, 2006.
8. M. I. Fuller, E. V. Brush, M. D. C. Eames, T. N. Blalock, J. A. Hossack, and W. F. Walker, The sonic window: Second generation prototype of low-cost, fully-integrated, pocket-sized medical ultrasound device, *Ultrasonics Symposium (IUS), 2005 IEEE International*, 167–173, September 2005.
9. I. Kim, H. Kim, F. Griggio, R. L. Tutwiler, T. N. Jackson, and S. Trolier-McKinstry, CMOS ultrasound transceiver chip for high resolution ultrasonic imaging systems, *IEEE Transactions on Biomedical Circuits and Systems*, 3(5), 293–303, 2009.
10. T. L. Szabo, *Wave Scattering and Imaging, Diagnostic Ultrasound Imaging: Inside Out*, Elsevier Academic Press, MA pp. 213–242, 2004.
11. C. J. Pavlin and F. S. Foster, *Ultrasound Biomicroscopy of the Eye*, Springer-Verlag, New York, Inc., NY, 1994.
12. M. E. Schafer and P. A. Lewin, The influence of front-end hardware on digital ultrasonic imaging, *IEEE Transactions on Sonics and Ultrasonics*, SU-31(4), 1984.
13. P. N. T Wells. *Advances in Ultrasound Techniques and Instrumentation*, Churchill Livingstone, New York, NY, 1993.
14. M. Karaman, A. E. Kolağasıoğlu, and A. Atalar, A VLSI receive beamformer for digital ultrasound imaging, *Proceedings of IEEE International Conference on Acoustic, Speech, Signal Processing*, pp. 657–660, San Francisco, CA, 1992.
15. A. Kassem, J. Wang, A. Khouas, M. Sawan, and M. Boukadoum, Pipelined sampled-delay focusing CMOS implementation for ultrasonic digital beamforming, *Proceedings of the third IEEE Workshop on SoC for Real-Time Application*, pp. 247–250, 2003.
16. I. G. Mina, H. Kim, I. Kim, S. K. Park, K. Choi, T. N. Jackson, R. L. Tutwiler, and S. Trolier-McKinstry, High frequency piezoelectric MEMS ultrasound transducers, *IEEE Transactions on Ultrasonics, Ferroelectrics, and Frequency Control*, 54(12), 2422–2430, 2007.
17. S. Triger, J. Wallace, J. Saillant, S. Cochran, and D. R. S. Cumming, MOSAIC: An integrated ultrasonic 2D array system, *2007 IEEE Ultrasonics Symposium*, New York, NY, October 2007.
18. R. Reeder and C. Petersen, The AD9271—A revolutionary solution for portable ultrasound. Available at: http://www.analog.com/library/analog Dialogue/archives/41–07/ultrasound.pdf.
19. B. Murmann, ADC performance survey 1997–2008. Available at: http://www.stanford.edu/~murmann/adcsurvey.html.
20. B. Murmann, A/D converter trends: Power dissipation, scaling and digitally assisted architectures, *IEEE 2008 Custom Integrated Circuits Conference (CICC)*, San Jose, CA, September 21–24, pp. 105–112, 2008.
21. A. C. Kak and K. A. Dines, Signal processing of broad-band pulsed ultrasound: Measurement of attenuation of soft biological tissues, *IEEE Transactions on Biomedical Engineering*, BME-25, 321–344, 1978.
22. H. B. Meire and P. Farrant, *Basic Ultrasound*, John Wiley & Sons, Chichester, England 1995.
23. R. J. Baker, Data converter SNR, *CMOS Mixed-Signal Circuit Design*, Vol. 2, IEEE Press, NJ, pp. 63–148, 2002.
24. B. Razavi, Differential amplifiers, in *Design of Analog CMOS Integrated Circuits*, McGraw-Hill Companies, Inc., New York, NY, pp. 100–132, 2001.
25. C. Wu, C. Liu, and S. Liu, A 2 GHz CMOS variable-gain amplifier with 50 dB linear-in-magnitude controlled gain range for 10GBase-LX4 Ethernet, *ISSCC 2004*, 1, 484–541, 2004.
26. C. E. Shannon, Communication in the presence of noise, *Proceedings of the Institute of Radio Engineers*, 37(1), 10–21, 1949.
27. J. Yoo, D. Lee, K. Choi, and A. Tangle, Future-ready ultrafast 8-bit CMOS ADC for system-on-chip applications, in *14th Annual IEEE International ASIC/SOC Conference*, September 2001, pp. 455–459.

28. J. Yoo, K. Choi, and D. Lee, Comparator generation and selection for highly linear CMOS flash analog-to-digital converter, *Journal of Analog Integrated Circuits and Signal Processing*, 35, 179–187, 2003.
29. I. Kim, J. Yoo, J. Kim, and K. Choi, Highly efficient comparator design automation for TIQ flash A/D converter, *IEICE Transactions on Fundamentals*, E91-A(12), 3415–3422, 2008.
30. UC Berkeley Device Group, BSIM. Available at: http://www-device.eecs. berkeley.edu/~bsim3/.
31. J. H. Kim, T. K. Song, and S. B. Park, Pipeline sampled-delay focusing in ultrasound imaging systems, *Journal of Ultrasonic Imaging*, 9, 75–91, 1987.

17 Smart Eye Tracking Sensors Based on Pixel-Level Image Processing Circuits

Dongsoo Kim

CONTENTS

17.1 INTRODUCTION AND GENERAL ISSUES IN EYE TRACKERS

Examples of commonly used pointing devices in a computer system include the mouse and the pen digitizer. However, these interfaces are difficult to be used in a mobile environment wearing a head-mounted display (HMD). One of the alternative pointing devices is the eye tracker that acquires the point on the screen that the user gazes on [1–3]. Figure 17.1 shows the eye tracker in a HMD. The eye tracker gives information to the HMD that indicates the point on the screen that the user gazes on.

Infrared light is commonly used in the eye tracker because it eliminates the influence of ambient illumination and improves discrepancy between the pupil and the white of the eye [4]. Under infrared

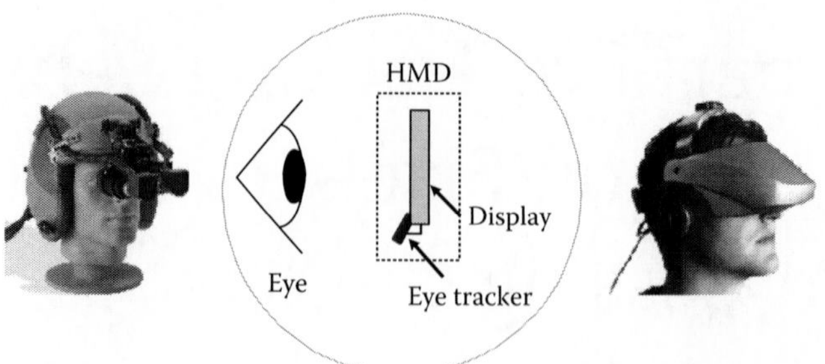

FIGURE 17.1 Eye tracker in an HMD.

illumination, the pupil is the biggest black region in the eye image. Therefore, the point that the eye gazes on can be obtained by finding the center point of the pupil in the eye image.

The common eye tracker uses a normal image sensor and an image processing algorithm [3–5]. However, this system needs A/D converter (ADC), interface circuit, and software computation. As the tracking resolution is increased, the tracking time is increased drastically due to the speed limitation of the ADC, data interface, and computation. To overcome these disadvantages, smart image sensors that include image processing and pattern recognition circuits on the same silicon chip have been reported in [6–11]. This chapter introduces three versions of the single-chip eye tracker with the smart complementary metal-oxide-semiconductor (CMOS) image sensor pixels.

17.1.1 Eye Movement

The oculomotor system can be analyzed more easily than most other movement control systems because it can be broken down functionally into smaller subsystems [12] that can be analyzed individually. Eye movements can generally be grouped into six types: saccades, smooth pursuit, vergence, optokinetic reflex, vestibule-ocular reflex, and fixation. Table 17.1 shows the velocity range and the angular range of these eye movements.

Saccades are the rapid eye movements occurring when we look around to examine our environment. Saccadic eye movements can vary considerably in magnitude, from less than 1° to more than 100° as the situation demands. The peak velocity during the movement depends on the size of the saccade. For large saccades it can reach 800°/s. because the velocity is so high, the movements are brief. The most frequently occurring saccades, which are smaller than 15°, take less than 50 ms from start to finish. Saccades are voluntary eye movements in the sense that we can consciously choose to look, or ignore, things in the visual scene. Once initiated, however, the execution of the movement is automatic. During the eye movement, when the retinal image is sweeping rapidly across the retina, vision is actively suppressed.

Smooth pursuit movements are visually guided movements in which the eye tracks a small object that is moving relative to a stationary background. The purpose of smooth pursuit movements is to

TABLE 17.1
Velocity and Angular Ranges for Various Eye Movements

Type of Movement	Velocity Range	Angular Range
Saccade	10–800°/s (2–170 mm/s)	0.1–100°
Smooth pursuit and optokinetic reflex	<40°/s (8 mm/s)	>1°
Vergence	10°/s (2 mm/s)	~15°
Vestibule-ocular reflex	100–400°/s (21–84 mm/s)	1–12°
Fixation	10–300°/s (0.03–1 mm/s)	0.003–0.2°

stabilize the retinal image of a moving object in order to allow it to be visually examined. Pursuit movements are voluntary only insofar as we can choose to look at a moving object or ignore it. The kinematics of pursuit movements are completely determined by the motion of the object that is being tracked. It has the peak velocity of 40°/s.

Vergence moves the eyes in opposite directions, causing the intersection point of the lines of sight of the two eyes to move closer or further away. The purpose of vergence eye movements is to direct the fovea (area of the retina with the highest resolution) of both eyes at the same object. The vergence movements have the angular range of about 15°. Under natural conditions vergence movements are accompanied by saccades or pursuit movements.

The optokinetic reflex is a visually guided reflex, the purpose of which is to compensate for body and head movements so that retinal image motion is minimized. The optokinetic reflex responds optimally if the stimulus is movement of all, or a large portion of, the retinal image. We have no voluntary control over these reflexive eye movements. If the retinal image of the whole field of view moves, our eyes invariably follow this motion. Just as in the case of pursuit movements, the kinematics of eye movements resulting from the optokinetic reflex are determined by the motion of the stimulus.

The vestibule-ocular reflex is similar to the optokinetic reflex in that its function is also to compensate for head motion and stabilize the retinal image. In contrast to the optokinetic reflex however, the vestibulo-ocular reflex is not guided visually, but is generated by receptors in the inner ear that detect acceleration and changes with respect to gravity. The vestibule-ocular reflex is also beyond our voluntary control. The kinematics of these eye movements are directly linked to the signals generated by the vestibular organs in the inner ear. The velocity range of the vestibular movements is 100–400°/s.

Fixation or visual fixation means maintaining the visual gaze on a location. Humans (and other animals with a fovea) typically alternate saccades and visual fixations. Visual fixation is never perfectly steady: this eye movement occurs involuntarily. The term "fixation" can also be used to refer to the point in time and space of the focus rather than to the act of fixating; a fixation in this sense is the point between any two saccades, during which the eyes are relatively stationary and virtually all visual input occurs. The fixation always lasts at least 100 ms. It is during these fixations that most visual information is acquired and processed. At least three types of small involuntary eye movements commonly occur during the fixations: Flicks are very rapid (perhaps as little as 30 ms apart), involuntary, saccade-like movements of less than 1°; drifts are very small and slow (about 0.1°/s), apparently random motions of the eye; and tremors are tiny (less than 30 arc seconds), high-frequency (30–150 Hz) eye vibrations [13].

17.1.2 Eye Tracking Technique

There exist four main methods for measuring eye movements in relation to head movements: electro-oculography (EOG), scleral contact lens/search coil, photo-oculography (POG) or video-oculography (VOG), and video-based combined pupil and corneal reflection [14].

17.1.2.1 Electro-Oculography

EOG is based on the electronic measurement of the potential created by differences between the cornea and the retina when the eye is rotated and is the most widely applied eye movement recording method. A picture of a subject wearing the EOG apparatus is shown in Figure 17.2. The recorded potentials exist in the range of 15–200 μV, with nominal sensitivities of the order of 20 μV/deg of eye movement. This technique measures eye movements relative to head position and hence is not generally suitable for point-of-regard measurements unless head position is also measured.

17.1.2.2 Scleral Contact Lens/Search Coil

Scleral contact lens/search coils involve attaching a mechanical or optical object to a large contact lens that is worn directly on the eye (covering both the cornea and scleral). Figure 17.3 shows a

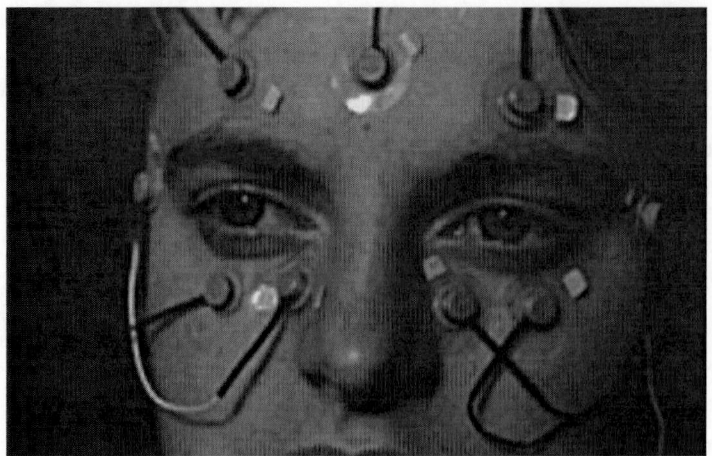

FIGURE 17.2 Example of EOG eye movement measurement. (Copyright © Metrovision, France. Available at: http://www.metrovision.fr.)

picture of the search coil embedded in a scleral contact lens and the electromagnetic field frame. Although the scleral search coil is the most precise eye movement measurement method, it is also the most intrusive method. Insertion of the lens requires care and practice. Wearing of the lens causes discomfort. This method also measures eye position relative to the head, and is not generally suitable for point-of-regard measurement.

17.1.2.3 Photo-Oculography or Video-Oculography

POG or VOG groups together a wide variety of eye movement recording techniques that involve the measurement of distinguishable features of the eyes under rotation/translation, such as the apparent shape of the pupil, the position of the limbus, and corneal reflections of a closely situated directed light source. Automatic limbus tracking often make use of photodiodes (PDs) mounted on spectacle frames as shown in Figure 17.4. This method requires the head to be fixed by using, for example, a head/chin rest or a bite bar.

17.1.2.4 Video-Based Combined Pupil/Corneal Reflection

Although the above techniques are in general suitable for eye movement measurements, they do not often provide point-of-regard measurement. Video-based combined pupil and corneal reflection is an eye movement measurement technique that is able to provide information about where the user is looking at in space, while taking the user's eye positions relative to the head into account.

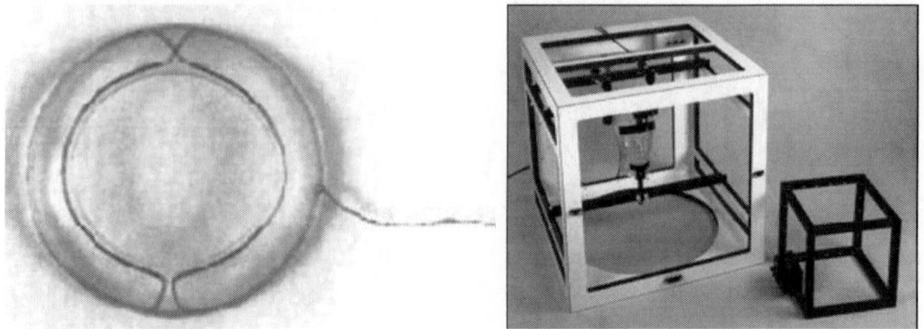

FIGURE 17.3 Example of search coil embedded in contact lens and electromagnetic field frames for search coil eye movement measurement. (Copyright © Skalar Medical, Netherlands, Available at: http://www.skalar.nl)

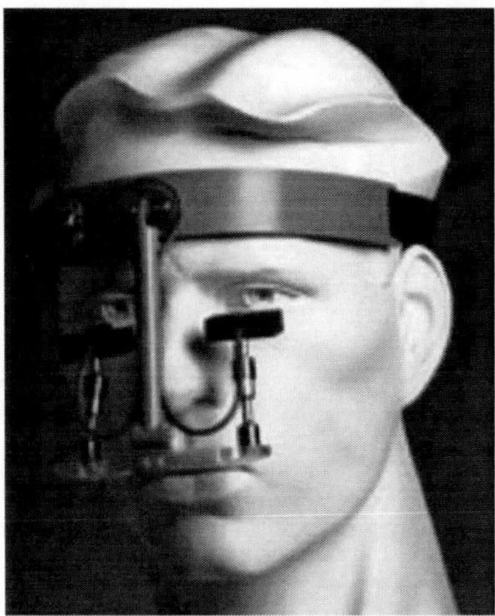

FIGURE 17.4 Example of infrared limbus tracker apparatus. (Copyright © Microguide, USA. Available at: http://www.eyemove.com)

Video-based trackers utilize inexpensive cameras and image processing hardware to compute the point-of-regard in real time. The apparatus may be table-mounted, as shown in Figure 17.5, or worn on the head, as shown in Figure 17.6. The optics of both table-mounted and head-mounted systems is essentially identical, with the exception of size. These devices, which are becoming increasingly available, are most suitable for use in interactive systems.

17.1.3 Illumination of the Eye Tracker

Figure 17.7 shows the eye image under visual and infrared illumination. An iris is the biggest black region under visual illumination and some region of it is covered by the eyelid. The boundary between the iris and the white of the eye is not distinct. However, under infrared illumination a pupil is the biggest black region and it is a circle with a clear boundary. Infrared illumination eliminates the influence of ambient illumination. Therefore, the common eye tracker uses infrared illumination

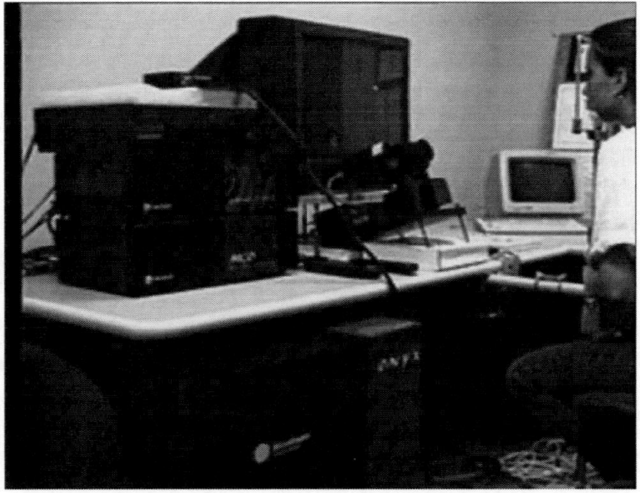

FIGURE 17.5 Example of the table-mounted video-based eye tracker.

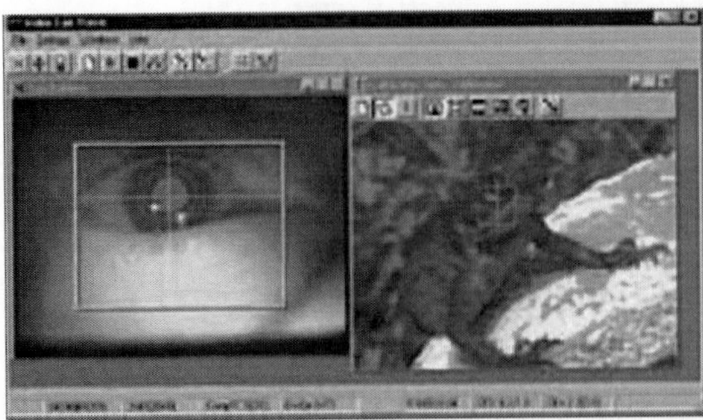

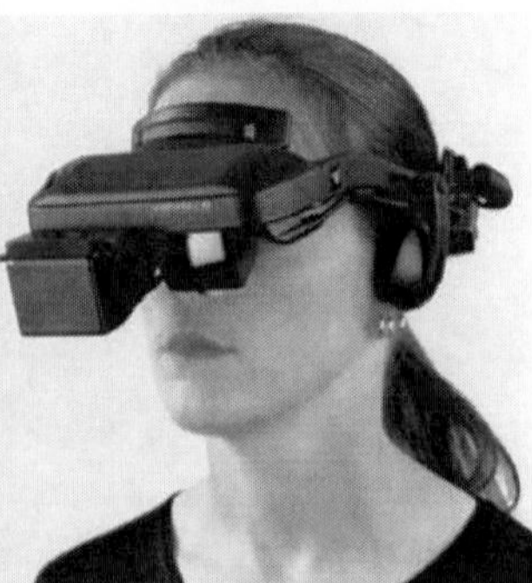

FIGURE 17.6 Example of the head-mounted video-based eye tracker. (Copyright © Iota AB. EyeTrace Systems, Sundsvall Business & Tech. Available at: Sweden: http://www.iota.se)

for finding the center of the eyeball. A diffuser can be used to spread out the bright spot caused by an infrared light source and the contact lens does not have a significant effect on the eye tracker.

17.1.4 Evaluation Criterion for the Eye Tracker

In this section, we discuss some of the evaluation criteria for the eye tracking system. The performance of the eye tracker can be evaluated by the resolution, speed (sampling rate), transport delay, accuracy, and other considerations. Table 17.2 lists several general application categories, the performance parameters that are probably most important, and the values for those parameters that are probably in an appropriate range.

17.1.5 Cellular Neural Networks

The basic circuit unit of cellular neural networks is called a *cell*. It contains linear and nonlinear circuit elements, which typically are linear capacitors, linear resistors, linear and nonlinear controlled sources, and independent sources. The structure of cellular neural networks is similar to that found in cellular automata; namely, any cell in a cellular neural network is connected only to its neighbor cells. The adjacent cells can interact directly with each other. Cells not directly connected together may affect each other indirectly because of the propagation effects of the continuous-time dynamics of cellular neural networks. An example of a two-dimensional (2D) cellular neural network is shown in Figure 17.8.

A typical example of a cell C_{ij} of a cellular neural network is shown in Figure 17.8, where the suffixes u, x, and y denote the *input*, *state*, and *output*, respectively. The node voltage v_{xij} of C_{ij} is called the state of the cell and its initial condition is assumed to have a magnitude less than or equal to 1. The node voltage v_{uij} is called the input of C_{ij} and is assumed to be a constant with magnitude less than or equal to 1. The node voltage v_{yij} is called the output.

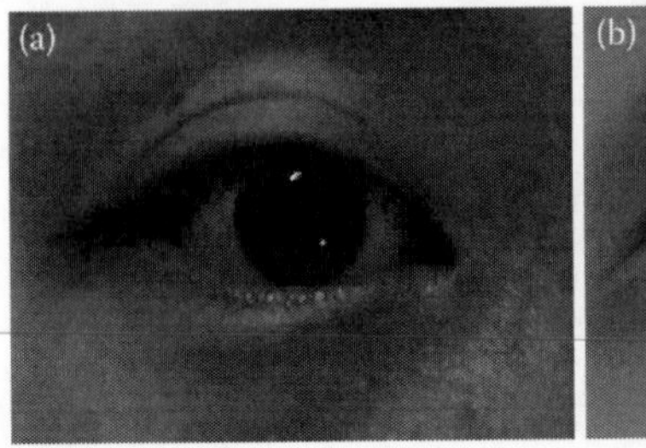

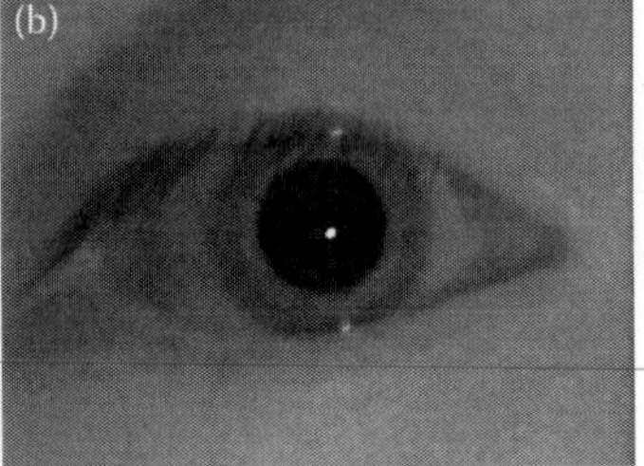

FIGURE 17.7 Eye image under (a) visual and (b) infrared illumination.

TABLE 17.2
Performance Parameters for the General Applications

Measure point-of-regard or scan path for offline analysis

- Accuracy = 1°. Visual angle
- Sample rate = 60 Hz

Real-time control using point-of-regard (switch selection, display control)

- Transport delay ≤50 ms
- Sample rate 60 Hz
- Accuracy 1°

Study saccadic velocity profiles, nystagmus

Sample rate ≥240 Hz

- Linearity ≤5%
- Resolution 0.25°

Study flicks, drifts

Sample rate ≥240 Hz

- Linearity ≤5%
- Resolution = 10 arc minutes

Measure tremor

Sample rate ≥1000 Hz

- Linearity ≤5%
- Resolution 1 arc second

Stabilize image on retina

- Accuracy = 2 arc minutes
- Sample rate ≥240 Hz
- Transport delay ≤10 ms

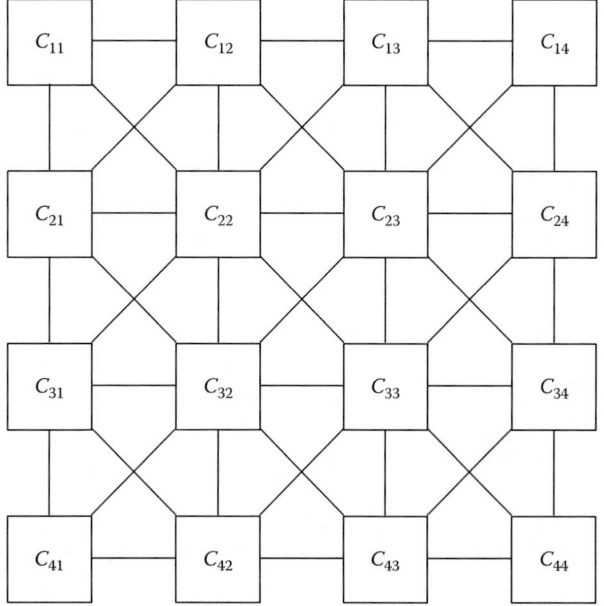

FIGURE 17.8 2D cellular neural network.

Observe from Figure 17.9 that each cell C_{ij} contains one independent voltage source E_{ij}, one independent current source I, one linear capacitor C, two linear resistors R_x and R_y, and at most $2m$ linear voltage-controlled current sources that are coupled to its neighbor cells via the controlling input voltage v_{ukl}, and the feedback from the output voltage v_{ykl} of each neighbor cell C_{kl}, where m is equal to the number of neighbor cells. In particular, $I_{xy}(i,j;k,l)$ and $I_{xu}(i,j;kl)$ are linear voltage-controlled current sources with the characteristics $I_{xy}(i,j;k,l) = A(i,j;kl)v_{ykl}$ and $I_{xu}(i,j;kl) = B(i,j;kl)v_{ukl}$ for all neighbor cells C_{kl}.

Applying Kirchhoff's Current Law (KCL) and Kirchhoff's Voltage Law (KVL), the circuit equations of a cell with an $M \times N$ cell array are easily derived as follows:.

State equation:

$$C\frac{dv_{xij}(t)}{dt} = -\frac{1}{R_x}v_{xij}(t) + \sum_{C_{kl};\text{neighbor cell of } C_{ij}} A(i,j;k,l)v_{ykl}(t)$$
$$+ \sum_{C_{kl};\text{neighbor cell of } C_{ij}} B(i,j;k,l)v_{ukl} + I, \quad 1 \le i \le M;\ 1 \le j \le N$$

Output equation:

$$v_{yij}(t) = \frac{1}{2}\left(\left|v_{xij}(t)+1\right| - \left|v_{xij}(t)-1\right|\right), \quad 1 \le i \le M;\ 1 \le j \le N$$

Input equation:

$$v_{uij} = E_{ij}, \quad 1 \le i \le M;\ 1 \le j \le N$$

Constraint conditions:

$$\left|v_{xij}(0)\right| \le 1, \quad 1 \le i \le M;\ 1 \le j \le N$$
$$\left|v_{uij}\right| \le 1, \quad 1 \le i \le M;\ 1 \le j \le N$$

Parameter assumptions:

$$A(i,j;k,l) = A(k,l;i,j), \quad 1 \le i,k \le M;\ 1 \le j,\ l \le N$$
$$C > 0,\ R_x > 0$$

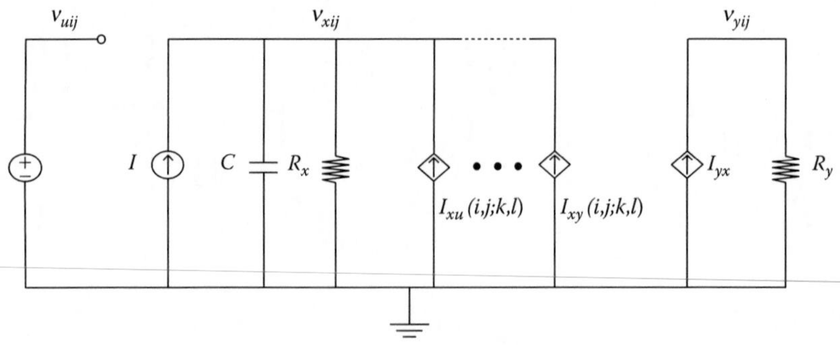

FIGURE 17.9 Example of a cell circuit.

17.1.6 Eye Tracker Calibration

When the eye tracker interacts with the display of the HMD or the graphical applications, the most important requirement is the mapping of the eye tracker coordinates to the display image coordinates.

In the monocular case, a typical 2D image-viewing application is expected, and the coordinates of the eye tracker are mapped to the 2D (orthogonal) viewport coordinates accordingly (the viewport coordinates are expected to match the dimensions of the image being displayed in the HMD). In the binocular (VR) case, the eye tracker coordinates are mapped to the dimensions of the near viewing plane of the viewing frustum. The following sections discuss the mapping and the calibration of the eye tracker coordinates to the display coordinates for the monocular applications.

For the calibration of the eye tracker, the data obtained from the tracker must be mapped to a range appropriate for the 2D display image coordinates as shown in Figure 17.10 [14].

A linear mapping between two coordinate systems can be adopted. In general, if $u \in [u_0, u_1]$ needs to be mapped to the range $[0, x_1]$, we have

$$x = \frac{\left(u - u_0\right) x_1}{\left(u_1 - u_0\right)} \quad (17.1)$$

Equation 17.1 has a straightforward interpretation:

1. The value u is translated to its origin, by subtracting u_0.
2. The value $(u - u_0)$ is then normalized by dividing through by the range $(u_1 - u_0)$.
3. The normalized value $(u - u_0)/(u_1 - u_0)$ is then scaled to the new range (x_1).

The y-coordinate can be also obtained by the same linear mapping as follows:

$$y = \frac{(v - v_0) \cdot y_1}{\left(v_1 - v_0\right)} \quad (17.2)$$

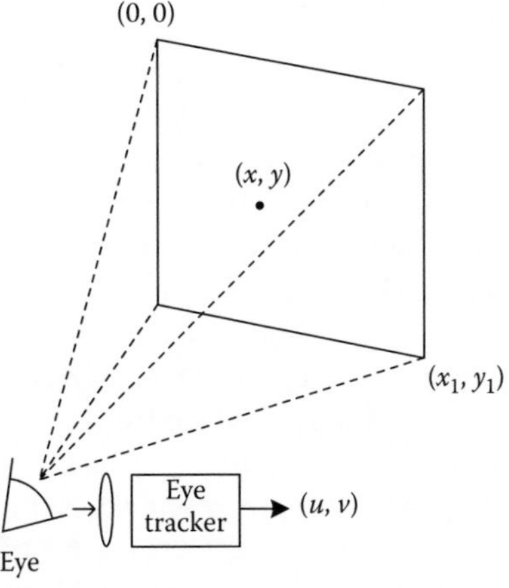

FIGURE 17.10 Calibration method of the eye tracker.

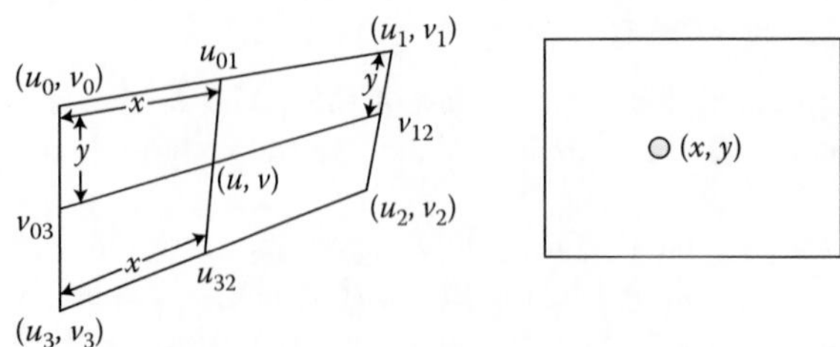

FIGURE 17.11 Bilinear transform for the calibration of the eye tracker.

To reduce the mapping error, a bilinear transform can be used. If the coordinates (u,v) of the eye tracker have a trapezoid shape as shown in Figure 17.11, u_{01}, u_{32}, v_{03}, and v_{12} can be obtained as

$$\begin{aligned} u_{01} &= u_0 + x(u_1 - u_0) \\ u_{32} &= u_0 + x(u_2 - u_3) \\ v_{03} &= v_0 + y(v_3 - v_0) \end{aligned} \tag{17.3}$$

The (u,v) can be also calculated as follows:

$$\begin{aligned} u &= u_{01} + y(u_{32} - u_{01}) \\ v &= v_{03} + x(v_{12} - v_{03}) \end{aligned} \tag{17.4}$$

The final coordinates (x,y) can be solved by the mathematical solve tools [18–19] from Equations 17.3 and 17.4.

17.2 FIRST VERSION OF THE EYE TRACKER

This section proposes the first version of the single-chip eye tracker that generates the address for the center point of the pupil. Section 17.2.1 proposes the eye tracker architecture and operation principle. Section 17.2.2 describes circuit implementation. Section 17.2.3 presents the simulation and the experimental results. Finally, Section 17.2.4 provides the conclusion.

17.2.1 Proposed Eye Tracker Architecture

The proposed eye tracker is composed of a smart CMOS Image Sensor (CIS) pixel array, Winner-Take-All (WTA) circuits, address encoders, and a stop criterion circuit, as shown in Figure 17.12. The pixel array includes a photosensor and an interpixel feedback circuit that captures the image and performs shrink operation that will be described below. The WTA circuit finds the winning current and the location from the horizontally/vertically summed current from the pixel array. The winning location is encoded by the encoder and it is latched by the trigger signal, V_{STOP}, from the stop criterion circuit.

Figure 17.12 shows the flow chart of the operation principle that is explained below. The image is captured by PD and then transferred as an initial state voltage. During the shrink phase the black region of the image is shrunk by interpixel positive feedback. Each pixel generates current, I_{ij}, that is inversely proportional to its state voltage and these current are summed column-wise and row-wise, respectively. These summed current (I_i, I_j) represent the number of black pixels present in each column and row, respectively. The WTA circuit detects the column and row that have the largest number of black pixels during the shrink operation. The operations ①, ②, ③, and ④ in Figure 17.13 are performed simultaneously by the analog circuits. This procedure is continuously repeated until

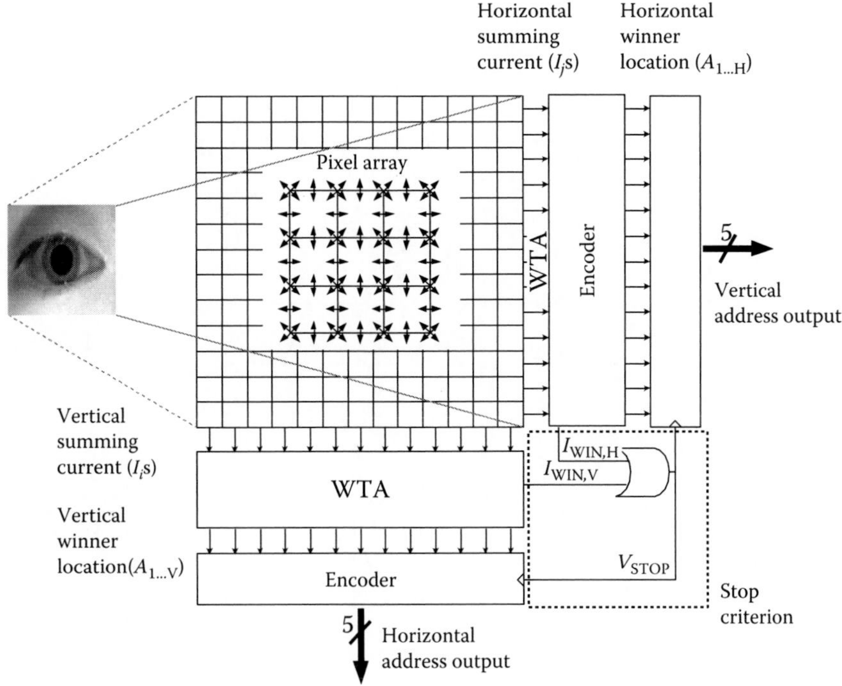

FIGURE 17.12 Block diagram of the proposed eye tracker. (Copyright © Kluwer 2005.)

the number of black pixels is less than 2. When the number of black pixels is less than 2, the winning column and row address is latched and read out. These addresses indicate coordinates of the remaining black pixels that correspond to the center of the pupil. Once the address is read out, a new image is captured and the above procedure is repeated with the new image.

The smart CIS pixel array performs shrink operation with continuous-time interpixel feedback as shown in Figure 17.13. The dynamics of the proposed smart pixel can be expressed as

$$\begin{cases} C_F \dfrac{dx_{ij}}{dt} = \displaystyle\sum_{k=-1}^{1}\sum_{l=-1}^{1} \varepsilon_{kl}\, y_{(i+k,j+l)}, \quad x_{ij}(0) = u_{ij} \\ y_{ij} = f(x_{ij}) \end{cases} \tag{17.5}$$

where C_F is the integration capacitor and u_{ij} is the initial state of the pixel (i, j) that is captured from the photosensor. The x_{ij} and y_{ij} represent the state voltage and the output current of pixel (i, j), respectively. $f(x_{ij})$ is a transconductor with saturation and ε_{kl} is the interpixel feedback gain coefficient as shown in Figure 17.14. Here, the feedback coefficients should satisfy $0 < \varepsilon_1 < \varepsilon_2 < 1$ and the self-feedback should be zero for isotropic shrink operation.

During the shrink operation, the current I_{ij} is generated by each pixel as $I_{ij} = g(x_{ij})$. I_{ij} is generated when the pixel is considered as a black pixel and it is inversely proportional to x_{ij}. The current I_{ij} are summed column-wise and row-wise as shown in Figure 17.13, and are denoted by I_i and I_j, where i and j are the row number and column number, respectively. Since the black pixel (low x_{ij}) generates high I_{ij}, the summed currents represent the number of black pixels remaining in each column and row.

Since each pixel gives positive feedback to its surrounding pixels, a white pixel forces its neighbor pixels to be white, while a dark pixel provides small amount of feedback to its neighbor pixels. This interpixel feedback causes the boundary black pixels to be changed to white continuously and

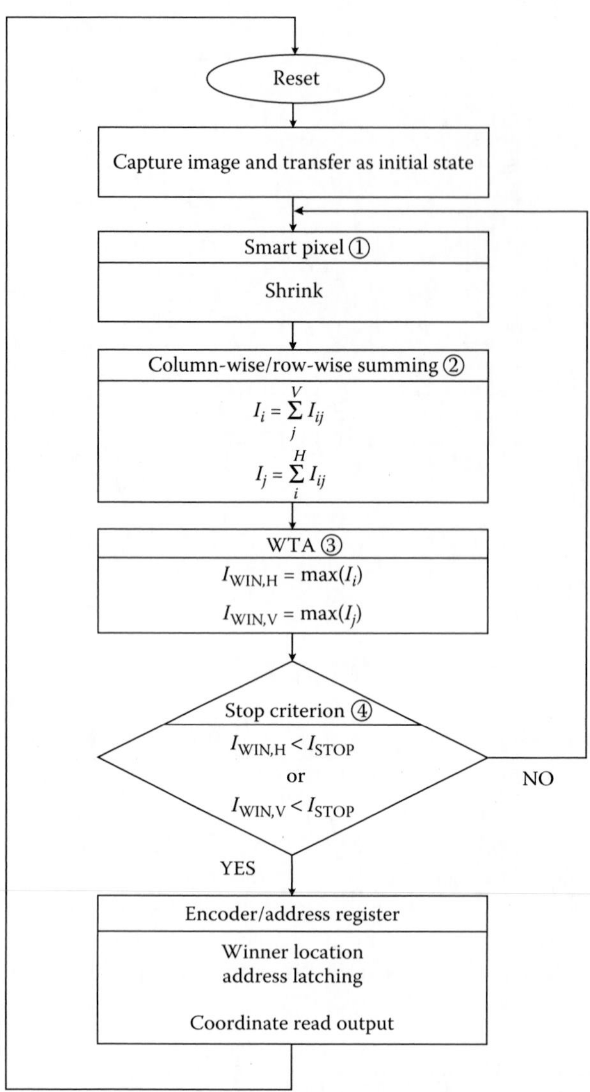

FIGURE 17.13 Flow chart of the operational principle. (Copyright © Kluwer 2005.)

the size of the black regions is shrunk as shown in Figure 17.14. The nonlinear function $f(x_{ij})$ causes the gray image to be gradually changed to the black and white image. This shrink operation (see Figure 17.15) continues and eventually all pixels become white.

Figure 17.16 shows the block diagram of the WTAs, stop criterion circuit, address encoder, and address latch. Each WTA detects continuously the column/row that has the highest summed current (I_i or I_j) during the shrink operation. The WTA generates winner location logic output A_1, and only one node out of A_l is logic-high that represents the winning column/row. The WTA circuit not only identifies the location of the winner, but also it selects the winning current I_{WIN} as well. The I_{WIN} is used by the stop criterion circuit to decide whether the shrink operation is completed.

The address encoder continuously encodes the winning row/column during the shrink operation. If the wining current (I_{WIN}) is smaller than a certain limit (I_{STOP}) that corresponds to two black pixels, it means that the largest black region is completely shrunk down to 2 pixels that is located at the center of the largest black object. In this situation, the winner location logic output represents the location of the center of the remaining pixels. The stop criterion circuit generates logic-high signal

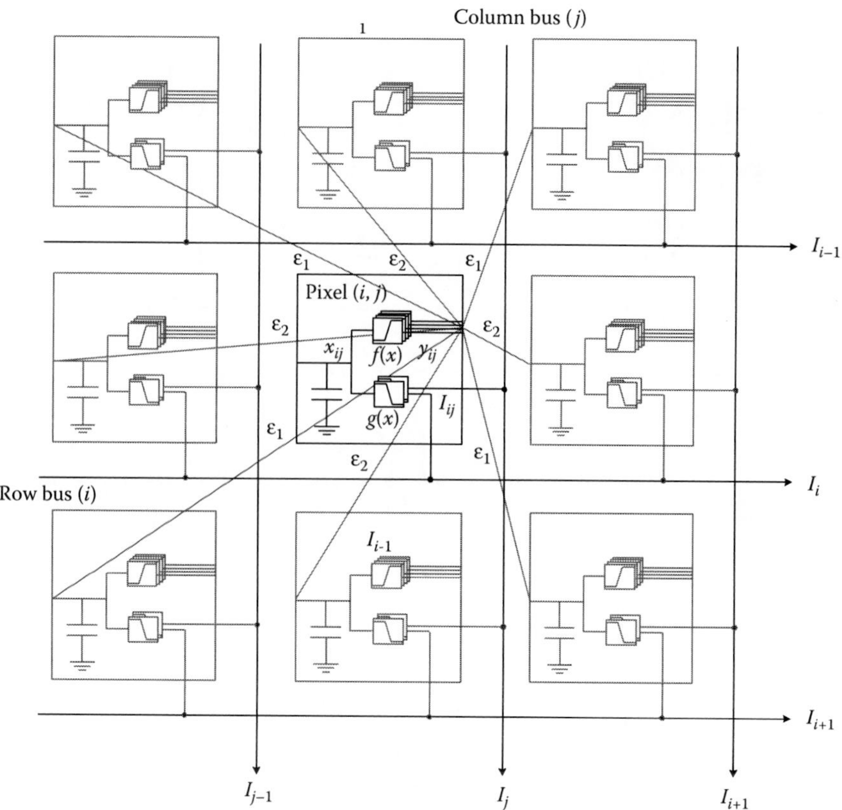

FIGURE 17.14 Block diagram of the smart CIS pixels array: interconnections are depicted only for the pixel (i, j). (Copyright © Kluwer 2005.)

when either the horizontal or the vertical winning current reaches I_{STOP} and it causes that the address registers latch the winning address from the encoders. This latched address corresponds to the center of the pupil.

17.2.2 Circuits Implementation

A schematic diagram of the proposed smart CIS pixel is shown in Figure 17.17a. Figure 17.17b represents the timing diagram for one frame. First, the PD capacitor C_S is precharged to V_{REF1} and C_F is reset during the *reset* phase by turning on TX and RST switches. Second, the TX switch is turned off and C_S is discharged corresponding to the incident light during the *capture* phase. In the *transfer* phase, the charge in C_S is transferred to C_F by turning on the TX switch and turning off the RST switch. The C_S is reset to V_{REF1} again at this moment. Once the PD charge is transferred into C_F, x_{ij} represents the light intensity (u_{ij}) of the pixel (i, j). The transistors M_Y generate feedback currents εy_{ij} corresponding to the pixel state voltage x_{ij}. In *shrink* phases, the *STR* switch is turned on and the current to the surrounding pixels is summed and integrated in C_F causing x_{ij} to be increased.

Here, C_F is chosen four times larger than C_S because C_S is in the range of several tens of femtofarads and the use of such a small capacitance for C_F causes high sensitivity to parasitic capacitance. This ratio causes x_{ij} to be one-fourth of u_{ij}. Figure 17.18 shows the implementation of $f(x_{ij})$ and $g(x_{ij})$ by careful arrangement of V_{REF1} and V_{REF2} considering the operating region of M_Y and M_S. Since the dynamic range of u_{ij} is bounded as $0 < u_{ij} < V_{REF1}$, and $x_{ij} = 1/4u_{ij}$, the V_{REF1} is chosen about $4/5V_{DD}$ considering the dynamic range and the implementation of the saturation function

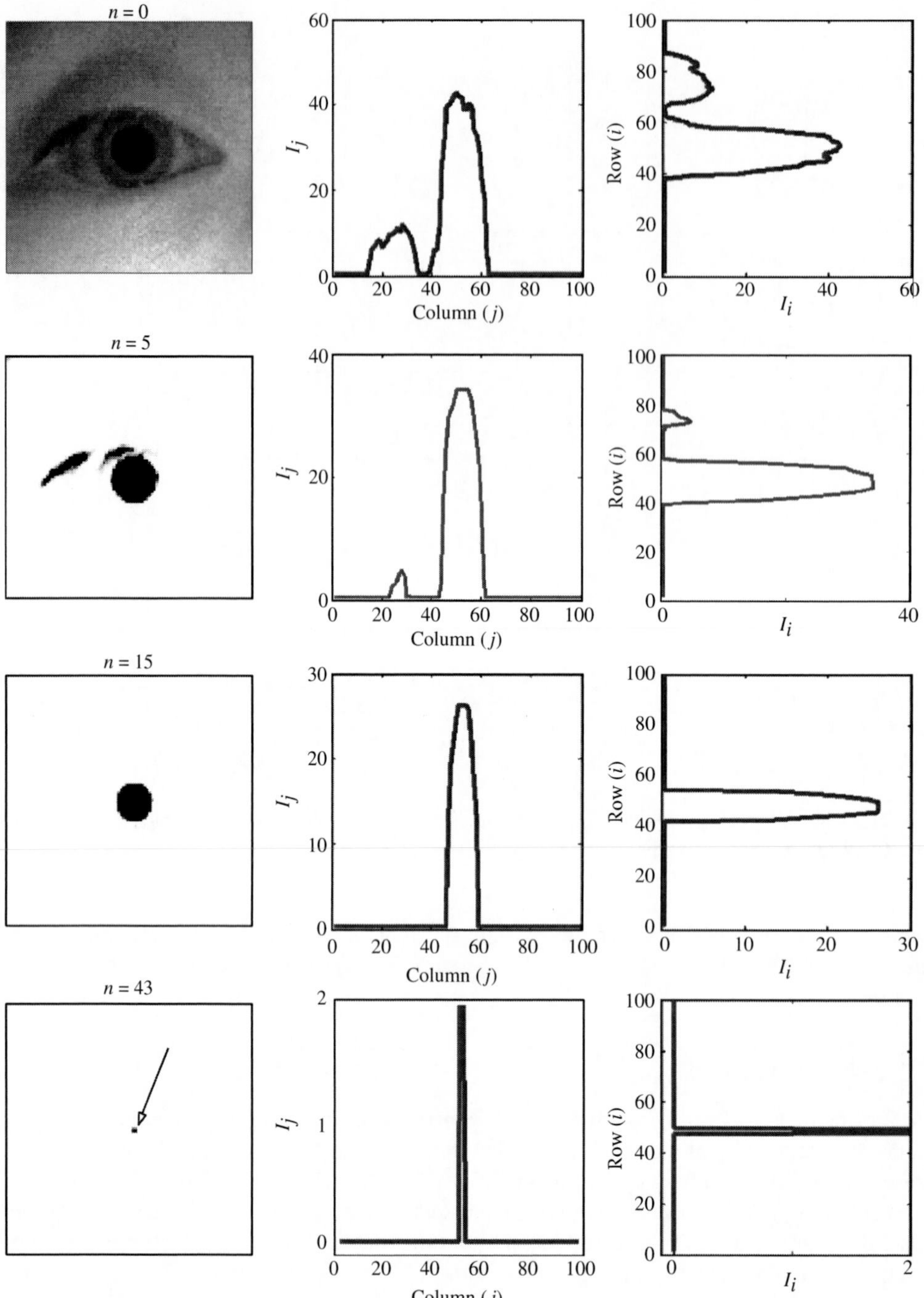

FIGURE 17.15 System-level simulation results of shrink operation: the image size is 100 × 100, n is the iteration number, ε_1 =0.1 and ε_2 =0.15. (Copyright © Kluwer 2005.)

$f(x_{ij})$. The V_{REF2} is chosen so that M_Y is operated in cutoff when the x_{ij} is low. The $g(x_{ij})$ is realized by M_S's threshold voltage. M_S is turned on when x_{ij} is sufficiently low that it is considered as a black pixel.

Figure 17.19 presents a schematic diagram of the WTA [20–23] and the stop criterion circuit. The common source voltage V_S is decided to turn on only the winning transistor out of $M_{1...H}$ that has the

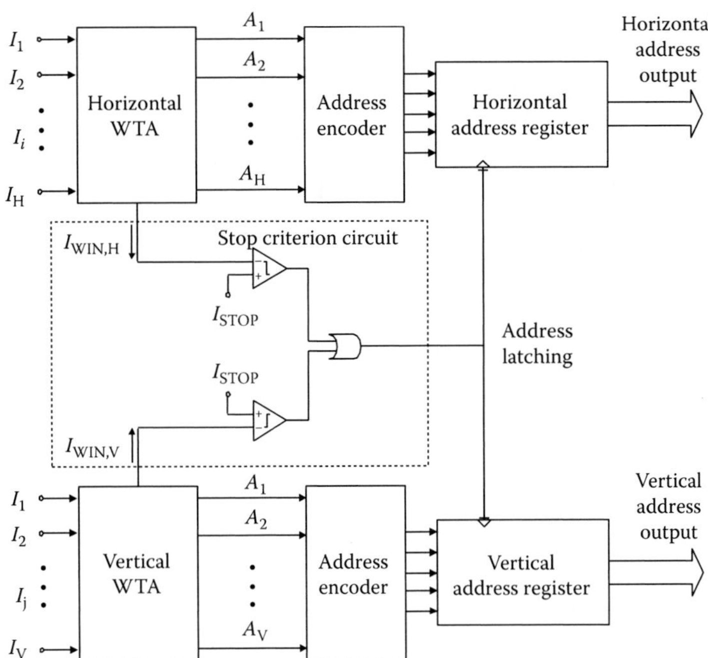

FIGURE 17.16 Block diagram of the WTA, address encoder, and stop criterion. (Copyright © Kluwer 2005.)

highest input current and all others are turned off. The bias current I_{BIAS} is chosen to be twice the maximum I_{ij} generated by one black pixel. The winner current I_{WIN} is equal to the highest input current and it is copied to the stop criterion circuit.

Since only the winning transistor is turned on and allows current flow (see Figure 17.20b), only the winner generates logic-high winning location logic output ($A_{1...H}$) and all others are low. The $A_{1...H}$ outputs are connected to the address encoder. Although the WTA deals with a large number of inputs, the mismatch among transistors is not critical because eventually the WTA identifies the winner from two adjacent inputs that correspond to the remaining two black pixels in shrink operation. In the stop criterion circuit, the address latching signal V_{STOP} is generated by comparing I_{WIN} and I_{STOP}. The V_{STOP} is changed to logic high when I_{WIN} is smaller than I_{STOP}.

17.2.3 Simulation and Experimental Results

Figure 17.20 shows the transistor-level simulation result for a 32 × 32 array with the test image shown in Figure 17.20a. Figure 17.20b shows the row-wise and column-wise summed currents (I_is and I_js), the outputs of row and column WTAs (A_{1V} and $A_{1...H}$), and V_{STOP}. As the shrink operation is started at 55 μs, I_is and I_js start to decrease continuously as shown in Figure 17.20b. The currents that correspond to a smaller circle located at (21, 22) are completely reduced to zero at 60 μs. This means that the smaller circle disappears in the image. The logic output of the WTA changes to low as time elapses and only the winning row and column are kept logic high. When the current of the 11th row and the 9th column that corresponds to the center of the bigger circle is lower than I_{STOP}, the V_{STOP} changes to high, causing the winning address to be latched at 67 μs. The operation time of shrinking is about 12 μs and it is decided automatically by the stop criterion circuit.

The proposed single-chip eye tracker was fabricated with a 0.35-μm CMOS process. Figure 17.21 shows the microphotograph of the fabricated chip. The fabricated pixel array is 32 × 32 and one pixel occupies 50 × 50 μm^2. The PD is realized with n^+/p^--substrate junction whose area is 10 × 10 μm^2.

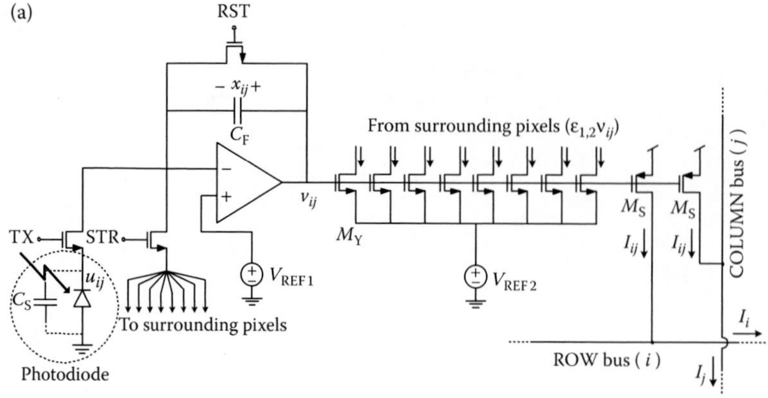

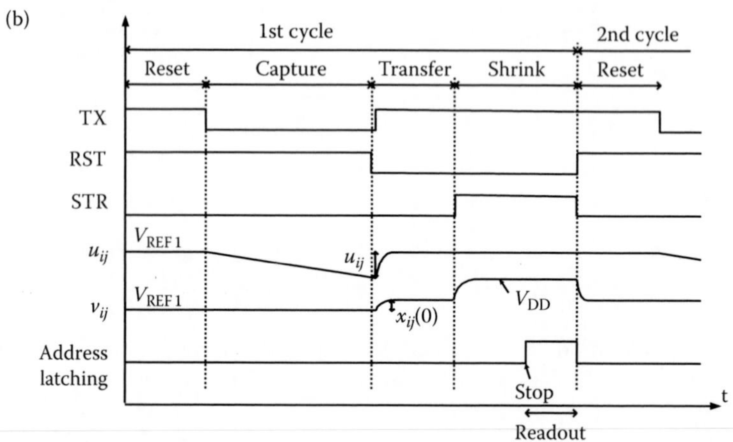

FIGURE 17.17 Block and timing diagrams of the smart CIS pixel. (a) Schematic diagram of the smart CIS pixel. (b) Timing diagram of the proposed eye tracker. (Copyright © Kluwer 2005.)

Figure 17.22 shows the testing setup for the error performance measurement with the fabricated prototype chip. The eye image captured under the infrared illumination is projected on the prototype chip through the beam projector and microscope. The light intensity of the image is decreased to a realistic intensity level by optical attenuation filters. The projected image on the chip is monitored by a digital camera instantaneously. The image on the pixel array is aligned precisely with the image displayed on the computer.

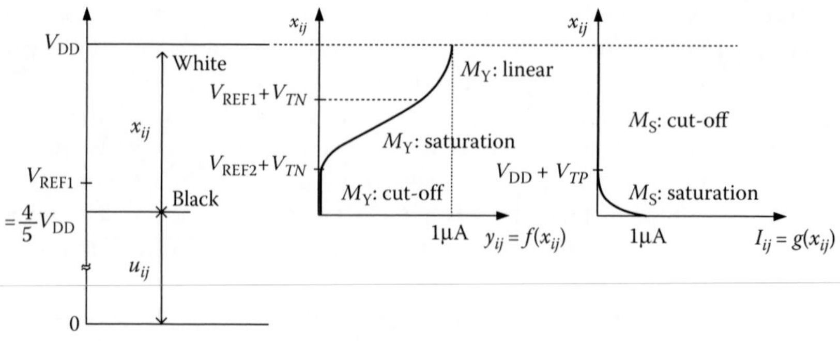

FIGURE 17.18 Implementation of $f(x_{ij})$ and $g(x_{ij})$. (Copyright © Kluwer 2005.)

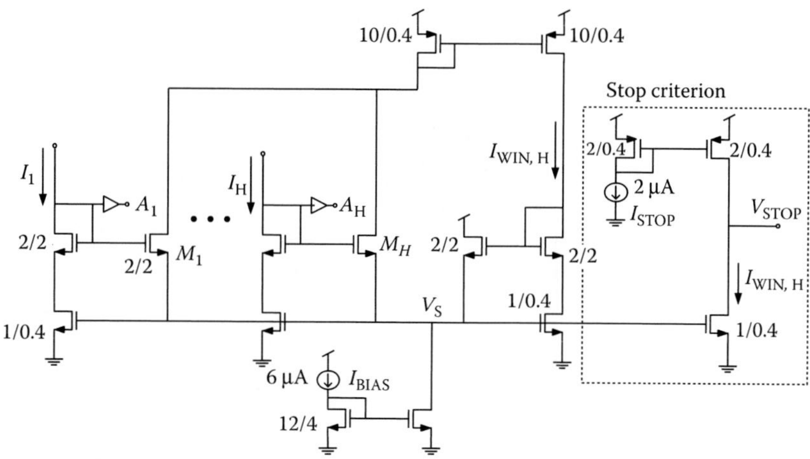

FIGURE 17.19 Circuit diagram of the WTA circuit and stop criterion. (Copyright © Kluwer 2005.)

Figure 17.23 shows the microphotograph of the projected test images on the fabricated chip. The measurement results that were read out from the fabricated chip are marked as × and the expected results from the simulation are marked as □. Figure 17.24 shows the measured error map of the fabricated eye tracker. The error of the fabricated eye tracker was tested with test images that are similar to the test image shown in Figure 17.20a. The center of the black circle is changed pixel by pixel and the output address from the chip is compared with the ideal one. The test result shows that the error is within ±1 pixel. Error distribution in the upper-right side of the array is slightly higher than that of the lower-left side of the array due to process variation. The frame rate is 125 frames/second (fps) and the power consumption is 260 mW with 3.3 V power supply. The specification of the prototype eye tracker is summarized in Table 17.3.

17.3 SECOND VERSION OF THE EYE TRACKER

This section proposes the second version of the single-chip eye tracker that eliminates the glint effect and generates the digital address for the center of the pupil. Section 17.3.1 proposes an eye tracking algorithm and architecture that can eliminate the effect of glints. Section 17.3.2 describes circuit implementation. Section 17.3.3 presents the simulation and experimental results. Finally, Section 17.3.4 provides the conclusion.

17.3.1 Proposed Eye Tracking Algorithm and Architecture

Figure 17.25 describes the algorithmic processes of the eye tracking. The *shrink* operation is the process that each white pixel gives feedbacks to surrounding pixels that force them to be white, whereas the black pixel gives negligible feedbacks. As the shrink operation is performed repeatedly, the boundary black pixels are changed to white continuously and the size of the black region shrinks, eliminating the small black regions such as iris, eyelashes, eyelid, and various shadows as shown in Figure 17.25a. This process is repeated until only a few pixels remain. Then, the location of the remaining pixel represents the center of the pupil.

Although the shrink operation is an effective way to eliminate other objects and find the center of the pupil, the glint generated by the corneal reflection of the light source is inevitable as shown in Figure 17.25b. Since this glint is expanded during the shrink operation and causes wrong center address as shown in Figure 17.25b, the white hole should be filled with black pixels to eliminate the effect of the glint. The hole filling can be performed by the *expand* operation as shown in

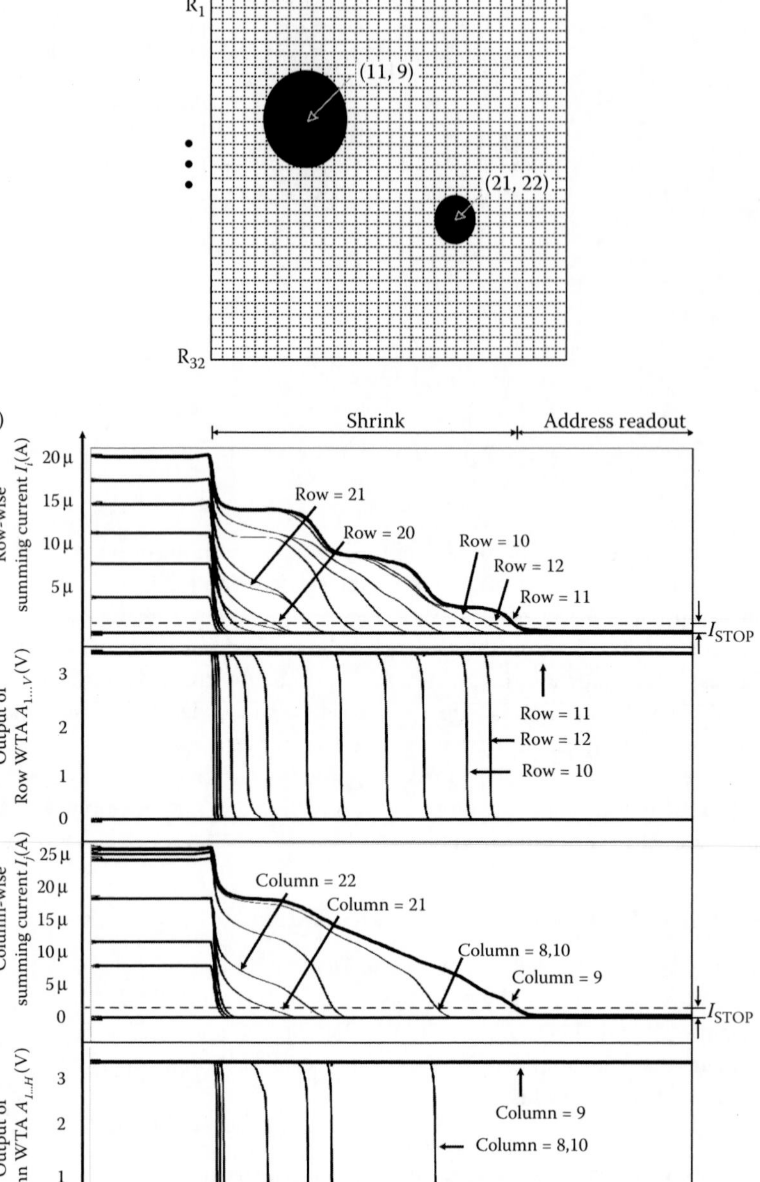

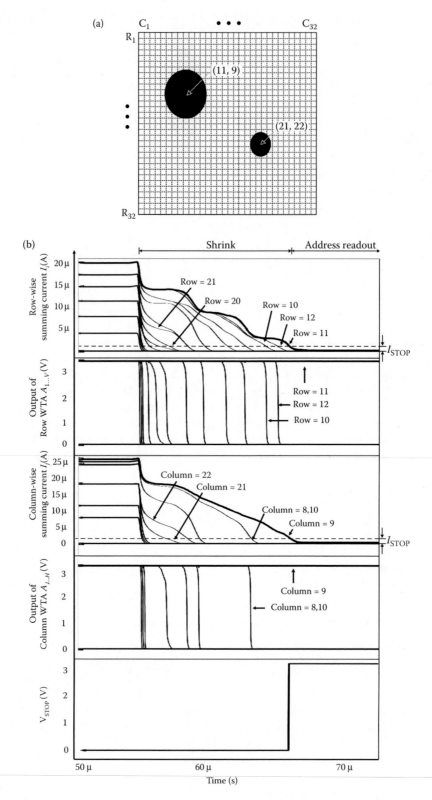

FIGURE 17.20 Transistor-level simulation results. (a) Input image for simulation. (b) Simulated waveforms during the shrink operation. (Copyright © Kluwer 2005.)

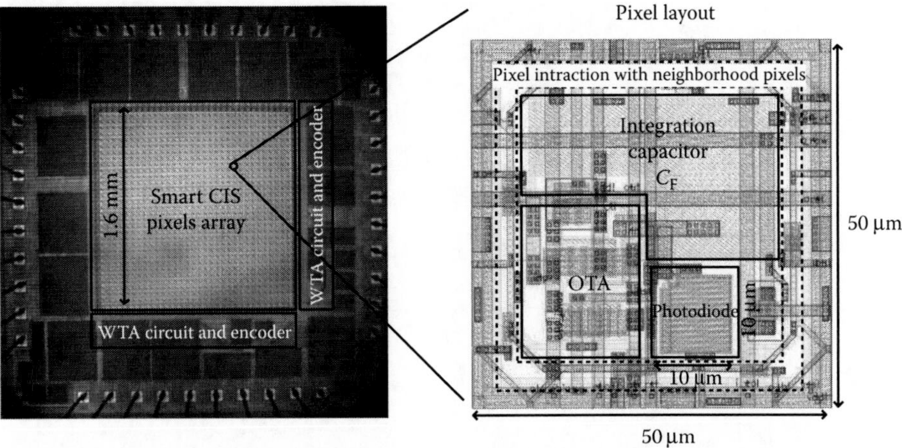

FIGURE 17.21 Chip microphotograph of the fabricated eye tracker and the layout of the smart pixel. (Copyright © Kluwer 2005.)

Figure 17.25c. During the expand operation, the black pixels force its neighbor pixels to be black and these interactions cause that the boundary white pixels are changed to black continuously. After a certain number of iterations of the shrink operation to eliminate noisy black objects, the expand operation is executed to fill the hole caused by the glint. Once the hole is filled with black pixels, the shrink operation resumes and continues until the last pixel remains. Although the number of iterations for expansion should be decided empirically, the introduction of the expand operation provides accurate center location.

The proposed eye tracker is composed of a smart pixel array, WTA circuits, a stop criterion circuit, latches, and address encoders as shown in Figure 17.26. The smart pixel array captures the image and performs the shrink and the expand operations. The number of black pixels is counted vertically and horizontally by summing the currents from pixels in each row or in each column, respectively. The WTA circuit not only finds the location of the largest current out of the column-wise summed current I_i^V or the row-wise summed current I_j^H, but also copies the winning current value I_w^V or I_w^H. The stop criterion circuit generates the *latch* signal when either I_w^V or I_w^H is smaller than the reference current I_{STOP} that corresponds to two black pixels. The WTA circuit generates logic high only for the winning column or row, while all other logic outputs (A_i or A_j) are logic low. Each latch stores the corresponding WTA logic output when the *latch* signal is generated by the stop criterion circuit. Then, the winning addresses are encoded and read out.

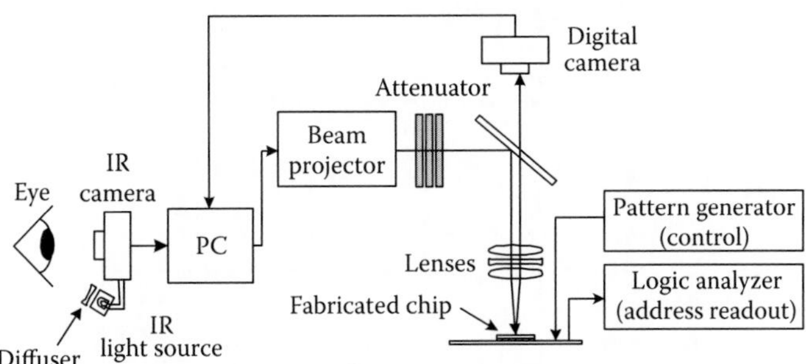

FIGURE 17.22 Testing environment for error measurement with the fabricated chip. (Copyright © Kluwer 2005.)

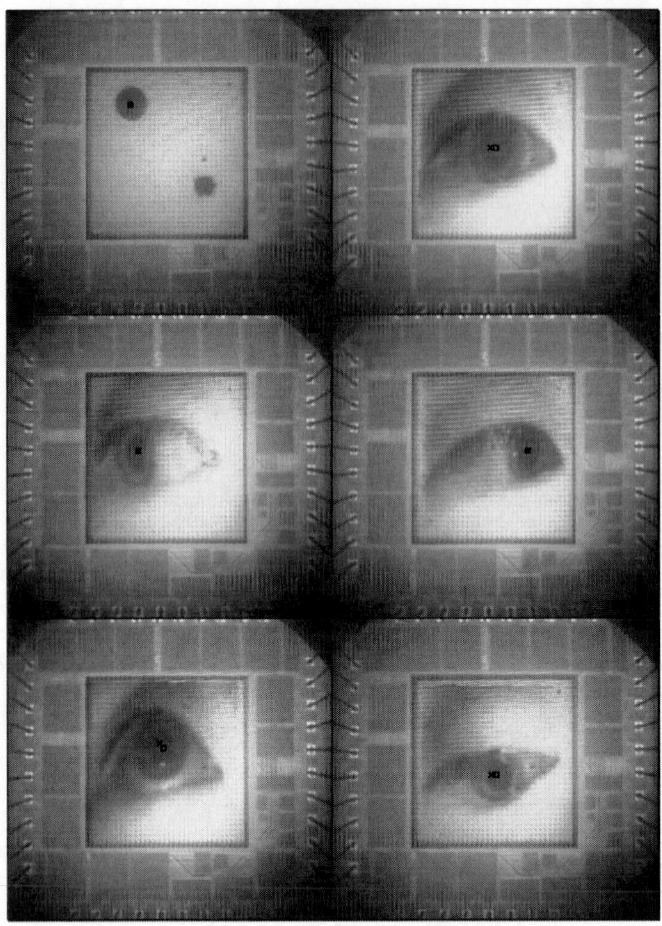

FIGURE 17.23 Image of the prototype chip and measurement results: the measurement results are marked with × and the expected results are marked with □. (Copyright © Kluwer 2005.)

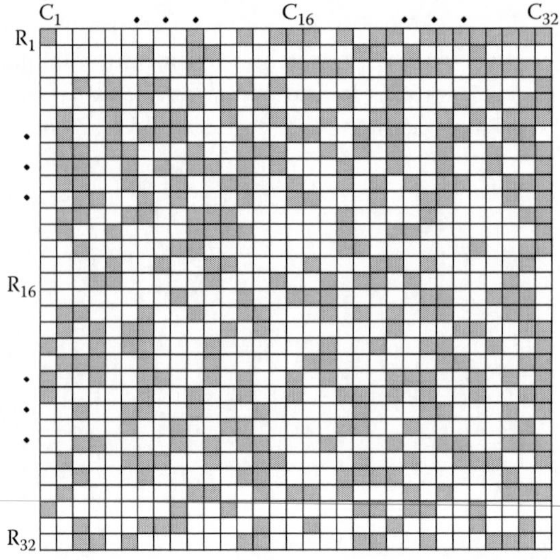

FIGURE 17.24 The measured error map of the fabricated eye tracker. (Copyright © Kluwer 2005.)

TABLE 17.3
Performance Summary of the First Version Eye Tracker

Process	0.35-μm CMOS 2-Poly 4-Metal
Power supply	3.3 V
Power consumption	260 mW
Chip size	1.95 × 1.95 mm²
Smart CIS cells array	32 × 32
Smart CIS cell size	50 × 50 μm²
PD size	10 × 10 μm²
Quantum efficiency	0.19 at 1000 nm
PD signal range	1.9 V
Frame rate	125 fps
Integration time	1 ms
Error	±1 pixel

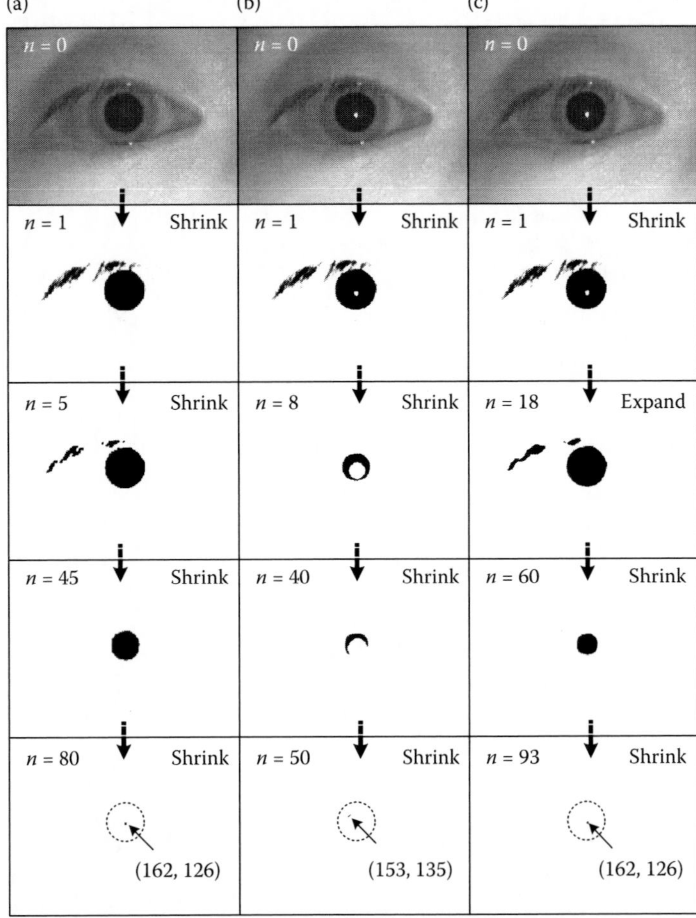

FIGURE 17.25 Algorithmic processes of eye tracking: image size is 320 × 240, *n* is the iteration number, and the dashed circle indicates the shape of the pupil. (a) Eye tracking without glint using shrink operation (From D. Kim, S. Lim, and G. Han, *Analog Integr. Circuits Signal Process.*, 45, 131–141, 2005. With permission.). (b) Eye tracking with glint using shrink operation only. (c) Eye tracking with glint using the shrink and expand operations. (Copyright © IEEE 2009.)

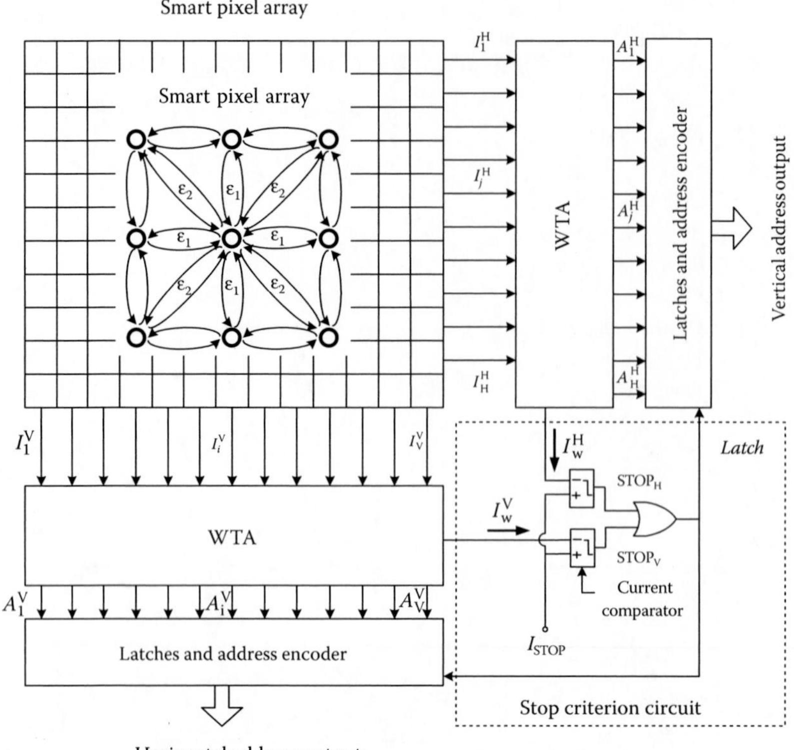

FIGURE 17.26 Block diagram of the proposed eye tracker. (Copyright © IEEE 2009.)

17.3.2 Circuits Implementation

The smart CIS pixel array performs the shrink and the expand operations with continuous-time interpixel feedback. Figure 17.27a presents the functional block diagram of the proposed smart pixel whose dynamics can be expressed as

$$\begin{cases} y_{ij} = f(x_{ij}) \\ n_{ij} = \sum_{k=-1}^{1}\sum_{l=-1}^{1} \varepsilon_{kl}\, y_{(i+k,\ j+l)} \\ C_{PD}\dfrac{dx_{ij}}{dt} = h_{s,e}(n_{ij}) \end{cases} \tag{17.6}$$

where C_{PD} is the parasitic capacitance of the PD and x_{ij} represents the state voltage whose initial value is decided from the captured image. Here, x_{ij} is lower for brighter light. $f(x_{ij})$ is an inverted saturation function that discriminates the black pixel from the white pixel. The n_{ij} is the weighted sum of feedbacks from the neighboring pixels as shown in Figure 17.28. Here, the weights for diagonal neighbors should be smaller than that for vertical and horizontal neighbors to guarantee the isotropic shrink and expansion. $h_s(n_{ij})$ and $h_e(n_{ij})$ are nonlinear transconductance functions for generating feedback currents, I_{FB}, respectively for the shrink and the expand operations.

Each pixel counts the number of neighboring white pixels by calculating n_{ij}. When the control signal is set to perform the shrink operation, I_{FB} is generated based on $h_s(n_{ij})$ as shown in Figure

17.27a. If more than three white pixels exist in the neighborhood, then the pixel is considered to be located at the boundary of the black pixels. The transconductor takes out current from the C_{PD}, causing the x_{ij} to be lowered, which corresponds to a becoming white pixel. On the contrary, when the control signal is set to perform the expand operation, I_{FB} is generated based on $h_e(n_{ij})$. If less than five white pixels exist in the neighborhood, then the pixel is considered to be located at the boundary

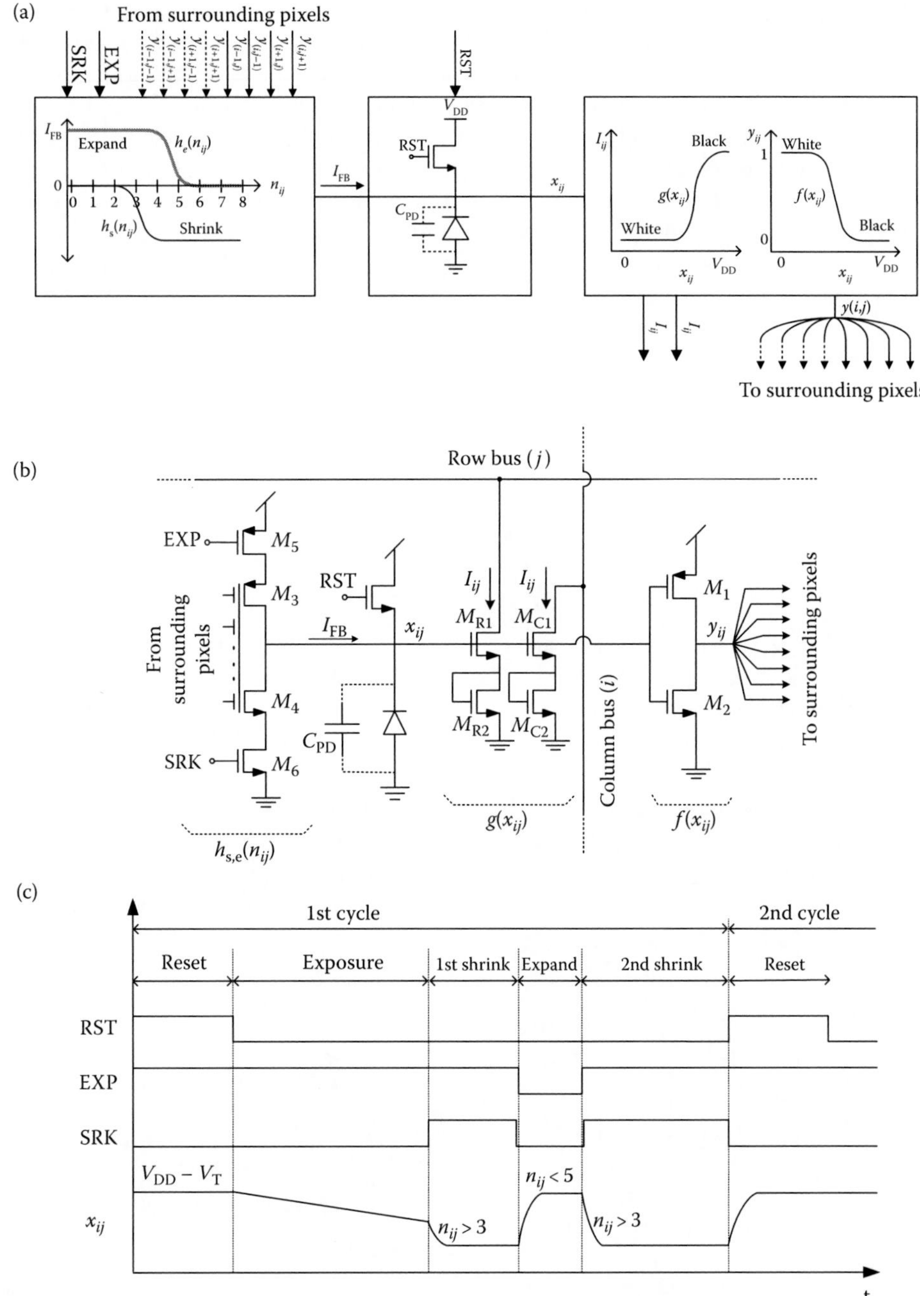

FIGURE 17.27 (a) Functional, (b) schematic, and (c) timing diagrams of the smart CIS pixel. (Copyright © IEEE 2009.)

of the white pixels. The transconductor supplies current to the C_{PD}, causing the x_{ij} to be increased, which corresponds to becoming black pixel.

Each pixel generates I_{ij} when the pixel is considered as a black pixel by the saturation function $g(x_{ij})$ as shown in Figure 17.27a. The currents from pixels are summed column-wise and row-wise using the column-bus line and the row-bus line, respectively, as shown in Figure 17.26. The summed currents I_i^{V} and I_j^{H} represent the number of black pixels present in each column and in each row, respectively.

The schematic diagram and timing diagram of the proposed smart pixel are shown in Figures 17.27b and c. First, the PD capacitor C_{PD} is precharged to $(V_{DD} - V_T)$ during the reset phase by turning on the RST switch. Once the RST switch is off, light-generated electrons are accumulated in C_{PD}, lowering the potential x_{ij} during the exposure phase. The transistors M_1 and M_2 form the nonlinear function $f(x_{ij})$ whose output voltage is distributed to surrounding pixels. $M_{3,4,5,6}$ form the nonlinear transconductors $h_s(n_{ij})$ and $h_e(n_{ij})$. It works as a current source that realizes $h_e(n_{ij})$ when M_5 is on and M_6 is off. On the contrary, it works as a current sink that realizes $h_s(n_{ij})$ when M_5 is off and M_6 is on. Both M_5 and M_6 are off and no interpixel interaction occurs during the exposure phase. $M_{R1,2}$ or $M_{C1,2}$ forms a nonlinear transconductor $g(x_{ij})$. Two stacked transistors are turned on and generate output current I_{ij} only when x_{ij} exceeds $2V_T$, which corresponds to the black pixel.

The weighted sum of feedbacks from the neighboring pixels is obtained by a floating gate associated with M_3 and M_4. Figure 17.28 shows the schematic and layout diagrams of the weighted-sum circuit using floating gate capacitors. The floating gate voltage v_{fg} is obtained as follows:

$$v_{fg} = \sum_{k=-1}^{1}\sum_{l=-1}^{1}\left(\frac{C_{kl}}{C_{tot}} \cdot y_{(i+k,j+l)}\right) \tag{17.7}$$

where C_{kl} is the floating gate capacitance and C_{tot} is the sum of the floating gate capacitances and the parasitic gate capacitances of M_3 and M_4. Feedback coefficients $\epsilon_{k,l}$ in Equation 17.6 are decided by C_{kl} that is defined by the electrode area overlaid on the floating gate as shown in Figure 17.28b.

Figure 17.29 presents a schematic diagram of the current-mode WTA [20–24] circuit and the current comparator. The input currents of WTA are column-wise or row-wise summed currents, I_i^{V} or I_j^{H}. The common source voltage V_S is decided to turn on only the winning transistor that has the highest input current out of $M_{1...H}$ and all others are turned off. Then the highest input current is copied to the current comparator. Since only the winning transistor is turned on and allows current flow, the logic output $(A_{1...H})$ is high only for the winner and all others are low. Each logic

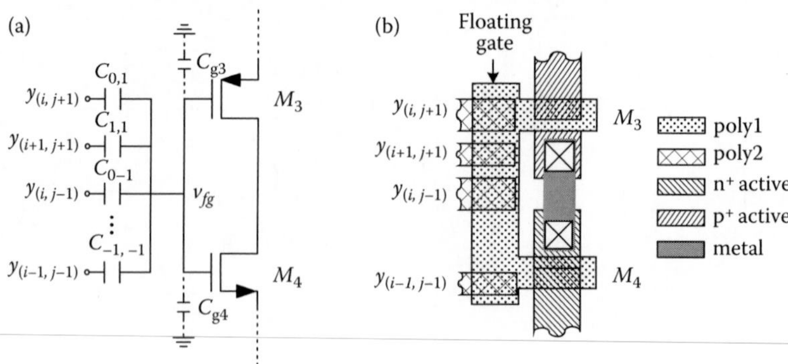

FIGURE 17.28 Schematic and layout diagrams of the weighted-sum circuit using floating gate capacitors. (a) Schematic diagram. (b) Layout diagram. (Copyright © IEEE 2009.)

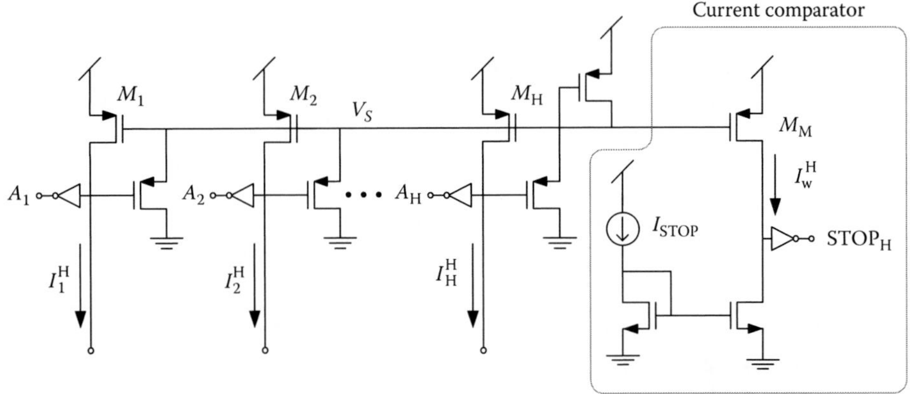

FIGURE 17.29 Circuit diagram of the WTA and current comparator. (Copyright © IEEE 2009.)

output A_i is connected to the corresponding latch. The current comparator compares the winning current I_w^H with the reference current I_{STOP} and generates logic-high output $STOP_H$ when I_w^H is smaller than I_{STOP}.

An identical WTA circuit is used for the horizontal and vertical WTAs. The stop criterion circuit generates logic-high *latch* signal when any of the horizontal or vertical current comparator generates logic-high $STOP_{H,V}$ signal as shown in Figure 17.26. The *latch* signal generated by the stop criterion circuit makes the latches store the winning locations from the WTA circuits. The wining addresses are read out through the address encoder that is implemented with the counter and the latch array. The counter counts the number of clocks until the shifted latch array output is high. Then, the counter contents represent the winner address.

17.3.3 Simulation and Experimental Results

Figure 17.30 shows the transistor-level simulation results for a 50 × 40 pixel array. Figure 17.30a shows the images taken at $T_{0,1,...,5}$ and Figure 17.30b shows the waveforms. After 1 ms of exposure time, the first shrink operation is started at T_0. I_i^V s and I_j^H s continuously decrease because the small black regions around the pupil caused by iris, eyelashes, eyelids, and various shadows shrink and disappear. The size of the glint is slightly increased until the expand operation is started at T_2. As the black region expands during the expand phase, I_i^V and I_j^H at (31, 23) that is the address of the glint increase. The glint is eliminated completely at T_3. The second shrink operation resumes at T_3 and the pupil shrinks again. The currents that correspond to the center of the pupil at (28, 20) remain as the winner and reach I_{STOP} at T_5, while all other currents become zero in advance. The *latch* signal is changed to high, causing the winning address to be latched.

The logic outputs of the WTA, A_is or A_js change to low as time elapses and only the winning row and column pixels are kept logic high. The *shifted column latch output* and the *shifted row latch output* show the pulses that correspond to the winning location. The operation time to find the center of the pupil is about 100 μs.

The proposed single-chip eye tracker was fabricated with a 0.35-μm CMOS process. Figure 17.31 shows the microphotograph of the fabricated chip. The fabricated chip has an array of 80 × 60 pixels with 24.4-μm pixel pitch and the core area is 2.9 × 2.6 mm^2. The PD is realized with the n$^+$/p$^-$-substrate junction whose fill factor is about 20%. The image readout circuit that is composed of a 3-Transistor (TR) pixel circuit and column-parallel single-slope ADC including correlated double sampling [25–27] are implemented as well for testing purpose.

Figure 17.32 shows the testing setup for the performance measurement with the fabricated prototype chip. The fabricated eye tracker is mounted in an HMD. IR illumination and IR filter are also

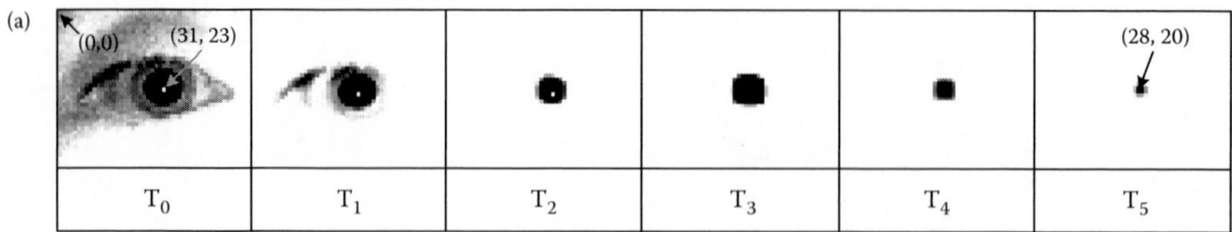

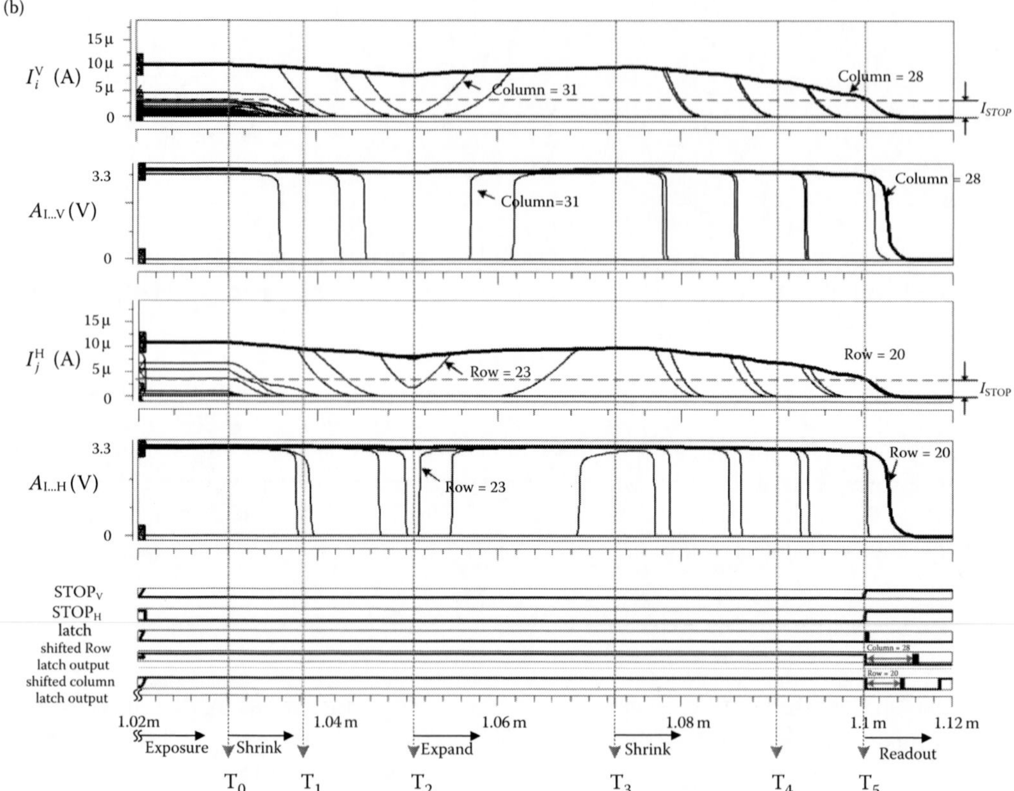

FIGURE 17.30 Transistor-level simulation results. (a) Image transitions extracted from transistor simulation results: the input eye image has a pupil center at (28,20) and a glint near at (31,23). (b) Simulated waveforms for one frame. (Copyright © IEEE 2009.)

assembled. The user gazes at a point on the screen of the HMD and the eye image is captured by the fabricated chip through a half-mirror of the HMD. The captured image is sent to the PC for testing purpose. At the same time, the eye tracking output address from the fabricated chip is monitored by the logic analyzer.

Figure 17.33 shows the sample images taken from the fabricated chip and the detected center of the pupils. Besides the detected center output address from the fabricated sensor, the center of the pupil is also obtained by software computation. Results of software computation are marked with □ and the output addresses obtained from the fabricated chip are marked with ×. The error is defined by the difference between the software computation result and the sensor output. Figure 17.34 shows the measured error map of the fabricated eye tracker that is obtained by gazing at a target at various locations on the screen. The test result shows that the error is within $\pm\sqrt{2}$ pixel pitch. The error in the lower region of the array is slightly higher than that in the other regions of the array because the pupil is slightly covered by the eyelash when the eye gazes toward the lower direction. The eye

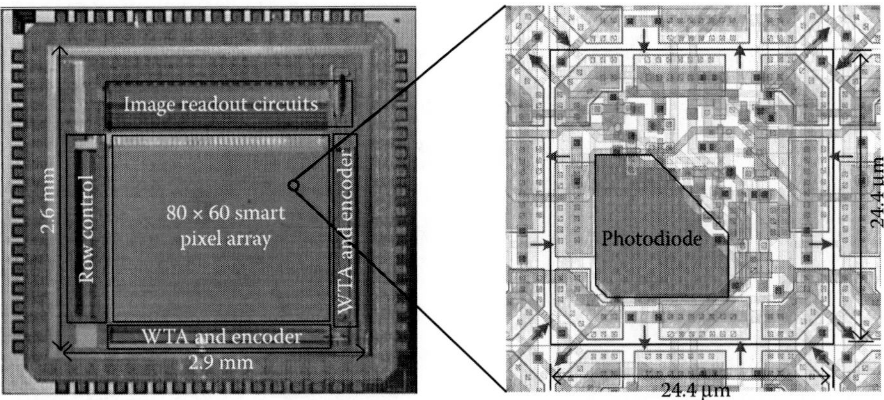

FIGURE 17.31 Chip microphotograph of the fabricated eye tracker and the layout of the smart pixel. (Copyright © IEEE 2009.)

tracking time is 200 μs excluding the exposure time and the power consumption is 100 mW with 3.3-V power supply. The specification of the prototype eye tracker is summarized in Table 17.4.

17.4 THIRD VERSION OF THE EYE TRACKER

This section proposes the third version of the single-chip eye tracker that has a 512 × 256 improved smart pixel array. Section 17.4.1 describes circuit implementation. Section 17.4.2 presents the simulation and experimental results. Finally, Section 17.4.3 provides the conclusion.

17.4.1 Proposed Eye Tracking Architecture

The third version of the eye tracker has the same structure as the second version of the eye tracker as shown in Figure 17.26. The eye tracker is composed of a smart pixel array, WTA circuits, a stop criterion circuit, latches, and address encoders. The smart pixel array captures the image and performs the shrink and the expand operations. The number of black pixels is counted vertically and horizontally by summing the currents from pixels in each row or in each column, respectively. The WTA circuit not only finds the location of the largest current out of column-wise summed current I_i^V or row-wise summed current I_j^H, but also copies the winning current value I_w^V or I_w^H. The stop criterion circuit generates the *latch* signal when either I_w^V or I_w^H is smaller than the reference current I_{STOP} that corresponds to two black pixels. The WTA circuit generates logic high only for the winning column or row, while all other logic outputs (A_i or A_j) are logic low. Each latch stores the

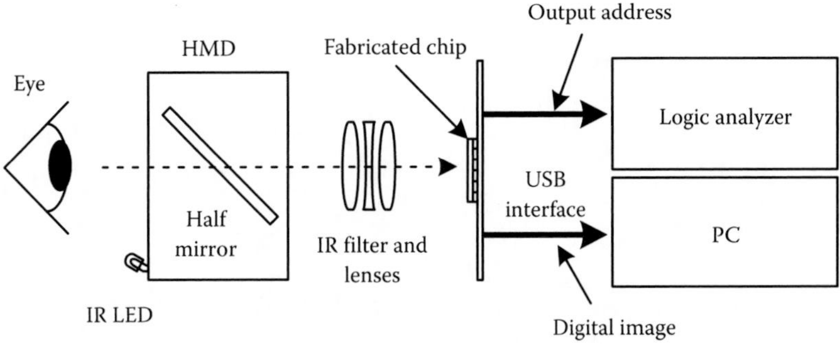

FIGURE 17.32 Testing environments with the fabricated chip.

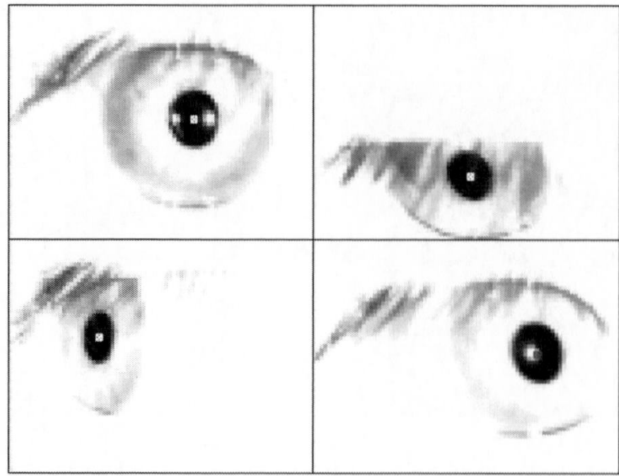

FIGURE 17.33 Sample image and the center location from the fabricated sensor. (Copyright © IEEE 2009.)

corresponding WTA logic output when the *latch* signal is generated by the stop criterion circuit. Then, the winning addresses are encoded and readout.

17.4.2 Circuit Implementation

The smart CIS pixel array performs the shrink and the expand operations with continuous-time interpixel feedback. Figure 17.35a presents the functional block diagram of the proposed smart pixel whose dynamics can be expressed as

$$\begin{cases} y_{ij} = f(x_{ij}) \\ n_{ij} = \sum_{k=-1}^{1}\sum_{l=-1}^{1} \varepsilon_{kl} y_{(i+k,j+l)} + \alpha \cdot OPC \\ C_{PD}\dfrac{dx_{ij}}{dt} = h_{s,e}(n_{ij}) \end{cases} \tag{17.8}$$

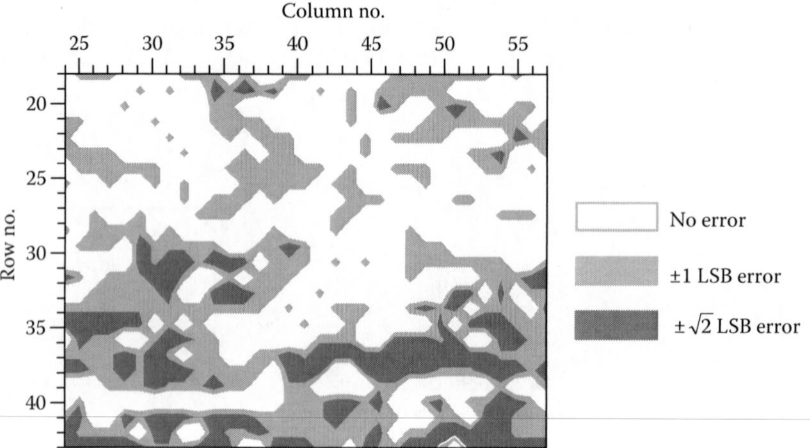

FIGURE 17.34 The measured error map from the fabricated eye tracker and the software computation. (Copyright © IEEE 2009.)

TABLE 17.4
Performance Summary of the Second Version Eye Tracker

Process	0.35-μm CMOS 2-Poly 3-Metal
Power supply	3.3 V
Power consumption	100 mW
Chip size	2.9×2.6 mm^2
Array size	80×60
Pixel size	24.4×24.4 μm^2
Photodetector	n^+/p^--substrate
Fill factor	20 %
Conversion gain	1.6 μV/e$^-$
Full well capacity	1.19×10^6 e$^-$
Sensitivity at 950 nm	5.6 V/s · (μW/cm^2)
Sampling rate (tracking time)	5000 fps (200 μs)
Error	Less than $\pm\sqrt{2}$ pixel pitch

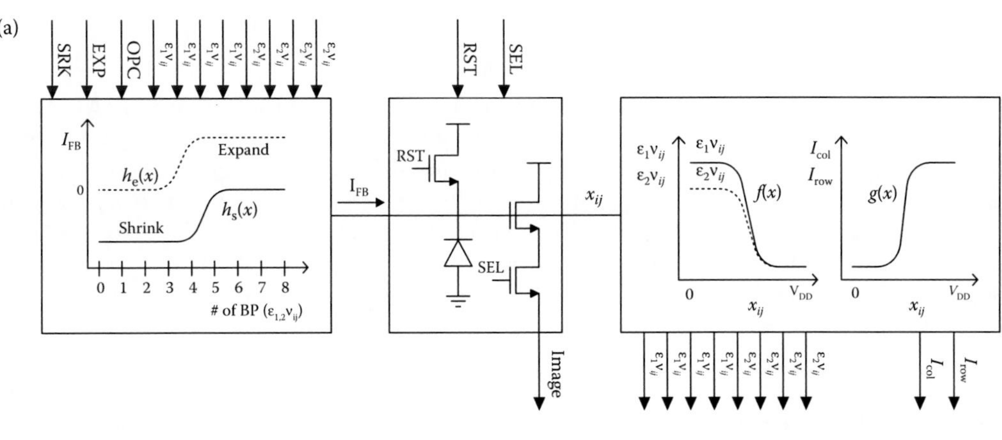

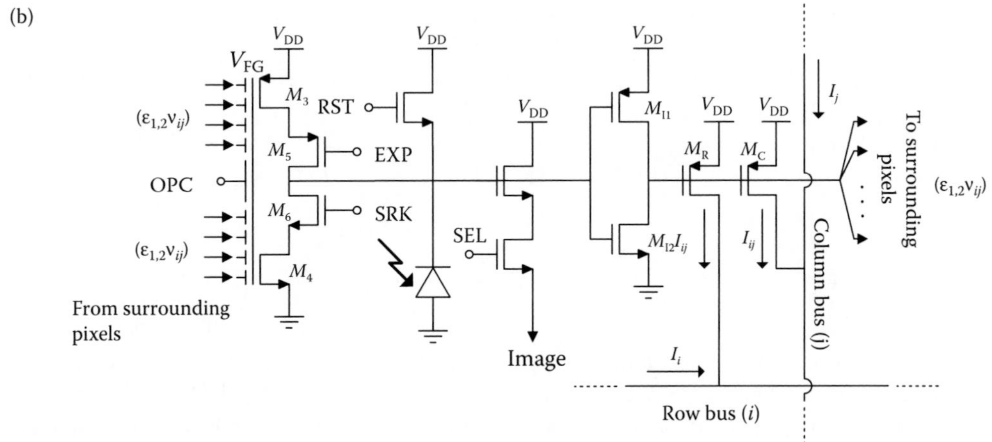

FIGURE 17.35 Functional and schematic diagrams of the proposed smart pixel. (a) Functional diagram. (b) Schematic diagram.

where C_{PD} is the parasitic capacitance of the PD and x_{ij} represents the state voltage whose initial value is decided from the captured image. Here, x_{ij} is lower for brighter light. $f(x_{ij})$ is an inverted saturation function that discriminates the black pixel from the white pixel. n_{ij} is the weighted sum of feedbacks from the neighboring pixels. Here, the weights for diagonal neighbors should be smaller than that for vertical and horizontal neighbors to guarantee the isotropic shrink and expansion. $h_s(n_{ij})$ and $h_e(n_{ij})$ are nonlinear transconductance functions to generate feedback currents, I_{FB}, respectively for the shrink and the expand operations.

Each pixel counts the number of neighboring white pixels by calculating n_{ij}. When the control signal is set to perform the shrink operation, I_{FB} is generated based on $h_s(n_{ij})$ as shown in Figure 17.35a. If more than three white pixels exist in the neighborhood, then the pixel is considered to be located at the boundary of the black pixels. The transconductor takes out current from the C_{PD} causing the n_{ij} to be lowered, which corresponds to becoming white pixel. On the contrary, when the control signal is set to perform the expand operation, I_{FB} is generated based on $h_e(n_{ij})$. If less than five white pixels exist in the neighborhood, then the pixel is considered to be located at the boundary of the white pixels. The transconductor supplies current to the C_{PD}, causing the x_{ij} to be increased, which corresponds to becoming black pixel.

Each pixel generates I_{ij} when the pixel is considered as a black pixel by the saturation function $g(x_{ij})$ as shown in Figure 17.35a. The currents from pixels are summed column-wise and row-wise using the column-bus line and the row-bus line, respectively, as shown in Figure 17.26. The summed currents I_i^V and I_j^H represent the number of black pixels present in each column and in each row, respectively.

The schematic diagram of the proposed smart pixel is shown in Figure 17.35b. First, the PD capacitor C_{PD} is precharged to $(V_{DD} - V_T)$ during the reset phase by turning on the RST switch. Once the RST is off, light-generated electrons are accumulated in C_{PD}, lowering the potential x_{ij} during the exposure phase. The transistors M_{11} and M_{12} form the nonlinear function $f(x_{ij})$ whose output voltage is distributed to surrounding pixels. $M_{3,4,5,6}$ form the nonlinear transconductors $h_s(n_{ij})$ and $h_e(n_{ij})$. It works as a current source that realizes $h_e(n_{ij})$ when M_5 is on and M_6 is off. On the contrary, it works as a *current* sink that realizes $h_s(n_{ij})$ when M_5 is off and M_6 is on. Both M_5 and M_6 are off and no interpixel interaction occurs during the exposure phase. M_R or M_C forms a nonlinear transconductor $g(x_{ij})$. Two stacked transistors are turned on and generate output current I_{ij} only when the pixel is black.

If I_{FB} is large, the shrink and expand operations perform too fast because the parasitic capacitance of the PD is very small. I_{FB} must be controlled as a small value to latch the last winner location. Therefore, the M_5 and M_6 of the second version smart pixel in Figure 17.27 are operated in the subthreshold region by the EXP and SRK. The EXP and SRK are about $(V_{DD} - V_T)$ and V_T values, respectively. However, the third version of the eye tracker does not need these analog controls. The operation control (OPC) and operation capacitor C_{OPC} enable M_5 and M_6 transistors to operate in the subthreshold region.

The weighted sum of feedbacks from the neighboring pixels is obtained by a floating gate associated with M_3 and M_4. The floating gate voltage v_{fg} is obtained as follows:

$$v_{fg} = \sum_{k=-1}^{1}\sum_{l=-1}^{1}\left(\frac{C_{kl}}{C_{tot}} \cdot y_{(i+k,j+l)}\right) + \frac{C_{OPC}}{C_{tot}} \cdot OPC \tag{17.9}$$

where C_{kl} is the floating gate capacitance, C_{OPC} is the operation capacitance, and C_{tot} is the sum of the floating gate capacitances and the parasitic gate capacitances of M_3 and M_4. Feedback coefficients $\epsilon_{k,l}$, α in Equation 17.8 are decided by C_{kl} that is defined by the electrode area overlaid on the floating gate. The voltage of the floating gate is shown in Figure 17.36.

Figure 17.37 presents the schematic diagram of the current-mode WTA [21–24] circuit and the current comparator. The input currents of WTA are column-wise or row-wise summed currents

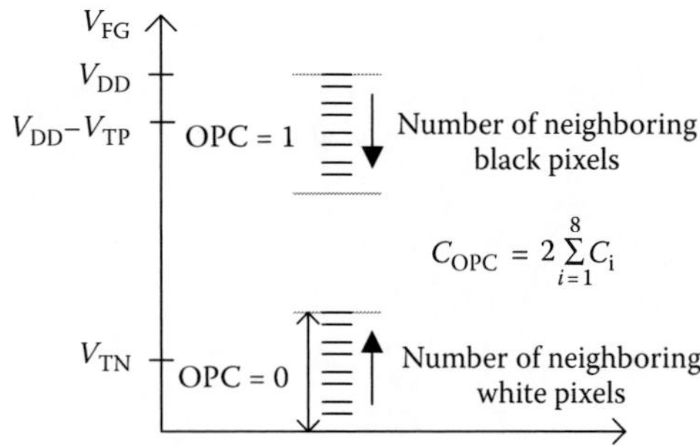

FIGURE 17.36 Potential of the floating gate.

I_i^V or I_j^H. The common source voltage V_S is decided to turn on only the winning transistor that has the highest input current out of $M_{1...H}$ and all others are turned off. Then the highest input current is copied to the current comparator. Since only the winning transistor is turned on and allows current flow, the logic output ($A_{1...H}$) is high only for the winner and all others are low. Each logic output A_i is connected to the corresponding latch. The current comparator compares the winning current I_w^H with the reference current I_{STOP} and generates logic-high output $STOP_H$ when I_w^H is smaller than I_{STOP}.

Identical WTA circuit is used for the horizontal and vertical WTAs. The stop criterion circuit generates logic-high *latch* signal when any of the horizontal or vertical current comparator generates logic-high $STOP_{H,V}$ signal as shown in Figure 17.26. The *latch* signal generated by the stop criterion circuit makes the latches store the winning locations from the WTA circuits. The wining addresses are read out through the address encoder that is implemented with the counter and the latch array. The counter counts the number of clock until the shifted latch array output is high. Then, the counter contents represent the winner address.

17.4.3 Experimental Results

The proposed single-chip eye tracker was fabricated with a 0.35-μm CMOS process. Figure 17.38 shows the microphotograph of the fabricated chip and the core area is 9.3 × 2.6 mm². The fabricated pixel array is 512 × 256 and one pixel occupies 15.8 × 18.0 μm². The PD is realized with the n^+/p^--substrate junction whose fill factor is about 31%. The fabricated third version eye tracker is under testing.

Figure 17.39 shows the proposed testing setup for the performance measurement with the fabricated prototype chip and HMD. The user looks at the screen of the HMD and the eye image under the infrared illumination is captured through a half-mirror of the HMD, IR filter, and lenses. The captured image is converted to the digital image in image sensor mode and the eye tracking address is outputted in eye tracking mode.

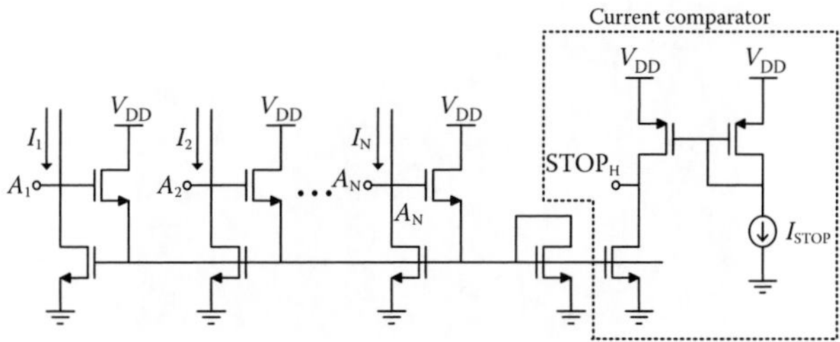

FIGURE 17.37 Circuit diagram of the WTA and current comparator.

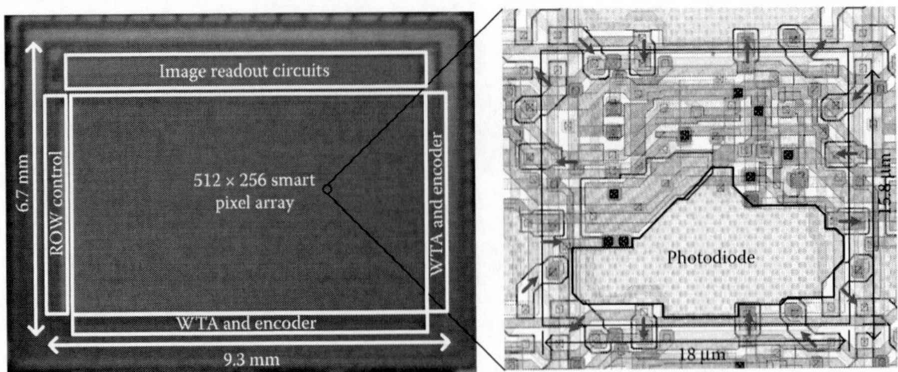

FIGURE 17.38 Chip microphotograph of the fabricated eye tracker and layout of the smart pixel; the pixel interaction line with neighborhood pixels are indicated by arrows.

The proposed measurement results of the fabricated chip linked with an HMD are presented in Figure 17.40. A landscape is shown to a user in the HMD, and then the eye movement is tracked during 3 s. The expected results are accomplished with eye-gazing location and time, which are outputted from the eye tracker every 2 ms. Circles on the image indicate the visual fixations and the size of circles indicates the fixation time. Arrows show the saccadic eye movements.

17.5 CONCLUSION

This chapter introduced three versions of high-speed single-chip eye trackers using smart CIS pixels that do not require any additional peripherals. The proposed sensors detect the center of the pupil using shrink/expand operations and WTA that were realized with compact analog circuits. The shrink operation effectively removes noisy objects, whereas the expand operation effectively removes the glints providing the center of the pupil.

The first version eye tracker was designed and fabricated with 0.35-μm CMOS process having a 32 × 32 smart CIS pixels array and the core size is 3.8 mm^2. As the frame rate of the proposed eye tracker is 125 fps and the conventional eye tracker is commonly 30 fps, the prototype chip test

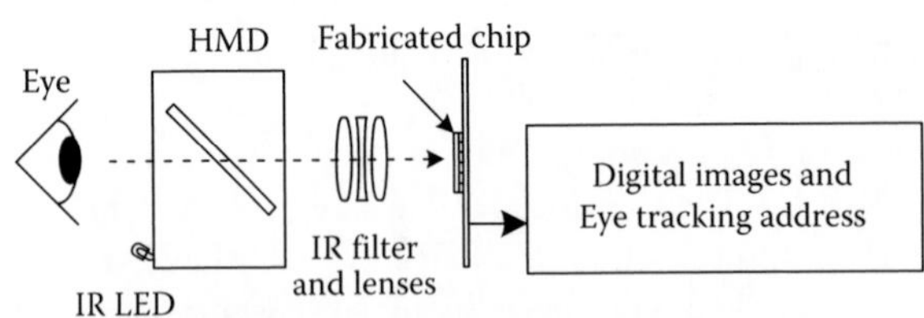

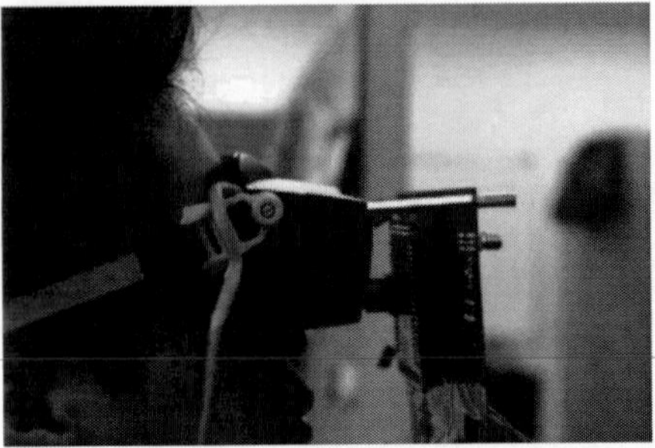

FIGURE 17.39 Expected testing environment for error measurement with the fabricated chip.

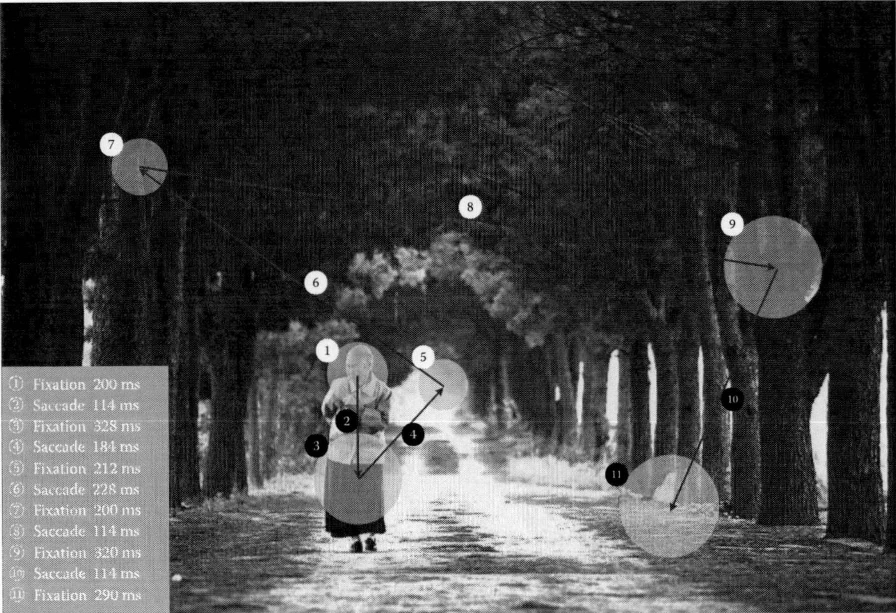
7
8
9
6
1
5
2
4
3
10
11
① Fixation 200 ms
② Saccade 114 ms
③ Fixation 328 ms
④ Saccade 184 ms
⑤ Fixation 212 ms
⑥ Saccade 228 ms
⑦ Fixation 200 ms
⑧ Saccade 114 ms
⑨ Fixation 320 ms
⑩ Saccade 114 ms
⑪ Fixation 290 ms

FIGURE 17.40 The expecting measurement results of the fabricated chip: circles on the image indicate visual fixations and the size of the circle indicates the fixation time; the arrows show the saccades.

results demonstrated that the proposed system can generate information indicating where the user gazes on at higher speed than the conventional eye tracker. Measurement results show ±1 pixel error and the power consumption is 260 mW. The pixel size and power consumption of the first version eye tracker are still large and there is a possibility to improve the pixel size.

The second version eye tracker was designed and fabricated with the 0.35-μm CMOS process having a 80 × 60 smart CIS pixels array and the core size is 7.5 mm^2. The second version of the eye tracker eliminates the glint effect caused by the illumination light. The test results show $\pm\sqrt{2}$ pixel error at the rate of 5000 fps. The power consumption is 100 mW with 3.3 V supply voltage. Even though the smart pixel of the second version performs more complex functions, the pixel area of the second version eye tracker is decreased to 23.8% compared to the pixel area of the first version eye tracker The power consumption is reduced to 38% of the power consumption of the first version. However, the pixel array is still small and there is a possibility to improve the resolution.

The third version eye tracker was designed and fabricated with the 0.35-μm CMOS process having a 512 × 256 smart CIS pixels array and the core size is 62.3 mm^2. The third version of the eye tracker has a higher specification than that of the commercial eye tracker. The proposed test results show $\pm\sqrt{2}$ pixel error at the rate of 1000 fps. The power consumption is 200 mW with 3.3 V supply voltage. The pixel area of the third version eye tracker is 47.7% of the second version eye tracker and 11% of the first version eye tracker, respectively.

The introduced eye trackers are intended to be used as a pointing device in conjunction with an HMD and an input device for the handicapped. Therefore, the handicapped can give instructions to a computer just by gazing at the location and the more interactive video game can be accomplished by the HMD including the eye tracker.

REFERENCES

1. T. Miyoshi and A. Murata, Input device using eye tracker in human–computer interaction, *Proc. 10th IEEE Int. Workshop on Robot and Human Interactive Communication*, Paris, France, September 2001, pp. 18–21, 1998.

2. G. Beach, C. J. Cohen, J. Braun, and G. Moody, Eye tracker system for use with head mounted displays, *IEEE Int. Conf. Syst. Man Cybern.*, 5, 4348–4352, 1998.
3. K. Iwamoto, S. Katsumata, and K. Tanie, An eye movement tracking type head mounted display for virtual reality system: Evaluation experiments of a prototype system, *IEEE Int. Conf. Syst., Man Cybern.*, 1, 13–18, 1994.
4. Z. Zhiwei, J. Qiang, K. Fujimura, and L. Kuangchih, Combining Kalman filtering and mean shift for real time eye tracking under active IR illumination, *Proc. 16th Int. Conf. Pattern Recognit.*, 4, 318–321, 2002.
5. T. Oya, H. Hashimoto, and F. Harashima, Active eye sensing system-predictive filtering for visual tracking, *Proc. Int. Conf. Ind. Electron., Control Instrum.*, 3, 1718–1723, 1993.
6. A. Graupner, J. Schreiter, S. Getzlaff, and R. Schüffny, CMOS image sensor with mixed-signal processor array, *IEEE J. Solid-State Circuits*, 38, 948–957, 2003.
7 Y. Muramatsu, S. Kurosawa, M. Furumiya, H. Ohkubo, and Y. Nakashiba, A signal-processing CMOS image sensor using a simple analog operation, *IEEE J. Solid-State Circuits*, 38, 101–106, 2003.
8. S. Espejo, A. Rodríguez-Vázquez, R. Domínguez-Castro, J. L. Huertas, and E. Sánchez-Sinencio, Smart-pixel cellular neural networks in analog current-mode CMOS technology, *IEEE J. Solid-State Circuits*, 29, 895–905, 1994.
9. M. Schwarz, R. Hauschild, B. J. Hosticka, J. Huppertz, T. Kneip, S. Kolnsberg, L. Ewe, and H. K. Trieu, Single-chip CMOS image sensors for a retina implant system, *IEEE Trans. Circuits Syst. II*, 46, 870–877, 1999.
10. L. O. Chua and L. Yang, Cellular neural networks: Theory, *IEEE Trans. Circuits Syst. I*, 35, 1257–1272, 1988.
11. L. O. Chua and L. Yang, Cellular neural networks: Applications, *IEEE Trans. Circuits Syst. I*, 35, 1273–1290, 1988.
12. D. A. Robinson, The use of control system analysis in the neurophysiology of eye movements, *Ann. Rev. Neurosd.* 4, 463–503, 1981.
13. Iota AB. EyeTrace Systems, Sundsvall Business & Tech. Available at: Sweden: http://www.iota.se.
14. A. T. Duchowski, *Eye Tracking Methodology: Theory and Practice*, Springer-Verlag, 2002.
15. Metrovision, France. Available at: http://www.metrovision.fr.
16. Skalar Medical, Netherlands, Available at: http://www.skalar.nl.
17. Microguide, USA. Available at: http://www.eyemove.com.
18. S. Wolfram, *MATHEMATICA: A System for Doing Mathematics by Computer*. Addison-Wesley, 1988.
19. B. W. Char et al., *Maple V Library Reference Manual*. New York, NY: Springer-Verlag, 1991.
20. A. Fish, D. Turchin, and O. Yadid-Pecht, An APS with 2-D winner-take-all selection employing adaptive spatial filtering and false alarm reduction, *IEEE Trans. Electron Dev.*, 50, 159–165, 2003.
21. T. Serrano-Gotarredona and B. Linares-Barranco, A high-precision current-mode WTA-MAX circuit with multichip capability, *IEEE J. Solid-State Circuits*, 33, 280–286, 1998.
22. I. E. Opris, Analog rank extractors, *IEEE Trans. Circuits Syst. I*, 44(12), 1114–1121, 1997.
23. J. Choi and B. J. Sheu, A high-precision VLSI winner-take-all circuit for self-organizing neural networks, *IEEE J. Solid-State Circuits*, 28(5), 576–584, 1993.
24. D. Kim, S. Lim, and G. Han, Single-chip eye tracker using smart CMOS image sensor pixels, *Analog Integr. Circuits Signal Process.*, 45, 131–141, 2005.
25. P. Lee, R. Gee, M. Guidash, T. Lee, and E. R. Fossum, An active pixel sensor fabricated using CMOS/CCD process technology, *IEEE Workshop on CCD's and Advanced Image Sensors*, Dana Point, CA, April 20–22, 1995.
26. W. Yang, O. Kwon, J. Lee, G. Hwang, and S. Lee, An integrated 800×600 CMOS imaging system, *ISSCC Dig. Tech. Pap.*, 304–305, February 1999.
27. T. Sugiki, S. Ohsawa, H. Miura, M. Sasaki, and N. Nakamura, A 60-mW 10-b CMOS image sensor with column-to-column FPN reduction, *ISSCC Dig. Tech. Pap.*, 108–109, February 2000.

18 Design and Manufacturing of CNT-Based Nanodevices for Optical Sensing Applications

Ning Xi, King Wai Chiu Lai, Jiangbo Zhang, Carmen Kar Man Fung, Hongzhi Chen, and T. J. Tarn

CONTENTS

18.1 INTRODUCTION

Carbon nanotube (CNT) has some unique properties that are superior to some conventional semiconducting materials. We have developed a spectrum infrared (IR) sensor using a CNT which is capable to sense IR from near IR (NIR) middle-wave IR (MWIR) radiation in room temperature environment. This chapter gives an idea to design and fabricate CNT-based IR sensors. In addition, we have developed a series of processes to manufacture the devices. The process starts with the microfluidic-based delivery and separation of the nanomaterials. A precision assembly can be achieved by the atomic force microscopy-based nanorobotic system. It is capable of manipulating the nanomaterial at the desired position efficiently. The band gap of the semiconducting material is an important property for many applications, such as optical detectors and solar cells. We have developed an electrical breakdown control method to adjust the band structure of a CNT; this process has provided a steady and high-yield on-chip band gap engineering approach in batch electronics fabrication. Therefore, the spectral response of the devices can be adjusted. Finally, thermal annealing process and packaging process have been developed to maintain stability and reliability of nanodevices. The integration of the above technologies has provided an effective and efficient nanomanufacturing process for fabrication of nanosensors and electronic devices.

18.1.1 Characterization of CNTs

As the traditional silicon-based semiconductor industry faces increasing technological and financial challenges on the way to further scaling down, new technologies and concepts have to be developed and assessed. CNTs represent such a candidate and are likely to create breakthroughs in the fields of nanoelectronics. Since the discovery of CNTs in 1991 [1], their mechanical and electrical properties have been intensively studied. Due to their unique hollow cylindrical structure, CNTs have promising potential applications in nanoelectronics [2,3] and nanomechanics [4]. They are capable of working as fundamental building blocks of nanoelectronic devices with their excellent one-dimensional (1D) material properties [5]. They are also extremely strong materials and have good thermal conductivity [6] . Moreover, CNTs photobehavior has attracted lots of attention due to their well-defined 1D structure [7–14]. A single-walled carbon nanotube (SWCNT) is formed by rolling a sheet of graphene into a cylinder along a lattice vector (m,n) in the graphene plane. The (m,n) vector determines the diameter and the particular roll orientation of a CNT, which is called the chirality. The (m,n) vector is also called a chiral vector. The angle between the roll orientation and the axis of the tube is termed the chiral angle. The chirality (or chiral angle) determines the electronic properties of a CNT. Depending on the chirality, CNTs with the same diameter can be either metallic or semiconducting. There are three types of rolls: armchair, zigzag, and chiral [15]. Armchair CNTs are formed when $m = n$. The chiral angle of an armchair CNT is 30°, and the armchair CNTs display metallic properties. Zigzag CNTs are formed when either n or m equals zero, where the chiral angle is 0°. All other lattice vectors result in nanotubes that are termed chiral CNTs. Both zigzag and chiral CNTs are semiconducting. The diameter of a SWCNT is determined by the vector (m,n) using the equation [16]

$$d_{\text{CNT}} = \frac{a\sqrt{3\left(m^2 + mn + n^2\right)}}{\pi} = \frac{C_\text{h}}{\pi} \tag{18.1}$$

where a is the carbon-to-carbon bond length (1.42 Å), or the length between consecutive carbon atoms. C_h is the length of the chiral vector (m,n).

A metallic CNT has a much higher conductivity than the best metals, and semiconducting CNTs have mobilities and transconductances that meet or exceed the best semiconductors [5]. Hence the metallic CNTs have the potential to work as nanowires for interconnection in nanodevices. And the semiconducting CNTs have the potential to be the future material for field-effect transistor (FET) channels. The band gap of a semiconducting CNT is given by [16–19]

$$E_\text{gap} = \frac{4\hbar v_\text{f}}{3d_{\text{CNT}}} \tag{18.2}$$

where v_f is the fermi velocity, and $\hbar$ is the Dirac constant. The unique electrical properties of SWCNTs are caused by the confinement of electrons in the two directions and the requirements for energy and momentum conservation. These constrains reduce the scattering processes of electrons and result in a ballistic transport.

As rolling a single graphene into a SWCNT, a multiwalled carbon nanotube (MWCNT) can be formed by rolling multiple layers of graphene sheets into a cylinder shape. Hence an MWCNT consists of multiple tubes [16,20] with spacing between consecutive tubes of 3.4 Å [21]. Each layer of the MWCNT can have different chirality and can be metallic or semiconducting. It has been reported that the concentric tubes of an MWCNT have poor electrical contact with each other [22]. Theoretical and experimental studies have also shown that the outermost layer of an MWCNT dominates the electrical conduction of the MWCNT [23]. The band gap of a SWCNT varies inversely with its diameter and the outermost layer of an MWCNT normally has a large diameter exceeding 10 nm [21]. The band gap of the outermost nanotube of an MWCNT is very small.

With their outstanding properties, CNTs have potential applications in a wide range of fields. MWCNTs have been studied as very-large-scale integration interconnectors because of their high thermal stability, high thermal conductivity, and high current conductivity [24]. Semiconducting CNTs have been used as the channels of CNTFETs because of their superior electrical characteristics [25–30].

18.1.2 History of the Development of CNT-Based IR Sensors

As a 1D nanostructural material, CNTs have potential applications in solar collection and IR sensing due to their unique properties such as direct band gap, wide range of band gaps [5], and reduced carrier scattering [31]. Many researchers are looking into CNT optoelectronics, and the photoconductivity of CNTs has been studied in thin SWCNT films [9,10,32] and single SWCNT transistors [12]. It has also been demonstrated that both semiconducting and metallic SWCNTs can function as photodetectors over a wide spectral range using capacitive photocurrent measurement [14]. Moreover, a single SWCNT p–n junction diode was built in [15] to demonstrate its photovoltaic effect.

The CNT-based photosensing devices can be classified into three categories based on their structures. The first category is the basic structure with a pair of microelectrodes bridged by a CNT or CNT bundle/film [10,32]. The second type of the CNT photosensing device is featured with the gate structure. Gate electrodes are employed to electrically control the photoconducting of the CNT channel [11,12], and two bottom gate electrodes were used to electrically shift the fermi level of the CNT at both ends to create a p–n junction in the middle of the CNT [13]. The third type of the CNT photosensing device is a metal–insulator–semiconductor photodetector [14] and photons are detected by measuring the displacement photocurrent on the semiconductor.

The first structure is simple and easy to implement. The other two structures may lead to a better performance, but the complicated design makes it difficult to fabricate, especially for the device arrays. In this research, we first fabricate the single CNT-based IR sensors using the basic structure (two microelectrodes bridged by a CNT) to study the photobehaviors of single CNTs. After that, new designs enhanced by additional structures are employed to improve the performance of the single CNT-based IR sensors.

18.1.3 Challenges and Difficulties in Manufacturing of CNT-Based Devices

The techniques for manufacturing nanodevices can be generally classified into bottom-up and top-down methods. The fabrication process of CNT devices normally includes both methods, where top-down methods are used to fabricate supporting structures such as contacting electrodes, and bottom-up methods are used to assemble CNTs with the supporting structures. Current available methods in fabricating single-CNT devices include direct growth of CNT across microelectrodes [13,33–35]. The direct growth method is able to fabricate multiple single-CNT devices at one time. Thus, it is good for making CNT-based nanodevice arrays. But limitation of this method is that the properties of the CNTs cannot be effectively controlled. Different CNTs may have different properties even though they were produced at one batch. Moreover, the production process may generate impurities around the microelectrodes and CNTs, which will affect the electronic properties of the CNT device. The third limitation is that it is difficult to grow only a single CNT between the microelectrodes. Since CNT bundles or films lose the unique properties brought by the 1D structure of CNTs, this limitation limits the performance of the CNT device. Deposition of as-grown CNTs on electrodes by dielectrophoresis is another typical method [36–39]; although the number of CNTs attracted to the electrodes can be roughly controlled by varying the AC voltage and the concentration of the CNT solution, it is very difficult to deposit a single CNT with this method. Another approach for a CNT-based device assembly is to fabricate electrodes on top of as-deposited CNTs either by electron beam lithography (EBL) [40–42] or by shadow masks [43,44]; this fabrication method provides a best contact condition between the CNT and microelectrodes among these fabrication methods. But due to the low efficiency of the EBL fabrication process, this method is inefficient. More importantly, since the CNTs are randomly distributed on the substrate surface, it is impossible to fabricate a CNT device array which aligns in a desired pattern. Hence, the EBL fabrication method is only good for prototyping individual devices. Other methods such as self-assembly by functionalizing CNTs and electrodes with different chemicals or even DNA molecules [45,46] have been introduced. To a certain extent, these methods have their shortcomings in terms of repeatability, mass production, and ability in eliminating uncertainties.

Another controllable assembly process for fabricating CNT devices is to mechanically manipulate CNTs to bridge the microelectrodes. Atomic force microscope (AFM), or scanning force microscope, was invented in 1986 by Binnig et al. [47]. Figure 18.1 shows the schematic diagram of a head scanning AFM system. Like all other scanning probe microscopes, the AFM utilizes a sharp probe moving over the surface of a sample in a raster scan. In the case of the AFM, the probe is a tip at the end of a cantilever which bends in response to the force between the tip and the sample. The surface topography is acquired by recording the bending of the cantilever at each sampling point. A single CNT attached at the tip end of an AFM cantilever were manipulated using focused ion beam [48]. But the nanotube has to be metal coated for manipulation. Hence this technology is not good for building nanoelectronic devices. A 3D manipulation of CNTs has been studied in [49], but the manipulation has to be performed under scanning electron microscopy, which limited the applications. A more general way is to manipulate CNTs using the AFM tip such that CNTs can be positioned on the substrate surface in a bare environment [50–52], but all these works limited to manipulating CNTs and none of them built nanoelectronic devices through manipulating CNTs. In short, no single process can manufacture CNT-based nanodevices nowadays. In order to overcome the difficulties to fabricate nanodevices, we have developed a hybrid manufacturing process for building CNT-based nanodevices using a DEP deposition system and AFM manipulation, the DEP deposition system can approximately deposit CNTs to metal electrodes, followed by fine manipulation by an AFM nanorobotic system. As a result, CNT-based nanodevices can be made effectively.

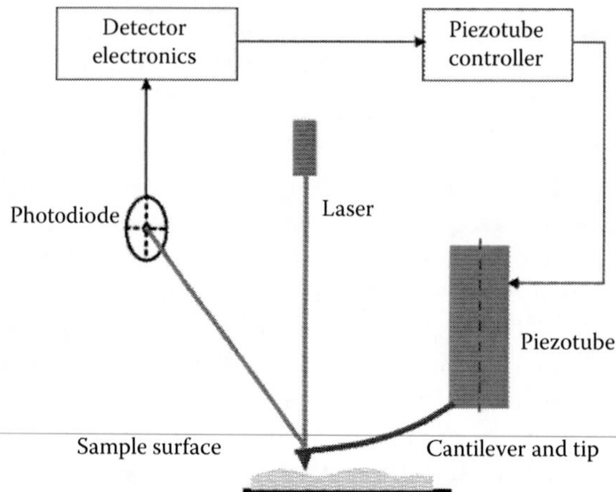

FIGURE 18.1 Schematic diagram of a head scanning AFM.

18.2 DESIGN OF THE CNT-BASED IR SENSORS

The challenges of development of single-CNT-based IR sensors lie in two aspects, design [53,54] and fabrication [53,55]. Since the diameter of a CNT can be as small as subnanometer, the design of the sensor structure is essential for the fabrication process. An appropriate design can make it easier to assemble a single CNT onto the microelectrodes. Another challenge is how to improve the performance of the CNT sensors. Since the impedance of CNTs (especially semiconducting CNTs) is very huge in general, the current signal will be very small. How to increase the photocurrent signal and effectively read it out are the main difficulties to consider during the design of the CNT sensors.

18.2.1 Schottky Diode-Based CNT Sensors

A semiconducting CNT can work as a photoconductor or a photodiode for photodetection. Due to its high dark current and big noise, a photoconductor normally has a lower sensitivity than a photodiode. Therefore, a CNT Schottky diode will be designed for the IR detection. Figure 18.2 shows the energy band diagrams of the CNT–metal contact for n-type and p-type CNTs respectively. For n-type CNTs, a Schottky barrier is formed at the CNT–metal interface when $\phi_M > X_{CNT}$, where ϕ_M is the work function of the metal electrode, and X_{CNT} is the electron affinity of the CNT. For p-type CNTs, a Schottky barrier is formed at the CNT–metal interface when $\phi_M < X_{CNT} + E_g$, where E_g is the band gap of the CNT. Since semiconducting CNTs normally are p-type in air due to the oxygen doping, the case of Figure 18.2b is considered in this research. As shown in Figure 18.2b, there is a Schottky barrier at the CNT–metal interface which blocks the transportation of holes.

By choosing metals with different work functions as the microelectrodes, we can adjust the Schottky barrier at the CNT–metal interface. Two different designs are developed in this research to study the dependence of the photocurrent on the CNT–metal contact conditions. Figure 18.3 shows the structure and the energy band diagram of CNT sensors with symmetric contacts, where both of the microelectrodes are made from the same material. As IR photons hits the SWCNT, the photons with energy higher than the band gap will excite electrons and holes inside the CNT to form electron–hole pairs. The electron–hole pairs will be separated by an external electrical field or the built-in field and contribute to the photocurrent. Since there is no built-in field outside the depletion regions, the electron–hole pairs will recombine quickly and do not contribute to the photocurrent. Only the electron–hole pairs generated at the depletion regions can form photocurrent. Hence, the total photocurrent under zero bias is calculated by $I = I_1 - I_2$. As shown in Figure 18.3b, the holes generated at one Schottky barrier have to tunnel through another Schottky barrier to form current. This significantly limits the magnitude of the photocurrents I_1 and $I_1 - I_2$. Moreover, since the CNT–metal contacts are symmetric, I_1 is very close to I_2 if the incident IR power intensity is the same on both the electrodes. Thus, the total photocurrent will be very small and becomes difficult to measure.

Figure 18.4 shows the structure and the energy band diagram of CNT sensors with asymmetric contacts. By using different materials as the contact electrodes, asymmetric CNT–metal contacts

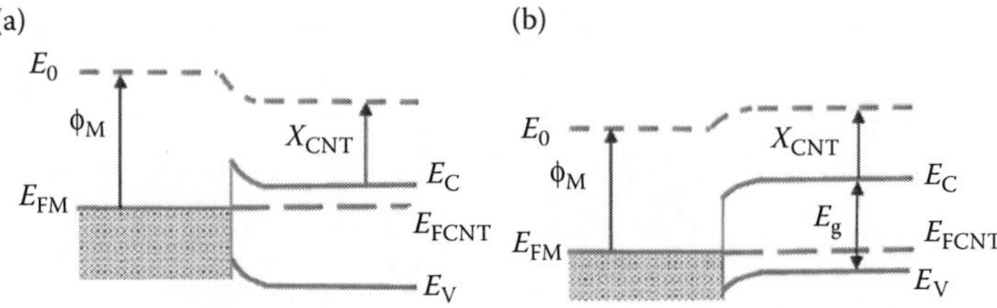

FIGURE 18.2 The energy band diagrams of the CNT–metal contact for (a) n-type CNTs and (b) p-type CNTs.

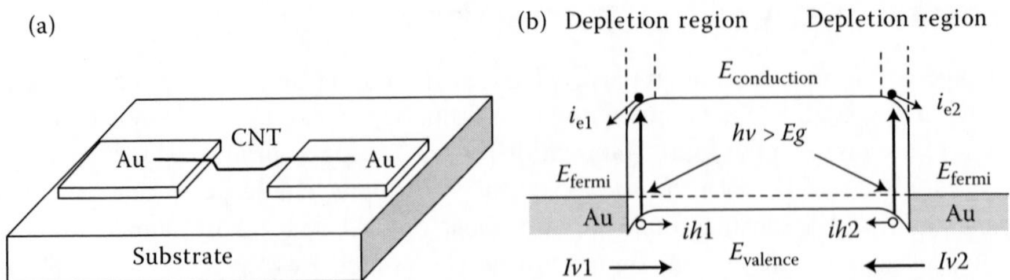

FIGURE 18.3 The single CNT-based IR sensors with symmetric contacts. (a) Structure of the CNT sensors. (b) Energy band diagram of the CNT sensors.

are created to maximize the total photocurrent *I*. By lowering one of the Schottky barrier, the photo-generated holes at another barrier will be able to tunnel through this barrier easier. Thus the total photocurrent will be increased. Moreover, the total photocurrent will also be increased by enlarging the difference between the photocurrents generated at the two barriers due to the asymmetry of the CNT–metal contacts. For example, as shown in Figure 18.4b, since many people have reported that palladium (Pd) is the best materials to form an ohmic CNT–metal contact [40,56], when silver (Ag) and Pd are used as the contact materials, a Schottky contact is formed at the CNT–Ag interface and an ohmic contact is formed at the CNT–Pd interface. In this way, the photocurrent $I_2 = 0$ and the total photocurrent *I* is maximized to I_1. With the asymmetric CNT–metal contacts, the sensitivity and other performance of individual CNT-based IR detectors are expected to be further improved.

18.2.2 FET on CNT-Based IR Sensors

We designed a CNT FET-based IR detector with asymmetric contacts (Au–CNT–Ag) that can repress dark current and enhance photocurrent simultaneously by applying a proper electrical field, highly improving the performance of the detector [57,58]. In addition, it is found that detecting open-circuit voltage (V_{oc}) instead of photocurrent is more efficient in these 1D detectors. A CNT photodetector typically has much smaller photocurrent than traditional bulk detectors due to smaller absorption area and depth. Whereas it can generate a large V_{oc}, since V_{oc} depends on the on/off ratio and the off-state current can be extremely small due to its nanoscale size and quantum confinement. We investigated a CNTFET IR detector with Ag contacts, which shows a huge Voc with the value of ~0.3 V. CNTs may become important building blocks for future nano-optoelectronics sensors. The CNT IR sensor based on the asymmetric FET structure is shown in Figure 18.5. A CNT bridges an Au electrode and an Ag electrode on the top of a heavily doped Si/SiO_2 substrate, which serves as a back gate. The fabrication process starts from a Si/SiO_2 substrate, an Au electrode will be fabricated on the top through standard photolithography and followed by an Ag electrode after fine alignment to form a gap of around 1 μm.

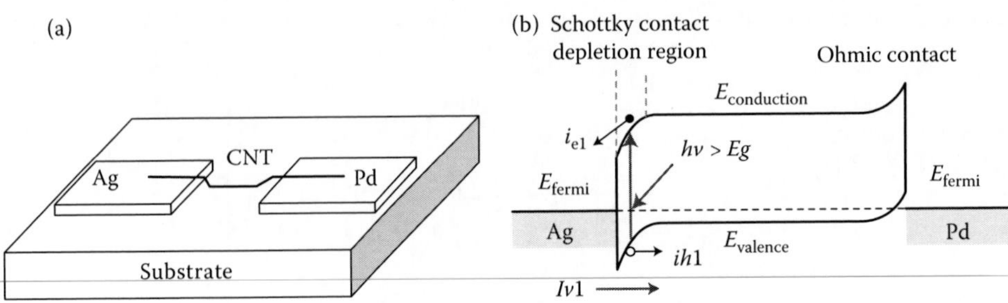

FIGURE 18.4 The single CNT-based IR sensors with asymmetric contacts. (a) Structure of the CNT sensors. (b) Energy band diagram of the CNT sensors.

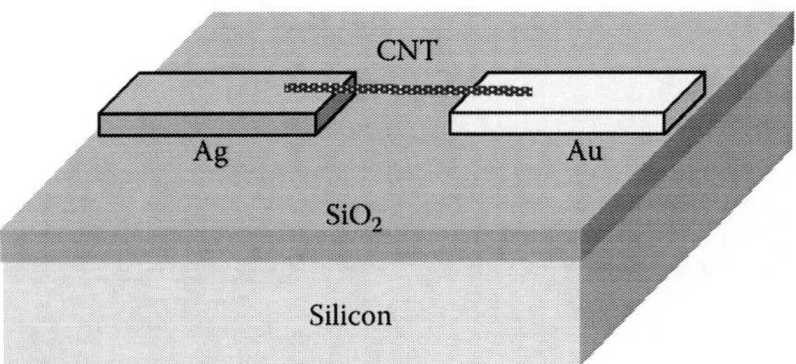

FIGURE 18.5 Structure of the CNTFET IR detector.

The final step is depositing a single CNT to connect two electrodes by our DEP deposition system and AFM manipulation system are discussed in Sections 18.3.1 and 18.3.2, respectively.

The CNT transistor shows p-type characteristics due to the oxygen doping in the air. The transfer characteristic at zero bias is shown in Figure 18.6a. The dark current (IR OFF) increases with negative gate voltage and decreases with positive gate voltage. The current difference between the IR ON and OFF is the photocurrent. It is observed that the on/off ratio is around 10^3 with proper positive gate voltage. Figure 18.6b shows the photocurrent measurement with three different gate voltages. It is found that +8 V gate voltage can decrease dark current and increase photocurrent, resulting in on/off ratio improvement.

18.2.3 Nanoantennas for CNT-Based IR Sensors

Since the photocurrent responses of CNT detectors are relatively low because of the small sensing area the enhancement technology has been developed to increase the electric field at the sensing area [59]. Since the size of the CNT is in nanoscale, the technique to enhance the electric field that is incident on such small sensing element is challenging. A nanoantenna was designed for our system as depicted in Figure 18.7 which consists of two symmetric thin metal wires that are separated by a nanometric gap. When the antenna is illuminated with an IR source, a standing-wave current pattern is generated along two metal wires. The field in the vicinity of the electrically conducting object is enhanced; The CNT sensing element is then aligned to the position of the maximum estimated field near the antenna. The maximum radiation occurs at the point that is perpendicular to the antenna axis.

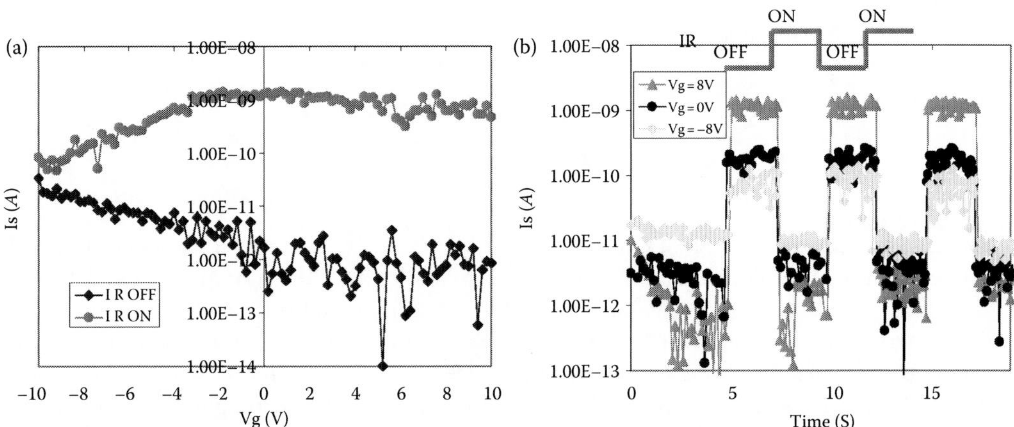

FIGURE 18.6 (a) Transfer characteristics of the CNTFET IR detector with IR signal OFF and ON. (b) Current signal measurement by switching the IR ON and OFF of 0.2 HZ at gate voltage 8 V, 0 and –8 V.

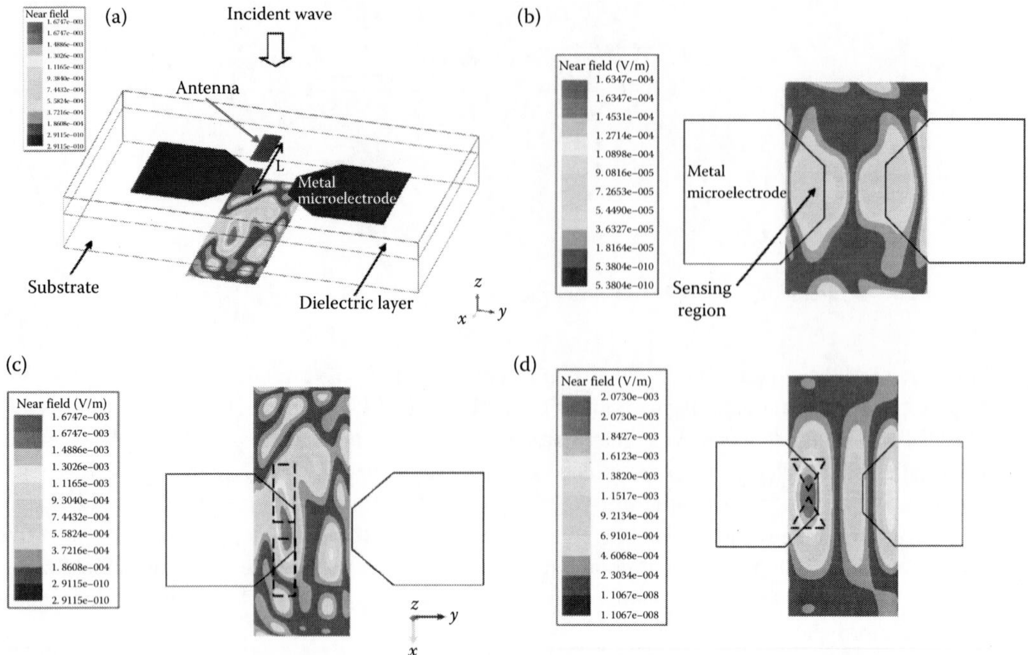

FIGURE 18.7 (a) Geometry of the structure for analysis, L is the length of the antenna arm; amplitude of the Y component of the electric field calculated for (b) no antenna, (c) dipole antenna, and (d) bowtie antenna under the incident plane wave excitation (wavelength $\lambda = 800$ nm).

In keeping with the goal of creating a locally resonant structure, we hypothesize that a metallic pattern (antenna) acting in concert with the metallic electrode can create necessary resonant structure. This hypothesis leaves room for several parameters that can be optimized, namely, location, specific pattern, multiplayer metallization, size of metallization, and so on. As shown in Figure 18.7, the antenna structures are placed over the CNT-based sensor such that resonant enhancement can be obtained. Here, two different antenna topologies, dipole and bowtie, were studied and their enhancement factors were estimated by the following theoretical analysis.

Imposing the boundary condition that the tangential component of the total electric field, $\mathbf{E}^{\text{total}}(\mathbf{r}) = \mathbf{E}^{\text{i}}(\mathbf{r}) + \mathbf{E}^{\text{s}}(\mathbf{r})$, on the metallic structures vanishes results in an integral equation that may be solved to obtain the current $\mathbf{J}(\mathbf{r})$, viz,

$$\begin{aligned} \hat{z} \times (\mathbf{E}^{\text{i}} + \mathbf{E}^{\text{s}}) &= 0 \\ \mathbf{E}^{\text{s}} &= \bar{\bar{G}}(\mathbf{r}) * \mathbf{J}(\mathbf{r}) \end{aligned} \tag{18.3}$$

where $\bar{\bar{G}}(\mathbf{r})$ is the layered medium Green's function and $\hat{z}$ denotes the vector that is normal to the interface. Details of this derivation can be obtained from [60]. Once the currents are found, the field in the entire structure can be easily found as well. The configuration is tested for different geometries of the nanoantenna, and the magnitude of the electric field is plotted in the plane of the microelectrode. As is evident from Figure 18.7, the field depends on the length and shape of the antenna. When the length of the arm is zero (Figure 18.7b), the field near the sensing region is an order of magnitude smaller than when the arm is 4 μm. In addition, the field from the bowtie antenna (Figure 18.7d) is higher than the field from the dipole antenna (Figure 18.7c). These results indicate that the antenna topology and its location are parameters that can be optimized.

18.3 MANUFACTURING PROCESSES OF CNT-BASED DEVICES

In this section, we focus on the major processes to fabricate the CNT-based nanodevices. We have developed a series of processes (Figure 18.8) to manufacture nanodevices using nanoparticles, nanorods, and nanowires such as CNTs. First, a microfluidic device has been developed to separate the CNTs. A precisions assembly can be achieved by the atomic force microscopy-based nanorobotic system. It is capable of manipulating the nanomaterial at the desired position efficiently. The band gap of the semiconducting material is an important property for many applications, such as optical detectors and solar cells. We have developed an electrical breakdown control method to adjust the band structure of a CNT; this process has provided a steady and high-yield on-chip band gap engineering approach in batch electronics fabrication. Therefore the spectral response of the devices can be adjusted. Finally, thermal annealing process and packaging process have been developed to maintain stability and reliability of nanodevices. The integration of the above technologies has provided an effective and efficient nanomanufacturing process for fabrication of nanosensors and electronic devices.

18.3.1 Dielectrophoretic-Based Manipulation and Separation of CNTs

In order to manipulate CNTs precisely and effectively, a novel and automotive CNT deposition system was designed and described in this section. We considered the essential process and designed a CNT deposition system based on DEP force. Especially, this system enables to classify specific types of CNTs and manipulates single CNTs to desired position. It proves the CNT-based nanodevices manufactured is more reliable and consistent. As a result, an automated computer-controllable system can be developed to realize the deposition of single CNTs. This system benefits CNTs to be used for manufacturing nanodevices in commercial application.

Our CNT deposition system employed dielectrophoretic (DEP) force to manipulate CNT on microelectrode structure. DEP manipulation induces movement of the CNT in nonuniform electric

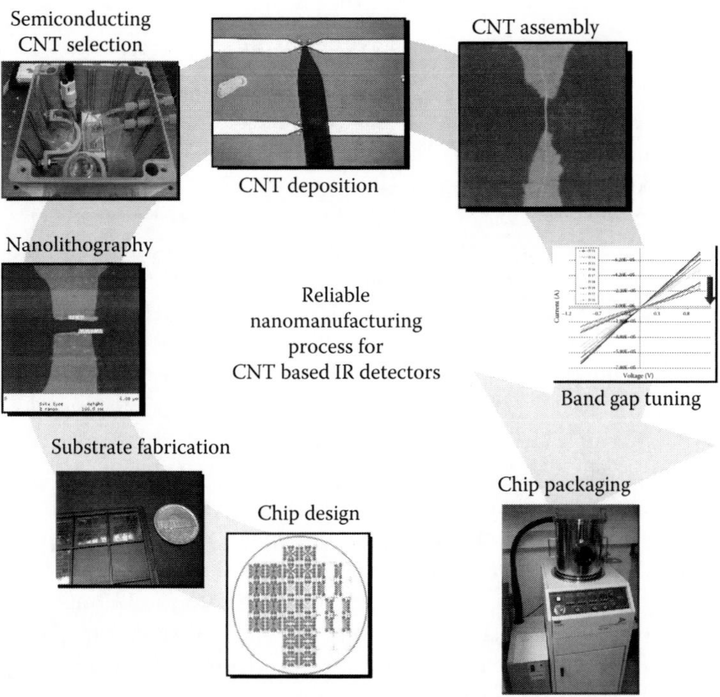

FIGURE 18.8 The nanomanufacturing process for CNT-based devices.

fields. It is supposed that the CNT is suspended in liquid medium. A particle is induced with effective dipole moment in nonuniform electric fields, and this effective dipole moment produced the movement of the particle [61]. The particle and the medium are polarized by the electric field, but their polarizabilities are different due to their properties. When the polarizability of particle is higher than that of the medium, a net dipole is induced across the particle and it is parallel to the applied electric field. On the contrary, the net dipole is induced opposite to the electric field when the polarizability of the medium is higher. The direction of force to push the particle to a high-electric field region or low electric field region is depended on the comparison of the polarizability between the particle and the medium. Indeed, the polarization of the particle is frequency dependent. Complex permitivity (ε^*) of the particle or medium is defined as [61,62],

$$\varepsilon^* = \varepsilon - i\frac{\sigma}{\omega} \tag{18.4}$$

where ε is the real permittivity, σ is the conductivity of the particle and the medium, and ω is the angular frequency of the applied electric field. Clausius–Mossotti factor ($K(\omega)$) is defined as a complex factor, describing a relaxation in the effective permitivity or polarizability of the particle with a relaxation time described in [61,62]

$$K(\omega) = \frac{\varepsilon_p^* - \varepsilon_m^*}{\varepsilon_p^* + 2\varepsilon_m^*} \tag{18.5}$$

where ε_m^* and ε_p^* are complex permittivities of the medium and the particle, respectively. A well-known equation describing time-averaged DEP force acting on the particle is given as [61,62]

$$F_{DEP} = \tfrac{1}{2} V \,\mathrm{Re}[K(\omega)] \nabla |E|^2 \tag{18.6}$$

where V is the volume of the particle and E is the electric field.

Based on this equation, the direction of DEP force is determined by the real part of $K(\omega)$. When $\mathrm{Re}[K(\omega)] > 0$, it is called positive DEP force, resulting in the movement of the particle toward microelectrodes (high-electric field region). When $\mathrm{Re}[K(\omega)] < 0$, it is called negative DEP force, resulting in the movement of the particle away from microelectrodes. Since we dispensed the CNT into alcohol, and we considered different kinds of CNTs in suspension, the plot of $\mathrm{Re}[K(\omega)]$ against frequency for different cases is shown as Figure 18.9, this result indicated that the semiconducting CNT undergoes positive DEP force in low-frequency range (<1 MHz) and it is changed to undergo negative DEP force when the applied frequency is larger than 10 MHz. Moreover, a metallic CNT always undergo positive DEP force in different frequencies (from 10 to 10^{10} Hz) of the applied AC voltage. This result provides a better understanding of manipulation of CNTs in a microelectrode structure. If DEP force is used to separate and identify different electronic types of CNTs (metallic and semiconducting), it can selectively attract metallic CNTs only to microelectrodes by applying an electric field in relatively high frequency range (>10 Mhz). However, it cannot attract semiconducting CNTs by using the same frequency range based on the result shown in Figure 18.9.

In order to overcome this problem, we proposed to integrate a microchamber to filter metallic CNTs before CNT dilution is spotted on microelectrodes as shown in Figure 18.10 [63]. A microchamber was fabricated with a lot of finger-like microelectrodes on a substrate. As shown in Figure 18.10, the fabricated chamber consisted of one inlet and one outlet to control the flow of the CNT sample solution. When CNT suspension flows into the chamber, high-frequency AC voltage is applied to the microelectrodes, so metallic CNTs are attracted toward the microelectrodes and stay in the microchamber. Then, semiconducting CNTs remain in the suspension. Finally, the suspension

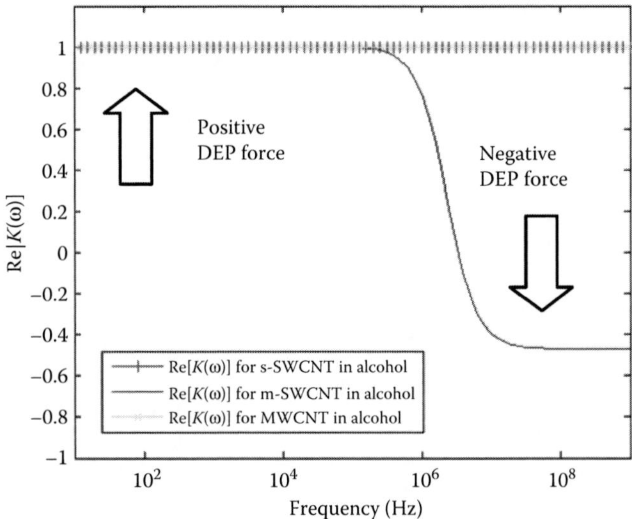

FIGURE 18.9 Plot of Re[$K(\omega)$] indicated positive and negative DEP force on different CNTs.

(with semiconducting CNTs only) is transferred to spotting probe and spotted on the microelectrode for the later CNT deposition process.

In order to apply DEP manipulation precisely and deposit CNT suspension effectively, a novel CNT deposition system was developed as shown in Figure 18.11. This system consisted of a microspotting probe, three micromanipulators, a DC microdiaphragm pump, a microchamber, and a microprobe station. In order to spot micron-sized CNT dilution droplets on the microelectrodes, micron-sized spotting probes with a diameter of 10–50 μm were fabricated from a micropipette using a mechanical puller. This spotting probe was connected with a DC microdiaphragm pump through a flexible polypropylene tube. This pump was used to deliver CNT dilution to the probe tip. The spotting probe was also mounted with a computer-controllable micromanipulator which could move the probe to the desired position of microelectrodes automatically. On the other hand, electrical circuit was made and connected to other micromanipulators. The electrical circuit provided AC voltage with different magnitudes and frequencies. The micromanipulators were also able to be moved to different locations of a microchip, and so the electric field can be applied to different microelectrodes. A microchip with arrays of microelectrodes was fabricated and placed on the stage of a microprobe station. The micromanipulators, DC microdiaphragm, and electrical circuit were connected with a computer, so that all components could be controlled simultaneously during the deposition process. By controlling the position of micromanipulators, the magnitude and frequency of AC voltage, the flow rate and applied time of the micropump, CNTs could be manipulated and attracted to microelectrodes on the microchip. This CNT deposition system integrated all essential

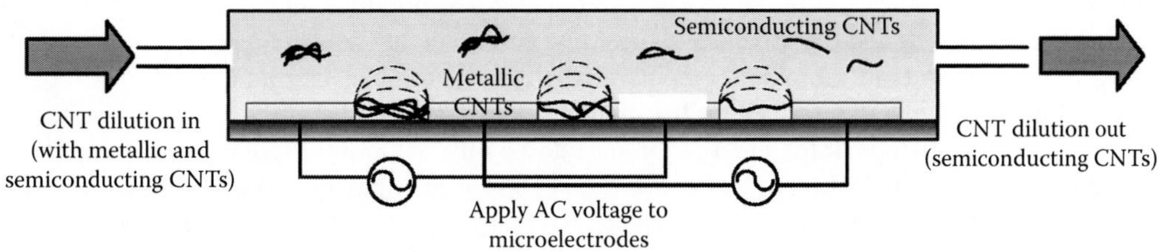

FIGURE 18.10 Illustration of microchamber to filter metallic CNT. Metallic CNTs are attracted on microelectrodes. Only semiconducing CNTs flow to the outlet.

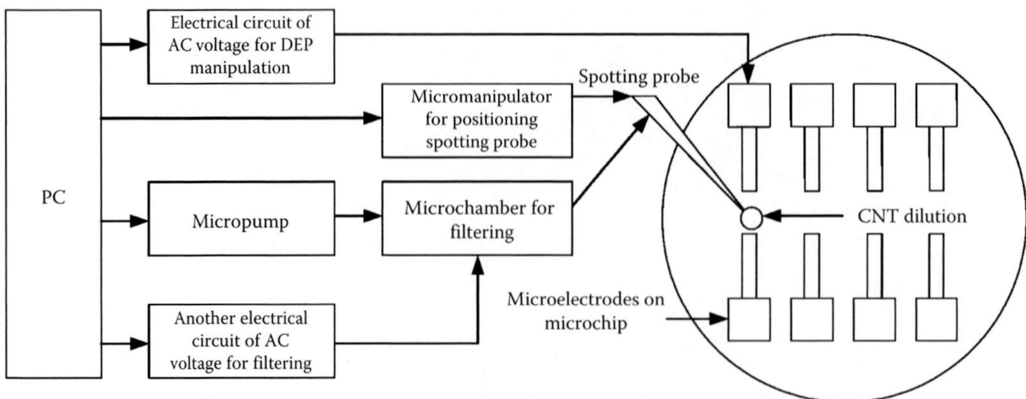

FIGURE 18.11 Illustration of CNT deposition system.

components to manipulate CNTs to desired positions precisely by DEP force, the development of this system benefits to the assembling and manufacturing of CNT-based devices.

During the deposition experiment, the fabricated microchip substrate was put on the stage of a microprobe station of the CNT deposition system. Microchips were fabricated using standard photolithography process. An array of gold microelectrodes was fabricated on a substrate, and a small gap distance of 2–3 μm was designed so as to form the CNT across the microelectrodes. The microelectrodes on the chip were applied by AC voltage (1.5 Vpp, 1 kHz) by the micromanipulator. CNTs were suspended in acetone solution (which has similar properties as alcohol). The CNT suspension was transferred to the probe tip by the micropump. The probe was then commanded and moved to the desired position of the microelectrodes by using the computer-controllable micromanipulator automatically. The CNT suspension was deposited on each pair of microelectrodes precisely. When each droplet of the CNT suspension deposited on the microelectrodes, the CNT was attracted and connected across the electrodes by activating the AC voltage. AFM was also used to observe the formation. The frequency and the amplitude of the AC voltage were experimentally optimized to achieve optimal possibility to attract an individual CNT between two electrodes, and the process was done by our CNT DEP workstation [64]. However, some impurities or more than one CNT were trapped between the electrodes in some cases. Therefore, an AFM-based nanomanipulation system has been developed to manipulate the nanoobjects and clean up the middle area of the electrode gap.

18.3.2 Atomic Force Microscopy-Based Nanorobotic Assembly

The AFM-based nanorobotic manipulation system with the augmented reality interface can provide the operator with real-time visual display and force feedback during nanomanipulations [65–71]. It consists of three subsystems: the AFM system, the augmented reality interface, and the real-time adaptable end effector controller. The AFM system includes the AFM head, signal access module (SAM), AFM controller, and the main computer. The SAM provides interfaces among the AFM head, AFM controller, and other devices. The AFM controller controls the AFM head through the SAM. It also connects to the main computer, which is responsible for running the main control program and providing an interface for the imaging. The augmented reality interface consists of a haptic device and a nanomanipulation program running on a Windows PC. The nanomanipulation program provides an interactive interface for users. During manipulation, operators use the haptic device to input the tip position command and feel the real-time interaction force between the tip and the nanoobjects. The real-time visual display is dynamic AFM images locally updated in video frame rate. The augmented reality interface also sends tip position command to the main computer. The real-time adaptable end effector controller subsystem includes a real-time linux system and a

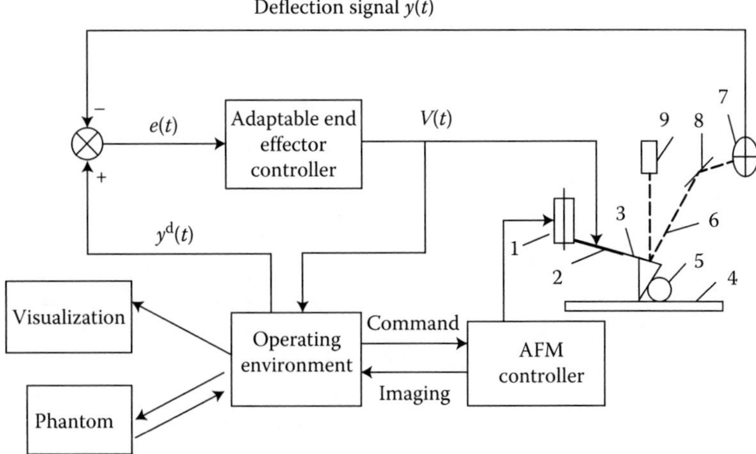

FIGURE 18.12 The control scheme of the AFM-based nanomanipulation system using adaptable end effector. 1: Piezo tube. 2: Piezoceramic layer of the adaptable end effector. 3: Adaptable end effector. 4: Substrate surface. 5: Object. 6: Laser beam. 7: Quad-photodiode detector. 8: Mirror. 9: Laser gun.

DAQ card. The adaptable end effector controller running in the real-time linux samples deflection signal of the cantilever through DAQ card and then outputs control signal to the adaptable end effector. At the same time, the control signal is also rendered to the haptic device to display the interaction force. These three subsystems communicate with each other through the Ethernet.

The details of the control scheme of the nanomanipulation system using the adaptable end effector are shown in Figure 18.12. The operating environment sends position command to the AFM controller which controls the tip position. An active probe is used as the adaptable end effector and a control loop is introduced into the system to keep the adaptable end effector rigid during manipulation. During pushing, the adaptable end effector is controlled to keep straight by feeding back the deflection signal from the photodiode detector. At the same time, the control signal is also sent to the haptic device Phantom™ as a force signal through the operating environment.

The effectiveness and reliability of the AFM-based nanomanipulation method using the adaptable end effector have also been proved by practical applications. This system has been employed to manipulate the CNT onto some microelectrode to build nanosensors. The process of manipulating a CNT onto a pair of gold electrodes to form a connection is shown in Figure 18.13. Figure 18.13a shows the AFM image before manipulation: there are two CNTs in the image, a longer one and a

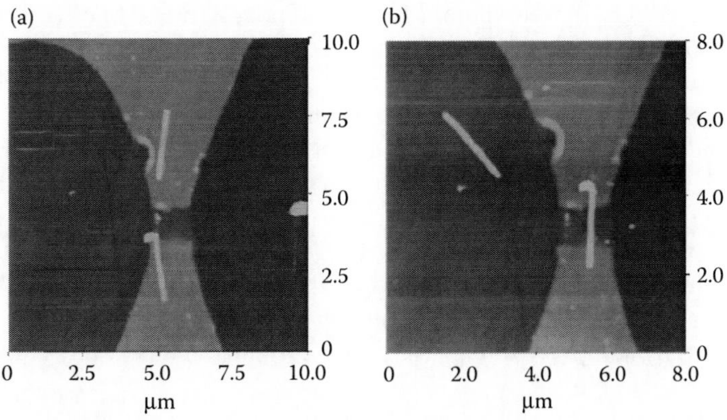

FIGURE 18.13 Manipulating a CNT onto a pair of gold electrodes. (a) The AFM image before manipulation. (b) The image from a new AFM scan after manipulations.

shorter one. The longer one will be pushed onto the electrodes to form the connection, and the shorter one will be pushed away as shown in Figure 18.13b which is a new AFM scan image after manipulation. With this system, the nanomanipulations and nanoassembly are not difficult anymore. It becomes more deterministic and more reliable.

18.3.3 On-Chip Band Gap Engineering

Controlling band gap of a CNT is crucial to its applications, but the processes is challenging. Some people consider various CNT synthesis processes, Li et al. [72] grew nearly 90% of semiconducting CNTs by a plasma-enhanced chemical vapor deposition method, but the band gaps cannot be controlled. Some synthesis methods control to grow narrow distribution of CNTs, for example, HiPco process (grew in high-pressure carbon monoxide) [73] and CoMoCAT process (using a silica-supported Co–Mo catalyst) [74], but the diameters of the CNTs are small (~0.5–1.5 nm), so the band gap of the CNT is limited which is not suitable for MWIR sensing applications. On the other hand, several approaches were pursued to separate different electronic types of CNTs. Arnold et al. [75] demonstrated a method using sonication and centrifugation to separate functionalized CNTs with different diameters, which are roughly inversely proportional to their band gaps. An on-chip band gap engineering method was proposed to breakdown multiwalled CNT (MWCNT) electrically [76]. When endure current beyond the breakdown limits, the outer carbon shells of an MWCNT can be electrically removed. A gate electrode under the CNTs is implemented to deplete the transport carriers in the semiconducting shell; the gate electrode increases the effectiveness to convert a metallic tube into a semiconductor one. However, this method remains uncontrolled which may result in cascade breakdown and destroy the CNT device.

Therefore, a novel CNT breakdown system has been developed to control the band gap of the CNT; it involves development of a real-time CNT electrical breakdown controller and the breakdown detection by extended Kalman filter for fault detection [77]. The controller is designed based on a quantum electron transport model to generate the optimal electron transmission inside the nanotube for the breakdown process. An extended Kalman filter is used to estimate the system state, and it detects the rapid change of the states caused by the electron movement in a CNT. This kind of system fault usually represents the status of the electrical breakdown. Our experimental results have shown that the band gap of a semiconducting MWCNT depends on the diameter of its outermost layer. If we can control the diameter of an MWCNT, we can generate a semiconductor material with a prespecified band gap. The basic idea is that we can start with an MWCNT with relative large diameter and small band gap, and then we can use the electrical breakdown process to remove the outer layers of the MWCNT. When the breakdown process can be controlled precisely, a semiconducting CNT with a desired band gap can be produced. In order to verify the breakdown process experimentally, the MWCNTs were illuminated by different NIR and MWIR signals, and then we measured the photocurrent of the MWCNTs after each breakdown process. Since the band gaps of the MWCNTs were changed during the process, the sensitivity of different wavelength IR signals were affected. As a result, a spectrum IR sensor can be made by the MWCNT.

First, we considered the electrical current model of a CNT. An electron transmission model calculated from the self-consistence nonequilibrium Green's functions (NEGFs) method gives the optimal estimation of the current–voltage characteristic of a specific device; it is utilized as the state-space model for breakdown current control [78]. The quantum energy states and electron wave function inside the CNT can be modeled by the Hamiltonian matrix (H) which is derived from Schrodinger's equation. The numerical solution of electron transport model for CNT conduction can be obtained by iteratively solving the NEGF formulas and Poisson's equation as shown in Figure 18.14.

The self-consistence algorithm for solving the electron transport model is computationally intensive. In order to calculate the numerical solution in real-time, the state-space model is derived based on the optimal fitting by the effective-mass transport model for the self-consistence result [79].

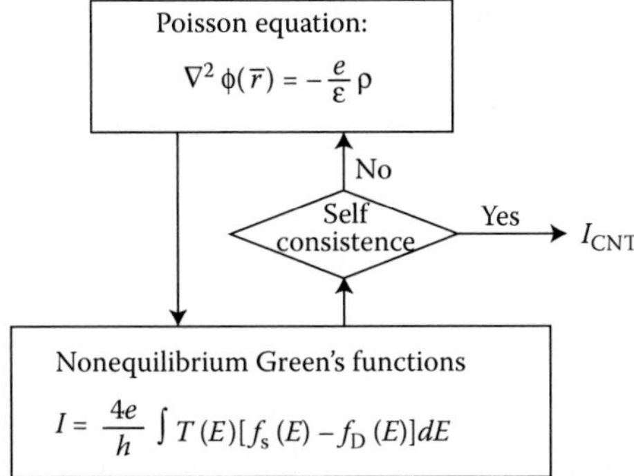

FIGURE 18.14 Self-consistence loop for the numerical calculation of the NEGF formulists and Poisson's equation.

Although the semiclassical model may lose accuracy for large drain voltage due to the simplification of quantum effect [80], it follows the characteristic features of curvature, which is critical to estimate the breakdown voltage. After combining the NEGF result and effective-mass equation, the modeling error is tolerable for the breakdown application. The current in the CNT device (I_{CNT}) is given by

$$I_{CNT} = \left(\frac{4e}{h}\right)k_B T\left\{\ln\left[\frac{1+\exp(\eta_{FS}/k_B T)}{1+\exp(\eta_{FD}/k_B T)}\right]\right\} \tag{18.7}$$

where e is the electron charge. h is the Planck constant. $\eta_{F,S(D)} = \phi_{S(D)} - \phi_{barr}$ denotes the potential difference between the source(drain), $\phi_{S(D)}$ and the barrier height of the metal–semiconductor contact, ϕ_{barr}. T is the temperature in Kelvin. And k_B is the Boltzmann constant. In experiment, the source is grounded and ϕ_S equals to zero. And ϕ_{barr} can be calculated by the optimal fitting from the NEGF result. Thus, I_{CNT} is completely determined by the drain voltage ϕ_{D}.

The quantum current controller design is based on an extended Kalman filter. The extended Kalman filter is a real-time nonlinear recursive algorithm to estimate the state of a dynamic system from discrete and noisy measurements [81]. The iterative process of the extended Kalman filter includes two steps. The time update step projects the current system state and its statistical information forward in time according to system plant. The measurement update step adjusts the propagated estimate by an actual measurement based on statistical decision theory and the least-square method. Figure 18.15 demonstrates the ongoing extended Kalman filtering loop.

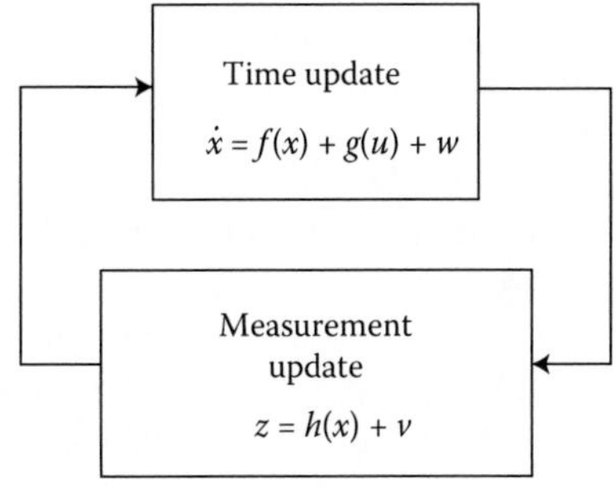

FIGURE 18.15 The recursive iteration for an extended Kalman filter: Time update and measurement update.

The controller is developed as follows. The system state, x is defined using the potential difference between the source and drain, U_{SD}. The polynomial quantum electron transport model, $h(x)$, is integrated in the measurement update stage. During the electrical breakdown process, the voltage across the CNT electrodes is increased by system input, u. Thus, in continuous-time form, the extended Kalman filter loop can be derived as

$$\dot{x} = u \tag{18.8}$$

$$z = h(x) \tag{18.9}$$

For real-time control, the discrete extended Kalman filter is derived according to the above dynamic system. The time update of the extended Kalman filter is obtained as

$$\hat{x}_k^- = \hat{x}_{k-1} + u_{k-1} \tag{18.10}$$

$$P_k^- = P_{k-1} + Q \tag{18.11}$$

where $\hat{x}$ is the system state for the source drain potential difference generated by the controller. The control variable u_k is the potential change in each iteration step. P is the error covariance matrix. Q is the covariance of the modeling error. The measurement update is modeled as

$$K_k = P_k^- H^{\mathrm{T}}(\mathrm{HP}_k^- H^{\mathrm{T}} + R)^{-1} \tag{18.12}$$

$$\hat{x}_k = \hat{x}_k^- + K_k(z_k - H\hat{x}_k^-) \tag{18.13}$$

$$P_k = (I - K_k H)P_k^- \tag{18.14}$$

where K is the optimal feedback gain, R is the measurement noise covariance, z is the current measurement of the CNT, and H is the observation matrix, which can be derived as a Jacobean matrix from the quantum electron transport model; see (18.15).

$$H = \left.\frac{\partial h}{\partial x}\right|_{\hat{x}_{k-1}, u_k} = -\frac{4q\exp(\varsigma_{\mathrm{DB}})}{h\{\exp(1+\varsigma_{\mathrm{DB}})\}} \tag{18.15}$$

$$\varsigma_{\mathrm{DB}} = \hat{x}_k^- - \phi_{\mathrm{barr}} \tag{18.16}$$

Based on the EKF scheme, the breakdown voltage is optimally propagated based on the statistical information from the previous data, while the incoming measurement of CNT current is utilized to adjust the projected estimation. The Gaussian random noise in modeling and measurement is filtered iteratively. The fault detect algorithm is embed into the real-time scheme of EKF. The rapid change in current, which usually represents the occurrence of a breakdown status, can be detected as the system fault based on the robust parameter estimation approaches [82]. The fault observer is modeled by generating the Mahalanobis distance. The breakdown voltage is stopped immediately once r exceeds the fault threshold to prevent cascade breakdowns.

$$r = (z_k - H\hat{x}_{\bar{k}})^{\mathrm{T}} P_k^{-1}(z_k - H\hat{x}_{\bar{k}}) \tag{18.17}$$

After the MWCNT was deposited on the electrodes by our DEP deposition system and AFM nanorobotic system, the band gap of the MWCNT was tuned by controlling the electrical breakdown process. The quantum Kalman fault detector algorithm was implemented in computer by controlling the Agilent's 4156C Precision Semiconductor Parameter Analyzer to generate the optimal breakdown voltage and measure the current through the CNT as feedback in real-time. The extended Kalman filter was used to provide the optimal breakdown voltage. The fault detection algorithm detects the current sudden change, which indicates the beginning of the breakdown process, and the system can stop it immediately. Finally, a desired band gap of a semiconducting CNT can be obtained through the breakdown process.

In order to study the breakdown effect on CNT-based IR detectors, a CNT-based IR sensor was tested by the IR radiation from a blackbody (Newport Corporation, Oriel Blackbody). The temperature of the blackbody was configured at 1050°C, the emission peak wavelength was around 2.2 μm. Bandpass filters (3.2 μm, 4 μm, and 5 μm, Spectrogon US, Inc) were inserted between the blackbody and the sensor to ensure specific wavelength of photon radiated on the sensor. The photocurrent responses of the sensor were measured with different bandpass filters before and after each breakdown process as shown in Figure 18.16. The sensor was not able to detect the IR signal with a wavelength of 5 μm after the sixth breakdown process. Since the band gap of the CNT was increased after the breakdown process, the sensing range was limited between 3.2 and 4 μm. After the eighth breakdown process, the detector was not able to detect the signal with wavelengths beyond 3.2 μm. This result further proves that the band gap of the CNT was increased through each CNT breakdown process. As a result, a photovoltaic material with a desired band gap can be tuned in the range of 3–5 μm by using this method.

18.3.4 Thermal Annealing Process and Packaging Process

Heterogeneous electrodes have been considered to improve the sensitivity, as discussed in the previous section. However, it was found that the stability of the CNT device was influenced by oxygen contamination. The exposure of SWCNT samples to oxygen appeared to have a strong influence on their electronic transport properties [83,84]. Besides, it was reported that the oxygen adsorption of CNTs modified the barriers at the CNT–metal interfaces [85]. In an ideal case, if CNT forms a Schottky contact at one of the CNT–metal interface and it forms an ohmic contact at another CNT–metal interface, the photocurrent should be maximized. Since CNTs are influenced by oxygen molecules in ambient environment, the contact condition would be affected. Therefore, in order to maximize the sensitivity of a CNT-based IR detector, it is important to control the oxygen doping

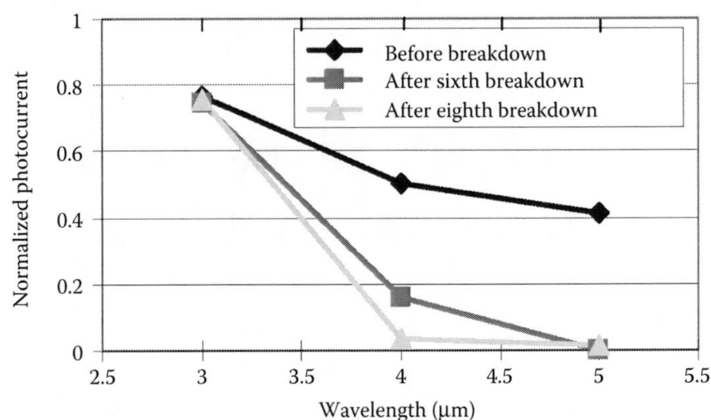

FIGURE 18.16 Photocurrent responses of the CNT-based sensor at specific wavelengths.

of the CNT device. We found that it is possible to remove the oxygen molecules (dedoped process) by annealing the CNTs in a vacuum furnace [86].

Gold (Au) and titanium (Ti) are chosen as the heterogeneous electrodes because they have different work functions (Au = 5.2 eV and Ti = 4.3 eV), so the Schottky barriers and the contact resistances at two CNT–metal interfaces are different, and the measured photocurrent can be increased. We first deposited a single MWCNT on the heterogeneous Au–Ti electrodes, and *I–V* characteristic of the MWCNT-based IR detector was measured. Then, the MWCNT-based IR detector was annealed at 400°C in a vacuum furnace for 1 h. Photonic effects of the oxygen-doped and the dedoped MWCNT-based IR detector were studied. The MWCNT-based IR detector was tested under an IR laser source (UH5–30G-830-PV, World Star Tech, optical power: 30 mW; wavelength: 830 nm). The temporal photoresponses of the dedoped MWCNT-based IR detector and the oxygen-doped MWCNT-based IR detector were compared as shown in Figure 18.17. For the oxygen-doped MWCNT-based IR detector, the signal noises of the dark current and the photocurrent were about 0.4 nA. Moreover, it exhibited signal drifting during the experiment. For the dedoped MWCNT, the signal noises of the dark current and the photocurrent were <0.1 nA and 0.2 nA, respectively. They were smaller after the thermal annealing process. This result clearly indicated that the photocurrent of the dedoped MWCNT-based IR detector had a more stable performance.

On the other hand, we tried to prevent the oxygen-doping effect on a dedoped SWCNT-based IR detector. We deposited another single SWCNT on a pair of heterogeneous electrodes. Similarly, this SWCNT-based IR detector was annealed at 400°C in a vacuum furnace for 1 h, and hence the oxygen molecules were removed. Then, we tried to package it by a layer of parylene C thin film with a thickness of 1 μm. Parylene C is used as an oxygen barrier of the fabricated device based on its barrier properties [87]. In Figure 18.18, it showed *I–V* characteristics of a CNT-based IR detector over different states of the processes. Before the thermal annealing process, curves 1–3 indicted the fluctuation and the unstable performance of the detector. After the thermal annealing process (Curve 4), the current of the detector increased significantly. Finally, the *I–V* characteristics of the detector became very stable after the parylene C packaging process. The signals were repeated over a couple of days. The results indicated a method to maintain, control, and prevent the oxygen

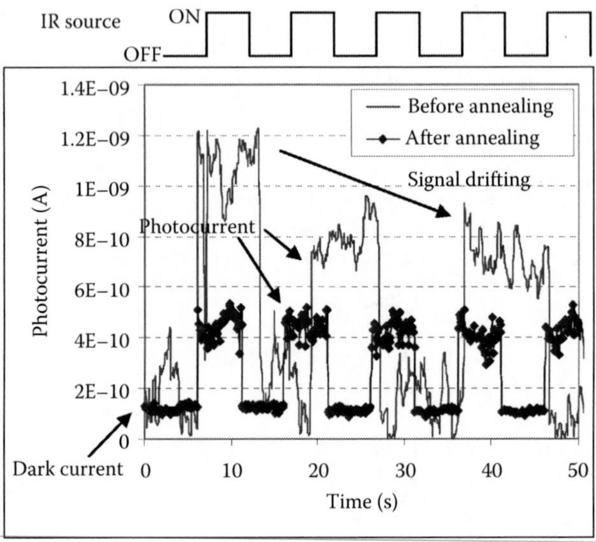

FIGURE 18.17 Temporal photoresponses of the dedoped (after annealing) and the oxygen-doped (before annealing) MWCNT-based IR detector. The oxygen-doped MWCNT-based IR detector exhibited signal drifting before the annealing process; it is a very unstable performance.

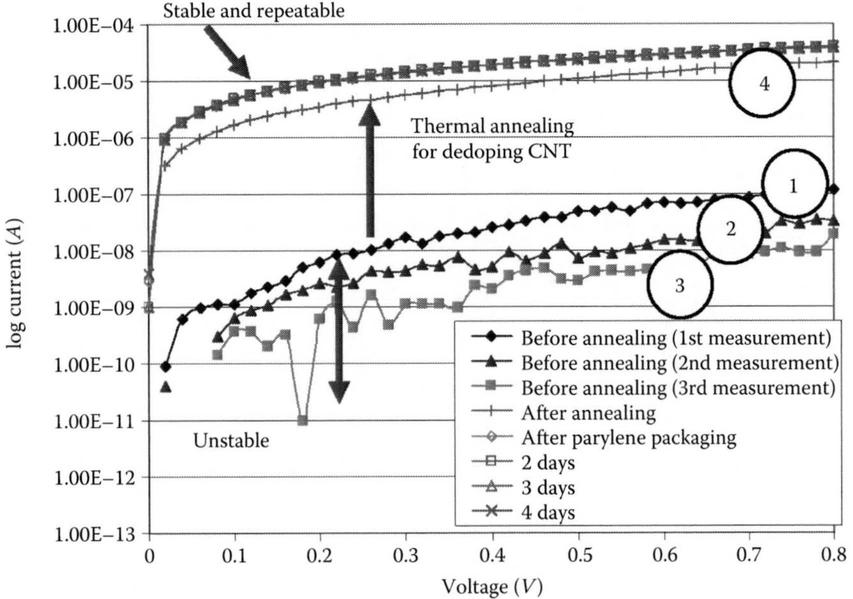

FIGURE 18.18 *I–V* characteristic of a CNT IR detector during the thermal annealing process and the parylene C packaging process.

doping of a CNT device. This method included two steps: (1) oxygen removal by the vacuum thermal annealing process and (2) oxygen prevention by parylene C packaging process.

18.4 PERFORMANCE EVALUATION AND ANALYSIS FOR CNT-BASED IR SENSORS

18.4.1 Temperature Dependency and Thermal Noise

As a 1D material, a CNT has some unique properties such as wide range of band gaps, and reduced carrier scattering, and so on. As a result, CNT-based IR sensors have the potential to work at room temperature or moderate low temperature with high quantum efficiency, which is difficult for other MWIR sensing materials to implement. Hence it is important to characterize the CNT sensors at different temperatures. We tested the temperature dependence of CNT detectors. The detectors were made from MWCNTs. A single MWCNT was deposited on a heterogeneous electrode structure. The detector was put in the vacuum cooler. The temperature was controlled from room temperature to −180°C. The *I–V* curves were measured every 10°C. We found the changes of the *I–V* characteristics of the CNT-based IR detector were small when the temperatures were changed as shown in Figure 18.19. When comparing the result with other photoconductive materials, it indicated that CNT is a less temperature-dependent material as shown in Table 18.1.

18.4.2 Quantum Efficiency

The quantum efficiency is defined as

$$QE = \frac{n_E}{n_P} \tag{18.18}$$

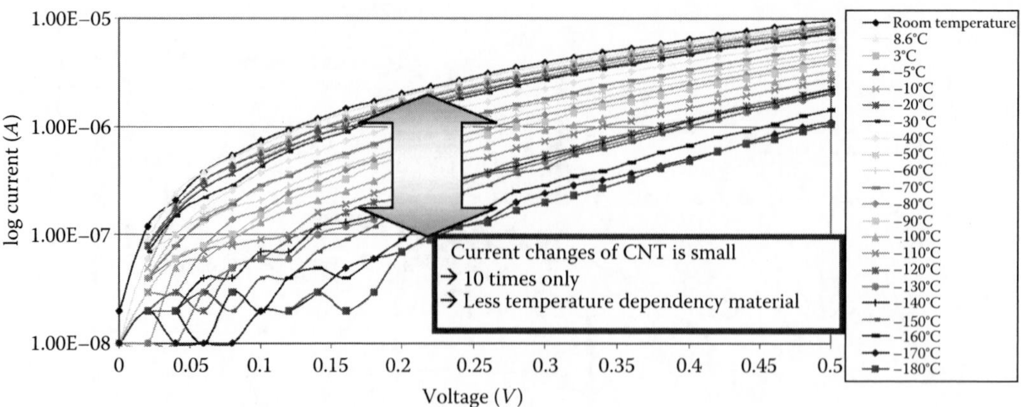

FIGURE 18.19 The *I–V* characteristics of the IR detector which was kept in the vacuum cooler under different temperatures.

where n_E is the number of collected electrons and n_p is the number of absorbed photons. The number of collected electrons can be calculated by

$$n_E = \frac{I_{ph}}{q} \tag{18.19}$$

where I_{ph} is the photocurrent and q is the electron charge. Using the photocurrent measured in the experiment, n_E can be calculated as

$$n_E = \frac{I_{ph}}{q} = \frac{1.3 \times 10^{-10}}{1.6022 \times 10^{-19}} = 8.114 \times 10^{8}\ S^{-1} \tag{18.20}$$

The number of photons absorbed by CNT is given by

$$n_p = \frac{P/A \times A_S}{E_{photon}} \tag{18.21}$$

where $P = 30$ mW is the total power of the IR source, $A = \pi(100\ \mu m)^2$ is the area of the IR spot, A_s = (length of CNT), X (diameter of CNT) is the sensing area of the CNT sensor, and E_{photon} is the photon energy and is given by

$$E_{photon} = h \times \frac{C}{\lambda} \tag{18.22}$$

TABLE 18.1
Temperature Dependency of Different Materials

Materials	Temperature Change	Current Change
CNT (Carbon nanotube)	200°C	<10
HgCdTe (Mercury Cadmium Telluride)	60°C	$\times 10^4$
InGaAsP (Indium Gallium Arsenide Phosphide)	120°C	$\times 10^4$
(Cs)Na2KSb (Cesiated Sodium Potassium Antimony)	110°C	$\times 10^2$
Na2KSb	120°C	$\times 10^3$

TABLE 18.2
Quantum Efficiency of Different IR Materials

Materials	Wavelength (μm)	QE
Quantum well IR photodetector	3–20	0.32
Quantum dot IR photodetector	4.7–5.2	0.0002
InSb	3–5	0.3–0.8
CNT	2.2	0.054

where $h = 6.626 \times 10^{-34}$Js is Plank's constant. $C = 3 \times 10^{8}$ ms^{-1} is the light velocity. $\lambda = 830$ nm is the wavelength of the IR light. Hence, the number of absorbed photon is $n_p = 1.495 \times 10^{10}$ S^{-1}.

Then the quantum efficiency can be calculated as

$$\text{QE} = \frac{n_E}{n_P} = \frac{8.114 \times 10^{8}\, S^{-1}}{1.495 \times 10^{10}\, S^{-1}} = 5.43\% \tag{18.23}$$

This value is consistent with the previous reported results [12,88,89]. The quantum efficiency of different IR materials is shown in Table 18.2. It can be seen that the quantum efficiency of SWCNT is still lower than other well-developed IR materials. The low quantum efficiency of the SWCNT is due to its thin diameter. Most of the photons which reach the SWCNT surface will pass through the SWCNT wall without exciting the electron–hole pairs. Hence, further study on the structure of CNT-based IR sensors is expected for improving the quantum efficiency.

18.5 CONCLUSIONS

Design and fabrication of the single CNT-based nanodevices for optical sensing has been discussed in this chapter. The CNT-based devices have been used for IR-sensing. The devices with symmetric and asymmetric contacts have also been considered to achieve maximum photocurrent under illumination of IR signal, photocurrent. Besides, the photocurrent and signal ON/OFF are enhanced by integrating nanoantennas and CNTFET devices. The nanomanufacturing process has been presented which includes several key developments: (1) CNT filtering and DEP deposition, (2) AFM-based nanoassembly, (3) on-chip band gap engineering, and (4) thermal annealing and packing of the devices. The development of CNT-based spectrum sensors has been investigated and studied, experimental result show that the CNTs can effectively sense NIR and MWIR signal at room temperature environment. The DEP manipulation and AFM assembly are not limited to be used for CNTs, they can be widely used for other nanoobjects such as nanoparticles, nanowires, DNA molecules, and so on. Besides a quantum electron transport controller based on the quantum state model and the extended Kalman filter is developed for real-time CNTs electrical breakdown control. Optimal breakdown electron transport through the CNT is generated by the controller based on the statistic information of the previous data, and so the rapid current change can be detected immediately. The results from the on-chip CNT band gap engineering experiment indicate that the desired band gap of as MWCNT can be tuned by the electrical breakdown process, and so the sensor can be adjusted to have high sensitivity in different wavelengths. Our breakdown control method can adjust the band structure of CNTs and provides a steady and high-yield on-chip band gap engineering approach which is important to manufacture the next generation of nano-IR sensors. These methods provide a way to fabricate and maintain optoelectronic properties of CNT-based nanodevices. As a result, high efficiency, high sensitivity, stable and reliable CNT-based IR detector can be fabricated.

ACKNOWLEDGMENTS

This research work is partially supported under NSF Grants IIS-0713346 and DMI-0500372, and ONR Grants N00014–04–1–0799 and N00014–07–1–0935.

REFERENCES

1. S. Iijima, Helical microtubules of graphitic carbon, *Nature*, 354, 56–58, 1991.
2. A. Bachtold, P. Hadley, T. Nakanishi, and C. Dekker, Logic circuits with carbon nanotube transistors, *Science*, 294, 1317–1320, 2001.
3. V. Derycke, R. Martel, J. Appenzeller, and Ph. Avouris, Carbon nanotube inter- and intramolecular logic gates, *Nano Lett.*, 1, 453–456, 2001.
4. D. Qian, G. J. Wagner, W. K. Liu, M. Yu, and R. S. Ruoff, Mechanics of carbon nanotubes, *Appl. Mech. Rev.*, 55, 495–533, 2002.
5. P. L. McEuen, M. S. Fuhrer, and H. Park, Single-walled carbon nanotube electronics, *IEEE Trans. Nanotechnol.*, 1, 78–85, 2002.
6. Q. Z. Xue, Model for the effective thermal conductivity of carbon nanotube composites, *Nanotechnology*, 17, 1655–1660, 2006.
7. M. S. Dresselhaus, G. Dresselhaus, A. Jorio, A. G. Souza Filho, and R. Saito, Raman spectroscopy on isolated single wall carbon nanotubes, *Carbon*, 40, 2043–2061, 2002.
8. R. J. Chen, N. R. Franklin, J. Kong, J. Cao, T. W. Tombler, Y. Zhang, and H. Dai, Molecular photodesorption from single-walled carbon nanotubes, *Appl. Phys. Lett.*, 79, 2258–2260, 2001.
9. A. Fujiwara, Y. Matsuoka, H. Suematsu, N. Ogawa, K. Miyano, H. Kataura, Y. Maniwa, S. Suzuki, and Y. Achiba, Photoconductivity in semiconducting single-walled carbon nanotubes, *Jpn. J. Appl. Phys.*, 40, L1229–L1231, 2001.
10. I. A. Levitsky and W. B. Euler, Photoconductivity of single-wall carbon nanotubes under continuous-wave near-infrared illumination, *Appl. Phys. Lett.*, 83, 1857–1859, 2003.
11. K. Balasubramanian, Y. Fan, M. Burghard, K. Kern, M. Friedrich, U. Wannek, and A. Mews, Photoelectronic transport imaging of individual semiconducting carbon nanotubes, *Appl. Phys. Lett.*, 84, 2400–2402, 2004.
12. M. Freitag, Y. Martin, J. A. Misewich, R. Martel, and Ph. Avouris, Photoconductivity of single carbon nanotubes, *Nano Lett.*, 3, 1067–1071, 2003.
13. J. U. Lee, Photovoltaic effect in ideal carbon nanotube diodes, *Appl. Phys. Lett.*, 87, 073101, 2005.
14. A. Mohite, S. Chakraborty, P. Gopinath, G. U. Sumanasekera, and B. W. Alphenaar, Displacement current detection of photoconduction in carbon nanotubes, *Appl. Phys. Lett.*, 86, 061114, 2005.
15. H. Dai, Carbon nanotubes: Synthesis, integration, and properties, *Acc. Chem. Res.*, 35, 1035–1044, 2002.
16. M. Dresselhaus, G. Dresselhaus, and Ph. Avouris, *Carbon Nanotubes: Synthesis, Structure, Properties and Application*, Springer, Berlin, 2001.
17. J. W. Mintmire, B. I. Dunlap, and C. T. White, Are fullerene tubules metallic? *Phys. Rev. Lett.*, 68, 631–634, 1992.
18. M. S. Dresselhaus, G. Dresselhaus, and R. Saito. Carbon fibers based on c60 and their symmetry, *Phys. Rev. B*, 45, 6234–6242, 1992.
19. Ph. Avouris, Carbon nanotube electronics, *Chem. Phys.*, 281, 429–445, 2002.
20. P. G. Collins and Ph. Avouris, Carbon fibers based on c60 and their symmetry, *Sci. Am.*, 283, 62–29, 2000.
21. H. Dai, Carbon nanotubes: Opportunities and challenges, *Surf. Sci*, 500, 218–241, 2002.
22. M. Ahlskog, P. Hakonen, M. Paalanen, L. Roschier, and R. Tarkiainen, Multiwalled carbon nanotubes as building blocks in nanoelectronics, *J. Low Temp. Phys.*, 124, 335–352, 2001.
23. B. Q. Wei, R. Vajtai, and P. M. Ajayan, Reliability and current carrying capacity of carbon nanotubes, *Appl. Phys. Lett.*, 79, 1172–1174, 2001.
24. N. Srivastava and K. Banerje, Performance analysis of carbon nanotube inter-connects for VLSI applications, *In Proc. 2005 IEEE/ACM Int. Conf. Computer-Aided Design*, pp. 383–390, San Jose, CA, 2005.
25. S. J. Wind, J. Appenzeller, and Ph. Avouris, Lateral scaling in carbon-nanotube field-effect transistors, *Phys. Rev. Lett.*, 91(5), 058301, 2003.
26. S. Hasan, S. Salahuddin, M. Vaidyanathan, and M. A. Alam, High-frequency performance projections for ballistic carbon-nanotube transistor, *IEEE Trans. Nanotechnol.*, 5, 14–22, 2006.

27. J. Appenzeller, Y.-M. Lin, J. Knoch, Z. Chen, and Ph. Avouris Comparing carbon nanotube transistors—The ideal choice: A novel tunneling device design, *IEEE Trans. Electron Devices*, 52, 2568–2576, 2005.
28. S. J. Wind, J. Appenzeller, R. Martel, V. Derycke, and Ph. Avouris, Vertical scaling of carbon nanotube field-effect transistors using top gate electrodes, *Appl. Phys. Lett.*, 80, 3817–3819, 2002.
29. D. V. Singh, K. A. Jenkins, J. Appenzeller, D. Neumayer, A. Grill, and H.-S. P. Wong, Frequency response of top-gated carbon nanotube field-effect transistors, *IEEE Trans. Nanotechnol.*, 3, 383–387, 2004.
30. Z. Chen, J. Appenzeller, Y.-M. Lin, J. Sippel-Oakley, A. G. Rinzler, J. Tang, S. J. Wind, P. M. Solomon, and Ph. Avouris, An integrated logic circuit assembled on a single carbon nanotube, *Science*, 311, 1735, 2006.
31. M. Freitag, V. Perebeinos, J. Chen, A. Stein, J. C. Tsang, J. A. Misewich, R. Martel, and Ph. Avouris, Hot carrier electroluminescence from a single carbon nanotube, *Nano Lett.*, 4, 1063–1066, 2004.
32. S. Lu and B. Panchapakesan, Photoconductivity in single wall carbon nanotube sheets. *Nanotechnology*, 17, 1843–1850, 2006.
33. N. R. Franklin, Q. Wang, T. W. Tombler, A. Javey, M. Shim, and H. Dai, Integration of suspended carbon nanotube arrays into electronic devices and electromechanical systems, *Appl. Phys. Lett.*, 81, 913–915, 2002.
34. P. Qi, O. Vermesh, M. Grecu, A. Javey, Q. Wang, H. Dai, S. Peng, and K. J. Cho, Toward large arrays of multiplex functionalized carbon nanotube sensors for highly sensitive and selective molecular detection, *Nano Lett.*, 3, 347–351, 2003.
35. A. Nojeh, A. Ural, R. F. Pease, and H. Dai, Electric-field-directed growth of carbon nanotubes in two dimensions, *J. Vac. Sci. Technol. B*, 22, 3421–3425, 2004.
36. J. Li, Q. Zhang, D. Yang, and J. Tian, Fabrication of carbon nanotube field effect transistors by ac dielectrophoresis method, *Carbon*, 42, 2263–2267, 2004.
37. S. Taeger, D. Sickert, P. Atanasov, G. Eckstein, and M. Mertig. Self-assembly of carbon nanotube field-effect transistors by ac-dielectrophoresis, *Phys. Stat. Sol. (b)*, 243, 3355–3358, 2006.
38. S. Banerjee, B. White, L. Huang, B. J. Rego, S. O'brien, and I. P. Herman, Precise positioning of carbon nanotubes by ac dielectrophoresis using floating posts, *Appl. Phys. A*, 86, 415–419, 2007.
39. P. Makaram, S. Selvarasah, X. Xiong, C.-L. Chen, A. Busnaina, N. Khanduja, and M. R. Dokmeci, Three-dimensional assembly of single-walled carbon nanotube interconnects using dielectrophoresis, *Nanotechnology*, 18, 395204, 2007.
40. Z. Chen, J. Appenzeller, J. Knoch, Y. Lin, and Ph. Avouris, The role of metal–nanotube contact in the performance of carbon nanotube field-effect transistors, *Nano Lett.*, 5, 1497–1502, 2005.
41. C. Lu, L. An, Q. Fu, J. Liu, H. Zhang, and J. Murduck, Schottky diodes from asymmetric metal–nanotube contacts, *Appl. Phys. Lett.*, 88, 133501, 2006.
42. D. Perello, M. J. Kim, D. Cha, G. H. Han, D. J. Bae, S. Y. Jeong, Y. H. Lee, and M. Yun, Schottky barrier engineering in carbon nanotube with various metal electrodes, *In Proc. 7th IEEE Int. Conf. Nanotechnolgy*, pp. 189–193, Hong Kong, August 2007.
43. J. Lefebvre, M. Radosavljevic, and A. T. Johnson, Fabrication of nanometer size gaps in a metallic wire, *Appl. Phys. Lett.*, 76, 3828–3830, 2000.
44. M. M. Deshmukh, D. C. Ralph, M. Thomas, and J. Silcox, Nanofabrication using a stencil mask, *Appl. Phys. Lett.*, 75, 1631–1633, 1999.
45. S. G. Rao, L. Huang, W. Setyawan, and S. Hong, Large-scale assembly of carbon nanotubes, *Nature*, 425, 36–37, 2003.
46. M. Hazani, F. Hennrich, M. Kappes, R. Naaman, D. Peled, V. Sidorov, and D. Shvarts, DNA-mediated self-assembly of carbon nanotube-based electronic devices, *Chem. Phys. Lett.*, 391, 389–392, 2004.
47. G. Binnig, C. F. Quate, and C. Gerber, Atomic force microscope, *Phys. Rev. Lett.*, 56(9), 930–933, 1986.
48. Z. Deng, E. Yenilmez, A. Reilein, J. Leu, H. Dai, and K. A. Moler, Nanotube manipulation with focused ion beam, *Appl. Phys. Lett.*, 88, 023119, 2006.
49. M. Yu, M. J. Dyer, G. D. Skidmore, H. W. Rohrs, X. Lu, K. D. Ausman, J. R. Von Ehr, and R. S. Ruoff, Three-dimensional manipulation of carbon nanotubes under a scanning electron microscope, *Nanotechnology*, 10, 244–252, 1999.
50. T. Hertel, R. Martel, and Ph. Avouris, Manipulation of individual carbon nanotubes and their interaction with surfaces, *J. Phys. Chem. B*, 102, 910–915, 1998.
51. Ph. Avouris, T. Hertel, R. Martel, T. Schmidt, H.R. Shea, and R.E. Walkup, Carbon nanotubes: Nanomechanics, manipulation, and electronic devices, *Appl. Surf. Sci.*, 141, 201–209, 1999.

52. H. W. C. Postma, A. Sellmeijer, and C. Dekker, Manipulation and imaging of individual single-walled carbon nanotubes with an atomic force microscope, *Adv. Mater.*, 12, 1299–1302, 2000.
53. J. Zhang, N. Xi, and K. Lai, Fabrication and testing of a nano infrared Detector using a single carbon nanotube (CNT), SPIE Newsroom (2007). Available at: http://spie.org/x8489.xml
54. J. Zhang, N. Xi, H. Chen, K. W. C. Lai, and G. Li, Photovoltaic effect in single carbon nanotube based Schottky diodes, *Int. J. Nanoparticles*, 1(2), 108–118, 2008.
55. J. Zhang, N. Xi, H. Chen, K. W. C. Lai, and G. Li, Design, manufacturing and testing of single carbon nanotube based infrared sensors, *IEEE Trans. Nanotechnol.*, 8(2), 245–251, 2009.
56. A. Javey, J. Guo, Q. Wang, M. Lundstrom, and H. Dai, Ballistic carbon nanotube field-effect transistors, *Nature*, 424, 654–657, 2003.
57. H. Chen, N. Xi, K. W. C. Lai, and J. Zhang, Infrared detection using carbon nanotube field effect transistor, *In Proc. IEEE Conf. Nanotechnology 2008*, Arlington, TX, pp.88–91, August 18–21, 2008.
58. H. Chen, N. Xi, K. W. C. Lai, C. K. M. Fung, and R. Yang, CNT infrared detectors using Schottky barriers and p–n junctions based FETs, *IEEE Nanotechnol*ogy. *Mate*rials and *Devices Conference*, Traverse City, MI, June 2–5, 2009.
59. C. K. M. Fung, N. Xi, B. Shanker, and K. W. C. Lai, Nano resonant signal booster for carbon nanotube based infrared detectors, *Nanotechnology*, 20, 185201, 2009.
60. K. A. Michalski and D. Zheng, Electromagnetic scattering and radiation by surfaces of arbitrary shape in layered media, *IEEE Trans. Antennas Propag.*, 38, 335–344, 1990.
61. H. Morgan and N. G. Green, *AC Electrokinetics: Colloids and Nanoparticles*, Research Studies Press Ltd, England, 2003.
62. T. B. Jones, *Electromechanics of Particles*, Cambridge University Press, New York, 1995.
63. K. W. C. Lai, N. Xi, and U. C. Wejinya, Automated process for selection of carbon nanotube by electronic property using dielectrophoretic manipulation, *J. Micro-Nano Mechatronics*, 4(1), 37–48, 2008.
64. K. W. C. Lai, N. Xi, C. K. M. Fung, J. Zhang, H. Chen, Y. Luo, and U. C. Wejinya, Automated nanomanufacturing system to assemble carbon nanotube based devices, *Int. J. Robot. Res. (IJRR)*, 28, 523–536, 2009.
65. G. Li, N. Xi, M. Yu, and W. K. Fung, Augmented reality system for real-time nanomanipulation, *In Proc. IEEE Int. Conf. Nanotechnology*, San Francisco, CA, August 12–14, 2003.
66. G. Li, N. Xi, and M. Yu, Development of augmented reality system for afm based nanomanipulation, *IEEE/ASME Trans. Mechatronics*, 9, 358–365, 2004.
67. G. Li, N. Xi, H. Chen, C. Pomeroy, and M. Prokos, "Videolized" atomic force microscopy for interactive nanomanipulation and nanoassembly, *IEEE Trans. Nanotechnol.*, 4, 605–615, 2005.
68. H. Chen, N. Xi, and G. Li, CAD-guided automated nanoassembly using atomic force microscopy-based nonrobotics, *IEEE Trans. Autom. Sci. Eng.*, 3(3), 208–217, 2006.
69. J. Zhang, Ni. Xi, G. Li, H. Chan, and U. C. Wejinya, Adaptable end effector for atomic force microscopy based nanomanipulation, *IEEE Trans. Nanotechnol.*, 5(6), 628–642, 2006.
70. L. Liu, Y. Luo, N. Xi, Y. Wang, J. Zhang, and G. Li, Sensor referenced real-time videolization of atomic force microscopy for nanomanipulations, *IEEE/ASME Trans. Mechatronics*, 13(1), 76–85, 2008.
71. J. Zhang, N. Xi, L. Liu, H. Chen, K. W. C. Lai, and G. Li, Atomic force yields a master nanomanipulator, *IEEE Nanotechnol. Mag.*, 2(2), 13–17, 2008.
72. Y. Li, D. Mann, M. Rolandi, W. Kim, A. Ural, S. Hung, A. Javey et al. Preferential growth of semiconducting single-walled carbon nanotubes by a plasma enhanced CVD method, *Nano Lett.*, 4, 317–321, 2004.
73. S. M. Bachilo, M. S. Strano, C. Kittrell, R. H. Hauge, R. E. Smalley, and R. B. Weisman, Structure-assigned optical spectra of single-walled carbon nanotubes, *Science*, 298, 2361–2366, 2002.
74. S. M. Bachilo, L. Balzano, J. E. Herrera, F. Pompeo, D. E. Resasco, and R. B. Weisman, Narrow (n,m)-distribution of single-walled carbon nanotubes grown using a solid supported catalyst, *J. Am. Chem. Soc*, 125, 11186–11187, 2003.
75. M. S. Arnold, A. A. Green, J. F. Hulvat, S. I. Stupp, and M. C. Hersam, Sorting carbon nanotubes by electronic structure using density differentiation, *Nature Nanotechnol.*, 1, 60–65, 2006.
76. P. G. Collins, M. S. Arnold, and Ph. Avouris, Engineering carbon nanotubes and nanotube circuits using electrical breakdown, *Science*, 292, 706–709, 2001.
77. K. W. C. Lai, N. Xi, C. K. M. Fung, H. Chen, and T.-J. Tarn, Engineering the band gap of carbon nanotubes for infrared sensors, *Appl. Phys. Lett.*, 95(22), 221107, 2009.
78. S. Datta, *Quantum Transport: Atom to Transistor*, New York, NY: Cambridge University Press, 2005.
79. R. Tamura and M. Tsukada, Analysis of quantum conductance of carbon nanotube junctions by the effective-mass approximations, *Phys. Rev. B*, 58, 8120–8124, 1998.

80. S. Koswatta, N. Neophytou, D. Kienle, G. Fiori, and M. Lundstrom, Dependence of DC characteristics of CNT MOSFETs on bandstructure models, *IEEE Trans. Nanotechnol.*, 5, 368–372, 2006.
81. R. E. Kalman, A new approach to linear filtering and prediction problems, *Transactions of the ASME–J. Basic Eng.*, 82, 35–45, 1960.
82. P. M. Frank, Fault diagnosis in dynamic systems using analytical and knowledge-based redundancy—A survey and some new results, *Automatica*, 26(3), 459–474, 1990.
83. P. G. Collins, K. Bradley, M. Ishigami, and A. Zettl, Extreme oxygen sensitivity of electronic properties of carbon nanotubes, *Science*, 287, 28012804, 2000.
84. L. Valentinia, I. Armentanoa, L. Lozzib, S. Santuccib, and J. M. Kenny, Interaction of methane with carbon nanotube thin films: Role of defects and oxygen adsorption, *Mater. Sci. Eng.: C*, 24, 527–533, 2004.
85. V. Derycke, R. Martel, J. Appenzeller, and Ph. Avouris, Controlling doping and carrier injection in carbon nanotube transistors, *Appl. Phys. Lett.*, 80(15), 2273–2275, 2002.
86. K. W. C. Lai, N. Xi, C. K. M. Fung, H. Chen, J. Zhang, and Y. Luo, Photonic effect on oxygen-doped and de-doped carbon nanotubes, *In Proc. 8th IEEE Conf. Nanotechnology*, pp. 251–254, 18–21, August 2008.
87. K. W. C. Lai, N. Xi, J. Zhang, G. Li, and H. Chen, Packaging carbon nanotube based infrared detector, *In Proc. 7th IEEE Conference on Nanotechnology*, pp. 778–781, 2–5, August 2007.
88. D. A. Stewart and F. Leonard, Energy conversion effciency in nanotube optoelectronics, *Nano Lett.*, 5, 2005, 219–222.
89. G. Y. Guo and K. C. Chu, Linear and nonlinear optical properties of carbon nanotubes from first-principles calculations, *Phys. Rev. B*, 69, 205416, 2004.

19 Acoustically Controlled All-Fiber Lasers

Christian Cuadrado-Laborde, Antonio Diez, José L. Cruz, and Miguel V. Andrés

CONTENTS

19.1 INTRODUCTION

The interest of all-fiber lasers is stimulated by the inherent advantages they have over bulk lasers in aspects such as heat dissipation and robustness. The performance of Q-switched and mode-locked fiber lasers can benefit highly from the development of all-fiber configurations, since when a bulk-intracavity component is used, many interesting features are lost [1]. Earlier and subsequent demonstrations of active Q-switching (QS) [2–5] or mode-locking (ML) [6–8] of fiber lasers were based on the use of bulk external modulators; however, this procedure has important drawbacks. On the one hand, it may not fulfill the requirements for mechanical stability that most practical systems need due to alignment problems, and on the other hand, it increases the cavity losses, which reduces the laser efficiency. A fiber laser with strictly all-fiber components can fulfill the requirements for increasing mechanical stability, low maintenance, enhanced power efficiency, high peak power damage, and a simplified assembly process. In this framework, recently developed in-fiber acoustooptic devices have demonstrated new possibilities for actively Q-switched distributed feedback

TABLE 19.1
Nomenclature

CW	Continuous wave
QS	*Q*-switching
ML	Mode-locking
AM	Amplitude modulation
FM	Frequency modulation
QML	*Q*-switching mode-locking
FBG	Fiber Bragg grating
EDF	Erbium-doped fiber
DFB	Distributed feedback
AOSLM	Acoustooptic superlattice modulator

fiber (QS-DFB) lasers [9–11], continuous-wave mode-locking (CW-ML) lasers [12–17] and doubly active *Q*-switched mode-locking (QML) [18–19]. Here we illustrate the new possibilities arising from the interaction of light with acoustic pulses and harmonic acoustic waves.

This chapter is organized as follows. In Section 19.2 we describe a QS-DFB all-fiber laser that uses a novel in-line acoustic pulse generator. The use of this DFB all-fiber laser as a compact light source for Brillouin sensing applications is also discussed. In Section 19.3 we describe a CW-ML all-fiber laser. In Section 19.3.1 we review the acoustooptic superlattice modulator (AOSLM), since this mechanism was used to actively mode-lock the laser. Sections 19.3.2 and 19.3.3 describe two different all-fiber mode-locked lasers by driving the AOSLM by either standing or traveling acoustic waves. Section 19.4 describes two different mechanisms to actively *Q*-switch and mode-lock simultaneously an all-fiber laser. The conclusions are presented in Section 19.5. Finally, a list of common acronyms used throughout this chapter is given in Table 19.1.

19.2 ACTIVE QS OF A DFB ALL-FIBER LASER

The development of single-mode narrow-linewidth lasers is of great interest as they have wide applicability in fields such as high-resolution interferometry, distributed Brillouin sensing, optical coherent communication, wavelength division multiplexing, light detection and ranging, laser Doppler velocimeters, spectroscopy, instrumentation, and so on. DFB lasers based on semiconductor technology have linewidths typically in the megahertz domain, because the cavity length is short, and thermal dissipation low, leading to broader spectral properties [1]. On the contrary, fiber lasers usually operate in a multimode regime and have a broad spectrum. To make efficient single-mode narrow-linewidth fiber lasers, different approaches have been implemented. Fiber ring lasers fulfill the requirement and produce narrow-linewidth outputs; most importantly, they can be made widely tunable [1]. However, they are more complex and—because of their long cavities—susceptible to mode hopping. Distributed Bragg reflector (DBR) fiber lasers are another option; however, temperature stabilization is still required in order to prevent mode hopping and, in the short laser cavity, the pump wave absorption is low; as a consequence, the DBR fiber laser is not efficient, and external optical amplifiers are generally needed [20]. DFB fiber lasers can overcome part of these problems. They have the simplest, robust, and compact design providing operation without mode hopping. Their fabrication is relatively simple, and involves the writing of a grating structure—that is, a fiber Bragg grating (FBG)—with ultraviolet light into an active fiber. A single-mode pump leads to an alignment-free resonator with optimum overlap of pump and signal light [21]. For these FBG-based DFB lasers, the distributed reflection occurs in the grating when a phase shift has been generated within it. A number of techniques have been proposed for this; however, statics phase shifts only allow CW operation [11], which translates into low power emission. Recently, some approaches have been reported for obtaining single-frequency pulsed all-fiber lasers, based on active QS of DFB fiber cavities [9–11]. The pulsed operation of a DFB laser is interesting because certain applications (e.g., Brillouin sensing) require not only a narrow linewidth but also a peak power about a minimum threshold, which otherwise could not be reached by a CW operation. Here we describe an acoustically QS-DFB strictly all-fiber laser that provides transform-limited pulses. In the following, we describe the laser setup together with a characterization of the QS technique (Section 19.2.1). In Section 19.2.2 we describe the operation of this laser and a characterization of its output when different control parameters are varied. Finally, in Section 19.2.3 we discuss its use as a source for Brillouin sensing applications.

19.2.1 Laser Setup and QS Technique

Figure 19.1 shows the scheme of the proposed DFB all-fiber laser. The FBG was 100 mm long, and was written in a 1500 ppm erbium hydrogen-loaded fiber (codoped with germanium and aluminum) of the same length using a doubled argon laser and a uniform period mask. The FBG shows more than 30 dB attenuation at the Bragg wavelength (λ_B = 1532.45 nm) and a 3-dB bandwidth of 88 pm. The FBG was pumped through a 980/1550-nm wavelength division multiplexer (WDM) with a 980-nm semiconductor laser, providing a maximum pump power of 130 mW. A square-shaped rod of a magnetostrictive material (Terfenol-D, 15 mm long and 1 mm^2 section) was bonded outside the FBG to a free section of fiber at 88 mm from the center of the grating, and placed inside a small coil, see Figure 19.1.

The dynamic defect in the FBG was induced through a magnetostrictive device, because it has a superior performance as compared with piezoelectric devices, which have a frequency-dependent response characterized by strong mechanical resonances. On the contrary, a magnetostrictive device has a lower frequency range but its frequency response is basically flat [22,23]. The magnetostrictive rod can be bonded directly over the FBG, but this has some detrimental consequences. First, any external actuator bonded directly on the fiber is likely to exhibit long-term instabilities [22]. Second, once the magnetostrictive rod is fixed to the fiber, any temperature change generates a differential expansion between the fiber and the magnetostrictive rod, producing a local static perturbation of the FBG that may cause CW emission. Because of this, we avoided these drawbacks by attaching he magnetostrictive rod outside the FBG and generating the dynamic defect through an acoustic axially propagating pulse. Thereby, when a pulse of electric current is applied to the coil, the small rod lengthens and stretches the section of fiber attached to it, generating in this way a longitudinal acoustic pulse that propagates toward the FBG [9]. The pulse propagating along the grating generates a phase shift opening a transmission peak within the reflection band of the grating; as a consequence, a high Q resonance is produced and a laser pulse is emitted [10,11]. Otherwise, if no

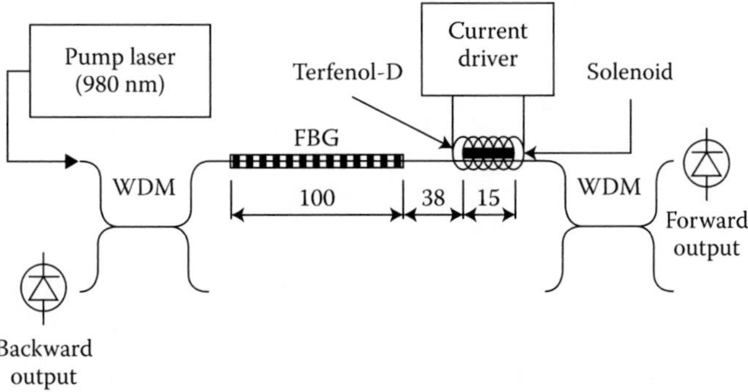

FIGURE 19.1 QS-DFB all-fiber laser setup; the backward and forward outputs make reference to the pump direction, whereas WDM stands for wavelength division multiplexer.

perturbation is present within the FBG, there is no efficient feedback for the optical signal, and the laser emission is not allowed. Since the defect is not fixed, but induced by a traveling acoustic pulse with a time-varying position along the FGB, one could think that this might have important consequences on the spectral position of the transmission peak. However, this is not the case, as it was recently demonstrated [22]. The spectral position of the resonance is constant, no matter the actual spatial location of the acoustic pulse, although some short transients are produced when the pulse overlaps the extremes of the FBG. This property ensures that the laser will emit with a narrow linewidth, preserving one of the most attractive properties of DFB fiber lasers.

The transmission properties of the passive FBG—that is, without pumping—interacting with the acoustic pulses were investigated by illuminating the FBG with a tunable laser at λ_B and detecting the reflected signal. When the coil current is zero, the reflectance is maximal; but when a current pulse of 220 mA and 5 μs temporal width is applied to the coil, a transmission peak opens the reflection band, being as narrow as 2 μs (full-width at half-maximum (FWHM)); see Figure 19.2a. Figure 19.2b shows a detail of the current pulse applied to the coil. The rise and fall times of the current pulse are according to the characteristics of the electrical circuit (1 mH for the coil inductance in series with a 1 kΩ resistance, that is, a time constant of 1 μs). This new in-line acoustooptic modulator allows continuous tuning of the repetition rate plus easy access to both outputs of the DFB all-fiber laser.

19.2.2 The QS-DFB All-Fiber Laser Characteristics

Figure 19.3a–c show the voltage pulses applied to the current driver, the backward output of the DFB laser, and a detail of the optical pulse, respectively. The observed delay time between the voltage signal and the optical pulses—compare Figure 19.3a and b—is mainly due to the distance that pulses have to travel from the magnetostrictive device to the FBG; see Figure 19.1. Finally, the spatial position of the acoustic pulse, at the instant when the laser emission is produced, was estimated by dumping the acoustic pulse with a drop of oil displaced longitudinally over the grating starting at the backward output side. There was no laser emission when the drop was at 123 mm from the magnetostrictive transducer; this indicates that laser emission takes places around the last third of the grating; see Figure 19.1.

One key characteristic in this setup is its versatility, which is given by the possibility of selecting a variety of peak powers and time widths just by varying the coil current. Figure 19.4 shows the peak power and pulse width for backward and forward outputs as a function of the coil current for two different repetition rates: 500 Hz and 2 kHz, Figure 19.4a,b and c,d, respectively. There is a low threshold value for the coil current (I); below this value there is no laser emission, since the Q value

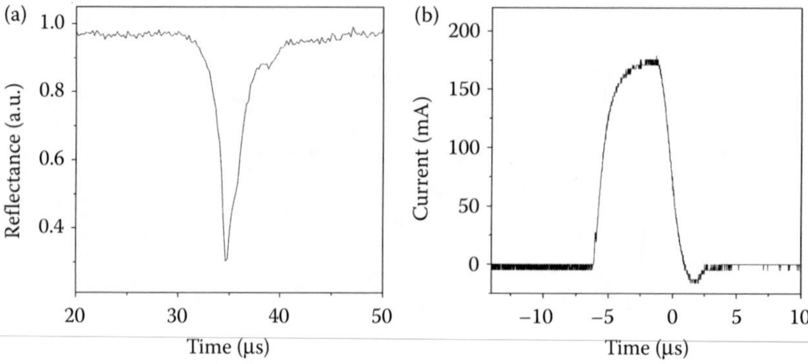

FIGURE 19.2 Passive characterization of the QS-DFB all-fiber laser. (a) Reflection at the Bragg wavelength when an acoustic pulse travels within the FBG. (b) Detail of the single current pulse applied to the coil.

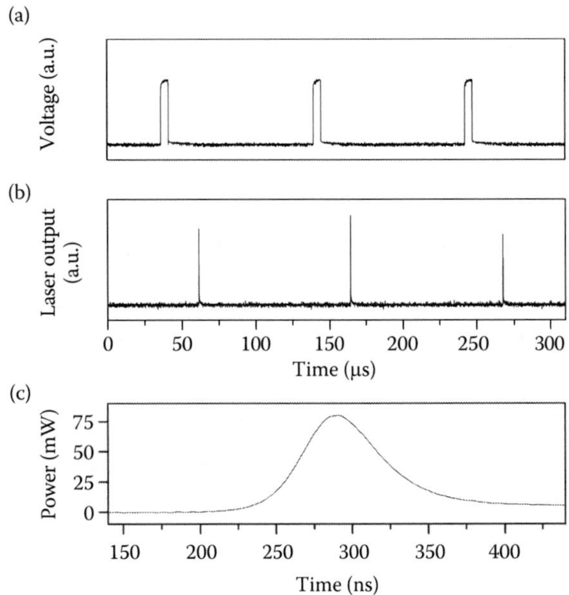

FIGURE 19.3 QS-DFB all-fiber laser. Behavior at 10 kHz repetition rate and 80 mW of pump power. (a) Voltage signal applied to the current driver. (b) Emitted optical train of pulses. (c) Detail of a single optical pulse of the train.

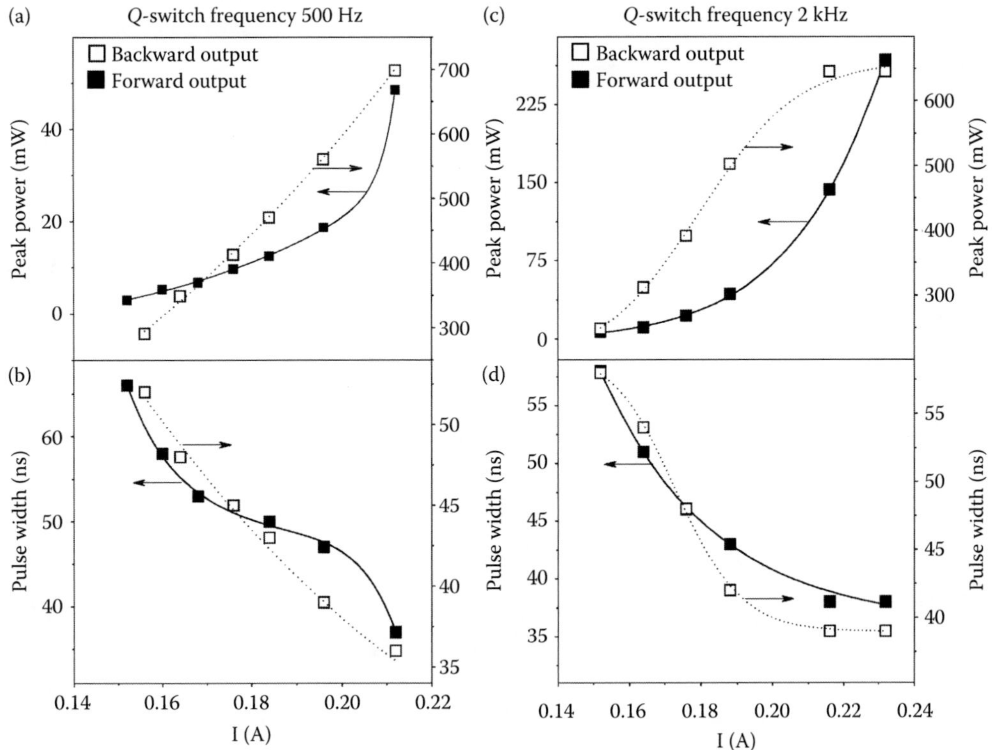

FIGURE 19.4 QS-DFB all-fiber laser. Peak power and pulse width for backward and forward outputs as a function of the coil current for two different QS repetition rates: 500 Hz (a, b) and 2 kHz (c, d), respectively, and 55 mW of pump power.

is not high enough (i.e., $I < 150$ mA). Above this value, the laser emission is allowed and one optical pulse per cycle is emitted; at higher electric currents (i.e., $I > 230$ mA) there are two optical pulses per current pulse. At different repetition rates the peak power and time width values change but the general trend is preserved. The effect of pump power on the optical pulses, for repetition rates ranging from 200 Hz to 20 kHz, is shown in Figure 19.5a–d, for the backward and forward outputs, respectively. A fixed coil current of 200 mA amplitude was used in all cases. At each different frequency, there is a corresponding pump power threshold. Above the threshold, the peak power increases with pump power and there is a corresponding reduction of the pulse width. Pulses of 800 mW peak power and 32 ns time width were obtained at 500 Hz repetition rate and 46 mW pump power for the backward output. If the pump power is high enough, the laser emits more than one pulse per cycle, defining in this way an upper limit also. One can observe the differences in peak powers between backward and forward outputs, being higher in the first case. Temporal widths and peak power jitters were measured to be below 5%.

The emission linewidth $\Delta\nu_{DFB}$ was measured, using a classical heterodyne configuration [24]. A tunable laser was used as the local oscillator (LO), with $\Delta\nu_{LO} = 100$ kHz. The output of this laser was superimposed on the optical pulses of the DFB laser (backward output), through a 1550 nm 20 dB coupler. The beat signal at the coupler output was detected with a 1-GHz bandwidth photodetector, and analyzed with a 500-MHz bandwidth oscilloscope. The beating between both fields is centered at frequency $\nu_{DFB} - \nu_{LO}$, and has the same spectrum as the laser under test, provided that $\Delta\nu_{LO} \ll \Delta\nu_{DFB}$ [24]. In the example of Figure 19.6, the DFB laser frequency rate was 10 kHz and pumped with 80 mW, whereas the LO wavelength was selected close enough to the DFB laser emission wavelength. Figure 19.6 shows the spectrum of the beat signals, resulting in a DFB laser linewidth of $\Delta\nu_{DFB} = 6$ MHz (i.e., 43 fm at λ_{DFB}), measured directly in the spectrum at −3 dB. The inset

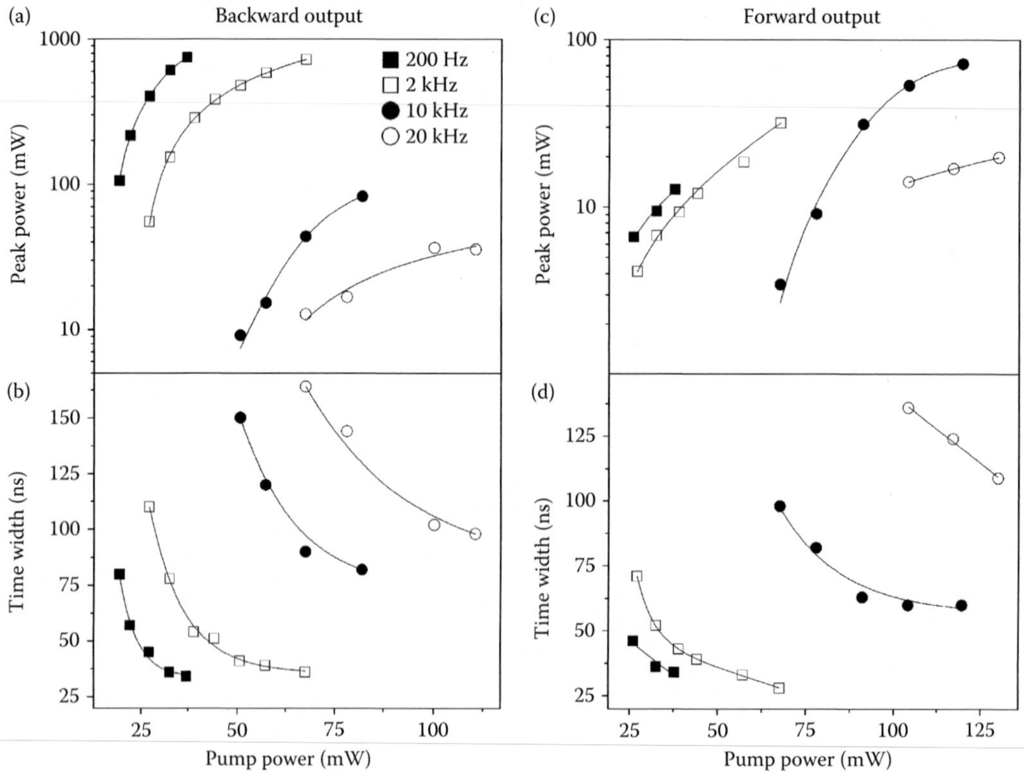

FIGURE 19.5 QS-DFB all-fiber laser. Peak power (a) and temporal width (b) for the backward laser output as a function of the pump power, for several repetition rates; (c, d) same as before but for the forward laser output.

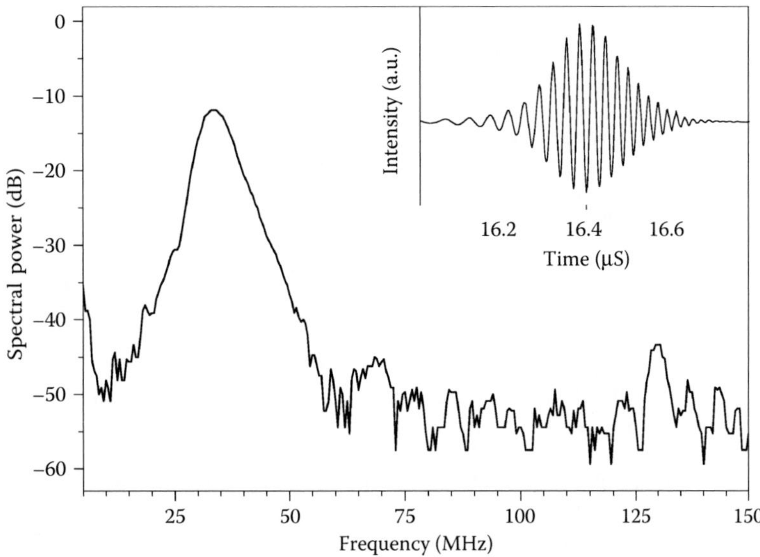

FIGURE 19.6 QS-DFB all-fiber laser. Spectrum corresponding to the heterodyning between the backward output and a tunable narrow linewidth laser used as the LO. The inset shows the original beating signal in the time domain. The frequency rate was 10 kHz and the pump power was of 80 mW.

of Figure 19.6 shows the characteristic heterodyne beating. The optical pulses from the DFB all-fiber laser had a temporal width of 80 ns; see Figure 19.5; hence, according to the time–frequency uncertainty principle [25], its bandwidth cannot be lower than 5.5 MHz. From the comparison between this last value and the linewidth measurement for $\Delta\nu_{DFB}$, we conclude that the optical pulses of our DFB are transform limited.

19.2.3 The QS-DFB All-Fiber Laser in Brillouin Sensing Applications

Brillouin scattering essentially refers to the scattering of a light wave by an acoustic wave [25]. When a coherent pulse of light propagates through a medium, part of its energy is backscattered due to a nonelastic interaction with the acoustic phonons. This backscattered light is composed of a frequency downshifted Stokes light and an upshifted anti-Stokes light, whose spectral positions are dependent on temperature and strain environment of the fiber, in this way allowing its use as a sensing mechanism [25–30]. Fiber optics distributed temperature, and/or strain, sensors have becoming very attractive for applications requiring sensing lengths of many kilometers, principally due to their inexpensiveness and availability. Optical fiber-based distributed sensor systems normally make use of the principle of optical time-domain reflectometry [27,28,31]. Therefore, an optical pulse is launched into one end of the fiber system and the variation of the scattered light is detected as a function of time, giving in this way information about the temperature or strain as a function of distance. A key requirement in this measurement system is a stable light source with a narrow enough spectral linewidth [27]. In addition, for time-domain reflectometry applications, the sensor spatial resolution proportionally depends on the optical pulse width and so it must also be considered [28]. In order to fulfill all these requirements, solid state lasers with external cavities—plus amplifiers and amplitude modulators—are currently used in these systems [27]. Here we propose using this compact all-fiber pulsed light source as a relatively simpler alternative.

Figure 19.7a shows the backscattered light spectrum after illuminating a 10.5 km length optical fiber spool (Corning SMF-28) with the backward output of our DFB all-fiber laser (4 kHz repetition rate and 74 mW pump power). The Brillouin spectrum was registered with an optical spectral analyzer (resolution of 20 pm). The extreme of the fiber optic spool was terminated with a matching

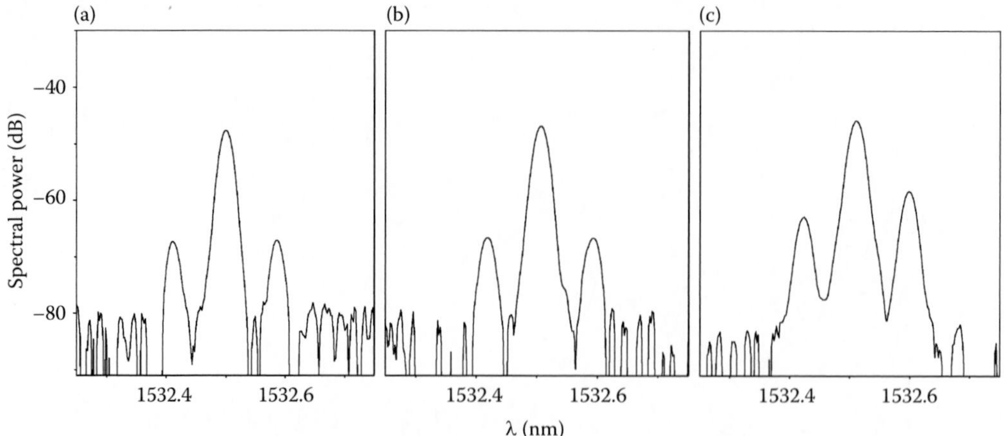

FIGURE 19.7 QS-DFB all-fiber laser. Brillouin spectra at room temperature for a 10.5-km length SMF-28 optical fiber spool. (a) 4 kHz repetition rates and 74 mW pump power, (b) 20 kHz repetition rate and 120 mW pump power, and (c) 4 kHz repetition rate and 120 mW pump power.

refractive index liquid ($n = 1.46$). The central (highest) peak corresponds to the proper laser beam reflections after successive connections and splices together with Rayleigh scattering. Peaks symmetrically positioned on both sides correspond to the Brillouin backscattering by Stokes and anti-Stokes processes [27]. The measured Brillouin shift results in 88 pm (i.e., 11.24 GHz at 1532.4 nm), which correspond to the expected value in this fiber [25]. Figure 19.7b shows another backscattered light spectrum when a different repetition rate is used (20 kHz and 120 mW of pump power). Finally, if we use the same QS repetition rate of the example shown in Figure 19.7a (4 kHz) but increases the pump power up to 120 mW, the Stokes peak increases with respect to the anti-Stokes peak; see Figure 19.7c; this behavior agrees with previous results [27].

19.3 ACTIVE ML OF ALL-FIBER LASERS THROUGH AOSLM

Over the years, mode-locked lasers have evolved from being a technologically promising source for ultrashort pulses into a reality. Indeed, many ML configurations developed earlier as a pure subject of research became later commercially available products. Such progress—surely induced by the increasing commercial demand—arises from the vast number of possible applications. A comprehensive—and chronological—review on ML lasers may be found in [32]. The areas that have benefited from these ultrashort pulse optical sources range from the telecommunications industry to medical surgery. As an example, mode-locked lasers are a solution for ultrafast phenomenon research, nonlinear optical research, optical communications, multiphoton microscopy, and pumping of parametric devices [33–36]. The shortest pulses are obtained by passive ML schemes. However, passive mode-locked lasers have some drawbacks, among them, they are generally unstable, they have higher timing-jitter between pulses, and usually self-starting cannot be ensured. An alternative to using passive ML schemes that reduces jitter and allows for synchronization is to use an active ML scheme. To this end, a modulator is driven at the cavity's fundamental repetition rate (or at a multiple, in which case the technique is called harmonic ML). Therefore, timing-jitter is reduced since each pulse is triggered by the modulator, which in turn is accurately driven by an electrical signal. In this way, in active ML, one is able to synchronize a laser to an external clock or electronic signal [37], which undoubtedly improves its applicability for the communications industry. Among all these lasers, the all-fiber solution has been the subject of intensive research due to their compact structure, free from alignment problems, and low cost, besides other merits. Earlier and subsequent active mode-locked fiber lasers were not strictly all-fiber lasers, since they included a bulk modulator [6–8]. This not only induces extra loss into the laser cavity but of course also destroys the benefits of an all-fiber configuration. On the contrary, a strictly all-fiber modulator can overcome these limitations and it can be used for actively mode-locked rare-earth-doped silica fiber lasers [12–17,38].

In the following, we start by reviewing the key element that allows the construction of a strictly all-fiber cavity: the AOSLM, together with an experimental analysis of its performance (Section 19.3.1). Since an AOSLM can be driven by either standing or traveling acoustic waves, we describe first a CW-ML laser driven by standing acoustic waves, and later its counterpart driven by traveling acoustic waves, in Sections 19.3.2 and 19.3.3, respectively.

19.3.1 The Acoustooptic Superlattice Modulation

When a traveling axially propagating acoustic wave is launched through an FBG, the periodic strain field of the acoustic wave perturbs the grating in two different ways. First, the average index changes in response to the stress-optical effect. Second, the grating pitch is periodically modulated, causing a spatial frequency modulation of the grating [39]. As a consequence of both effects, the reflectivity changes—although separately they have opposite sign. The main features of these changes depend on the ratio between the acoustical wavelength and the grating length [22]. Thus, we can distinguish two very different situations: the long-wavelength and the short-wavelength regimes. In the first, the pitch of the grating is homogeneously perturbed along its length. The successive cycles of compression and expansion generated by the longitudinal wave will shift periodically in time the spectral response of the grating as a whole to longer and shorter wavelengths [22,40]. On the contrary, in the short-wavelength regime, the acoustic wave generates many compressed and expanded sections, which gives rise to a superstructure within the grating. In this case, the spectral response of the original FBG shows new—and narrow—reflection bands symmetrically on both sides of the original Bragg wavelength [41,42]. The position of these sidebands can be controlled by varying the frequency at a slope of 0.15 and 0.30 nm/MHz for the first and second order sidebands, respectively. The strength of the reflection bands, on the other hand, can be controlled independently by varying the voltage applied to the piezoelectric. Since these sidebands can be regarded as weak ghosts of the strong permanent Bragg grating, its FWHM bandwidth is that of a weak Bragg grating of the same length [41], namely $\Delta\lambda_{AOSLM} = 1.39\ \lambda^2/(\pi L n_0)$, where L is the fiber length and n_0 is the modal effective index; which can be translated to the frequency domain as a spectral bandwidth of $\Delta\nu_{AOSLM} = 1.39c/(\pi L n_0)$.

Figure 19.8 shows the setup for a typical reflectivity measurement on an AOSLM. The AOSLM in turn is composed of a radio-frequency (RF) source, an electrical RF amplifier, a piezoelectric disk, a silica horn, and an FBG. The tip of the silica horn was reduced by chemical etching to the same diameter of FBG—125 μm—and subsequently fusion spliced to the grating. The uniform and

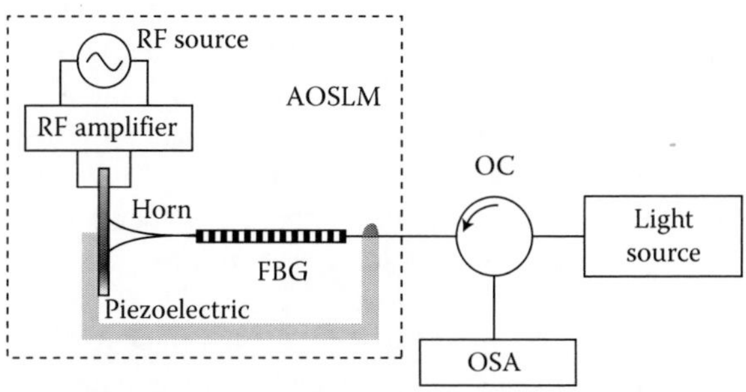

FIGURE 19.8 AOSLM setup; OSA stands for optical spectrum analyzer, OC for optical circulator, FBG for fiber Bragg grating, and RF for radiofrequency.

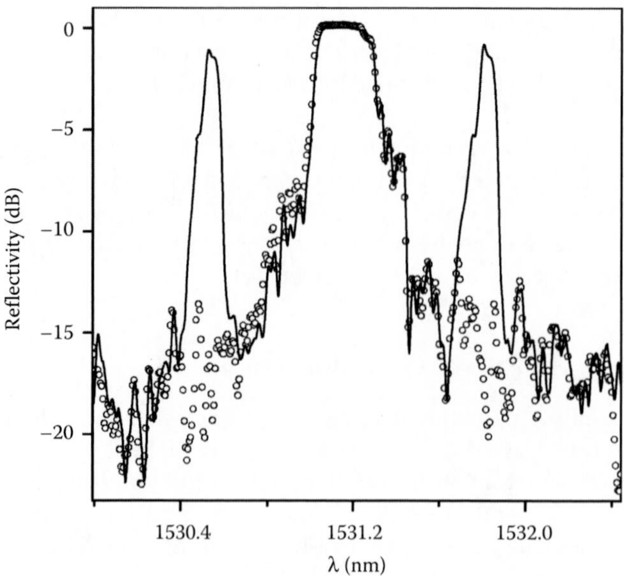

FIGURE 19.9 Reflectivity of the FBG with an electrical signal applied to the piezoelectric (4.55 MHz and 16 V peak-to-peak) and without electrical signal, solid curve and scatter points, respectively.

nonapodized grating was written in photosensitive fiber using a doubled argon laser and a uniform period mask; the FBG was 120 mm long. The reflection properties of the AOSLM were investigated by illuminating the FBG through an optical circulator with a broadband light source, and detecting the reflected light with an optical spectrum analyzer (OSA). Figure 19.9 shows the reflectivity of the unperturbed FBG—that is, without electrical signal applied to the piezoelectric—and with an electrical signal applied to the piezoelectric of 4.55 MHz and 16 V (whenever we refer to voltages throughout this chapter, it is a peak-to-peak measurement). The presence of the sidebands symmetrically positioned around the Bragg wavelength is clearly discernible. Further, these sidebands are produced by either standing or traveling acoustic waves. However, the light reflected by the sidebands in each case behaves differently. When traveling acoustic waves are used—by dumping the end of the FBG opposite to the silica horn for example with a drop of oil—the light reflected on these sidebands is completely downshifted or upshifted by ν_s—with ν_s the frequency of the acoustical signal—depending on whether the reflection was in the long- or short-wavelength sideband, respectively [41,42]. Together with this and depending on the operating conditions, there is also an amplitude modulation at the frequency of the acoustical signal ν_s. Figure 19.10 shows the measurement performed by tuning a laser diode to the center of the short-wavelength sideband and measuring the reflected light. As expected, the amplitude modulation is at the same frequency of the electrical signal used to drive the piezoelectric. On the other hand, when standing acoustic waves are used—by clamping the end of the FBG opposite to the silica horn—the sidebands raise and fall at twice the frequency of the electrical signal [12]. Further, in principle, for a perfect acoustical reflection, the light reflected by the sidebands does not experiment any Doppler shift, as opposed to the previous case when traveling acoustic waves are used. Figure 19.11 shows the measurement performed by tuning a laser diode to the center of the short-wavelength sideband and measuring the reflected light. Now the optical modulation frequency is two times the acoustical signal frequency. To summarize, an AOSLM can be driven in two different regimes, by using either traveling or standing acoustic waves. In both cases we can use it as an amplitude modulator. However, in the first case—traveling waves—the light reflected on the sidebands is modulated at the same frequency of the acoustical signal, whereas in the second case—standing waves—it is modulated at two times this frequency, respectively.

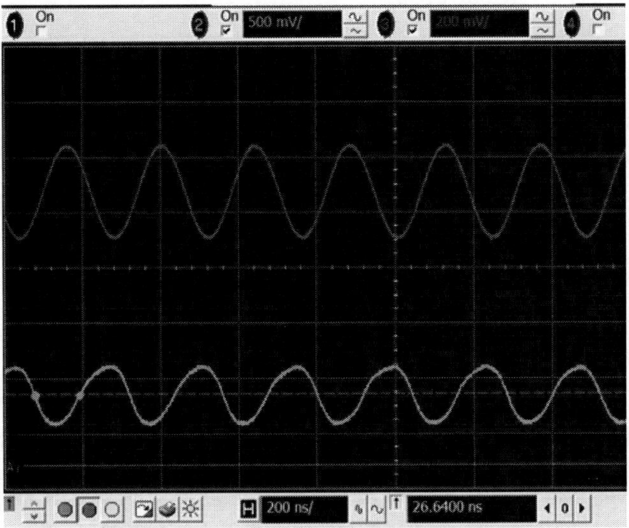

FIGURE 19.10 Optical signal reflected by the short-wavelength sideband when traveling acoustic waves are used (lower trace) and RF voltage applied to the piezoelectric (4.11 MHz and 16 V, upper trace).

19.3.2 The CW-ML Laser with an AOSLM Driven by Standing Acoustic Waves

Now, we show the use of the amplitude modulation induced by standing acoustic waves in the AOSLM to mode-lock an all-fiber laser [12]. The setup proposed for the CW-ML laser is schematically illustrated in Figure 19.12. The gain was provided by an erbium-doped fiber (EDF) containing 300 parts per million (ppm) of Er^{3+}, with a cutoff wavelength of 939 nm and a numerical aperture of 0.24. The active fiber was pumped through a WDM coupler by a pigtailed laser diode emitting at 976 nm, providing a maximum pump power of 160 mW. The AOSLM and a short delay line followed by a second fiber Bragg grating FBG_2 were fusion spliced at each end of the active fiber. FBG_2 (10 mm long and with a Bragg wavelength of 1530.2 nm) was written with a uniform period in a photosensitive fiber using a doubled argon laser and a uniform period mask. The Fabry–Perot cavity was established once the reflection band of FBG_2 is made to match the short-wavelength sideband of the FBG of the AOSLM, that is, 1530.5 nm, by straining it with a translational stage (see Figure 19.9).

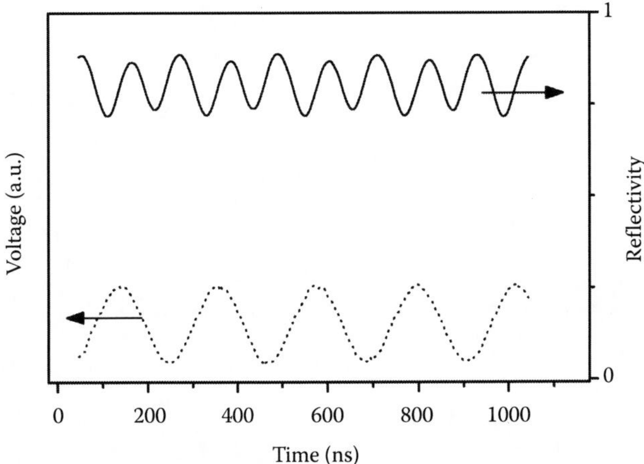

FIGURE 19.11 Optical signal reflected by the short-wavelength sideband when standing acoustic waves are used (solid curve) and RF voltage applied to the piezoelectric (4.55 MHz and 16 V, dotted curve).

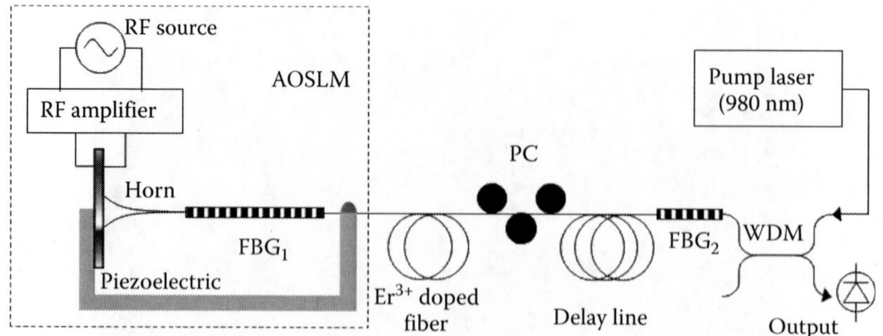

FIGURE 19.12 Setup of the CW-ML all-fiber laser; PC stands for polarization controller.

The delay line length (see Figure 19.12) must be selected to match the round-trip time τ with the reciprocal of the optical modulation frequency ν_{AM}, which in turn is twice the electrical frequency applied to the piezoelectric ν_{PZT}, that is, $2L = c\ (n2\nu_{PZT})^{-1}$, with c the speed of light in vacuum, n the modal index (~1.447), and L the cavity length. Since the selected piezoelectric operation point was $\nu_{PZT} = 4.55$ MHz, this results in a cavity length of $L = 11.4$ m. However, fine-tuning of ν_{PZT} was required in order to achieve ML. Figure 19.13a exemplifies the laser behavior showing the train of optical pulses generated, at a frequency rate of 9 MHz (50 GHz bandwidth oscilloscope). Figure 19.13b shows a single optical pulse; the timing-jitter was measured to be 40 ps root mean square (RMS). The pulses of this laser are best fitted by a hyperbolic secant squared function (sech^2); see Figure 19.13b. An attempt to fit the experimental data with a Gaussian function results in a worst fitting, with a higher deviation coefficient. According to earlier AM-ML theory, in a laser devoid of dispersion and nonlinearity, AM-ML produces unchirped Gaussian pulses [43]. Later, it was realized that the pulse shapes produced by actively mode-locked lasers were frequently more consistent with a sech^2 envelope than with a Gaussian envelope. It was realized then that the effects of dispersion and nonlinearity within the laser cavity were playing a role in the pulse shaping. In light of this, our time-domain measurements suggest that cavity dispersion and fiber nonlinearity are determining in the shaping of these laser pulses. Further, the dispersion measurements of the different fibers we used to form the laser cavity show that both kinds of dispersion coexist, from the anomalous dispersion of the delay line to the normal dispersion of the EDF. For this type of dispersion-mixed

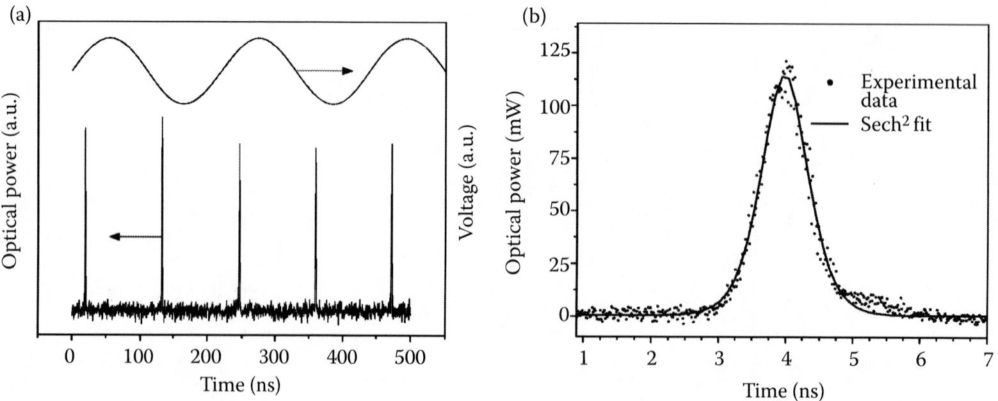

FIGURE 19.13 CW-ML all-fiber laser driven by standing acoustic waves. (a) RF voltage applied to the piezoelectric at 4.55 MHz and 16 V, and its corresponding mode-locked train of pulses generated at twice this frequency with a pump power of 160 mW (upper and lower trace, respectively). (b) A single optical pulse and its corresponding fitting by a sech^2 function (scatter points and solid curve, respectively).

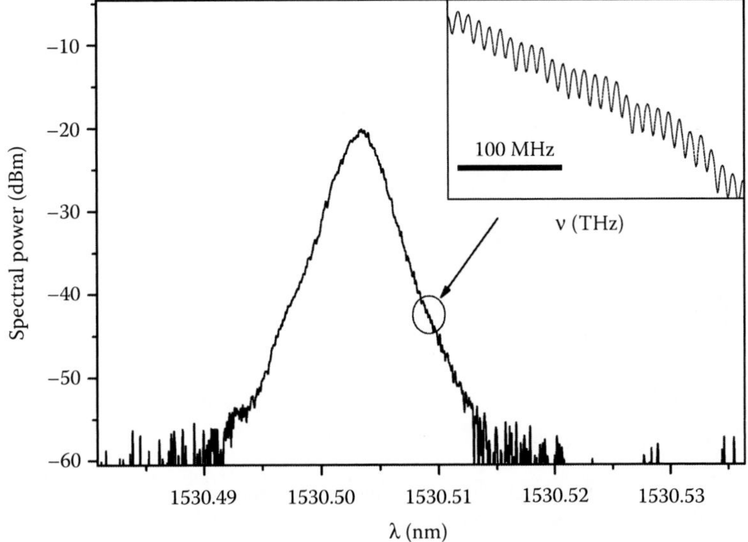

FIGURE 19.14 CW-ML all-fiber laser driven by standing acoustic waves. High-resolution optical spectrum of the output pulses shown in Figure 19.13; the inset shows the cavity modes spaced by ~9 MHz.

cavities, the analytical steady-state solution is expected to be also of the $sech^2$ type [44], which adds further evidence in the same direction.

The emission linewidth $\Delta\lambda_{ML}$ was measured using a high-resolution optical spectrum analyzer (BOSA-C, Aragón Photonics, resolution of 80 fm). Figure 19.14 shows the spectrum of the optical pulses shown in Figure 19.13. The high resolution of the OSA permits a direct observation of the individual cavity modes separated by 9 MHz (see the inset of Figure 19.14). The measured 3-dB linewidth results in $\Delta\lambda_{ML} = 2.8$ pm, that is, $\Delta\nu_{ML} = 360$ MHz at 1530.5 nm. On the other hand, the optical pulses have a temporal width of $\Delta\tau_{ML} = 780$ ps; hence, according to the Fourier-transform-limited relation for a $sech^2$ pulse, that is, $\Delta\tau_{ML}\,\Delta\nu_{ML} \geq 0.315$ [45], its bandwidth cannot be lower than 380 MHz. From the comparison between this last value and the linewidth measurement, we conclude that the optical pulses of our mode-locked laser are transform-limited, that is, unchirped. A brief digression is in order here, the Fourier-transform-limited relation for Gaussian pulses—that is, $\Delta\tau_{ML}\,\Delta\nu_{ML} \geq 0.44$ [43,45]—would result in a much higher linewidth (564 MHz), which is in contradiction with our spectral measurements. As a consequence, the fitting of the temporal pulses, see Figure 19.13b, the application of the Fourier-transform-limited relations, and dispersion measurements together with previous theoretical work [44] seem to corroborate a $sech^2$ nature for the emitted pulses.

The optical pulse's peak power and temporal width as a function of the pump power are shown in Figure 19.15. A smooth variation of the pulse width with pump power can be observed, before reaching the gain saturation. This kind of variation has been reported before for homogeneously broadened mode-locked lasers [46]. A higher available pump power would allow additional axial modes to contribute, increasing the spectral bandwidth, and thereby decreasing the pulse's width.

19.3.2.1 ML Dependence with the Frequency Detuning

Within the ML context, detuning is mathematically defined as the frequency shift from the ideal ML frequency. From an experimental point of view, it is difficult to guarantee the permanent synchronization between the modulator frequency and the cavities' fundamental repetition rate—unless, of course, regenerative ML is used through a feedback loop [47]. Detuning rarely occurs because the electrical signal used to drive the modulator drifts, but more often because any

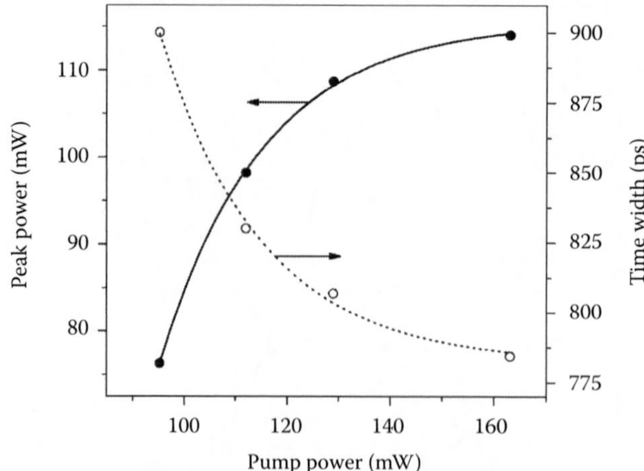

FIGURE 19.15 CW-ML all-fiber laser driven by standing acoustic waves. Peak power and temporal width (FWHM) of the optical pulses as a function of the pump power (solid and dotted curves, respectively) for the CW-ML laser.

mechanical or thermal variation modifies the optical path length of the cavity, thereby changing its fundamental repetition rate. Primarily, detuning is a function of the modulation technique, that is, ML by amplitude nodulation (AM) or frequency modulation (FM) shows different behaviors, mainly because AM-ML cannot introduce any frequency shift to compensate any frequency change of the modulator [43]. Theoretical studies of detuning in AM-ML reported that the higher the bandwidth and lower the modulation depth, the lower the detuning the laser can tolerate [48]. In this way, it is important to quantify how the ML process is affected by detuning in a given configuration. The adjustment between the frequency of the RF signal applied to the piezoelectric and the cavity round-trip did not require a high accuracy in this setup. Other ML configurations relying on interferometric modulation show a higher sensitivity to frequency detuning due to a very low modulation depth [38]. To analyze the consequences of detuning, in this case we have preferred to do it in the frequency domain through an RF spectrum analyzer (2 GHz bandwidth), because of its higher sensitivity. Figure 19.16 shows the spectrum of the optical pulses once ML is reached; in this regime, successive harmonics appears at integer multiples of $1/\tau = 9$ MHz. The amplitude of the Fourier components are 13 dB above the noise level when an accurate matching is achieved, that is, $1/\tau = 2\nu_{PZT}$. A small frequency detuning at this stage (e.g., by hundreds of Hertz) does not appreciably change the pulse's characteristics, but becomes easily measurable in the frequency domain. Eventually, if the detuning is increased enough (e.g., a mismatch of ±5 kHz), the laser is no longer able to form well-defined pulses and enter into an oscillatory regime, with the clearly deteriorated pulse's temporal parameters, whereas the harmonics shown by the electrical spectral analyzer smoothly decrease. When the detuning is higher (e.g., a mismatch of ±11 kHz), as a result of the modulator's driving frequency and the cavity's repetition rate no longer coinciding, the pulse essentially passes through the modulator at different temporal locations for each round trip, and we do not obtain standard CW-ML. Beyond this point, the harmonic components are no longer present and the pulses drop out. These results confirm the predicted theoretical trend in AM-ML detuning [48]; in this ML setup we have both a relatively low modulation bandwidth and a relatively high modulation depth, and both effects induce this relatively high tolerance to frequency detuning.

19.3.2.2 ML Dependence with the Modulation Voltage

The intensity of the reflection sidebands of the AOSLM can be dynamically controlled by varying the voltage applied to the piezoelectric as we explained in Section 19.3.1. This voltage controls the amplitude of the propagating acoustic wave and the amplitude of the standing wave, as a function of

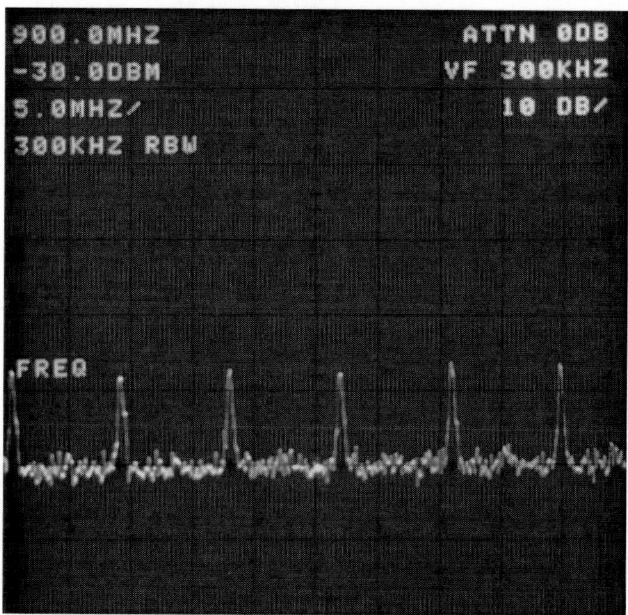

FIGURE 19.16 CW-ML all-fiber laser driven by standing acoustic waves. Electrical spectrum of the optical pulses showing discrete frequency components spaced by 9 MHz.

the reflection at the clamp. Thus, as opposed to ML by bulk acoustooptic or electrooptic modulators, here the reflectivity (R) and the modulation depth are intrinsically linked. Figure 19.17 shows R and δR_{pp} [$\delta R_{pp} = (R_{Max} - R_{Min})/R_{Max}$, i.e., the relative peak-to-peak modulation amplitude of R] as a function of voltage. In the range of voltage available in our experimental setup—between 0 and 18 V—when the applied voltage increases, both the reflectivity and the modulation amplitude increase. Figure 19.18 shows the peak power and time width, respectively, as a function of the voltage applied to the piezoelectric. At lower reflectivity and modulation amplitude, the peak power

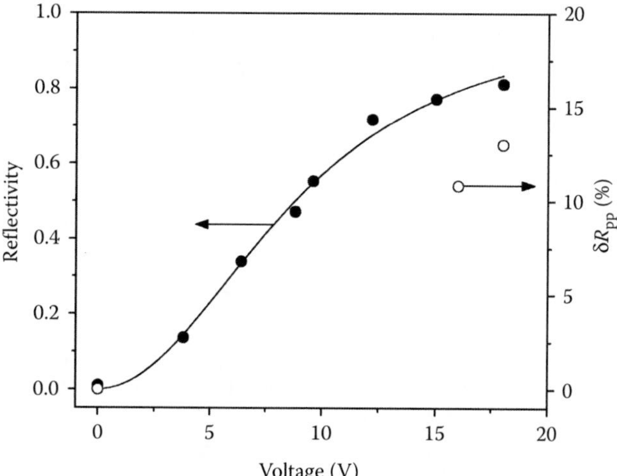

FIGURE 19.17 CW-ML all-fiber laser driven by standing acoustic waves. Measured reflectivity of the short-wavelength sideband (solid scatter points) together with its corresponding theoretical fitting (solid curve), and the peak-to-peak modulation amplitude (open scatter points) as a function of the voltage applied to the piezoelectric.

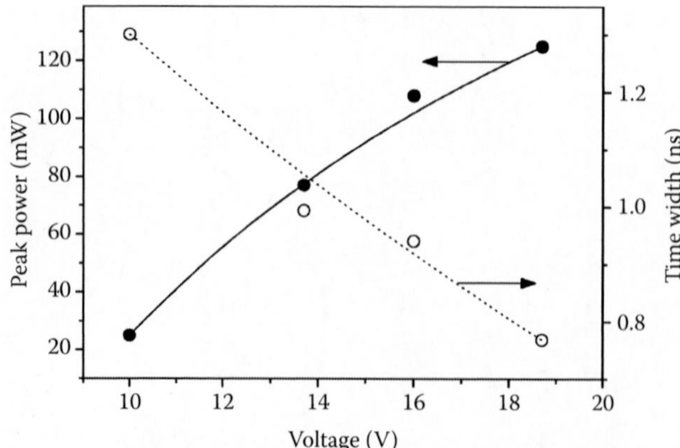

FIGURE 19.18 CW-ML all-fiber laser driven by standing acoustic waves. Peak power (solid scatter points) and time width (open scatter points) of the output light pulses as a function of the voltage applied to the piezoelectric. Pump power of 160 mW.

diminishes, whereas the time width increases. According to the pioneering AM-ML model for homogeneously broadened lasers developed by Kuizenga and Siegman [43], the pulse duration τ_{AM} can be expressed—except for a numerical constant—by $\tau_{AM} \propto (g/\delta)^{1/4}(\nu_m \Delta\nu_g)^{-1/2}$, where g is the saturated amplitude gain, δ is the modulation amplitude (i.e., $\delta = \delta R_{pp}$), ν_m is the modulation frequency, and $\Delta\nu_g$ is the gain bandwidth (which could be replaced in our setup by the modulator bandwidth $\Delta\nu_{AOSLM}$ that is considerably narrower). The pulse width is inversely proportional to $\delta^{1/4}$, and in turn δ increases with the applied voltage; see Figure 19.17. However, the pulses shorten very slowly with the increased modulation strength; hence this shortening procedure is generally discouraged [43]. From Figure 19.18, one can conclude that further increase in the voltage might improve the pulse parameters, but it is not likely to lead to a great enhancement in terms of either peak power or temporal width. From Kuizenga and Sigeman's model and previous works, both a higher modulation frequency and a modulator bandwidth should be more efficient narrowing mechanisms in this setup [43].

19.3.2.3 ML Dependence with Different Delay Lines

In this section we analyze experimentally the operation of the laser when the fiber that forms the delay line is changed [13]. The strong influence that dispersion has on the behavior of mode-locked lasers has been recognized earlier [32,43–47]. In Section 19.3.2 we discussed that a non-Gaussian pulse envelope for the output pulses is an indication of the effect of dispersion on the pulse formation mechanism. Thus, we analyze here the ML mechanism of pulse formation when the average dispersion of the cavity is changed. To this end, it is of special significance tracing the dispersion maps of the cavity. The dispersion for each type of optical fiber used throughout this chapter was measured by the frequency-domain modulated-carrier method. Figure 19.19 shows a dispersion map for every case studied in this section. In this way, different kinds of dispersions that light pulses experience through its build up within the cavity, as well as its average value, can be easily followed. Figure 19.19a shows the dispersion map for the standard cavity studied throughout this subsection. It is composed of three different types of fiber, with the following dispersions: Fibercore SM980 ($D = -4.09$ ps/nm/km), EDF ($D = -18.8$ ps/nm/km), and Corning LEAF ($D = 2$ ps/nm/km), which correspond to the pigtails of the FBGs, the active fiber, and the delay line, respectively. Thus, the resulting average dispersion of this cavity is normal and its value is −1.2 ps/nm/km. According to previous theoretical models [44], as this is a dispersion-mixed cavity, a sech^2 function for the light pulses is expected, as is depicted in Figure 19.13b. Further, it was shown that soliton propagation can be formed in the normal dispersion regime also. As soliton formation is induced purely by the existence of gain, the soliton was named as a gain-guided soliton [49]. Next, the optical fiber of the delay

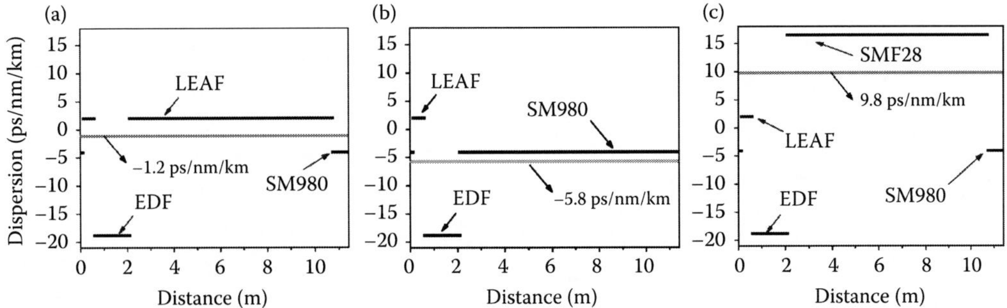

FIGURE 19.19 CW-ML all-fiber laser driven by standing acoustic waves. Dispersion maps when three different optical fibers are used for the delay line, with a constant length of EDF L_{EDF} = 1.5 m: (a) LEAF, (b) SM980, and (c) SMF28. In all cases the gray line represents the average dispersion of the cavity.

line—the Corning LEAF fiber—was replaced by a normal dispersion fiber—Fibercore SM980—leading to a lower (normal) overall dispersion of −5.8 ps/nm/km; see Figure 19.19b. Figure 19.20 shows the peak power and time width of both configurations, that is, the cavities with the LEAF and the SM980 delay lines, as a function of the pump power. With the new delay line, a higher pump reaches the EDF, since a better effective area compatibility is ensured throughout the different fibers of the system—in fact, unlike LEAF fiber, the SM980 ensures single-mode propagation of the pump power. As a result, output pulses have higher peak power and shorter time width than in the previous configuration. In this way, optical pulses with temporal width and peak power of 640 ps and 160 mW, respectively, were obtained. These pulse parameters represent an improvement of 18% and 28% with respect to the previous configuration. Finally, in order to reverse the sign of the average dispersion of the cavity, we used an SMF28 optical fiber for the delay line, resulting in an average—anomalous—dispersion of 9.8 ps/nm/km; see Figure 19.19c. In this case, we did not observe ML lasing. One reason for this could be motivated by the large average dispersion introduced within the cavity, since mode-locked fiber lasers usually work with close-to-zero average dispersion cavities.

19.3.2.4 ML Dependence with the EDF Length

The change of the pulse parameters was measured as a function of the length of EDF—ranging from 0.5 to 3.3 m, but keeping a constant cavity length of 11.4 m, by adjusting each time the length

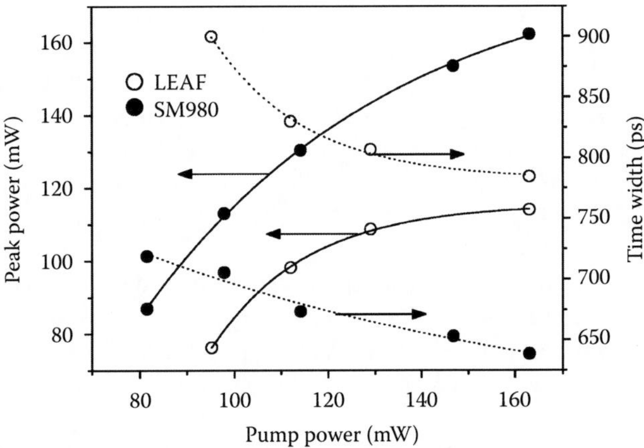

FIGURE 19.20 CW-ML all-fiber laser driven by standing acoustic waves. Peak power (solid curves) and time width (dotted curve) of the output light pulses, as a function of the pump power for two different delay lines: LEAF (open circles) and SM980 (solid circles).

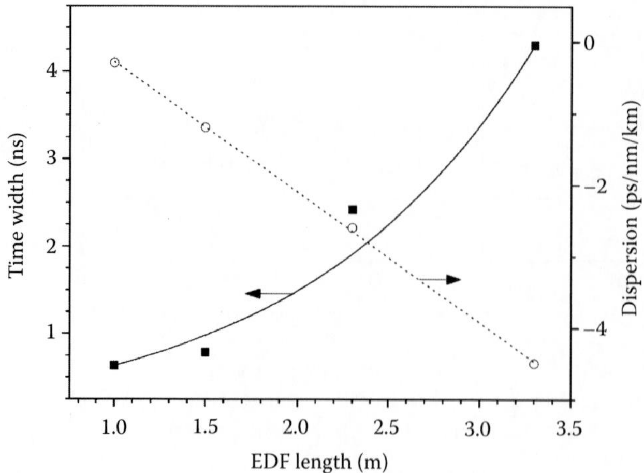

FIGURE 19.21 CW-ML all-fiber laser driven by standing acoustic waves. Time width of the output light pulses (solid curve), as a function of the EDF length, for a fixed pump power of 160 mW. Additionally, the average dispersion of the cavity is also shown for each EDF length (dotted curve).

of LEAF fiber. The average dispersion remains normal—regardless of the amount of EDF used—for each case, and it was −0.3 ps/nm/km, −2.6 ps/nm/km, and −4.5 ps/nm/km, respectively. The temporal pulse width as a function of the EDF length is shown in Figure 19.21, for a fixed pump power of 160 mW. This figure includes the average dispersion of the cavity as a function of the EDF length. A direct relationship can be observed between the EDF length, the dispersion, and the time width of the pulses, with a minimum of 630 ps obtained for an EDF length of 1 m. This kind of interplay between gain and time width agrees with the theoretical results given by Kuizenga and Siegma's model [43]. Further narrowing of the optical pulses could not be reached by this trend, since no ML lasing was observed with 0.5 m of EDF and the available pump power, as a result of insufficient cavity gain.

19.3.3 The CW-ML Laser with an AOSLM Driven by Traveling Acoustic Waves

The setup of the CW-ML laser driven by traveling acoustic waves is essentially the same as described earlier in Section 19.3.2—see Figure 19.12—but with two important differences. First, the pigtailed laser diode emitting at 976 nm provides now a—higher—maximum pump power of 410 mW. Second, the modulation frequency is now at the same frequency of the acoustical signal [19], since we use traveling acoustic waves; see Section 19.3.1. Then, the delay line length is much larger, because we must match the round-trip time with this frequency, which is lower, that is, $2L = c(n\nu_s)^{-1}$. Since the selected piezoelectric operation point was $\nu_s = 4.1$ MHz, this results in a cavity length of 25 m—compare this with the 11.4 m of cavity length used before. Apart from the 1.4 m of EDF, the cavity was constructed entirely with Fibercore SM980 fiber; this results in a dispersion map with an average value of −4.9 ps/nm/km (i.e., normal).

Figure 19.22 exemplifies the laser behavior showing the sinusoidal electrical signal applied to the piezoelectric at a frequency rate of 4.1 MHz and the train of optical pulses generated at the same frequency. The inset shows a detail of a single optical pulse with a temporal width (FWHM) of 720 ps. Once ML was reached, the polarization controllers were adjusted in order to obtain the minimum pulse width.

This time the emission linewidth $\Delta\nu_{ML}$ was measured using a classical heterodyne configuration [24]. To this end, a tunable laser was used as the LO, with $\Delta\nu_{LO} = 100$ kHz. The output of this laser was superimposed on the optical pulses of the mode-locked laser, through a 1550 nm 50/50 coupler. The beat signal at the coupler output was detected with a 45 GHz bandwidth photodetector, and

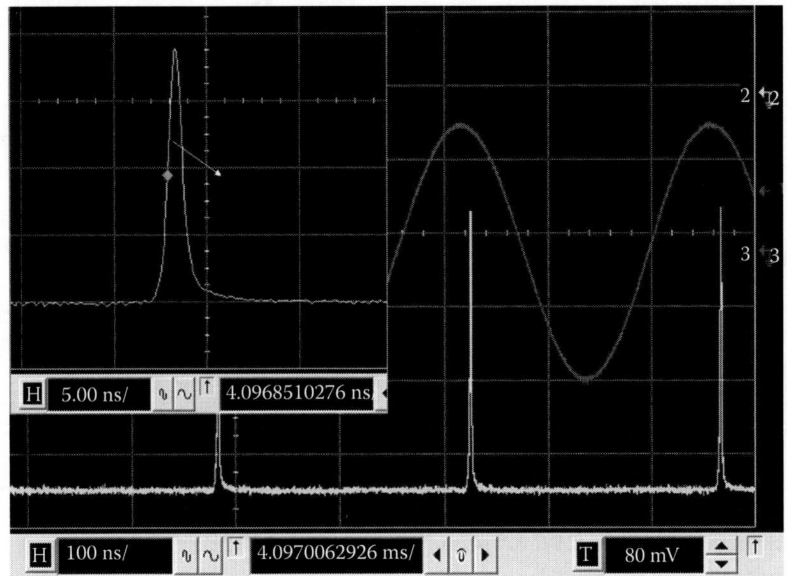

FIGURE 19.22 CW-ML all-fiber laser driven by traveling acoustic waves. Oscilloscope traces of the sinusoidal electrical signal applied to the piezoelectric at 4.1 MHz repetition rate and 16 V (upper trace), and the train of optical pulses generated (lower trace); a pump power of 230 mW was used. The inset shows the detail of a single pulse of the optical train, with an FWHM of 720 ps and a peak power of 500 mW.

analyzed with a 2.5 GHz oscilloscope. This results in a CW-ML linewidth of $\Delta\nu_{ML} = 560$ MHz for a 900 ps (FWHM) pulse, measured directly in the spectrum at −3 dB. Again, we found that the output pulses of this laser are best fitted by a sech^2 function rather than with a Gaussian function. From the Fourier-transform-limited relation for a sech^2 pulse, its time-bandwidth product cannot be lower than 0.315 (FWHM) [45]. Since we obtain 560 MHz × 900 ps = 0.504, we conclude that the optical pulses of our mode-locked laser have now some moderate degree of chirp.

It is known that the pulse duration is limited by a variety of factors in an active mode-locked laser, among them, modulation frequency, gain of the active medium, modulator bandwidth, and modulation strength [43]. From these parameters, we believe the narrow spectral bandwidth of the AOSLM $\Delta\lambda$ plays a key role in this setup. These sidebands can be regarded as weak ghosts of the strong permanent Bragg grating; its FWHM bandwidth is that of a weak Bragg grating of the same length [41], namely $\Delta\lambda = 1.39\lambda^2/(\pi L n_0)$, where L is the fiber length and n_0 is the modal effective index. For the grating used in this chapter, with $L = 120$ mm, at $\lambda = 1530$ nm, this translates into $\Delta\lambda = 6$ pm, which is equivalent to 770 MHz at the operation wavelength of this laser (1530.5 nm). As a rough estimation, since the cavity modes are separated by 4.1 MHz, it is easily seen that this AOSLM only is able to lock a few percent of the axial modes available by the medium gain, namely 770 MHz/4.1 MHz = 192 modes (FWHM). If we assume for the output pulses of this laser a sech^2 envelope, then this parameter alone determines a lower limit for the pulse width around 0.315/770 MHz = 410 ps. Therefore, we believe that narrower pulses can be reached by broadening the sidebands of the AOSLM in order to lock additional axial modes. The optical pulse's peak power and temporal width as a function of the pump power are shown in Figure 19.23. A smooth variation of the pulse width with pump power can be observed, before reaching the gain saturation.

19.3.3.1 ML Dependence with the Frequency Detuning

Figure 19.24 shows the time width as a function of the frequency detuning. The behavior was asymmetric, that is, it depends on whether the detuning was positive or negative. Once ML is reached and the PC is adjusted to get the minimum pulse width, a small detuning in either direction does not

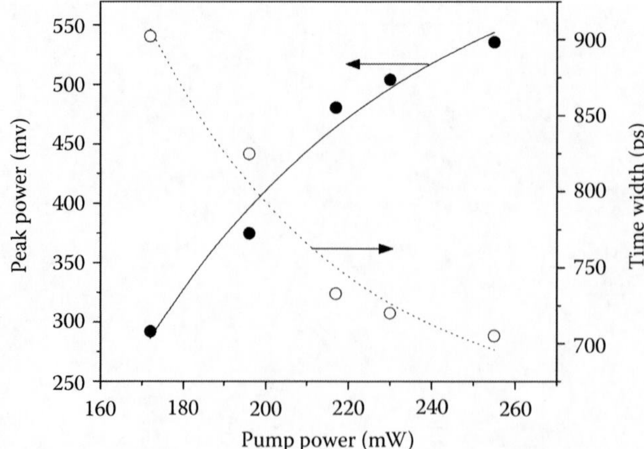

FIGURE 19.23 CW-ML all-fiber laser driven by traveling acoustic waves. Peak power and temporal width (FWHM) of the optical pulses as a function of the pump power (solid and dotted curves, respectively).

modify the pulse width—for example, up to a few tens of Hertz, as expected for AM-ML [43]. However, when the detuning is considerably higher, a positive detuning continuously broadens the time width, whereas for a negative detuning, the ML is rapidly lost, and the pulses drop out. We believe that this asymmetry could be caused by the nonflat frequency response of the piezoelectric.

19.3.3.2 ML Dependence with the Applied Voltage

We conclude this section by analyzing the behavior of this laser under CW-ML regime when the voltage applied to the piezoelectric changes. Figure 19.25 shows the influence on the time width of the optical pulses with the voltage applied to the piezoelectric. For higher voltages, the time width decreases; further narrowing by this trend appears to finish when the reflectivity of the sideband approaches the maximum (in addition, 20 V was the maximum voltage provided by the electrical amplifier used to drive the piezoelectric). Within the range of voltages available in our experiments, both the reflectivity and the modulation amplitude increase continuously. This is consistent with

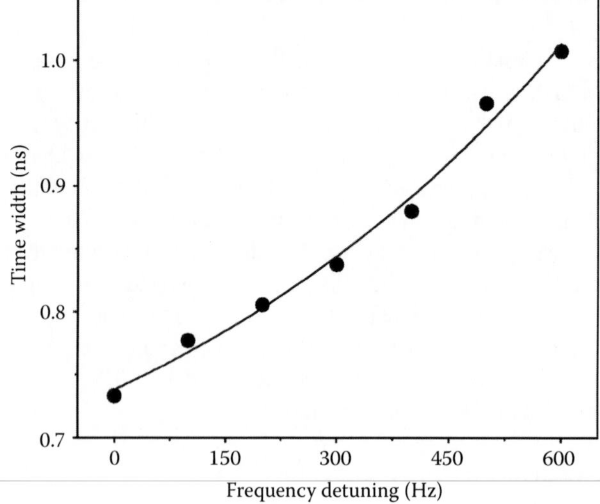

FIGURE 19.24 CW-ML all-fiber laser driven by traveling acoustic waves. Time width of the optical pulses as a function of the frequency detuning of the electric signal.

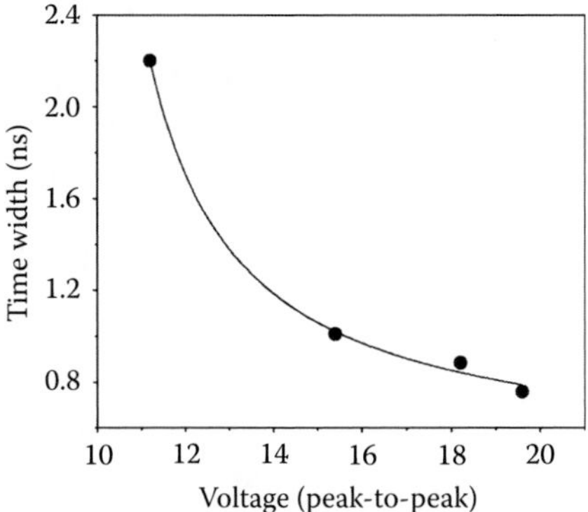

FIGURE 19.25 CW-ML all-fiber laser driven by traveling acoustic waves. Time width of the optical pulses as a function of the applied voltage to the piezoelectric.

previous theoretical models of active mode-locked lasers, in which the time width is inversely related to both, the modulation depth and the reflectivity [43].

19.4 DOUBLE ACTIVE QML OF ALL-FIBER LASERS

Although ML is the history of how new methods were developed to generate increasingly shorter pulses, there are also applications in which attention must be paid also to the simultaneous increment in the peak power. Among these applications, micromachining by ultrashort laser pulses has shown to be a successful high-quality processing tool for various materials [50,51]. The actual requirements of such laser systems are determined by the special application, but generally the power density of the focused laser light at the work plane should be above—but close to—the ablation threshold. The additional complexity of fs lasers is not essential for such tasks, as laser sources with output pulses of μJ energies in the ten of ps width are generally enough [52,53]. The first beneficial consequence of this is the relaxation in the laser design; for example, dispersion effects are less critical as we move away from the fs regime. There is also another interesting advantage, which is determined by the higher processing speed because of the higher pulse energy and average power. One method to increase the pulse energy with the same pump power—but simultaneously retaining the short pulse width—is by increasing the cavity length of a mode-locked laser, even up to several kilometers; in this way, the pulse repetition rate severely decreases [54]. However, since the power density has to be close to the ablation threshold, the ablation rate per pulse, and thus the processing speed, is rather limited in these cases. In order to increase the ablation rate, laser sources with bursts of mode-locked pulses can be applied. In fact the material processing with such bursts confirmed both the processing speed and good quality [55,56]. This can be done by the QS of a mode-locked train of pulses [57–59]. Thus, the peak power of the central pulses of the mode-locked train, underneath the QS envelope, can be greatly enhanced. It is important to differentiate this regime from the instabilities in passively mode-locked lasers [60], where the intracavity pulse energy undergoes large oscillations. Therefore the pulse energy becomes small for a number of subsequent pulses before the next burst of pulses is generated. This effect is undesired, since it is uncontrollable and it should be avoided because optical laser components can be easily damaged due to the increased pulse power and energy. However, stable and controlled QML could indeed provide higher pulse energies as compared to CW-ML laser sources. There are also other methods that produce pulses with the required characteristics, such as cavity dumping [61] and regenerative amplifier [62], but their configurations are more complicated than the QML technique. We describe the QML operation of the mode-locked lasers described in the preceding sections by driving the AOSLM with either standing or traveling acoustic waves, in Sections 19.4.1 and 19.4.2, respectively.

19.4.1 QML All-Fiber Laser with an AOSLM Driven by Standing Acoustic Waves

In Section 19.3.2 we presented CW-ML by driving the AOSLM with standing acoustic waves. Here we demonstrate the possibility to simultaneously Q-switch and mode-lock, actively and independently. It is worth mentioning that a passive mechanism is used in this setup neither for QS nor for ML. To this end, we design a solution for actively QS, while simultaneously ML, preserving the all-fiber configuration. This solution is based on FBG fast modulation using a magnetostrictive device [63]. This feature provides a direct control of the repetition rate and a fully modulated train of mode-locked pulses. To the best of our knowledge, this is the first doubly active QML strictly all-fiber laser presented [18].

The setup of our doubly active QML all-fiber laser is basically the same as the one described in Section 19.3.2 for the CW-ML and shown in Figure 19.12, with the same length of EDF and delay line, except by the magnetostrictive device controlling the FBG_2; see Figure 19.26. This device is essentially the same as the one we used in the QS-DFB all-fiber laser presented in Section 19.2. It is composed of a 15-mm-long (1 mm^2 cross section) magnetostrictive rod of Terfenol-D bonded to the FBG_2. The rod and the fiber were placed inside a small coil driven by an electronic circuit designed to drive square current pulses with amplitudes up to 260 mA of any required duty cycle. Figure 19.27 shows the spectral positions of both FBGs—that is, the FBG of the AOSLM and FBG_2, which helps understand the operation principle of this laser also. When the magnetic pulses are generated in the solenoid stretch FBG_2, its central wavelength is brought to match the short-wavelength sideband of FBG_1 for a short period of time, which results in an increased Q-value. In this way, by modulating the coil current with a frequency ν_{QS}, the Q-factor is actively modulated at the same frequency. The magnetostriction presents the advantage to permit a continuous tuning of both the QS repetition rate and the duty cycle of the modulation pulses. The dependence of the wavelength shift on the coil current was measured by illuminating FBG_2 with a tunable laser source and detecting the reflected light. A quasilinear behavior was observed as a result of using moderate magnetic fields.

Now we discuss the QML laser operation. The laser emission wavelength is 1530.55 nm, since the overlapping between the short-wavelength sideband of FBG_1 and the shifted position of FBG_2 takes place at this wavelength; see Figure 19.27. Figure 19.28a exemplifies the QML laser behavior showing the train of optical pulses generated for a pump power of 70 mW. The optical QML pulses are 2 ms apart, since the repetition rate of the train of voltage pulses applied to the current driver was of $\nu_{QS} = 500$ Hz. Figure 19.28b shows a single QS envelope with an FWHM of 550 ns; it has between 12 and 14 fully modulated mode-locked pulses, with the expected temporal separation $1/\nu_{ML} = 110$ ns. As observed, the QML pulses of this laser have excellent interpulse characteristics. However, the individual short pulses are broadened due to the limited bandwidth and sampling rate of the oscilloscope. In order to measure the FWHM of the individual short pulses, a 50 GHz sampling oscilloscope was used. In this case, the large difference between the independent

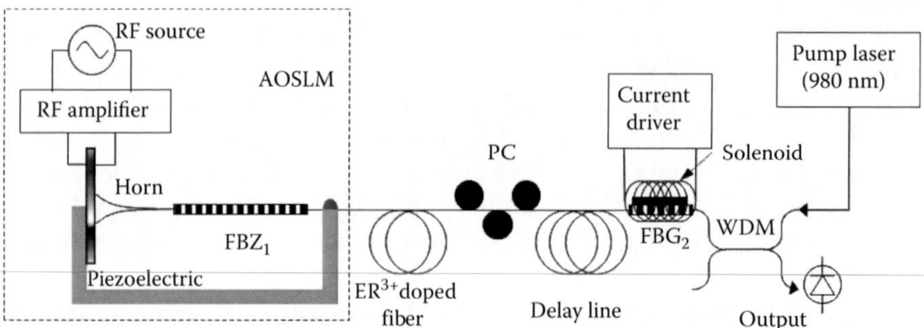

FIGURE 19.26 QML all-fiber laser setup, when the AOSLM is driven by standing acoustic waves.

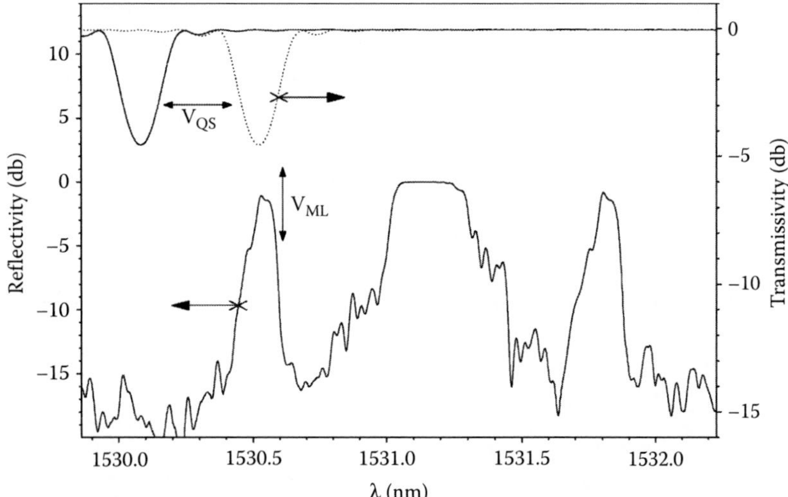

FIGURE 19.27 QML all-fiber laser with an AOSLM driven by standing acoustic waves. Reflection spectrum of the AOSLM when an RF signal of 4.55 MHz and 16 V (peak-to-peak) is applied to the piezoelectric (left ordinate). Transmissivity of FBG_2 (solid curve) for zero coil current; the dotted curve shows the new spectral position of FBG_2 for a DC coil current of 100 mA (right ordinate).

frequencies ν_{QS} and ν_{ML} makes it difficult to trigger properly the oscilloscope. Even so, relatively good traces were recorded as the one depicted in the inset of Figure 19.28b. As we discussed before when we presented the CW-ML in Section 19.3.2, the tuning sensitivity between the RF signal applied to the piezoelectric and the cavity round trip is not too critical in this setup; see Section 19.3.2.1. Only when the detuning is considerable—for example, by a few kilohertz—the pulse clearly deteriorates. Figure 19.28c shows the QS pulse obtained by avoiding the ML pulse formation, just by detuning ν_{PZT} by 10 kHz; in this way, only the QS operation is allowed within the cavity. As expected, the QS pulse reproduces the waveform of the envelope of the QML pulses shown in Figure 19.28b, but with a much lower peak power (by a factor of ~4×10^{-3}) and an increased temporal

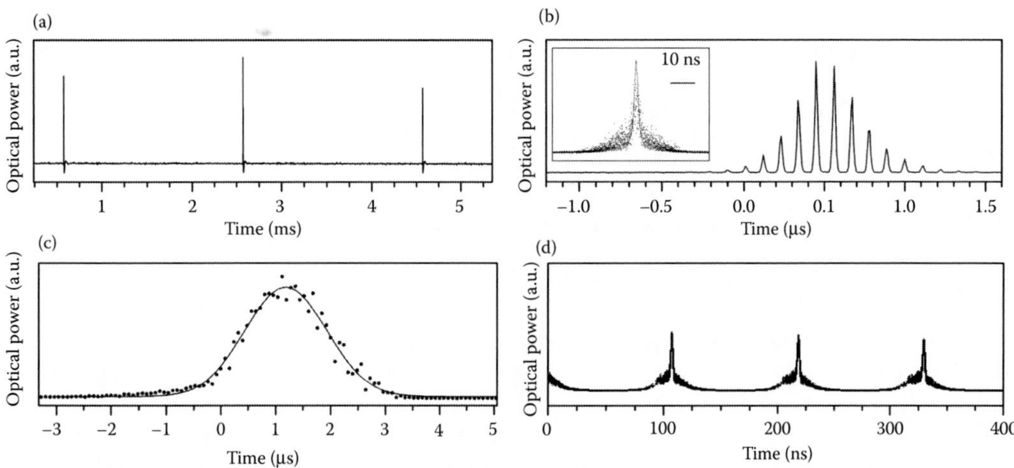

FIGURE 19.28 QML all-fiber laser with an AOSLM driven by standing acoustic waves. (a) QML train of pulses at a QS frequency of 500 Hz. (b) Single *Q*-switched pulse enveloping a train of 12–14 mode-locked pulses; the inset shows a single mode-locked pulse. (c) Single *Q*-switched pulse with no ML. (d) CW-ML operation of the laser without QS. In all cases, the pump power was 70 mW.

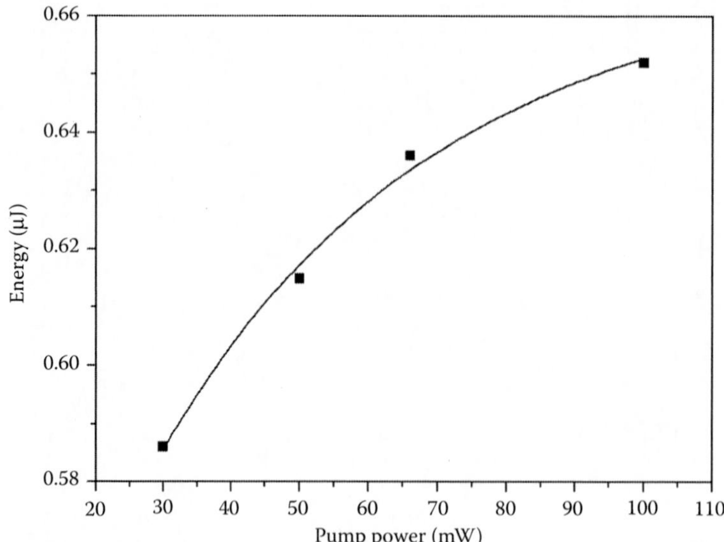

FIGURE 19.29 QML all-fiber laser with an AOSLM driven by standing acoustic waves. Energy of QML pulses as a function of the pump power for a repetition rate of 500 Hz.

width. The transition from the fully modulated QML pulses to the pure QS operation—that is, from Figures 19.28b and c—is progressive as we detune ν_{PZT}. Finally, Figure 19.28d shows the behavior of this laser when turning off the active QS, that is, CW-ML operation of the laser. To this end, a DC current was driven to the coil of the magnetostrictive device in order to achieve a stationary overlap with the short-wavelength sideband of the AOSLM. The trace of Figure 19.28d was recorded with the 1 GHz oscilloscope. In this case, the thermal effects produced by the DC current made difficult an optimum and stable adjustment of FBG_2. The comparison of Figures 19.28b and d illustrates the improved performance of the laser in terms of peak power when both QS and ML are operating.

The energy of a Q-switched train of pulses, as that reported in Figure 19.28b, as a function of the pump power is shown in Figure 19.29. This energy was measured directly with a pyroelectric detector. At high pump powers, the energy of the QML train of pulses reaches gain saturation. Thus, a peak power higher than 250 W can be calculated for the central pulses of a train with an energy of 0.65 μJ, assuming that the mode-locked pulses are 1 ns width. This result demonstrates a dramatic enhancement in comparison with the peak power achieved when the laser was operated in CW-ML regime [12], since the ratio is higher than 2×10^3.

19.4.2 QML All-Fiber Laser with an AOSLM Driven by Traveling Acoustic Waves

The most significant advantage of using traveling acoustic waves instead of standing acoustic waves is determined by the possibility to actively Q-switch this mode-locked laser simply by launching to the grating a burst acoustical wave [19]. Therefore, the setup is exactly the same as that reported before for CW-ML driven by traveling acoustic waves in Section 19.3.3, that is, Figure 19.12. The burst signal consists of an integer number of sinusoidal acoustical cycles N. Figure 19.30a shows the burst voltage signal applied to the piezoelectric together with the QML train of pulses generated, at a frequency rate of 1 kHz. Figure 19.30b shows several QML pulses as a function of N. When N is low, QML is not reached. For higher N, QML is reached and the emission is allowed. For example, the left bottom corner of Figure 19.30b shows a single QS envelope with an FWHM of 1.4 μs for $N = 25$; it has between 16 and 18 fully modulated mode-locked pulses, with the expected temporal separation given by 1/4.1 MHz = 244 ns. The inset shows a

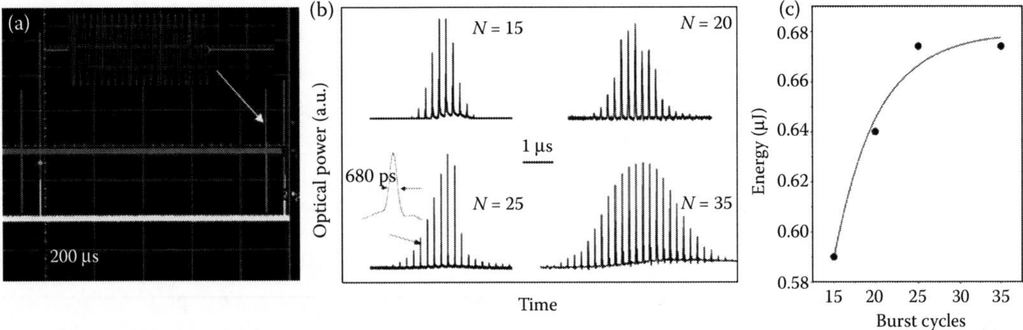

FIGURE 19.30 QML all-fiber laser with an AOSLM driven by an acoustical burst signal. (a) Voltage signal applied to the piezoelectric (upper trace) and QML train of pulses generated (lower trace) for a 1 kHz QS repetition rate; the inset shows a detail of the burst signal. (b) Single QML pulses enveloping a train of mode-locked pulses for different burst cycles; the inset shows a single-shot capture of a single mode-locked pulse with an FWHM of 680 ps. (c) Energy of the QML pulses as a function of the cycles contained in the burst for a fixed QS frequency of 500 Hz and a pump power of 270 mW.

single-shot capture of a mode-locked pulse within this train with a temporal width of 680 ps. As observed, the QML pulses of this laser have excellent interpulse characteristics. The energy of a QS train of pulses as a function of N is shown in Figure 19.30c. This energy was measured directly with a pyroelectric detector. As expected, for a longer burst signal, the energy of the QML train of pulses increases, until it reaches saturation. Thus, a peak power higher than 200 W can be calculated for the central pulses of a train with an energy of 0.68 μJ, assuming that the mode-locked pulses are of 680 ps width. This result clearly demonstrates the degree of enhancement in comparison with the peak power achieved when the laser was operated in the CW-ML regime, since the ratio is higher than 4×10^2; see Section 19.3.3.

19.5 CONCLUSIONS

The use of intracavity bulk elements in fiber lasers has important drawbacks as reduced mechanical stability and high insertion losses. In this chapter we have shown how lasers can benefit from a strictly all-fiber configuration by using the interaction of light with acoustic pulses and harmonic acoustic waves. In this way, we first showed an actively QS-DFB all-fiber laser driven by acoustic pulses generated by a novel in-line acoustic pulse generator based on a magnetostrictive device. Both outputs of the laser were available and transform-limited optical pulses of up to 800 mW peak power and 32 ns pulse width were generated at variable frequencies in the kilohrtz range. The measured emission linewidth was as low as 6 MHz at 10 kHz frequency. We also discussed its promising use as a compact source for Brillouin sensing applications.

Next, we proposed the use of an AOSLM to actively mode-lock a laser in a strictly all-fiber configuration. Since an AOSLM can be driven in two different ways either by standing or traveling acoustic waves; we discussed first the construction of a CW-ML laser driven by standing acoustic waves. In this configuration we obtained transform-limited optical pulses of up to 120 mW peak power and 780 ps pulse width generated at a fixed repetition rate of 9 MHz, with an emission linewidth of 2.8 pm at 1530.5 nm. We also study the influence of different parameters on the ML process such as frequency detuning, EDF length, amplitude modulation, and dispersion. In this case, narrower pulses were obtained at higher modulation depths, normal dispersion, and shorter lengths of active fiber. Best results were reached when the CW-ML laser was optimized according to these variables (160 mW peak power and 630 ps temporal width at 9 MHz repetition rate). Then, we discussed the construction of a CW-ML laser when the AOSLM is driven by traveling acoustic waves. In this case, the modulation frequency is half the frequency obtained when standing acoustic waves are used. Optical pulses were obtained of 530 mW peak power, 700 ps temporal width, at a repetition rate of 4.1 MHz.

We also presented simultaneous doubly active QML using strictly all-fiber modulation techniques in both CW-ML configurations, that is, when the AOSLM was driven by standing or traveling acoustic waves. In the first case, it is necessary to slightly modify the setup as compared with its CW-ML counterpart. To this end, we attached a magnetostrictive rod to the output FBG to modulate the Q factor of the Fabry–Perot cavity. Fully modulated QML trains of optical pulses were obtained for a wide range of pump powers and repetition rates. For a Q-switched repetition rate of 500 Hz and a pump power of 100 mW, the laser generates trains of 12–14 mode-locked pulses of about 1 ns each, within an envelope of 550 ns, an overall energy of 0.65 μJ, and a peak power higher than 250 W for the central pulses of the train. On the contrary, we demonstrated that it is not necessary to modify the setup when traveling acoustic waves are used to drive the AOSLM. In this case, the commutation between the CW-ML and QML regimes is remarkably simple; we need to use a different electrical signal to drive the piezoelectric of the AOSLM, namely from a sinusoidal to a burst-sinusoidal electrical signal. In this case, fully modulated 10–25 mode-locked pulses around 700 ps each within a QS envelope around 1 μs and a maximum overall energy of 0.68 μJ were obtained.

The optimization of the techniques presented here require the development of new strictly all-fiber modulation techniques. Specifically, in the CW-ML lasers presented, we have identified the relatively narrow modulator bandwidth of the AOSLM as one of the key limiting factors that precludes reaching narrower pulses. In this way, one possible alternative is to broaden the sidebands of the AOSLM. Together with this, the study of new mechanisms to modulate at higher frequencies is important, since this parameter has been mentioned also as another narrowing mechanism of the optical pulses.

ACKNOWLEDGMENTS

The results presented in this chapter are part of the research activity supported by the Ministerio de Educación y Ciencia and the Generalitat Valenciana of Spain (projects TEC2008–05490 and PROMETEO/2009/077, respectively). C. Cuadrado-Laborde acknowledges also the Secretaría de Estado de Universidades e Investigación del Ministerio de Investigación y Ciencia (Spain).

REFERENCES

1. J. Canning, Fibre lasers and related technologies, *Opt. Laser Eng.*, 44, 2006, 647–676.
2. I. P. Alcock, A. C. Tropper, A. I. Ferguson, and D. C. Hanna, Q-switched operation of a neodymium-doped monomode fibre laser, *Electron. Lett.*, 22, 1986, 84–85.
3. P. R. Morkel, K. P. Jedrzejewski, E. R. Taylor, and D. N. Payne, Short-pulse, high-power Q-switched fiber laser, *IEEE Photon. Technol. Lett.*, 4, 1992, 545–547.
4. O. Schmidt, J. Rothhardt, F. Röser, S. Linke, T. Schreiber, K. Rademaker, J. Limpert et al., Millijoule pulse energy Q-switched short-length fiber laser, *Opt. Lett.*, 32, 2007, 1551–1553.
5. W. Shin, B. A. Yu, Y. L. Lee, T. J. Yu, T. J. Eom, Y. C. Noh, J. Lee, and D. K. Ko, Tunable Q-switched erbium-doped fiber laser based on digital micro-mirror array, *Opt. Express*, 14, 2006, 5356–5364.
6. M. W. Phillips, A. I. Ferguson, and D. C. Hanna, Frequency-modulation mode locking of a Nd^{3+}-doped fiber laser, *Opt. Lett.*, 14, 1989, 219–221.
7. G. Geister and R. Ulrich, Neodymium-fibre laser with integrated-optic mode locker, *Opt. Commun.*, 68, 1988, 187–189.
8. D. D. Hudson, K. W. Holman, R. J. Jones, S. T. Cundiff, J. Ye, and D. J. Jones, Mode-locked fiber laser frequency-controlled with an intracavity electro-optic modulator, *Opt. Lett.*, 30, 2005, 2948–2950.
9. C. Cuadrado-Laborde, P. Pérez-Millán, M. V. Andrés, A. Díez, J. L Cruz, and Yu. O. Barmenkov, Transform-limited pulses generated by an actively Q-switched distributed fiber laser, *Opt. Lett.*, 33, 2008, 2590–2592.
10. M. Delgado-Pinar, A. Díez, J. L. Cruz, and M. V. Andrés, Single-frequency active Q-switched distributed fiber laser using acoustic waves, *Appl. Phys. Lett.*, 90, 2007, 171110.

11. P. Pérez-Millán, J. L. Cruz, and M. V. Andrés, Active Q-switched distributed feedback erbium-doped fiber lasers, *Appl. Phys. Lett.*, 87, 2005, 011104.
12. C. Cuadrado-Laborde, A. Díez, M. Delgado-Pinar, J. L. Cruz, and M. V. Andrés, Mode locking of an all-fiber laser by acousto-optic superlattice modulation, *Opt. Lett.*, 34, 2009, 1111–1113.
13. C. Cuadrado-Laborde, A. Díez, J. L. Cruz, and M. V. Andrés. Experimental study of an all-fiber laser actively mode-locked by standing-wave acousto-optic modulation, *Appl. Phys. B—Lasers Opt.*, 99, 2010, 95–99.
14. D. O. Culverhouse, D. J. Richardson, T. A. Birks, and P. St. J. Russell, All-fiber sliding-frequency Er^{3+}/Yb^{3+} soliton laser, *Opt. Lett.*, 20, 1995, 2381–2383.
15. M. Y. Jeon, H. K. Lee, K. H. Kim, E. H. Lee, W. Y. Oh, B. Y. Kim, H. W. Lee, and Y. W. Koh, Harmonically mode-locked fiber laser with an acousto-optic modulator in a Sagnac loop and Faraday rotating mirror cavity, *Opt. Commun.*, 149, 1998, 312–316.
16. C. Cuadrado-Laborde, A. Díez, J. L. Cruz, and M. V. Andrés, Actively Mode-locked fiber laser with an acousto-optic in-fiber superlattice modulator, in *CLEO/Europe and EQEC 2009 Conference Digest (Optical Society of America* 2009*)*, paper CJ_P24.
17. M. W. Phillips, A. I. Ferguson, G. S. Kino, and D. B. Patterson, Mode-locked fiber laser with a fiber phase modulator, *Opt. Lett.*, 14, 1989, 680–682.
18. C. Cuadrado-Laborde, A. Díez, J. L. Cruz, and M. V. Andrés, Doubly active Q switching and mode locking of an all-fiber laser, *Opt. Lett.*, 34, 2009, 2709–2711.
19. C. Cuadrado-Laborde, A. Diez, J. L. Cruz, and M. V. Andrés, Actively Q-switched and modelocked all-fiber lasers, *Laser Phys. Lett.*, 7, 2010, 870–875.
20. S. A. Babin, D. V. Churkin, A. E. Ismagulov, S. I. Kablukov, and M. A. Nikulin, Single frequency single polarization DFB fiber laser, *Laser Phys. Lett.*, 4, 2007, 428–432.
21. A. Schülzgen, L. Li, D. Nguyen, Ch. Spiegelberg, R. Matei Rogojan, A. Laronche, J. Albert, and N. Peyghambarian, Distributed feedback fiber laser pumped by multimode laser diodes, *Opt. Lett.*, 33, 2008, 614–616.
22. M. V. Andrés, J. L. Cruz, A. Díez, P. Pérez-Millán, and M. Delgado-Pinar, Actively Q-switched all-fiber lasers, *Laser Phys. Lett*, 5, 2008, 93–99.
23. J. L. Cruz, A. Díez, M. V. Andrés, A. Segura, B. Ortega, and L. Dong, Fibre Bragg gratings tuned and chirped using magnetic fields, *Electron. Lett.*, 33, 1997, 235–236.
24. A. Galtarossa, E. Nava, and G. Valentini, in *Single-Mode Optical Fiber Measurement: Characterization and Sensing*, G. Cancellieri (Ed.), Artech Pub., Boston, 1993.
25. G. P. Agrawal, *Nonlinear Fiber Optics*, Academic Press, California, 2001.
26. Y. Li, F. Zhang, and T. Yoshino, Wide-range temperature dependence of Brillouin shift in a dispersion-shifted fiber and its annealing effect, *J. Lightwave Technol.*, 21, 2003, 1663–1667.
27. T. R. Parker, M. Farhadiroushan, R. Feced, V. A. Handerek, and A. J. Rogers, Simultaneous distributed measurement of strain and temperature from noise-initiated Brillouin scattering in optical fibers, *IEEE J. Quantum Electron.*, 34, 1998, 645–659.
28. X. Bao, J. Dhliwayo, N. Heron, D. J. Webb, and D. A. Jackson, Experimental and theoretical studies on a distributed temperature sensor based on Brillouin scattering, *J. Lightwave Technol.*, 13, 1995, 1340–1348.
29. D. Culverhouse, F. Farahi, C. N. Pannell, and D. A. Jackson, Potential of stimulated Brillouin scattering as a sensing mechanism for distributed temperature sensors, *Electron. Lett.*, 25, 1989, 913–915.
30. D. Culverhouse, F. Farahi, C. N. Pannell, and D. A. Jackson, Stimulated Brillouin scattering: A means to realize tunable microwave generator or distributed temperature sensor, *Electron. Lett.*, 25, 1989, 915–916.
31. K. Brown, A. W. Brown, and B. G. Colpitts, Characterization of optical fibers for optimization of a Brillouin scattering based fiber optic sensor, *Opt. Fiber Technol.*, 11, 2005, 131–145.
32. H. A. Haus, Mode-locking of lasers, *IEEE J. Sel. Top. Quantum Electron*, 6, 2000, 1173–1185.
33. S. W. Chu, T. M. Liu, C. K. Sun, C. Y. Lin, and H. J. Tsai, Real-time second-harmonic-generation microscopy based on a 2-GHz repetition rate Ti:sapphire laser, *Opt. Express*, 11, 2003, 933–938.
34. C. B. Schaffer,J. F. García, and E. Mazur, Bulk heating of transparent materials using a high-repetition-rate femtosecond laser, *Appl. Phys. A—Mater.*, 76, 2003, 351–354.
35. C. X. Yu, H. A. Haus, E. P. Ippen, W. S. Wong, and A. Sysoliatin, Gigahertz-repetition-rate mode-locked fiber laser for continuum generation, *Opt. Lett.*, 25, 2000, 1418–1420.
36. N. H. Bonadeo, W. H. Knox, J. M. Roth, and K. Bergman, Passive harmonic mode-locked soliton fiber laser stabilized by an optically pumped saturable Bragg reflector, *Opt. Lett.*, 25, 2000, 1421–1423.
37. P. M. W. French, The generation of ultrashort laser pulses, *Rep. Prog. Phys*, 58, 1995, 169–267.
38. N. Myrén andW. Margulis, All-fiber electrooptical mode-locking and tuning, *IEEE Photon. Technol. Lett.*, 17, 2005, 2047–2049.

39. P. St. J. Russell and W. F. Liu, Acousto-optic superlattice modulation in fiber Bragg gratings, *J. Opt. Soc. Am. A*, 17, 2000, 1421–1429.
40. C. Cuadrado-Laborde, M. Delgado-Pinar, S. Torres-Peiró, A. Díez, and M. V. Andres, Q-switched all-fibre laser using a fibre-optic resonant acousto-optic modulator, *Opt. Commun.*, 274, 2007, 407–411.
41. W. F. Liu, P. St. J. Russell, and L. Dong, Acousto-optic superlattice modulator using a fiber Bragg grating, *Opt. Lett.*, 22, 1997, 1515–1517.
42. W. F. Liu, P. St. J. Russell, and L. Dong, 100% efficient narrow-band acoustooptic tunable reflector using fiber Bragg grating, *J. Lightwave Technol.*, 16, 1998, 2006–2009.
43. D. J. Kuizenga and A. E. Siegman, FM and AM mode locking of the homogeneous laser-Part I: Theory, *IEEE J. Quantum Electron.*, 6, 1970, 694–708.
44. P. A. Bélanger, On the profile of pulses generated by fiber lasers, *Opt. Express*, 13, 2005, 8089–8096.
45. K. Wada, J. Fujita, J. Yamada, T. Matsuyama, and H. Horinaka, Simple method for estimating shape functions of optical spectra, *Opt. Commun.* 281, 2008, 368–373.
46. F. Shohda, T. Shirato, M. Nakazawa, K. Komatsu, and T. Kaino, A passively mode-locked femtosecond soliton fiber laser at 1.5 μm with a CNT-doped polycarbonate saturable absorber, *Opt. Express*, 16, 2008, 21191–21198.
47. M. Nakazawa, Ultrafast mode-locked fiber lasers for high-speed OTDM transmission and related topics, *J. Opt. Fiber. Commun. Rep.*, 2, 2005, 462–496.
48. Y. Li, C. Lou, and Y. Gao, Theoretical study on a detuned AM mode-locked laser, *Proc. IEEE Lasers Electro-Optics Society*, 2, 1999, 838–839.
49. L. M. Zhao, D. Y. Tang, and J. Wu, Gain-guided soliton in a positive group-dispersion fiber laser, *Opt. Lett* 31, 1788–1790, 2006.
50. A. Ruf, and F. Dausinger, *Femtosecond Technology for Technical and Medical Applications*, Springer, Berlin, 2004.
51. D. Breitling, A. Ruf, and F. Dausinger, Fundamental aspects in machining of metals with short and ultrashort laser pulses, *Proc. SPIE*, 5339, 2004, 49–63.
52. M. S. Amer, M. A. El-Ashry, L. R. Dosser, K. E. Hix, J. F. Maguire, and B. Irwin, Femtosecond versus nanosecond laser machining: comparison of induced stresses and structural changes in silicon wafers, *Appl. Surf. Sci.*, 242, 2005, 162–167.
53. C. Theobald, M. Weitz, R. Knappe, R. Wallenstein, and J. A. L'Huillier, Stable Q-switch mode-locking of Nd:YVO4 lasers with a semiconductor saturable absorber, *Appl. Phys. B—Lasers Opt.*, 92, 2008, 1–3.
54. S. Kobtsev, S. Kukarin, and Y. Fedotov, Ultra-low repetition rate mode-locked fiber laser with high-energy pulses, *Opt. Express*, 16, 2008, 21936–21941.
55. S. Camacho-Lopez, R. Evans, C. Greenhalgh, C. Torti, J. Robertson, R. S. Marjoribanks, P. R. Herman, M. Nantel, and L. Lilge, Single-pulse and 'pulsetrain-burst' (>100 MHz) effects in ultrafast laser processing of metals, glasses, and bio-tissues, *Proc. Conf. Lasers Electro-Optics*, 2, 2003, 1–6.
56. M. Nantel, R. Evans, S. Camacho-López, C. Greenhalgh, L. Lilge, P. R. Herman, and R. S. Marjoribanks, Laser-matter interactions of pulsetrain bursts with solids and tissues, in *Frontiers in Optics, OSA Technical Digest*, 2003, ThP4.
57. Y. Gan, W. H. Xiang, and G. Z. Zhang, Studies on CW and Q-switched mode-locked in passive mode-locked ytterbium-doped fibre laser, *Laser Phys.*, 19, 2009, 445–449.
58. J. K. Jabczyński, W. Zendzian, and J. Kwiatkowski, Q-switched mode-locking with acousto-optic modulator in a diode-pumped Nd:YVO_4 laser, *Opt. Express*, 14, 2006, 2184–2190.
59. J. H. Lin, H. R. Chen, H. H. Hsu, M. D. Wei, K. H. Lin, and W. F. Hsieh, Stable Q-switched mode-locked Nd^{3+}:$LuVO_4$ laser by Cr^{4+}:YAG crystal, *Opt. Express*, 16, 2008, 16538–16545.
60. F. J. Grawert, F. Ö. Ilday, D. F. Kielpinski, J. T. Gopinath, G. S. Petrich, L. A. Kolodziejski, E. P. Ippen, and F. X. Kärtner, Automatic feedback control of an Er-doped fiber laser with an intracavity loss modulator, *Opt. Lett.*, 30, 2005, 1066–1068.
61. A. Killi, J. Dörring, U. Morgner, M. J. Lederer, J. Frei, and D. Kopf, High speed electro-optical cavity dumping of mode-locked laser oscillators, *Opt. Express*, 13, 2005, 1916–1922.
62. A. Beyertt, D. Nickel, and A. Giesen, Femtosecond thin-disk Yb:KYW regenerative amplifier, *Appl. Phys. B—Lasers Opt.*, 80, 2005, 1–6.
63. P. Pérez-Millán, A. Díez, M. V. Andrés, D. Zalvidea, and R. Duchowicz, Q-switched all-fiber laser based on magnetostriction modulation of a Bragg grating, *Opt. Express*, 13, 2005, 5046–5051.

20 Ultrafast Fiber Lasers

Jian Liu and Lihmei Yang

CONTENTS

20.1 INTRODUCTION

The ability to directly write predesigned engineering structures on the micron and nanometer scales is an exciting theme in materials processing and manufacturing. While many applications for such structures in microsystems (e.g., optical devices and sensors) have been envisioned, the engineering challenges needing the greatest research attention require the development of innovative approaches to micro- and nanostructurally engineered materials. Fashioning these structures requires a tool capable of highly localized transformations in preselected regions of a material so that sharp well-defined architectures can be "written" at will. A promising and rapidly emerging processing tool for achieving these goals is the use of focused ultrashort pulses of light of very short duration (picoseconds (ps) or femtoseconds (fs)). From an engineering and manufacturing perspective, fs laser processing is attractive because it is deterministic, repeatable and allows the fabrication of truly three-dimensional (3D) structures of any desired shape. While this technique has already been used for the fabrication of optical devices [1–17] and lab-on-chip components [18–27], it is expected to grow further in importance with applications in optical data storage, telecommunications, and bio-imaging and -sensing.

The mechanism of ultrashort laser pulse modification of materials can be divided into two parts: absorption of the fs laser energy by the materials (such as metal, glass, and polymer) and the subsequent dissipation of the absorbed energy. The energy absorption process has been studied in the context of fs-laser ablation. Absorption of the fs laser pulse takes place via the following sequence of steps: (1) production of initial seed electrons through either nonlinear photoionization of free electrons or excitation of impurity defects, (2) avalanche photoionization, and (3) plasma formation. Note that the laser energy is only absorbed in the small focal volume of the laser since only there the intensity is high enough for multiphoton ionization to occur.

The second part of the mechanism involves the transfer of the energy from the hot plasma created by the laser pulses to the lattice, resulting in the modified regions in the bulk material. The energy dissipation process is less well understood than the energy absorption process. It is known that the dissipation process occurs on a timescale of hundreds of nanoseconds to microseconds; this is substantially longer than the hundreds of fs required for the energy absorption process. It is believed that the primary dissipation mechanisms are a combination of thermal diffusion and shock-wave generation, although it is uncertain which process is dominant and this probably depends on the precise writing conditions (pulse fluence and repetition rate). The final results of the fs laser–metal interaction are physical, chemical, and structural changes of the material after exposure to the laser beam. Figure 20.1 shows a summary of the mechanism generally guiding the laser microstructuring process. A rule of thumb is that when the pulse width is less than 1 ps, the thermal diffusion can be confined to micron dimension and heat affected zone (HAZ) can be eliminated.

Figure 20.1 also gives a comparison of material processing between femtosecond and nanosecond pulses. It clearly shows that the fs process provides much better quality in terms of smoothness, cleanness, and surrounding damage. Ultrashort laser provides a vital solution to fine material processing due to its superior performance (less heat-affected zone, no damage to surrounding materials or structures, nanometer feature precision) over long pulsed lasers.

Five major variables control the fs microstructuring process: the laser pulse energy, the beam quality and focusing conditions, the laser repetition rate, and the speed and direction with which the sample is moved. Laser pulse duration is also very important [28], but for many laser systems this parameter is difficult to vary. Of the five variables used to control the fs modification process, the laser pulse energy together with the beam quality and focusing conditions determines the laser pulse fluence (J/cm^2) that is typically the most influential experimental variable for all of the writing configurations. The high repetition rates (e.g., MHz) increase the production rate, since the scan speed can be increased.

Present-day fs laser manufacturing systems using ultrashort pulses of light are based on solid-state oscillator/amplifier technology designed originally for use in the scientific research market.

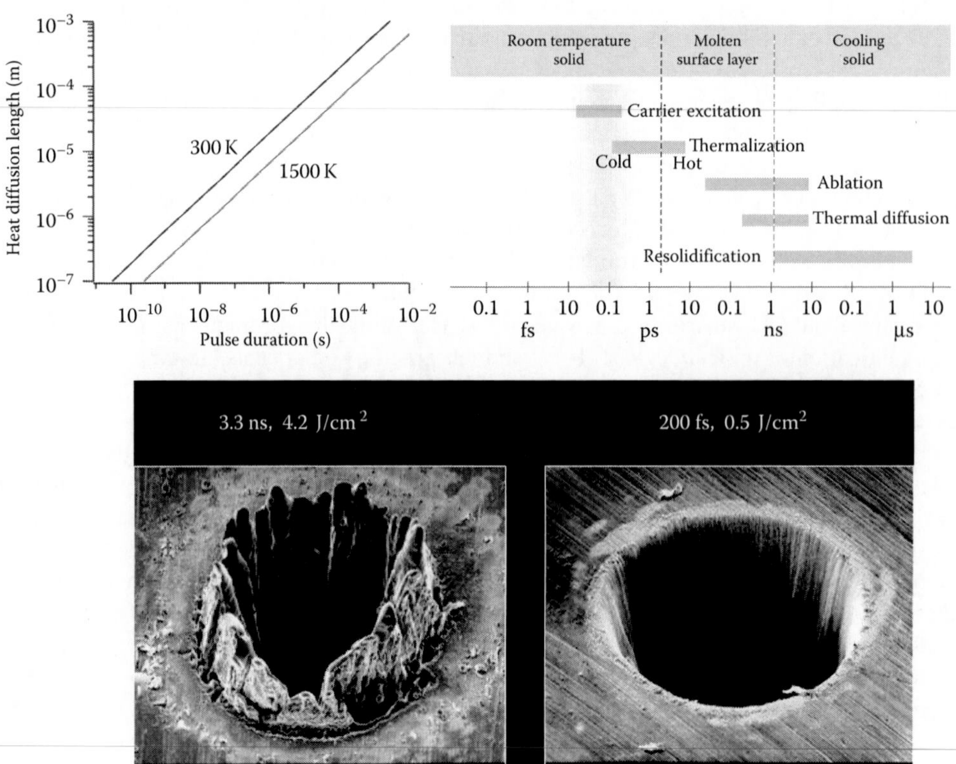

FIGURE 20.1 Material process mechanism for pulsed laser and a comparison of material processing between femtosecond laser and nanosecond laser.

Solid-state-based fs lasers and amplifiers using Ti:sapphire or Nd- and Yb- doped crystalline materials are operating at repetition rates of kHz level and are usually bulky and lack robustness for practical applications. Furthermore, they have low wall plug efficiency and serious thermal distortion of beam quality at high power operation [29–36]. This system architecture is suboptimal for producing the highest quality results at high material modification rates and makes this technology less viable when manufacturing low-cost components.

Yb-doped fiber lasers/amplifiers offer efficient, reliable, and compact solutions for high power amplification with less thermal management and maintenance [37–54]. Over 1 kW output power continuous wave (CW) and pump light conversions of 85% (normally 60–70%) and peak powers over 1 MW (pulsed) have been reported for fiber lasers/amplifiers. However, based on an in-depth survey of the literature over the last 10 years, it was concluded that there has been no commercial product achieving over 100 W average power among fs fiber lasers/amplifiers at repetition rates in the megahertz range. At high repetition rates (e.g., MHz), the production rate is higher, since the scan speed can be increased. So, innovative approaches must be conceived for the development of a high-throughput fs laser microstructuring system.

There are a number of applications for the ultrashort laser system:

- Material processing. This includes (1) photonic device fabrication, such as waveguide, coupler, WDM, modulator, and switching; (2) all types of precision metal processing such as welding, cutting, annealing, and drilling; (3) semiconductor and microelectronics manufacturing such as lithography, inspection, control, defect analysis and repair, and via drilling; (4) marking different materials including plastic, metals, and silicon; and (5) other types of material processing such as rapid prototyping, desktop manufacturing, micromachining, photofinishing, embossed holograms, and grating manufacturing.
- Medical equipment and biomedical instrumentation. The high-power laser can be applied to ophthalmology, refractive surgery, photocoagulation, general surgery, therapeutic, imaging, and cosmetic applications. Biomedical instruments include those involved in cells or proteins, cytometry, and DNA sequencing; laser Raman spectroscopy, spectrofluorimetry, and ablation; and laser-based microscopes.
- Military/aerospace. The proposed fiber laser can be directly used in military applications, and space, aircraft, and satellite applications such as LIDAR systems, the remote sensing system, the illuminator system, and the phase array antenna system.

20.2 FIBER LASERS

A fiber laser is a laser in which the active gain medium is an optical fiber doped with rare-earth elements such as erbium, ytterbium, neodymium, dysprosium, praseodymium, and thulium. Fiber nonlinearities, such as stimulated Raman scattering or four wave mixing, can also provide gain and thus serve in effect as gain media. Unlike most other types of lasers, the laser cavity in a fiber laser is constructed monolithically by fusion splicing the different types of fibers; most notably fiber Bragg gratings replace conventional dielectric mirrors to provide optical feedback. To pump fiber lasers, semiconductor laser diodes or other fiber lasers are used almost exclusively. Fiber lasers can have several-kilometers-long active regions and provide very high optical gain. They can support kilowatt level continuous output power because the fiber's high surface area-to-volume ratio allows efficient cooling. The fiber waveguiding properties reduce or remove completely thermal distortion of the optical path, thus resulting in typically diffraction-limited high-quality optical beams. Fiber lasers also feature compact layout compared to rod or gas lasers of comparable power, as the fiber can be bent to small diameters and coiled. Other advantages include high vibrational stability, extended lifetime, and maintenance-free turnkey operation.

Many high-power fiber lasers are based on double-clad fiber. The gain medium forms the core of the fiber, which is surrounded by two layers of cladding. The lasing mode propagates in the core, while a multimode pump beam propagates in the inner cladding layer. The outer cladding keeps this pump light confined. This arrangement allows the core to be pumped with a much higher power beam than could otherwise be made to propagate in it, and allows the conversion of pump light with relatively low brightness into a much higher-brightness signal. As a result, fiber lasers and amplifiers are occasionally referred to as "brightness converters." A doped optical fiber is an essential component that is used as a gain medium to generate and amplify an optical signal for fiber lasers and amplifiers. In general, the signal to be amplified and a pump laser are multiplexed into the doped fiber, and the signal is amplified through interaction with the doping ions. The most common example is the erbium-doped fiber (EDF), where the core of a silica fiber is doped with trivalent erbium ions and can be efficiently pumped with a laser at a wavelength of 980 nm or 1480 nm, and exhibits gain in the 1,550 nm region; the ytterbium-doped fiber, where the core of a silica fiber is doped with trivalent ytterbium ions and can be efficiently pumped with a laser at a wavelength of 980 nm or 915 nm, and exhibits gain in the 1064 nm region; and the thulium-doped fiber, where the core of a silica fiber is doped with trivalent thulium ions and can be efficiently pumped with a laser at a wavelength of 790 nm or 1560 nm, and exhibits gain in the 2000 nm region. By using glasses with a composition ZrF_4-BaF_2-LaF_3-AlF_3-NaF (ZBLAN) fibers (Er doped, Ho doped, or Tm doped), the wavelengths can be extended to visible and mid-infrared (IR) regions such as 2.7 and 3 μm.

20.3 ULTRAFAST FIBER LASERS AND APPLICATIONS

Ultrafast fiber lasers, by definition, should be a thoroughly fiber-based laser system or with minimum nonfiber-based components. At least the seed laser, stretcher, and amplifiers should be fiber based. Those lasers using only one or two pieces of fibers in the amplifier stages shall not be counted as fiber lasers.

The development and commercialization of ultrafast fiber lasers have evolved into a new era over the last few of years and companies such as PolarOnyx (San Jose, CA) and IMRA (Ann Arbor, MI) have series of products covering 1 and 1.55 μm spectral regions and energy level beyond 10 μJ and average power level over 10 W. Cornell University (Frank Wise Group) has pioneered high-energy and high-power seed oscillators.

The seed mode-locked fiber laser oscillator is the heart of the ultrafast fiber lasers and its performance is critical to the chirped pulse amplification and compression. At wavelengths in the 1550 nm region, due to the demand of fiber telecommunication, a variety of fibers are commercially available in terms of nonlinear properties, dispersions and dispersion slopes, and doping levels of EDF or Er–Yb codoped fibers. This has caused many companies (including PolarOnyx and IMRA) and universities to develop many different types of ultrafast fiber lasers.

Things are a little different when working at the 1 μm region. Conventionally, ultrashort pulse mode-locked fiber lasers operating at wavelengths below 1.3 μm pose a challenge in that there is no simple all-fiber-based solution for dispersion compensation in this wavelength regime. Dispersion is a phenomenon that causes the separation of a wave into spectral components with different wavelengths, due to the dependence of the component's speed on its wavelength (i.e., wavelength-dependent index of refraction). Normal dispersion is the dispersion in which the refractive index decreases monotonically and continuously with increasing wavelength; anomalous dispersion is the opposite. For wavelengths above 1.3 μm, several types of fibers exist exhibiting either normal or anomalous dispersion; by splicing different lengths of fibers together, one can obtain a cavity with adjustable overall dispersion. Below 1.3 μm, only normal dispersion fibers existed; so previous researchers used bulk devices (e.g., grating pairs and prisms) to provide an adjustable amount of dispersion for the cavity. Unfortunately, these devices require the coupling of the fiber into a bulk device, which results in a laser that is highly sensitive to alignment and thus the environment.

Photonics crystal fibers (PCFs) show novel properties by manipulating its structure, such as hollow lattice shapes and filling factors, to obtain both normal and anomalous dispersion below the 1.3 μm range [38–43]. It can be designed and used to compensate both the dispersion and its slope in the cavity to generate a short-pulsed fiber laser by selecting various PCFs. Furthermore, due to one of its unique features of smaller effective area, strong nonlinear effects such as self-phase modulation (SPM) can be caused in the fiber. This allows shorter cavities by selecting appropriate PCFs.

Most recently, PolarOnyx and Cornell University have independently developed several types of seed oscillators by using fibers without dispersion compensation or with minimum dispersion compensation. PolarOnyx even introduced a seed oscillator operating at 1 MHz pulse repetition rate.

In the following sections, we will discuss high-energy ultrafast fiber lasers (Section 20.3.1) and their applications (Section 20.3.2) and high-power ultrafast fiber lasers (Section 20.3.3) and their applications (Section 20.3.4). For high-energy ultrafast fiber lasers, we talk about low repetition rate (<2 MHz) and high energy (>1 μJ). For the high-power ultrafast fiber lasers, we discuss high repetition rate (tens of MHz) and low energy (tens of nJ to hundreds of nJ).

20.3.1 High-Energy Ultrafast Fiber Lasers

Figure 20.2 shows a schematic diagram of the high-energy fiber laser system by several fiber laser groups, such as PolarOnyx, Cornell University, and IMRA. It includes a seed mode-locked fs fiber laser operating in the 1030–1064 nm spectral region, fiber stretcher, an acoustic–optic modulator (pulse picker) reducing the repetition rate from tens of MHz to a range of 10 kHz to 2 MHz, and high-energy/power fiber amplifier systems. Up to 100 μJ has been developed into product (www.polaronyx.com). However, due to the nonlinearity, gain narrowing, and third-order dispersion (TOD) mismatch, the pulse width is limited to sub-ps level.

Researchers at Cornell University have shown that the nonlinear phase shift accumulated by a pulse in amplification can actually be compensated for to some degree by the cubic spectral phase [51–53]. Two effects that are separately detrimental to pulses can thus combine to improve linear propagation. This conclusion has important consequences for short-pulse fiber amplifiers. First, *the performance of a chirped pulse amplification (CPA) system with a fiber stretcher and a grating compressor actually improves with nonlinearity.* This behavior contrasts with that of a CPA system with a grating stretcher and a compressor, where the pulse fidelity decreases monotonically with nonlinear phase shift. Second, near the optimal value of the nonlinear phase, *a fiber stretcher can perform better than a grating stretcher.* Of course, a fiber stretcher offers overwhelming practical advantages over a grating stretcher, so the improved performance comes with no practical trade-off.

A qualitative explanation of the compensation is the following: After stretching, the pulse develops a slightly asymmetric intensity profile owing to the TOD of the fiber. The peak of the pulse

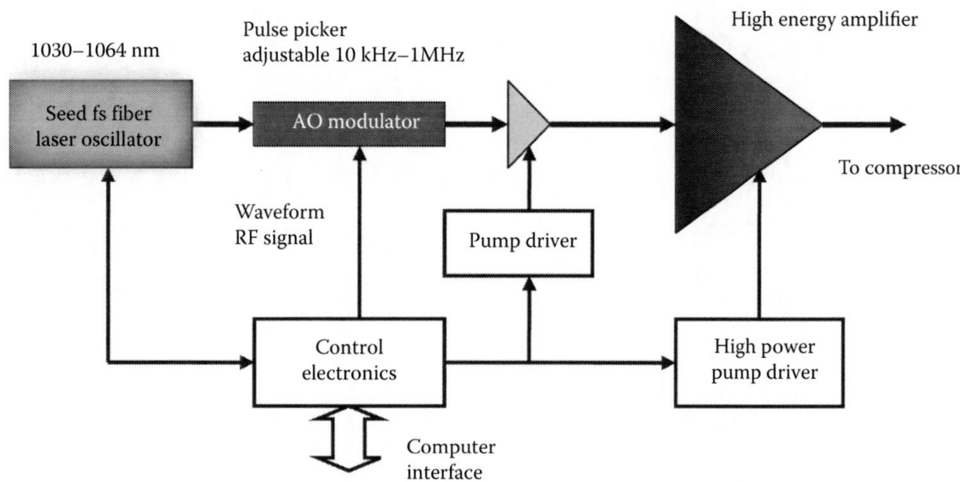

FIGURE 20.2 Schematic diagram of the ultrafast high-energy fiber laser system.

moves to slightly earlier (negative) time, while the asymmetric tail extends to later time, for $d^3\phi/d\omega^3 > 0$. The nonlinear phase shift accumulated by the stretched pulse is then also peaked at slightly negative time, and the temporal phase has negative slope at the center of the pulse. In the compressor, the large quadratic phase from group velocity dispersion (GVD) is subtracted off, while the positive TOD counters the negative phase slope. This intuitive explanation seems to be consistent with theory and initial experiments (below), but more work is needed to clarify the process completely.

Numerical simulations clearly show that TOD and nonlinearity can compensate each other. CPA with a fiber stretcher, a fiber amplifier, and a grating compressor was modeled. 150-fs pulses are stretched to 180 ps in 400 m of SMF. The amplifier consists of 2 m of Yb-doped gain fiber. The magnitude of the nonlinear phase shift is adjusted by varying the gain of the amplifier. The compressor is a pair of gratings. The nonlinear Schrödinger equations that govern propagation in each section are solved by the standard split-step technique.

A pulse that propagates through the amplifier with small nonlinear phase shift (Figure 20.3, left panel) exhibits the signature asymmetric broadening and secondary structure from TOD. The full-width at half-maximum pulse duration has increased to 420 fs. Increasing the nonlinear phase shift improves the quality of the output pulse. For the modeled configuration, best results are obtained with $\Phi^{NL} \approx 15\pi$. With this nonlinear phase shift, the compressed pulse (Figure 20.3, right panel) duration is reduced to 280 fs, and the trailing "wing" of the pulse is suppressed. For larger nonlinear phase shifts, the pulse quality degrades. Thus, for a given amount of cubic phase, there is an optimal value of Φ^{NL}.

The results of a series of similar calculations with varying nonlinear phase shift are summarized in Figure 20.4. The relative peak power is defined as the ratio of the peak power of the output pulse to the ideal peak power that would be obtained in the absence of TOD and nonlinear phase shift. With a grating stretcher, the relative peak power decreases monotonically with Φ^{NL}, as is well known. The relative peak power with a fiber stretcher increases until $\Phi^{NL} \sim 12\pi$, and then decreases. For $\Phi^{NL} > \mathbf{4\pi}$ the fiber stretcher performs better than the grating stretcher.

PolarOnyx used a novel fiber-based dispersion management stretcher (patents 7,430,224; 7,430,226; 7,477,667; and 7,440,173; granted to PolarOnyx, Inc.) in dechirping the pulse and reducing TOD to the minimum. One of the key pulse-shaping techniques is to manipulate the TOD of the fiber. Basically, the dispersion in the fiber is controlled by both material dispersion and waveguide dispersion. In the 1020–1090 nm spectral region, material dispersion shows a positive dispersion slope. With traditional fiber designs such as that for Corning's (Corning, NY) SMF-28, the TOD is always a positive number around 0.3 ps/nm^2 km, which does not match the TOD of the grating compressor used. However, by manipulating the fiber waveguide structure (with a depressed cladding), waveguide dispersion can be introduced to modify the material dispersion such that the TOD and dispersion slope of the whole fiber system are matched, especially with the grating compressor.

The bulk grating pair is used as a compressor. If photonic band gap fiber (PBF) can be used in the compression stage, a truly all-fiber solution is provided for the high-energy fiber laser without any discrete free-space components. This is significant for many industrial applications.

In the high-power PCF amplifier, first, a PCF is used to provide large mode field diameter (60 μm) for signal amplification in the core and large numerical aperture (NA) as high as 0.8 in the cladding

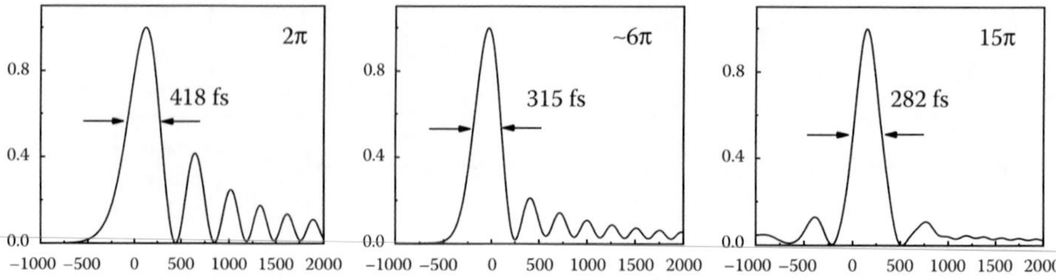

FIGURE 20.3 Results of numerical simulations that demonstrate that SPM and TOD can compensate for each other. The nonlinear phase shift is indicated in each panel.

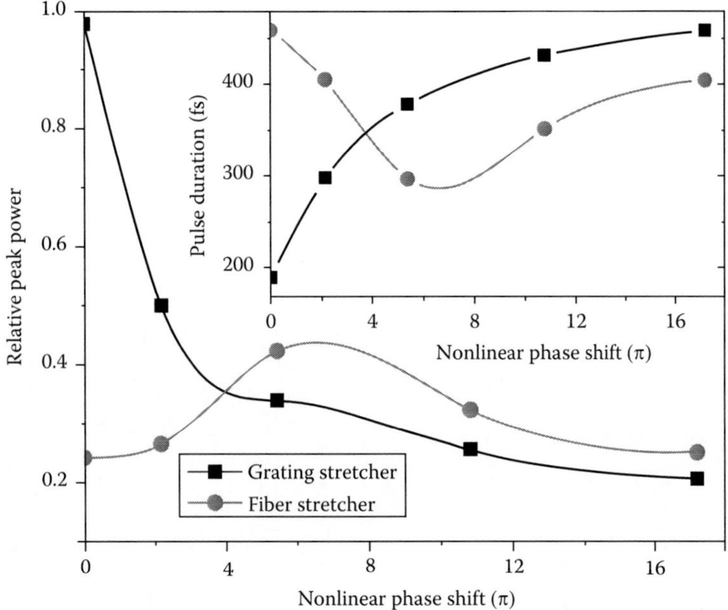

FIGURE 20.4 Variation of relative peak power with Φ^{NL} for CPA with grating (square symbols) and fiber (round symbols) stretchers. The inset shows the variation of the pulse duration with Φ^{NL}.

for coupling more pump power into the fiber. This enables the use of a short length of fiber to increase average output power and to reduce the effect of nonlinearity for high-energy pulse. Second, the PCF is highly doped, so more power extraction can be accomplished. Figure 20.5 shows detailed design of the PCF high-power amplifier with integrated pump solution. It has a total of 200 W pump power launched into the PCF amplifier. An experiment at 100 μJ level energy (100 W average power) with a pulse width < 600 fs has been demonstrated at a pulse repetition rate of 1 MHz.

Figure 20.6 shows the pulse train and autocorrelation trace for 100 μJ level energy (100 W average power) operation. The contrast ratio (peak voltage/valley voltage) is higher than 36 dB, which indicates very clean pulse amplification. The pulse width is 600 fs. The satellite pulse comes with the nonperfect PM fiber design (PM: polarization maintaining). Figure 20.6 shows the beam quality with M2 < 1.3.

20.3.2 High-Energy Ultrafast Fiber Laser Applications

20.3.2.1 Dependence on Laser Processing Parameters

Several variables control the fs microstructuring process: the laser pulse energy, the beam quality and focusing conditions, the laser repetition rate, and the speed and direction with which the sample

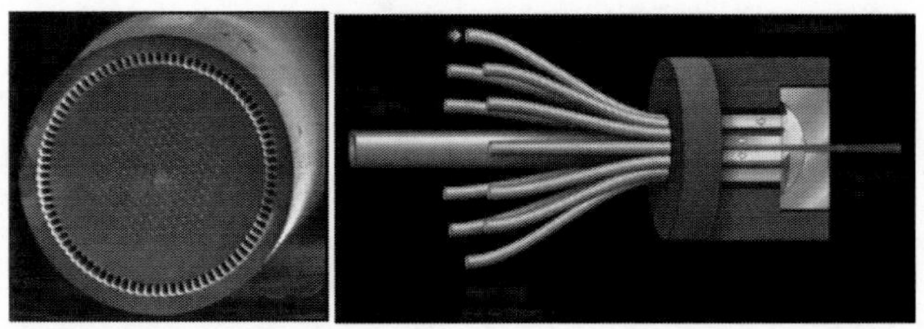

FIGURE 20.5 PCF fiber and pump coupling package (NKT).

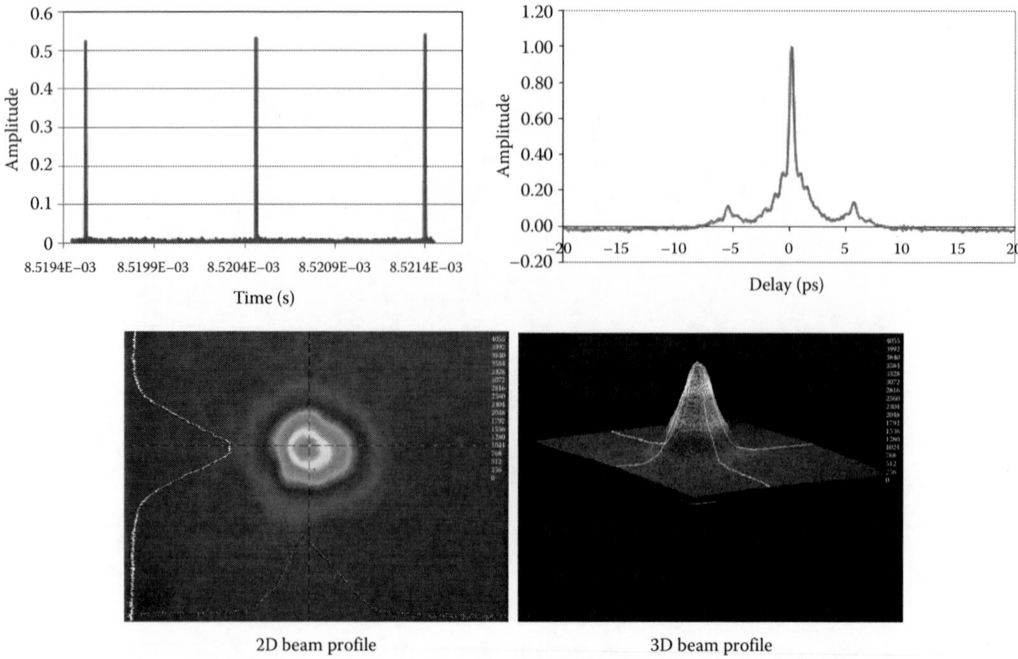

FIGURE 20.6 Pulse train, autocorrelation trace, and beam quality of the compressed pulse for 100 W and 100 μJ operation.

is moved. The laser fluence, which is determined by the laser pulse energy, the beam quality, and focusing conditions, is typically the most influential experimental variable for all of the writing configurations [55–67]. Adjusting the laser fluence by an order of magnitude can cause dramatically different results: from no modification, to the controlled modification used for producing microstructured devices, to uncontrolled damage as shown in Figure 20.7.

This sensitivity results from the modification process having a highly nonlinear dependence on the peak intensity (I), which is directly proportional to the fluence (F) for a fixed pulse width (τ). Since most fs laser systems have pulse widths of ~100 fs, the laser fluence (J/cm^2) has become the

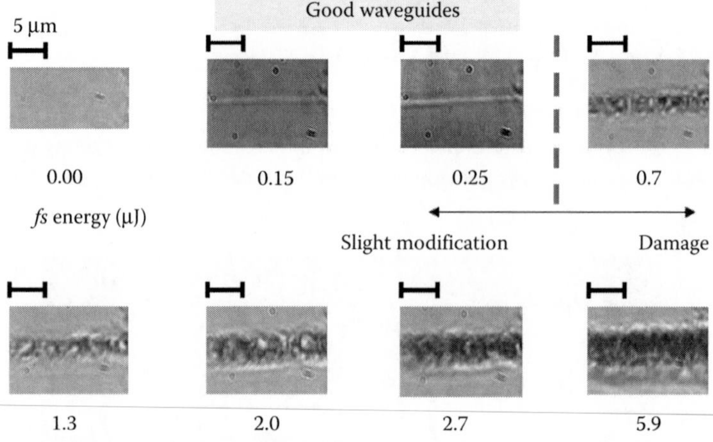

FIGURE 20.7 White-light microscopy images showing the morphology of waveguides and damage lines using different fs pulse energies through a 50 × objective.

standard parameter for describing experimental conditions. Pulse intensity, pulse fluence, and pulse width are related by

$$I = \frac{F}{\tau} = \frac{E}{\tau A} \tag{20.1}$$

$$A = \frac{\pi w_0^2}{4} \tag{20.2}$$

$$w_0 = \frac{2M^2\lambda}{\pi N} \tag{20.3}$$

where I is the intensity, F the pulse fluence, E the pulse energy, τ pulse duration, A the beam area, w_0 the beam waist diameter, λ the laser wavelength, M the beam quality factor, and N the NA.

Figure 20.8 shows the ablation depth under the radiation of laser pulses with durations from 70 fs to less than 1 ps. In Figure 20.5 (left), the laser pulse duration is 70 fs, and most model prediction points are close to the experimental measurement points. The ablation depth increases from around 30 nm at 1 J/cm^2 to around 250 nm at 10 J/cm^2, indicating that increasing laser pulse fluence in this range can increase the laser ablation depth very effectively. The differences between model predictions and measurements get a little bit larger for longer pulses as shown in Figure 20.8 (middle and right). However, the agreement is still reasonably good. Figure 20.9 illustrates the plume development under 100-fs laser pulse ablation in a depth of 400 nm and a time interval of 1 ns. These modelings help in understanding the laser–material interaction and are critical for process optimization.

The laser repetition rate is another important experimental parameter. There are clear advantages of using a high repetition rate laser system. The high repetition rates increase the production rate of the marking, and so the scan speed of the material can be increased.

20.3.2.2 Material Microstructuring and Processing

An fs fiber laser (Uranus Series, PolarOnyx, Inc.) was used to write waveguide in glass samples with the transverse writing configuration. Figure 20.10 shows examples of various waveguide structures: 2D structures (two parallel waveguides) and 3D structures obtained by writing waveguides at different depths in glass. The writing speed is 100 mm/s and a 50 × microscopic lens was used. The power was adjusted to get the optimized results. It shows that the fs fiber laser can write waveguide for photonic devices with the unique features of flexibility in structure shapes, 2D and 3D dimensions,

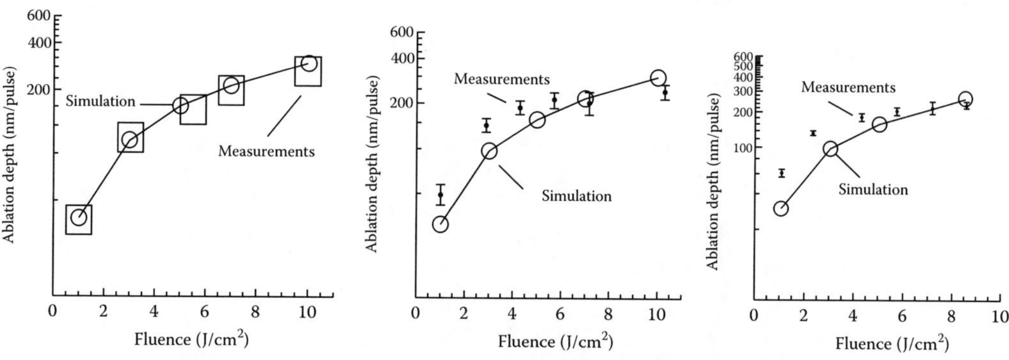

FIGURE 20.8 The variation of ablation depth with laser fluence, at varying laser pulse duration: 70 fs (left), 150 fs (middle), and 500 fs (right).

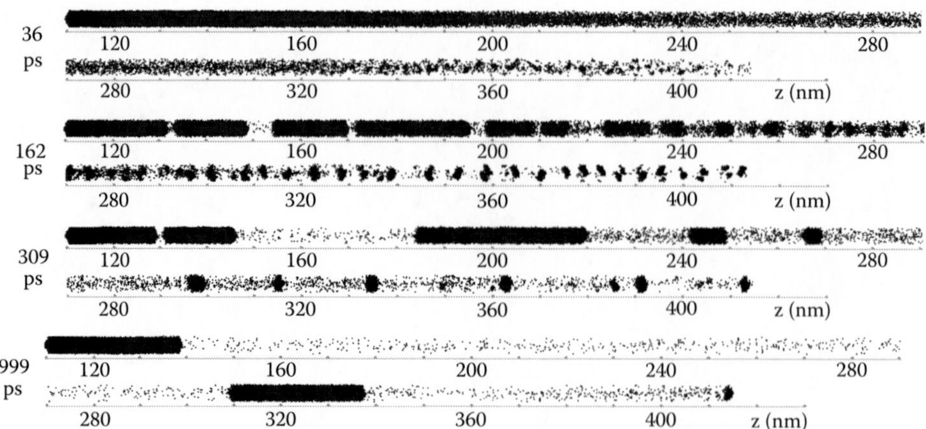

FIGURE 20.9 Plume development within 1 ns.

and writing materials. This provides a solid foundation for 3D photonic device fabrication, which is the future for next-generation telecommunication components.

To further demonstrate the capability of the fs fiber lasers and compare the performance with other types of nanosecond (ns) lasers, we have performed microstructuring on silicon and copper. Our fs fiber laser was adjusted to have similar energy and repetition rate as those of the ns laser to make a comparable testing. Figure 20.11 shows the experimental results with parameters listed in the figures. It does show that the fs fiber laser has little HAZ and finer structure.

An fs fiber laser system has also been used to drill through holes with the trepanning drilling strategy. The laser system consists of a high-energy fs fiber laser, a high-precision three-axis positioning system, and a high-speed scanner. The laser parameters used are as follows: pulse duration 0.8 ps, wavelength 1030 nm, average power 0.7 W, and repetition rate 100 kHz. The laser beam is directed by two successive mirrors inside the scanner and thus holes larger than the laser focal spot diameter (20 μm) can be drilled. The advantage of the trepanning method is that it allows for drilling holes of various sizes and shapes without changing the setup. Noncircular holes can be easily attained.

Figures 20.12 shows the entrance and side view of a through hole drilled on a steel plate. The steel plate has a thickness of 812.8 μm. The roundness of the hole on the entrance side and exit side was quite good. The diameter of the hole entrance is 290 μm, and that of the exit is 150 μm. The taper angle is less than 5°, which reveals that the conicity is very small, that is, the taper angle is about 4°.

20.3.3 High-Power Ultrafast Fiber Lasers

In biomedical applications, achieving 100 fs pulse widths has long been conceived as a barrier for high-power fs fiber lasers to compete with solid-state lasers (such as 80 MHz, 1 W Ti:sapphire

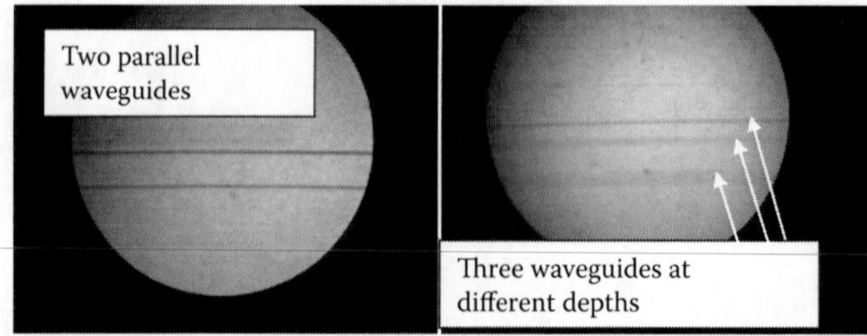

FIGURE 20.10 Glass waveguide fabrication with 2D and 3D configurations.

Silicon wafer: comparison of heat effect

fs laser

Pav = 1.4 W, f = 30 mm, S.S. 0.1 mm/s, line width = 22 um

SHG laser

Pav = 1.66 W, f = 100 mm, S.S. = 200 mm/s, line width = 36 um

Heat affected zone

LP-V10

Pave = 2.1 W, f = 100 mm, S.S. = 200 mm/s, line width = 30 um

Comparison conditions
- Average power approx. same

※ V10: least marking power
※ same magnification photographs

Laser	Rep rate	Pulse width	Wave-length
FS	10 kHz	350 fs	1030 nm
SHG	40 kHz	12 ns	532 nm
LP-V10	40 kHz	30 ns	1064 nm

Copper: comparison of heat effect

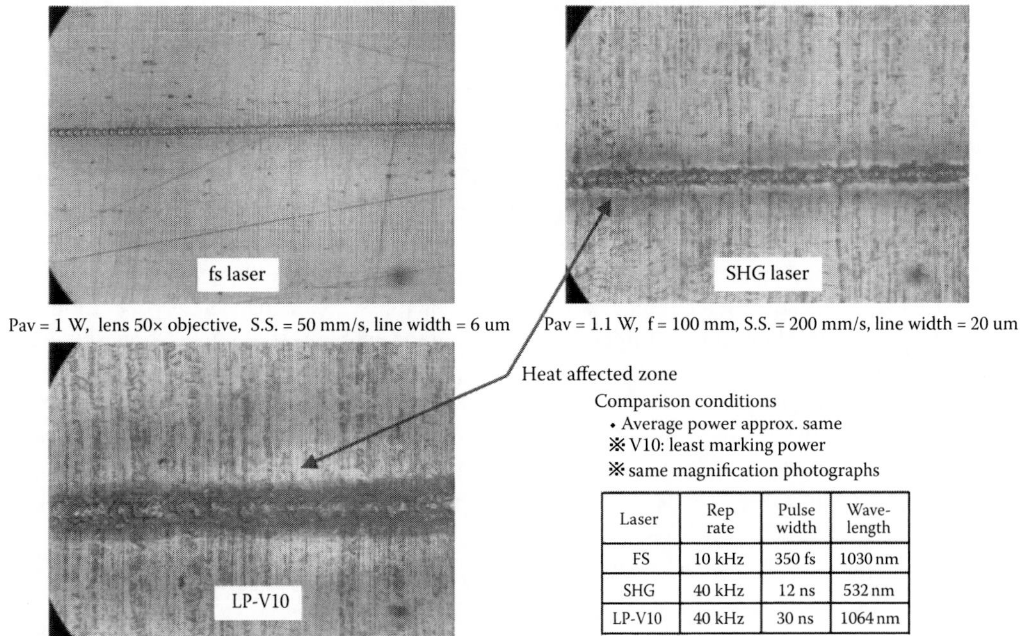

Laser	Rep rate	Pulse width	Wave-length
FS	10 kHz	350 fs	1030 nm
SHG	40 kHz	12 ns	532 nm
LP-V10	40 kHz	30 ns	1064 nm

Pav = 4.7 W, f = 100 mm, S.S. = 200 mm/s, line width = 37 um

FIGURE 20.11 Experimental results of femtosecond fiber laser microstructuring and comparison.

lasers), since most ultrafast laser applications such as nonlinear imaging, tissue ablation, and coherent supercontinuum generation require pulse widths down to that level. Over the past several years, high-power fs fiber lasers have been intensively investigated both in industry and academia. Although average power as high as 200 W has been reported for many fs fiber lasers, 100 fs pulse widths are still a technical barrier for the ultrafast fiber laser community.

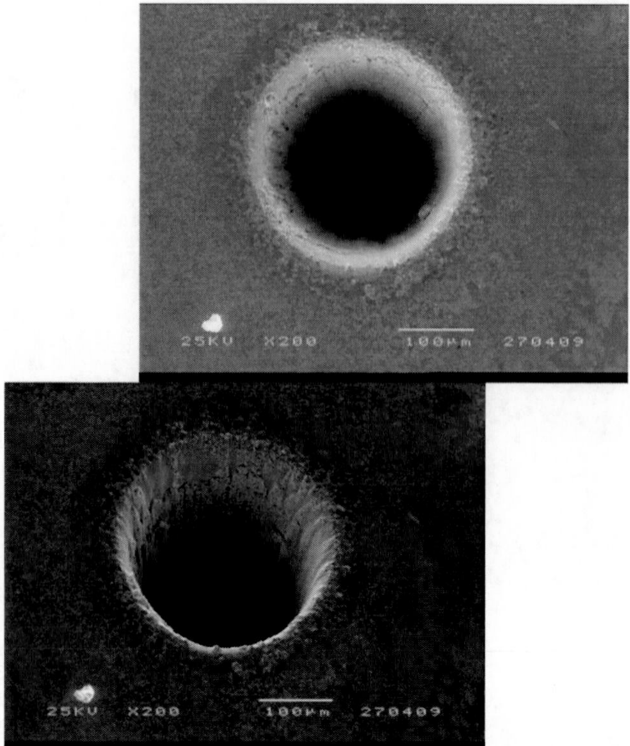

FIGURE 20.12 The entrance and side view of a hole. The diameter of the hole entrance is 290 μm.

At Photonics West 2010 in San Francisco, CA, PolarOnyx broke the 100 fs bottleneck using a novel development in high-power fs fiber laser technology. Using our proprietary pulse-shaping and spectral-shaping technologies, the pulse width of our high-power fs fiber lasers was compressed to 100 fs. This significant improvement (100 fs versus 200 fs) opens a wide range of applications for fs fiber lasers and will enable the aggressive replacement of solid-state lasers in addition to the already well-known fiber laser features of compactness, maintenance-free operation, and cost-effectiveness (see table). The fs fiber lasers are now the enabling technology for many industrial and clinical applications.

The challenges to pulse-width reduction of fs fiber lasers are the management of dispersion, nonlinearity, and gain narrowing. Compared to solid-state lasers, due to the relatively long length of fibers and gain medium, fiber lasers experience severe nonlinearity and gain-narrowing effects. These impact the pulse shape and spectral bandwidth and limit the compressed pulse width to typically 200 fs for 1 W operation. Moreover, the high-order dispersion (HOD) mismatch between the fiber and the grating compressor used in the fs fiber laser makes this cancellation or compensation even more difficult.

To resolve these issues, researchers at Cornell University investigated a high-power mode-locked fiber laser oscillator that exploits dissipative-soliton pulse shaping along with cladding pumping for high average power [68]. By properly selecting the optical filter bandwidth and adjusting the polarization, stable mode locking can be achieved. The fiber laser generates 31 nJ chirped pulses at 70 MHz repetition rate, for an average power of 2.2 W. After dechirping outside the laser, 15 nJ, 80 fs pulses with 200 kW peak power are obtained (see Figure 20.13).

This approach is a breakthrough in fs fiber laser research that overcomes the pulse-width bottleneck. With proper control of the energy propagation and filtering effect, HOD and gain narrowing can be mitigated. However, due to the complexity of operation and involvement of free-space components, significant effort is required to develop a practical product.

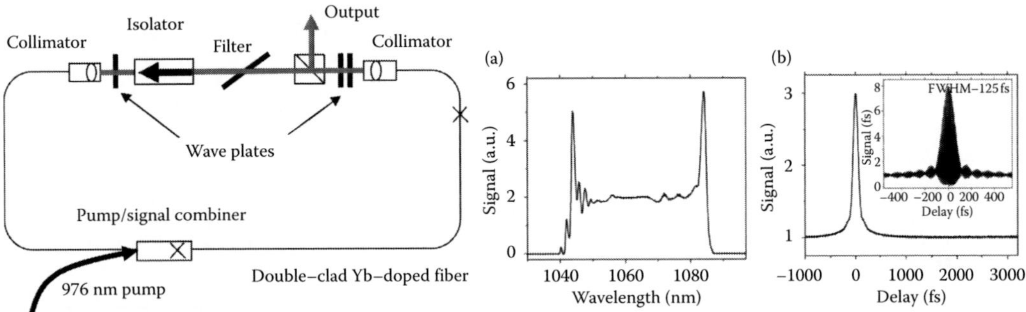

FIGURE 20.13 High-power femtosecond fiber laser oscillator configuration (a) and its performance of spectrum (b) and autocorrelation (c).

A master oscillator power amplifier (MOPA) design has proven to be a reliable approach for fs fiber lasers and has been adopted in current products from companies such as PolarOnyx (San Jose, CA) and IMRA (Ann Arbor, MI). As an example, PolarOnyx's fs fiber lasers operate at 30–100 MHz repetition rate, 100 fs pulse widths, and greater than 1 W compressed output power using the MOPA design (see Figure 20.14). By using polarization, pulse, and spectral-shaping technologies to properly design the fiber laser oscillator and amplifier, the pulse generation and amplification can have an excellent balance among the HOD, dispersion, nonlinear distortion, and gain narrowing (United States patents: 7,430,224; 7,440,173; 7,555,022; 7,477,666; 7,593,434; 7,529,278; 7,526,003; and 7,430,226. Granted to PolarOnyx, Inc.).

One of the key pulse-shaping techniques is to manipulate the TOD of the fiber. Basically, the dispersion in the fiber is controlled by both material dispersion and waveguide dispersion. In the 1020–1090 nm spectral region, material dispersion shows a positive dispersion slope. With traditional fiber designs such as that for Corning's (Corning, NY) SMF-28, the TOD is always a positive number around 0.3 ps/nm^2 km, which does not match the TOD of the grating compressor used. However, by manipulating the fiber waveguide structure (with a depressed cladding), waveguide dispersion can be introduced to modify the material dispersion such that the TOD and dispersion slope of the whole fiber system are matched, especially with the grating compressor.

Another key spectral-shaping technique used for reducing the pulse width is to obtain enough pulse spectral bandwidth by taking advantage of the SPM that may take place after the amplification stage such that the broadening spectrum will not be limited by the gain spectrum or narrowing effect of the amplifier. The fiber implemented in the amplification stage should have appropriate length in order to generate the required spectrum bandwidth. The SPM effect causes spectral broadening when the peak power of the pulse reaches a certain level. Depending on the pulse energy level and pulse width (that defines the peak power), the broadening factor can be optimized by selecting the right length and fiber type. Moreover, proper control of SPM can balance the TOD mismatch between the fiber stretcher and bulk-grating compressors.

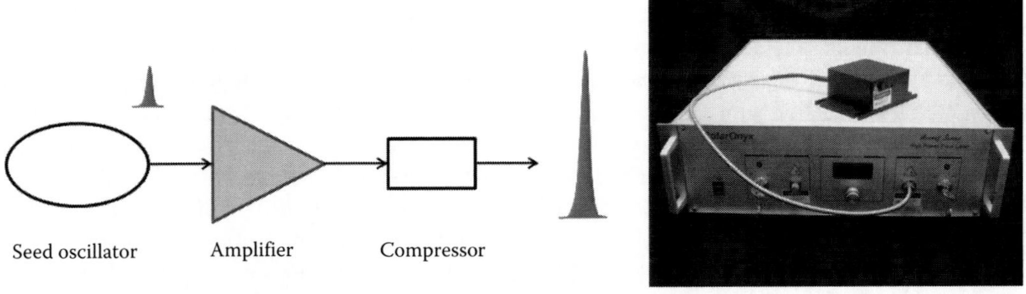

FIGURE 20.14 High-power femtosecond fiber laser with MOPA configuration and product photograph.

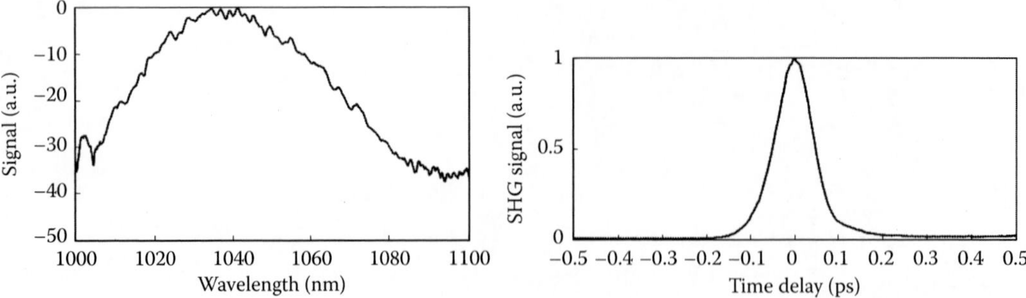

FIGURE 20.15 Spectrum and pulse width of a 1 W fs fiber laser.

These techniques resolve the trade-off between power scaling and pulse-width broadening, in which the amplified spectral bandwidth can support the 100 fs pulse width without significant residual TOD and gain-narrowing effects. Assuming transform-limited pulse quality, a 100 fs pulse is supported by a 15-nm spectral bandwidth.

The 1 W, 100 fs fiber laser has a pulse repetition rate of 33 MHz, compressed pulse energy of 30 nJ, and an average power of 1.4 W. With an operating wavelength around 1035 nm, the actual measured pulse width is 90 fs with a Gaussian shape assumption (see Figure 20.15). It has a compact compressor integrated with the fiber laser for ease of operation and reliability. For a pulse width of 200 fs, output power levels as high as 5 W compressed have been achieved. Further optimization can be performed toward a pulse width of 100 fs. And by adding an optical parametric oscillator as a supplement, the wavelength can cover from the visible to mid-IR range, further extending the capability of fs fiber lasers.

20.3.4 High-Power Ultrafast Fiber Laser Applications

The fs fiber lasers provide clear advantages in terms of price, reliability, and maintenance, and are becoming a driving force for clinical applications [69].

Recently, efforts to develop compact multiphoton systems for *in vivo* imaging and clinical applications use fs pulses from ultrafast lasers coupled into double-clad PCFs or hollow-core PBFs. Fiber-connected miniature scanning probes have been developed to provide flexible access to tissue and to acquire multiphoton microscopy (MPM) images. While the probes are becoming smaller and smaller, the sources they use are often traditional solid-state Ti:sapphire lasers that are bulky, expensive, not portable, and require precise alignment. Finding new ultrafast laser sources that are low-cost, compact, and portable is expected to enhance the impact of MPM in research and particularly in clinical studies.

Subcellular laser ablation (SLA) has emerged as a powerful tool for the measurement of mechanical properties of load-bearing cytoskeletal elements in their living, intracellular context [70]. In SLA, high-energy laser pulses of ultrashort (100 fs) duration are focused through a high-NA objective lens onto an intracellular target, such as an organelle or a cytoskeletal element. Using an ultrashort pulse, material at the laser focus undergoes nonlinear multiphoton absorption leading to optical breakdown and material destruction with minimal heat transfer or collateral damage to surrounding structures. Proof-of-principle studies demonstrate that these ultrafast systems are capable of destroying a single mitochondrion in a living cell without compromising the plasma membrane.[4]

But despite this progress, compact, fiber-delivered, user-friendly, and economical instruments are needed if fs lasers are to proliferate outside of research environments and find application in multiuser biology facilities, medical clinics, manufacturing environments, and even in mobile facilities. Improved instruments will also greatly facilitate the use of fs techniques in a variety of scientific research projects and industrial applications, particularly if the cost can be reduced. The approximately $150,000 price tag for a Ti:sapphire laser places it beyond the reach of many research groups and applications.

20.4 FUTURE PERSPECTIVES ON ULTRAFAST FIBER LASERS

Ultrafast fiber lasers are being rapidly adopted in diverse fields and applications and have proved to be promising candidates for many applications in defense, biomedical imaging and surgery processing, material microstrucuring and processing, and spectroscopy. Fiber lasers exhibit a range of advantages over solid-state sources, including: compact size, diffraction-limited beam quality, high efficiency, and extremely low-noise and maintenance-free operation. PolarOnyx, Inc. is the worldwide leader in driving research and development of high-power and high-energy ultrafast fiber-based lasers. (The company has twice been recognized for excellence with the receipt of PhAST/Laser Focus World Innovation Awards at CLEO 2006 and CLEO 2007.) IMRA is another company pushing for industrial deployment of ultrafast fiber lasers and successfully integrate their product into the eye surgery system by working with Carl Zeiss.

Over the next few years, we will witness an explosive expansion of the use of ultrafast fiber lasers both in existing fields by replacing traditional solid-state lasers and in unexplored new fields. In addition to present-day 1.55 and 1 μm wavelength regions, more wavelength regions such as 2 μm, 2.7 μm, 3 μm, mid-IR (MIR) and long-wave IR (LWIR), visible, and UV will emerge to find applications everywhere. High-energy and high-power fiber lasers will be continuously pushing for higher energy (>mJ), higher power (>kW), and shorter pulse (<100 fs). The future of ultrafast fiber lasers is beyond our imagination and without boundary.

REFERENCES

1. K. Itoh, W. Watanabe, S. Nolte, and C. B. Schaffer, Ultrafast processes for bulk modification of transparent materials, *MRS Bull.* 31, 620, 2006.
2. M. Davis, K. Miura, N. Sugimoto, and K. Hirao, Writing waveguides in glass with a femtosecond laser, *Opt. Lett.* 21, 1729, 1996.
3. K. Miura, J. R. Qiu, H. Inouye, T. Mitsuyu, and K. Hirao, Photowritten optical waveguides in various glasses with ultrashort pulse laser, *Appl. Phys. Lett.* 71, 3329, 1997.
4. E. N. Glezer, M. Milosavljevic, L. Huang, R. J. Finlay, T.-H. Her, J. P. Callan, and E. Mazur, Three-dimensional optical storage inside transparent materials, *Opt. Lett.* 21, 2023, 1996.
5. E. N. Glezer and E. Mazur, Ultrafast-laser driven micro-explosions in transparent materials, *Appl. Phys. Lett.* 71, 882, 1997.
6. D. Homoelle, S. Wielandy, A. L. Gaeta, N. F. Borrelli, and C. Smith, Infrared photosensitivity in silica glasses exposed to femtosecond laser pulses, *Opt. Lett.* 24, 1311, 1999.
7. A. M. Streltsov and N. F. Borrelli, Fabrication and analysis of a directional coupler written in glass by nanojoule femtosecond laser pulses, *Opt. Lett.* 26, 42, 2001.
8. K. Minoshima, A. M. Kowalevicz, I. Hartl, E. P. Ippen, and J. G. Fujimoto, Photonic device fabrication in glass by use of nonlinear materials processing with a femtosecond laser oscillator, *Opt. Lett*, 26, 1516, 2001.
9. S. Nolte, M. Will, J. Burghoff, and A. Tuennermann, Femtosecond waveguide writing: A new avenue to three-dimensional integrated optics, *Appl. Phys.* A77, 109, 2003.
10. J. Liu, Z. Zhang, S. Chang, C. Flueraru, and C. P. Grover, Directly writing of 1-to-N optical waveguide power splitters in fused silica glass using a femtosecond laser, *Opt. Commun.* 253, 315, 2005.
11. Y. Sikorski, A. A. Said, P. Bado, R. Maynard, C. Florea, and K. A. Winick, Optical waveguide amplifier in Nd-doped glass written with near-IR femtosecond laser pulses, *Electron. Lett.* 36, 226, 2000.
12. R. Osellame, S. Taccheo, G. Cerullo, M.Marangoni, D. Polli, R. Ramponi, P. Laporta, and S. De Silvestri, Optical gain in Er-Yb doped waveguides fabricated by femtosecond laser pulses, *Electron. Lett.* 38, 964, 2002.
13. S. Taccheo et al., Er:Yb-doped waveguide laser fabricated by femtosecond laser pulses, *Opt. Lett.* 29, 2626, 2004.

14. R. Osellame, N. Chiodo, G. Della Valle, G. Cerullo, R. Ramponi, P. Laporta, A.Killi, U. Morgner, and O. Svelto, Waveguide Lasers in the C-Band Fabricated by Laser Inscription With a Compact Femtosecond Oscillator, *IEEE J. Sel. Top. Quantum Electron.* 12, 277, 2006.
15. Y. Kondo, K. Nouchi, T. Mitsuyu, M. Watanabe, P. G. Kazansky, and K. Hirao, Fabrication of long-period fiber gratings by focused irradiation of infrared femtosecond laser pulses, *Opt. Lett.* 24, 646, 1999.
16. H.-B. Sun, Y. Xu, S. Juodkazis, K. Sun, M. Watanabe, S. Matsuo, H. Misawa, and J. Nishii, Arbitrary-lattice photonic crystals created by multiphoton microfabrication, *Opt. Lett.* 26, 325, 2001.
17. S. J. Mihailov, C. W. Smelser, P. Lu, R. B. Walker, D. Grobnic, H. Ding, G. Henderson, and J. Unruh, Fiber Bragg gratings made with a phase mask and 800-nm femtosecond radiation, *Opt. Lett.* 28, 995, 2003.
18. M. Masuda, K. Sugioka, Y. Cheng, N. Aoki, M. Kawachi, K. Shihoyama, K. Toyoda, H. Helvajian, and K. Midorikawa, 3D microstructuring inside photosensitive glass by femtosecond laser excitation, *Appl. Phys. A* 76, 857, 2003.
19. Y. Cheng, K. Sugioka, K. Midorikawa, M. Masuda, K. Toyoda, M. Kawachi, and K. Shihoyama, Control of the cross-sectional shape of a hollow microchannel embedded in photostructurable glass by use of a femtosecond laser, *Opt. Lett.* 28, 55, 2003.
20. Y. Cheng, K. Sugioka, K. Midorikawa, M. Masuda, K. Toyoda, M. Kawachi, and K. Shihoyama, Three-dimensional micro-optical components embedded in photosensitive glass by a femtosecond laser, *Opt. Lett.* 28, 1144, 2003.
21. Y. Cheng, Z. Xua, K. Sugioka, and K. Midorikawa, Femtosecond laser microfabrication of 3D structures in Foturan glass *Proc. SPIE* 6400, 640001, 2006.
22. A. Marcinkevicius, S. Juodkazis, M. Watanabe, M. Miwa, S. Matsuo, H.Misawa, and J. Nishii, *Opt. Lett.*, 26, 277, 2001.
23. Y. Bellouard, A. Said, M. Dugan, and P. Bado, Scanning thermal microscopy and Raman analysis of bulk fused silica exposed to low energy femtosecond laser pulses, *Opt. Express* 12, 2120, 2004.
24. C. Hnatovsky, R. S. Taylor, E. Simova, P. P. Rajeev, D. M. Rayner, V. R. Bhardwaj, and P. B. Corkum, Fabrication of microchannels in glass using focused femtosecond laser radiation and selective chemical etching, *Appl. Phys. A: Mater. Sci. Process.* 84, 47, 2006.
25. V. Maselli, R. Osellame, G. Cerullo, R. Ramponi, P. Laporta, L. Magagnin, and P. L. Cavallotti, Fabrication of long microchannels with circular cross section using astigmatically shaped femtosecond laser pulses and chemical etching, *Appl. Phys. Lett.*, 88, 191107, 2006.
26. T. N. Kim, K. Campbell, A. Groisman, D. Kleinfeld, and C. B. Schaffer, Femtosecond laser-drilled capillary integrated into a microfluidic device, *Appl. Phys. Lett.* 86, 201106, 2005.
27. R. An, Y. Li, Y. Dou, D. Liu, H. Yang, and Q. Gong, Picosecond and low-power all-optical switching based on an organic photonic-bandgap microcavity, *Appl. Phys. A: Mater. Sci. Process.* 83, 27, 2006.
28. C. Hnatovsky, R. S. Taylor, P. P. Rajeev, E. Simova, V. R. Bhardwaj, D. M. Rayner, and P. B. Corkum, Pulse duration dependence of femtosecond-laser-fabricated nanogratings in fused silica, *Appl. Phys. Lett.* 87, 014104, 2005.
29. A. Killi et al., High peak power pulses from a cavity dumped Yb: KY(WO4)2 oscillator, *Opt. Lett.* 30(14), 1891–1893, 2005.
30. C. P. J. Barty et al., Generation of 18 fs multiterawatt pulses by regenerative pulse shaping and chirped pulse amplification, *Opt. Lett.* 21(9), 668–670, 1996.
31. R. J. Jones and J. Ye, Femtosecond pulse amplification by coherent addition in a passive optical cavity, *Opt. Lett.* 27, 1848–1850, 2002.
32. W. F. Krupke, Ytterbium solid state lasers—The first decade, *J. Sel. Top. Quantum Electron.* 6(6), 1287–1296, 2000.
33. H. Hemmati, M. Wright, and C. Esproles, High efficiency pulsed laser transmitters for deep space communications, *SPIE* 3932, 188–195, 2000.
34. D. C. Brown, Ultrahigh average power diode pumped Nd: YAG and Yb: YAG lasers, *IEEE J. Quantum Electron.* 33, 861–873, 1998.
35. D. C. Browns, Nonlinear thermal distortion in YAG rod amplifiers, *IEEE J. Quantum Electron.* 34, 2383, 1998.
36. D. C. Browns, Nonlinear thermal and stress effects and scaling behavior of YAG slab amplifiers, *IEEE J. Quantum Electron.* 34, 2392, 1998.
37. J. Nilsson et al., High power fiber lasers: New developments, *SPIE* 4974, 50–59, 2003.
38. D. Gapontsev Fiber lasers VI: Technology, systems, and applications, *SPIE*, 7195, 2009.

39. J. Limpert et al., High power rod-type photonic crystal fiber laser, *Opt. Express* 13, 1055–1058, 2005.
40. J. Limpert et al., Low nonlinearity single transverse mode Yb doped photonic crystal fiber amplifier, *Opt. Express* 12, 1313–1319, 2004.
41. Y. Jeong, J. Sahu, D. Payne, and J. Nilsson, Ytterbium-doped large-core fiber laser with 1.36 kW continuous-wave output power, *Opt. Express* 12, 6088–6092, 2004.
42. J. Limpert et al., Thermo-optical properties of air-clad photonic crystal fiber lasers in high power operation, *Opt. Express* 11, 2982–2990, 2003.
43. A. Tunnermann et al., Large mode area fibers for high power laser operation based on solid and air microstructured cores, *SPIE* 5709, 301–309, 2005.
44. P. Russell, Photonic crystal fibers, *Science 299*, 358, 2003.
45. G. P. Lee et al., Q switched erbium doped fiber laser utilizing a novel large mode area fiber. *Electron. Lett.* 33(5), 393–394, 1998.
46. A. Galvanauskes, High power fiber laser, *Opt. Photonics News*, 42–44, 2004.
47. B. Desthieux, R. L. Laming, and D. N. Payne, 111 kW Pulse amplification, *Appl. Phys. Lett.* 63(5), 585–588, 1993.
48. D. Taverner et al., Generation of high energy pulses using a large mode area erbium doped fiber amplifier, *Proc. CLEO'*, 96, 496–497, 1996.
49. J. Limpert et al., High average power femtosecond fiber CPA system, *Opt. Lett.* 28, 1984, 2003.
50. D. Strickland and G. Mourou, Compression of amplified chirped optical pulses, *Opt. Commun.* 56, 219, 1985.
51. S. Zhou, L. Kuznetsova, A. Chong, and F. Wise, Compensation of nonlinear phase shifts with third-order dispersion in short-pulse fiber amplifiers, *Opt. Express* 13, 4869–4877, 2005.
52. L. Kuznetsova, S. Zhou, A. Chong, and Frank W. Wise, Single -mode fiber source of 0.8 μJ, 150-fs pulses at 1 μm, *Proceedings of the Conference on Lasers and Electro-Optics* (Baltimore, May 2005), paper CTuCC7.
53. Z. Liu, L. Shah, I. Hartl, G. C. Cho, and M. E. Fermann, High-energy fiber chirped-pulse amplification system based on cubicons, *Proceedings of the Conference on Lasers and Electro-Optics* (Baltimore, May 2005), paper CThG4.
54. F. O. Ilday, K. Beckwitt, H. Lim, Y.-F. Chen, and F. W. Wise, Controllable Raman-like nonlinearities from non-stationary cascaded quadratic processes, *J. Opt. Soc. Am. B* 21, 376, 2004.
55. S. C. Jones, P. Braunlich, R. T. Casper, X. A. Shen, and P. Kelly, Recent progress on laser-induced modifications and intrinsic bulk damage of wide-gap optical-materials, *Opt. Eng.* 28, 1039, 1989.
56. C. B. Schaffer, A. Brodeur, and E. Mazur, Laser-induced breakdown and damage in bulk transparent materials induced by tightly focused femtosecond laser pulses, *Meas. Sci. Technol.* 12, 1784, 2001.
57. C. W. Carr, H. B. Radousky, and S. G. Demos, Wavelength dependence of laser-Induced damage: Determining the damage initiation mechanisms, *Phys. Rev. Lett.* 91, 1274021, 2003.
58. B. C. Stuart, M. D. Feit, S. Herman, A. M. Rubenchik, B. W. Shore, and M. D. Perry, Nanosecond-to-femtosecond laser-induced breakdown in dielectrics, *Phys. Rev. B* 53, 1749, 1996.
59. X. Liu, D. Du, and G. Mourou, Laser ablation and micromachining with ultrashort laser pulses, *IEEE J. Quantum Electron.* 33, 1706, 1997.
60. D. Du, X. Liu, G. Korn, J. Squier, and G. Mourou, Laser-induced breakdown by impact ionization in SiO_2 with pulse widths from 7 ns to 150 fs, *Appl. Phys. Lett.* 64, 3071, 1994.
61. T. Q. Jia, Z. Z. Xu, R. X. Li, D. H. Feng, X. X. Li, C. F. Cheng, H. Y. Sun, N. S. Xu, and H. Z. Wang, Mechanisms in fs-laser ablation in fused silica, *J. Appl. Phys.* 95, 5166, 2004.
62. C. H. Fan and J. P. Longtin, Modeling optical breakdown in dielectrics during ultrafast laser processing, *Appl. Opt.* 40, 3124, 2001.
63. S. Juodkazis, K. Nishimura, S. Tanaka, H. Misawa, E. G. Gamaly, B. Luther-Davies, L. Hallo, P. Nicolai, and V. T. Tikhonchuk, Laser-induced microexplosion confined in the bulk of a sapphire crystal: Evidence of multimegabar pressures, *Phys. Rev. Lett.* 96, 166101, 2006.
64. E. G. Gamaly, S. Juodkazis, K. Nishimura, H. Misawa, B. Luther-Davies, L. Hallo, P. Nicolai, and V. T. Tikhonchuk, Laser-matter interaction in the bulk of a transparent solid: Confined microexplosion and void formation, *Phys. Rev. B* 73, 214101, 2006.
65. J. W. Chan, T. Huser, S. Risbud, and D. M. Krol, Structural changes in fused silica after exposure to focused femtosecond laser pulses, *Opt. Lett.* 26, 1726, 2001.
66. C. B. Schaffer, A. Brodeur, J. F. Garcia, and E. Mazur, Micromachining bulk glass by use of femtosecond laser pulses with nanojoule energy, *Opt. Lett.* 26, 93, 2001.
67. L. Shah, A. Y. Arai, S. M. Eaton, and P. R. Herman, Waveguide writing in fused silica with a femtosecond fiber laser at 522 nm and 1 MHz repetition rate, *Opt. Express* 13, 1999, 2005.

68. K. Kieu et al., Sub-100 fs pulses at watt-level powers from a dissipative-soliton fiber laser, *Opt. Lett. 34*, 5, 593–595, 2009.
69. S. Tang et al., Developing compact multiphoton systems using femtosecond fiber lasers, *J. Biomed. Opt.* 14(3), 1–3, 2009.
70. N. Shen et al., Ablation of cytoskeletal filaments and mitochondria in live cells using a femtosecond laser nanoscissor, *Mech. Chem. Biosyst.* 2, 17–25, 2005.

21 High-Speed Directly Modulated Injection-Locked VCSELs

Xu Wang and Lukas Chrostowski

CONTENTS

21.1 INTRODUCTION

21.1.1 Vertical-Cavity Surface-Emitting Lasers

First proposed in 1977 and demonstrated in continuous-wave at room temperature in 1988 [1], vertical-cavity surface-emitting lasers (VCSELs) are now a mature technology with a demonstrated applicability in short-reach optical communications. VCSELs are a type of semiconductor laser with a very short cavity length (typically one or several lasing wavelengths long), and with laser beam emission in the vertical direction, perpendicular to the wafer. The small cavity allows the laser to operate at very low current levels, typically low milliamperes. These lasers are mass fabricated—a 1 cm^2 die may contain 2500 individual lasers—and can be tested on-wafer without the need for dicing and packaging, desirable for low-cost and high-density integration applications. Other advantages include easy fiber coupling due to the circular beam profile, and a single longitudinal mode emission. Finally, VCSELs can be directly modulated for digital and analog communications. It is this last property that makes them interesting for optical interconnect applications, and is the topic of this chapter.

21.2 DIRECT MODULATION OF VCSELs

21.2.1 Introduction

Semiconductor lasers are typically pumped by electrical injection; the electrical current can be modulated using digital or analog data. This is known as direct modulation. The modulation bandwidth (typically in gigahertz) is the most important figure-of-merit for directly modulated lasers, which determines the maximum data rate in optical communication systems (typically in Gb/s) for a given coding scheme. Since the 1990s, tremendous effort has been directed toward optimizing the VCSEL materials, the fabrication processes, and the device structure in order to obtain the highest possible direct current (DC) modulation rates. We have witnessed a steady progress in the increasing trend of data rates. As shown in Figure 21.1, the 3-dB modulation

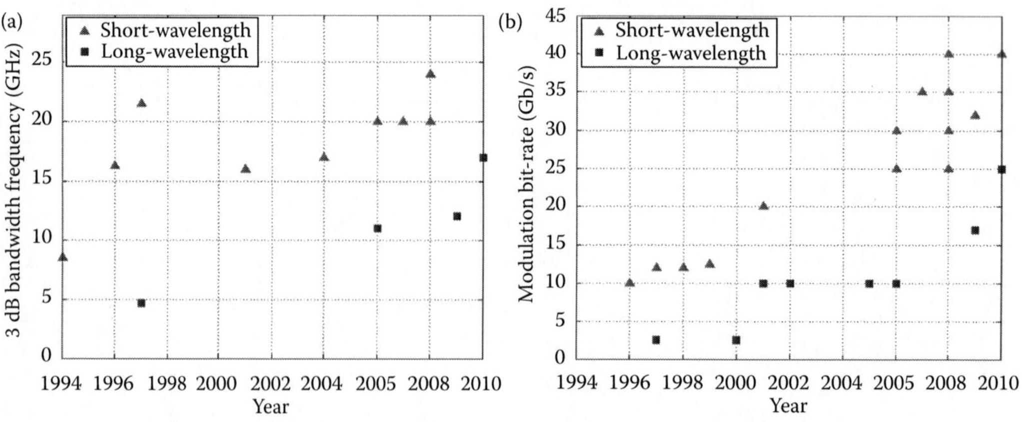

FIGURE 21.1 Historical VCSEL direct modulation records. (a) 3 dB bandwidth and (b) maximum bit rate. Selected representative VCSEL modulation records are shown for research 850 nm VCSELs [3–9], 980 nm VCSELs [10–16], 1100 nm VCSELs [2,17], 1310 nm VCSELs [18–20], and 1550 nm VCSELs [21–28]. Commercially available VCSELs at 10 Gb/s are manufactured at most of these wavelengths.

bandwidth of VCSELs has gradually increased to beyond 20 GHz; this has been followed by an increase in the transmission bit rates demonstrated with VCSELs, up to a record 40 Gb/s [2]. Since different wavelength VCSELs are fabricated with different materials with varying optical and electrical properties, the performance of VCSELs varies with wavelength. Factors such as optical gain and thermal and electrical resistance affect the high-speed performance. In general, the short-wavelength VCSELs (850–1100 nm) have the highest performance, while the long-wavelength ones (1310–1550 nm) have more material challenges [29] and thus have a lower bandwidth, as shown in Figure 21.1.

21.2.2 Applications: Short-Reach Optical Interconnects

VCSELs have emerged as cost-effective light source candidates for a wide range of applications in the last decade [30]. They have replaced edge-emitting lasers in commercial applications such as Gigabit Ethernet and Fibre Channel. In this section, we will focus on some aspects of current and future applications of VCSEL in short-reach optical interconnects.

21.2.2.1 Optical Fiber Data Communication

VCSELs are now low-cost and reliable light sources for high-speed local area networks/storage area networks [31]. The exploding demand for Internet access has fuelled the need for higher bandwidth networks, leading us from 10/100 Mb/s to 1 Gb/s, and followed soon by 10 Gb/s. Commercial 850 nm GaAs VCSELs with multimode fibers (MMFs) have been widely deployed in Gigabit Ethernet. For the 10 Gigabit Ethernet, the fundamental limitations of copper-based electrical links make fiber-based data communication indispensable. As defined in the IEEE 802.3ae, the 10 GBASE-SR ("short-range") standard uses 850 nm lasers (specifically VCSELs) to deliver data up to 300 m over MMFs. The 10 GBASE-LR ("long-range") standard uses 1310 nm lasers and has a specified reach of 10 km over single-mode fibers (SMFs); therefore low-cost and high-performance 1310 nm VCSELs are also attracting much interest for use in such high-speed links of over several kilometers with SMFs.

Fibre Channel, as the premier technique for SAN, is another major market for VCSELs, where 850 nm VCSELs are most commonly used. The latest Fibre Channel FC16G (14 Gb/s, 2009) and FC32G (28 Gb/s, 2012) are being standardized on the road map, and high-speed VCSELs are expected to play an increasingly important role.

21.2.2.2 Active Optical Cables

Active optical cable (AOC) links for short-reach computer and consumer applications are increasingly based on VCSELs operating in the near-infrared spectral range [31].

The term "active cable" refers to copper cables with power amplification to reduce the signal degradation in traditional passive copper cables. This active boosting makes them more compact and portable than passive cables; therefore, they are ideal for use in consumer electronics, such as smartphones, high-definition televisions (HDTVs), and the latest DisplayPort, as well as enterprise and storage network applications. AOCs [32] take this one step further, using fiber as the medium in order to take further advantage of common optical transport benefits, such as extended reach, lower bit error rates, higher transmission speeds, smaller size, and lower weight. The electrical–optical–electrical conversion is implemented inside the cables, allowing users to build electronic equipment without having to redesign their internal electrical designs to support full optical I/O connections. Currently, the major AOC markets include InfiniBand, USB, HDMI, and DisplayPort [32], and are expected to build significant revenue growth over the next few years.

VCSELs are, and expected to continue to be, the core laser source serving AOC designs. The current AOC VCSEL distribution is dominated by 5 Gb/s devices; however, commercial 10 Gb/s serial AOC designed with 850 nm VCSEL has been used for 1/10 Gigabit Ethernet and 1/2/4/8x Fibre Channel. Parallel AOC based on VCSEL array technology has also been used for 40/100 Gigabit Ethernet and InfiniBand QDR/12 × QDR.

21.2.2.3 Optical Interconnects for Supercomputers and Silicon Chips

The performance of supercomputers has exponentially increased in the last two decades. As the scaling of the performance is primarily achieved by increasing the number of cores, a corresponding increase in the intrasystem (rack-to-rack, board-to-board, and chip-to-chip) interconnects bandwidth is necessary, and the aggregate bandwidth per chip is projected to hit ~10 TB/s by 2015 [33]. On the other hand, however, the power consumption should not scale with the performance. Interconnects have been a major source of power consumption and will become an increasingly significant factor. Due to physical limitations, electrical interconnects have difficulty in keeping pace with such bandwidth and power consumption requirements, while optical interconnects offer potential solutions and have been already used in practice to help remove electronic bottlenecks in supercomputers and high-performance servers.

The first application of optical interconnects in supercomputers started with rack-to-rack communications, in the Roadrunner Petaflop supercomputer now running at Los Alamos National Laboratory, which was built by IBM. Its thousands of connections were based on both InfiniBand and Gigabit Ethernet, using VCSELs and MMFs. Although the Roadrunner does not have any intra-rack optical interconnects, the new Sequoia, targeting at 20 petaflop which is about 20 times faster than Roadrunner, is being constructed by IBM and expected to take advantage of optical interconnects at all levels. There is little doubt that high-speed VCSELs will continue playing a substantial role as optical sources for the interconnects.

As can be seen from IBM's plan, it is essential for optics to enter the board-level and chip-level systems. Recently, much effort has focused on integrating optics into printed circuit boards. The IBM Terabus program [34–36] aimed to develop a complete technology set to support terabit/second chip-to-chip parallel data transfers through polymer waveguides, where two-dimensional (2D) arrays of high-speed 985 nm bottom-emitting VCSELs [37] were used as transmitter modules.

There are many reasons why VCSELs appear to be the optical source most suitable for such extremely short-reach interconnects. To compete with the current state of the art in electrical off-chip interconnects, the energy per bit of the optical source should be less than 1 pJ (1 pJ/bit is the same as 1 mW/(Gb/s)) [38]. Due to its inherent advantage of low power consumption and high-speed modulation, VCSELs are the only device that can meet this requirement, with 286 fJ/bit demonstrated at 35 Gb/s in an oxide aperture VCSEL [16]. Small-sized and large-scale 2D arrays are also crucial features for the integration of VCSELs into the circuit board. Furthermore, wavelength division multiplexing (WDM) technology is an additional option that in the future might be particularly useful for the guided-wave optical interconnects and could also be used in free-space interconnects [38]. Since their lasing wavelength can be adjusted during epitaxial growth or lithography [39], VCSELs are well suited for WDM transmission.

21.2.3 High-Speed Performance VCSELs

The following sections describe the high-speed performance and the bandwidth limitations of VCSELs, including (1) the laser dynamics (resonance frequency and damping), (2) the electrical parasitics, and (3) the carrier dynamics. Improvements using the injection locking technique [40,41] will be discussed in Section 21.3.

21.2.3.1 Laser Dynamics

The first limitation on the laser's bandwidth arises from the lasing process itself, originating from the dynamics between the photons and carriers in the laser cavity. For a simple Fabry–Perot cavity, as shown in Figure 21.2, the round-trip gain of the electric field A is given by

$$A(\tau_r) = A(0) r_1 r_2 e^{-i\kappa \times 2L} e^{(\frac{g}{2} - \frac{\alpha_i}{2})2L} \tag{21.1}$$

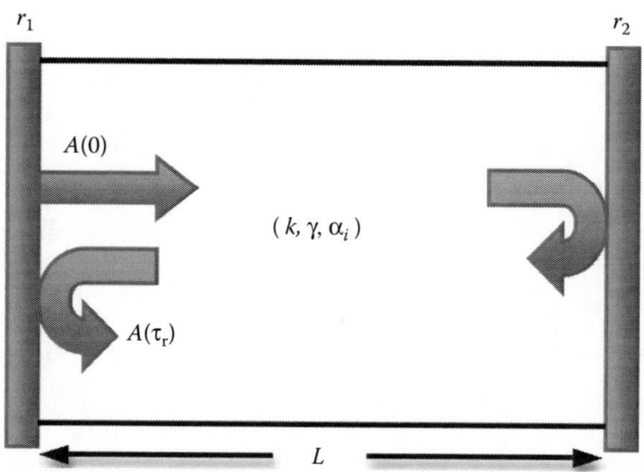

FIGURE 21.2 The Fabry–Perot laser.

where τ_r is the cavity round-trip time, r_1 and r_2 are the reflection coefficients of the two facets, κ is the propagation constant, g is the optical gain, α_i is the internal optical loss, and L is the cavity length. The cavity round-trip time is

$$\tau_r = \frac{2L}{\upsilon_g} \tag{21.2}$$

where υ_g is the group velocity. The mirror losses, although occurring at the facets, can be modeled as being uniformly distributed:

$$\alpha_m = -\frac{1}{L}\ln(r_1 r_2) \tag{21.3}$$

Rewriting Equation 21.1:

$$A(\tau_r) = A(0)e^{-i\kappa \times 2L}e^{(g-\alpha_{total})L} \tag{21.4}$$

where the total cavity loss is

$$\alpha_{total} = \alpha_i + \alpha_m \tag{21.5}$$

The lasing condition requires the round-trip gain to be unity at steady state; therefore,

$$e^{-i\kappa \times 2L} = 1, \quad g = \alpha_{total} \tag{21.6}$$

Neglecting the spontaneous emission, the derivative of the electric field can be approximated based on Equation 21.4:

$$\begin{aligned}\frac{dA}{dt} = \frac{\Delta A}{\Delta t} &= \frac{A(e^{-i\kappa \times 2L}e^{(g-\alpha_{total})L} - 1)}{\tau_r} \\ &\approx A\frac{(-i2\Delta\kappa + g - \alpha_{total})L}{2L/\upsilon_g} \\ &\approx A\left[-i\Delta\kappa + \frac{1}{2}(g - \alpha_{total})\right]\upsilon_g\end{aligned} \tag{21.7}$$

Taking into account the linewidth enhancement factor α [42]:

$$\alpha = -\frac{4\pi}{\lambda}\frac{\mathrm{d}n/\mathrm{d}N}{\mathrm{d}g/\mathrm{d}N} \tag{21.8}$$

where λ is the lasing wavelength, n is the index of refraction, and N is the carrier number; and remembering the definition of the propagation constant:

$$\kappa = \frac{2\pi n}{\lambda} \tag{21.9}$$

we obtain

$$\begin{aligned}\Delta\kappa &= \frac{2\pi}{\lambda}\Delta n = \frac{2\pi}{\lambda}\frac{\mathrm{d}n}{\mathrm{d}g}\Delta g \\ &= \frac{2\pi}{\lambda}\alpha\left(-\frac{\lambda}{4\pi}\right)(g-\alpha_{\mathrm{total}}) \\ &= -\frac{\alpha\cdot(g-\alpha_{\mathrm{total}})}{2}\end{aligned} \tag{21.10}$$

Substituting Equation 21.10 into Equation 21.7 yields

$$\frac{\mathrm{d}A}{\mathrm{d}t} = A\cdot\frac{1}{2}(1+i\alpha)(g-\alpha_{\mathrm{total}})\upsilon_{\mathrm{g}} \tag{21.11}$$

This can also be written as the following:

$$\frac{\mathrm{d}A}{\mathrm{d}t} = \frac{1}{2}(1+i\alpha)G_0(N-N_{\mathrm{th}})\cdot A \tag{21.12}$$

where G_0 is the linear gain coefficient, and N_{th} is the threshold carrier number. The linear gain coefficient is defined by

$$G_0 = \frac{\Gamma\cdot g\cdot\upsilon_{\mathrm{g}}}{V(1+\epsilon\cdot S)} \tag{21.13}$$

where Γ is the optical confinement factor, V is the active volume, and ϵ is the gain compression factor. Since $G_0(N-N_{\mathrm{th}}) = G_0(N-N_0) - 1/\tau_{\mathrm{p}}$, where N_0 is the transparency carrier number, $G_0(N-N_0)$ is the modal gain, and τ_{p} is the photon lifetime; we can also write Equation 21.12 as follows:

$$\frac{\mathrm{d}A}{\mathrm{d}t} = \frac{1}{2}(1+i\alpha)\left[G_0(N-N_0)\frac{1}{\tau_{\mathrm{p}}}\right]\cdot A \tag{21.14}$$

Whereas the differential equations above govern the complex field of a free-running laser, the photon number S is more preferable for numerical simulation. Assuming that A is normalized field and $|A|^2 = S$, it can be written as $A = \sqrt{S}\exp i\theta$, where θ is the phase. The photon number rate equations can be found by writing

$$\frac{\mathrm{d}S}{\mathrm{d}t} = \frac{\mathrm{d}A^*A}{\mathrm{d}t} = \frac{\mathrm{d}A^*}{\mathrm{d}t}A + \frac{\mathrm{d}A}{\mathrm{d}t}A^* \tag{21.15}$$

and based on Equation 21.14

$$\frac{dS}{dt} = \left(G_0(N - N_0) - \frac{1}{\tau_p} \right) \cdot S + \beta \frac{N}{\tau_s} \quad (21.16)$$

where τ_s is the carrier lifetime, and β is the spontaneous emission factor. It is worth noting that the spontaneous emission is included here, providing the seed for the lasing. The rate equation governing the carrier number is given as

$$\frac{dN}{dt} = \eta_i \frac{I}{q} - \frac{N}{\tau_s} - G_0(N - N_0) \cdot S \quad (21.17)$$

where η_i is the carrier injection efficiency, I is the electrical current injection, and q is the electron charge, respectively. Equations 21.16 and 21.17 are the well-known laser rate equations that clearly demonstrate the dynamic coupling between photons and carriers. These equations are for S and N as quantities (e.g., 10^5 photons in the cavity). Alternatively, they can be expressed as densities (see, e.g., ref. [43]).

The rate equations can be solved analytically or numerically for the steady-state optical output power, or when modulated. To gain insights into the modulation properties of the laser, the small-signal sinusoidal modulation is considered with the laser response linearized for a particular DC bias current. The current applied to the laser is $I(t) = I_0 + \Delta I \cos(\omega t)$, where I_0 is the DC bias current; ΔI and ω are the amplitude and frequency of the (small) modulation signal. The frequency response, known as the intrinsic response, can be written in a normalized form relative to the input:

$$H_{\text{intrinsic}}(\omega) = \frac{\Delta S(\omega)}{\Delta I(\omega)} = \frac{\eta_i / q}{1 + j\gamma\omega/\omega_R^2 - (\omega/\omega_R)^2} \quad (21.18)$$

where γ is the damping, and ω_R is the resonance frequency:

$$\omega_R = \sqrt{\frac{G_0 S_0}{\tau_p}} \quad (21.19)$$

$$\gamma = \frac{1}{\tau_s} + K\omega_R^2 \quad (21.20)$$

where the K factor is

$$K = \tau_p \frac{\epsilon}{\upsilon_g \cdot g} \quad (21.21)$$

The 3-dB modulation bandwidth can be approximated as [43]

$$f_{3dB} = 1.55 f_R = 1.55 \frac{\omega_R}{2\pi} \quad (21.22)$$

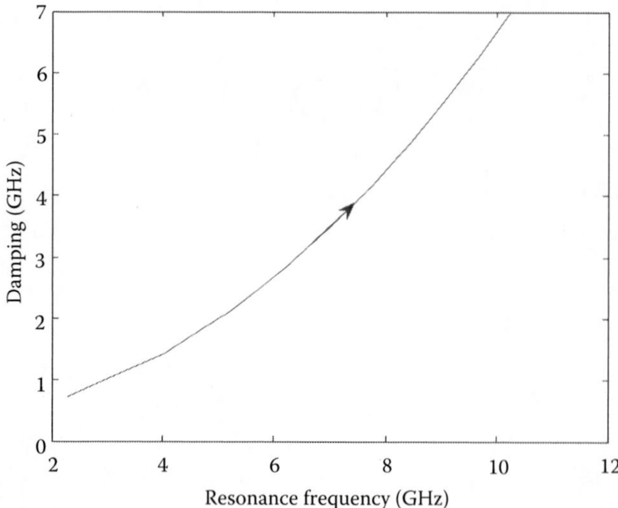

FIGURE 21.3 The intrinsic relationship between the resonance frequency and damping of a free-running semiconductor laser. The arrow indicates an increasing DC bias current I_0.

A high resonance frequency is required in order to obtain a large modulation bandwidth, and is obtained for high photon densities, and for materials with large differential gain. Early pulsed measurements demonstrated the potential for achieving a high resonance frequency in VCSELs, up to 71 GHz [44]. In practice, however, the resonance frequency is much lower due to self-heating and reduced differential gain for high photon densities. Also the damping factor γ increases for high resonance frequencies as the photon density increases, as shown in Figure 21.3. This leads to an overdamped modulation response $|H(\omega)|^2$, which ultimately limits the 3-dB bandwidth.

21.2.3.2 Electrical Parasitics

The second limitation in high-speed laser performance is the device parasitics. The resistance and capacitance of the laser lead to a low-pass filter, which limits the modulation bandwidth. VCSELs typically have a high resistance due to the Bragg reflectors [45]. In the oxide confined VCSEL, the capacitance is a result of the oxide current confinement layer. This low-pass effect is typically modeled as a parasitic pole added to the intrinsic response in Equation 21.18, and the laser response is expressed as

$$H_{\text{total}}(\omega) = \frac{1}{1 + j\omega/\omega_{RC}} H_{\text{intrinsic}}(\omega) \tag{21.23}$$

where ω_{RC} is the parasitic pole frequency. For oxide confined VCSELs, ω_{RC} is typically below 10 GHz, greatly limiting the modulation bandwidth. Many researchers have reported methods for reducing parasitic resistances and capacitances associated with VCSELs [5], such as oxidation-implantation [46], and buried-tunnel junction [23].

21.2.3.3 Carrier Dynamics

In Section 21.2.3.1 we neglected the effects of carrier dynamics, including spectral hole burning (SHB), carrier heating (CH), carrier transport effects, diffusion, and so on. For cases where the intrinsic region of the PIN diode and the active region are one and the same, such as for simple bulk double heterostructure structures, this assumption is generally good. However, modern high-speed lasers utilize separate-confinement heterostructures with quantum-well (QW) active regions, and these effects should be considered [26]. Their influence on the modulation performance can be summarized as follows:

- SHB, which can be alleviated with a fast carrier–carrier scattering rate, introduces a gain compression factor ϵ_{SHB}, and increases the K factor and damping rate through Equations 21.20 and 21.21.
- CH (the redistribution of the carriers to a Fermi distribution with higher temperature, due to carrier–optical photon interaction) introduces a gain compression factor ϵ_{CH} and also increases the K factor and damping rate through Equations 21.20 and 21.21.
- Transport of carriers from the bulk material into the QWs is not instantaneous and can be described by the capture and escape lifetimes τ_{cap} and τ_{esc}. They effectively reduce the differential gain, the resonance frequency, and the damping rate, thus reducing the bandwidth. Capture time also adds a low-pass filtering effect with a cutoff frequency of $1/2\pi\tau_{cap}$ [43].
- Carrier diffusion further reduces the resonance frequency and bandwidth.

21.3 OPTICAL INJECTION LOCKING

21.3.1 Introduction

Optical injection locking (OIL) of semiconductor lasers was first demonstrated in 1976 using edge-emitting Fabry–Perot lasers [47], in 1991 using distributed feedback lasers (DFBs) [48], and in 1996 using VCSELs [49]. The conventional injection locking technique uses one laser (master) to optically lock another laser (slave or follower), that is, the frequency and phase of the slave laser are locked to light injection from the master laser. The coupling between the master and the slave laser is highly unidirectional so that the slave laser does not provide optical feedback to the master laser. Both the master and the slave laser can be operated in continuous-wave mode, or under current modulation.

This section will focus on the discussion of modulation characteristics by applying a modulation signal to the slave laser, with the master laser operating in continuous-wave mode, as shown in Figure 21.4b. In this case, the slave laser is directly modulated, and the simultaneous injection locking leads to significant improvements: single-mode performance and enhanced side-mode suppression [50], suppressed nonlinear distortion [51], reduced frequency chirp [52], reduced relative intensity noise (RIN) and linewidth [53], and most importantly, enhanced resonance frequency and modulation bandwidth [40,41,54].

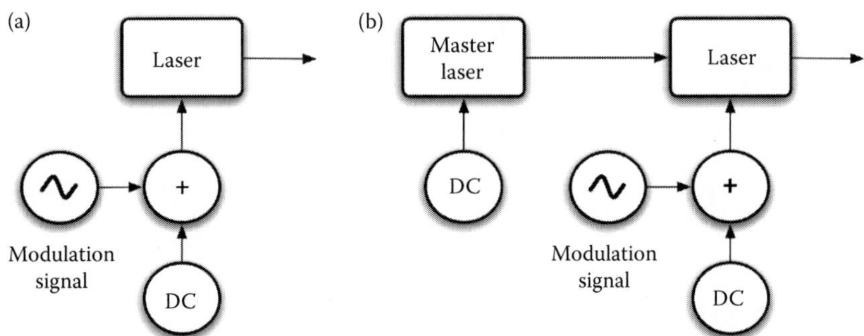

FIGURE 21.4 (a) Direct modulation of a laser, with the bias current and modulation electrical signal applied directly to the laser. (b) Direct modulation, with injection locking, of a laser, with the bias current and modulation electrical signal applied directly to the laser, and the master laser light optically injected into the slave laser.

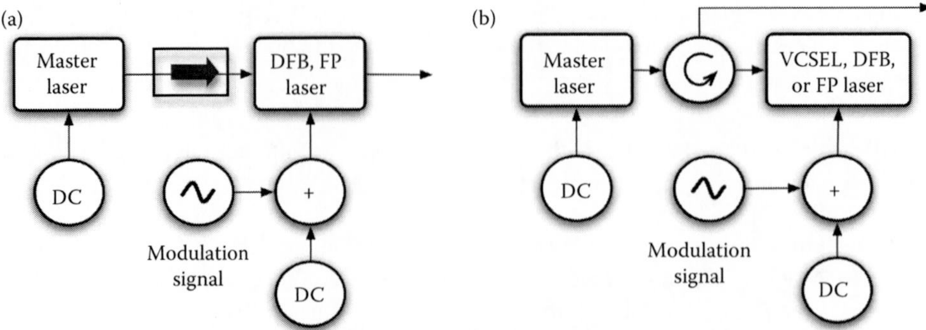

FIGURE 21.5 Diagram for injection locking modulation: (a) in the transmission mode, where the injected light is incident on one facet of the slave laser, the output is collected from the other facet, and the isolator is used to eliminate light coupling back to the master; (b) in the reflection mode, where the optical circulator allows only one facet of the slave laser to be used for both master laser light input and slave laser light output.

Figure 21.5 shows two experimental diagrams of an injection-locked laser system, both using extra optical components to realize the isolation between the master and the slave laser. In transmission-mode injection locking, as shown in Figure 21.5a, both facets of the slave laser are used: one for the injection light input and the other for the output. An isolator is placed between the master and slave lasers to prevent light from coupling back to the master. In reflection-mode injection locking, as shown in Figure 21.5b, a circulator is used to collect the output from the same facet as the input of the injection light; therefore, only one facet of the slave laser is used. In either mode, the integration of the two separate lasers onto one platform is challenging due to the need for isolation. However, a recently proposed method is to integrate a master laser with a semiconductor ring laser on one chip, without the use of an isolator or circulator [55–57]. When injection-locked, the ring laser only operates in one rotation direction and the lasing in reverse direction is significantly suppressed; hence, the isolation is achieved without additional components, allowing the realization of monolithic integration. Researchers have also considered integrating two distributed-Bragg-reflector lasers without isolation, demonstrating effects similar to injection locking [58].

21.3.2 Analytic Model

To analyze the OIL system, the most commonly used model based on rate equations will be discussed in this section [59–62].

21.3.2.1 Injection Locking Rate Equations

The derivation of the injection locking rate equations begins with the differential equation governing the complex electric field of the free-running slave laser Equation 21.12, with the addition of the injection light electrical field:

$$\frac{\mathrm{d}A}{\mathrm{d}t} = \left\{ \frac{1}{2}(1+i\alpha)G_0(N-N_{\mathrm{th}}) - i2\pi\Delta f \right\} \cdot A + \kappa_c A_{\mathrm{inj}} \tag{21.24}$$

where Δf is the difference between the master laser frequency f_m and the free-running slave laser frequency f_s: $\Delta f = f_m - f_s$ (defined as the detuning frequency). A_{inj} is the complex field of the master laser injected into the slave laser cavity, A is the complex field of the slave laser under injection locking; and both of them are at an optical frequency equal to that of the master laser. κ_c is the internal coupling rate, which was historically defined by the longitudinal mode spacing [60], or the reciprocal of the cavity round-trip time τ_r:

$$\kappa_c = \frac{1}{\tau_r} = \frac{\upsilon_g}{2L} \tag{21.25}$$

This can be used to explain why the injection light adds to the internal field by distributing itself across the entire cavity. Equation 21.24 can be written in terms of photon number and phase, for the purpose of numerical simulation. Assuming that A and A_{inj} are normalized fields, they can also be written as $A = \sqrt{S}\exp(i\theta)$ and $A_{inj} = \sqrt{S_{inj}}\exp(i\theta_{inj})$, where S and S_{inj}, θ and θ_{inj} are the photon number and phase of the slave laser and the injection light from the master laser, respectively. Similar to the free-running case, the injection-locked photon number rate equation can be found using Equation 21.15, and based on Equation 21.24:

$$\frac{dS}{dt} = G_0(N - N_{th})\cdot S + 2\kappa_c\sqrt{S_{inj}\cdot S}\cos(\theta - \theta_{inj}) \tag{21.26}$$

The phase equation can be found by writing

$$\begin{aligned}
\frac{dA}{dt} &= \frac{d|A|}{dt}e^{i\theta} + i|A|\frac{d\theta}{dt}e^{i\theta} \\
&= \left\{\frac{1}{2}(1 + i\alpha)G_o(N - N_{th}) - i2\pi\Delta f\right\}\cdot A + \kappa_c A_{inj} \\
\frac{dA^*}{dt} &= \frac{d|A|}{dt}e^{-i\theta} - i|A|\frac{d\theta}{dt}e^{-i\theta} \\
&= \left\{\frac{1}{2}(1 - i\alpha)G_o(N - N_{th}) + i2\pi\Delta f\right\}\cdot A^* + \kappa_c A_{inj}^*
\end{aligned} \tag{21.27}$$

and solving for $d\theta/dt$ yields

$$\frac{d\theta}{dt} = \frac{\alpha}{2}G_o(N - N_{th})2\pi\Delta f - \kappa_c\sqrt{\frac{S_{inj}}{S}}\cdot\sin(\theta - \theta_{inj}) \tag{21.28}$$

Equations 21.26 and 21.28, along with the carrier number rate equation 21.17, constitute the three differential rate equations of an injection-locked laser. They can be solved analytically or numerically, in steady-state operation, or when modulated by small-signal sinusoidal or large-signal digital input currents.

21.3.2.2 Locking Range

From the steady-state solutions [62], the locking range, which is defined as the range of detuning frequencies that satisfy stable locking conditions, can be approximately determined by [63]

$$-\kappa_c\sqrt{\frac{S_{inj}}{S_0}}\sqrt{1+\alpha^2} \le 2\pi\Delta f \le \kappa_c\sqrt{\frac{S_{inj}}{S_0}} \tag{21.29}$$

where S_0 is the steady-state injection-locked photon number. Injection locking of VCSELs is easily achievable with a large possible detuning range due to its relatively low power and hence large

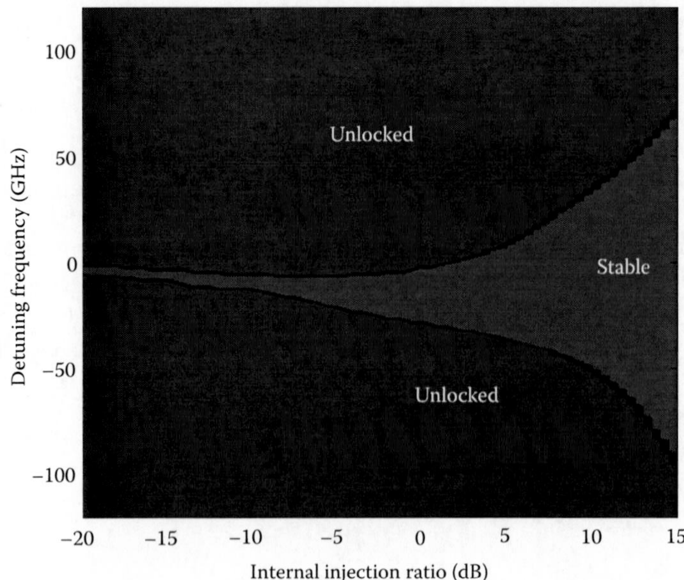

FIGURE 21.6 Locking range as a function of internal injection ratio and detuning frequency.

achievable injection ratio. Figure 21.6 shows a simulated locking range of a typical VCSEL, based on solving the above rate equations. It is asymmetric, due to the linewidth enhancement factor ($\alpha = 3$ in the modeling). However, it should be noted that the negative detuning side is less than three times larger than the positive side, because S_0 changes over the locking range. As discussed in [63], S_0 can be much larger on the negative side, hence reducing the frequency of the negative detuning edge.

21.3.2.3 Injection Ratio and Coupling Rate

As shown in Figure 21.6, the injection ratio and detuning frequency are the two basic parameters commonly used in injection locking. There are two definitions of injection ratio in the literature [64]: since the laser power is proportional to the photon number, the internal and external injection ratios are often defined in terms of power:

$$R_{\text{int}} = \frac{P_{\text{inj,int}}}{P_{\text{fr,int}}}, \quad R_{\text{ext}} = \frac{P_{\text{inj,ext}}}{P_{\text{fr,ext}}}, \tag{21.30}$$

respectively, where $P_{\text{inj,int}}$ and $P_{\text{inj,ext}}$ are the injected power internal to the cavity and incident on the slave laser facet, and $P_{\text{fr,int}}$ and $P_{\text{fr,ext}}$ are the internal and output power of the free-running slave laser. In Figure 21.6, the internal injection ratio is used, as well as the internal coupling rate defined by Equation 21.25. Again, it should be noted that S_{inj}/S_0 in Equation 21.29 is not constant and does not represent the injection ratio. The internal injection ratio was commonly used in theoretical papers, while the external injection ratio is experimentally measurable. For injection-locked VCSELs (reflection-mode only), assuming that the back-side mirror reflectivity is 100%, the two definitions of injection ratio can be related using the power reflectivity of the injection facet R [64]:

$$R_{\text{int}}/R_{\text{ext}} = \frac{(1-R)^2}{R} \tag{21.31}$$

While a VCSEL has a cavity much shorter than edge-emitting lasers, the photon round-trip time can be very small and the internal coupling rate predicted by Equation 21.25 can be very high. However, taking into account the facet power reflectivity, the external coupling rate can be defined as [55]

$$\kappa_{\mathrm{c,ext}} = \frac{\ln(1/R)}{\tau_{\mathrm{r}}} \approx \frac{\upsilon_{\mathrm{g}}}{2L}\frac{1-R}{\sqrt{R}} \tag{21.32}$$

The quality factor Q of an optical resonator is defined as [65]

$$Q = \omega_0 \times \frac{\text{Field energy stored by resonator}}{\text{Power dissipated by resonator}} = \omega_0 \tau_{\mathrm{p}} \tag{21.33}$$

For a lossless Fabry–Perot resonator, the photon lifetime is given by

$$\tau_{\mathrm{p}} = (\alpha_{\mathrm{m}} c / n_{\mathrm{g}})^{-1} = (\alpha_{\mathrm{m}} \upsilon_{\mathrm{g}})^{-1} \tag{21.34}$$

For injection-locked VCSELs here, the mirror losses can by approximated by

$$\alpha_{\mathrm{m}} = -\frac{1}{L}\ln(r_1 r_2) = -\frac{1}{L}\ln(\sqrt{R}) \approx \frac{1}{2L}\frac{1-R}{\sqrt{R}} \tag{21.35}$$

Thus

$$\kappa_{\mathrm{c,ext}} = \frac{1}{\tau_{\mathrm{p}}} = \frac{\omega_0}{Q} \tag{21.36}$$

which indicates that the external coupling rate is only dependent on the photon lifetime or the cavity quality factor; hence VCSELs will have similar external coupling rates as other lasers when injection-locked. As will be discussed further, the maximum resonance frequency enhancement can be simply determined by the external injection ratio and the quality factor.

21.3.3 Physical Mechanism of Injection Locking

The injection locking rate equations have been derived in the previous section; however, the physical mechanism is still a subject of debate, that is, why the slave laser is locked and having the same frequency as the master laser. This section will focus on several theoretical models that attempted to explain the mystery of injection-locked lasers.

21.3.3.1 Gain Competition Model

An intuitive gain competition model developed by Henry [61] in 1985 was the first model reported. As shown in Figure 21.7, the injection locking process is the competition of the amplified spontaneous emission (ASE) and the amplified master laser signal, as well as the beating between them. Outside the locking range, the ASE dominates the slave laser by capturing much more gain than the injected light; therefore the slave laser still lases at its natural cavity mode. If the detuning frequency steps into the locking range, the injected light wins the competition with ASE and dominates the slave laser by suppressing the ASE inside the cavity.

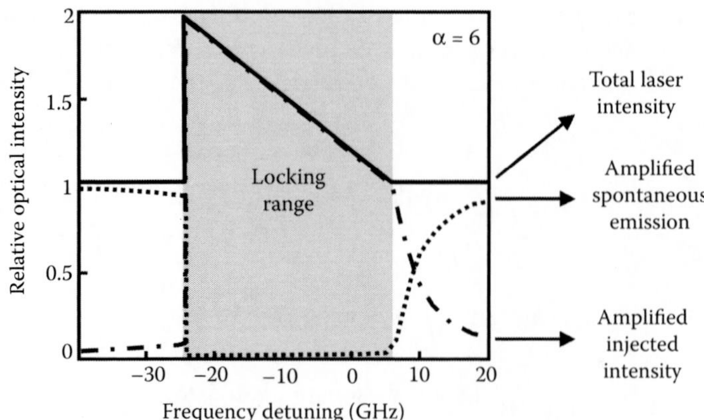

FIGURE 21.7 Gain competition model of injection locking. (From C. H. Henry, N. A. Olsson, and N. K. Dutta, *IEEE J. Quantum Electron.*, QE-21(8), 1152–1156, 1985. With permission.)

21.3.3.2 Amplifier Model

Recently, a new amplifier model was established for injection-locked lasers by Zhao and Chang-Hasnain [66]. By recognizing that the injection-locked slave laser is a gain-clamped amplifier with a red-shifted cavity mode, it explains the injection locking process based on but in more detail than the previous gain competition model. Furthermore, the frequency response properties, such as resonance frequency enhancement and damping, can also be intuitively explained, or even calculated using this model, which will be discussed in the next sections. In this model, when injection-locked, the stimulated emission introduced by the injection light depletes the carriers of the slave laser. Therefore, the gain of the slave laser is lower than its threshold value, which makes the slave laser act essentially as an FP amplifier. Additionally, the gain amplitude of this amplifier depends on the detuning frequency. Although the slave laser is below threshold, the continuously injected light from the master compensates the gain reduction inside the cavity, and overall the slave laser appears to lase at the master laser's frequency.

21.3.3.3 Phasor Diagram

Henry also developed a phasor diagram model for injection-locked lasers by analyzing the injection effects on the slave laser field [61]. As shown in Figure 21.8, the phasor of the slave laser field is in the frame-of-reference of the master laser. The phase difference between the master and slave lasers ($\theta_0 - \theta_{inj}$) is the angle of the phasor. If the slave laser is locked to the master, that is, its lasing frequency is the same as the master; the phasor should be static and would not rotate with time at steady state. Therefore, all phasor vectors due to the injection are required to sum to zero to preserve the injection locking requirement [63,67]. The equation governing the slave laser field when injection-locked, Equation 21.24, should be modified to the form of vectors:

$$\frac{dA}{dt} = -i\left\{2\pi\Delta f - \frac{\alpha}{2}G_0(N - N_{th})\right\}\cdot A + \kappa_c A_{inj} + \frac{1}{2}G_0(N - N_{th})A \tag{21.37}$$

where $2\pi\Delta f - \frac{\alpha}{2}G_0(N - N_{th})$ can be defined as $\Delta\omega_R$, the difference between the master laser frequency and the slave laser's shifted-cavity mode frequency. As will be discussed further, $\Delta\omega_R$ is the resonance frequency enhancement. In Figure 21.8, vector 1, corresponding to the first term on the RHS of Equation 21.37, rotates the phasor by $\Delta\omega_R\Delta t$ in each time interval Δt. In the frame-of-reference of the master laser, vector 2, corresponding to the second term on the RHS of Equation 21.37, is a real vector

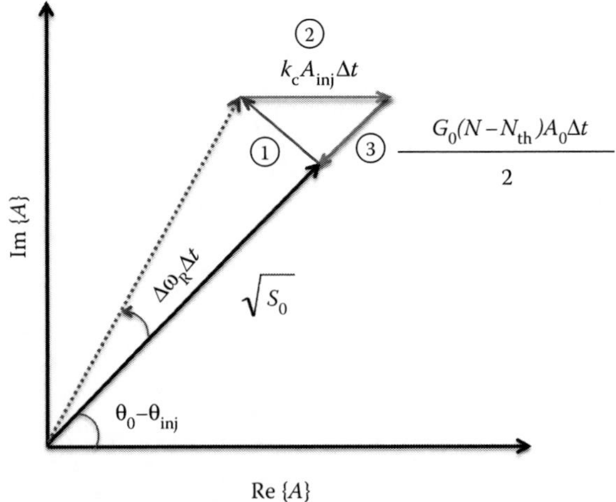

FIGURE 21.8 Phasor diagram of injection locking.

and adds the contribution of the injected light. Finally, vector 3, corresponding to the third term on the RHS of Equation 21.37, is negative because the carrier density is depleted below threshold by injection light, hence reducing the slave field to steady state.

21.3.4 Bandwidth Enhancement

As discussed in Section 21.2.3.1, the resonance frequency of a free-running laser, which basically limits its direct modulation bandwidth, depends on the dynamic coupling between photons and carriers. However, using the OIL technique, the resonance frequency and modulation bandwidth can be significantly enhanced above the theoretical limit for the free-running laser, which was first predicted in 1995 [68,69].

21.3.4.1 Transient Responses

By numerically solving the injection locking rate equations, Figure 21.9 gives an example of the transient response of an injection-locked laser in comparison with the free-running operation, for the same step function current.

For the free-running laser, since the gain compression effect is considered here, the steady-state carrier number is slightly increased due to the increasing power, to maintain the gain at threshold. The phase is also increased due to the linewidth enhancement factor, and this corresponds to a blue shift of lasing frequency (positive chirp).

For the injection-locked laser, the photon number is much higher than the free-running case, due to the strong light injection. Also it oscillates much faster, implying the enhancement of relaxation oscillation frequency. The carrier number, on the other hand, is lower than the free-running case, as explained in Section 21.3.3. It should be noted that the oscillation of the carrier is much more damped, also resulting from the carrier depletion due to the light injection. The phase, much different from the free-running case, is slightly decreased, and this results in a reduced and negative chirp. Intuitively, this phenomenon can be used to explain why the phase is modified not only by the cavity mode shift but also the injection light through Equation 21.28. Further research has experimentally shown that the chirp polarity and magnitude of injection-locked VCSELs can be adjusted by varying detuning frequency, and the negative chirp can be used to compensate for the fiber chromatic dispersion, leading to great enhancement of transmission distance [70].

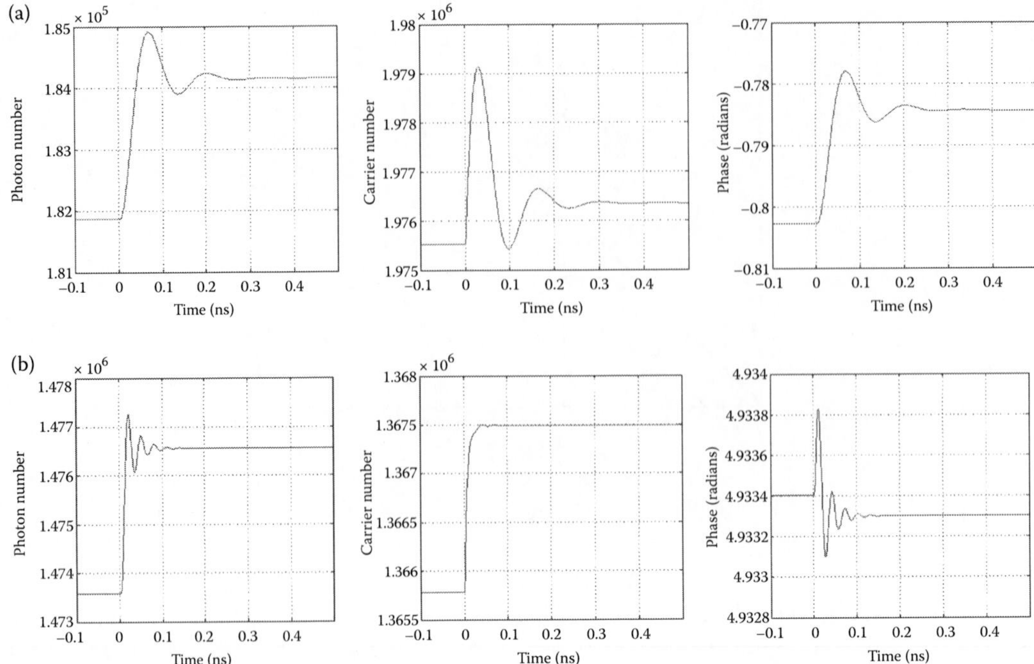

FIGURE 21.9 Transient responses to a step current: (a) free-running and (b) injection-locked.

The transient oscillations between photons, carriers, and phase are illustrated in Figure 21.10. For the free-running laser, the oscillation between photons and carriers is always counterclockwise, which is determined by the fact that the carrier number must rise/fall before the gain can begin to make a change in the photon number. The phase is proportional to the photon number, which agrees with the conventional positive chirp.

For the injection-locked laser, however, the oscillation between photons and carriers is no longer always counterclockwise. The irregularity corresponds to Figure 21.9b, where the increasing carrier is depleted too fast, not only by the increasing photon number inside but also by the injection light, to keep pace with the photon's oscillation. Another interesting observation is the oscillation between photons and phase, which contributes a new dynamics to the injection-locked laser and potentially leads to the enhancement of resonance frequency, as will be discussed further.

21.3.4.2 Small-Signal Analysis

Similar to the small-signal linear analysis of free-running laser, the frequency response of the injection-locked laser can also be derived. The differentials of the injection-locked rate equations can be written in matrix form [63]:

$$\begin{bmatrix} m_{SS}+j\omega & m_{S\theta} & m_{SN} \\ m_{\theta S} & m_{\theta\theta} & m_{\theta N} \\ m_{NS} & 0 & m_{NN}+j\omega \end{bmatrix} \begin{bmatrix} \Delta S \\ \Delta\theta \\ \Delta N \end{bmatrix} \begin{bmatrix} 0 \\ 0 \\ \eta_i \Delta I/q \end{bmatrix} \tag{21.38}$$

where the matrix terms are

$$\begin{aligned} &m_{SS}=z\cos(\theta_0-\theta_{inj}) \quad m_{S\theta}=2zS_0\cos(\theta_0-\theta_{inj}) \quad m_{SN}=-G_0S_0 \\ &m_{\theta S}=-z\sin(\theta_0-\theta_{inj}) \quad m_{\theta\theta}=z\cos(\theta_0-\theta_{inj}) \quad m_{\theta N}=-\alpha G_0/2 \\ &m_{NS}=1/\tau_p \quad m_{NN}=1/\tau_s+G_0S_0 \end{aligned} \tag{21.39}$$

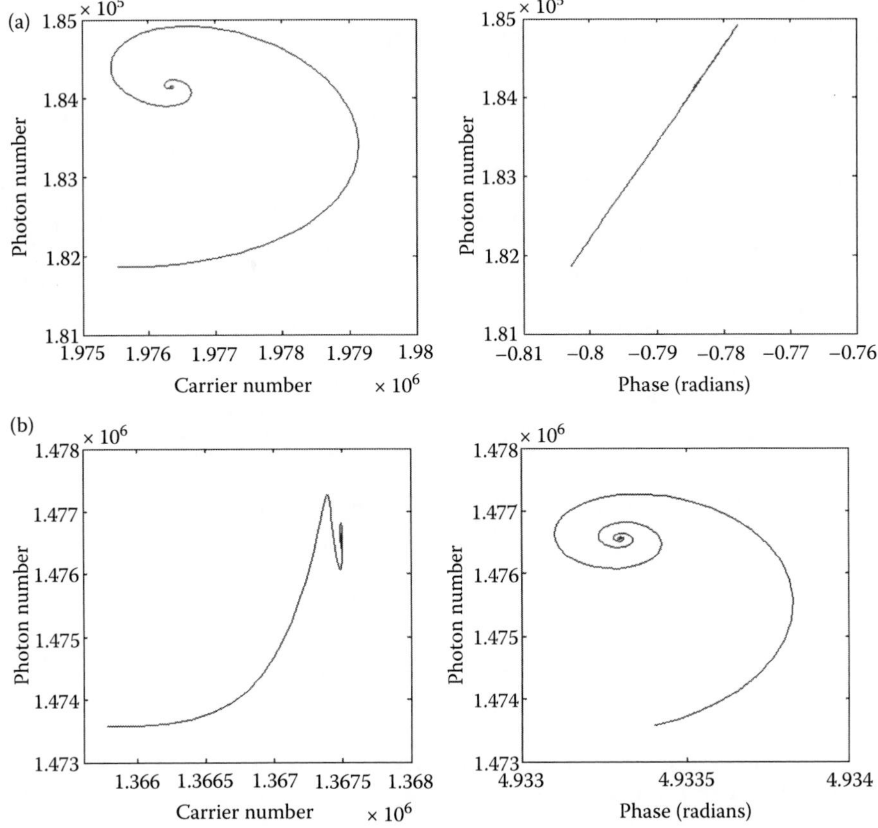

FIGURE 21.10 Transient oscillations: (a) free-running and (b) injection-locked.

and $z = \kappa_c \sqrt{S_{inj}/S_0}$. The frequency response is

$$H(\omega) = \frac{\Delta S}{\Delta I} = E \frac{j\omega + D}{(j\omega)^3 + A(j\omega)^2 + B(j\omega) + C} \tag{21.40}$$

where

$$\begin{aligned}
A &= m_{SS} + m_{\theta\theta} + m_{NN} \\
B &= m_{SS}m_{\theta\theta} + m_{SS}m_{NN} + m_{\theta\theta}m_{NN} - m_{S\theta}m_{\theta S} - m_{SN}m_{NS} \\
C &= m_{SS}m_{\theta\theta}m_{NN} + m_{S\theta}m_{\theta N}m_{NS} - m_{S\theta}m_{\theta S}m_{NN} \\
D &= (m_{S\theta}m_{\theta N} - m_{SN}m_{\theta\theta})/m_{SN} \\
E &= -m_{SN}\eta_i/q
\end{aligned} \tag{21.41}$$

Equation 21.40 can also be factored into its corresponding poles [63]:

$$H(\omega) \approx \frac{\mathrm{DE}}{(j\omega + \omega_p)(j\omega - j\omega_R + \frac{1}{2}\gamma)(j\omega + j\omega_R + \frac{1}{2}\gamma)} \tag{21.42}$$

where ω_R is the resonance frequency, γ is the damping, and ω_p is the real pole frequency.

21.3.4.3 Resonance Frequency

The resonance frequency can be approximated by [63]

$$\omega_R^2 = -m_{SN}m_{NS} - m_{S\theta}m_{\theta S} \tag{21.43}$$

where the first term is from the dynamic coupling between photons and carriers, which is actually the physical origin of relaxation oscillation of a free-running laser; the second term is from the dynamic coupling between photons and phase, which can be regarded as the physical origin of the resonance frequency enhancement, as described in Section 21.3.4.1. Expanding the first term using Equation 21.39:

$$\begin{aligned} -m_{SN}m_{NS} &\approx \omega_{R0}^2 = G_0 S_{fr}/\tau_p \\ \omega_{R0} &= \sqrt{G_0 S_{fr}/\tau_p} \end{aligned} \tag{21.44}$$

where ω_{R0} is the resonance frequency of the free-running laser [65]. Expanding the second term using Equation 21.39:

$$\begin{aligned} -m_{S\theta}m_{\theta S} = \Delta\omega_R^2 &= (z\sin(\theta_0 - \theta_{inj}))^2 = (\kappa_c\sqrt{S_{inj}/S_0}\,\sin(\theta_0 - \theta_{inj}))^2 \\ \Delta\omega_R &= \kappa_c\sqrt{S_{inj}/S_0}\,\sin(\theta_0 - \theta_{inj}) \end{aligned} \tag{21.45}$$

where $\Delta\omega_R$ is defined as the resonance frequency enhancement [63]. The resonance frequency in Equation 21.43 can be rewritten as

$$\omega_R^2 = \omega_{R0}^2 + \Delta\omega_R^2 \tag{21.46}$$

When $\Delta\omega_R$ is much larger than ω_{R0}, the resonance frequency ω_R approximates to the enhancement term.

To find the maximum resonance frequency enhancement, we use Equation 21.45 at the positive detuning edge of the locking range, where $\theta_0 - \theta_{inj}$ equals $-\pi/2$ [60], as well as the lowest photon number which is close to the free-running value [63]. For a given injection ratio, the maximum resonance frequency enhancement is [64]

$$\Delta\omega_{R,max} = \kappa_c\sqrt{S_{inj}/S_0} \approx \kappa_c\sqrt{S_{inj}/S_{fr}} = \kappa_c\sqrt{R_{int}} \tag{21.47}$$

It has been mentioned that VCSEL has very high internal coupling rate due to its short cavity; however, the short cavity requires mirrors with very high reflectivity, which in reverse reduces the internal injection ratio. To get more clear insights into the maximum resonance frequency enhancement, we rewrite Equation 21.47 in terms of the external coupling rate and external injection ratio [64]:

$$\Delta\omega_{R,max} \approx \kappa_{c,ext}\sqrt{R_{ext}} = \frac{\omega_0}{Q}\sqrt{R_{ext}} \tag{21.48}$$

which indicates that the maximum enhancement is proportional to the square root of the external injection ratio and is inversely proportional to the quality factor of the slave laser cavity.

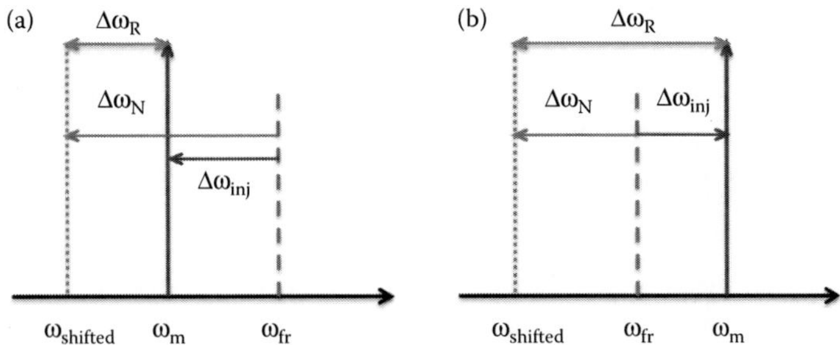

FIGURE 21.11 Cavity mode explanation of resonance frequency enhancement by injection locking: (a) negative frequency detuning and (b) positive frequency detuning.

21.3.4.4 Physical Origin of Resonance Frequency Enhancement

Together with the basic mechanism of injection locking, the physical origin of resonance frequency enhancement also remains an interesting subject. We have shown that the second term of Equation 21.43 is from the dynamic coupling between photons and phase, which can be regarded as the physical origin of the resonance frequency enhancement. However, there are some other explanations that will be discussed here. The steady-state condition of Equation 21.28 yields

$$0 = \frac{\alpha}{2} G_o (N - N_{th}) - 2\pi\Delta f - \kappa_c \sqrt{\frac{S_{inj}}{S}} \cdot \sin(\theta - \theta_{inj}) \tag{21.49}$$

where the first term $\Delta\omega_N = \frac{\alpha}{2} G_o (N - N_{th})$ is the slave laser's cavity mode red-shift due to the carrier reduction, and the second term $\Delta\omega_{inj} = 2\pi\Delta f$ is the frequency detuning. Using Equation 21.45, the resonance frequency enhancement can be rewritten as

$$\Delta\omega_R = \left|\Delta\omega_{inj} - \Delta\omega_N\right| = \left|\omega_m - \omega_{shifted}\right| \tag{21.50}$$

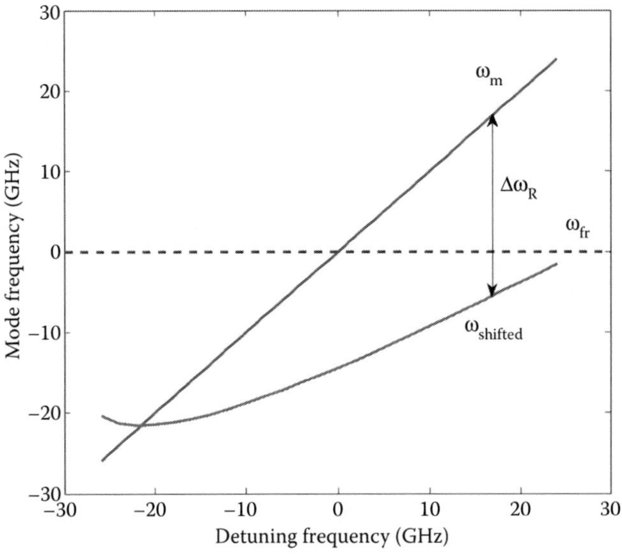

FIGURE 21.12 Mode frequency versus detuning frequency.

which is simply equal to the difference between the master laser frequency and the slave laser's shifted-cavity mode frequency, as shown in Figure 21.11. The relationship between the enhancement and the detuning frequency is clearly shown in Figure 21.12 that shows that the maximum enhancement occurs at the positive detuning edge.

Based on Equation 21.50, the resonance enhancement can be regarded as a cavity phenomenon, which was first predicted by Simpson et al. [69]. They attributed the enhancement to a dynamic competition between the injection-imposed operating frequency and the preferred frequency of the cavity; however, the underlying physics was not clear until Murakami et al. [62] framed a more detailed theory that the enhancement results from an interference beat between the transient field caused by the shifted-cavity mode and the injection-locked field.

The amplifier model, as previously mentioned, can also provide an intuitive explanation for the frequency response of injection-locked lasers. When injection-locked, although most of the slave laser's optical gain is given to the injection field, the cavity mode still exists and is red-shifted. If the slave laser is modulated at a frequency near $\Delta\omega_R$, the cavity mode will resonantly amplify the modulation sideband near it, thus causing a resonance peak at $\Delta\omega_R$ in its frequency response. This explanation agrees with Simpson and Murakami's theories, and has been experimentally verified by Lau and Zhao et al. [71], using both DFB lasers and VCSELs.

For a certain injection locking condition, that is, a certain injection ratio and detuning frequency, the frequency response can be calculated based on the amplifier model. The modeling approach [66] is to (1) first solve the OIL rate equations at steady-state operation, (2) extract important parameters such as the carrier density reduction and cavity mode red-shift from these solutions, and (3) simulate a conventional FP structure using these parameters obtained in step 2 to determine the optical spectrum as well as the modulation response. Note that the optical spectrum of the OIL laser includes not only the master laser frequency but also the red-shifted ASE spectrum from the slave laser cavity. For the reflection-mode setup, the ASE spectrum is the reflection spectrum of the FP etalon with clamped gain [65]. When a small-signal modulation signal is applied to the slave laser, the modulation sidebands scan over a certain frequency range beside the master laser frequency, as shown in Figure 21.13 [66]. The sidebands, acting as probes, replicate the features of the ASE spectrum; and in the radio frequency (RF) domain, the frequency response is the sum of the lower and upper sidebands' responses. If the modulation frequency equals $\Delta\omega_R$, the upper or lower sideband will overlap with the ASE peak, hence resulting in the resonance. It is also worth noting that the two sidebands are asymmetric, and single-sideband modulation can be obtained at large injection ratios [72].

In addition, the approximation of maximum resonance frequency enhancement using Equation 21.50 agrees with that using Equation 21.45, where $\Delta\omega_{inj} = \kappa_c\sqrt{R_{int}}$ is the upper bound of Equation 21.29, and $\Delta\omega_N \approx 0$ because the carrier number is close to the free-running value near the positive detuning locking edge [63]. It is also important to remember that the resonance frequency enhancement is the rotation speed of vector 1 in the phasor diagram.

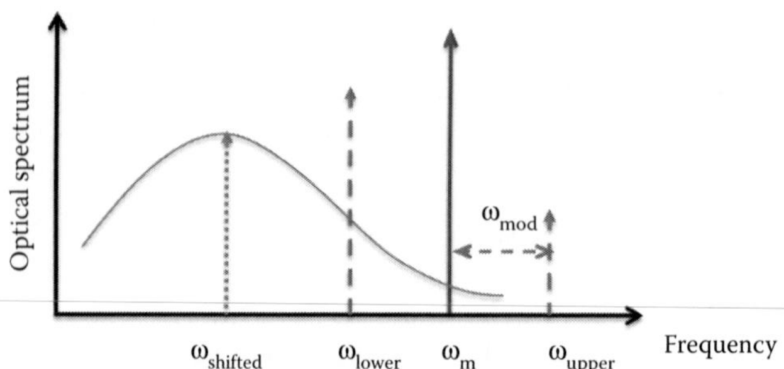

FIGURE 21.13 Optical spectrum of an injection-locked laser under small-signal modulation.

21.3.4.5 Damping and Real Pole

The injection-locked damping can be approximated by [67]

$$\begin{aligned}\gamma \approx A &= m_{SS} + m_{NN} + m_{\theta\theta} \\ &= 2\kappa_c\sqrt{\frac{S_{inj}}{S_0}}\cos(\theta_0 - \theta_{inj}) + 1/\tau_s + G_0S_0\end{aligned} \quad (21.51)$$

The steady-state condition of Equation 21.26 yields

$$0 = G_0(N - N_{th}) + 2\kappa_c\sqrt{S_{inj}/S_0}\cos(\theta - \theta_{inj}) \quad (21.52)$$

Therefore, the damping can be written as [67]

$$\gamma \approx \gamma_0 - G_0(N - N_{th}) \quad (21.53)$$

where $\gamma_0 = 1/\tau_s + G_0S_0$ is close to the free-running damping if the gain compression effect is neglected [73] and $S_0 \approx S_{fr}$. We can interpret that the injection-locked damping is enhanced by the reduction of gain below threshold, which is due to the carrier reduction. However, the approximation of Equation 21.53 is not accurate near the positive detuning edge and should be modified [67]:

$$\gamma\left(\theta_0 - \theta_{inj} \approx -\frac{\pi}{2}\right) \approx -\frac{\alpha G_0 S_0}{\Delta\omega_R \cdot \tau_p} - G_0(N - N_{th}) \quad (21.54)$$

which indicates that the carrier number needs to be adequately below threshold to keep a positive damping and the solution in the region of convergence. Briefly, with increasing detuning frequency, the damping becomes lower and hence sharpens the resonance, as shown in Figure 21.14. This can also be explained using the amplifier model. With increasing detuning frequency, the carrier reduction becomes smaller, resulting in a higher and sharper amplifier gain peak, which converts to a

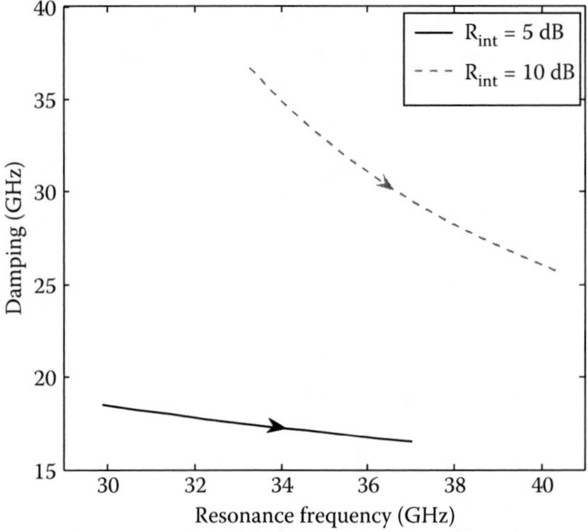

FIGURE 21.14 The relationship between the resonance frequency and damping, of an injection-locked semiconductor laser for the same bias current but two different injection ratios. The arrow indicates an increasing detuning frequency. Specifically, it is possible to obtain a reduced level of damping for high resonance frequency, thereby obtaining a high modulation bandwidth.

sharper resonance in the RF domain, or in other words, the damping is reduced [66]. For very large injection ratio and positive detuning, when high resonance frequency is desired, the real pole frequency can be approximated by [67]

$$\omega_p \approx \left(1+\frac{\alpha}{\omega_R \cdot \tau_p}\right)\cdot G_0 S_0 \tag{21.55}$$

which indicates that the real pole frequency is proportional to the stimulated emission inside the slave laser cavity.

21.3.4.6 Optimizing Bandwidth

The intrinsic modulation bandwidth of free-running lasers is determined by its resonance frequency and associated damping [74]. In OIL, however, the bandwidth is dominated not only by the resonance frequency and damping but also by the DC-to-resonance dip (see Figure 21.15) caused by the real pole in the transfer function of Equation 21.42, which makes optimizing bandwidth more complicated.

We have shown that the resonance frequency of injection-locked lasers is no longer limited by the coupling between photons and carriers as in free-running lasers. The maximum enhancement occurs at the positive detuning edge for a given injection ratio, and scales approximately as the square root of the external injection ratio. Also, the damping decreases as the resonance frequency is enhanced, contrary to the trend in free-running lasers, as shown in Figures 21.3 and 21.14. If the frequency response was governed only by this damped resonance, very large bandwidth could be achieved simply by increasing the injection ratio and detuning frequency.

However, the dip between DC and resonance in the frequency response can greatly limit the bandwidth. The smaller the real pole frequency, the larger the dip appears to be. With increasing detuning frequency, the resonance frequency increases and the photon number decreases, both leading to smaller real pole frequency through Equation 21.55, thus making the dip larger as shown in Figure 21.15.

Owing to this trade-off between the resonance frequency and real pole frequency, it is necessary to optimize the bandwidth. First, the resonance frequency should be enhanced as much as possible using positive detuning, as long as the dip caused by the real pole does not go 3 dB below DC. On the other hand, an effective method is to increase the slave laser's bias current while maintaining the injection ratio [63]. Using this method, the stimulated emission inside the cavity will be enhanced, therefore increasing the real pole frequency, while keeping the maximum resonance frequency enhancement constant throughout Equation 21.48. Actually, the real pole frequency does not need to be very high,

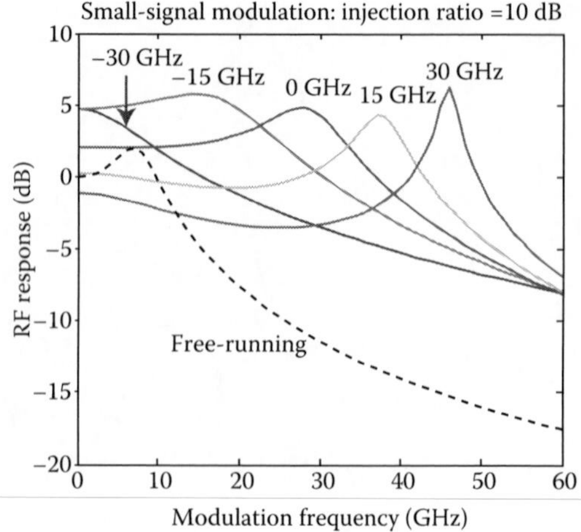

FIGURE 21.15 Frequency responses of injection-locked VCSELs for various detuning frequencies at an internal injection ratio of 10 dB. Responses are normalized such that the free-running DC response is 0 dB.

since the dip is being pulled up by the damped resonance. In conclusion, the detuning frequency should be somewhere in the middle positive locking range, and the slave laser's bias current and injection ratio should be optimized to engineer the frequency response. For injection-locked VCSELs, a very large intrinsic 3-dB bandwidth (80 GHz) has been achieved beyond the resonance frequency [71].

21.3.5 Optical Polarization Effects

One of the problems with VCSELs is that they typically have a quasicylindrical symmetry; hence the optical gain for transverse-electric modes in VCSELs is not dependent on the direction of the electric field vector in the plane of the active layer. Owing to this polarization independence, VCSEL cavities usually have two orthogonal polarization eigenstates. The absence of a well-defined polarization selection mechanism leads to the coexistence, switching, or bistability of lasing modes or even to the rotation of the polarization eigenstates with a change in the drive current or temperature [75]. Over the last two decades, significant effort has been directed to improving the VCSEL polarization stability.

In previous sections, the polarization state of injection light was assumed to be the same as the fundamental lasing mode of slave VCSEL. This section will discuss the polarization effects on the injection-locked VCSELs by intentionally misaligning the injection light polarization angle from the fundamental VCSEL polarization [76]. As shown in Figure 21.16, we define the VCSEL field component with the polarization angle of 0° to be the fundamental or first polarization mode, and the field component with the polarization angle of 90° to be the orthogonal (to fundamental) or second polarization mode. The master laser is polarized at an angle θ_p between 0° and 90° with respect to the fundamental VCSEL polarization mode. Intuitively, the injection light can be decomposed into both polarization modes, and the coupling rate for each mode depends on the polarization angle. The conventional injection locking rate equations should be modified to include the two polarization modes as follows:

$$\frac{dS_i}{dt} = \left(G_0(N - N_0) - \frac{1}{\tau_{pi}} \right) \cdot S_i + 2k_{ci}\sqrt{S_{inj} \cdot S_i}\cos(\theta_i - \theta_{inj}) \tag{21.56}$$

$$\frac{d\theta_i}{dt} = \frac{\alpha}{2}\left(G_0(N - N_0) - \frac{1}{\tau_{pi}} \right) - 2\pi\Delta f_i - k_{ci}\sqrt{\frac{S_{inj}}{S_i}} \cdot \sin(\theta_i - \theta_{inj}) \tag{21.57}$$

$$\frac{dN}{dt} = \eta_i \frac{I}{q} - \frac{N}{\tau_s} - G_0(N - N_0) \cdot S_{total} \tag{21.58}$$

where the index $i = 1, 2$ stands for the first and second polarization mode, and $S_{total} = S_1 + S_2$. Note that the photon lifetime of the first polarization mode (τ_{p1}) is longer than the second polarization mode (τ_{p2}) so that the free-running VCSEL is lasing at the first mode. Both modes are assumed to

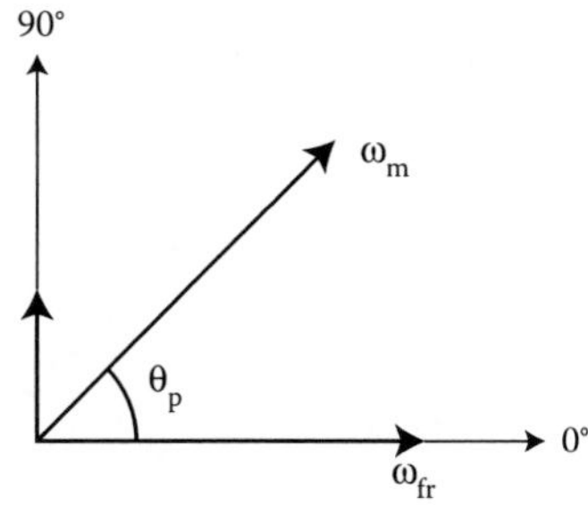

FIGURE 21.16 Polarization angle between master laser and slave VCSELs.

have the same optical confinement factor (i.e., the same G_0) and linewidth enhancement factor. The coupling rates and detuning frequencies for the two polarization modes are

$$k_{c1} = k_c \cos(\theta_p), \quad k_{c2} = k_c \sin(\theta_p) \tag{21.59}$$

$$\Delta f_1 = f_m - f_1, \quad \Delta f_2 = f_m - f_2, \tag{21.60}$$

and $\Delta f_{PMS} = f_1 - f_2$ is the free-running polarization mode spacing.

The frequency response of the system for different polarization angles can be numerically simulated, as shown in Figure 21.17. The internal injection ratio is 3 dB and the detuning frequency is

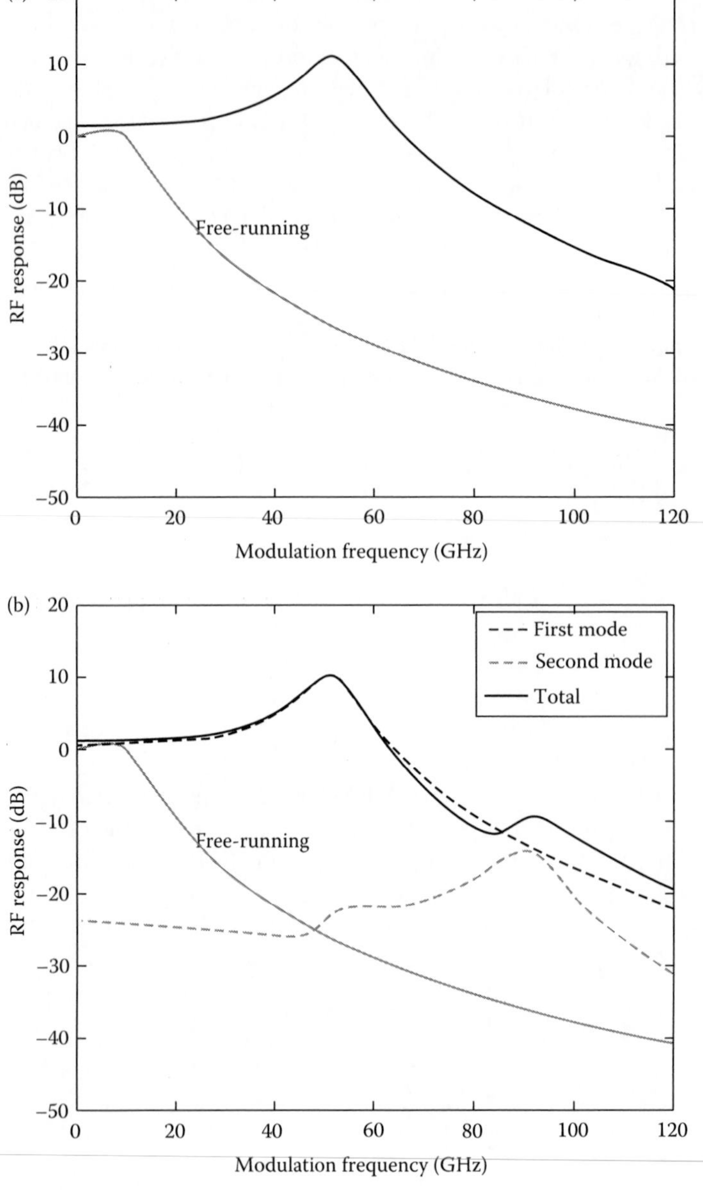

FIGURE 21.17 Frequency response of an injection-locked VCSEL for different polarization angles. (a) $\theta_P = 0°$, (b) $\theta_P = 30°$, (c) $\theta_P = 60°$, and (d) $\theta_P = 90°$. $R_{int} = 3$ dB, $\Delta f = 20$ GHz.

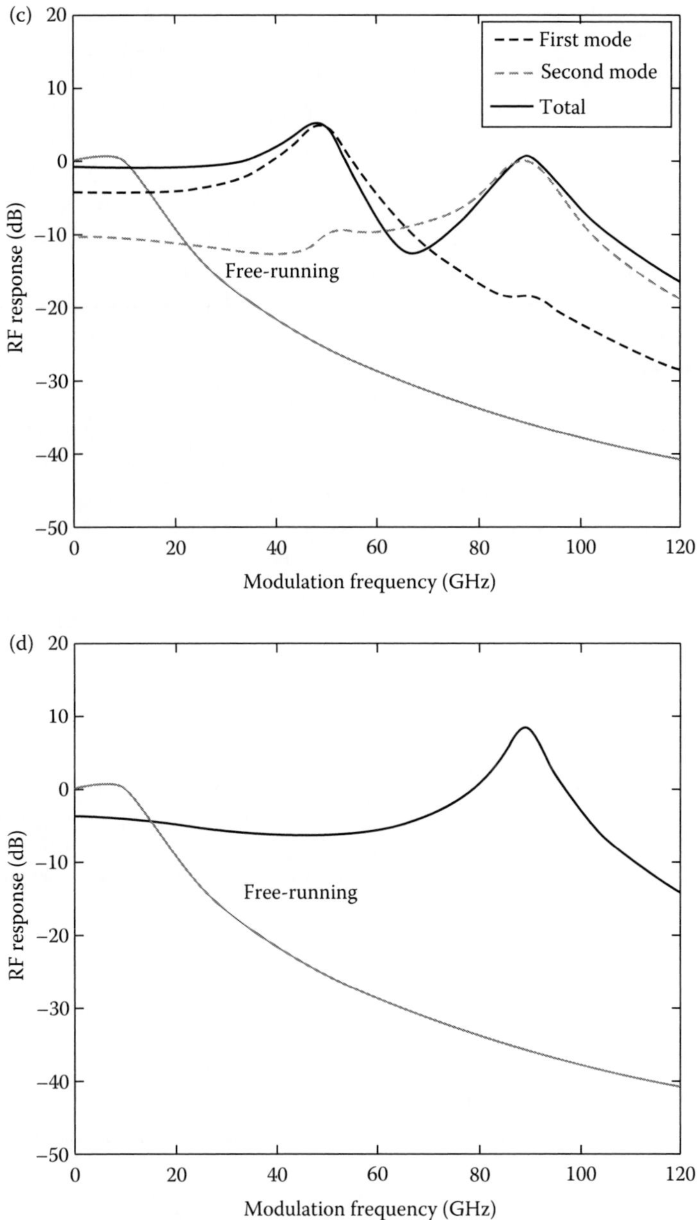

FIGURE 21.17 (Continued)

positive (20 GHz). The polarization mode spacing is assumed to be $\Delta f_{PMS} = 35$ GHz; that is, the fundamental mode is at a higher frequency than the orthogonal mode.

At 0° injection angle, the orthogonal polarization mode can be neglected and the system is simplified to the original model without the polarization effects. The frequency response agrees with previous results, showing a conventional single resonance in Figure 21.17a. For an injection angle of 30° and 60°, the frequency response of each mode is plotted in Figure 21.17b and c (thin dashed curves). Assuming that the detector is polarization insensitive, the total response can be obtained by vector addition of the two modes and a dual-resonance response is observed. As can be seen, the new resonance frequency introduced by the polarization is approximately 35 GHz higher than the original resonance frequency, corresponding to the polarization mode spacing. For an injection angle of 90°, only the orthogonal polarization mode is injection-locked; therefore the frequency response is similar to 0° injection angle where only one resonance is observed, as shown in Figure 21.17d.

The physical origin of the dual-resonance frequency response can be similarly explained using the theory for the single-polarization injection locking system. As discussed in Section 21.3.4.4, the resonance frequency depends on the frequency difference between the injection light and the slave laser's shifted-cavity mode. Similarly, in the dual-polarization injection locking system, the two resonances are due to the beating between the injection light and the two shifted-cavity polarization modes, as shown in Figure 21.18. As long as the master laser frequency is outside the range between the frequencies of the two polarization modes, the difference between the two resonances is equal to the polarization mode spacing. Because the two modes share the one carrier population, the carrier-induced cavity mode shift is the same for both modes; therefore the polarization mode spacing is constant, independent of the injection ratio and detuning.

The dual-resonance frequency response has been experimentally demonstrated in [76]. Figure 21.19 gives a set of measured extrinsic frequency responses (including all the device parasitics) of an injection-locked VCSEL for an injection angle of 45°, showing resonance peaks separated by ~10 GHz, which is the polarization mode spacing. By varying the polarization angle and the frequency difference between the two VCSEL polarization modes, it is possible to engineer the shape of the dual resonance to optimize the maximum modulation bandwidth. This could allow larger freedom in the design of the frequency response of injection-locked VCSELs. Using this approach, a record extrinsic 3-dB bandwidth of 49 GHz has been achieved [76].

21.3.6 Analog Modulation Enhancements

In digital optical fiber communication systems, the modulation bandwidth is one of the most important figures-of-merit for directly modulated semiconductor lasers that determine the maximum data rate. In previous sections, we have demonstrated that OIL can significantly enhance the modulation bandwidth of directly modulated VCSELs. However, for analog fiber-optic transmission, some other

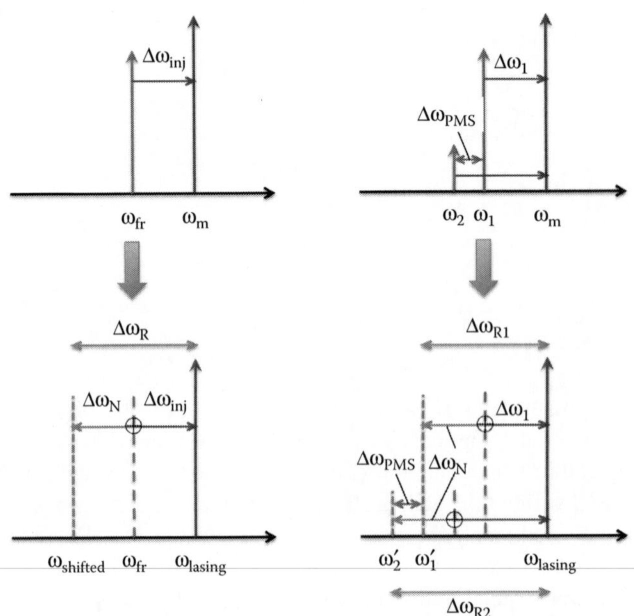

FIGURE 21.18 Illustration of two resonance frequencies.

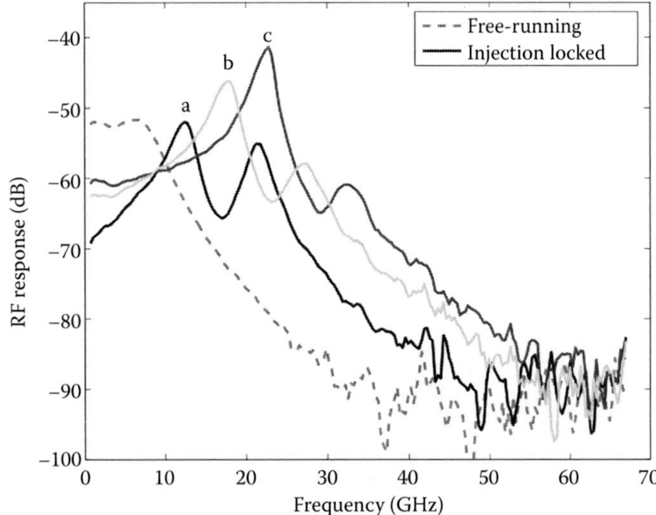

FIGURE 21.19 Experimental frequency response of an injection-locked VCSEL showing dual resonance separated by the polarization mode spacing. (a) $\Delta\lambda = -0.04$ nm, $R_{int} = 2$ dB, (b) $\Delta\lambda = -0.05$ nm, $R_{int} = 5$ dB, and (c) $\Delta\lambda = -0.11$ nm, $R_{int} = 6.5$ dB. (From L. Chrostowski et al. *IEEE J. Sel. Top. Quantum Electron.*, 13(5), 1200–1208, 2007. With permission.)

strict requirements are set for the optical transmitter to reproduce the signal, such as high RF link gain, negligible distortion, and low noise. External optical modulators are capable of meeting such requirements and have been used for high-performance links, but still costly and bulky. Directly modulated lasers, especially VCSELs, are very promising due to low cost, small size, and low power dissipation. However, large distortion near the resonance frequency limits directly modulated lasers only to be used at very low RF frequencies [77] (e.g., <1 GHz).

The distortion physically originates from the nonlinear characteristics of the laser, dominated by the carrier–photon interaction, which is also the origin of the laser resonance frequency. The intensity noise also depends on such interaction and the noise peak is at the resonance frequency. To avoid performance degradation due to the distortion, it is desirable to have the laser resonance frequency greatly exceed the highest RF frequency of use. Naturally, using OIL could be an effective method by which to greatly increase the resonance frequency. In this section, we will show that OIL can indeed reduce the nonlinear distortion and noise, and another microwave performance improvement is the RF gain enhancement.

21.3.6.1 RF Gain

As can be seen in Figure 21.15, the low-frequency modulation response can oftentimes be higher than the free-running response, and this typically occurs for negative frequency detuning. This RF gain enhancement was first experimentally observed in injection-locked VCSELs [78]. Figure 21.20a shows the de-embedded experimental frequency response of an injection-locked VCSEL at a fixed injection ratio of 13.8 dB, and the RF gain enhancement as a function of wavelength detuning is given in Figure 21.20b [79]. The minimum RF gain is at a blue detuning associated with frequency response showing a sharp resonance peak. On the other hand, the maximum RF gain is obtained at red detuning accompanied by a highly damped frequency response. Hence, there exists a trade-off between the resonance frequency and RF gain. The free-running modulation efficiency of the VCSEL used is 0.22 W/A [23]. As can be seen, the RF gain enhancement is up to 20 dB at large positive wavelength detuning (1.25 nm in Figure 21.20b), resulting in a modulation efficiency of 2.2 W/A, or an equivalent 2.75 photons generated per electron–hole pair. Furthermore, the maximum RF gain enhancement becomes larger with increasing injection ratio, as shown in Figure 21.21 [79].

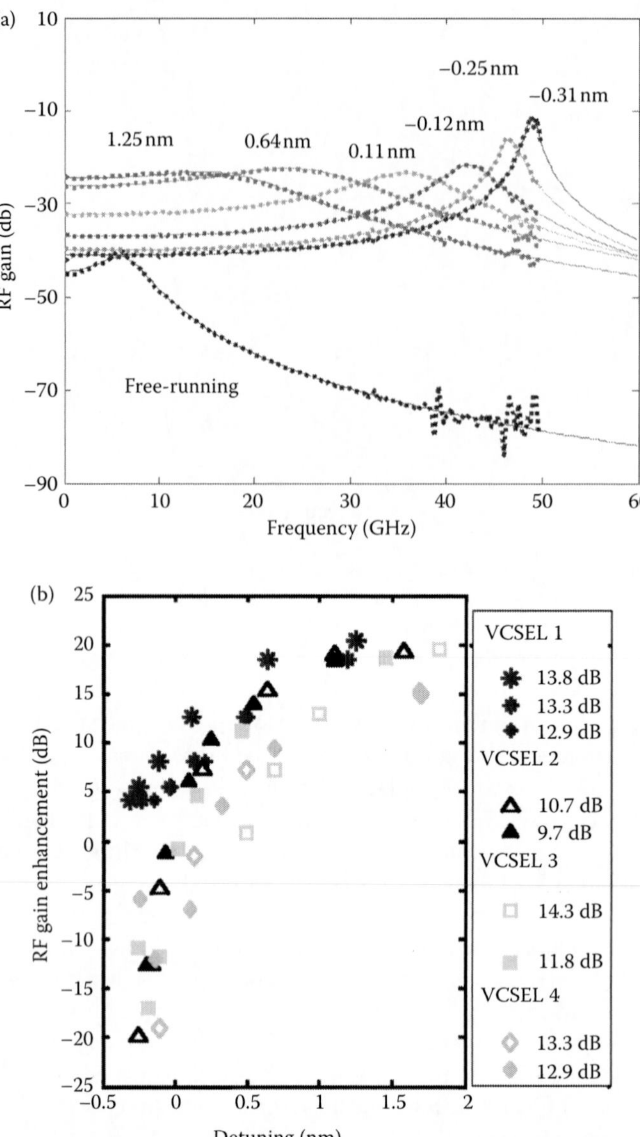

FIGURE 21.20 Experimental illustration of RF gain enhancement for an injection-locked VCSEL at a fixed injection ratio of 13.8 dB. (a) De-embedded frequency response for various wavelength detunings. (b) RF gain measured at 1 GHz for four VCSELs versus wavelength detuning. (From L. Chrostowski, X. Zhao, and C. Chang-Hasnain, *IEEE Trans. Microw. Theory Tech.*, 54(2), 788–796, 2006. With permission.)

The RF gain enhancement dependence on detuning can be intuitively explained using the same theory for the resonance frequency enhancement, as discussed in Section 21.3.4.4. As shown in Figure 21.13, the upper and lower modulation sidebands move closer to the master laser frequency with decreasing modulation frequency, and will overlap each other at DC. By decreasing the detuning frequency, the master laser frequency approaches the red-shifted cavity mode (see Figure 21.12); hence low-frequency signals can get more amplification by the ASE spectrum. In contrast, for positive frequency detunings, the master laser frequency is far from the shifted cavity mode, hence reducing the RF gain. The trade-off between high resonance frequency and high RF gain can be simply understood as due to their opposite demands for the spacing between the master laser frequency and the red-shifted cavity mode.

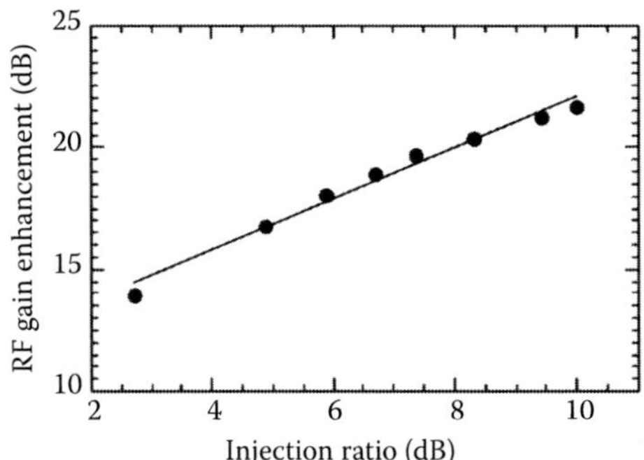

FIGURE 21.21 Maximum RF gain enhancement versus injection ratio. (From L. Chrostowski, X. Zhao, and C. Chang-Hasnain, *IEEE Trans. Microw. Theory Tech.*, 54(2), 788–796, 2006. With permission.)

21.3.6.2 Distortion and Dynamic Range

In analog links, high linearity is desirable in order to reproduce the source information with minimal distortion. The nonlinear distortion comes from several sources, including second and higher-order harmonics of the signal, and the intermodulation distortion (IMD). In actual applications of multichannel signal transmission where baseband signals from different channels are carried by a number of well-separated high-frequency carriers, second- (or higher-) order harmonic distortions generated by signals in a channel are actually of little concern since they generally do not fall within the frequency band of that particular channel or any other channels [77]. However, the third-order intermodulation (IMD3) product of the laser transmitter (for two-tone modulation at ω_1 and ω_2, the IMD3 are at frequencies ($2\omega_1-\omega_2$ and $2\omega_2-\omega_1$)) may lie within the frequency band and is thus not desirable. For device studies, the standard technique is to characterize the IMD3 using two-tone modulation. The spurious-free dynamic range (SFDR) is a useful measure to characterize how IMD3 can limit system performance [80]. It is defined as the ratio of the fundamental to the intermodulation product at the point where the system noise floor equals the intermodulation product [81].

As has been mentioned, the nonlinear distortion becomes severe when the laser is modulated at frequencies close to the resonance frequency, where the nonlinear coupling is the strongest. Hence, with the increased resonance frequency, injection-locked lasers are promising for exhibiting reduced nonlinear distortion and improved dynamic range. Figure 21.22a shows a significant SFDR enhancement of 20 dB for an injection-locked VCSEL measured at 1 GHz two-tone modulation. The frequency response of both the fundamental tone and the two-tone IMD3 distortion is shown in Figure 21.22b. For each injection ratio, the wavelength detuning was chosen to be close to the red edge where the RF gain tends to be larger. On the other hand, the IMD3 power is reduced due to the resonance frequency enhancement. The SFDR enhancement is a combination of the RF gain enhancement plus one-third of the distortion reduction. Since both effects become stronger with increasing injection ratio, the SFDR enhancement is proportional to the injection ratio, as shown in Figure 21.23.

21.3.6.3 Relative Intensity Noise

OIL has been reported to reduce the RIN for FP edge-emitting lasers [82], and VCSELs [83]. As mentioned, the intensity noise is also caused by the carrier–photon interaction (random component), so its peak is at the resonance frequency of the free-running laser [43]. In OIL lasers, the intensity and phase fluctuations of the injection light also contribute noises to the system [53,83]. However, the RIN peak keeps with the resonance frequency, which is moved to much higher frequencies; hence the noise at low frequencies can be suppressed. Besides, the carrier reduction due to the injection locking can reduce the spontaneous emission of the laser, therefore reducing the noise further.

Figure 21.24 shows an experimental RIN spectrum of an injection-locked VCSEL at different injection conditions [79]. As can be seen, the RIN peaks of both free-running and injection-locked

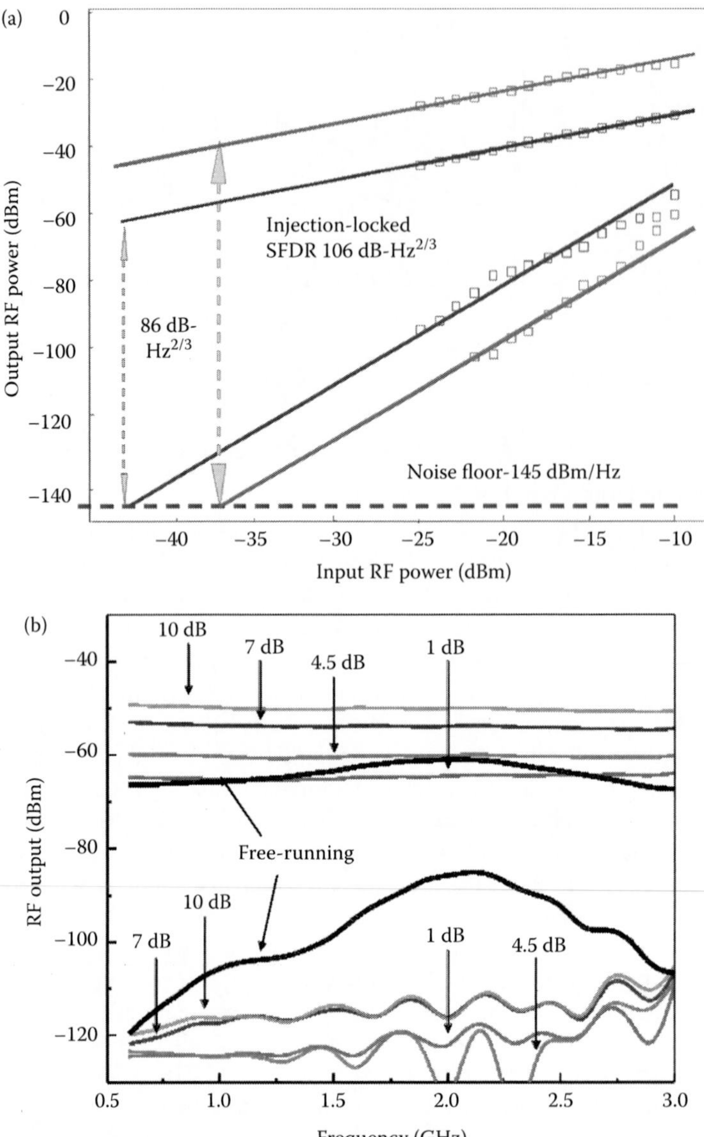

FIGURE 21.22 Distortion and dynamic range of OIL-VCSELs. (a) SFDR enhancement at 1 GHz two-tone modulation with frequency spacing of 10 MHz (inner lines are for free-running and outer lines are for injection-locked). (b) Experimental frequency response of the fundamental tone and the IMD3 distortion. Data were taken for free-running as well as injection-locked at different injection ratios. (From L. Chrostowski, X. Zhao, and C. Chang-Hasnain, *IEEE Trans. Microw. Theory Tech.*, 54(2), 788–796, 2006. With permission.)

conditions are in agreement with resonance frequencies in the small-signal modulation response of the laser. For the injection ratio of 8 dB, the RIN peak is moved to higher frequencies and becomes less damped with decreasing wavelength detuning. A large RIN reduction is observed at the low frequency range (0–13 GHz).

21.3.7 Bidirectional Communication

With greatly improved modulation performance as discussed above, the injection locking system can serve as the transmitter in both digital and analog transmission systems [85]. Recently, a novel

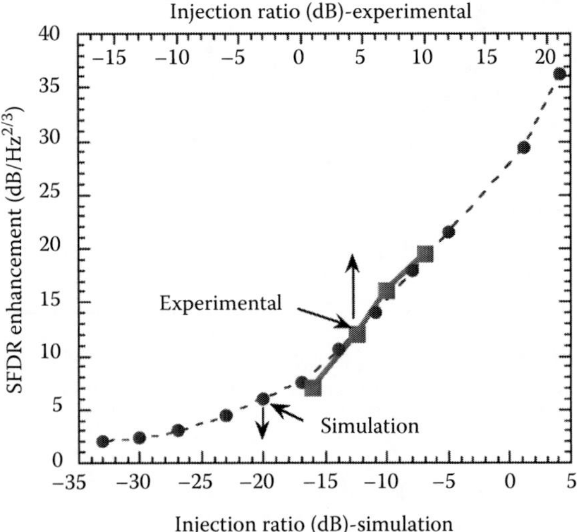

FIGURE 21.23 Experimental SFDR enhancement versus injection ratio. (From L. Chrostowski, X. Zhao, and C. Chang-Hasnain, *IEEE Trans. Microw. Theory Tech.*, 54(2), 788–796, 2006. With permission.)

communication scheme with an OIL-VCSEL functioning both as a transmitter and as a receiver was reported [86,87]. The proposed system uses a full-duplex VCSEL in the home and a conventional transmitter/receiver in the central office (CO), as depicted in Figure 21.25. To act as a receiver, the VCSEL is forward-biased, in contrast to the reverse-biased operation in photodetectors [88]. The CO master laser's frequency needs to be within the locking range of the temperature-stabilized VCSEL. When injection-locked, the carrier density of the VCSEL is affected by the modulated injection light, leading to a measurable electrical signal at the VCSEL contacts. Figure 21.26 shows

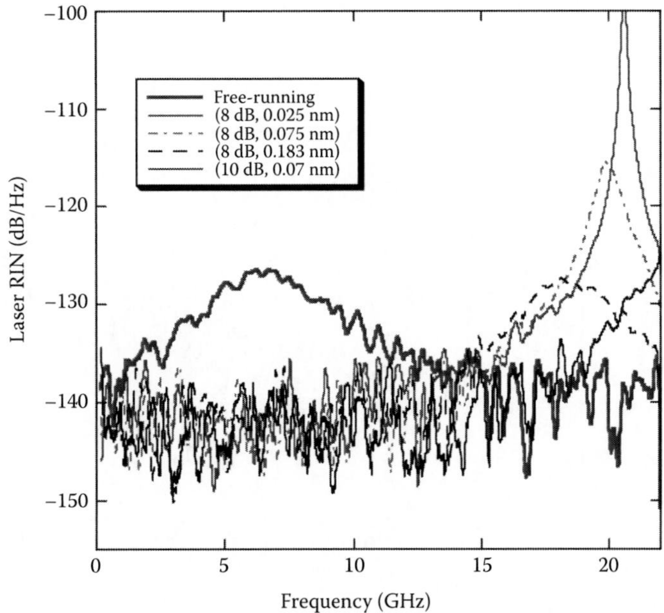

FIGURE 21.24 Experimental RIN spectrum of an injection-locked VCSEL. The legend indicates values of (injection ratio, wavelength detuning). (From L. Chrostowski, X. Zhao, and C. Chang-Hasnain, *IEEE Trans. Microw. Theory Tech.*, 54(2), 788–796, 2006. With permission.)

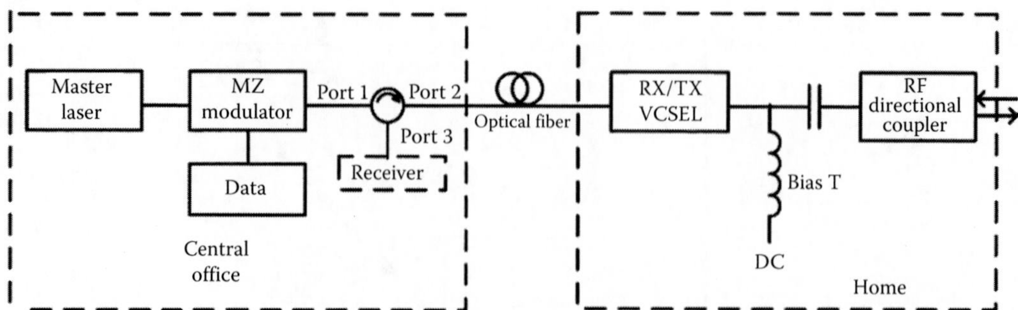

FIGURE 21.25 Proposed full-duplex system with an OIL-VCSEL at home. (From Q. Gu, W. Hofmann, M. C. Amann, and L. Chrostowski, *IEEE Photon. Technol. Lett*, 20, 7, 463–465, 2008. With permission.)

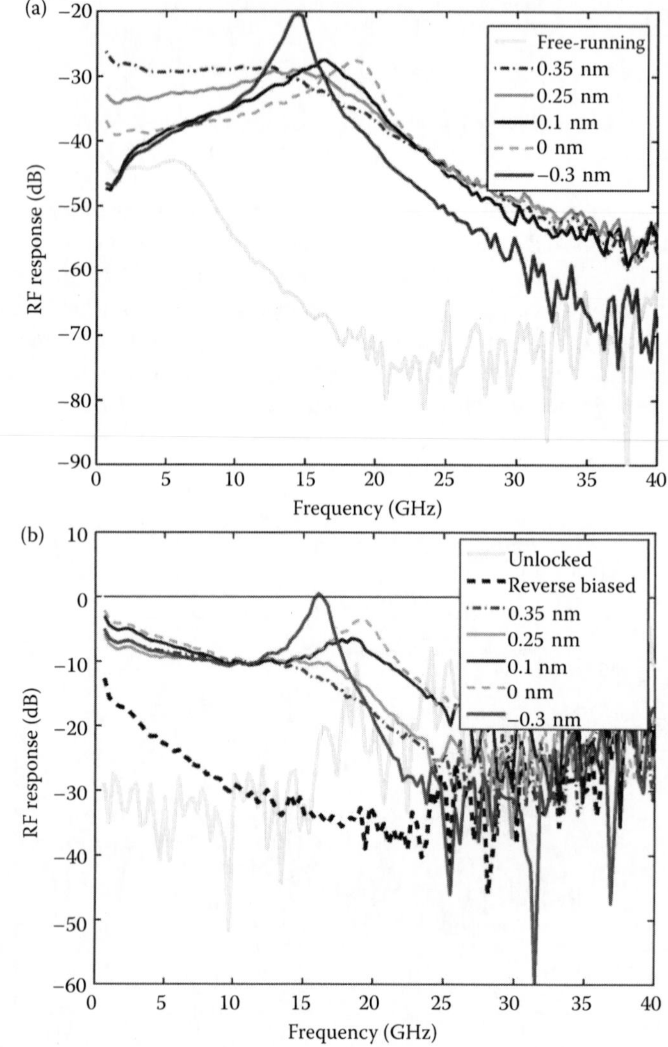

FIGURE 21.26 Experimental frequency response of the OIL-VCSEL as a transmitter (a) and as a receiver (b). When injection-locked, the VCSEL is forward-biased at 2 mA with an injection ratio of 0.6 dB. (From Q. Gu, W. Hofmann, M. C. Amann, and L. Chrostowski, *IEEE Photon. Technol. Lett*, 20, 7, 463–465, 2008. With permission.)

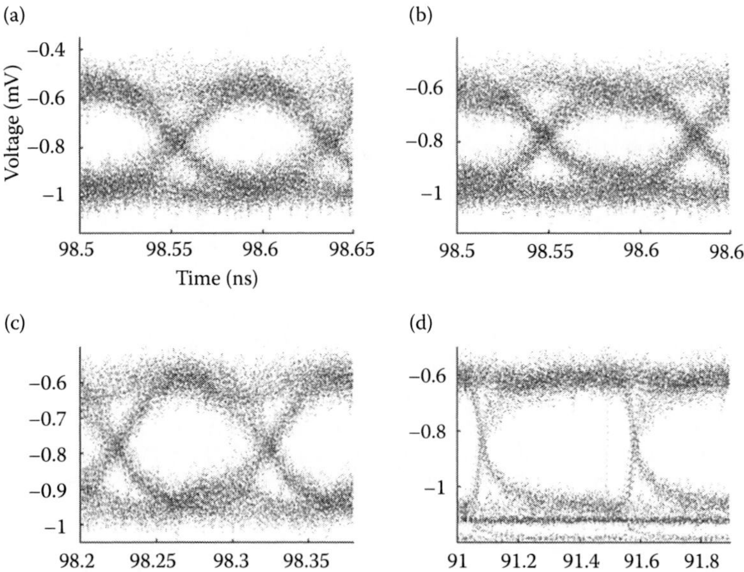

FIGURE 21.27 Experimental eye diagrams of the OIL-VCSEL as a receiver. (a) 12 Gb/s, 0.6 dB, 0.25 nm, 2 mA, (b) 12 Gb/s, 5.1 dB, −0.2 nm, 4 mA, (c) 10 Gb/s, 0.6 dB, −0.1 nm, 2 mA, and (d) 2 Gb/s, 5.1 dB, −0.2 nm, 4 mA (indicating values of the bit rate, injection ratio, detuning, and forward bias). (From Q. Gu, W. Hofmann, M. C. Amann, and L. Chrostowski, *IEEE Photon. Technol. Lett*, 20, 7, 463–465, 2008. With permission.)

the experimental frequency response of the OIL-VCSEL in both transmitter and receiver configurations. Similar trends are observed by varying the detuning because they are both based on the injection locking rate equations: in the transmitter case, the current is the input and the photon is the output; and vice versa in the receiver case. Large-signal digital modulation was also performed using the OIL-VCSEL as a receiver, as shown in Figure 21.27.

This duplex transmitter/receiver based on OIL has the potential to enable high-speed bidirectional communication with reduced cost, particularly in fiber-to-the-home (FTTH) networks.

21.4 CONCLUSION

VCSELs are a mature type of lasers that are suitable for optical interconnect applications. Directly modulated, their performance enables 10–40 Gb/s digital communications. Research with VCSELs using the OIL technique has revealed that their performance can be further improved. This allows VCSELs to be used for even higher frequency modulation formats with lower distortion and noise. This may become important for higher spectral efficiency and high-bit-rate coding schemes using a larger number of constellation points, such as QAM. The OIL technique has also been used with VCSELs for experiments in alternative communication schemes, such as full-duplex communication using a single optical interface. Such approaches may be useful for low-cost FTTH communications.

ACKNOWLEDGMENTS

The authors acknowledge Xiaoxue Zhao, Chih-Hao Chang, Erwin Lau, and Connie Chang-Hasnain for discussions and for their significant contributions to the field of VCSEL OIL; Behnam Faraji, Qing Gu, Orion Chan, Wei Shi, and Nicolas A. F. Jaeger for discussions and experimental contributions; Werner Hofmann, Michael Mueller, and Markus-Christian Amann for providing high-speed long-wavelength VCSELs for the experiments; and the Natural Sciences and Engineering Research Council (NSERC) of Canada and the Canadian Foundation for Innovation (CFI) for funding this research.

REFERENCES

1. K. Iga, Surface-emitting laser—Its birth and generation of new optoelectronics field, *IEEE J. Sel. Top. Quantum Electron.*, 6(6), 1201–1215, 2000.
2. T. Anan, N. Suzuki, K. Yashiki, K. Fukatsu, H. Hatakeyama, T. Akagawa, K. Tokutome, and M. Tsuji, High-speed 1.1-μm-range InGaAs VCSELs, in *Optical Fiber Communication Conference*, 2008, paper OThS5.
3. K. Lear, V. Hietala, H. Hou, J. Banas, B. Hammons, J. Zolper, and S. Kilcoyne, Small and large signal modulation of 850 nm oxide-confined vertical-cavity surface-emitting lasers, in *Conference on Lasers and Electro-Optics*, 11, 193–194, 1997.
4. F. Mederer, C. Jung, R. Jager, M. Kicherer, R. Michalzik, P. Schnitzer, D. Wiedenmann, and K. Ebeling, 12.5 Gbit/s data rate fiber transmission using single-mode selectively oxidized GaAs VCSELs at $\lambda = 850$ nm, in *Proceedings of IEEE LEOS 12th Annual Meeting*, 2, 697–698, 1999.
5. A. AL-Omari and K. Lear, Polyimide-planarized vertical-cavity surface-emitting lasers with 17.0-GHz bandwidth, *IEEE Photon. Technol. Lett.*, 16(4), 969–971, 2004.
6. P. Westbergh, J. Gustavsson, A. Haglund, H. Sunnerud, and A. Larsson, Large aperture 850 nm VCSELs operating at bit rates up to 25 Gbit/s, *Electron. Lett.*, 44(15), 907–908, 2008.
7. R. Johnson and D. Kuchta, 30 Gb/s directly modulated 850 nm datacom VCSELs, in *Conference on Lasers and Electro-Optics/Quantum Electronics and Laser Science Conference and Photonic Applications Systems Technologies*, 2008, paper CPDB2.
8. P. Westbergh, J. S. Gustavsson, Å. Haglund, A. Larsson, F. Hopfer, D. Bimberg, and A. Joel, 32 Gb/s transmission experiments using high speed 850 nm VCSELs, in *Conference on Lasers and Electro-Optics/International Quantum Electronics Conference*, 2009, paper CMGG6.
9. J. A. Lott, N. N. Ledentsov, V. A. Shchukin, S. A. Blokhin, A. Mutig, G. Fiol, A. M. Nadtochiy, and D. Bimberg, 850 nm VCSELs for up to 40 Gbit/s short reach data links, in *Conference on Lasers and Electro-Optics*, 2010, paper CME2.
10. J. W. Scott, B. J. Thibeault, C. J. Mahon, L. A. Coldren, and F. H. Peters, High modulation efficiency of intracavity contacted vertical cavity lasers, *Appl. Phys. Lett.*, 65(12), 1483–1485, 1994.
11. U. Fiedler, G. Reiner, P. Schnitzer, and K. Ebeling, Top surface-emitting vertical-cavity laser diodes for 10-Gb/s data transmission, *IEEE Photon. Technol. Lett.*, 8(6), 746–748, 1996.
12. K. Lear, A. Mar, K. Choquette, S. Kilcoyne, J. Schneider, R.P., and K. Geib, High-frequency modulation of oxide-confined vertical cavity surface emitting lasers, *Electron. Lett.*, 32(5), 457–458, 1996.
13. N. Hatori, A. Mizutani, N. Nishiyama, A. Matsutani, T. Sakaguchi, F. Motomura, F. Koyama, and K. Iga, An over 10-Gb/s transmission experiment using a p-type delta-doped InGaAs-GaAs quantum-well vertical-cavity surface-emitting laser, *IEEE Photon. Technol. Lett.*, 10(2), 194–196, 1998.
14. D. Kuchta, P. Pepeljugoski, and Y. Kwark, VCSEL modulation at 20 Gb/s over 200 m of multimode fiber using a 3.3 v SiGe laser driver IC, in *Technical Digest LEOS Summer Topical Meetings*, 49–50, 2001.
15. Y.-C. Chang, C. Wang, and L. Coldren, High-efficiency, high-speed VCSELs with 35 Gbit/s error-free operation, *Electron. Lett.*, 43(19), 1022–1023, 2007.
16. Y.-C. Chang and L. Coldren, Optimization of VCSEL structure for high-speed operation, in *Proc. IEEE 21st ISLC*, 2008, 159–160.
17. N. Suzuki, H. Hatakeyama, K. Fukatsu, T. Anan, K. Yashiki, and M. Tsuji, 25-Gbps operation of 1.1 μm-range InGaAs VCSELs for high-speed optical interconnections, in *Optical Fiber Communication Conference*, Anaheim, CA, USA, 2006, paper OFA4.
18. N. Nishiyama, C. Caneau, S. Tsuda, G. Guryanov, M. Hu, R. Bhat, and C.-E. Zah, 10 Gb/s error-free transmission under optical reflection using isolator-free 1.3-μm InP-based vertical-cavity surface-emitting lasers, *IEEE Photon. Technol. Lett.*, 17(8), 1605–1607, 2005.
19. G. Steinle, F. Mederer, M. Kicherer, R. Michalzik, G. Kristen, A. Egorov, H. Riechert, H. Wolf, and K. Ebeling, Data transmission up to 10 Gbit/s with 1.3 μm wavelength InGaAsN VCSELs, *Electron. Lett.*, 37(10), 632–634, 2001.
20. K. Adachi, K. Shinoda, T. Shiota, T. Fukamachi, T. Kitatani, Y. Matsuoka, D. Kawamura, T. Sugawara, and S. Tsuji, 100°C, 25 Gbit/s direct modulation of 1.3-μm surface emitting laser, in *Conference on Lasers and Electro-Optics*, 2010, paper CME4.
21. S. Zhang, N. Margalit, T. Reynolds, and J. Bowers, 1.54 μm vertical-cavity surface-emitting laser transmission at 2.5 Gb/s, *IEEE Photon. Technol. Lett.*, 9(3), 374–376, 1997.
22. W. Yuen, G. Li, R. Nabiev, J. Boucart, P. Kner, R. Stone, D. Zhang et al., High-performance 1.6 μm single-epitaxy top-emitting VCSEL, *Electron. Lett.*, 36(13), 1121–1123, 2000.

23. M. Ortsiefer, R. Shau, F. Mederer, R. Michalzik, J. Rosskopf, G. Bohm, F. Kohler, C. Lauer, M. Maute, and M.-C. Amann, High-speed modulation up to 10 Gbit/s with 1.55 μm wavelength InGaAlAs VCSELs, *Electron. Lett.*, 38(20), 1180–1181, 2002.
24. W. Hofmann, N. H. Zhu, M. Ortsiefer, G. Bohm, J. Rosskopf, L. Chao, S. Zhang, M. Maute, and M. C. Amann, 10-Gb/s data transmission using BCB passivated 1.55 μm InGaAlAs-InP VCSELs, *IEEE Photon. Technol. Lett.*, 18(2), 424–426, 2006.
25. W. Hofmann, N. H. Zhu, M. Ortsiefer, G. Bohm, Y. Liu, and M. C. Amann, High speed (>11 GHz) modulation of BCB-passivated 1.55 μm InGaAlAs-InP VCSELs, *Electron. Lett.*, 42(17), 976–977, 2006.
26. W. Hofmann, M. Mueller, G. Bohm, M. Ortsiefer, and M. Amann, 1.55-μm VCSEL with enhanced modulation bandwidth and temperature range, *IEEE Photon. Technol. Lett.*, 21, 13, 923–925, 2009.
27. M. Mueller, W. Hofmann, M. Horn, G. Boehm, and M. Amann, Low-parasitics 1.55μm VCSELs with modulation bandwidths beyond 17 GHz, in *Conference on Lasers and Electro-Optics*, 2010, paper CME5.
28. W. Hofmann, High-speed buried tunnel junction vertical-cavity surface-emitting lasers, *IEEE Photonics J.*, 1(5), 1–14, 2010.
29. C. Chang-Hasnain, Progress and prospects of long-wavelength VCSELs, *IEEE Opt. Commun.*, S30–S34, 2003.
30. F. Koyama, Recent advances of VCSEL photonics, *J. Lightwave Technol.*, 24(12), 4502–4513, 2006.
31. P. Moser, A. Mutiga, J. A. Lottb, S. Blokhina, G. Fiola, A. M. Nadtochiya, N. N. Ledentsovb, and D. Bimberga, Oxide confined 850 nm VCSELs for high speed datacom applications, in *Proc. SPIE*, 7720, 1W1–IW7, 2010.
32. T. Rossi, Active optical cables 2010 market report, *Fiber Integr. Opt.*, 29(3), 149–153, 2010.
33. M. W. Haney, D. K. Sparacin, and J. Hodiak, The transition to chip-level optical interconnects, in *Optical Fiber Communication Conference*, 2010, paper OMV2.
34. L. Schares, J. A. Kash, F. E. Doany, C. L. Schow, C. Schuster, D. M. Kuchta, P. K. Pepeljugoski et al., Terabus: Terabit/second-class card-level optical interconnect technologies, *IEEE J. Sel. Top. Quantum Electron.*, 12(5), 1032–1044, 2006.
35. F. E. Doany, C. L. Schow, C. W. Baks, D. M. Kuchta, P. Pepeljugoski, L. Schares, R. Budd, F. Libsch, R. Dangel, F. Horst, B. J. Offrein, and J. A. Kash, 160 Gb/s bidirectional polymer-waveguide board-level optical interconnects using CMOS-based transceivers, *IEEE Trans. Adv. Packag.*, 32(2), 345–359, 2009.
36. C. L. Schow, F. E. Doany, C. W. Baks, Y. H. Kwark, D. M. Kuchta, and J. A. Kash, A single-chip CMOS-based parallel optical transceiver capable of 240-Gb/s bidirectional data rates, *J. Lightwave Technol.*, 27(7), 915–929, 2009.
37. C.-K. Lin, A. Tandon, K. Djordjev, and S. W. Corzine, High-speed 985 nm bottom-emitting VCSEL arrays for chip-to-chip parallel optical interconnects, *IEEE J. Sel. Top. Quantum Electron.* 13(5), 1332–1339, 2007.
38. D. A. B. Miller, Device requirements for optical interconnects to silicon chips, in *Proc. IEEE*, 97(7), 1166–1185, 2009.
39. V. Karagodsky, B. Pesala, C. Chase, W. Hofmann, F. Koyama, and C. J. Chang-Hasnain, Monolithically integrated multi-wavelength VCSEL arrays using high-contrast gratings, *Opt. Express*, 18(2), 694–699, 2010.
40. J. M. Liu, H. F. Chen, X. J. Meng, and T. B. Simpson, Modulation bandwidth, noise, and stability of a semiconductor laser subject to strong injection locking, *IEEE Photon. Technol. Lett.*, 9(10), 1325–1327, 1997.
41. X. J. Meng, C. Tai, and M. C. Wu, Experimental demonstration of modulation bandwidth enhancement in distributed feedback lasers with external light injection, *Electron. Lett.*, 34(21), 2031–2032, 1998.
42. C. H. Henry, Theory of the linewidth of semiconductor lasers, *IEEE J. Quantum Electron.*, QE-18(2), 259–264, 1982.
43. L. A. Coldren and S. W. Corzine, *Diode Lasers and Photonic Integrated Circuits*. John Wiley & Sons, Inc., 1995.
44. D. Tauber, G. Wang, R. S. Geels, J. E. Bowers, and L. A. Coldren, Large and small signal dynamics of vertical cavity surface emitting lasers, *Appl. Phys. Lett.*, 62(4), 325–327, 1993.
45. M.-C. Amann, M. Ortsiefer, R. Shau, J. Roßkopf, F. Köhler, and G. Böhm, *Long-Wavelength Buried-Tunnel-Junction Vertical-Cavity Surface-Emitting Lasers*. Springer, Berlin/Heidelberg, 41, 75–85, 2001.
46. C. H. Chang, L. Chrostowski, and C. Chang-Hasnain, Parasitics and design considerations on oxide-implant VCSELs, *IEEE Photon. Technol. Lett.*, 13(12), 1274–1276, 2001.
47. R. Lang and K. Kobayashi, Suppression of the relaxation oscillation in the modulated output of semiconductor lasers, *IEEE J. Quantum Electron.*, QE-12(3), 194–199, 1976.

48. R. Hui, A. D'Ottavi, A. Mecozzi, and P. Spano, Injection locking in distributed feedback semiconductor lasers, *IEEE J. Quantum Electron.*, 27(6), 1688–1695, 1991.
49. H. Li, T. L. Lucas, J. G. McInerney, M. W. Wright, and R. A. Morgan, Injection locking dynamics of vertical cavity semiconductor lasers under conventional and phase conjugate injection, *IEEE J. Quantum Electron.*, 32(2), 227–235, 1996.
50. K. Iwashita and K. Nakagawa, Suppression of mode partition noise by laser diode light injection, *IEEE J. Quantum Electron.*, QE-18(10), 1669–1674, 1982.
51. X. J. Meng, T. Chau, and M. C. Wu, Improved intrinsic dynamic distortions in directly modulated semiconductor lasers by optical injection locking, *IEEE Trans. Microw. Theory Tech.*, 47(7), 1172–1176, 1999.
52. S. Mohrdiek, H. Burkhard, and H. Walter, Chirp reduction of directly modulated semiconductor lasers at 10 Gb/s by strong CW light injection, *J. Lightwave Technol.*, 12(3), 418–424, 1994.
53. N. Schunk and K. Petermann, Noise analysis of injection-locked semiconductor injection lasers, *IEEE J. Quantum Electron.*, QE-22(5), 642–650, 1986.
54. J. Wang, M. K. Haldar, L. Li, and F. V. C. Mendis, Enhancement of modulation bandwidth of laser diodes by injection locking, *IEEE Photon. Technol. Lett*, 8(1), 34–36, 1996.
55. L. Chrostowski and W. Shi, Monolithic injection-locked high-speed semiconductor ring lasers, *J. Lightwave Technol.*, 26(19), 3355–3362, 2008.
56. M. I. Memon, B. Li, G. Mezosi, Z. Wang, M. Sorel, and S. Yu, Modulation bandwidth enhancement in optical injection-locked semiconductor ring laser, *IEEE Photon. Technol. Lett.*, 21(24), 1792–1794, 2009.
57. M. A. Osinski, O. K. Qassim, N. J. Withers, and G. A. Smolyakov, Light-emitting device having injection-lockable semiconductor ring laser monolithically integrated with master laser, U.S. Patent 0 034 223 A1, 2010.
58. W. W. Chow, Z. S. Yang, G. A. Vawter, and E. J. Skogen, Modulation response improvement with isolator-free injection-locking, *IEEE Photon. Technol. Lett.*, 21(13), 839–821, 2009.
59. R. Lang, Injection locking properties of a semiconductor laser, *IEEE J. Quantum Electron.*, QE-18(6), 976–983, 1982.
60. F. Mogensen, H. Olesen, and G. Jacobsen, Locking conditions and stability properties for a semiconductor laser with external light injection, *IEEE J. Quantum Electron.*, QE-21(7), 784–793, 1985.
61. C. H. Henry, N. A. Olsson, and N. K. Dutta, Locking range and stability of injection locked 1.54 μm InGaAsP semiconductor lasers, *IEEE J. Quantum Electron.*, QE-21(8), 1152–1156, 1985.
62. A. Murakami and K. Kawashima, Cavity resonance shift and bandwidth enhancement cavity resonance shift and bandwidth enhancement in semiconductor lasers with strong light injection, *IEEE J. Quantum Electron.*, 39(10), 1196–1204, 2003.
63. E. K. Lau, L. J. Wong, and M. C. Wu, Enhanced modulation characteristics of optical injection-locked lasers: A tutorial, *IEEE J. Sel. Top. Quantum Electron.*, 15(3), 618–633, 2009.
64. E. K. Lau, H.-K. Sung, and M. C. Wu, Scaling of resonance frequency for strong injection-locked lasers, *Opt. Lett.*, 32(23), 3373–3375, 2007.
65. A. Yariv, *Optical Electronics in Modern Communications*, 5th edn, Oxford University Press, 1997.
66. X. Zhao and C. Chang-Hasnain, A new amplifier model for resonance enhancement of optically injection-locked lasers, *IEEE Photon. Technol. Lett.*, 20(6), 395–397, 2008.
67. E. K. Lau, H. K. Sung, and M. C. Wu, Frequency response enhancement of optical injection-locked lasers, *IEEE J. Quantum Electron.*, 44(1), 90–99, 2008.
68. T. B. Simpson, J. M. Liu, and A. Gavrielides, Bandwidth enhancement and broadband noise reduction in injection-locked bandwidth enhancement and broadband noise reduction in injection-locked semiconductor lasers, *IEEE Photon. Technol. Lett.*, 7(7), 709–711, 1995.
69. —T. B. Simpson, J. M. Liu, and A. Gavrielides, Small-signal analysis of modulation characteristics in a semiconductor laser subject to strong optical injection, *IEEE J. Quantum Electron.*, 32(8), 1456–1468, 1996.
70. X. Zhao, B. Zhang, L. Christen, D. Parekh, F. Koyama, W. Hofmann, M. C. Amann, A. E. Willner, and C. Chang-Hasnain, Data inversion and adjustable chirp in 10-Gbps directly-modulated injection-locked 1.55-μm VCSELs, in *Conference on Lasers and Electro-Optics/Quantum Electronics and Laser Science Conference and Photonic Applications Systems Technologies*, 2008, paper CMW5.2001.
71. E. K. Lau, X. Zhao, H.-K. Sung, D. Parekh, C. Chang-Hasnain, and M. C. Wu, Strong optical injection-locked semiconductor lasers demonstrating > 100-GHz resonance frequencies and 80-GHz intrinsic bandwidths, *Opt. Express*, 16(9), 6609–6618, 2008.
72. E. K. Lau, High-speed modulation of optical injection-locked semiconductor lasers, PhD dissertation, UC Berkeley, 2006.
73. S. L. Chuang, *Physics of Optoelectronic Devices*, John Wiley & Sons, Inc, 1995.

74. R. S. Tucker, High-speed modulation of semiconductor lasers, *IEEE Trans. Electron. Devices*, ED-32(12), 2572–2584, 1985.
75. C. W. Wilmsen, H. Temkin, and L. A. Coldren, Eds., *Vertical-Cavity Surface-Emitting Lasers.*, Cambridge University Press, 1999.
76. L. Chrostowski, B. Faraji, W. Hofmann, M. C. Amann, and W. Chow, 40 GHz bandwidth and 64 GHz resonance frequency in injection-locked 1.55 μm VCSELs, *IEEE J. Sel. Top. Quantum Electron.*, 13(5), 1200–1208, 2007.
77. K. Y. Lau and A. Yariv, Intermodulation distortion in a directly modulated semiconductor injection laser, *Appl. Phys. Lett.*, 45(10), 1034–1036, 1984.
78. L. Chrostowski, C. H. Chang, and C. Chang-Hasnain, Enhancement of dynamic range in 1.55-μm VCSELs using injection locking, *IEEE Photon. Technol. Lett.*, 15(4), 498–501, 2003.
79. L. Chrostowski, X. Zhao, and C. Chang-Hasnain, Microwave performance of optically injection-locked VCSELs, *IEEE Trans. Microw. Theory Tech.*, 54(2), 788–796, 2006.
80. H. L. T. Lee, R. V. Dalal, R. J. Ram, and K. D. Choquette, Dynamic range of vertical-cavity surface-emitting lasers in multimode links, *IEEE Photon. Technol. Lett.*, 11(11), 1473–1475, 1999.
81. R. V. Dalal, R. J. Ram, R. Helkey, H. Roussell, and K. D. Choquette, Low distortion analogue signal transmission using vertical cavity lasers, *Electron. Lett.*, 34(16), 1590–1591, 1998.
82. X. Jin and S. L. Chuang, Relative intensity noise characteristics of injection-locked semiconductor lasers, *Appl. Phys. Lett.*, 77(9), 1250–1252, 2000.
83. L. Chrostowski, C. H. Chang, and C. Chang-Hasnain, Reduction of relative intensity noise and improvement of spur-free dynamic range of an injection locked VCSEL, in *Proc. IEEE LEOS 16th Annual Meeting*, pp. 706–707, 2003.
84. P. Spano, S. Piazzolla, and M. Tamburrini, Frequency and intensity noise in injection-locked semiconductor lasers: Theory and experiments, *IEEE J. Quantum Electron.*, QE-22(3), 427–435, 1986.
85. E. Wong, X. Zhao, C. Chang-Hasnain, W. Hofmann, and M. C. Amann, Optically injection-locked 1.55-μm VCSELs as upstream transmitters in WDM-PONs, *IEEE Photon. Technol. Lett.*, 18(22), 2371–2373, 2006.
86. Q. Gu, W. Hofmann, M. C. Amann, and L. Chrostowski, Optically injection-locked VCSEL for bi-directional optical communication, in *Conference on Lasers and Electro-Optics/Quantum Electronics and Laser Science Conference and Photonic Applications Systems Technologies*, 2008, paper CMW6.
87. Q. Gu, W. Hofmann, M. C. Amann, and L. Chrostowski, Optically injection-locked VCSEL as a duplex transmitter/receiver, *IEEE Photon. Technol. Lett*, 20, 7, 463–465, 2008.
88. K. Kishino, M. Unlu, J. I. Chyi, J. Reed, L. Arsenault, and H. Morkoc, Resonant cavity-enhanced (RCE) photodetectors, *IEEE J. Quantum Electron.*, 27(8), 2025–2034, 1991.

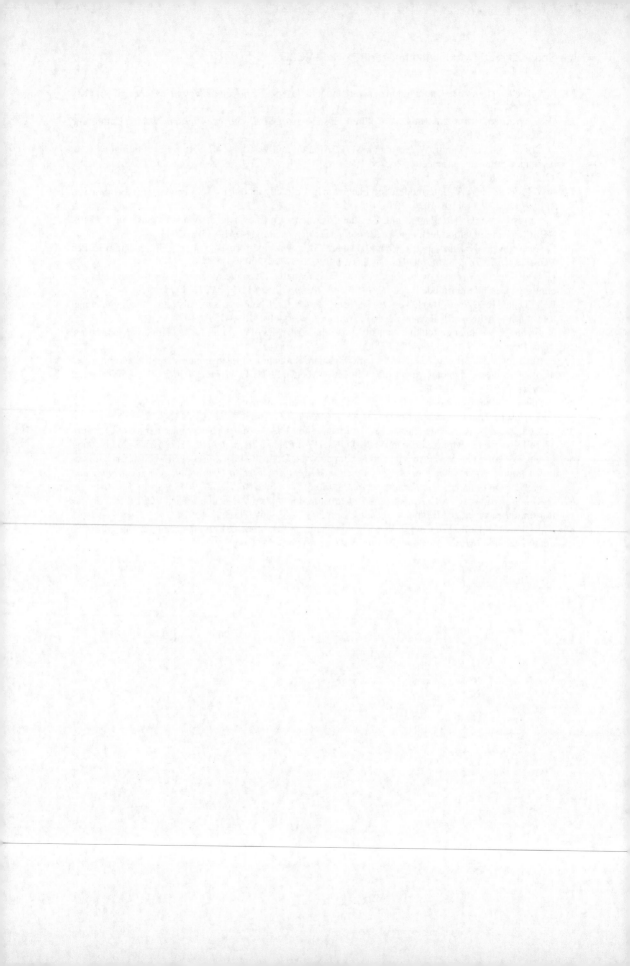

22 High-Speed Si/Ge-Based Photodiodes for Optical Interconnect Applications

J.-W. Shi and F.-M. Kuo

CONTENTS

22.1 INTRODUCTION

Owing to the ever-increasing need for higher bandwidths, optical interconnect (OI) technologies for rack-to-rack, board-to-board, and chip-to-chip signal transmission have received a great deal of attention in recent years [1,2]. The MAUI project (funded in part by the DARPA, United States) has successfully demonstrated a 500-Gbps parallel wavelength-division multiplexed OI [1] with 48 channels of 10.42-Gbps data transmitted over a parallel 12-fiber ribbon at 4 wavelengths per fiber. This device was developed in order to carry the bandwidth load needed for board-to-board and processor-to-processor capabilities in high-end computer systems. High-speed, high-efficiency, and low-power-consumption vertical-cavity surface-emitting lasers (VCSELs) [3–5], modulators, and photodiodes (PDs) [6,7] that operate at a wavelength of 850 nm or around 1000 nm have lately attracted much attention due to their suitability for applications in the OI system. Silicon (Si) photonic technology [8,9], which includes Si-based light sources, modulators, and PDs, can be used to realize these key active components in the OI system, because Si-based optoelectronic (OE) devices have the potential to be monolithically integrated with Si-based integrated circuits (ICs). Figure 22.1 depicts a 4 × 10-Gb/s, 0.13 μm complementary metal-oxide-semiconductor (CMOS) silicon-on-insulator (SOI) integrated OE transceiver chip copackaged with a single, externally modulated continuous-wave (CW) laser [10].

As can be seen in the figures, the Si-based waveguide, modulator, coupler, and electronic amplifiers are all monolithically integrated on a single chip. These integrated active/passive components (i.e., Si- or germanium(Ge)-based high-speed PDs [11–14] that operate at optical wavelengths of 850 and 1550 nm) constitute one of the most important active components needed in Si photonic

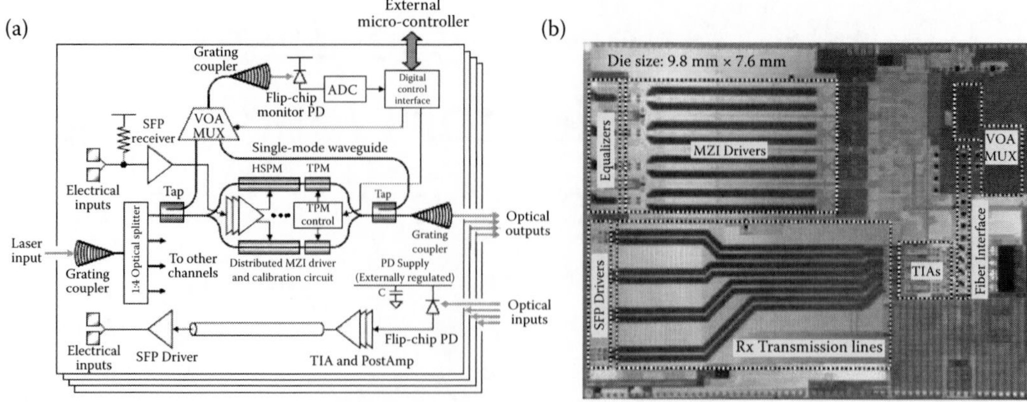

FIGURE 22.1 (a) Conceptual diagram of a 4 × 10-Gb/s, 0.13 μm CMOS SOI integrated OE transceiver chip copackaged with a single, externally modulated CW laser; (b) photograph of the same. (Data from A. Narasimha, et al., A 40-Gb/s QSFP optoelectronic transceiver in a 0.13 μm CMOS silicon-on-insulator technology, in *Proc. OFC 2008*, San Diego, CA, USA, March 2009, pp. OMK7. Copyright 2008 IEEE.)

technology. Figure 22.2 shows a Ge-based waveguide PD, which is monolithically integrated with CMOS ICs to form a single chip, for application to OI or in short-reach fiber communication [14]. In this chapter, we will review several kinds of high-speed Si-, Ge-, and SiGe-based high-speed PDs, introduce their working principles, and discuss the factors that limit their bandwidth. Finally, we will also introduce their applications in next-generation OI systems.

22.2 Si-BASED HIGH-SPEED PDs: 850 NM WAVELENGTH

22.2.1 The Fundamental Problems with Si-Based High-Speed PDs

Owing to the maturity of high-speed 850 nm VCSELs [3–5], the application of 850 nm high-speed PDs in OI systems has attracted much attention. Figure 22.3 shows the absorption coefficients and penetration depths versus wavelength for several different kinds of semiconductor materials [15], which include Si and Ge. As can be seen, Si has a much weaker absorption coefficient than that of

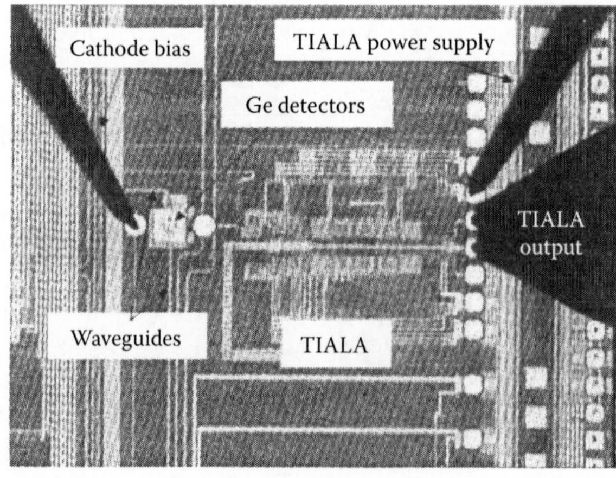

FIGURE 22.2 Photograph of a Ge-based waveguide PD monolithically integrated with a CMOS IC. (Data from G. Masini et al., A four-channel. 10Gbps monolithic optical receiver in 130 nm CMOS with integrated Ge waveguide photodetectors, *Postdeadline Paper, OFC* 2007, Anaheim, CA, USA, March 2007, pp. PDP31. Copyright 2007 IEEE.)

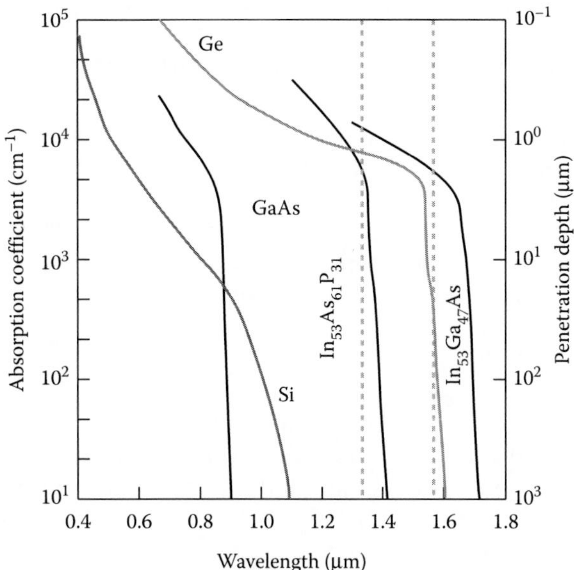

FIGURE 22.3 Photoabsorption coefficients versus wavelengths of different semiconductor materials. (Data from M. Morse et al., State of the art Si-based receiver solutions for short reach applications, in *Proc. OFC 2009*, San Diego, CA, USA, March 2009, pp. OMR5. Copyright 2009 IEEE.)

GaAs under 0.8 μm wavelength excitation (1 μm^{-1} versus 0.1 μm^{-1}), which corresponds to a 10 times larger penetration depth into Si material (10 μm versus 1 μm). A larger penetration depth indicates a longer carrier drift time and lower speed performance for Si-based PDs. Furthermore, the depth of the p–n junction is usually on the order of ~1 μm, which means that most of the photogenerated carriers will be concentrated in the neutral Si substrate without an electrical field inside. Poor speed performance can thus be expected. There are several reported methods for overcoming this fundamental problem with Si-based PDs. Figure 22.4a shows the cross-sectional view of a

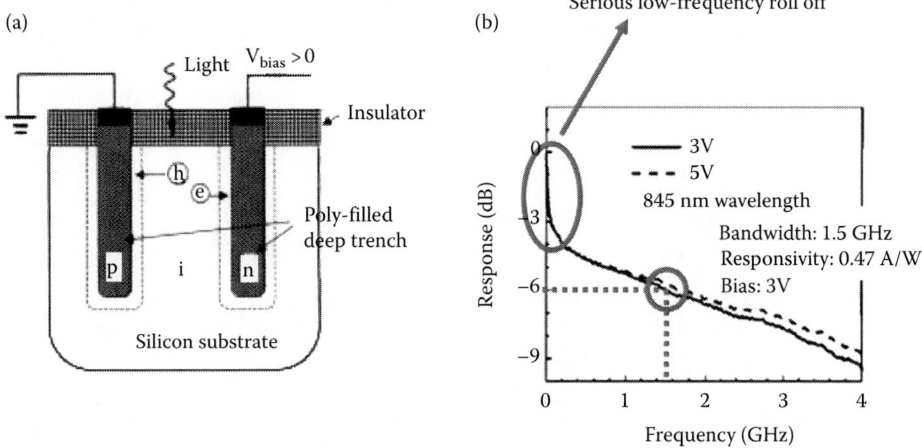

FIGURE 22.4 (a) Conceptual cross-sectional view of a deep-trench p–i–n photodiode; (b) its measured O–E frequency response under 850 nm wavelength excitation. (Data from M. Yang et al., *IEEE Electron Device Lett.*, 23, 395–397, 2002. Copyright 2002 IEEE.)

Si-based PD with a deep trench and lateral p–n junction structure [16]. The p–n junction depth (trench depth) is around 7 μm, which is much larger than that of a Si diode with a vertical p–n junction. Figure 22.4b shows its measured optical-to-electrical (O–E) frequency response under excitations of 845 nm optical wavelength [16]. As can be seen, under 845 nm wavelength excitation, a serious low-frequency roll-off exists and a poor 3-dB bandwidth (<100 MHz, 1.5 GHz 6 dB bandwidth) has been measured. We may thus conclude that even with a deep-trench p–n junction structure (7 μm junction depth) under ~850 nm optical wavelength excitation, the slow diffusion current from the Si substrate seriously limits the 3-dB O–E bandwidth. A larger junction depth (>7 μm) may minimize this phenomenon; however, it will result in a large junction capacitance and poor RC-limited bandwidth. In the following sections, we will discuss some methods for further overcoming such problems.

22.2.2 Spatial Modulation Si-Based PDs at 850 nm Wavelength

It has been demonstrated that the spatial modulation of Si-based PDs, which are fully compatible with the modern CMOS process, diminishes the low-frequency roll-off of Si-based PDs under 850 nm wavelength excitation [17]. Figure 22.5 shows a conceptual cross-sectional view and block diagram of the implementation process. As can be seen, the shaded PD also suffers from a slow diffusion current from the illuminated PD, which results in a low tail in the transient response of the PD. However, using a differential amplifier, we can get differential signals for two such PDs (shaded and illuminated) which partially cancel the long tail (low-frequency roll-off) during the transient response. However, the magnitude of the differential signal is less than that of a single photodiode. The long tail of the illuminated PDs cannot be 100% cancelled out due to the nonequal distribution of substrate photocurrents from the illuminated and shaded PDs. A 2 Gb/s data transmission at an optical wavelength of 850 nm has been demonstrated using such a technique.

22.2.3 Si-Based High-Speed Avalanche PDs that Operate at the 850 nm Wavelength

Recently, several research groups have fabricated high-speed Si-based PDs on standard Si substrates by biasing these PDs under avalanche operation [18–20]. The high-speed and high-gain avalanche current screens the slow diffusion current that arises from the Si substrate (as discussed above), leading to improvement in the bandwidth. Figure 22.6 shows a conceptual cross-sectional view of Si-based PDs with an interdigitated p–n junction structure and its bias-dependent speed performance [18]. As can be seen, the speed performance of the PDs increases significantly with the

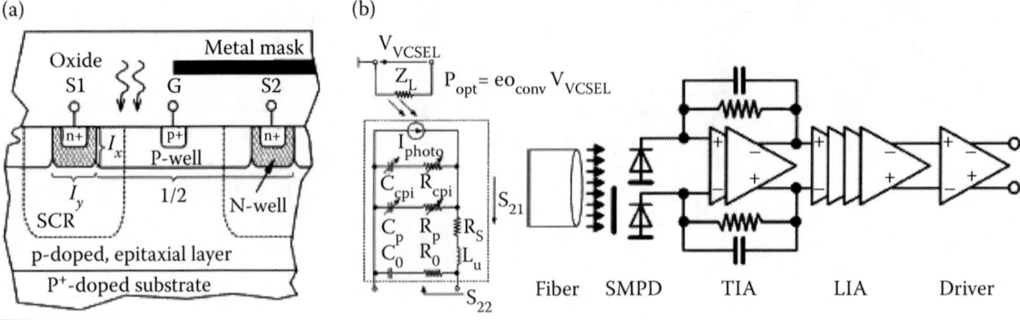

FIGURE 22.5 (a) Conceptual cross-sectional view of the spatial modulation of a Si-based p–i–n photodiode; (b) its setup for high-speed operation. (Data from M. Jutzi et al., *IEEE Photon. Technol. Lett.*, 17, 1268–1270, 2005. Copyright 2005 IEEE.)

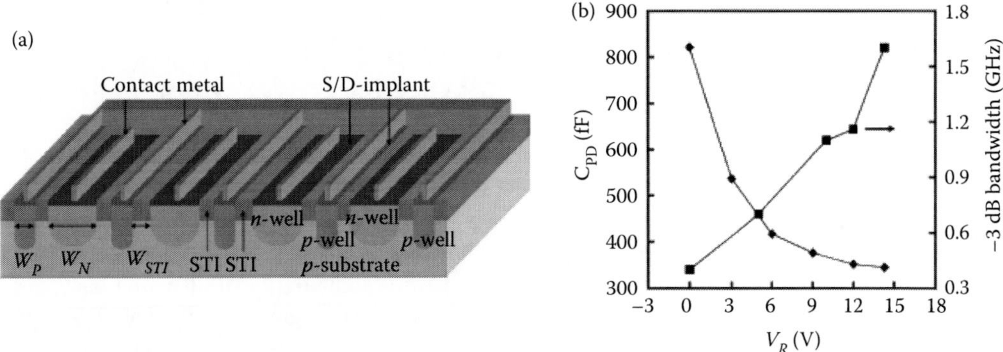

FIGURE 22.6 (a) Conceptual cross-sectional view and top view of interdigitated CMOS-based PDs; (b) measured 3-dB bandwidth and junction capacitance versus reverse bias voltage. (Data from W.-K. Huang et al., *IEEE Photon. Technol. Lett.*, 19, 197–199, 2007. Copyright 2007 IEEE.)

reverse bias voltage once the bias voltage reaches the breakdown point. Furthermore, under avalanche operation, a resonant phenomenon may appear in the measured O–E frequency response, which induces a further increase in the measured O–E bandwidth [19–21]. This phenomenon has been attributed to the space charge effect [21] or the traveling space charge wave [19]; ultrahigh gain-bandwidth products have also been reported [19,21]. Figure 22.7 shows the measured O–E frequency response reported for Si/SiGe-based avalanche photodiodes (APDs) under avalanche operation and 850 nm optical wavelength excitation.

A significant resonant phenomenon can be observed. By using this phenomenon, clear 10 Gb/s eye-opening with reasonable sensitivity performance (−11 dBm) for error-free operation can be achieved under 850 nm optical wavelength excitation [19]. Recently, another research group utilized the structure of Si-based spatial modulation PDs [17], as discussed above, operated in the avalanche region, to realize monolithic Si-based photoreceiver circuits that operate at the 850 nm optical wavelength. These circuits have improved responsivity and speed performance. 10 Gb/s eye-opening and error-free operation can also be achieved [22].

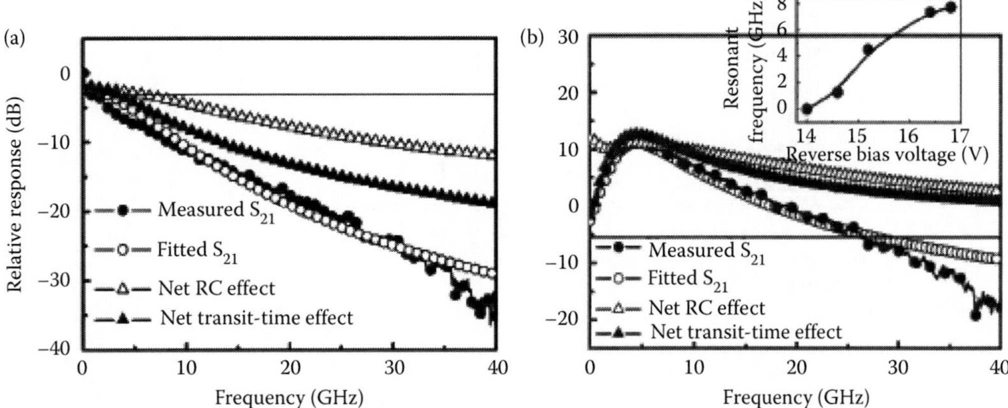

FIGURE 22.7 Measured O–E frequency responses of Si/SiGe APD (a) below and (b) above breakdown voltage operation. (Data from J.-W. Shi et al., *IEEE Electron Device Lett.*, 30, 1164–1166, 2009. Copyright 2009 IEEE.)

22.3 GERMANIUM AND GE/SI-BASED HIGH-SPEED PHOTODIODES FOR 1.3–1.55 μM WAVELENGTH OPERATION

22.3.1 The Fundamental Problems of Ge and Ge/Si-Based High-Speed PDs

The 1.3 and 1.55 μm wavelengths attract more attention than the 850 nm optical wavelengths due to the fact that, in that wavelength regime, the propagation loss and dispersion in the optical fiber is lower. As shown in Figure 22.3, the absorption of the bulk Si material is negligible in that wavelength (1.3–1.55 μm) regime. Using Ge is a promising way to extend the capability of Si-based high-speed PDs to perform long-wavelength detection. As can be seen in Figure 22.3, the photoabsorption constant of the bulk Ge material is comparable to that of the III–V-based semiconductor material (InGaAsP), under 1.3 μm wavelength operation. However, when the operating wavelength reaches 1.55 μm, the absorption constant of Ge dramatically decreases and becomes much smaller than that of the III–V-based material (InGaAs). The absorption edge of the bulk Ge material seems to be around 1.5 μm. In addition, there is a large difference between the lattice constants of the Ge and Si materials, which results in problems with the growth of high-quality Ge thin films on Si substrates. In the following sections, we will describe several reported technologies for overcoming the aforementioned problems.

22.3.2 High-Speed Ge-Based PDs

Ge substrates can be used to fabricate high-speed Ge-based metal–semiconductor–metal (MSM) or p–i–n PDs. Figure 22.8 shows the top view, the cross-sectional view and measured external quantum efficiency versus wavelength of Ge PDs [23]. One of the major problems with Ge-based PDs compared with InP-based PDs is their higher dark current density. The proper choice of contact metal, such as silver as is shown in Figure 22.8, is one possible solution for enhancing the barrier height and reducing the dark current density. In addition, dopant segregation in MSM Ge-based PDs has been demonstrated to lead to a higher Schottky barrier height and a lower dark current [24]. Apart from the high dark current, another problem with Ge-based PDs is the cutoff of the photoabsorption under 1.55 μm wavelength excitation. As can be seen in Figure 22.8, serious external efficiency roll-off is measured when the wavelength reaches 1.55 μm. Applying strain to the Ge epi-layer is one possible way of further extending the cutoff wavelength [25].

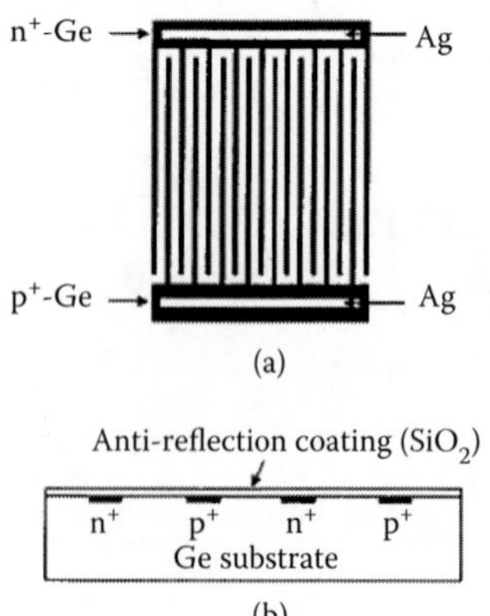

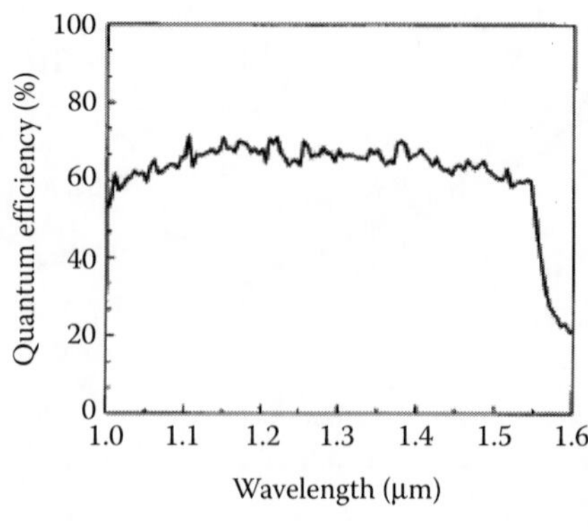

FIGURE 22.8 (a) Top view and (b) cross-sectional view of Ge-based PDs, showing measured external quantum efficiency versus wavelength. (Data from J. Oh et al., *IEEE Photon. Technol. Lett.*, 14, 369–371, 2002. Copyright 2002 IEEE.)

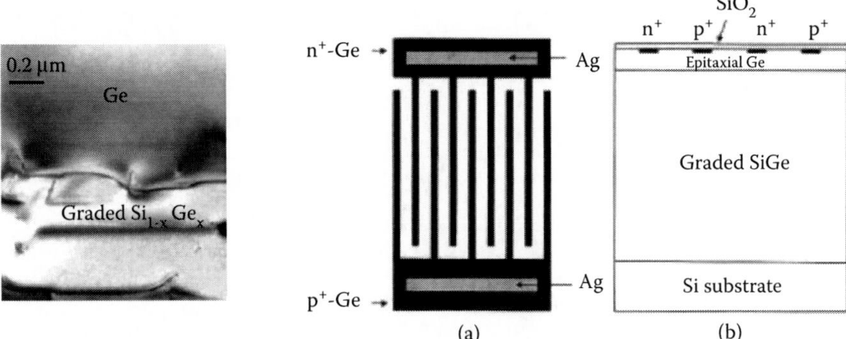

FIGURE 22.9 Cross-sectional view of Ge-based PDs with a graded SiGe buffer on a Si substrate. (Data from J. Oh et al., *IEEE J. Quantum Electron*, 38, 1238–1241, 2002. Copyright 2002 IEEE.)

This kind of PD will be discussed in more detail in the following section. Another important issue with the Ge-based PD is its capability to integrate with Si-based ICs. Figure 22.9 shows the cross-sectional view of a Ge-based PD grown on a Si substrate [26]. As can be seen, a thick SiGe buffer (several microns) is necessary due to the large lattice mismatch between the Ge and Si layers. This thick buffer layer impedes the monolithic integration of Si-based ICs on the bottom layer and Ge-based PDs on the top. The growth of a high-speed selective area of the Ge layer on the Si substrate is one promising solution to overcome this problem. We will discuss this issue in the following section.

22.3.3 High-Speed Selective-Area Growth on Ge-on-Si-Based PDs

As discussed in Figure 22.9, due to the large lattice mismatch (4%) between the Si and Ge materials, a thick SiGe buffer layer is necessary for full Si wafer growth. The selective-area growth technique is one attractive solution for the realization of a high-quality buffer-free Ge epi-layer on the Si substrate. During the selective-area growth process, the growth temperature is lowered down to around ~300°C to produce a thin (several nanometers), flat Ge seed layer covering the patterned Si substrate followed by a thick Ge epi-layer (several micrometers in thickness) grown at a high temperature (500–700°C) [8]. After that, cyclical high–low temperature hydrogen gas annealing (900–700°C) was performed to reduce the threading dislocation and grow a high-quality Ge layer grown on the Si substrate [8]. Ge on Si should be compressively strained when grown coherently because of the larger lattice constant. However, the thick Ge epi-layer on Si shows tensile strain in the epi-layers of the PDs. This is because the linear lattice expansion coefficient of Ge is larger than that of Si, provided the epi-layer is not relaxed during growth cooling [8]. This tensile-strained Ge epi-layer can extend the absorption cutoff wavelength of Ge layer to around 1.55 μm. Figure 22.10 shows the measured absorption coefficient versus wavelengths for the Ge layer, with and without tensile strain [25]. As can be seen, the area of selective growth in the Ge layer will have residual tensile strain (0.141%) and enhanced photoabsorption on the long wavelength side compared to that of the full-relaxed Ge layer. The value of the absorption constant for the strained Ge layer is comparable to that of the III–V-based $In_{0.53}Ga_{0.47}As$ layer. Very-high-speed performance (~40 GHz) has been demonstrated by the selective-area Ge PD growth on a Si substrate at a 1.55 μm wavelength [12]. Another advantage of the selective-area growth technique is that it makes possible the realization of high-quality Ge–Si heterostructures. One of the most important motivations for the realization of Ge–Si heterostructures is for application in high-performance APDs at approximately the 1.55 μm wavelength

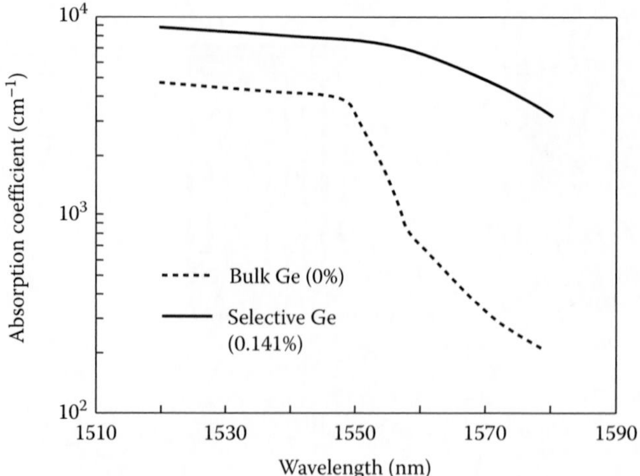

FIGURE 22.10 The absorption constants of tensile-strained Ge film and full-relaxed Ge film on Si substrate. (Data from M. Piels et al., Microwave nonlinearities in Ge/Si avalanche photodiodes having a gain bandwidth product of 300 GHz, in *Proc. OFC 2009*, San Diego, CA, USA, March 2009, pp. OMR1. Copyright 2009 IEEE.)

regime. This is because the Si material has the largest difference in ionization coefficients between electrons and holes among all the III–V-based semiconductor materials. However, the band gap of Si restricts its application as high-performance APDs in the fiber communication wavelength regime. By combining the selective-area-grown strained Ge photoabsorption layer, which has reasonable photoabsorption at the 1.55 μm wavelength, and the Si-based multiplication layer, a high-performance telecommunication APD can thus be expected. Figure 22.11 shows the conceptual cross-sectional view of a Ge–Si APD [27]. As can be seen, the high-quality Ge absorption layer is directly grown on the Si-based multiplication layer. This kind of APD has demonstrated a very high gain–bandwidth product at the 1.3 μm wavelength [27].

22.3.4 Ge-on-Insulator (GOI) and SOI-Based PDs

An alternative to the fabrication of high-speed Si-based PDs on the standard Si substrate is the fabrication of high-speed PDs on SOI or Ge-on-insulator (GOI) substrates, both of which show some unique advantages. Figures 22.12 and 22.13 show the conceptual cross-sectional view of high-speed PDs on SOI and GOI substrates, respectively [11,13]. The major advantage of SOI and GOI PDs compared to those on the standard Si substrates is that the slow diffusion current from the Si substrate (under 850 nm optical wavelength excitation) is blocked by the buried insulator layer. The shaded PDs' structure and avalanche operation of the PD on a standard Si substrate, as discussed in Sections 22.2.2 and 22.2.3, may not be necessary for minimizing the influence of slow substrate current on the speed performance, in the case of SOI and GOI substrates. Furthermore, SOI and GOI substrates also play important roles in the realization of chip-level OIs and Si-based photonic-integrated circuits (PICs). As shown in Figure 22.1, integration of active PDs and Si-based modulators with passive optical waveguides on the same Si chip to form Si-based PICs is necessary. SOI or GOI substrates offer a promising solution for the realization of such systems. This is because there is a huge difference in the index between the buried oxide layer and active Ge or Si epi-layers. A strong index guided ride waveguide on SOI or GOI substrates can thus be expected. Figure 22.14 shows conceptual top views and cross-sectional views of a GOI waveguide PD for chip-level OI applications. As can be seen, the topmost Ge layer serves as a photoabsorption layer to absorb photons propagating at the 1.55 μm wavelength in the SOI waveguide [28].

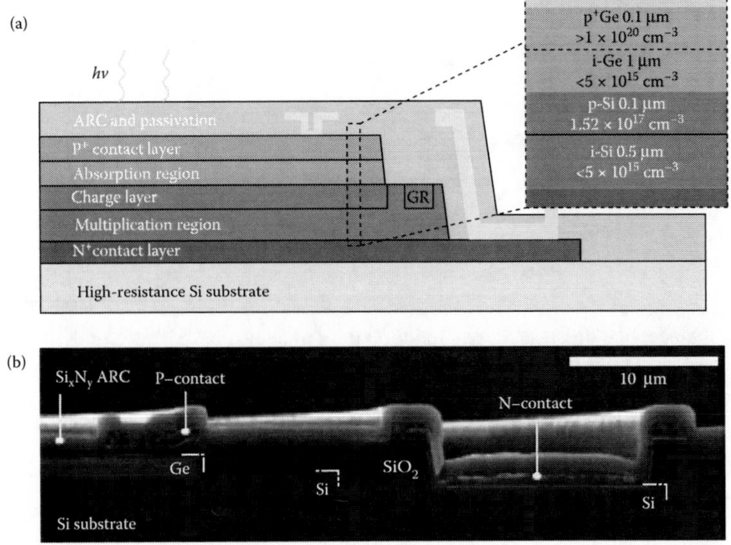

FIGURE 22.11 (a) Conceptual cross-sectional view; (b) scanning electron microscope image of the Ge-on-Si APD. (Data from B. Yang et al., *IEEE Photon. Technol. Lett.*, 15, 745–747, 2003. Copyright 2003 IEEE.)

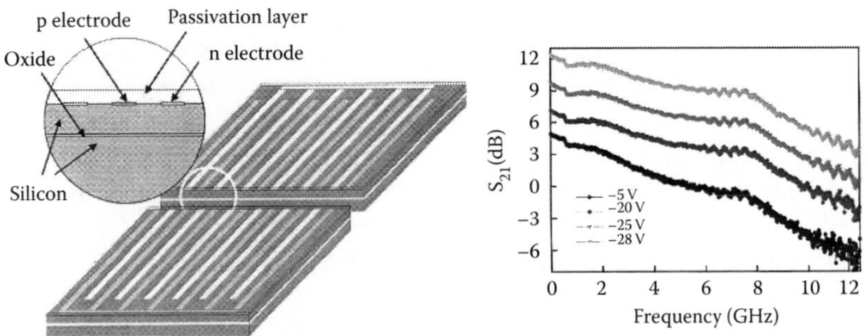

FIGURE 22.12 Conceptual cross-sectional view of an SOI PD and its measured O–E frequency response under 850 nm wavelength excitation. As can be seen, there is no low-frequency roll-off. (Data from B. Yang et al., *IEEE Photon. Technol. Lett.*, 15, 745–747, 2003. Copyright 2003 IEEE.)

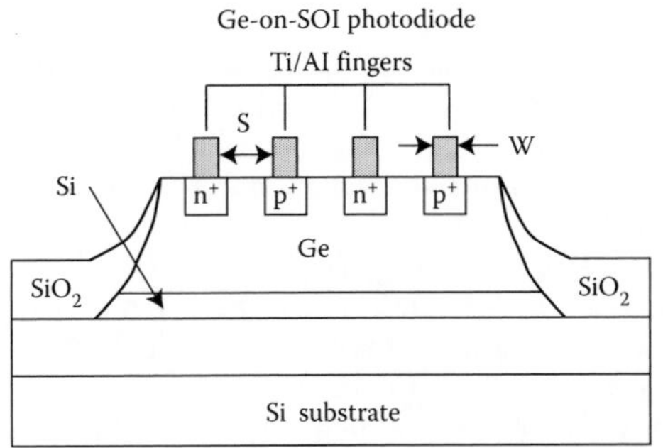

FIGURE 22.13 Conceptual cross-sectional view of the GOI PD. (Data from C. L. Schow et al., *IEEE Photon. Technol. Lett.*, 18, 1981–1983, 2006. Copyright 2006 IEEE.)

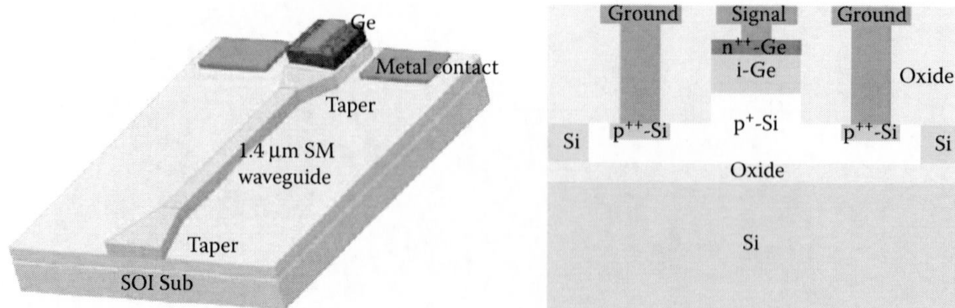

FIGURE 22.14 Conceptual cross-sectional and top views of a GOI-based waveguide PD. (Data from T. Yin et al., *Opt. Express*, 15(21), 13965–13971, 2007. Copyright 2007 OSA.)

22.4 CONCLUSION

In this chapter, we have reviewed several kinds of Si (Ge)-based high-speed PDs for OI applications. Under 850 nm wavelength excitation, the main problem is the slow diffusion current from the Si substrate, which will seriously degrade the speed performance of the PD. In order to overcome this problem, a shaded PD structure, avalanche operation, and SOI substrates are utilized to block or screen this slow substrate photocurrent. A Ge-based epi-layer can be incorporated into the Si substrate for 1.3–1.55 μm wavelength detection. A selective-area growth and cycling temperature annealing process is necessary in order to overcome the problem caused by the 4% lattice mismatch between the Ge and Si layers, to process and to improve the material quality of Ge thin film. Very-high-speed performance of Ge-on-Si-based PDs and GOI PDs and APDs has been demonstrated at 1.3 and 1.55 μm. Among these reported technologies, the Ge PDs on Si (or SOI) substrates show the most promising result for applications in short (850 nm) or long (~1300 nm) wavelength communication and detection. The product of selective-area-grown Ge-based high-speed discretized PDs has been released. Compared with III–V-based PDs, the major advantage of the Si-based PD is that it can be integrated with the mature CMOS ICs. Recently, IBM and Luxtera have demonstrated the integration of GOI waveguide PDs with CMOS ICs. It seems likely that Si (Ge)-based PDs will play an important role in the fabrication of Si-based PICs in the near future.

REFERENCES

1. B. E. Lemoff, M. E. Ali, G. Panotopoulos, G. M. Flower, B. Madhavan, A. F. J. Levi, and D. W. Dolfi, MAUI: Enabling fiber-to-processor with parallel multiwavelength optical interconnects, *IEEE/OSA J. Lightwave Technol.*, 22, 2043–2054, 2004.
2. L. Schares, J. A. Kash, F. E. Doany, C. L. Schow, C. Schuster, D. M. Kuchta, P. K. Pepeljugoski et al., Terabus: Terabit/second-class card-level optical interconnect technologies, *IEEE J. Sel. Top. Quantum Electron.*, 12, 1032–1044, 2006.
3. K. Yashiki, N. Suzuki, K. Fukatsu, T. Anan, H. Hatakeyama, and M. Tsuji, 1.1-μm-Range high-speed tunnel junction vertical-cavity surface-emitting lasers, *IEEE Photon. Technol. Lett.*,19, 1883–1885, 2007.
4. C.-K. Lin, A. Tandon, K. Djordjev, S. W. Corzine, and M. R. T. Tan, High-speed 985 nm bottom-emitting VCSEL arrays for chip-to-chip parallel optical interconnects, *IEEE J. Sel. Top. Quantum Electron.*, 13, 1332–1339, 2007.
5. J.-W. Shi, C.-C. Chen, Y.-S. Wu, S.-H. Guol, and Y.-J Yang, The influence of Zn-diffusion depth on the static and dynamic behaviors of Zn-diffusion high-speed vertical-cavity surface-emitting lasers at a 850 nm wavelength, *IEEE J. Quantum Electron.*, 45, 800–806, 2009.
6. J.-W. Shi, F.-M. Kuo, T.-C. Hsu, Ying-Jay Yang, A. Joel, M. Mattingley, and J.-I. Chyi, The monolithic integration of GaAs/AlGaAs based uni-traveling-carrier photodiodes with Zn-diffusion vertical-cavity surface-emitting lasers with extremely high data-rate/power-consumption ratios, *IEEE Photon. Technol. Lett.*, 21, 1444–1446, 2009.

7. K. Fukatsu, K. Shiba, Y. Suzuki, N. Suzuki, T. Anan, H. Hatakeyama, K. Yashiki, and M. Tsuji, 30 Gbs Over 100 m MMFs using 1.1 μm range VCSELs and photodiodes, *IEEE Photon. Technol. Lett.*, 20(11), 2008.
8. K. Wada, S. Park, and Y. Ishikawa, Si photonics and fiber to the home, *IEEE Proc.*, 97(7), 1329–1336, 2009.
9. L. Tsybeskov, D. J. Lockwood, M. Ichikawa, Si photonics: CMOS going optical, *IEEE Proc.*, 97(7), 1161–1165, 2009.
10. A. Narasimha et al., A 40-Gb/s QSFP optoelectronic transceiver in a 0.13 μm CMOS silicon-on-insulator technology, in *Proc. OFC 2008*, San Diego, CA, USA, March 2009, pp. OMK7.
11. B. Yang, J. D. Schaub, S. M. Csutak, D. L. Rogers, and J. C. Campbell, 10-Gb/s All-silicon optical receiver, *IEEE Photon. Technol. Lett.*, 15, 745–747, 2003.
12. M. Jutzi, M. Berroth, G. Wohl, M. Oehme, and E. Kasper, Ge-on-Si vertical incidence photodiodes with 39-G Hz bandwidth, *IEEE Photon. Technol. Lett.*, 17, 1510–1512, 2005.
13. C. L. Schow, L. Schares, S. J. Koester, G. Dehlinger, R. John, and F. E. Doany, A 15-Gb/s 2.4-V optical receiver using a Ge-on-SOI photodiode and a CMOS IC, *IEEE Photon. Technol. Lett.*, 18, 1981–1983, 2006.
14. G. Masini, G. Capellini, J. Witzens, and C. Gunn, A four-channel. 10Gbps monolithic optical receiver in 130 nm CMOS with integrated Ge waveguide photodetectors, *Postdeadline Paper, OFC* 2007, Anaheim, CA, USA, March 2007, pp. PDP31.
15. M. Morse, T. Yin, Y. Kang, O. Dosunmu, H.D. Liu, M. Paniccia, G. Sarid, E. Ginsburg, R. Cohen, Y. Saado, R. Shnaiderman, and M. Zadka, State of the art Si-based receiver solutions for short reach applications, in *Proc. OFC 2009*, San Diego, CA, USA, March 2009, pp. OMR5.
16. M. Yang, K. Rim, D. L. Rogers, J. D. Schaub, J. J. Welser, D. M. Kuchta, D. C. Boyd et al., A high-speed, high-sensitivity silicon lateral trench photodetector, *IEEE Electron Device Lett.*, 23, 395–397, 2002.
17. M. Jutzi, M. Grözing, E. Gaugler, W. Mazioschek, and M. Berroth, 2-Gb/s CMOS optical integrated receiver with a spatially modulated photodetector, *IEEE Photon. Technol. Lett.*, 17, 1268–1270, 2005.
18. W.-K. Huang, Y.-C. Liu, and Y.-M. Hsin, A high-speed and high-responsivity photodiode in standard CMOS technology, *IEEE Photon. Technol. Lett.*, 19, 197–199, 2007.
19. J.-W. Shi, F.-M. Kuo, F.-C. Hong, and Y.-S. Wu, Dynamic analysis of a Si/SiGe based impact ionization avalanche transit time photodiode with an ultra-high gain-bandwidth product, *IEEE Electron Device Lett.*, 30, 1164–1166, 2009.
20. M.-J. Lee, H.-S. Kang, and W.-Y. Choi, Equivalent circuit model for Si avalanche photodetectors fabricated in standard CMOS process, *IEEE Electron Device Lett.*, 29, 1115–1117, 2008.
21. W. S. Zaoui, H.-W. Chen, J. E. Bowers, Y. Kang, M. Morse, M. J. Paniccia, A. Pauchard, and J. C. Campbell, Origin of the gain-bandwidth-product enhancement in separate-absorption-charge-multiplication Ge/Si avalanche photodiodes, in *Proc. OFC 2009*, San Diego, CA, USA, March 2009, pp. OMR6.
22. S.-H. Huang and W.-Z. Chen, A 10-Gbps CMOS single chip optical receiver with 2-D meshed spatially-modulated light detector, *IEEE 2009 Custom Integrated Circuits Conference*, San Jose, CA, pp. 129–132, September 2009.
23. J. Oh, S. Csutak, and Joe C. Campbell, High-speed interdigitated Ge PIN photodetectors, *IEEE Photon. Technol. Lett.*, 14, 369–371, 2002.
24. H. Zang, S. J. Lee, W. Y. Loh, J. Wang, M. B. Yu, G. Q. Lo, D. L. Kwong, and B. J. Cho, Application of dopant segregation to metal–germanium–metal photodetectors and its dark current suppression mechanism, *Appl. Phys. Lett.*, 92, 051110, 2008.
25. H.-Y. Yu, S. Ren, W. S. Jung, A. K. Okyay, D. A. B. Miller, and K. C. Sarawat, High-efficiency p-i-n photodetetcors on selective-area-grown Ge for monolithic integration, *IEEE Electron Device Lett.*, 30, 1161–1163, 2009.
26. J. Oh, Joe C. Campbell, S. G. Thomas, S. Bharatan, R. Thoma, C. Jasper, R. E. Jones, and T. E. Zirkle, Interdigitated Ge p–i–n photodetectors fabricated on a Si substrate using graded SiGe buffer layers, *IEEE J. Quantum Electron.*, 38, 1238–1241, 2002.
27. M. Piels, A. Ramaswamy, W. Sfar Zaoui, J. E. Bowers, Y. Kang, and M. Morse, Microwave nonlinearities in Ge/Si avalanche photodiodes having a gain bandwidth product of 300 GHz, in *Proc. OFC 2009*, San Diego, CA, USA, March 2009, pp. OMR1.
28. T. Yin, R. Cohen, M. M. Morse, G. Sarid, Y. Chetrit, D. Rubin, and M. J. Paniccia, 31 GHz Ge n-i-p waveguide photodetectors on silicon-on-insulator substrate, *Opt. Express*, 15(21), 13965–13971, 2007.

23 Patterned Sapphire and Chip Separation Technique in InGaN-Based LEDs

Jae-Hoon Lee

CONTENTS

23.1 INTRODUCTION

Group III–nitride semiconductors and their ternary solid solutions are very promising as the candidates for both short-wavelength optoelectronics and power electronic devices [1–6]. The AlGaN/GaN heterostructure field effect transistors have a great potential for future high-frequency and high-power applications because of the intrinsic advantages of materials such as a wide band gap, high breakdown voltage, and high electron peak velocity. These III–nitride materials are also suited for application such as the high-temperature piezoelectronics, the pyroelectric sensors, and the surface acoustic wave devices, due to the inherent strong polarization effects of hexagonal lattices [7–9]. AlN, GaN, and InN all crystallize in the wurtzite structure and have vastly different band gaps ranging from 6.0 eV for AlN down to 0.7 eV for InN [10]. Major developments in wide-gap III–nitride semiconductors have led to the commercial production of high-brightness light-emitting diodes (LEDs). The InGaN-based LEDs have already been extensively used in full-color displays, traffic displays, and various other applications such as projectors, automobile headlights, and general lighting. In particular, white LEDs based on InGaN/GaN are regarded as the most promising solid-state lighting devices to replace conventional incandescent.

In spite of their recent success, however, the output power of InGaN/GaN LEDs needs to be improved for commercial use. The limitation on light output power is mainly attributed to the low internal quantum efficiency and light extraction efficiency. The low internal quantum efficiency results from the high threading dislocation density of GaN films [11,12]. It is well known that high-density threading dislocations are inherent in epitaxial GaN films on sapphire substrates due to the large difference in lattice constant between the epitaxial layer and the sapphire substrate. Therefore, how to reduce the dislocation density is an important issue for fabricating high-performance LEDs. Epitaxial lateral overgrowth (ELOG) or pendeo epitaxy (PE) has been used to partially overcome the problems [13,14]. Although the ELOG and PE processes can dramatically decrease dislocation density, the related growth process is complicated and time consuming. Recently, it was reported that not only one can reduce the threading dislocation density in GaN films, but also one can enhance the light extraction efficiency by using a patterned sapphire substrate (PSS) [15–18]. The PSS technique has attracted much attention for its high production yield due to the single growth process without any interruption. Moreover, the refractive index of nitride films ($n = 2.5$) is higher than that of air ($n = 1$) and sapphire substrate ($n = 1.78$). The critical angle of the escape cone is about 23°, which indicates that only about 4% of the total light can be extracted from the surface [19]. Most of the light generated in the active layer is absorbed by the electrode at each reflection and gradually disappears, due to the total internal reflection, and is then converted to heat. There has been intensive research for the improvement of light extraction efficiency and the enhancement of brightness in the LED by using surface roughening, the PSS technique, flip-chip bonding, laser lift-off, and photonic crystal structure [20–27].

To further improve the extraction efficiency of devices, a method of die separation after chip fabrication on wafer is important. Sapphire is used as the substrate for many blue LED devices but this material is very difficult to dice using traditional diamond. The process of cutting the sapphire wafer is usually divided into three steps. First, the wafer is thinned to a thickness of about 80–150 μm. The wafer is scribed along the proper shapes using the diamond tips in the second step. Then, it is fractured and split using standard cleaving equipment. However, there are many problems in this final process, such as low depth of scribing and abrasion of the harder material itself. The low depth of scribing can also induce failure in breaking the wafer along the scribed line, including low throughput and high operating costs. The laser scribing process developed recently can eliminate most of the problems encountered in diamond tip scribing, which offers high-speed scribing with narrow kerfs, an increase in the chip density due to reduced street width, and hence a reduction in overall manufacturing costs. Various laser technologies, such as dry laser dicing, water jet-guided laser dicing, and stealth dicing, have already been developed and widely used in industrial applications [28–30]. However, some problems related to laser ablation, such as debris and thermal damage on the device, remain to be solved. Highly efficient peak power intensity, which strongly depends on both laser wavelength and pulse duration, is required for good laser scribing [31].

In this chapter, the history and important properties of group III–nitrides is briefly reviewed in Section 23.1. The characteristics of GaN film grown on PSS are discussed in Section 23.2. The effect of residual stress of InGaN/GaN films after sapphire lapping and polishing is described in Section 23.3. Section 23.4 deals with chip breaking using traditional diamond tip scribing. To improve the output power of LEDs through the reduction of both debris and thermal damage of sapphire substrate, a method of LED-chip separation using the 100 kHz femtosecond laser scribing technique is proposed and discussed in Section 23.5.

23.1.1 Evolution of III–Nitride Materials

GaN was first created in 1932 by Johnson at the University of Chicago by reacting ammonia gas with solid gallium at a temperature of 900–1000°C [32]. The GaN synthesis technique was also used to study the crystal structure and lattice constant by Juza et al. [33] in 1938 and to study the photoluminescence spectra by Grimmeiss and Koelmans [34] in 1959. Maruska and Tietjen [35] deposited the first large-area GaN layers on sapphire in 1969 using vapor-phase transport in chlorine. This earliest research on GaN was directed at understanding the properties of the material and learning how to design the material for specific uses. All the early GaN was very conductive as grown, and it was realized that these crystals were n-type with high carrier concentration owing to the highly defective nature of the crystal [36]. Because the work on GaN had earlier been focused on its potential for optical sources, p-type GaN was required in order to make p–n junction emitters, and hence much effort was focused on this area. Pankove et al. [37] were successful in fabricating the first blue GaN LED. It was a metal/insulating GaN:Zn/n-GaN (m-i-n or MIS) diode. The n-GaN layers contained different concentrations of Zn. The wavelength of the emitted light depended on the Zn concentration. Until the late 1970s the quality of GaN was not very good. The results of optical and electrical measurements were not reproducible. Yoshida et al. [38] deposited an AlN buffer layer to overcome the nucleation problems of GaN grown directly on a sapphire substrate in 1983. This buffer layer technique was very effective in improving the overall material quality of sapphire. The two-step method was investigated and perfected by Akasaki and coworkers in 1988/1989 [39]. In the first step, a thin buffer layer of AlN is grown on the sapphire substrate at the low temperature of ~500°C. The GaN layer is grown on the buffer layer. This important accomplishment allowed GaN to be grown with a much higher crystal quality than was previously available. The worldwide attention to research on group III–nitrides was stimulated by the success in material quality improvement using a low-temperature GaN nucleation layer attained by Nakamura [40] in the early 1990s and later by the success in blue LEDs and laser diodes (LDs) by Nakamura et al. [41], leading to a better understanding of the group III–nitride material system. The GaN-based field-effect transistors (FETs) were also fabricated about the same time, that is, in 1993 [42]. The fabrication of a heterostructure bipolar transistor (HBT) using p-type 6H SiC as the base and n-type GaN as the emitter was reported in 1994 [43]. Metalorganic chemical vapor deposition (MOCVD) has been the most popular growth technique for nitride growth and has been the choice for several electronic and optoelectronic devices such as high electron mobility transistors (HEMTs), HBTs, LEDs, and LDs.

23.1.2 Important Properties of III–Nitride Materials

The III–nitride group of materials includes GaN, AlN, InN, and their alloys. The band gap of the nitride group of materials is direct and has different band gaps ranging from 6.2 eV for AlN down to 0.7 eV for InN [10]. This gives a tremendous optical range for III–nitride materials, from yellow to ultraviolet (UV). The large band gap and strong termodynamical stability of the III–nitride material system point to promising high-power and high-temperature electronic device applications. Nitride materials are also extremely resilient to harsh chemical environments, giving the possibility for use in environments where the more traditional III–V materials are unable to perform. The most thermodynamically stable form of the nitride materials is the wurtzite or hexagonal form. This results in the familiar hexagonal close pack (HCP) model of alternating planes of Ga and N atoms stacked in an ABABAB sequence. The crystal planes in the wurtzite system are given using the Miller–Bravis index system of $[ijkl]$ with $k = -(i + j)$. Further details of HCP and hexagonal crystal notation can be found in the classic textbook *Introduction to Solid State Physics* by Charles Kittel [44]. Nitrides can also be forced to grow in a zinc blend form by using cubic substrates such as (001) Si and GaAs. The stacking sequence in this case is ABCABC. However, although the electrical properties of cubic III–nitrides are in theory expected to be better than for hexagonal GaN, in practice cubic III–nitrides are generally not as high quality as the wurtzite form and often contain a mixture of both cubic and wurtzite phases (mixed phase). The structural properties of the cubic nitrides can be found in Ref. [45].

The most common substrate for GaN epitaxial growth is sapphire. It was the substrate used during the first attempts at GaN epitaxy during the late 1960s and has remained the leading choice to this day. The attraction to sapphire for GaN epitaxy stems from its high melting point, chemical stability, availability of large wafer sizes, very-high-quality crystals, and low wafer cost. However, sapphire has a large lattice and thermal mismatch with GaN, leading to high defect density (~10^9/cm^2) in the GaN film and limiting the maximum layer thickness to less than 10 μm. In addition, the low thermal conductivity of sapphire limits heat dissipation through the substrate, imposing severe limits for power devices on this substrate. Despite these difficulties, sapphire remains the leading candidate for basic III–nitride epitaxy due to wide availability and low cost. In the case of growth on c-plane sapphire, a 30° rotation around the c-axis occurs for GaN epitaxy, resulting in an effective lattice constant that is $1/\sqrt{3}$ less than a sapphire. The resulting lattice mismatch is ~13%. In addition, on c-plane sapphire, the thermal expansion mismatch is −25.5%.

Table 23.1 lists some of the common electronic properties of the III–nitride group of materials (for comparison, the properties of Si, GaAs, and SiC are also included) [46]. As can be seen, both SiC and the nitride group have larger band gap energy than either Si or GaAs. The larger band gap and high breakdown field of these materials allow SiC- and nitride-based electronic devices to operate at higher temperatures and higher powers than Si- or GaAs-based devices. In addition, while SiC has a band gap near that of GaN, the III–nitrides group has three distinct advantages over SiC devices. First, the nitride group of materials has direct transition band gap, allowing its use in optical devices such as lasers and LEDs. Second, the nitride group has the structure of ternary (AlGaN, InGaN) and quaternary (AlInGaN) compounds, leading to a more versatile band gap range (0.7–6.2) than SiC alone and allowing for band gap engineering in both optical and electronic applications. Finally, the nitride ternary and quaternary compounds can be used for heterojunction (heterostructure field effect transistor (HEFT, HBT)) and quantum well-based devices. SiC does not have any alloy systems, relegating the use of SiC to native oxide-based devices (metal oxide semiconductor field effect transistor (MOSFETs)). As seen in Table 23.1, the undoped electron and hole mobility of the III–nitrides and SiC is relatively low compared to Si and GaAs. The electron mobility for unintentionally doped single GaN layers on either sapphire or SiC average about 300–400 cm^2/Vs. Undoped mobility in these materials are normally limited by defect-related scattering of defect hoping [47]. The highest reported mobility for MOCVD-grown GaN was ~900 cm^2/Vs [48]. The maximum calculated phonon-limited mobility in GaN is ~1350 cm^2/Vs for electrons and ~200 cm^2/Vs for holes [49]. Light n-type doping of GaN (~$1 \times 10^{17}/cm^3$) results in improved mobility due to the screening of dislocations and decreased defect-related conductivity. Further doping of the material leads to mobility degradation due to ionized impurity scattering [47]. It should be noted that much higher mobility is possible (1500–2000 cm^2/Vs) in GaN heterostructures by forming a high mobility two-dimensional electron gas channel. Another important property for high-frequency operation is the saturation electron drift velocity. This parameter gives the average electron velocity at high electric fields. The high saturated drift velocity of III–nitrides leads to applications at high frequencies than can be achieved from Si. As seen in Table 23.1, the calculated value of GaN electron velocity is 2.5×10^7 cm/s, although experimental evidence is closer to 2.0×10^7 cm/s [50] in bulk GaN and near 1.0×10^7 cm/s for submicron HFET devices [51]. The discrepancy between theory and experimental velocity saturation was accounted for in bulk GaN as due to high defect density not accounted for in theory and in the case of HFET devices as due to hot carrier effects. In addition, the wide band gap and high breakdown field give the possibility for nitride application at both high-frequency and much higher power levels than Si or traditional III–V materials.

23.2 GaN FILM ON PATTERNED SAPPHIRE SUBSTRATE

Figure 23.1 shows a scanning electron microscope (SEM) image of the fabricated cone-shape-patterned sapphire substrate (CSPSS) process. The preparation of the CSPSS is as follows [52]. After a photoresist (PR) with 3.5-μm thickness had been coated on a c-plane (0001) sapphire substrate, the PR was patterned first to be a rectangular shape (Figure 23.1a) with different intervals and reflowed during a hard-baking process at 140°C to make a cone shape as shown in Figure 23.1b. The sapphire substrate was then etched by using inductively coupled plasma reactive ion etching employing reactive Cl_2 gas. The diameter and interval of each cone-shaped pattern were 3 and 1 μm, respectively. The height of the cone shape was about 1.5 μm. The epitaxial layers were grown on both CSPSS and conventional sapphire substrate (CSS) by MOCVD. In the initial stage of the growth on CSPSS, the GaN layer starts to grow only on the etched flat basal sapphire surface, quite differently from the growth mode on the conventional PSS, because there is no preferential growth plane on the cone-shape-patterned region. Similarly to the ELOG, this selective growth on CSPSS prevents the dislocation generated during the initial stage of the growth from propagating further into the patterned

TABLE 23.1
Crystal and Electrical Properties of III–Nitrides, SiC, Si, and GaAs [32,44]

Material	Band gap (eV)	Lattice Constant (Å)	Lattice Mismatch with GaN (%)	Thermal Conductivity at 300 K (W/cm K)	Thermal Expansion Coefficient (10^{-6}/K)	Electron Mobility (cm^2/Vs)	Hole Mobility (cm^2/Vs)	Saturated Drift Velocity (10^7 cm/s)	Breakdown Field (MV/cm)	Melting Point (°C)
AlN	6.2	$a = 3.112$	2.48	2.0	4.2	135	14	1.4	4–12	3124
		$c = 4.982$			5.3					
GaN	3.44	$a = 3.1891$	0	1.3	5.59	300–1000	<200	2.5 (calc)	5.0	2518
		$c = 5.1855$			3.17			2.0 (exp)		
InN	0.7	$a = 3.548$	− 10.12	0.8	5.7	1000–1900	—	2.5	5.0	1873
		$c = 5.7034$			3.7					
6H SiC	3.03	$a = 3.081$	3.51	4.9	4.2	400	50	2.0	3–5	>2000
		$c = 15.117$			4.68					
Al_2O_3	9.0	$a = 5.431$	13.9	0.3	7.5	—	—	—	—	2015
		$c = 12.982$			8.5					
Si	1.12	$a = 5.431$	− 16.96	1.3	3.9	1500	450	1.0	0.3	1412
GaAs	1.42	$a = 5.653$	− 20.22	0.5	6.7	8500	400	1.0	0.4	1240

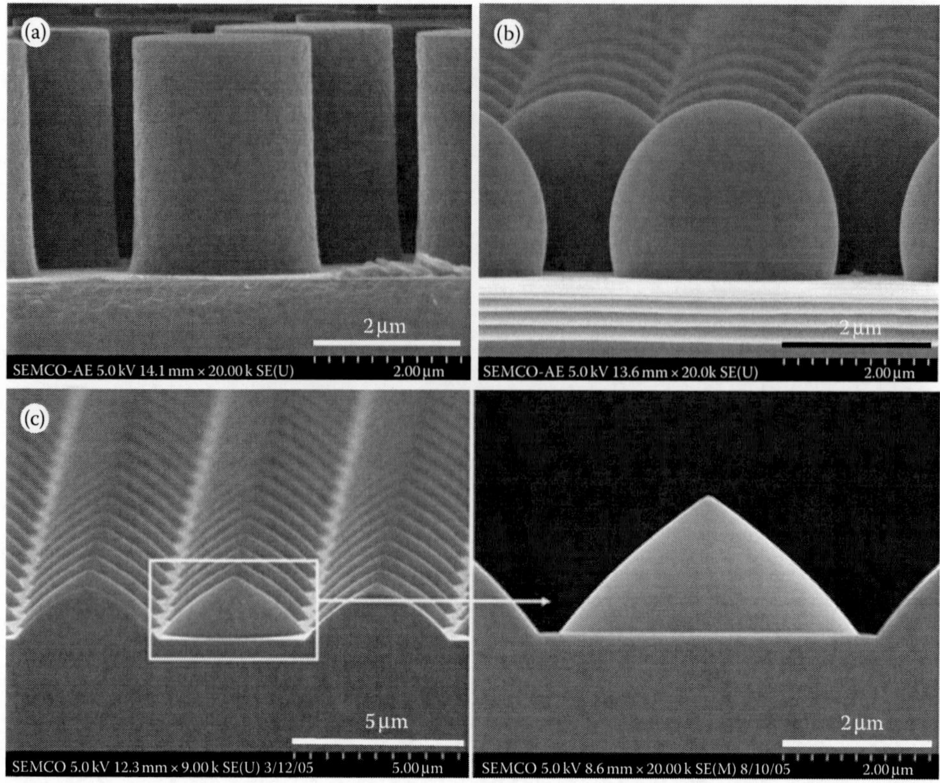

FIGURE 23.1 SEM images of the fabricated CSPSS process. (a) Rectangular-shaped PR on sapphire, (b) formation of cone-shaped PR after hard-baking process at 140°C, and (c) fabricated con-shape patterned sapphire substrate. (From Y. C. Chung, Y. C. Lin, M. Z. Shiu et al., *Lab on a Chip*, 3(4), 228–233, 2003. With permission.)

area when the growth proceeds laterally toward the cone region, decreases the dislocation density, and hence improves the crystal quality of the grown film.

The time evolution of interference micrographs for a GaN surface grown on a CSPSS is shown in Figure 23.2, that is, after the growth of the initial buffer layer at low temperature (Figure 23.2a), after temperature ramping (annealing the buffer layer) (Figure 23.2b), and after 10- and 30-min growth of the epitaxial layer (Figures 23.2c and d). In general, the III–nitride layer preferentially grows on the (0001) crystallographic *c*-plane of a sapphire substrate. Although there is no growth plane in the cone-shape-patterned region, the low-temperature GaN amorphous buffer layer is well formed on the plane and patterned sapphire region as shown in Figure 23.2a. When the temperature increases from low temperature (550°C) to high temperature (1020°C) in the ramping stage of the growth, the random recrystallized GaN islands are formed on the etched flat basal sapphire surface, which is similar to a typical growth mode on the CSS [53]. In the cone-shape-patterned region, however, the larger regular GaN islands are formed on the six corners of a hexagon-shaped cone as shown in Figure 23.2b, which explains why Ga species tend to migrate from the top region of the cone surface to the bottom region of the cone with increasing temperature [54–56]. In the initial stage of the high-temperature growth on the CSPSS, therefore, the coalescence starts on the etched flat basal sapphire surface, indicating that the growth mode on the CSPSS is considerably different from that on the conventional PSS such as stripe, hexagonal, or rectangular geometry. As expected, the growth of GaN on the CSPSS was only initiated from the etched basal surface with the (0001) crystallographic plane because there was no growth plane in the cone-shape-patterned region as shown in Figure 23.2c. As the growth proceeds, the growth also laterally propagates toward the

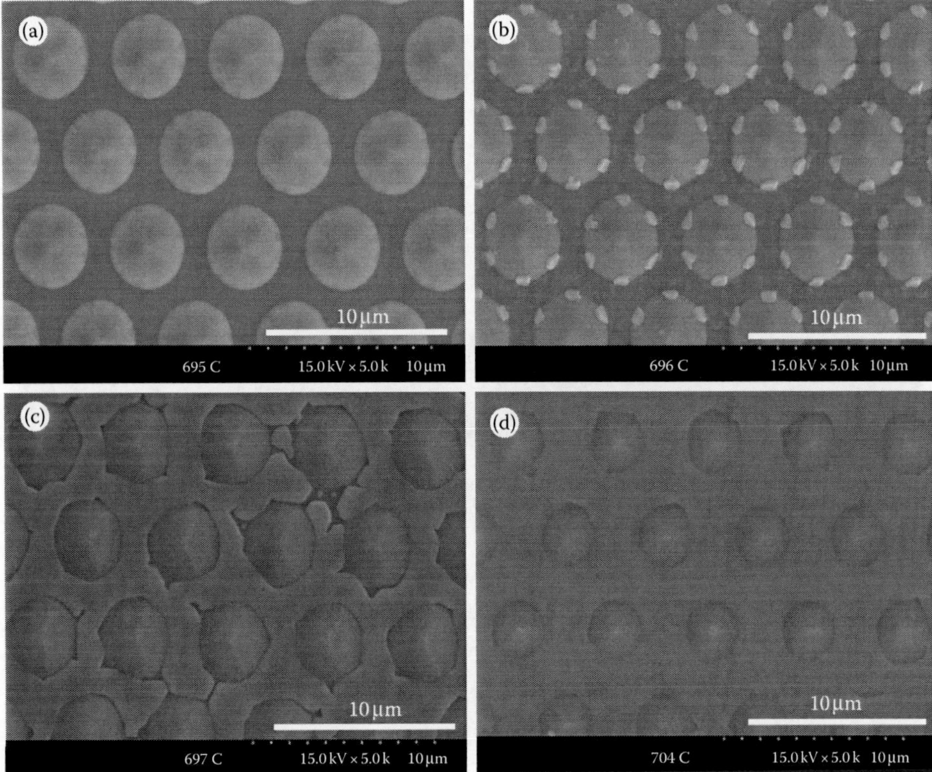

FIGURE 23.2 Time evolution of interference micrographs for a GaN surface grown on a CSPSS. (a) Buffer, (b) annealing, (c) 10 min, and (d) 30 min. (From C. W. Wei, J. Y. Cheng, C. T. Huang et al., *Nucleic Acids Research*, 33(8), 2005. With permission.)

peak of the cone as shown in Figure 23.2d. This lateral growth greatly decreases the dislocation density in the grown film, similarly to the ELOG mode [57]. This also enables reducing the time required for obtaining a smooth growth surface over the patterned region, compared to that for those grown on a conventional PSS, where the growth starts both on the etched and nonetched regions at the same time as shown in Figure 23.3 [58].

Figure 23.4a shows the cross-sectional transmission electron microscope (TEM) images under $g = 0002$ two-beam condition of the interface region between the CSPSS and a GaN layer grown on it, demonstrating that the ELOG-like mode on the CSPSS effectively suppresses the propagation of dislocation into the cone region, even though many dislocations were observed in the film grown on

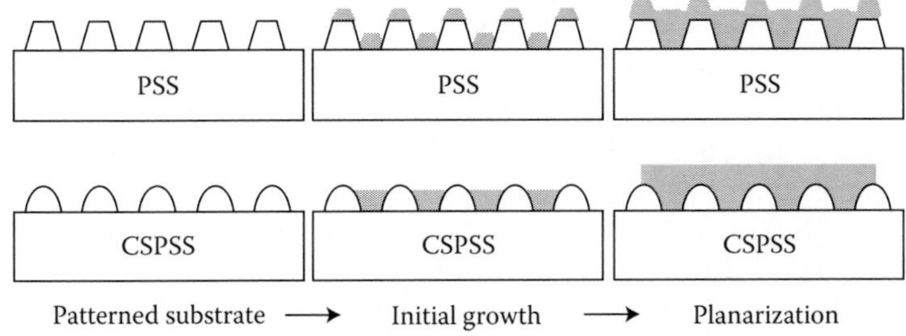

FIGURE 23.3 Schematic view of the planarization of GaN grown on the conventional PSS and on the proposed CSPSS. (From L. Wang and P. C. H. Li, *Journal of Agricultural and Food Chemistry*, 55(26), 10509–10516, 2007. With permission.)

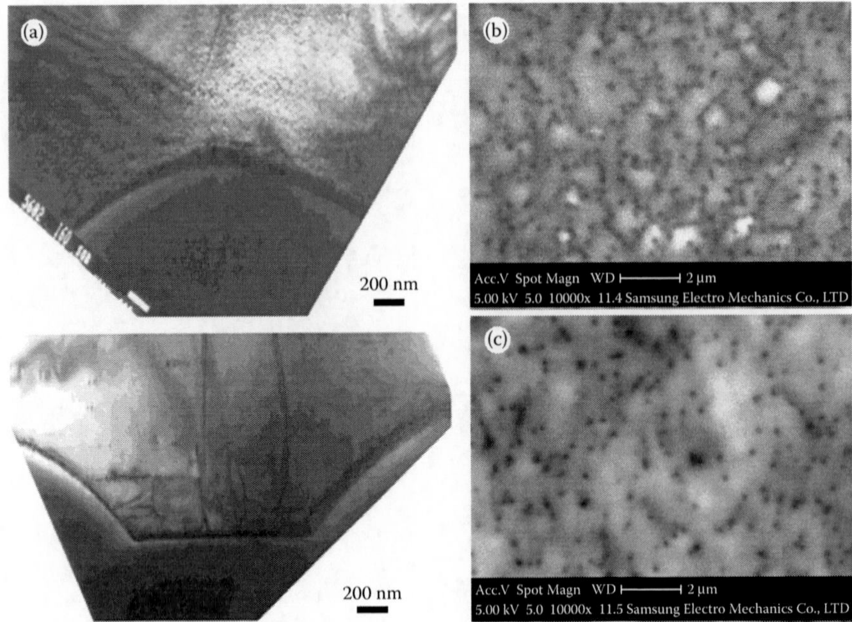

FIGURE 23.4 TEM image of a film grown on a CSPSS (a) and CL images of a film grown on a CSS (b) and a film grown on a CSPSS (c). (From L. Wang and P. C. H. Li, *Journal of Agricultural and Food Chemistry*, 55(26), 10509–10516, 2007. With permission.)

the basal plane of the sapphire. This reduction of dislocation was also confirmed by performing a cathodoluminescence (CL) measurement at room temperature as shown in Figures 23.4b and c. In bright regions, a radiative process dominates over a nonradiative process because of the lower density of structural defects. The dark spot density in the film grown on a CSS is roughly estimated to be about 7×10^8 cm^{-2}. Apparently, the dark spot density in the film grown on a CSPSS was decreased to about 2×10^8 cm^{-2} in number.

23.3 CHARACTERISTICS OF InGaN/GaN FILMS AFTER SAPPHIRE LAPPING AND POLISHING

To investigate the characteristics of InGaN/GaN films after sapphire lapping and polishing, samples were grown on 430-μm-thick 2-in. (0001) planar sapphire substrates using MOCVD [59]. The layer structures for LEDs with a total thickness of about 6 μm consist of undoped GaN/Si-doped n-GaN, five pairs of InGaN/GaN multiquantum well (MQW), and Mg-doped p-GaN. Devices of 260 μm × 670 μm dimensions were fabricated by a normal side view LED chip process using ITO transmittance for p-contact and Cr/Au metals for n-contact. After that, Sample A (430-μm thickness) was kept as a reference without thinning the substrate. The sapphire substrates for Samples B, C, and D were thinned to 200-, 150-, and 80-μm thickness by using backside lapping and polishing, respectively. Figure 23.5 shows the bowing of the sapphire wafers (samples A, B, C, and D). The curvature of the bowing increases as the sapphire substrate is thinned and is apparently observable when the thickness of the wafer reaches 80 μm, which is also observed in photography as in the inset of the figure. This is because the residual compressive stress in the GaN layer, caused by different thermal expansion coefficients between the GaN film and the sapphire substrate and accommodated during cooling down from growth temperature to room temperature, is released as the sapphire substrate thins down [60]. Therefore, caution is required after lapping and polishing to prevent chip breaking.

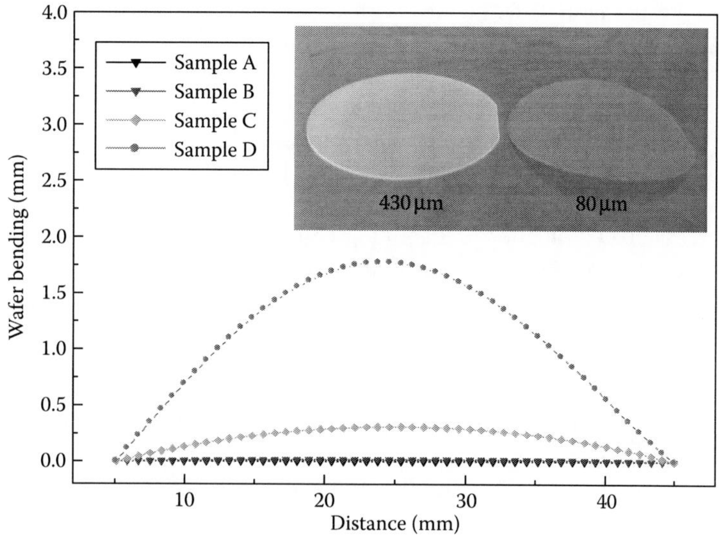

FIGURE 23.5 Bending of the wafer as a function of the sapphire thickness. (From C. A. Koch, P. C. H. Li, and R. S. Utkhede, *Analytical Biochemistry*, 342(1), 93–102, 2005. With permission.)

Figure 23.6 shows the median value for room-temperature electroluminescence (EL) peak position for Sample E over 10,000 chips in 2-in. dimension. The typical corresponding spectral EL peak wavelength (energy) from the InGaN/GaN MQWs was shifted from 467.1 nm (2.65 eV) to 466.0 nm (2.66 eV) as the sapphire substrate is thinned from 430- to 80-µm thickness as shown in the inset of Figure 23.6. These clearly indicate that the wafer bowing-induced mechanical stress can shift the wavelength of the light emitted from the InGaN/GaN MQWs in the device. The accommodated residual compressive stress in the GaN layer is released as the sapphire substrate is thinned as

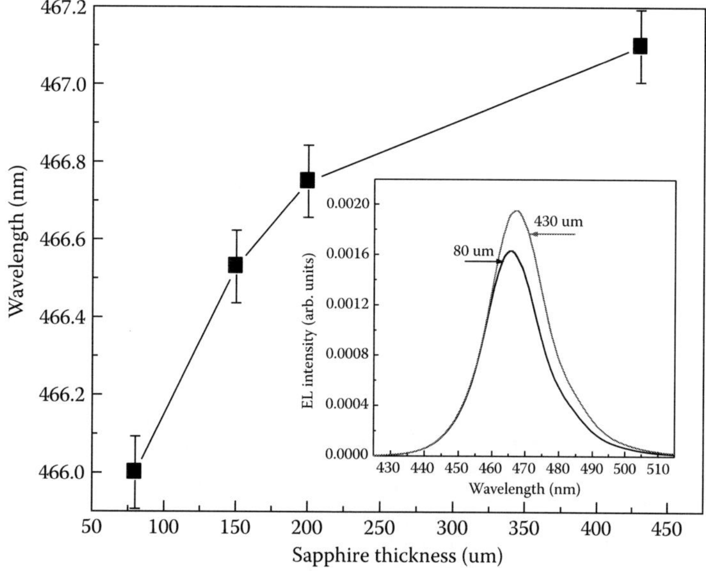

FIGURE 23.6 EL peak position median value of LED chips as a function of the sapphire thickness. The typical EL peak data for samples with 430 and 80 µm sapphire thickness are shown in the inset. (From R. Peytavi, F. R. Raymond, D. Gagne et al., *Clinical Chemistry*, 51(10), 1836–1844, 2005. With permission.)

mentioned above, resulting in wafer bowing with convex shape to balance the stress. However, the mechanical stress introduced by the wafer bowing, in turn, may change the piezoelectric field in the InGaN/GaN MQW active region and modify the energy band profile.

Figure 23.7 is an illustration of the transition energy in InGaN/GaN QWs under a piezoelectric field due to the wafer bowing-induced mechanical stress. The spatial separation of the electron and hole envelope wave functions increases due to the enhanced piezoelectric field-induced quantum-confined stark effect (QCSE), which would increase the optical transition energy of the MQW active region with decreased recombination probability [61]. This is the reason for the significant blue shift in emission wavelength from the samples with thinned sapphire substrates.

23.4 TRADITIONAL DIAMOND TIP SCRIBING IN InGaN-BASED LEDs

Figure 23.8 shows the sapphire unit cell with a hexagonal crystal structure and the typical diamond tip scribing process after lapping and polishing. The location and orientation of an *a*-plane, *c*-planes, and an *r*-plane of the sapphire unit cell are shown in Figure 23.8a. The *c*-planes form top and bottom *c*-faces of the sapphire unit cell and have (0001) orientations. All the current commercial products are fabricated via the *c*-orientation growth. The *a*-plane has a (1120) orientation and is perpendicular to the *c*-planes. The *r*-plane is oriented at an angle of 57.6° with respect to the *c*-planes [36]. The line of weakness extends in the *a*-plane direction of the *c*-face sapphire substrate. A force is applied to the bottom *c*-face to cleave the *c*-face sapphire substrate along the line of weakness in the *a*-plane direction. Figure 23.8b shows the typical LED-structure-grown *c*-face sapphire substrate including *a*-plane flat. The scribing process can be repeated to form any desired number of lines of weakness in the *a*-plane direction for cleaving as shown in Figure 23.8b. Figure 23.8c shows the cross-sectional SEM images of the sapphire after scribing. The width and depth of scribing are about 3 and 0.5 μm, respectively. When the scribing line is misaligned and not in the *a*-plane direction, the low depth of scribing can induce failure in breaking the wafer along the scribed line as shown in Figure 23.8d. When the chip separates using standard cleaving equipment, the breaking line progresses toward the *r*-plane direction because the *r*-plane is oriented at an angle of 57.6° with respect to the *c*-planes.

23.5 LASER SCRIBING IN InGaN-BASED LED

23.5.1 Theory of Laser

Material removal takes place through the ablation process where the target material under laser irradiation absorbs laser energy and transforms into either a liquid or a vapor [30,31]. The melted

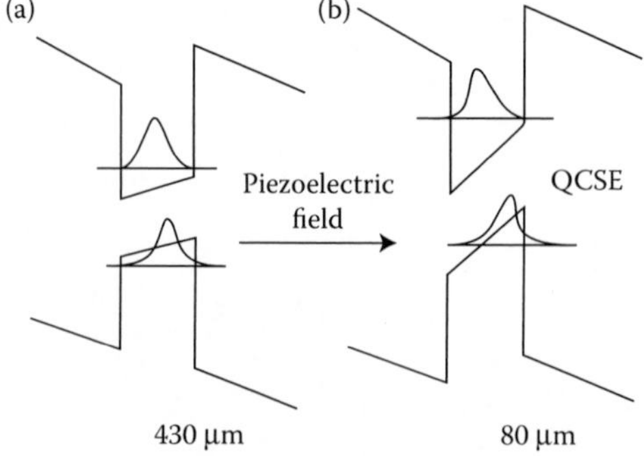

FIGURE 23.7 Schematic band diagrams of GaN/InGaN QWs under a piezoelectric field due to the wafer bowing-induced mechanical stress. (a) Band diagram of GaN/GaN QWs with 430 μm-thickness sapphire, (b) band diagram of GaN/GaN QWs with 80 μm-thickness sapphire. (From C. Y. Li, X. L. Dong, J. H. Qin et al., *Analytica Chimica Acta*, 640(1–2), 93–99, 2009. With permission.)

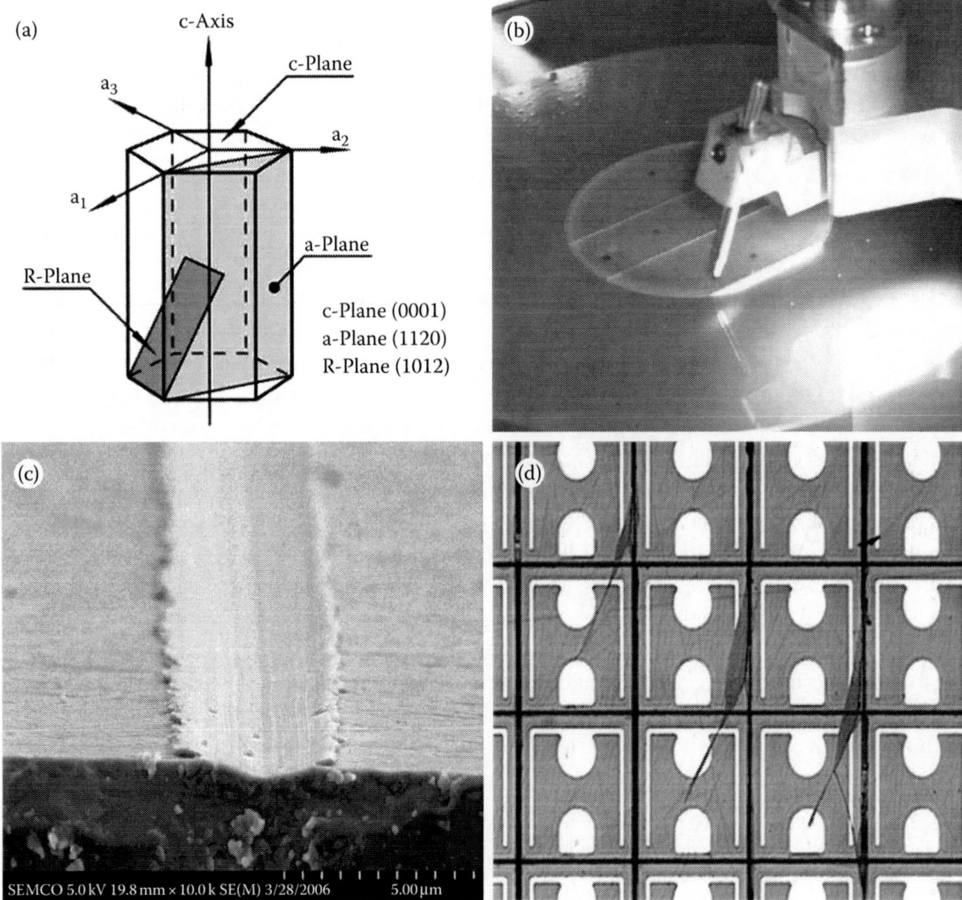

FIGURE 23.8 The unit cell of sapphire with a hexagonal crystal structure (a) and the typical diamond tip scribing process (b). The cross-sectional SEM image of the sapphire after scribing (c) and optical images of the top view after diamond tip scribing and breaking (d). (From L. Wang and P. C. H. Li, *Analytical Biochemistry*, 400(2), 282–288, 2010. With permission.)

liquid is expelled from the interaction region by the recoil action; and the vapor removes itself directly from the focus. Other processes associated with the laser–material interaction include heat conduction, radiation, and plasma expansion. The first step in laser ablation is the absorption of laser energy by the target material. This is accomplished by linear or nonlinear processes. The material in the focal region is heated to melting temperature and, depending on laser intensity and pulse width, subsequently to vaporization temperature. For non-UV wavelengths, the absorption mechanisms are different for absorbing materials such as metals and semiconductors and transparent dielectric materials such as glasses and plastics. For opaque materials, while linear absorption is the main absorption mechanism at long pulse widths with low intensity, nonlinear absorption can become dominant at ultrashort pulse widths with high intensity. For transparent materials, absorption has to come from nonlinear processes through laser-induced optical breakdown. Laser-induced breakdown is a process where a normally transparent material is first transformed into an absorbing plasma by the strong laser pulse. Subsequent absorption by the plasma of the laser energy causes heating that leads to irreversible damage to the host material. The nonlinear processes that cause breakdown are avalanche ionization and multiphoton ionization.

In a transparent dielectric material, the bound valence electrons have an ionization potential or band gap greater than the laser photon energy. The bound electrons do not absorb the laser light at low intensities. However, in any real materials there are always some free or conduction electrons present, and they are the seed electrons for avalanche ionization. These seed electrons can come from metallic impurities, thermal or linear optical ionization of shallow energy levels of inclusions. A free electron, when simply wiggling in the oscillating laser field, does not gain energy when averaged over an optical cycle, and thus does not absorb the laser energy. However, the free electron can absorb laser energy when it collides with the bound electrons and the lattice. This is the Joule heating process, also known as inverse Bremsstrahlung. The seed electron can be accelerated enough that its kinetic energy exceeds the ionization potential of the bound electron. Therefore the next collision with a bound electron will result in an ionization event if the free electron transfers nearly all its energy to the bound electron, resulting in two free electrons with low kinetic energies. This is called impact ionization. This process will repeat itself, leading to an avalanche where the free-electron density grows exponentially from the very low seed electron density. When enough bound electrons are ionized by this avalanche process, a plasma with a "critical density" is created, and the transparent material is broken down and becomes absorbing.

When the laser field strength is very high, as in the case of ultrashort-pulse laser–matter interaction, bound electrons of the transparent material can be directly ionized through multiphoton absorption. A bound electron can be lifted from its bound energy level or valence band to the free energy level or conduction band by simultaneously absorbing m photons in the laser pulse such that $mh\nu > U_I$, where $h\nu$ is the energy of the photon, and U_I is ionization potential or band gap. This is called multiphoton ionization. As this is an mth-order process, the cross section is extremely small. Only at very high field strength is multiphoton ionization significant. Therefore, for long pulse widths where the field strength at breakdown is lower, the multiphoton ionization contribution is negligible, and laser-induced breakdown is dominated by avalanche ionization. However, at ultrashort pulse widths, multiphoton ionization plays an important role: it determines the breakdown threshold behavior.

To study laser scribing, samples was grown on 430-μm-thick 2-in. (0001) sapphire substrates using MOCVD under the same growth conditions [62]. The layer structures for LEDs with a total thickness of about 6 μm consist of undoped GaN/Si-doped n-GaN, five pairs of InGaN/GaN MQW, and Mg-doped p-GaN. Devices of 260 μm × 670 μm dimensions were fabricated by a normal side view LED chip process using ITO transmittance for p-contact and Cr/Au metals for n-contact. After that, the sapphire substrate was thinned to about 80 μm thickness by using backside lapping and polishing. Two lasers, with nanosecond and femtosecond laser pulses, were used to scribe grooves on the back of the thinned sapphire substrates. The nanosecond pulse laser has a wavelength of 355 nm, a repetition rate of 50 kHz, a pulse duration of 30 ns, and an output power of 0.4 W. The corresponding values of the femtosecond pulse laser are 1045 nm, 100 kHz, 150 fs, and 0.45 W. During the laser scan, the wafer chuck moves 18 mm/s for nanosecond laser and 400 mm/s for femtosecond laser, respectively.

23.5.2 Nanosecond Laser Scribing

Figure 23.9a shows the schematics of a typical heat distribution in the sapphire substrate when the substrate is exposed to a focused long pulse laser beam. As the laser hits the wafer, the heat generated by the laser power greatly increases the temperature in the vicinity of the focused laser beam spot, locally melting the sapphire substrate, and further diffuses away into the material during the pulse duration, because the duration of laser pulse is longer than the heat diffusion time [63]. During the ablation process, the evaporated sapphire usually generates debris and particles on the surface with dimensions much larger than 50 μm as shown in Figure 23.9b. Figure 23.9c shows the cross-sectional optical images of the sapphire after scribing and separating the substrate. A fairly large amount of sapphire droplet remains and is strongly bound to the sidewall. Removal of these contaminants is very difficult, which prevents photons from being emitted to the air. In spite of this debris, the scribing depth of the laser (~20 μm) is much larger than that of diamond tip (~0.2 μm).

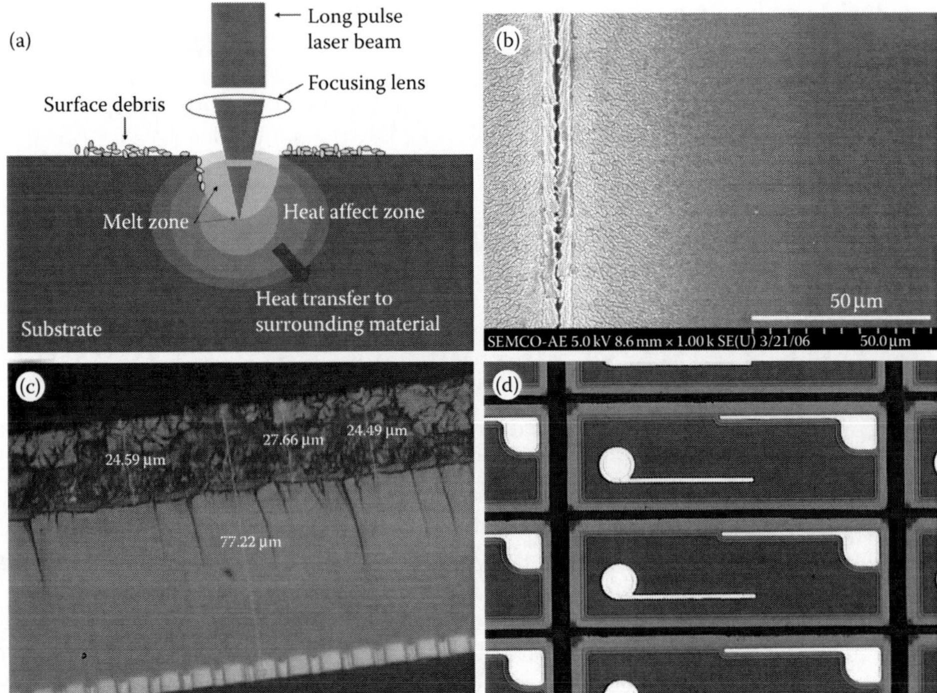

FIGURE 23.9 Schematics of the physical phenomena when long-pulse laser beams are present (Ref. [31]) (a). SEM and optical images of the top view (b, d) and the side view (c) after nanosecond laser scribing. (From L. Wang, P. C. H. Li, H. Z. Yu et al., *Analytica Chimica Acta*, 610(1), 97–104, 2008. With permission.)

This renders the chips to be easily separated with a standard cleaving process as shown in Figure 23.9d, which eliminates the cleaving failure encountered in scribing with a diamond tip.

Figure 23.10 shows the TEM and selected area electron diffraction pattern (SADP) images for the sample prepared by using the nanosecond laser scribing and then exposed to air by using the focused ion beam lift-out technique. The diffraction pattern of the sapphire substrate near the damaged region indicates combined polycrystalline and/or amorphous phase, while the

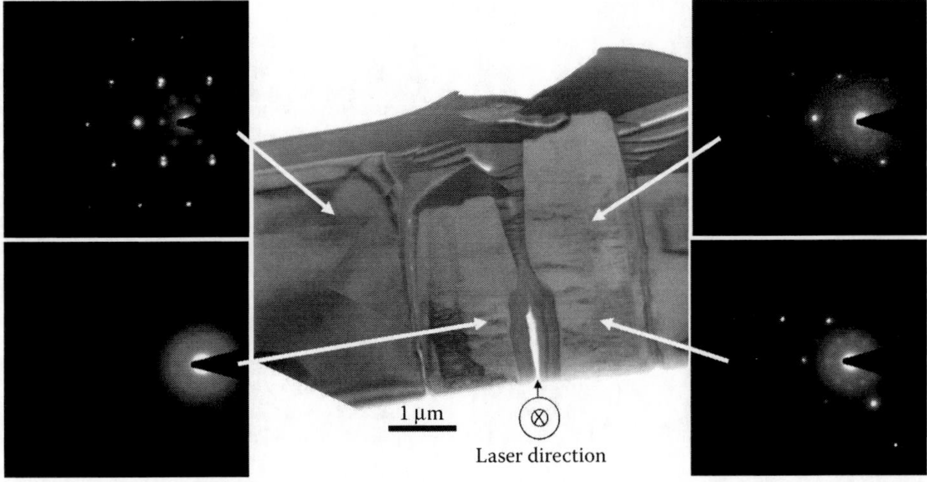

FIGURE 23.10 TEM and SADP images for the sample fabricated by using the nanosecond laser scribing. (From L. Wang and P. C. H. Li, *Analytical Biochemistry*, 400(2), 282–288, 2010. With permission.)

diffraction patterns far from the region damaged by the laser still maintain single crystalline phase. For long pulse widths where the field strength is lower, laser-induced breakdown is dominated by avalanche ionization [31]. The rate of heating is determined by the rate of laser energy absorption and the material is heated through Joule heating. Once the plasma of free electrons generated by avalanche ionization reaches a sufficiently high density, the material breaks down and ablation begins. At the same time, the electrons transfer energy to the ions and the lattice, and the material is heated up. The energy transfer from electrons to ions during the laser–matter interaction can be strong and heat diffusion can involve a much larger volume than the focus, which may result in the degraded transmittance by hindering the photon generated in MQW from being emitted to air.

23.5.3 Femtosecond Laser Scribing

Figure 23.11a shows schematics for the heat distribution in the sapphire substrate when an ultrafast laser beam is used for scribing, which is quite different from those of the long pulse laser beam. As the pulse widths decrease, the laser power intensity easily reaches hundreds of terawatts per square centimeter at the focused beam spot. The heat-affected volume is much smaller because the duration of the laser pulse is shorter than the heat diffusion time. Figure 23.11b shows the SEM image of the surface of sapphire after scribing with a femtosecond laser. There is no laser scribing line because the laser beam is focused inside the sapphire. Many scratch lines on the surface are due to lapping and polishing and are not related to the scribing. Figures 23.11c and d show the cross-sectional optical and SEM images. The central belt-shaped area (modified layer) is only affected by the laser power, which is responsible for the great decrease in amount of debris and particles on the sidewall of the sapphire.

Figure 23.12 shows that the TEM and SADP images for the sample prepared by using femtosecond laser scribing are very different from those obtained by using nanosecond laser. The diffraction

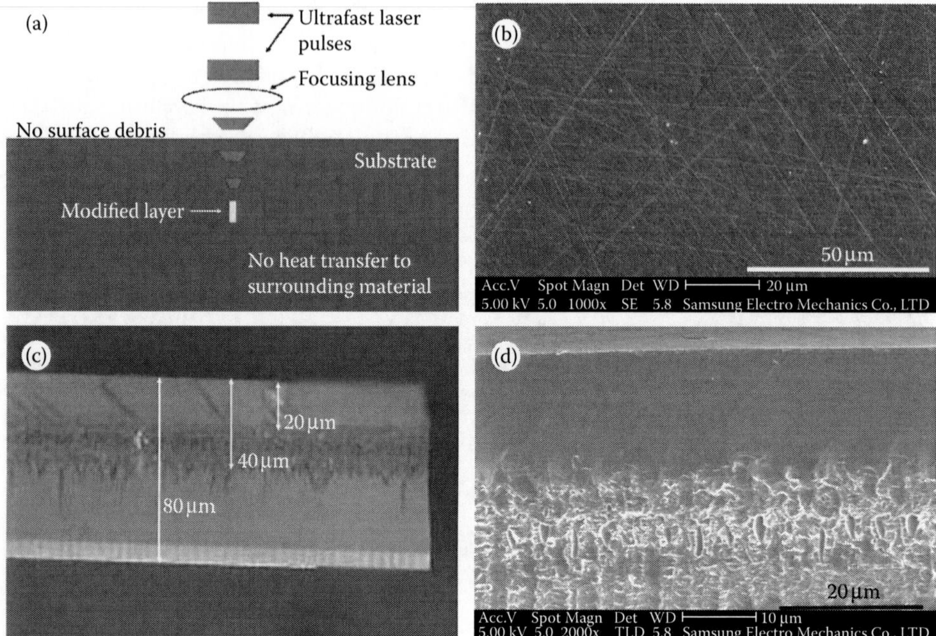

FIGURE 23.11 Schematics of the physical phenomena when ultrafast laser beams are present (Refs. [30,31]) (a). SEM and optical images of the top view (b) and the side view (c, d) after femtosecond laser scribing. (From L. Wang and P. C. H. Li, *Analytical Biochemistry*, 400(2), 282–288, 2010. With permission.)

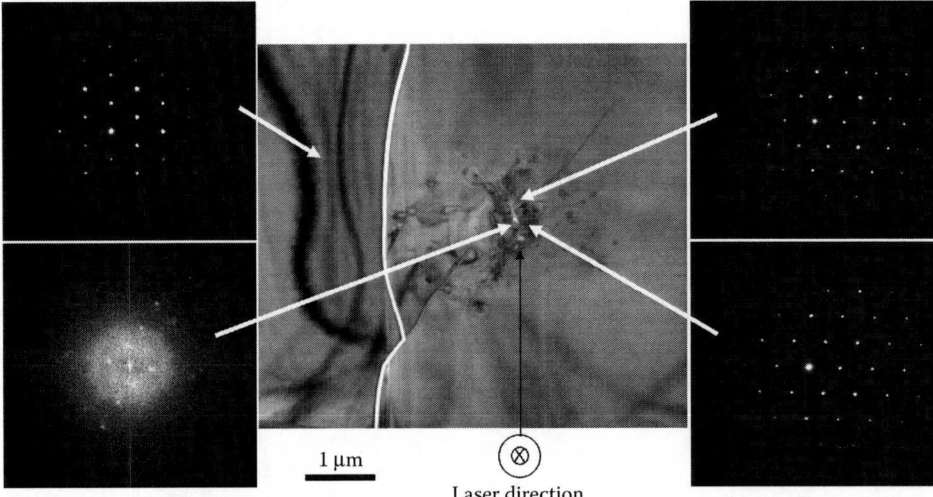

FIGURE 23.12 TEM and SADP images of the sample fabricated by using famtosecond laser scribing. (From H. Chen, L. Wang, and P. C. H. Li, *Lab on a Chip*, 8(5), 826–829, 2008. With permission.)

patterns indicate that most regions surrounding the laser-focused zone maintain a crystalline phase, except just right the focused spot zone where the diffraction patterns exhibit a combined polycrystalline and crystalline phase. For ultrashort pulse widths where the field strength is higher, laser-induced breakdown is dominated by multiple photon abortion [31]. The electrons are driven to much higher temperature, and the ion or lattice temperature is much lower than the electron peak temperature. The electron temperature can reach a few to tens of electronvolts during the duration of the laser pulse, while the ions remain relatively cold. Subsequent energy transfer between electrons and ions, mostly taking place after the laser pulse is off, will then rapidly heat the ions to much higher temperatures compared to the long pulse cases. Only a small fraction of the material in the interaction volume is vaporized and the heat-affected volume becomes much smaller because of the short interaction time.

23.5.4 Optical and Electrical Characteristics

Figure 23.13 shows the light output power for both NLS-LED (LED fabricated by using nanosecond laser scribing) and FLS-LED (LED fabricated by using femtosecond laser scribing) as a function of injection current. The total output power of the devices was measured by using side view PKG without phosphor to collect the light emitted in all directions from the LEDs. It should be noted that the output power at 20 mA was estimated to be 13.2 and 15 mW for NLS-LED and FLS-LED, respectively. This improved output power of FLS-LED is attributed to the increase of extraction efficiency, because the reduction in debris and thermal damage enhances the photon emission from the active MQW region in the sidewall direction, and also enhances the photon reflection from the Ag-coated bottom of PKG. The inset of Figure 23.5 shows the typical *I–V* characteristics for NLS-LED and FLS-LED. The forward voltage measured at a 20-mA current injection shows negligible difference, 3.16 and 3.15 V for each sample, respectively. The leakage currents of NLS-LED and FLS-LED at a reverse voltage of −5 V also show negligible differences of about −57 and −42 nA, respectively. It is shown that the method of laser scribing did not deteriorate the characteristics of LEDs.

23.6 CONCLUSIONS

The ELOG-like growth mode on the CSPSS effectively suppresses the probability dislocation propagation into the cone region and hence greatly improves the crystal quality of the GaN films. As the

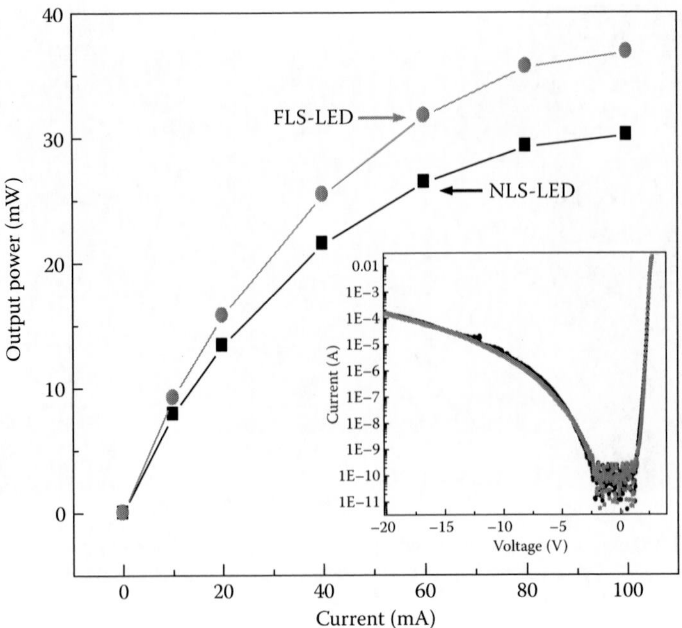

FIGURE 23.13 The output power for NLS-LED and FLS-LED as a function of injection current. The inset shows the typical *I–V* characteristics for NLS-LED and FLS-LED.

sapphire substrate is thinned down, the compressive stress strain in the GaN layer can be released and results in wafer bowing, which, in turn, may alter the piezoelectric field in the InGaN/GaN MQW active region of the device and increase the optical transition energy due to the enhanced QCSE. This is evidenced by the blue shift in the EL spectral peak wavelength with decreasing sapphire thickness. The enhanced output power of InGaN-based LED through reduction of both the debris and thermal damage of the sapphire substrate was demonstrated by using the femtosecond laser scribing. The SADP measurements confirmed that the heat-affected volume of the femtosecond laser scribing is much smaller than that of nanosecond laser scribing, which explains that the femtosecond laser scribed LED exhibits improved output power. This is because the laser intensity easily reaches hundreds of terawatts per square centimeters due to the extreme short pulse width and can minimize the heat-affected area.

ACKNOWLEDGMENTS

The author thanks Dr. Sang-Su Hong of Samsung Electro-Mechanics Company Ltd and Nam-Seoung Kim of Samsung LED Company Ltd for useful measurements and discussions.

REFERENCES

1. S. Nakamura, M. Senoh, S. Nagahama, N. Iwasa, T. Yamada, T. Mat-sushita, Y. Sugimoto, and H. Kiyoku, High-power, long-lifetime InGaN multi-quantum-well-structure laser diodes, *Jpn. J. Appl. Phys.*, 36, L1059, 1997.
2. S. Nakamura, M. Senoh, N. Iwasa, and S. Nagahama, High-brightness InGaN blue, green and yellow light-emitting diodes with quantum well structures, *Jpn. J. Appl. Phys.*, 34, L797, 1995.
3. A. Khan, Q. Chen, M. S. Shur, B. T. Dermott, J. A. Higgins, J. Birm, W. J. Schaff, and L. F. Eastman, GaN based heterostructure for high power devices, *Solid State Electron*, 41, 1555, 1997.
4. N. Vetury, Q. Zhang, S. Keller, and U. K. Mishra, The impact of surface states on the DC and RF characteristics of AlGaN/GaN HFETs, *IEEE Trans. Electron Devices*, 48, 560, 2001.

5. S. Shen, B. Heikman, R. Moran, N. Coffie, Q. Zhang, D. Buttari, I. P. Smorchova, S. Keller, S. P. DenBaars, and U. K. Mishra, AlGaN/AlN/GaN high-power microwave HEMT, *IEEE Electron Device Lett.*, 22, 457, 2001.
6. H. Youn, J. H. Lee, V. Kumar, K. S. Lee, J. H. Lee, and I. Adesida, The effects of isoelectronic Al doping and process optimization for the fabrication of high-power AlGaN-GaN HEMTs, *IEEE Trans. Electron Devices*, 51, 785, 2004.
7. A. F. Wright, Elastic properties of zinc-blende and wurtzite AlN, GaN, and InN, *J. Appl. Phys.*, 82, 2833, 1997.
8. M. S. Shur, A.D. Bykhovski, R. Gaska, Pyroelectric and piezoelectric properties of GaN-based materials, *MRS Internet J. Nitride Semicond. Res.* 4S1, G1.6, 1999.
9. S.-H. Lee, H.-H. Jeong, S.-B. Bae, H.-C. Choi, J.-H. Lee, Y.-H. Lee, Epitaxially grown GaN thin-film SAW filter with high velocity and low insertion loss, *IEEE Trans. Electron Devices*, 48, 524, 2001.
10. W. Wu, K. Walukiewicz, M. Yu, J. W. Ager III, E. E. Haller, H. Lu, W. J. Schaff, Y. Saito, and Y. Nanishi, Unusual properties of the fundamental band gap of InN, *Appl. Phys. Lett.*, 80, 3967, 2002.
11. S. D. Lester, F. A. Ponce, M. G. Craford, and D. A. Steigerwald, High dislocation densities in high efficiency GaN-based light-emitting diodes, *Appl. Phys. Lett*, 66, 1249, 1995.
12. B. Heying, X. H. Wu, S. Keller, Y. Li, D. Kapolnek, B. P. Keller, S. P. DenBaars, and J. S. Speck, Role of threading dislocation structure on the x-ray diffraction peak widths in epitaxial GaN films, *Appl. Phys. Lett.*, 68, 643, 1996.
13. A. Sakai, H. Sunakawa, and A. Usui, Defect structure in selectively grown GaN films with low threading dislocation density, *Appl. Phys. Lett.*, 71, 2259, 1997.
14. T. S. Zheleva, O. H. Nam, M. D. Bremser, and R. F. Davis, Dislocation density reduction via lateral epitaxy in selectively grown GaN structures, *Appl. Phys. Lett.*, 71, 2472, 1997.
15. M. Yamada, T. Mitani, Y. Narukawa, S. Shioji, I. Niki, S. Sonobe, K. Deguchi, M. Sano, and T. Mukai, InGaN-based near-ultraviolet and blue-light-emitting diodes with high external quantum efficiency using a patterned sapphire substrate and a mesh electrode, *Jpn. J. Appl. Phys.*, 41, L1431, 2002.
16. K. Tadatomo, H. Okagawa, Y. Ohuchi, T. Tsunekawa, Y. Imada, M. Kato, and T. Taguchi, High output power InGaN ultraviolet light-emitting diodes fabricated on patterned substrates using metalorganic vapor phase epitaxy, *Jpn. J. Appl. Phys.*, 40, L583, 2001.
17. D. S. Wuu, W. K. Wang, K. S. Wen, S. C. Huang, S. H. Lin, R. H. Horng, Y. S. Yu, and M. H. Pan, Fabrication of pyramidal patterned sapphire substrates for high-efficiency InGaN-based light emitting diodes, *J. Electrochem. Soc.*, 153, G765, 2006.
18. J. H. Lee, J. T. Oh, J. S. Park, J. W. Kim, Y. C. Kim, J. W. Lee, and H. K. Cho, Improvement of luminous intensity of InGaN light emitting diodes grown on hemispherical patterned sapphire, *Phys. Stat. Sol. (c)*, 3, 2169, 2006.
19. C. Huh, K. S. Lee, E. J. Kang, and S. J. Park, Improved light-output and electrical performance of InGaN-based light-emitting diode by microroughening of the p-GaN surface, *J. Appl. Phys.*, 93, 9383, 2003.
20. F. A. Kish, F. M. Steranka, D. C. DeFevere, D. A. Vanderwater, K. G.Park, C. P. Kuo, T. D. Osentowski, M. J. Peanasky, J. G. Yu, R. M. Fletcher, D. A. Steigerwald, and M. G. Craford, Very high-efficiency semiconductor wafer-bonded transparent substrate (AlxGa1-x) 0.5 In0. 5P/GaP light-emitting diodes, *Appl. Phys. Lett.*, 64, 2839, 1994.
21. S. S. Schad, M. Scherer, M. Seyboth, and V. Schwegler, Extraction efficiency of GaN-based LEDs, *Phys. Stat. Sol. (a)*, 188, 127, 2001.
22. S. H. Huang, R. H. Horng, K. S. Wen, Y. F. Lin, K. W. Yen, and D. S. Wuu, Improved light extraction of nitride-based flip-chip light emitting diodes via sapphire shaping and texturing, *IEEE Photon. Technol. Lett.*, 18(24), 2623, 2006.
23. J. H. Lee, J. T. Oh, S. B. Choi, Y. C. Kim, H. I. Cho, and J. H. Lee, Enhancement of InGaN-based vertical LED with concavely patterned surface using patterned sapphire substrate, *IEEE Photon. Technol. Lett.*, 20, 345, 2008.
24. W. Huang, C. C. Kao, J. T. Chu, H. C. Kuo, S. C. Wang, and C. C. Yu, Improvement of the luminous intensity of light-emitting diodes by using highly transparent Ag-indium tin oxide p-type ohmic contacts, *IEEE Photon. Technol. Lett.*, 17, 291, 2005.
25. T. Fujii, Y. Gao, R. Sharma, E. L. Hu, S. P. DenBaars, and S. Nakamura, Increase in the extraction efficiency of GaN-based light-emitting diodes via surface roughening, *Appl. Phys. Lett.*, 84, 855, 2004.
26. S. J. Wang, K. M. Uang, S. L. Chen, Y. C. Yang, S. C. Chang, T. M. Chen, and C. H. Chen, *Appl. Phys. Lett.*, Use of patterned laser liftoff process and electroplating nickel layer for the fabrication of vertical-structured GaN-based light-emitting diodes, 87, 011111, 2005.

27. W. K. Wang, S. Y. Huang, S. H. Huang, K. S. Wen, D. S. Wuu, and R. H. Horng, Fabrication and efficiency improvement of micropillar InGaN/Cu light-emitting diodes with vertical electrodes, *Appl. Phys. Lett.*, 88, 181113, 2006.
28. D. Karnakis, E. K. Illy, M.H. Knowles, E. Gu, and M. D. Dawson, High-throughput scribing for the manufacture of LED components, *Proc. SPIE*, 5366, 207, 2004.
29. T. Nilsson, F. Wagner, and B. Richerzhagen, Scribing of GaN wafer for white LED by water-jet-guided laser, *Proc. SPIE*, 5366, 200, 2004.
30. M. Kumagai, N. Uchiyama, E. Ohmura, R. Sugiura, K. Atsumi, and K. Fukumitsu, Advanced dicing technology for semiconductor waferStealth dicing, *IEEE Trans. Semicond. Manuf.*, 20, 259, 2007.
31. X. Liu, D. Du, and G. Mourou, *IEEE J. Quantum Electron.*, Laser ablation and micromachining with ultrashort laser pulses, 33, 1706, 1997.
32. W. C. Johnson, J. B. Parsons, and M. C. Crew, *J. Phys. Chem.*, 36, 2651, 1932.
33. R. Juza and H. Hahn, *Z. Anorg. Allg, Chem*, 239, 285, 1938.
34. H. Grimmeiss and Z. H. Koelmans, *Naturforsch*, 14a, 264, 1959.
35. H. P. Maruska and J. J. Tietjen, The preparation and properties of vapor-deposited single-crystalline GaN, *Appl. Phys. Lett.*, 15, 327, 1969.
36. J. I. Pankove, GaN and related materials, *GaN and Related Materials*, Gordon and Breach, New York, NY, 1997.
37. J. I. Pankove, E. A. Miller, and J. E. Berkeyheiser, GaN blue light-emitting diodes, *J. Limin.* 5, 84, 1972.
38. S. Yoshida, S. Misawa, and S. Gonda, Improvements on the electrical and luminescent properties of reactive molecular beam epitaxially grown GaN films by using AlN-coated sapphire substrates, *Appl. Phys. Lett.*, 42, 427, 1983.
39. H. Amano, N. Sawaki, I. Akasaki, and Y. Toyoda, Metalorganic vapor phase epitaxial growth of a high quality GaN film using an AlN buffer layer, *Appl. Phys. Lett.*, 48, 353, 1986.
40. S. Nakamura, GaN growth using GaN buffer layer, *Jpn. J. Appl. Phys.*, 30, L1705, 1991.
41. S. Nakamura, M. Senoh, S. Nagahoma, N. Iwasa, T. Yamada, T. Matsushita, H. Kiyoku, and S. Sugimoto, InGaN multi-quantum-well structure laser diodes grown on $MgAl_2O_4$ substrates, *Appl. Phys. Lett.*, 68, 2105, 1996.
42. M. A. Khan, J. N. Kuania, A. R. Bhattarai, and D.T. Olsen, Metal semiconductor field effect transistor based on single crystal GaN, *Appl. Phys. Lett*, 62, 1786, 1993.
43. J. I. Pankove, S. S. Chang, H. C. Lee, R. Molanar, T. D. Moustakas, and B. van Zeghbroeck, High-temperature GaN/SiC heterojunction bipolar transistor with high gain, *Tech. Dig. Int. Electron Devices Meet.*, 94, 389, 1994.
44. C. Kittel, Introduction to Solid state physics, *Introduction to Solid State Physics*, 7th Edn, Wiley, New York, 1995.
45. B. Gil, *Group III Nitride Semiconductor Compounds*, Clarendon, Oxford, 1998.
46. M. Levinshtein, S. Rumyantsev, and M. Shur, *Properties of Advanced Semiconductor Materials*, Wiley, New York, NY, 2001.
47. H. M. Ng, D. Doppalapudi, T. D. Moustakas, N. G. Weimann, and L. F. Eastman, The role of dislocation scattering in n-type GaN films, *Appl. Phys. Lett.*, 73, 821, 1998.
48. S. Nakamura and G. Fason, *The Blue Laser Diode*, Springer, Berlin, 1997.
49. D. C. Look and J. R. Sizelove, Predicted maximum mobility in bulk GaN, *Appl. Phys. Lett.*, 79, 1133, 2001.
50. M. Wraback, H. Shen, J. C. Carrano, T. Li, J. C. Campbell, M. J. Schurman, and I. T. Ferguson, Time-resolved electroabsorption measurement of the transient electron velocity overshoot in GaN, *Appl. Phys. Lett.*, 79, 1155, 2000.
51. B. K. Ridley, W. J. Schaff, and L. F. Eastman, Hot-phononinduced velocity saturation in GaN, *Appl. Phys. Lett.*, 96, 1499, 2004.
52. J. H. Lee, J. T. Oh, Y. C. Kim, and J. H. Lee, Stress reduction and enhanced extraction efficiency of GaN-based LED grown on cone-shape-patterned sapphire, *IEEE Photon. Technol. Lett.*, 20, 1563, 2008.
53. J. H. Lee, M. B. Lee, S. H. Hahm, Y. H. Lee, J. H. Lee, and H. K. Cho, Growth of semi-insulating GaN layer by controlling size of nucleation sites for SAW device applications, *MRS Internet J. Nitride Semicond. Res.*, 8(5), 1, 2003.
54. D. Simeonov, E. Fetin, J. F. Carlin, R. Butté, M. Ilegems, and N. Grandjean, GaN/AlN quantum dots grown by metal organic vapor phase Epitaxy, *J. Appl. Phys.*, 99, 083509, 2006.
55. L. Sugiura, K. Itaya, J. Nishio, H. Fujimoto, and Y. Kokubun, Effects of thermal treatment of low-temperature GaN buffer layers on the quality of subsequent GaN layers, *J. Appl. Phys.*, 82, 4877, 1997.

56. M. Sumiya, N. Ogusu, Y. Yotsuda, M. Itoh, S. Fuke, T. Nakamura, S. Mochizuki, T. Sano, S. Kamiyama, H. Amano, and I. Akasaki, Systematic analysis and control of low-temperature GaN buffer layers on sapphire substrates, *J. Appl. Phys.*, 93, 1311, 2003.
57. H. Gao, F. Yan, Y. Zhang, J. Li, Y. Zeng, and G. Wang, Fabrication of nano-patterned sapphire substrates and their application to the improvement of the performance of GaN-based LEDs, *J. Phys. D, Appl. Phys*, 41, 115106, 2008.
58. J. W. Lee, S. Y. Joon, J. H. Cho, and H. S. Paek, Light-emitting device and method of manufacturing the same, US, Patent no. 20060226431A, 2006.
59. J. H. Lee, N. S. Kim, D. Y. Lee, and J. H. Lee, Effect of residual stress and sidewall emission of InGaN-based LED by varying sapphire substrate thickness, *IEEE Photon. Technol. Lett*, 21, 1151, 2009.
60. M. Ohring, The Materials Science of Thin Films, New York, NY: Academic, 1991.
61. S. Chichibu, A. Abare, M. Minsky, S. Keller, S. Fleischer, J. Bowers, E. Hu, U. Mishra, L. Coldern, S. Denbaars, and T. Sota, Effective band gap inhomogeneity and pizoelectric field in InGaN/GaN multiquantum well structures, *Appl. Phys. Lett.*, 73, 2006, 1998.
62. J. H. Lee, N. S. Kim, S. S. Hong, and J. H. Lee, Enhanced extraction efficiency of InGaN-based light-emitting diodes using 100-kHz femtosecond-laser-scribing technology, *IEEE Photon. Technol. Lett.*, 31, 213, 2010.
63. J. P. Leonard, Determination of the absolute fluence profile in pulsed laser processing using melt-induced phase changes in an amorphous silicon thin film, *Rev. Sci. Instrum.*, 77, 053101, 2006.
64. Y. C. Chung, Y. C. Lin, M. Z. Shiu et al., Microfluidic chip for fast nucleic acid hybridization, *Lab on a Chip*, 3(4), 228–233, 2003.
65. C. W. Wei, J. Y. Cheng, C. T. Huang et al., Using a microfluidic device for 1 μ l DNA microarray hybridization in 500 s, *Nucleic Acids Research*, 33(8), 2005.
66. L. Wang and P. C. H. Li, Flexible microarray construction and fast DNA hybridization conducted on a microfluidic chip for greenhouse plant fungal pathogen detection, *Journal of Agricultural and Food Chemistry*, 55(26), 10509–10516, 2007.
67. C. A. Koch, P. C. H. Li, and R. S. Utkhede, Evaluation of thin films of agarose on glass for hybridization of DNA to identify plant pathogens with microarray technology, *Analytical Biochemistry*, 342(1), 93–102, 2005.
68. R. Peytavi, F. R. Raymond, D. Gagne et al., Microfluidic device for rapid (<15 min) automated microarray hybridization, *Clinical Chemistry*, 51(10), 1836–1844, 2005.
69. C. Y. Li, X. L. Dong, J. H. Qin et al., Rapid nanoliter DNA hybridization based on reciprocating flow on a compact disk microfluidic device, *Analytica Chimica Acta*, 640(1–2), 93–99, 2009.
70. L. Wang, and P. C. H. Li, Optimization of a microfluidic microarray device for the fast discrimination of fungal pathogenic DNA, *Analytical Biochemistry*, 400(2), 282–288, 2010.
71. L. Wang, P. C. H. Li, H. Z. Yu et al., Fungal pathogenic nucleic acid detection achieved with a microfluidic microarray device, *Analytica Chimica Acta*, 610(1), 97–104, 2008.
72. H. Chen, L. Wang, and P. C. H. Li, Nucleic acid microarrays created in the double-spiral format on a circular microfluidic disk, *Lab on a Chip*, 8(5), 826–829, 2008.

24 Assembly of Microscopic Three-Dimensional Structures and Their Applications in Three-Dimensional Photonic Crystals

Kanna Aoki

CONTENTS

24.1 INTRODUCTION

How straightforward and comfortable it would be if we could produce three-dimensional (3D) structures on a micrometer scale as we would build a bookcase in our normal life. Reality, however, is not nearly so simple. The fabrication of microscopic objects must be conducted without actual visualization of the process. We can view the outcome only after all fabrication steps are completed. A technology that enables us to handle microscopic components while watching the process in real time would enable us to explore the microscopic world more deeply than ever. This chapter introduces a micromanipulation system for the visually monitored assembly of components on the micrometer to nanometer scale, as established through the development of 3D photonic crystals.

24.2 MICROMANIPULATION

For objects smaller than micrometer scale, such as molecules and atoms, an atomic force microscope is widely used as a manipulation tool. For objects larger than micrometer scale, such as living tissue, a manipulator operated under observation with an optical microscope has been used intensively for various purposes such as artificial insemination. Issues related to the handling of objects ranging from micrometer to nanometer size have been left untouched, although many topics of current scientific interest—such as microelectromechanical systems, high-density memory structures, single photon/electron devices, living tissues, and lab-on-chips—are considered within this field. The micromanipulation system introduced in this chapter was developed with the intention of filling this gap [1]. The term "micromanipulation" is coined from "micro," which roughly indicates the scale length of target objects that are "manipulated" or handled.

24.2.1 System Components

The micromanipulation system comprises remotely operated multiaxial stages installed in the specimen chamber of a scanning electron microscope (SEM). Two multiaxial stages, one for an object sample and another for handling a probe, are arranged as mutually orthogonal; each is tilted at an angle of 45° to the axis of an objective lens. A probe, which functions as a "finger" to manipulate target objects, is usually made by wiredrawing a glass tube until it splits off. Then, the probe is coated with chromium and gold using an evaporator to avoid charge-up during assembly operations under SEM observation (Figure 24.1).

Among various operations, picking up an object is the most difficult because the handling probe is merely a thin rod with a sharp point, resembling a sewing needle. Below micrometer scale, electrostatic and van der Waals forces are more influential than gravity. Consequently, lifting an object is achieved by setting the system's condition such that a target object is likely to adhere to the tip of a probe by controlling the accelerating voltage of a SEM system. To remove an object from the tip, the object is fixed to a position with a stopper (microspheres and rectangular columns in this study); then the probe can be slid aside because no force is applied vertical to the probe's axis.

24.3 PHOTONIC CRYSTAL

Photonic crystals are often described as "semiconductors of light" because they can control the behavior of light. This capability originates from their fine structure, which has a length scale that is comparable to the wavelength of the target light. Commercially important wavelengths of light are the optical communication wavelengths of 1260–1625 nm. A photonic crystal operating in this region has fine structures of size 400–700 nm. To develop the equivalent of a semiconductor's energy band gap—a photonic band gap—the ratio of the refractive index between a crystal's material and its surroundings is expected to be larger than a certain value. In addition, the crystal's material is expected to be transparent in the working wavelength range. Common semiconductor materials such as silicon (Si), gallium arsenide (GaAs) and indium phosphide (InP) can fulfill these

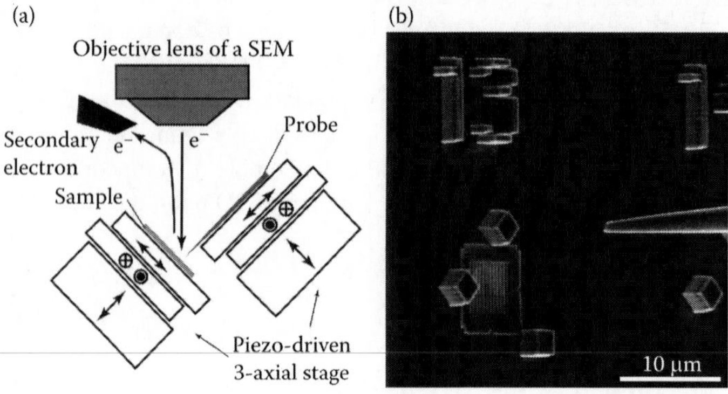

FIGURE 24.1 A micromanipulation system. (a) Schematic configuration of the system. (b) SEM image obtained during assembly.

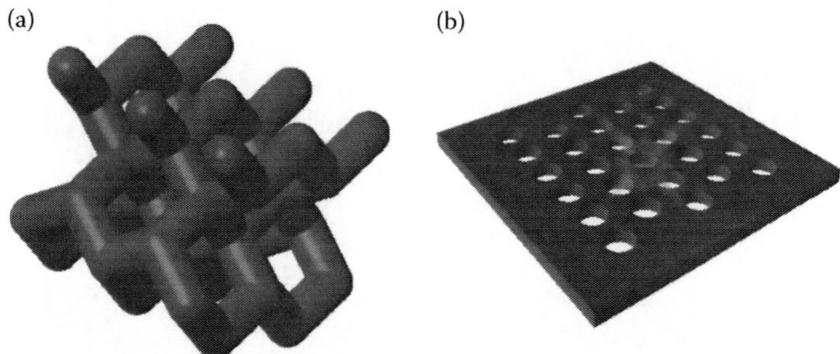

FIGURE 24.2 Opposing features of 2D and 3D photonic crystals. (a) A 3D photonic crystal can confine light completely, but it is difficult to make. (b) A 2D photonic crystal is sufficiently simple that it can be produced using conventional semiconductor fabrication techniques, but its light confining effect is imperfect.

requirements. Forming micrometer-scale patterns in these materials is easy using state-of-the-art semiconductor processing technologies, which are now used mainly for fabricating structures as narrow as several tens of nanometers on semiconductor wafers. However, because these technologies are developed for 2D processing, they cannot fabricate the 3D structures, which are crucial for full bandgap photonic crystals.

Consequently, instead of full bandgap photonic crystals, intensive study has been devoted to 2D photonic crystals that possess fine structures only within a plane. Therefore, a photonic bandgap affects only the area within the plane. A 2D photonic crystal confines light through the photonic bandgap effect in the plane direction, and uses total internal reflection to confine light in the direction vertical to the plane surface (Figure 24.2).

A crucial limitation of 2D photonic crystals is their limited light-confining effect: they are effective only on polarized light in a certain direction to a crystal. Light out of a controllable polarization direction freely escapes from its structure. This limit of its effectiveness is the greatest obstacle to the industrial use of 2D photonic crystals.

Aside from substituting a 2D photonic crystal for a full photonic bandgap crystal working around the resulting inconveniences, developing a new fabrication technique for micrometer- and nanometer-scale fine 3D structures is another way of addressing the situation. Micromanipulation is apparently the appropriate method for this purpose.

24.4 3D PHOTONIC CRYSTAL FOR MID-INFRARED (MID-IR) WAVELENGTH

It was not certain whether the micromanipulation technique was able to achieve a 3D photonic crystal that requires high precision because it was a pioneering approach; at that time, it had a poor record of high-precision assembly. Consequently, the micromanipulation technique was first applied on a trial basis to the fabrication of 3D photonic crystals operating in a longer wavelength range than optical communication wavelengths.

24.4.1 Unit Components

In this approach, the final 3D photonic crystal structure was considered as an ensemble of simple components. Unit components were prepared in the form of air-bridge plates using conventional semiconductor processing techniques for easy removal from a wafer during micromanipulation, and assembled into the designed 3D structure using a micromanipulation system. Here, InP was selected as the material for a 3D photonic crystal. Indium gallium arsenide (InGaAs) was deposited on an InP wafer using the metalorganic chemical vapor deposition (MOCVD) method as a sacrificial layer; then an InP layer was formed on it [2]. Subsequently, titanium and nickel layers, as a mask for dry etching processing, were formed using an evaporator, and a resist layer for electron-beam lithography was spin-coated onto the top (Figure 24.3).

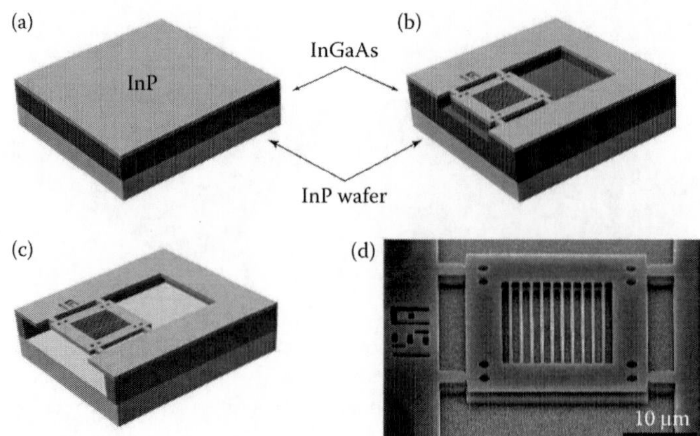

FIGURE 24.3 Fabrication process for a unit component. (a) InGaAs and InP layers were grown on an InP wafer using MOCVD. (b) Metal mask and resist layers were prepared on the crystal wafer in (a), and unit plate patterns drawn using electron-beam lithography were transferred to InP layer by dry etching. (c) An InGaAs sacrificial layer beneath an InP unit plate pattern was removed by wet etching to have the plate sustained in the air. (d) A SEM image of an air-bridge unit plate component.

The unit plate was designed so that photonic patterns were formed in the center of a unit plate and surrounded by a frame to sustain the structure. Circular holes to lock a planar component in a predefined position were also prepared in the frame.

24.4.2 Assembly Techniques

Precise combination of components is crucial to create an assembled structure to produce a 3D photonic bandgap effect. Here, plate components were aligned and fixed at the correct position by inserting polystyrene microspheres into circular holes in each plate's frame with diameters matching that of the microspheres. When the microspheres were inserted into the holes, their upper hemispheres protruded from the plane of the plate. When the subsequent plate is moved closer to the first plate, the upper hemisphere guides the second plate to the right position (Figure 24.4).

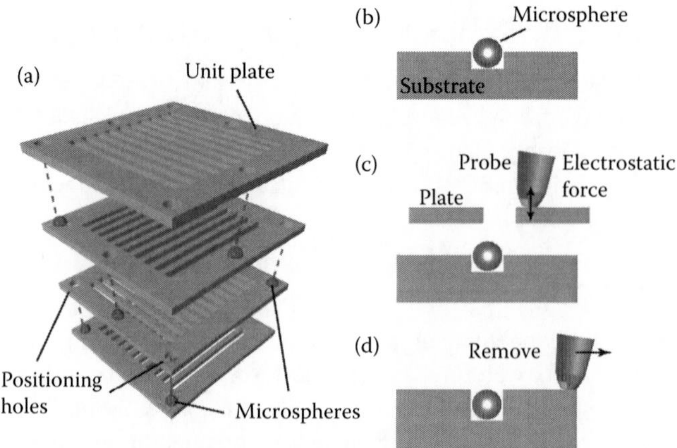

FIGURE 24.4 Schematic diagram of a lock-and-key approach for high-precision assembly. (a) Schematic diagram of the precise linking of a series of components. (b) At the beginning of an assembly, a microsphere was inserted in a hole prepared on a wafer, with a depth that is identical to the radius of the microsphere. (c) A unit plate was assembled above a set of microspheres. (d) The microsphere locks the plate in a right position; then a probe is slid aside.

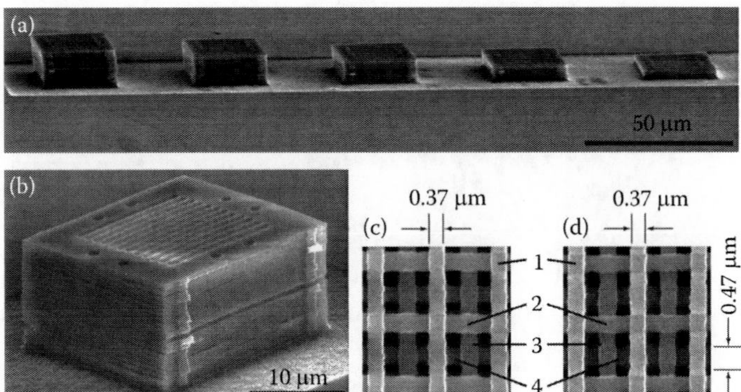

FIGURE 24.5 Assembled 3D photonic crystals operating in mid-IR. (a) 20-, 16-, 12-, 8-, and 4-layered crystals. (b) 20-layered crystal in (a). (c) Top view of a normal crystal. (d) Top view of a crystal with a planar defect. Defect layers were inserted in the 4th and 5th (not seen) layers from the top layer.

By repeating this procedure, arrays of 4-, 8-, 12-, 16-, and 20-layered 3D photonic crystals were assembled successfully in designated positions on a semiconductor chip (Figure 24.5). The fabricated crystals formed a so-called woodpile structure with an in-plane period length a of 1.4 μm, with 0.37 μm stripe width and 500 nm plate thickness, and exhibited a full photonic band gap between 3 and 4.5 μm, which corresponded to numerical simulations. The true value of a photonic crystal is exercised when a certain function, such as a resonator and a waveguide, is added to a crystal by introducing a defect structure in it. Consequently, the availability of a defect structure in a crystal is extremely important. Then, a crystal containing a planar defect was also fabricated to verify the technique's flexibility. The crystal with defect layers showed a clear resonant mode that originated from the defect structure. It matched well the results of numerical simulations. For details of the optical properties of the assembled crystals, see [3].

24.5 3D PHOTONIC CRYSTAL FOR OPTICAL COMMUNICATION WAVELENGTHS

The successful outcome of the pilot study ensured that this approach would function in the fabrication of a 3D photonic crystal operating at shorter wavelengths. In addition to reduction of the working wavelength, active 3D photonic crystals with a resonant cavity structure and luminescent materials were targeted in the following study [4].

24.5.1 Unit Components for an Active 3D Photonic Crystal

In this study, GaAs, another major material used for optoelectronic devices, was selected as the basis for active 3D photonic crystals. A unit component with a point defect structure contains an indium arsenide antimony quantum dot layer in the middle of a GaAs layer. With the decrease in the target wavelength down to around 1.5 μm, the plate component thickness and period length of stripe patterns, a, were also reduced, respectively, to 200 nm and 560–600 nm, almost half of those in the pilot study (Figure 24.6).

24.5.2 Advanced Assembly Technique

To extend operation to shorter wavelengths, major improvements in the alignment method were needed. In the first procedure, self-alignment of neighboring layers was achieved using a

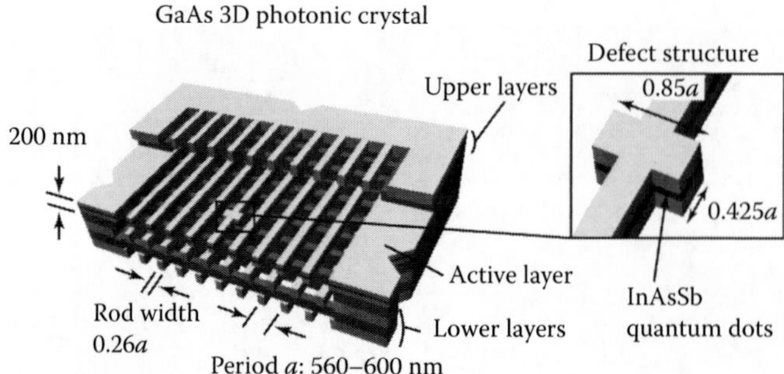

FIGURE 24.6 Schematic structure of an active 3D photonic crystal.

combination of polystyrene microspheres and planar components that contained matching circular holes. As the target wavelength decreases, the planar component thickness must also decrease, requiring smaller microspheres. To maintain high precision in its structure, it is important to maintain the tolerance limits of the component size within a small range. However, as the microspheres' necessary size shrinks, their commercial availability becomes severely limited. Furthermore, some concerns persist in relation to carbon contamination during the heat treatment process for wafer bonding. Most importantly, placing the microspheres in the planar component for every assembly is labor intensive.

To avoid these difficulties, a new alignment technique has been devised in which the microspheres are replaced by a set of columns formed on a semiconductor chip (Figure 24.7). Alignment

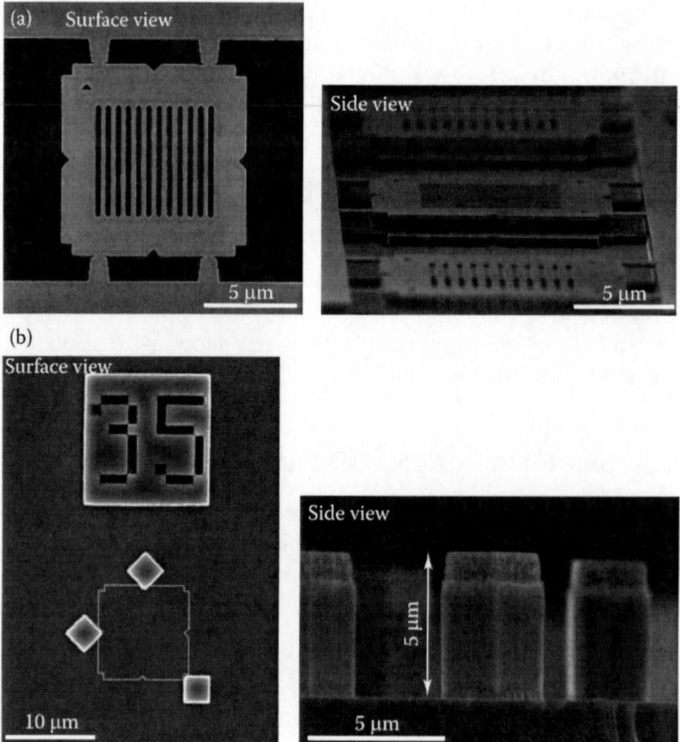

FIGURE 24.7 New lock-and-key design for high-precision assembly of components. (a) Unit components with positioning notches around a frame. (b) A set of positioning rods matching notches in a frame of a unit component in (a). The dotted frame in the surface view marks the plate position.

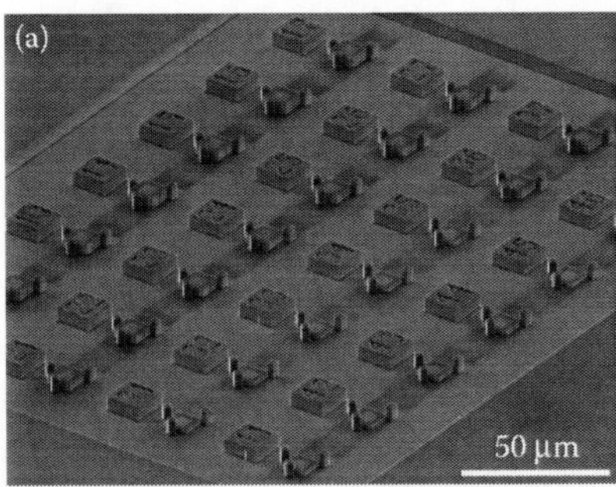

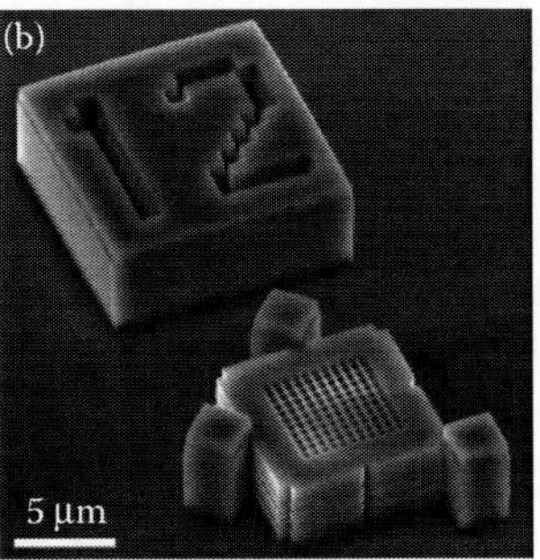

FIGURE 24.8 (a) Integrated 28 active 3D photonic crystals in the form of a 4 × 7 matrix. (b) Enlarged image of a 3D photonic crystal assembled in address number 12.

of the planar components while stacking was achieved by cutting notches at the corners and sides of each plate, which fit precisely to the set of rectangular columns on the substrate. Using this method, the microsphere assembly step was eliminated, thereby enabling continuous assembly of the plate components. This approach widens the range of sizes and positioning pattern designs, and the precision level of all components remains high because they are prepared using the same semiconductor processing procedures. Using the same material for components and alignment columns, deformation during heat treatment caused by a difference in thermal expansion coefficients can be avoided.

24.5.3 Integrated Active 3D Photonic Crystal Devices on a Chip

Positioning columns introduced in the previous section were prepared on a GaAs wafer in the form of a 4 × 7 matrix, with each position labeled with an address number (Figure 24.8). As a result of sequential assembly of normal and defect components, 28 active 3D photonic crystals were assembled with no failed structures. This is the first demonstration of an integrated 3D photonic crystal active device operating at optical wavelengths that comprises such a large number and variety of individual photonic crystal components. The shape of a point defect was fixed to a rectangle of $0.85a \times 0.425a$ throughout this study, but a varied between 560 and 600 nm (a is fixed to an identical value in one planar component and one crystal). Consequently, various crystals resonating at different wavelengths were achieved (Figure 24.9). Not only resonant

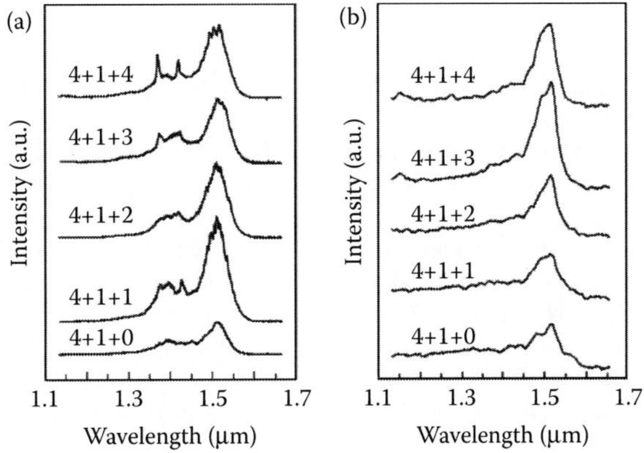

FIGURE 24.9 Emission spectra from 3D photonic crystals (a) with and (b) without a resonant cavity structure. Numbers assigned to each spectrum denote the numbers of lower layers, active layers, and upper layers, respectively.

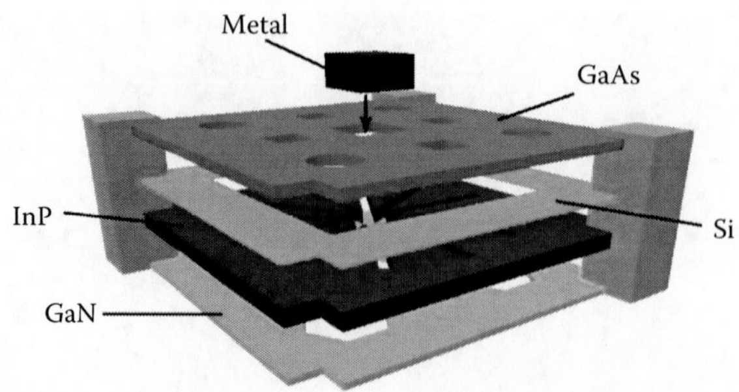

FIGURE 24.10 Micromanipulation provides high flexibility in the combination of materials and structure designs. An unlikely combination of materials is realizable using micromanipulation.

wavelengths, but also the quality factors of resonant peaks well matched numerical predictions. The quality factor marked 2300 at the maximum, which boosted the record for Q-factors of 3D photonic crystal cavity resonators by almost 10-fold; the value soon became greater than 8000 in a subsequent study [5].

Structural deviations in a crystal, which are surface roughness derived from fine structure processing and stacking errors during assembly, were determined to be as low as 50 nm using SEM observations. Consequently, high-precision and degradation-free materials in the crystal structures made it possible to achieve resonant emissions from crystals that showed good reproducibility of numerical prediction.

24.6 CONCLUSIONS

Micromanipulation is no longer a questionable technique. Precise assembly of objects on micrometer and nanometer scale is no longer a "mission impossible." This achievement expects to promote studies not only of 3D photonic crystals, but also of microchemical and microbiological reactions and analyses, optical devices, electronic devices, medical appliances, and so on.

A unique benefit of micromanipulation is the versatility it offers for assembly. The precision level of assembly is unaffected by the plate's pattern complexity and materials (Figure 24.10). Using this technique, structures and combinations of materials that cannot be realized using existing processing and crystal growth techniques can be achieved. Such exotic structures might yield as-yet-unforeseen devices and physical phenomena.

REFERENCES

1. H. Morishita and Y. Hatamura, Development of ultra micro manipulator system under stereo SEM observation, *Proc. 1993 IEEE/RSJ Int. Conf. Intelligent Robots and Systems* 3, 1717–1721, 1993.
2. K. Aoki, H.T. Miyazaki, H. Hirayama, K. Inoshita, T. Baba, N. Shinya, and Y. Aoyagi, Three-dimensional photonic crystals for optical wavelengths assembled by micromanipulation, *Appl. Phys. Lett.* 81, 3122–3124, 2002.
3. K. Aoki, H.T. Miyazaki, H. Hirayama, K. Inoshita, T. Baba, K. Sakoda, N. Shinya, and Y. Aoyagi, Microassembly of semiconductor three-dimensional photonic crystals, *Nature Mater.* 2, 117–121, 2003.
4. K. Aoki, D. Guimard, M. Nishioka, M. Nomura, S. Iwamoto, and Y. Arakawa, Coupling of quantum dot light emission with three-dimensional photonic crystal nanocavity, *Nature Photon.* 2, 688–692, 2008.
5. A. Tandaechanurat, S. Ishida, K. Aoki, D. Guimard, M. Nomura, S. Iwamoto, and Y. Arakawa, Demonstration of high-Q (>8,600) three-dimensional photonic crystal nanocavity embedding quantum dots, *Appl. Phys. Lett.* 94, 171115, 2009.

Part III

Biotechnology and MEMs

25 Surface Chemistry for Cell Capture in Microfluidic Systems

ShuQi Wang, Feng Xu, Alexander Chi Fai Ip, Mrudula Somu, Xiaohu Zhao, Altug Akay, and Utkan Demirci

CONTENTS

25.1 INTRODUCTION

Cell separation or sorting plays an important role in basic research and clinical applications such as the differentiation of stem cells [1,2], detection of circulating tumor cells (CTCs) [3,4] and quantification of CD4+ T lymphocytes in peripheral blood [5,6]. Conventionally, fluorescence-activated cell sorting or magnetic cell sorting methods have been widely used to separate cells of interest from a heterogeneous cell mixture. However, these methods require technical support, length sample preparation, and well-trained operators, which limit their applications in resource-limited and point-of-care settings. To address these drawbacks, various microfluidic devices have been designed and tested, targeting increased portability, reduced consumption of samples and reagents, decreased process complexity, and shortened sample-to-result time. In addition, the manufacturing of microfluidic devices can easily be scaled up, significantly reducing the cost of health care, even for developed countries. The microfluidic device can be further integrated into an automated system to reduce human errors. The advantages of microfluidic systems offer opportunities for improving health care in resource-limited settings, such as monitoring AIDS treatments using CD4 cell capturing devices [5,6].

Microfluidics-based cell separation or sorting often relies on cell capture using surface chemistry, mechanical filtering, dielectrophoresis, or a combination of these methods. Among these, the most popular method is antibody-based surface chemistry. The antigen–antibody affinity-based cell capture strategy can be employed in a microchannel, microarray, or column depending on the application. Recently, DNA/RNA aptamers have been utilized to capture cells due to high affinity between DNA/RNA aptamers and their corresponding biomarker proteins on the target cell surface [7,8]. In addition, barcode DNA technology has also come into the cell separation field [9]. This technology is based on highly specific nucleic acid hybridization between DNA probes and their complementary sequences, which are artificially conferred on the surface of target cells [10]. These microfluidics-based cell-sorting technologies can be combined with a variety of detection technologies, such as fluorescence [11,12], impedance measurements [13,14], lensless imaging [6,15], and polymerase chain reaction (PCR) [16], for further characterization in a miniaturized system.

In this chapter, we present recent advances in surface chemistry for cell capture in microfluidic systems, strategies to improve cell capture efficiency, and clinical applications of cell separation and quantification.

25.2 STRATEGIES TO CAPTURE CELLS

25.2.1 Antibody–Ligand-Based Cell Capture

Antibody–ligand-based cell capture is most commonly used to capture target cells from biological samples (e.g., whole blood) (Figure 25.1) [6,11,13,17]. Generally, the antibody against the surface protein of target cells is first immobilized on the microchannel surface of a microfluidic device by covalent linkage. A clinical sample is then flowed through the microchannels at a constant flow rate. If target cells are present in the clinical sample, and they will be captured by the immobilized antibody, enabling isolation and subsequent characterization of target cells (e.g., counting). Three major factors need to be considered for effective capture of target cells in a microfluidic device. First, the antibody/ligand should be specific to the antigen on the surface of target cells, such as monoclonal antibodies (MAbs), to minimize or avoid nonspecific binding. For example, Nouanthong et al. [18] reported that an anti-$CD4^+$ MAb was able to differentiate $CD4^+$ T lymphocytes from monocytes, which also express $CD4^+$ molecules on the cell surface. The use of such MAb can potentially increase the specificity of isolating $CD4^+$ T lymphocytes in the presence of monocytes. Second, the level of surface antigen on the target cells needs to be significantly higher than on other types of cells so that the antibody can bind most efficiently to the target cells [19,20]. For example, the expression of the epithelial cell adhesion molecule (EpCAM) on tumor-derived epithelial cells (one type of CTCs) is upregulated compared to normal epithelial cells [21]. This forms the basis for isolating CTCs from normal blood cells via anti-EpCAM antibody [3]. Third, the flow rate and corresponding shear stress need to be optimized. Because increased flow rate can increase the shear stress on the captured cells, this may detach the captured cells from the immobilized antibody. In addition, high flow rate decreases the antigen–antibody interaction time, resulting in reduced capture efficiency [3,20].

25.2.2 Aptamer-Based Cell Capture

Aptamers are also commonly used to capture target molecules from biological samples with high affinity and specificity (Figure 25.2) [7]. Aptamers are short strands of single-stranded DNA (ssDNA) or RNA, ranging from 25 to 40 nucleotides [7]. Under certain conditions, aptamers form secondary structures with an extremely high affinity for target molecules, such as membrane proteins found on cells of interest. Aptamers can be custom-selected *in vitro* using a library of up to 10^{15} different sequences via a reiterative screening process known as Systematic Evolution of Ligands by Exponential Enrichment [22]. Once a sequence is identified, the resulting aptamers can distinguish between isoforms of the same protein, for example, protein kinase C [23]. A small change in the

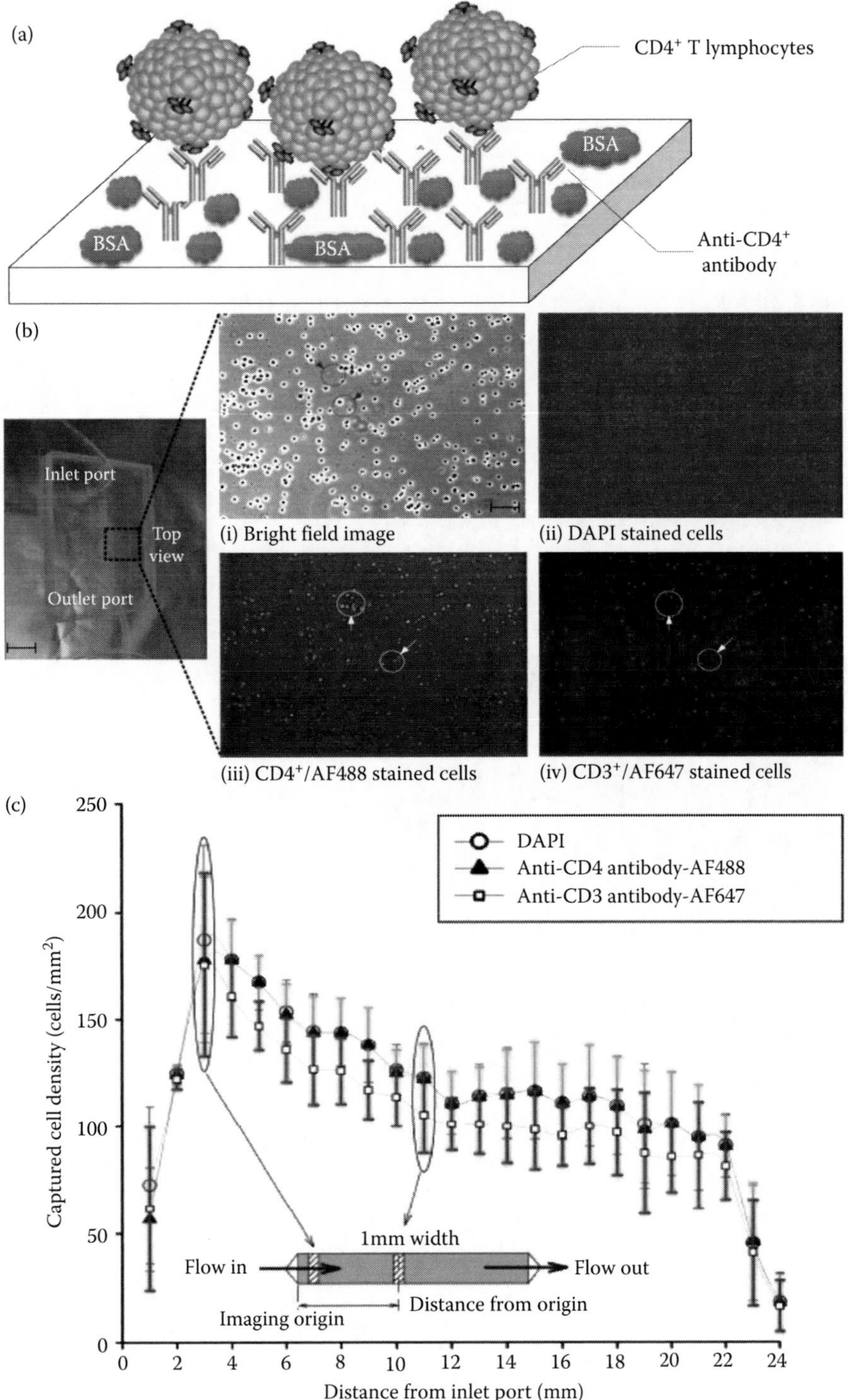

FIGURE 25.1 An example of antibody-based cell capture (e.g., CD4+ T lymphocytes). (a) Schematic of cell capture using antibody. (b) An example cell captured using anti-CD4 antibody surface immobilization. The captured cells were identified using optical and fluorescent images. Scale bars are 5 mm and 100 μm. (c) The cell capture efficiency is quantified as a function of the channel length from the inlet. (Adapted from S. Moon et al., *Biosens Bioelectron*, 24, 3208–3214, 2009.)

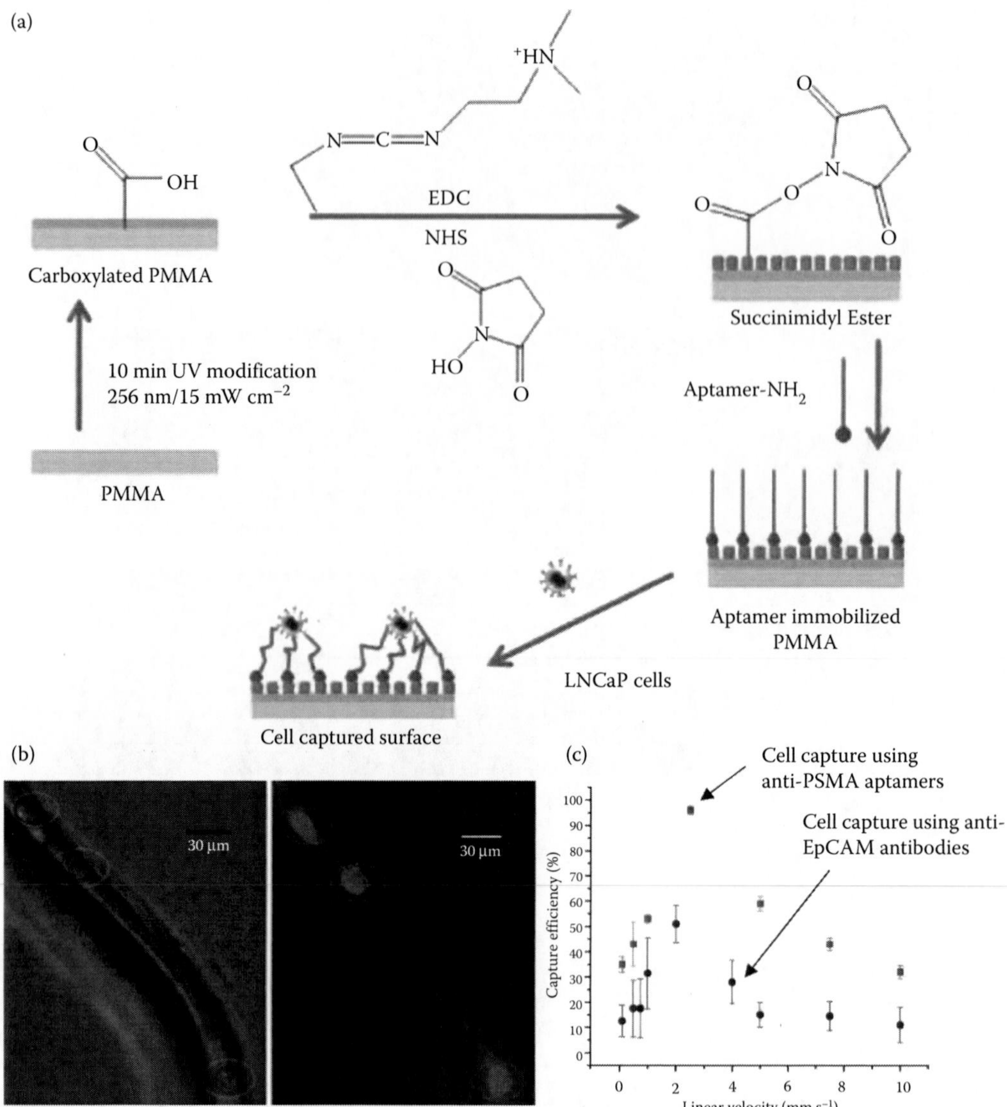

FIGURE 25.2 An example of aptamer-based cell capture (e.g., capture of CTCs). (a) Preparation of a high-throughput micro-sampling unit. PMMA is first irradiated with UV (15 mW cm-2) and then treated with l-ethyl-3-[3-dimethylaminopropyl] carbodimide hydrochloride (EDC). Aptamers are subsequently coated on the surface, allowing for specific capture of lymph node metastasis prostate cancer cells (LNCaP cells). (b) LNCaP cells (~1000 cells/mL suspended in PBS) infused into the HTMSU were positively selected as shown in brightfield and fluorescence images. (c) Comparison of LNCaP cell capture efficiencies under different cells' translational velocities using anti-PSMA aptamers or anti-EpCAM antibodies cell recognition elements. (Adapted from U. Dharmasiri et al., *Electrophoresis*, 30, 3289–3300, 2009. Copyright Wiley-VCH Verlag GmbH & Co. KGaA. Reproduced with permission.)

target chemical structure (e.g., the difference of a methyl group between theophylline and caffeine) can result in a 10,000-fold reduction in binding affinity [24]. In addition, aptamers can be further refined postselection by additional chemical modifications to reduce nonspecific binding, enhance binding affinity, and resist nuclease degradation [25].

When capturing cells, aptamers specifically interact with surface proteins such as receptors or ligands, which are specific to different cell types [8]. Cancerous cells tend to overexpress certain proteins, such as prostate-specific membrane antigen (PSMA) [26]. This overexpression can be utilized by aptamer-based capturing systems to immobilize, detect, and quantify CTCs expressing PSMA at a high level in blood samples [8]. The high specificity of aptamers can capture cancer cells with purity higher than 97% [27]. This high specificity of aptamers also allows multiple pathogen detection at once within a single system. It has been shown that simultaneous isolation of CTCs for lymphoblastic leukemia, Burkitt's lymphoma, and non-Hodgkin's B-cell lymphoma can be performed on the same device using corresponding CTC aptamers [28].

In addition to high affinity and specificity, aptamers possess many other advantages over antibodies, including *in vitro* synthesis, batch invariability, reversible conformation changes due to temperature variation, and extended shelf life [7]. Further, aptamers can be modified with fluorophores or biotin moieties and then attached to nanoparticles (NPs) as antibodies in various applications. This strategy can enhance the capture efficiency of aptamer-based surface chemistry and facilitate subsequent detection. Despite these advantages, aptamers also have limitations as capturing moieties. There are only a limited number of target molecules for which specific aptamers have been identified. Although a very large library of sequences (e.g., 10^{15} nucleotide sequences) can be created, the screening process for a suitable aptamer specific for a target cell marker is time consuming and may take a period of up to weeks [29].

25.2.3 DNA-Barcode-Directed Cell Capture

DNA-barcode technology was initially designed to detect low levels of protein or nucleic acid with the aid of gold NPs and magnetic microparticles [30]. Recently, this technology has also been utilized to capture single cells [10]. In this strategy, glycoproteins on the surface of living cells are modified by the incorporation of azide. The 5′-amine-modified ssDNA is then modified with a phosphine group by the administration of phosphine pentafluorophenyl ester, which allows for stable amide linkages between ssDNA and target cells. The ssDNA-bearing cells can then be captured on a DNA array in a sequence-dependent fashion. This strategy has enabled the capture of single cells and subsequent characterization with RT-PCR for gene expression [31] or with a microelectrode array for metabolic analysis [9]. Since target cells can be modified with any possible sequence, multiple cells can be patterned together via DNA hybridization, forming a complex network of living cells [10]. However, the target cells must be modified prior to DNA-barcode-based cell capture.

25.3 STRATEGIES TO IMPROVE THE EFFICIENCY OF CELL CAPTURE

25.3.1 NP Coating of Cell-Capture Surface

The capture efficiency of a device is dependent on the number of capture moieties (e.g., antibodies and nucleic acids) on the surface. NPs can potentially improve cell capture efficiency by increasing the cell-capture surface area in a microchannel, thereby increasing the number of capture moieties. To do so, Han et al. [32] coated positively charged colloidal silica NPs (10–15 nm) onto the channel surface via negatively charged poly-L-lysine (PLL) (Figure 25.3). Using this strategy, up to 35% additional capture moieties (e.g., P-selectin) were obtained as compared to adsorption in the uncoated channel. In addition, Han and colleagues used titanium (IV) butoxide as an adhesive to coat NPs on the channel surface. The results showed that titanium (IV) butoxide had comparable capture efficiency as PLL. In both cases, the increased roughness on the channel surface and the increased number of the capturing moiety, P-selectin, significantly enhanced the rolling velocity of cells [32]. Enhanced cell rolling, due to the interaction between cells and P-selectin, can initiate cell adhesion on a target issue such as in the process of leukocyte homing and cancer cell metastasis [33]. As expected, the enhanced cell rolling significantly increased the cell capture efficiency [32]. However, it should be noted that the amount of coated NPs needs to be optimized. Otherwise, excessive NPs coated on the channel surface may aggregate and occlude the microchannel.

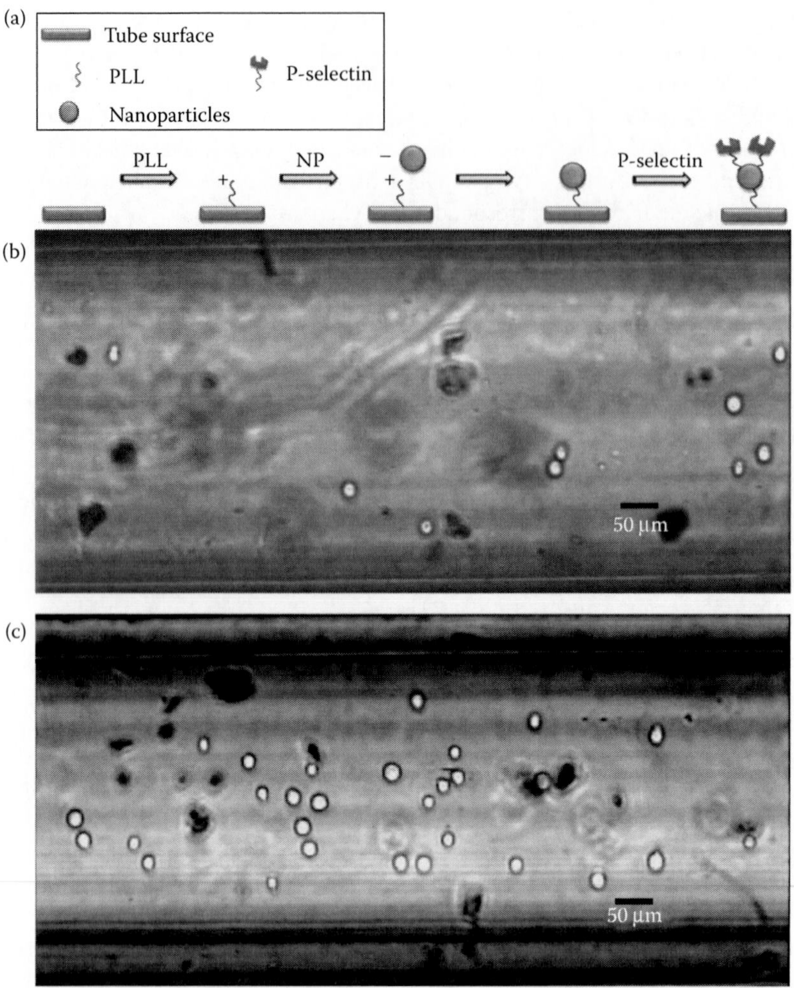

FIGURE 25.3 Improved capture efficiency based on nanoparticle-coating. (a) Illustration of conventional P-selectin coating in a microchannel using PLL as an adhesive. This increases the number of antibodies immobilized on the channel surface. (b) The total number of cells captured in a control channel, which was not coated with nanoparticles. (c) The total number of cells captured in a NP-coated channel. (Adapted from W. J. Han et al., *ACS Nano*, 4, 174–180, 2010.)

25.3.2 Geometry Optimization

For optimal cell capture in a microchannel, flow parameters such as shear stress and flow velocity must be optimized. One of the optimization strategies is to vary the geometry of the microchannel [34]. It is known that straight microchannels have a uniform flow velocity and hence have the most predictable cell adhesion pattern. In contrast, nonstraight microchannels may have different flow velocities, especially at turning points. As shown in Figure 25.4, the flow rate is the lowest (close to zero) at sharp turns, according to computational fluid dynamics analysis [34]. As the distance away from the sharp turn increases, flow velocity increases gradually. Due to the nonuniform flow velocities across the microchannel, nonuniform shear stress would be expected to be conferred on target cells, which may cause nonspecific adherence of cells, especially at the turning points. These cells cannot be dislodged with excess wash since the flow velocity is close to zero at this region (a dead corner) [34].

To remove dead corners, curved turns can be built in the nonstraight microchannels to favorably achieve a uniform flow rate and thus obtain uniform capture efficiency throughout the

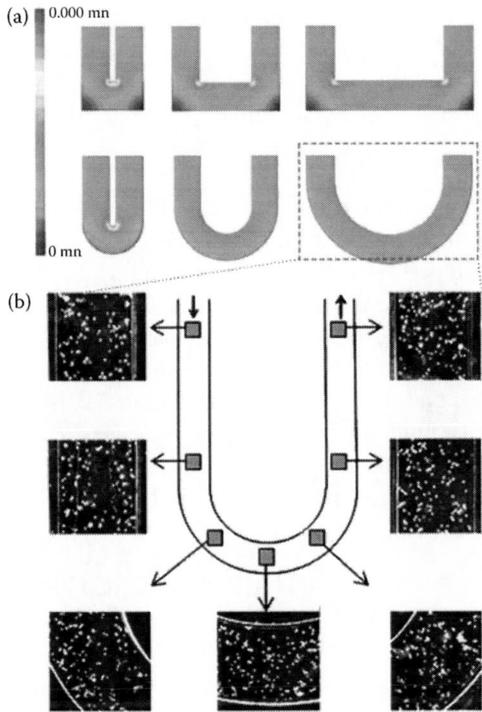

FIGURE 25.4 Effect of microchannel geometry on flow rate. (a) Schematic of flow velocity in sharp turns and curved turns. The flow rate in the microchannel is indicated in color according to a scaled indicator on the left. (b) Cell capture at 7 locations in a curved-turn device with a spacing of 3.7 mm between two vertical arms. (Adapted from J. V. Green et al., Effect of channel geometry on cell adhesion in microfluidic devices, *Lab Chip*, 9, 677–685 2009. Reproduced by permission of The Royal Society of Chemistry.)

microchannel [34]. As the gap between the two straight parallel parts in the curved channel is enlarged, the high flow rate zone becomes smaller and localized to the upper turns, and the velocity in the middle of the horizontal arm is at a level similar to that in the vertical arm (Figure 25.4). With this U-shape design, cell adhesion in sharp turn and curved turn channels showed essentially identical efficiency in capturing rat aortic smooth muscle cells as the straight channel had shown (around 50 cells/mm^2). In comparison, the cell adhesion was 53 cells/mm^2 in a curved turn channel with a gap spacing of 3.7 mm. As demonstrated, a curved turn channel can also be designed for providing uniform flow rates, thus giving predictable capture efficiency through the microchannel.

In addition, a micropost-based array can be utilized to increase cell capture in a microfluidic channel [3]. Nagrath et al. [3] tested three different micropost array distributions: a square array, a diagonal square array, and an equilateral triangular array. The results showed that the equilateral triangular micropost array had the highest cell capture efficiency as a function of the spacing between the microposts. The cell capture efficiency could be further improved with shorter spacing among microposts. However, target cells may physically be trapped by microposts if the center-to-center spacing is less than the diameter of target cells, which significantly limits the broad application of this technology.

25.3.3 Biotin–Streptavidin Affinity

Streptavidin, which is known to have high binding affinity for biotin, has also been widely used to improve antibody-based cell capture efficiency. Generally, up to four biotin molecules can be tightly bound to a streptavidin molecule simultaneously with an affinity constant of 2.5×10^{13} L/mol, which is one of the strongest noncovalent interactions [35]. The biotin–streptavidin affinity is generally used to control the orientation of coating antibodies on the surface, thus increasing the cell capture efficiency. In the adsorption method, antibodies can be immobilized onto the surface with its active antigen-binding site concealed. In addition, noncovalent linking between the antibody and the solid surface is reversible, which may lead to instability of the adsorbed antibody and loss of capture capability. The biotin–streptavidin interaction can be used to maximize the antibody orientation with exposed active binding sites. This interaction has been successfully implemented in various microfluidic devices, including for the capture of $CD4^+$ T lymphocytes [6,36].

The biotin–streptavidin interaction can be further improved to increase the number of biotinylated antibodies immobilized per streptavidin molecule. In this strategy, modification and polymerization of streptavidin are first performed on the surface of a 96-well plate (polystyrene) by introducing active thiol groups. The formation of thiolated streptavidin by covalent bonds clearly enhances the stability of streptavidin, compared to native streptavidin coating [35]. When using fluorescent europium-labeled biotin, the binding capability of the thiolated streptavidin surface was three times higher than the unmodified streptavidin surface. With a 40-fold molar excess of *N*-hydroxysuccinimide ester of *S*-acetylthioacetic acid, the biotin-binding capacity was further increased by 1.2 times compared to the native streptavidin coating.

25.4 APPLICATIONS OF CELL CAPTURE IN MICROFLUIDIC SYSTEMS

25.4.1 Capture of CTCs

Cancer causes approximately 13% of among all deaths annually, although one-third of the cancer patients can be cured if early diagnosis is made [37]. However, metastasis of cancer may cause subsequent relapse of the original tumor and spread the tumor to other organs within the patient via the circulatory system [38]. One of the methods to early diagnose metastasis is to detect CTCs in the peripheral blood of cancer patients [3,8,39]. CTCs are generally derived from the primary tumor and metastasize [40–43]. Early detection of these cancer-derived cells can help with clinical management of cancer patients and provide a better understanding of how metastasis occurs. However, CTCs are rare, at a ratio of one cell per 10^9 blood cells [3], and therefore it is a great challenge to capture and detect them reliably. Despite this difficulty, detection of CTCs has been achieved at both the cellular [8,39] and molecular levels [16].

At the cellular level, an enzyme-based fluorescent detection system is commonly used to achieve a direct visualization of captured cancer cells [44]. This method employs a fluorescent dye-conjugated antibody that is specific for different cancer cell types, allowing for quick fluorescence detection. Immunocytochemistry staining can also be used to confirm capture cells by targeting cell surface biomarkers [17]. Other physical properties of CTCs and normal tissue cells are also often used for CTC detection [45]. One such change is that the cancer cells become softer and more deformable [46]. This unique feature allows the detection of human kidney carcinoma cells using impedimetric transducers by monitoring the volume increase of cancer cells under hyposmotic pressure [47]. Human kidney cancer cells will swell under hyposmotic stress compared to the unchanging normal cells [47]. This application allowed the detection of cancer cells from whole blood without prelabeling or capturing. Alternatively, the size differences between cancer and noncancer cells can also be used to detect CTCs, based on the measurement of conductance [39].

At the molecular level, the detection and characterization of epidermal growth factor receptor gene (EGFR) can also be used to detect CTCs [16], since overexpression of EGFR has been confirmed to correlate with cancer incidence [48]. In a micropost-based CTC chip, nonsmall-cell lung cancer patient blood was made to flow through 78,000 EpCAM-coated microposts under optimized conditions. The captured CTCs were further analyzed by PCR, allowing for the identification of rare EGFR mutation [16]. With a better detection of EGFR mutations in cancer cells, the drug-resistant cancer cell mutations can be studied and potentially solved.

25.4.2 Capture of $CD4^+$ T Lymphocytes

Since the first case of AIDS was reported in 1981, HIV has caused approximately 60 million infections and 25 million deaths worldwide [49]. The number of $CD4^+$ T lymphocytes is needed in order to determine the immune state of HIV-infected individuals and his or her response to antiretroviral therapy (ART). To simplify ART monitoring in resource-limited settings, microfluidic devices have been developed to capture $CD4^+$ T lymphocytes from a small volume of whole blood [11,12]. This microdevice-based $CD4^+$ cell capture is realized using anti-$CD4^+$ antibody immobilized on the surface of a microchannel via biotin–streptavidin interaction. When whole blood is incubated in the microchannel, $CD4^+$ T lymphocytes are captured via surface molecule $CD4^+$ and anti-$CD4^+$ antibody. The captured $CD4^+$ T lymphocytes are then counted using fluorescence microscopy [11,12], light microscopy [5], or impedance measurement [50]. Alternatively, $CD4^+$ cell counts can be obtained using a lensless, ultrawide-field cell array based on shadow imaging [15], which enables rapid $CD4^+$ cell counting within 10 min using a portable battery-powered charge-coupled device camera [6].

25.4.3 Stem Cells

Stem cells have been attractive in medicine since they have the capability of self-renewal and of differentiating into lineages of multiple tissues [51,52]. However, efficient isolation of stem cells from a high background of other cell types is challenging and time consuming [1]. To address this, researchers have employed microfluidic devices to isolate stem cells with high efficiency and specificity [1,14,53]. Further, stem cells can be cultured in microfluidic devices in which microenvironments can be precisely controlled since they have essential effects on cell differentiation [54]. In addition, direct imaging of cultured stem cells can be achieved with transparent microfluidic devices, which facilitates the characterization of stem cells on the chip [54].

Endothelial progenitor cells (EPCs) originate from bone marrow and play an important role in neovascularization of ischemic tissues and in reendothelialization of vascular lesions. In addition, the number of EPCs can serve as a biomarker to predict clinical outcomes in the event of cardiovascular injury. However, the relative scarcity of circulating EPCs restricts its direct use for therapeutic and diagnostic applications. Efforts to isolate EPCs have been focused on density-gradient centrifugation [55] and the use of fluorescent or immunomagnetic beads in flow cytometry [56,57]. These methods are often associated with high-cost and complex isolation procedures. Plouffe et al. [1] have developed a microfluidic device (EPC chip) to capture EPCs. The EPC chip surface was coated with multiple antibodies targeting surface proteins such as $CD34^+$, $CD31^+$, vascular endothelial growth factor receptor-2 (VEGFR-2), $CD146^+$, $CD45^+$, and von Willebrand factor (vWF), which are consistent with the surface protein profile of EPCs. Under the same shear stress, the multiple antibody-coated surface achieved a cell capture efficiency 10 times higher than the single antibody-coated surface (anti-CD45) [1]. Recently, Ng et al. [14] developed impedance-based EPC detection on a microelectrode array for bed-side diagnosis.

Mesenchymal stem cells (MSCs) have the potential to differentiate into various cell types, such as osteoblasts, adipocytes, chondrocytes, astrocytes, and neurons [51]. However, it is challenging to isolate MSCs from multipotent derived from adult bone marrow, umbilical cords, blood, placentas, adipose tissues and amniotic fluid. Drop-based microfluidic devices [58,59] have recently been utilized to isolate MSCs [53]. By controlling fluid streams in microchannels, single cells can be separated, enabling the following characterization of cell-surface properties using a laser-based method. The following cell characterization in droplet microfluidic devices was highly correlated with flow cytometry. In addition, microfluidic devices employing louver-array structures have been explored [2]. The use of louver-array structures resulted in an optimal volume-flow-rates ratio, leading to a high separation efficiency of MSCs from amniotic fluids (82.8%). The increased separation efficiency was achieved by using a two-step process; on the first separation, the cells of interest are pipetted for a second separation trial, resulting in 97.1% separation efficiency.

25.5 CONCLUSIONS

Cell capture from biological samples is of great importance for basic research and clinical applications. However, this is challenging since the concentration of target cells can be fairly low (e.g., approximately 1 CTC out of 1 billion blood cells) and there exists a large amount of heterogeneity in the same sample. Therefore, methods offering highly selective capture of target cells with high efficiency are urgently needed. Microfluidic devices combined with surface chemistry-based cell capture, using capturing reagents such as antibody, aptamer, and DNA barcode, have demonstrated reliable capture and detection of rare types of cells in complex biological samples (e.g., whole blood). Further, modification of the device surface with NPs and optimization of geometric design of microfluidic devices can help achieve optimal cell capture efficiency. When combined with immunostaining or molecular biology detection methods, the cell-capture microfluidic devices can provide essential information for both scientific investigation and clinical applications. CTC and $CD4^+$ chips have been developed to investigate cancer metastasis and to monitor HIV treatment, respectively. Characteristics of these microchips such as low cost and short sample-to-result time may ultimately provide near-patient testing in both resource-rich and resource-limited settings.

ACKNOWLEDGMENTS

We would like to acknowledge the MIT Desphande Center Award, The W.H. Coulter Foundation Young Investigator Award, NIH RO1 A1081534, and NIH R21 AI087107. This work was supported by the Center for Integration of Medicine and Innovative Technology (CIMIT) under U.S. Army Medical Research Acquisition Activity Cooperative Agreements DAMD17-02-2-0006, W81XWH-07-2-0011, and W81XWH-09-2-0001. And this work was made possible by a research grant that was awarded and administered by the U.S. Army Medical Research & Materiel Command (USAMRMC) and the Telemedicine & Advanced Technology Research Center (TATRC), at Fort Detrick, MD.

REFERENCES

1. B. D. Plouffe et al., Development of microfluidics as endothelial progenitor cell capture technology for cardiovascular tissue engineering and diagnostic medicine, *FASEB J*, 23, 3309–3314, 2009.
2. H. W. Wu et al., A microfluidic device for separation of amniotic fluid mesenchymal stem cells utilizing louver-array structures, *Biomed Microdevices*, 11, 1297–1307, 2009.
3. S. Nagrath et al., Isolation of rare circulating tumour cells in cancer patients by microchip technology, *Nature*, 450, 1235–1239, 2007.
4. L. V. Sequist et al., The CTC-chip: An exciting new tool to detect circulating tumor cells in lung cancer patients, *J Thorac Oncol*, 4, 281–283, 2009.
5. X. Cheng et al., A microchip approach for practical label-free CD4+ T-cell counting of HIV-infected subjects in resource-poor settings, *J Acquir Immune Defic Syndr*, 45, 257–261, 2007.
6. S. Moon et al., Integrating microfluidics and lensless imaging for point-of-care testing, *Biosens Bioelectron*, 24, 3208–3214, 2009.
7. S. M. Nimjee et al., Aptamers: An emerging class of therapeutics, *Annu Rev Med*, 56, 555–583, 2005.
8. U. Dharmasiri et al., Highly efficient capture and enumeration of low abundance prostate cancer cells using prostate-specific membrane antigen aptamers immobilized to a polymeric microfluidic device, *Electrophoresis*, 30, 3289–3300, 2009.
9. E. S. Douglas et al., DNA-barcode directed capture and electrochemical metabolic analysis of single mammalian cells on a microelectrode array, *Lab Chip*, 9, 2010–2015, 2009.
10. R. A. Chandra et al., Programmable cell adhesion encoded by DNA hybridization, *Angew Chem Int Ed Engl*, 45, 896–901, 2006.
11. J. V. Jokerst et al., Integration of semiconductor quantum dots into nano-bio-chip systems for enumeration of CD4 + T cell counts at the point-of-need, *Lab Chip*, 8, 2079–2090, 2008.
12. W. R. Rodriguez et al., A microchip CD4 counting method for HIV monitoring in resource-poor settings, *PLoS Med*, 2, e182, 2005.

13. X. Cheng et al., Cell detection and counting through cell lysate impedance spectroscopy in microfluidic devices, *Lab Chip*, 7, 746–755, 2007.
14. S. Y. Ng et al., Label-free impedance detection of low levels of circulating endothelial progenitor cells for point-of-care diagnosis, *Biosens Bioelectron*, 25, 1095–1101, 2010.
15. A. Ozcan and U. Demirci, Ultra wide-field lens-free monitoring of cells on-chip, *Lab Chip*, 8, 98–106, 2008.
16. S. Maheswaran et al., Detection of mutations in EGFR in circulating lung-cancer cells, *N Engl J Med*, 359, 366–377, 2008.
17. Z. Du et al., Microfluidic-based diagnostics for cervical cancer cells, *Biosens Bioelectron*, 21, 1991–1995, 2006.
18. P. Nouanthong et al., A simple manual rosetting method for absolute CD4+ lymphocyte counting in resource-limited countries, *Clin Vaccine Immunol*, 13, 598–601, 2006.
19. K. Wang et al., Isolation and counting of multiple cell types using an affinity separation device, *Anal Chim Acta*, 601, 1–9, 2007.
20. Z. Du et al., Recognition and capture of breast cancer cells using an antibody-based platform in a microelectromechanical systems device, *Biomed Microdevices*, 9, 35–42, 2007.
21. P. T. Went et al., Frequent EpCam protein expression in human carcinomas, *Hum Pathol*, 35, 122–128, 2004.
22. C. Tuerk and L. Gold, Systematic evolution of ligands by exponential enrichment: RNA ligands to bacteriophage T4 DNA polymerase, *Science*, 249, 505–510, 1990.
23. R. Conrad and A. D. Ellington, Detecting immobilized protein kinase C isozymes with RNA aptamers, *Anal Biochem*, 242, 261–265, 1996.
24. R. D. Jenison et al., High-resolution molecular discrimination by RNA, *Science*, 263, 1425–1429, 1994.
25. A. A. Nery et al., Recognition of biomarkers and cell-specific molecular signatures: Aptamers as capture agents, *J Sep Sci*, 32, 1523–1530, 2009.
26. J. S. Vorhies and J. J. Nemunaitis, Nucleic acid aptamers for targeting of shRNA-based cancer therapeutics, *Biologics*, 1, 367–376, 2007.
27. J. A. Phillips et al., Enrichment of cancer cells using aptamers immobilized on a microfluidic channel, *Anal Chem*, 81, 1033–1039, 2009.
28. Y. Xu et al., Aptamer-based microfluidic device for enrichment, sorting, and detection of multiple cancer cells, *Anal Chem*, 81, 7436–7442, 2009.
29. M. Berezovski et al., Non-SELEX selection of aptamers, *J Am Chem Soc*, 128, 1410–1411, 2006.
30. J. M. Nam et al., Nanoparticle-based bio-bar codes for the ultrasensitive detection of proteins, *Science*, 301, 1884–1886, 2003.
31. N. M. Toriello et al., Integrated microfluidic bioprocessor for single-cell gene expression analysis, *Proc Natl Acad Sci USA*, 105, 20173–20178, 2008.
32. W. J. Han et al., Nanoparticle coatings for enhanced capture of flowing cells in microtubes, *ACS Nano*, 4, 174–180, 2010.
33. S. Hong et al., Covalent immobilization of p-selectin enhances cell rolling, *Langmuir*, 23, 12261–12268, 2007.
34. J. V. Green et al., Effect of channel geometry on cell adhesion in microfluidic devices, *Lab Chip*, 9, 677–685 2009.
35. J. Ylikotila et al., Improved surface stability and biotin binding properties of streptavidin coating on polystyrene, *Colloids Surf B Biointerfaces*, 70, 271–277, 2009.
36. X. Cheng et al., A microfluidic device for practical label-free CD4(+) T cell counting of HIV-infected subjects, *Lab Chip*, 7, 170–178, 2007.
37. World Health Organization, *World Health Organization: Cancer Key Facts*, Available at http://www.who.int/mediacentre/factsheets/fs297/en/index.html. Accessed on May 4, 2010, 2009.
38. B. R. Zetter, Angiogenesis and tumor metastasis, *Annu Rev Med*, 49, 407–424, 1998.
39. A. A. Adams et al., Highly efficient circulating tumor cell isolation from whole blood and label-free enumeration using polymer-based microfluidics with an integrated conductivity sensor, *J Am Chem Soc*, 130, 8633–8641, 2008.
40. M. Cristofanilli, Circulating tumor cells, disease progression, and survival in metastatic breast cancer, *Semin Oncol*, 33, S9–S14, 2006.
41. P. S. Steeg, Tumor metastasis: Mechanistic insights and clinical challenges, *Nat Med*, 12, 895–904, 2006.
42. G. P. Gupta and J. Massague, Cancer metastasis: Building a framework, *Cell*, 127, 679–695, 2006.

43. T. Reya et al., Stem cells, cancer, and cancer stem cells, *Nature*, 414, 105–111, 2001.
44. W. A. Bonner et al., Fluorescence activated cell sorting, *Rev Sci Instrum*, 43, 404–409, 1972.
45. S. E. Cross et al., Nanomechanical analysis of cells from cancer patients, *Nat Nanotechnol*, 2, 780–783, 2007.
46. C. Spagnoli et al., Atomic force microscopy analysis of cell volume regulation, *Phys Rev E Stat Nonlin Soft Matter Phys*, 78, 031916, 2008.
47. R. de la Rica et al., Label-free cancer cell detection with impedimetric transducers, *Anal Chem*, 81, 10167–10171, 2009.
48. H. Zhang et al., ErbB receptors: From oncogenes to targeted cancer therapies, *J Clin Invest*, 117, 2051–2058, 2007.
49. UNAIDS, Report on the global AIDS epidemic., pp. Available at http://data.unaids.org/pub/GlobalReport/2008/JC1510_2008GlobalReport_en.zip. Accessed on November 20, 2009, 2008.
50. X. H. Cheng et al., Enhancing the performance of a point-of-care CD4 + T-cell counting microchip through monocyte depletion for HIV/AIDS diagnostics, *Lab Chip*, 9, 1357–1364, 2009.
51. M. F. Pittenger et al., Multilineage potential of adult human mesenchymal stem cells, *Science*, 284, 143–147, 1999.
52. Y. Jiang et al., Pluripotency of mesenchymal stem cells derived from adult marrow, *Nature*, 418, 41–49, 2002.
53. M. Srisa-Art et al., Identification of rare progenitor cells from human periosteal tissue using droplet microfluidics, *Analyst*, 134, 2239–2245, 2009.
54. D. van Noort et al., Stem cells in microfluidics, *Biotechnol Progr*, 25, 52–60, 2009.
55. M. Vasa et al., Increase in circulating endothelial progenitor cells by statin therapy in patients with stable coronary artery disease, *Circulation*, 103, 2885–2890, 2001.
56. T. Asahara et al., Isolation of putative progenitor endothelial cells for angiogenesis, *Science*, 275, 964–967, 1997.
57. E. M. Van Craenenbroeck et al., Quantification of circulating endothelial progenitor cells: A methodological comparison of six flow cytometric approaches, *J Immunol Methods*, 332, 31–40, 2008.
58. A. Huebner et al., Microdroplets: A sea of applications?, *Lab Chip*, 8, 1244–1254, 2008.
59. S. Koster et al., Drop-based microfluidic devices for encapsulation of single cells, *Lab Chip*, 8, 1110–1115, 2008.

26 Two-Dimensional Microfluidic Bioarray for Nucleic Acid Analysis

Lin Wang and Paul C.H. Li

CONTENTS

26.1 INTRODUCTION TO MICROFLUIDIC DNA MICROARRAY HYBRIDIZATION

Nucleic acid hybridization techniques feature the use of a probe nucleic acid molecule to detect a target nucleic acid molecule. Here, probe molecules are usually short single-stranded nucleic acids (DNA or RNA) or oligonucleotides with known sequences; whereas target molecules are prepared from polymerase chain reaction (PCR) amplification of genomic extracts. Probe-target hybridization leads to the formation of a double-stranded molecule, called duplex. The concept of DNA microarray was evolved from Southern blotting technology based on solid-phase hybridization in the early 1990s [1]. This method relies on the immobilization of the probe molecules onto the solid surface to recognize their complementary DNA target sequence by hybridization. Up to millions of features have been integrated into a standard glass slide or silicon chip by microprinting or *in situ* synthesis of oligonucleotides [2,3]. The relative abundance of nucleic acid sequences in the target can be measured from chip-hybridization results optically, electrochemically, or radioactively, with proper detection labels [4]. DNA microarrays have dramatically accelerated many types of investigations including gene expression profiling, comparative genomic hybridization, protein–DNA interaction study (chromatin immunoprecipitation), single-nucleotide polymorphism (SNP) detection, and nucleic acid diagnostic applications. The advances in DNA microarray technology during the last couple of years have been summarized in many books and reviews [4–8].

With the recent growth of microelectromechanical systems (MEMS), microfluidic technology has been developing rapidly with many applications in the last decade. By combining the fields of microfluidics and DNA microarrays the advantages of both fields can be exploited simultaneously [9–11]. Microfluidics deals with the transfer and control of a small amount of fluids in microscale flow configurations. One obvious advantage of using a microfluidic system is the dramatic reduction in the sample volume. Instead of handling a volume of milliliter scale, a microfluidic system could deal with a volume as little as 1 pL [11]. Many interesting biological samples such as proteins and DNA extraction are rare or unavailable in large amounts; microfluidics therefore provides a way of studying these materials efficiently. The small volumes of the microfluidic system make it possible to develop compact and portable lab-on-a-chip systems that may be manufactured cheaply by mass production.

The second advantage of using microfluidic technology is that liquid movement in microchannels with a large surface-to-volume ratio facilitates target diffusion to the substrate surface. In conventional DNA microarray hybridization, ~30 μL samples are applied to the slide and the solutions are distributed across the probe arrays by covering them with a thin glass coverslip [12]. At first, this passive hybridization is characterized by a reaction-limited process. After the initial time period, probe depletion renders this process diffusion limited [13,14]. Because diffusion coefficients (D) for nucleic acids in aqueous solutions are on the order of 10^{-7} cm^2 s^{-1} [15], the typical distance ($L = \sqrt{Dt}$) moved by the target nucleic acid solely due to diffusion in 24 h is ~1 mm. Considering that the horizontal length scale of a microarray is on the order of a few centimeters, hemispherical depletion volumes form around each probe [16]. Pappaert et al. [17] found that for an analysis time of 24 h the maximum binding efficiency is less than 0.2%, and to increase that to 2% a six-day analysis would be required. Therefore, the conventional static method is a very inefficient means of achieving hybridization.

Microfluidics also offers the advantage of multisample capabilities on one chip. Conventional microarray experiments usually employ one sample on one glass slide [12]. However, in the application of genetic mutation analysis, clinical diagnostics or microorganism identifications, a direct comparison between different samples on the same chip would be preferable because the quality of slides with probe arrays varies from batch to batch [5]. Microfluidics allows for the delivery of controlled volumes of samples and reagents to the DNA microarray. By integrating multiple channels into one chip, a high-throughput multisample analysis has been achieved [18,19]. Moreover, DNA hybridization assays depend on different parameters such as temperature, stringency of the hybridization, and washing buffer conditions. The parameter space could be too large to be addressed efficiently using conventional approaches. On the contrary, because the microfluidic method has the capacity for multiple sample injection as well as accurate control of liquid flow and temperature, it has been developed for the automated selection of optimal assay parameters [20].

In conventional microarray hybridization protocols, sample solutions are loaded directly onto the glass slide surface and incubated for hours. Therefore, an intuitive way is to use a large microfluidic chamber covering the area with spotted probes, where sample DNA solutions are delivered to and hybridized with the probes. The chamber is usually detachable from the glass slide and is made with elastomer, such as polydimethylsiloxane (PDMS) [21]. The microfluidic chamber approach combined with a high-density microarray has been successfully used by different groups [16,22–25]. The hybridization time has been reduced from overnight to less than 2 h.

Although the microfluidic system offers significant improvement over the conventional bulk solution method, two inherent problems come with the large chamber hybridization on high-density microarrays. First, because a huge amount of probe features is packed into a small area, a great deal of effort is needed for data processing, normalization, and interpretation in high-density microarray hybridizations [26]. In addition, hybridization is most efficient when each target nucleic acid can move throughout the solution and encounter every probe. If the size of the microfluidic chamber is comparable to the size of a standard microscope slide, liquid flows have to be carefully designed to achieve an equally distributed liquid movement over the chamber as well as a lower amount of trapped air bubbles during filling [16,17,22,23,27–33].

In gene expression analysis, many thousands of genes are to be simultaneously monitored to create a global picture of cellular function, and high-density microarrays are thus needed. In contrast, in many gene diagnostic applications, once a relatively small number of genes are identified using high-density DNA microarray, low-density microarrays can be designed to screen these genes across many patients or to detect SNPs [34]. The approach has been proved to be reliable, cost effective, and much faster in data analysis and interpretation [35–41].

26.2 MICROFLUIDIC DNA HYBRIDIZATION WITH LOW-DENSITY PROBE ARRAYS

26.2.1 The Low-Density Microfluidic Microarray Method with Pin-Spotted Probes

The microfluidic method is suitable for being incorporated into low-density DNA microarray analysis. With micromachining techniques, the hybridization microchannels are aligned to the rows of probe spots. As shown in Figures 26.1 and 26.2, both straight [42–48] and serpentine microchannels have been designed [20,49–52]. In Figure 26.1, Chung et al. [44] found an up to sixfold increase in signal with the microchannel flow hybridization, as compared with the passive hybridization. The authors also found that the hybridization efficiency was further improved by introducing extensional strain to the sample DNA molecules (Figure 26.1c). Wei et al. [52] proposed a microchannel hybridization method with microtrenched serpentine channels, as shown in Figure 26.2. The sample consumption was reduced to 1 μL and hybridization time was as low as 500 s. The signal-to-noise ratio has been improved by 30-fold in the discrimination of two oligonucleotides with one-base difference (Figure 26.2b). In terms of probe spotting, either commercialized small arrayers [46,49–51] or even micropipettors [42,43,47] have been used. The use of microchannels instead of large hybridization chambers has alleviated the need for complicated design for homogeneous hybridization across the chamber area.

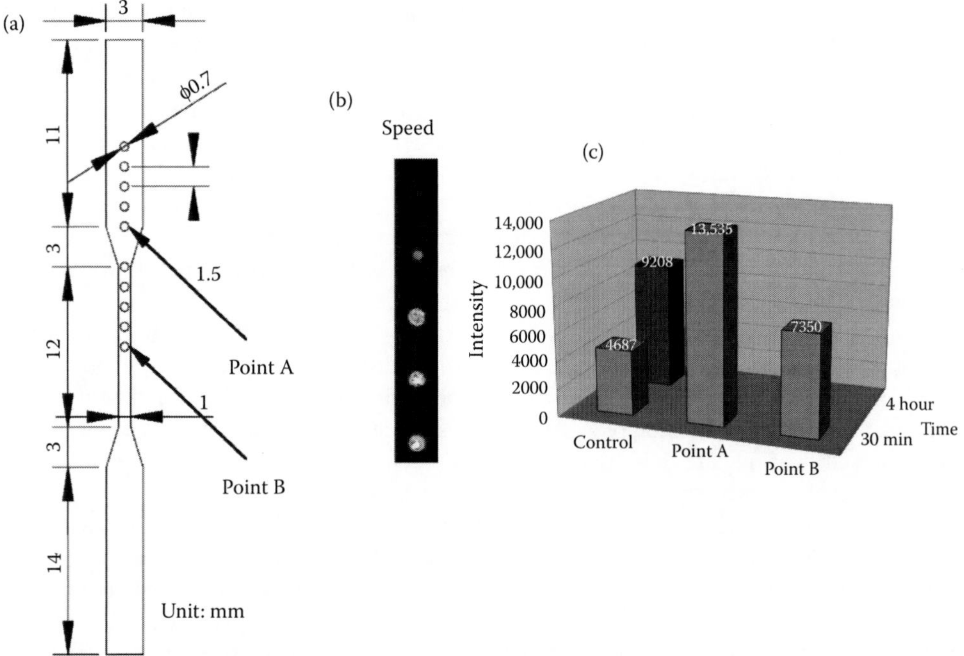

FIGURE 26.1 (a) Schematic drawing of a straight hybridization channel in Chung's work. Points A and B are two positions used for monitoring the effect of flow velocity on hybridization efficiency. The flow direction was from top to bottom. (b) Part of the fluorescence images after 30-min hybridization at a flow rate of $u = 1$ cm s^{-1}. (c) Comparison of fluorescence intensity at different velocity regions and hybridization times. (From Y. C. Chung, Y. C. Lin, M. Z. Shiu et al., *Lab on a Chip*, 3(4), 228–233, 2003. With permission.)

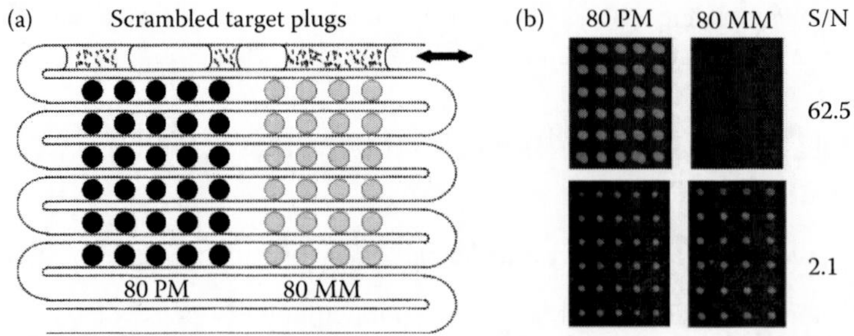

FIGURE 26.2 (a) An illustration showing that scrambled discrete plugs sweep over probe rows in the serpentine channel. The black arrow denotes the shuttle flow inside the microchannel. (b) Fluorescence images from microfluidic channel hybridization (top row) or conventional hybridization (bottom row) in 500 s. The left column presents the results from perfect-matched (PM) probes, and the right column presents the results from mismatched (MM) probes. The sample volumes are 1 and 30 μL for microfluidic hybridization and conventional hybridization, respectively. (From C. W. Wei, J. Y. Cheng, C. T. Huang et al., *Nucleic Acids Research*, 33(8), e78, 2005. With permission.)

26.2.2 The Low-Density Microfluidic Microarray Method with the Two-Dimensional (2D) Intersection Approach

In low-density DNA microarray analysis, the conventional pin-spotting method has been used to create dot-like probe arrays. The performance of the subsequent hybridization assay is thus heavily influenced by the quality of immobilized probe spots. In practice, because the spotting solutions are open to air and the spotting pins are very close to each other, the pin-spotting method may suffer from splashing, evaporation, and cross contamination [53]. In addition, probe spots of high homogeneity are beneficial, since they simplify image analysis and considerably enhance the accuracy of signal detection. When a spotting buffer such as saline sodium citrate solution is used, spot uniformity is often poor due to the hydrophobic properties of the chemically modified glass surface. Supplementary chemicals such as dimethyl sulfoxide can improve spot uniformity, but could introduce new problems such as spot size increase [54]. Moreover, during the blocking and cleaning procedures after spotting on the glass surface, the remaining unreacted probe molecules could diffuse away and smear the slide to form a comet-like spot [12]. Furthermore, if microchannel hybridization is going to be used later with a spotted microarray, additional devices such as steel clamps have to be used to ensure that the entire hybridization microchannel is well aligned to probe rows [52].

A simple and effective microspotting method is to use the microfluidic network to create probe line arrays on a surface. Biomolecules on a variety of solid substrates (gold, glass, or polymer) have been patterned successfully with PDMS-based microchannel plates [55–59]. Because the immobilization reaction between the biomolecules and the surface is confined in microchannels, solution evaporation and splashing are thus prevented. In our practice, less than 1 μL of reagent is needed to fill into each microchannel and the solution can be kept at room temperature for hours without dry-out [60]. Figure 26.3a shows an example of a PDMS microchannel plate assembled with a glass slide, in which an individual channel is shown in Figure 26.3b. Chemically modified DNA probes are introduced into the microchannels and are immobilized on the glass chip. The bonding between the polymer channel plate and the glass slide is reversible. After peeling off the PDMS layer, a homogeneous distribution of the probe molecules along the area enclosed by microchannels is achieved with high resolution, with the fluorescent image shown in Figure 26.3c. Because flow operation in each microchannel can be manipulated individually, the probe immobilization step and subsequent processes such as washing and blocking can be independently conducted, and the individual channels can thus be used for condition optimization tests (Figure 26.3d). Moreover, cross

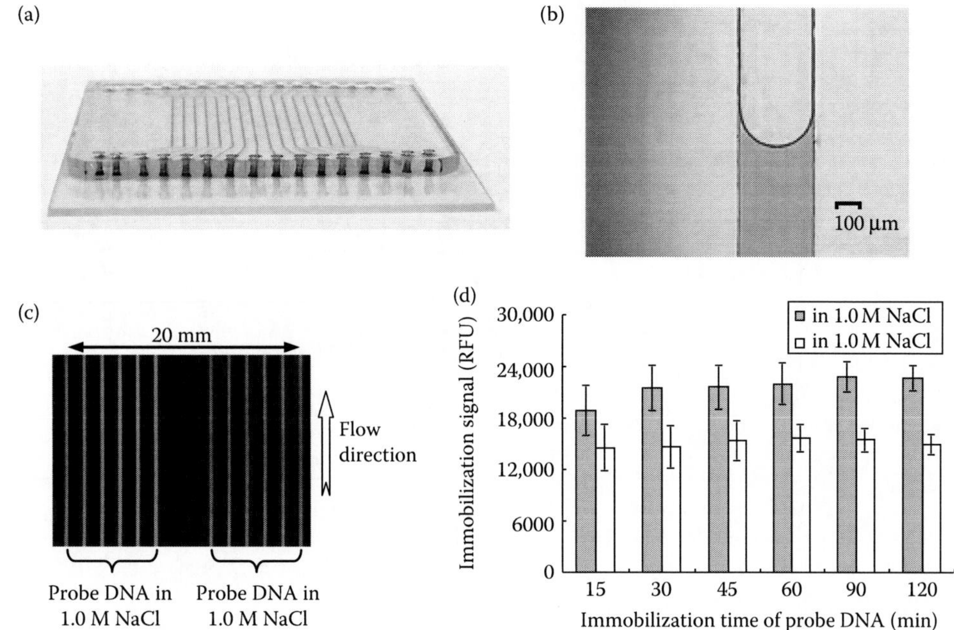

FIGURE 26.3 (a) The image of an assembly of a 2″ × 2″ PDMS channel plate on a 3″ × 2″ glass slide. The 16 channels filled with blue dye solutions. (b) A microscopic view of a straight channel partially filled with the dye solution. (c) The fluorescent image of immobilized DNA probe lines (vertical green stripes) printed on the glass slide at different incubation times and in two different buffer solutions. In this case, all the DNA probe molecules were labeled with the fluorescein dye. (d) The corresponding fluorescent signals from the immobilized DNA probe lines in (c). (From L. Wang, and P. C. H. Li, *Journal of Agricultural and Food Chemistry*, 55(26), 10509–10516, 2007. With permission.)

contamination from diffusion of unreacted agents is avoided during washing steps. The microfluidic approach is simple and flexible for the spotting of low-density probe arrays.

Low-density probe line arrays created from microfluidic methods have been used successfully for nucleic acid analysis [59–67]. In these applications, a two-dimensional (2D) intersection approach was used, and this approach resembled the microfluidic immunoassays proposed by Ligler and coworkers [68–70]. As shown in Figure 26.4, probe lines were printed onto a chemically modified glass slide with the first microchannel plate as depicted before. After peeling off plate 1, channel plate 2 used for hybridization is then assembled with the same glass slide. Here, microfluidic channels were arranged horizontally and were orthogonal to the preprinted probe lines. Sample DNA molecules that flow through the microchannels will intersect with the probe line arrays. If complementary probe molecules were encountered, the target molecules were retained and rectangular hybridization patches were thus formed. These patches can be detected by surface plasmon resonance imaging [59], or more often, by a fluorometric flatbed scanner [60–67]. Compared with a pin-spotted microarray (in Figure 26.5), the final hybridization results obtained from the microfluidic microarray are much cleaner and organized for later image analysis.

The 2D microfluidic microarray format is well suited for parallel sample hybridizations. Unlike a pin-spotted low-density DNA microarray, the use of long and narrow probe line arrays alleviates the need for alignment between hybridization channels and probe dots [20]. Parallel hybridization can be used not only for the investigation or comparison of optimal assay conditions, but also for high-throughput multisample analysis. Benn et al. [61] modeled the hybridization rates of 60-mer oligonucleotides in eight concentrations from 10 pM to 10 nM. Situma et al. [62] used a 16 × 16 array to detect two different low-abundant DNA point mutations in oncogenes. Wang and Li [60]

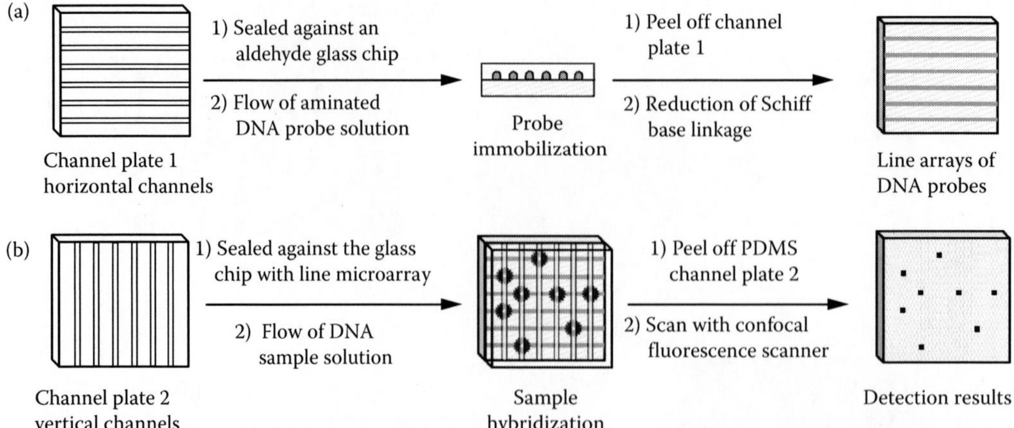

FIGURE 26.4 The 2D microfluidic microarray method using straight microchannels. (a) The creation of a DNA probe line array on an aldehyde-modified glass slide via straight microchannels. (b) The hybridization of DNA samples in straight channels orthogonal to the straight probe lines printed on the glass slide. (From L. Wang and P. C. H. Li, *Journal of Agricultural and Food Chemistry*, 55(26), 10509–10516, 2007. With permission.)

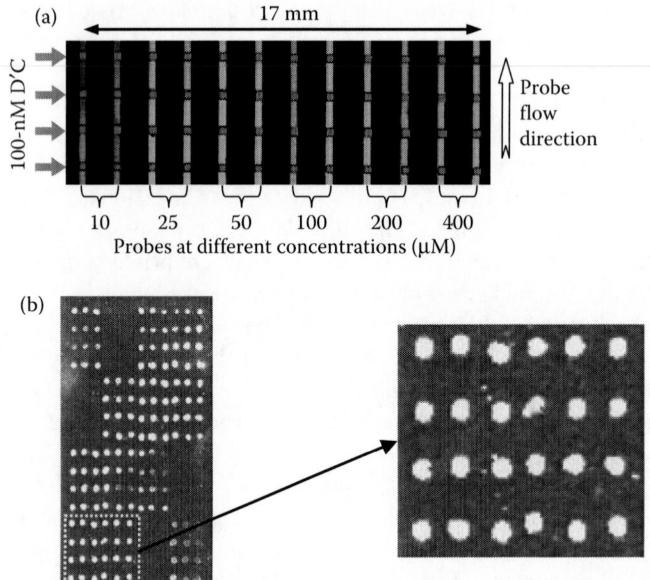

FIGURE 26.5 (a) Dual-channel fluorescent images of DNA hybridization results with the 2D microfluidic microarray method. The overlaid images from the same glass slide show both printed probe lines (vertical green lines) and square hybridization patches (red) at intersections [60]. (b) Fluorescent images of DNA hybridization results on a low-density pin-spotted microarray [41]. A hand-held arrayer with eight pins was used in spotting probe arrays. (From L. Wang and P. C. H. Li, *Journal of Agricultural and Food Chemistry*, 55(26), 10509–10516, 2007; C. A. Koch, P. C. H. Li, and R. S. Utkhede, *Analytical Biochemistry*, 342(1), 93–102, 2005. With permission.)

also used a 16 × 16 microfluidic microarray device to test the effect of salt concentrations as well as hybridization times on the same chip. With optimized conditions, they successfully discriminated PCR product samples from two fungal pathogen genomes at room temperature [118].

26.2.3 High-Throughput Parallel Hybridization with Centrifugal Force-Driven Microflows

Implementation of parallel sample hybridizations in multiple microchannels raises the question of finding an effective way of simultaneous liquid delivery. The conventional liquid pumping method used in microfluidics is pressure-driven flow by syringe pumping or vacuum suction. Because each microchannel has to be connected to a pump tubing and synchronization has to be considered in order to ensure parallel flows, this arrangement could be complicated in case many channels are to be used in this method. Another drawback of this pumping method is that a high pressure is required for liquid delivery in long and narrow microchannels, and this in turn requires a very tight sealing between the microfluidic channel plate and the substrate. For example, a steel clamp was used to tighten a microfluidic microarray assembly [52]. Electroosmotic flow (EOF) is another microflow-driven method and it has been used for parallel pumping of multiple channels [71,72]. However, the flow control of the EOF method depends not only on the applied voltage across the microchannel, but also on the surface physicochemical properties of the microchannel as well as the ionic strength of the buffered solutions [73]. The high ionic concentration typical of DNA hybridization buffer [12,74,75] may result in excessive Joule heating and electrolysis [42,76–78]. These effects will result in dynamic changes in the liquid temperature and pH value [79], causing instability of hybridization and SNP discrimination performance. Therefore, only a few reports were published in terms of applying EOF flow to microfluidic DNA microarray analysis [42].

An alternative liquid pumping method is to utilize the body force of the liquid column itself, and such a force can be created under a centrifugal force field. As compared with other methods, centrifugal pumping is easy to implement and is not sensitive to the physiochemical properties of the liquid. It can move fluids in a parallel manner in multiple channels of a wide range of sizes. Moreover, compact disk (CD) and related industries including disk materials, disk fabrication, signal reading and error correction, as well as the rotor-driven/control system, have been well developed over the last few decades. Combined with MEMS technology, the centrifugal microfluidic platform could fit in this CD system to develop a portable and point-of-care analysis system [80–82].

A centrifugal microfluidic platform has been developed in many applications including environmental assays, cell lysis, separation and extraction, immunoassay in biomedical diagnosis, and nucleic acid analysis [16,46–48,83–100]. Flow dynamics studies as well as microfluidic operation of the liquid in rotating radial microchannels were also investigated [101–111,117]. More studies on the application of centrifugal pumping to microfluidics can be found in several reviews [82,112–114].

Although centrifugal pumping has been successfully exploited in many microfluidic assays, its application to DNA microarray analysis is still rare [16,46–48]. Bynum and Gordon used extra rotors on a centrifugal platform to induce reciprocal flows inside hybridization chambers [16]. After 17-h reaction, the signals were measured to be 10 times higher than those from the conventional passive method [16]. Peytavi et al. [46] developed a chamber hybridization system, where the assembly of a glass slide and a PDMS microfluidic chamber is placed on a CD support that can hold up to five slides. As shown in Figure 26.6, low-density spotted probe arrays were used and the hybridization reagents were positioned to be pumped sequentially. The authors demonstrated the discrimination of four clinically relevant *Staphylococcus* species by using a 15-min automated hybridization process performed at room temperature [46]. Li et al. [48] presented a CD-like microfluidic device capable of generating the reciprocating flow of DNA samples within the microchannels and demonstrate its application in the rapid DNA hybridization assay [48]. Here, the centrifugal force was used to drive the sample solution to flow through the hybridization channel

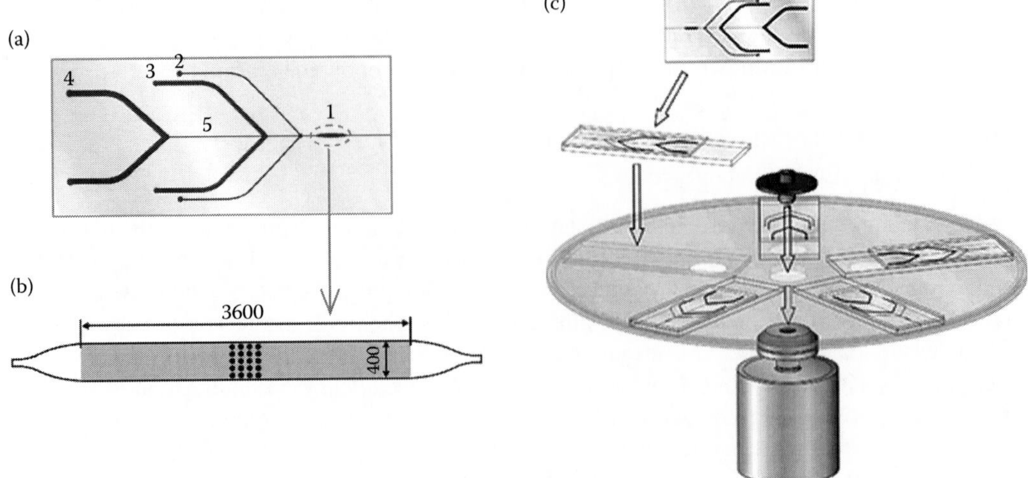

FIGURE 26.6 Schematic representation of the centrifugal microfluidic system for the microarray hybridization in [46] and [82]. (a) PDMS microfluidic unit: The test sample (chamber 2) is released first and flows over the hybridization chamber (chamber 1) where the oligonucleotide capture probes are spotted onto the glass support. The wash buffer in chamber 3 and the rinsing buffer in chamber 4 then start to flow at a higher angular velocity. (b) Schematic view of the hybridization chamber showing the dimensions in μm and the area of the chamber (shaded section) that can accommodate up to 150 microarray spots. (c) Engraved PDMS is applied to a glass slide on which are arrayed nucleic acid capture probes. The glass slide is placed on a CD support that can hold up to five slides. (From M. Madou et al., *Annual Review of Biomedical Engineering*, 8, 601–628, 2006. With permission.)

into a temporary collection reservoir while the capillary force pulled the solution back into the hybridization channel during the stopping period (Figure 26.7). The sample hybridization time was reduced to 90 s and the sample volume was as low as 350 nL with the proposed centrifugal microfluidic platform [48].

The limited applications of centrifugal pumping to nucleic acid microarray analysis could be attributed to the radial-direction structure design. Currently, almost all of the fluidic patterns in centrifugal microfluidic platforms are fabricated in the radial orientation. Due to the mechanical strength of materials and the demand of miniaturization, the length of the microfluidic structure in the radial direction is limited. For example, if a centrifugal platform is built on a 120-mm regular CD with a 15-mm center spindle hole, the length of a microfluidic structure cannot be more than 53 mm. Therefore, the applicable space is very limited and the capillary effect may dominate the liquid flow process in microchannels. Furthermore, the centrifugal force increases with increasing radius. As characterized in the work of Duffy et al. [90] and Madou et al. [82], the average velocity of the liquid is proportional to the radial extent of the fluid in a microchannel. Such an increasing flow velocity in the microchannel puts forward challenges and difficulties in the design of fluidic structure [101,104,109]. In 2D low-density microarray analysis, the probe molecules are spotted in line arrays and the orientation of the sample flows has to be orthogonal to the probe lines. The radial-like microfluidic structure cannot be applied to this intersection method because centrifugal pumping can only be exploited in one direction. Therefore, spotted probe arrays have to be used for microchannel hybridization, which limited sample throughput, and a lot of disk space was wasted.

Recently, a new microfluidic DNA microarray method has been reported. Here, the centrifugal advantages were exploited two times, first in the radial microchannels and then in the spiral channels [64]. As shown in Figure 26.8, the microarray assembly consists of two CD-like PDMS chips as microchannel plates and one 92-mm glass wafer as the substrate [64–66]. In the first step, channel

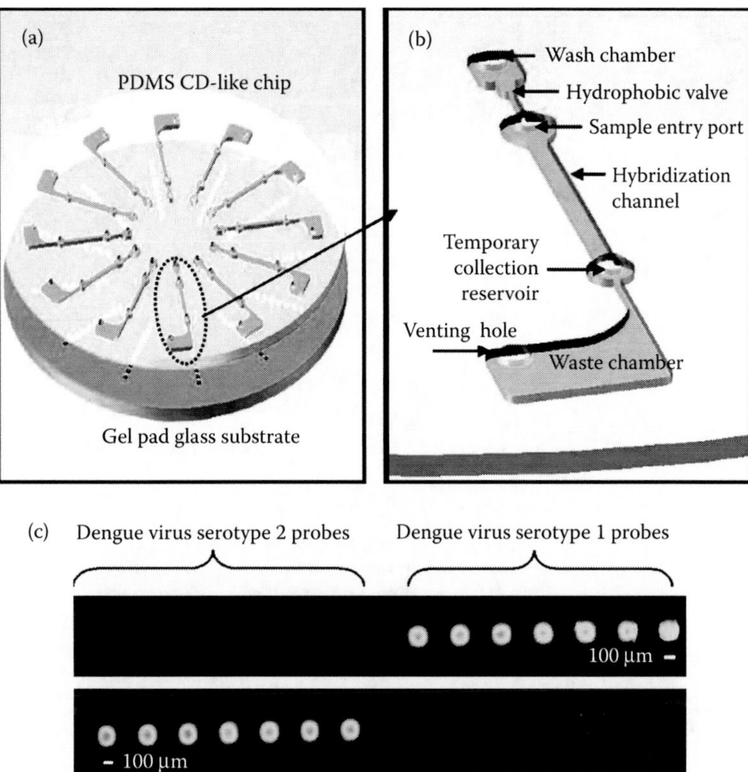

FIGURE 26.7 (a) Schematic representation of a CD microfluidic device for DNA hybridization. It consists of a PDMS CD slab containing 12 DNA hybridization assay units sealed with a glass substrate with immobilized DNA probe arrays. (b) Schematic diagram of a single DNA hybridization assay unit. (c) Hybridization specificity tests with the CD microfluidic device. Top: Dengue virus serotype 1 targets. Bottom: Dengue virus serotype 2 targets. The CD device was rotated at 22 Hz for 3 s and then stopped for 3 s during the reciprocating process. Duration of the reciprocating process was 90 s. (From C. Y. Li, X. L. Dong, J. H. Qin et al., *Analytica Chimica Acta*, 640(1–2), 93–99, 2009. With permission.)

plate 1 is assembled with the glass wafer for printing the radial probe line arrays, whereas during the second step, spiral channel plate 2 is sealed against the wafer with printed probe lines after removing channel plate 1. In both steps, liquid flows in the channels are driven by centrifugal pumping obtained from spinning the assembly. Because the spiral channels are nearly orthogonal to the radial direction, sample flows thus intersect with probe lines printed on the disk and result in hybridization patches after complementary target molecules were applied. The spiral channel design has been reported in detail elsewhere [115]. Figure 26.9 shows the fluorescent images from 3-min hybridization of oligonucleotide samples of different concentrations [65]. The hybridization patches are in a rectangular shape and easy to be analyzed. As shown in the insets of Figure 26.9b, DNA molecules were not retained by the noncomplementary probe lines at the intersection areas. For a disk with 92 mm diameter, up to 100 samples could be analyzed in parallel and each sample volume is less than 1 μL [64–66].

The characterization of centrifugal flow hybridization in spiral microchannels was also studied [66]. Figure 26.10a shows a fluorescent image comparing the hybridization results under two conditions, continuous-flow and stop-flow. Hybridization intensities from 3-min continuous-flow are very close to those from the 2-h stop-flow [66]. Moreover, as shown in Figure 26.10a, nonspecific binding is negligible in the continuous-flow method because the sample flow from centrifugal pumping continually removed unhybridized DNA molecules to prevent them from

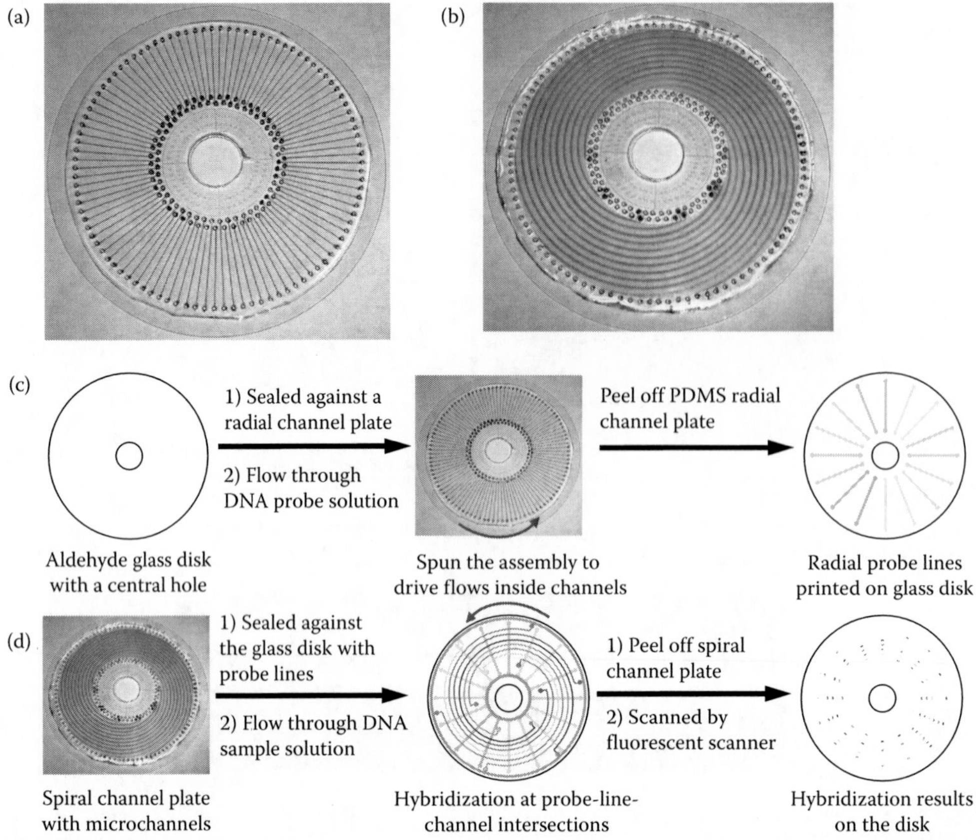

FIGURE 26.8 (a) Images of the assembly of a radial PDMS channel plate with a glass disk. Each channel was filled with blue dye solutions. (b) Images of the assembly of a spiral PDMS channel plate with a glass disk. Ten groups of channels, three in each group, were filled with blue dye solutions. (c) Probe line printing with a radial channel plate. (d) Hybridization procedure with the spiral channel plate. Hybridization occurring at the intersections of the spiral channels and radial probe lines, shown as colored patches in the rightmost disk. (From L. Wang and P. C. H. Li, *Analytical Biochemistry*, 400(2), 282–288, 2010. With permission.)

accumulating and binding nonspecifically onto the glass surface. On the contrary, in the stop-flow method, when DNA samples were incubated in microchannels for a longer time (2 h), non-specific binding of DNA was observed along the spiral channels shown as strips and post-hybridization channel washing is thus required (Figure 26.10a). The hybridization time was determined by the rotation speeds of the assembly during the hybridization test. A lower rotation speed (or a higher residence time in the microchannel) would result in stronger hybridization signals (Figure 26.10b). It was also found that the shallower microchannel gave a better sensitivity [66]. The signal-to-noise ratios from the 24-μm microchannel chip are twice as high as those from the 75-μm microchannel chip. The reduction of microchannel height enhanced mass transport of target DNA to the capture probes and thus generated higher hybridization signals. Moreover, DNA molecules were stretched in microflows, which offered further advantages for hybridization efficiency [44,45,116].

Thereafter, PCR product samples from the genomic extraction of three fungal pathogens were successfully detected with the CD-like microfluidic microarray assembly under optimized conditions [66]. Although a higher hybridization temperature resulted in improved sensitivity, 0.2-ng PCR products already gave a signal-to-noise ratio of ~20 at room temperature, as shown in Figure 26.11a.

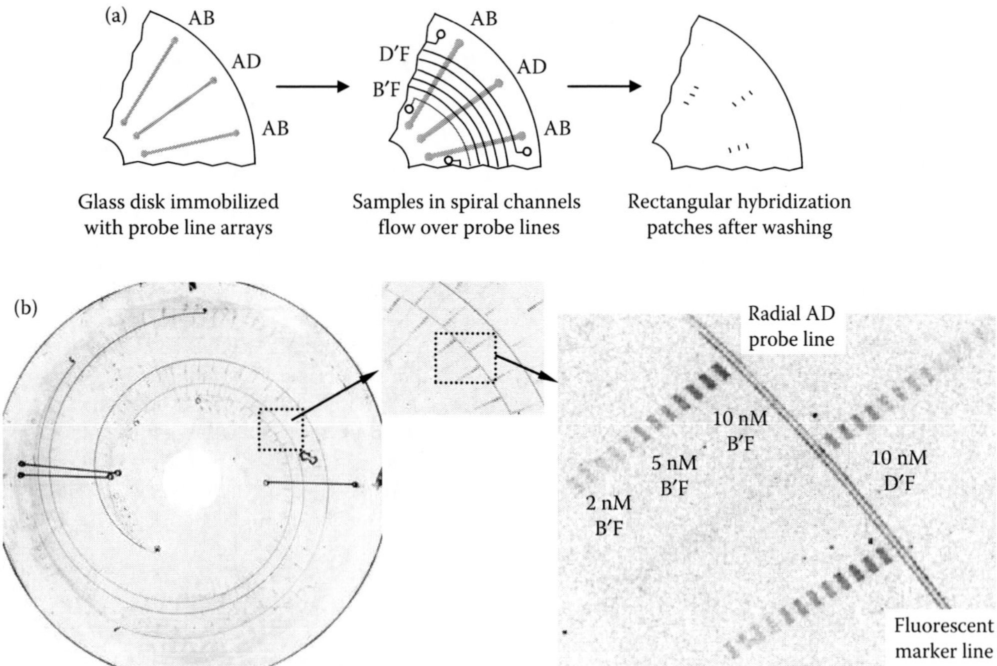

FIGURE 26.9 DNA hybridization on a CD-like glass chip. (a) The schematic diagram showing hybridization patches formed at the intersections between three probe lines (in radial) and six sample channels (in curve). (b) The fluorescent image of a glass disk with hybridization patches. The radial or spiral traces resulted from the flow of marker solutions for easy positioning. The two right insets show the magnified images of rectangular patches formed near the disk center, which resulted from the hybridization of different concentrations of oligonucleotide samples with their complementary probe lines. Oligonucleotides hybridizations were achieved at room temperature in 3-min spinning at 700 rpm and then dried out at 3600 rpm. (From L. Wang, P. C. H. Li, H. Z. Yu et al., *Analytica Chimica Acta*, 610(1), 97–104, 2008. With permission.)

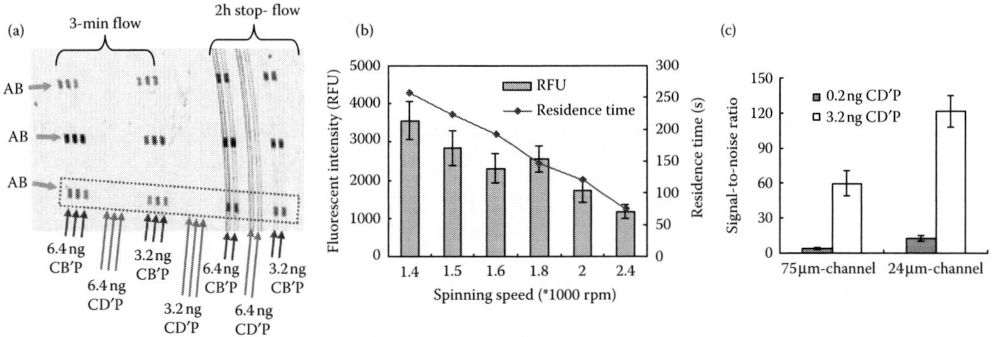

FIGURE 26.10 (a) The fluorescent images show the PCR product hybridizations conducted with two different flow methods. The dark rectangular patches represent the specific binding of the complementary targets. CD'P and CB'P are two PCR products, and only the latter is complementary to the probe AB molecule. (b) The bar graph showing the hybridization signals from the same amount of DNA samples hybridized under different rotation speeds. The line graph shows the corresponding sample residence time in the spiral microchannels. (c) The effect of channel depth on hybridization signal intensities is shown. (From L. Wang, and P. C. H. Li, *Analytical Biochemistry*, 400(2), 282–288, 2010. With permission.)

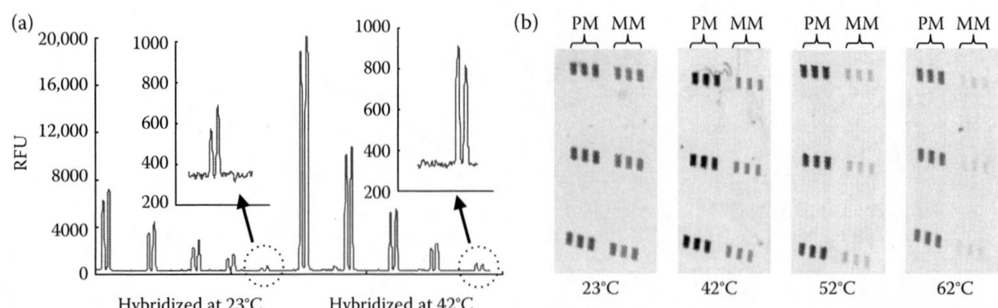

FIGURE 26.11 (a) Fluorescent intensities along a probe line. Five PCR product samples of different amounts were detected and each sample was conducted in duplicate. From left to right, five samples (6.4, 3.2, 1.6, 0.8, and 0.2 ng) were first hybridized at room temperature for 3 min. After dry-out of these channels, another group of five samples was hybridized at 42°C for 3 min. In all cases, the volume of sample solutions was 1.0 μL. The insets show the magnified graphs of the hybridization signals of 0.2 ng PCR product samples. (b) Differentiation of *Botrytis* species with single-base-pair difference at various hybridization temperatures. Each image was obtained from the hybridization of sample solutions in three spiral channels intersecting with three probe lines at the specified temperature. Two PCR products, perfect matched (PM) and mismatched (MM), were tested in the experiment. (From L. Wang and P. C. H. Li, *Analytical Biochemistry*, 400(2), 282–288, 2010. With permission.)

In addition, the method has been used for the discrimination of two related fungal subspecies, *Botrytis cinerea* and *Botrytis squamosa*. The two PCR amplicons differ in only one base pair in the middle of the 264-bp long sequence. With temperature control, the two DNA samples were discriminated in 3-min flow hybridization as shown in Figure 26.11b.

In addition to the radial–spiral approach where the 360°-spiral channels intersect with the radial probe lines, Chen et al. [67] also developed a new double-spiral format in which the 180°-clockwise-spiral channels intersect with the 180°-anticlockwise-spiral probe lines. In this manner, a higher spot density was achieved for high-throughput microarray assay on a 92-mm circular glass disk, which is of the same size as the one used previously. The arrangement that each inlet channel branches into four spiral channels helps the microarray experiment to be self-corrected (Figure 26.12a inset). For instance, when one spiral channel was blocked and the sample solution could not flow through it to produce the hybridization spots (a false negative error), this error could be corrected by observing the hybridization spots in the other three spiral channels. Moreover, because the group of 16 spots comes from the same batches of probe and sample solutions, fake signals from small surface defects, which are common in the conventional microarray method, can also be corrected [12]. The design increases the confidence of target detection. Using this double-spiral format, up to 384 assays (on 96 different samples) can be performed at the same time onto 384 probe lines (96 probes in four replicates) [67].

26.3 SUMMARY AND CONCLUSIONS

DNA microarray hybridization has been an important technique in genomic research. Because of their flexibility and low production cost, microarrays with low-density probes have been used in SNP detection as well as nucleic acid diagnostic applications. Recently, microfluidic technology was combined with the DNA microarray method through covering the spotted probe area with chambers or microchannels for sample hybridization. As summarized in this chapter, the microfluidic microarray method shows the advantages of less sample usage, fast reaction kinetics, as well as multiple sample capabilities for high-throughput analysis.

(a)

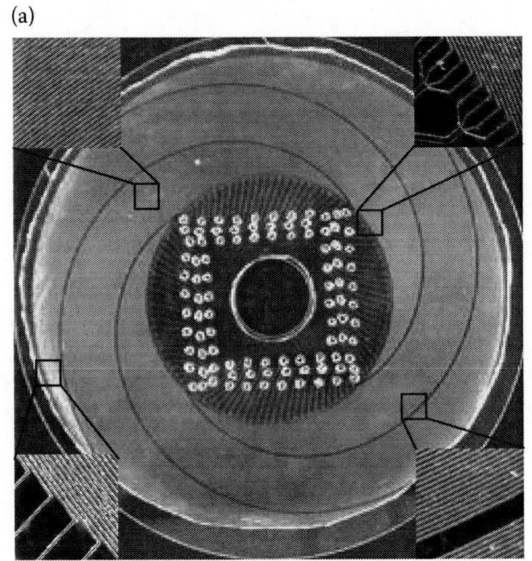

(b)

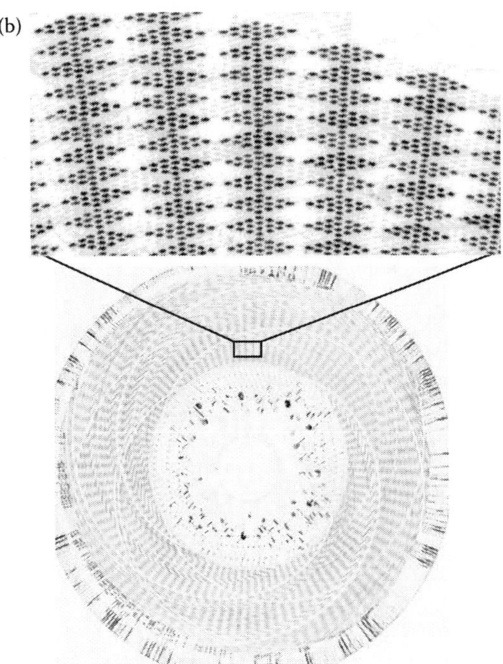

FIGURE 26.12 The double-spiral microfluidic microarray method. (a) The anticlockwise spiral channel plate, as imaged by a camera. The four anticlockwise lines represent the gap zone in which there are no channels. The four insets zoom in the regions near the inlet zone, gap zone, channel zone, and outlet zone. The clockwise spiral channel plate differs only in the channel direction. (b) Pattern of 384 × 384 hybridizations achieved on one glass disk. The inset shows the close-up of the hybridization spots. (From H. Chen, L. Wang, and P. C. H. Li, *Lab on a Chip*, 8(5), 826–829, 2008. With permission.)

Probe molecules could also be spotted by the microfluidic method and line arrays thus formed on the solid support. Hybridization microchannels are orthogonal to these line arrays and complementary DNA molecules will be retained at the intersection areas. This 2D microfluidic microarray method alleviates the need of the exact alignment of the hybridization microchannels and probe rows from the pin-spotted method. The spot shape is much regular for later image analysis. We have used a 16 × 16 microfluidic microarray device to successfully discriminate multiple PCR product samples from two fungal pathogen genomes.

In the microfluidic microarray method, different techniques have been developed to generate microflows, including electroosmosis, vacuum suction, and syringe pumping. The latter two pressure-driven methods are more widely used without the need for considering the physicochemical properties of solutions. Recently, the centrifugal force was employed to drive liquid movement in microchannels. This method utilizes the body force from the liquid itself and it is free of additional solution interface contacts such as from electrodes or syringes and tubing. Centrifugal force-driven flow also features the ease of parallel reactions. However, due to the radial-direction structure design, the applications of centrifugal pumping to nucleic acid microarray analysis are limited. To address this problem, CD-like PDMS chips with radial or spiral microchannels were reported. This design enabled centrifugal pumping for the 2D microfluidic DNA microarray method and the centrifugal advantages were exploited two times, first in the radial microchannels and then in the spiral channels. Reaction time and flow rate could be controlled by using different rotation speeds. The technique has been successfully applied to fast detection and discrimination of up to 100 DNA samples. The method was also developed further in a double-spiral way to get a higher probe/sample density with self-correction benefits.

REFERENCES

1. U. Maskos, and E. M. Southern, Oligonucleotide hybridizations on glass supports—A novel linker for oligonucleotide synthesis and hybridization properties of oligonucleotides synthesized *in situ*, *Nucleic Acids Research*, 20(7), 1679–1684, 1992.
2. T. R. Hughes, M. Mao, A. R. Jones et al., Expression profiling using microarrays fabricated by an ink-jet oligonucleotide synthesizer, *Nature Biotechnology*, 19(4), 342–347, 2001.
3. R. J. Lipshutz, S. P. A. Fodor, T. R. Gingeras et al., High density synthetic oligonucleotide arrays, *Nature Genetics*, 21, 20–24, 1999.
4. A. Sassolas, B. D. Leca-Bouvier, and L. J. Blum, DNA biosensors and microarrays, *Chemical Reviews*, 108(1), 109–139, 2008.
5. S. Russell, L. A. Meadows, and R. R. Russell, *MicroarrayTechnology in Practice*, Amsterdam, Boston, MA: Academic Press/Elsevier, 2009.
6. M. Schena, *Microarray Analysis*, Hoboken, NJ: John Wiley & Sons, 2003.
7. M. J. Buck, and J. D. Lieb, ChIP-chip: Considerations for the design, analysis, and application of genome-wide chromatin immunoprecipitation experiments, *Genomics*, 83(3), 349–360, 2004.
8. J. D. Hoheisel, Microarray technology: Beyond transcript profiling and genotype analysis, *Nature Reviews Genetics*, 7(3), 200–210, 2006.
9. A. Khademhosseini, Chips to hits: Microarray and microfluidic technologies for high-throughput analysis and drug discovery, *Expert Review of Molecular Diagnostics*, 5(6), 843–846, 2005.
10. C. Situma, M. Hashimoto, and S. A. Soper, Merging microfluidics with microarray-based bioassays, *Biomolecular Engineering*, 23(5), 213–231, 2006.
11. R. H. Liu, K. Dill, H. S. Fuji et al., Integrated microfluidic biochips for DNA microarray analysis, *Expert Review of Molecular Diagnostics*, 6(2), 253–261, 2006.
12. D. Bowtell, and J. Sambrook, *DNA Microarrays: A Molecular Cloning Manual*, Cold Spring Harbor, NY: Cold Spring Harbor Laboratory Press, 2003.
13. K. Pappaert, P. Van Hummelen, J. Vanderhoeven et al., Diffusion–reaction modelling of DNA hybridization kinetics on biochips, *Chemical Engineering Science*, 58(21), 4921–4930, 2003.
14. H. Y. Dai, M. Meyer, S. Stepaniants et al., Use of hybridization kinetics for differentiating specific from non-specific binding to oligonucleotide microarrays, *Nucleic Acids Research*, 30(16), e86, 2002.
15. G. L. Lukacs, P. Haggie, O. Seksek et al., Size-dependent DNA mobility in cytoplasm and nucleus, *Journal of Biological Chemistry*, 275(3), 1625–1629, 2000.
16. M. A. Bynum, and G. B. Gordon, Hybridization enhancement using microfluidic planetary centrifugal mixing, *Analytical Chemistry*, 76(23), 7039–7044, 2004.
17. K. Pappaert, J. Vanderhoeven, P. Van Hummelen et al., Enhancement of DNA micro-array analysis using a shear-driven micro-channel flow system, *Journal of Chromatography A*, 1014(1–2), 1–9, 2003.
18. J. Hong, J. B. Edel, and A. J. deMello, Micro- and nanofluidic systems for high-throughput biological screening, *Drug Discovery Today*, 14(3–4), 134–146, 2009.
19. G. Keramas, G. Perozziello, O. Geschke et al., Development of a multiplex microarray microsystem, *Lab on a Chip*, 4(2), 152–158, 2004.
20. M. Dufva, J. Petersen, and L. Poulsen, Increasing the specificity and function of DNA microarrays by processing arrays at different stringencies, *Analytical and Bioanalytical Chemistry*, 395(3), 669–677, 2009.
21. J. C. McDonald, D. C. Duffy, J. R. Anderson et al., Fabrication of microfluidic systems in poly(dimethylsiloxane), *Electrophoresis*, 21(1), 27–40, 2000.
22. J. Liu, B. A. Williams, R. M. Gwirtz et al., Enhanced signals and fast nucleic acid hybridization by microfluidic chaotic mixing, *Angewandte Chemie—International Edition*, 45(22), 3618–3623, 2006.
23. R. H. Liu, R. Lenigk, R. L. Druyor-Sanchez et al., Hybridization enhancement using cavitation microstreaming, *Analytical Chemistry*, 75(8), 1911–1917, 2003.
24. R. C. Anderson, X. Su, G. J. Bogdan et al., A miniature integrated device for automated multistep genetic assays, *Nucleic Acids Research*, 28(12), e60, 2000.
25. M. Noerholm, H. Bruus, M. H. Jakobsen et al., Polymer microfluidic chip for online monitoring of microarray hybridizations, *Lab on a Chip*, 4(1), 28–37, 2004.
26. P. Stafford, *Methods in Microarray Normalization*, Boca Raton, FL: CRC Press, 2008.
27. N. B. Adey, M. Lei, M. T. Howard et al., Gains in sensitivity with a device that mixes microarray hybridization solution in a 25-mu m-thick chamber, *Analytical Chemistry*, 74(24), 6413–6417, 2002.
28. J. Vanderhoeven, K. Pappaert, B. Dutta et al., Comparison of a pump-around a diffusion-driven, and a shear-driven system for the hybridization of mouse lung and testis total RNA on microarrays, *Electrophoresis*, 26(19), 3773–3779, 2005.

29. J. Vanderhoeven, K. Pappaert, B. Dutta et al., DNA microarray enhancement using a continuously and discontinuously rotating microchamber, *Analytical Chemistry*, 77(14), 4474–4480, 2005.
30. P. K. Yuen, G. S. Li, Y. J. Bao et al., Microfluidic devices for fluidic circulation and mixing improve hybridization signal intensity on DNA arrays, *Lab on a Chip*, 3(1), 46–50, 2003.
31. M. K. McQuain, K. Seale, J. Peek et al., Chaotic mixer improves microarray hybridization, *Analytical Biochemistry*, 325(2), 215–226, 2004.
32. J. M. Hertzsch, R. Sturman, and S. Wiggins, DNA microarrays: Design principles for maximizing ergodic, chaotic mixing, *Small*, 3(2), 202–218, 2007.
33. H. H. Lee, J. Smoot, Z. McMurray et al., Recirculating flow accelerates DNA microarray hybridization in a microfluidic device, *Lab on a Chip*, 6(9), 1163–1170, 2006.
34. A. Bouchie, Shift anticipated in DNA microarray market, *Nature Biotechnology*, 20(1), 8–, 2002.
35. J. P. Gillet, T. J. Molina, J. Jamart et al., Evaluation of a low density DNA microarray for small B-cell non-Hodgkin lymphoma differential diagnosis, *Leukemia & Lymphoma*, 50(3), 410–418, 2009.
36. G. Meneses-Lorente, F. de Longueville, S. Dos Santos-Mendes et al., An evaluation of a low-density DNA microarray using cytochrome P450 inducers, *Chemical Research in Toxicology*, 16(9), 1070–1077, 2003.
37. F. de Longueville, D. Surry, G. Meneses-Lorente et al., Gene expression profiling of drug metabolism and toxicology markers using a low-density DNA microarray, *Biochemical Pharmacology*, 64(1), 137–149, 2002.
38. J. P. Gillet, T. Efferth, D. Steinbach et al., Microarray-based detection of multidrug resistance in human tumor cells by expression profiling of ATP-binding cassette transporter genes, *Cancer Research*, 64(24), 8987–8993, 2004.
39. D. Tejedor, S. Castillo, P. Mozas et al., Reliable low-density DNA array based on allele-specific probes for detection of 118 mutations causing familial hypercholesterolemia, *Clinical Chemistry*, 51(7), 1137–1144, 2005.
40. P. Alvarez, P. Saenz, D. Arteta et al., Transcriptional profiling of hematologic malignancies with a low-density DNA microarray, *Clinical Chemistry*, 53(2), 259–267, 2007.
41. C. A. Koch, P. C. H. Li, and R. S. Utkhede, Evaluation of thin films of agarose on glass for hybridization of DNA to identify plant pathogens with microarray technology, *Analytical Biochemistry*, 342(1), 93–102, 2005.
42. D. Erickson, X. Z. Liu, U. Krull et al., Electrokinetically controlled DNA hybridization microfluidic chip enabling rapid target analysis, *Analytical Chemistry*, 76(24), 7269–7277, 2004.
43. Y. Wang, B. Vaidya, H. D. Farquar et al., Microarrays assembled in microfluidic chips fabricated from poly(methyl methacrylate) for the detection of low-abundant DNA mutations, *Analytical Chemistry*, 75(5), 1130–1140, 2003.
44. Y. C. Chung, Y. C. Lin, M. Z. Shiu et al., Microfluidic chip for fast nucleic acid hybridization, *Lab on a Chip*, 3(4), 228–233, 2003.
45. J. H. S. Kim, A. Marafie, X. Y. Jia et al., Characterization of DNA hybridization kinetics in a microfluidic flow channel, *Sensors and Actuators B—Chemical*, 113(1), 281–289, 2006.
46. R. Peytavi, F. R. Raymond, D. Gagne et al., Microfluidic device for rapid (<15 min) automated microarray hybridization, *Clinical Chemistry*, 51(10), 1836–1844, 2005.
47. G. Y. Jia, K. S. Ma, J. Kim et al., Dynamic automated DNA hybridization on a CD (compact disc) fluidic platform, *Sensors and Actuators B—Chemical*, 114(1), 173–181, 2006.
48. C. Y. Li, X. L. Dong, J. H. Qin et al., Rapid nanoliter DNA hybridization based on reciprocating flow on a compact disk microfluidic device, *Analytica Chimica Acta*, 640(1–2), 93–99, 2009.
49. Y. J. Liu, C. B. Rauch, R. L. Stevens et al., DNA amplification and hybridization assays in integrated plastic monolithic devices, *Analytical Chemistry*, 74(13), 3063–3070, 2002.
50. Y. C. Chung, Y. C. Lin, C. D. Chueh et al., Microfluidic chip of fast DNA hybridization using denaturing and motion of nucleic acids, *Electrophoresis*, 29(9), 1859–1865, 2008.
51. R. Lenigk, R. H. Liu, M. Athavale et al., Plastic biochannel hybridization devices: A new concept for microfluidic DNA arrays, *Analytical Biochemistry*, 311(1), 40–49, 2002.
52. C. W. Wei, J. Y. Cheng, C. T. Huang et al., Using a microfluidic device for 1 μl DNA microarray hybridization in 500 s, *Nucleic Acids Research*, 33(8), e78, 2005.
53. M. Campas, and I. Katakis, DNA biochip arraying, detection and amplification strategies, *Trac-Trends in Analytical Chemistry*, 23(1), 49–62, 2004.
54. V. Le Berre, E. Trevisiol, A. Dagkessamanskaia et al., Dendrimeric coating of glass slides for sensitive DNA microarrays analysis, *Nucleic Acids Research*, 31(16), e88, 2003.
55. E. Delamarche, A. Bernard, H. Schmid et al., Microfluidic networks for chemical patterning of substrate: Design and application to bioassays, *Journal of the American Chemical Society*, 120(3), 500–508, 1998.

56. M. Geissler, E. Roy, G. A. Diaz-Quijada et al., Microfluidic Patterning of Miniaturized DNA Arrays on Plastic Substrates, *Acs Applied Materials & Interfaces*, 1(7), 1387–1395, 2009.
57. E. Delamarche, D. Juncker, and H. Schmid, Microfluidics for processing surfaces and miniaturizing biological assays, *Advanced Materials*, 17(24), 2911–2933, 2005.
58. E. Delamarche, A. Bernard, H. Schmid et al., Patterned delivery of immunoglobulins to surfaces using microfluidic networks, *Science*, 276(5313), 779–781, 1997.
59. H. J. Lee, T. T. Goodrich, and R. M. Corn, SPR imaging measurements of 1-D and 2-D DNA microarrays created from microfluidic channels on gold thin films, *Analytical Chemistry*, 73(22), 5525–5531, 2001.
60. L. Wang, and P. C. H. Li, Flexible microarray construction and fast DNA hybridization conducted on a microfluidic chip for greenhouse plant fungal pathogen detection, *Journal of Agricultural and Food Chemistry*, 55(26), 10509–10516, 2007.
61. J. A. Benn, J. Hu, B. J. Hogan et al., Comparative modeling and analysis of microfluidic and conventional DNA microarrays, *Analytical Biochemistry*, 348(2), 284–293, 2006.
62. C. Situma, Y. Wang, M. Hupert et al., Fabrication of DNA microarrays onto poly(methyl methacrylate) with ultraviolet patterning and microfluidics for the detection of low-abundant point mutations, *Analytical Biochemistry*, 340(1), 123–135, 2005.
63. Y. C. Li, Z. Wang, L. M. L. Ou et al., DNA detection on plastic: Surface activation protocol to convert polycarbonate substrates to biochip platforms, *Analytical Chemistry*, 79(2), 426–433, 2007.
64. X. Y. Peng, P. C. H. Li, H. Z. Yu et al., Spiral microchannels on a CD for DNA hybridizations, *Sensors and Actuators B—Chemical*, 128(1), 64–69, 2007.
65. L. Wang, P. C. H. Li, H. Z. Yu et al., Fungal pathogenic nucleic acid detection achieved with a microfluidic microarray device, *Analytica Chimica Acta*, 610(1), 97–104, 2008.
66. L. Wang, and P. C. H. Li, Optimization of a microfluidic microarray device for the fast discrimination of fungal pathogenic DNA, *Analytical Biochemistry*, 400(2), 282–288, 2010.
67. H. Chen, L. Wang, and P. C. H. Li, Nucleic acid microarrays created in the double-spiral format on a circular microfluidic disk, *Lab on a Chip*, 8(5), 826–829, 2008.
68. C. A. Rowe, L. M. Tender, M. J. Feldstein et al., Array biosensor for simultaneous identification of bacterial, viral, and protein analytes, *Analytical Chemistry*, 71(17), 3846–3852, 1999.
69. C. A. Rowe, S. B. Scruggs, M. J. Feldstein et al., An array immunosensor for simultaneous detection of clinical analytes, *Analytical Chemistry*, 71(2), 433–439, 1999.
70. K. E. Sapsford, P. T. Charles, C. H. Patterson et al., Demonstration of four immunoassay formats using the array biosensor, *Analytical Chemistry*, 74(5), 1061–1068, 2002.
71. G. Krishnamoorthy, E. T. Carlen, H. L. deBoer et al., Electrokinetic lab-on-a-biochip for multi-ligand/multi-analyte biosensing, *Analytical Chemistry*, 82(10), 4145–4150, 2010.
72. S. C. Jacobson, T. E. McKnight, and J. M. Ramsey, Microfluidic devices for electrokinetically driven parallel and serial mixing, *Analytical Chemistry*, 71(20), 4455–4459, 1999.
73. P. C. H. Li, Microfluidic lab-on-a-chip for chemical and biological analysis and discovery, Boca Raton, FL: Taylor & Francis/CRC Press, Boca Raton, FL, 2006.
74. P. Gong, and R. Levicky, DNA surface hybridization regimes, *Proceedings of the National Academy of Sciences of the United States of America*, 105(14), 5301–5306, 2008.
75. R. Levicky, and A. Horgan, Physicochemical perspectives on DNA microarray and biosensor technologies, *Trends in Biotechnology*, 23(3), 143–149, 2005.
76. G. Y. Tang, D. G. Yan, C. Yang et al., Assessment of Joule heating and its effects on electroosmotic flow and electrophoretic transport of solutes in microfluidic channels, *Electrophoresis*, 27(3), 628–639, 2006.
77. X. C. Xuan, B. Xu, D. Sinton et al., Electroosmotic flow with Joule heating effects, *Lab on a Chip*, 4(3), 230–236, 2004.
78. I. Rodriguez, and N. Chandrasekhar, Experimental study and numerical estimation of current changes in electroosmotically pumped microfluidic devices, *Electrophoresis*, 26(6), 1114–1121, 2005.
79. B. J. Kirby, and E. F. Hasselbrink, Zeta potential of microfluidic substrates: 1. Theory, experimental techniques, and effects on separations, *Electrophoresis*, 25(2), 187–202, 2004.
80. R. A. Potyrailo, W. G. Morris, A. M. Leach et al., Analog signal acquisition from computer optical disk drives for quantitative chemical sensing, *Analytical Chemistry*, 78(16), 5893–5899, 2006.
81. S. A. Lange, G. Roth, S. Wittemann et al., Measuring biomolecular binding events with a compact disc player device, *Angewandte Chemie-International Edition*, 45(2), 270–273, 2006.
82. M. Madou, J. Zoval, G. Y. Jia et al., Lab on a CD, *Annual Review of Biomedical Engineering*, 8, 601–628, 2006.
83. A. S. Watts, A. A. Urbas, E. Moschou et al., Centrifugal microfluidics with integrated sensing microdome optodes for multiion detection, *Analytical Chemistry*, 79(21), 8046–8054, 2007.

84. R. D. Johnson, I. H. A. Badr, G. Barrett et al., Development of a fully integrated analysis system for ions based on ion-selective optodes and centrifugal microfluidics, *Analytical Chemistry*, 73(16), 3940–3946, 2001.
85. I. H. A. Badr, R. D. Johnson, M. J. Madou et al., Fluorescent ion-selective optode membranes incorporated onto a centrifugal microfluidics platform, *Analytical Chemistry*, 74(21), 5569–5575, 2002.
86. J. Steigert, M. Grumann, T. Brenner et al., Fully integrated whole blood testing by real-time absorption measurement on a centrifugal platform, *Lab on a Chip*, 6(8), 1040–1044, 2006.
87. M. Gustafsson, D. Hirschberg, C. Palmberg et al., Integrated sample preparation and MALDI mass spectrometry on a microfluidic compact disk, *Analytical Chemistry*, 76(2), 345–350, 2004.
88. J. Steigert, T. Brenner, M. Grumann et al., Integrated siphon-based metering and sedimentation of whole blood on a hydrophilic lab-on-a-disk, *Biomedical Microdevices*, 9(5), 675–679, 2007.
89. J. L. Zhang, Q. Q. Guo, M. Liu et al., A lab-on-CD prototype for high-speed blood separation, *Journal of Micromechanics and Microengineering*, 18(12), 125025, 2008.
90. D. C. Duffy, H. L. Gillis, J. Lin et al., Microfabricated centrifugal microfluidic systems: Characterization and multiple enzymatic assays, *Analytical Chemistry*, 71(20), 4669–4678, 1999.
91. P. Andersson, G. Jesson, G. Kylberg et al., Parallel nanoliter microfluidic analysis system, *Analytical Chemistry*, 79(11), 4022–4030, 2007.
92. S. W. Lee, J. Y. Kang, I. H. Lee et al., Single-cell assay on CD-like lab chip using centrifugal massive single-cell trap, *Sensors and Actuators A—Physical*, 143(1), 64–69, 2008.
93. S. Haeberle, T. Brenner, R. Zengerle et al., Centrifugal extraction of plasma from whole blood on a rotating disk, *Lab on a Chip*, 6(6), 776–781, 2006.
94. S. Lai, S. N. Wang, J. Luo et al., Design of a compact disk-like microfluidic platform for enzyme-linked immunosorbent assay, *Analytical Chemistry*, 76(7), 1832–1837, 2004.
95. A. Penrose, P. Myers, K. Bartle et al., Development and assessment of a miniaturised centrifugal chromatograph for reversed-phase separations in micro-channels, *Analyst*, 129(8), 704–709, 2004.
96. A. P. Wong, M. Gupta, S. S. Shevkoplyas et al., Egg beater as centrifuge: Isolating human blood plasma from whole blood in resource-poor settings, *Lab on a Chip*, 8(12), 2032–2037, 2008.
97. B. S. Lee, J. N. Lee, J. M. Park et al., A fully automated immunoassay from whole blood on a disc, *Lab on a Chip*, 9(11), 1548–1555, 2009.
98. L. G. Puckett, E. Dikici, S. Lai et al., Investigation into the applicability of the centrifugal microfluidics development of protein-platform for the ligand binding assays incorporating enhanced green fluorescent protein as a fluorescent reporter, *Analytical Chemistry*, 76(24), 7263–7268, 2004.
99. M. Grumann, J. Steigert, L. Riegger et al., Sensitivity enhancement for colorimetric glucose assays on whole blood by on-chip beam-guidance, *Biomedical Microdevices*, 8(3), 209–214, 2006.
100. Y. K. Cho, J. G. Lee, J. M. Park et al., One-step pathogen specific DNA extraction from whole blood on a centrifugal microfluidic device, *Lab on a Chip*, 7(5), 565–573, 2007.
101. J. M. Chen, P. C. Huang, and M. G. Lin, Analysis and experiment of capillary valves for microfluidics on a rotating disk, *Microfluidics and Nanofluidics*, 4(5), 427–437, 2008.
102. S. Haeberle, T. Brenner, H. P. Schlosser et al., Centrifugal micromixer, *Chemical Engineering & Technology*, 28(5), 613–616, 2005.
103. T. Glatzel, C. Litterst, C. Cupelli et al., Computational fluid dynamics (CFD) software tools for microfluidic applications—A case study, *Computers & Fluids*, 37(3), 218–235, 2008.
104. T. Brenner, T. Glatzel, R. Zengerle et al., Frequency-dependent transversal flow control in centrifugal microfluidics, *Lab on a Chip*, 5(2), 146–150, 2005.
105. M. Liu, J. Zhang, Y. Liu et al., Modeling of flow burst, flow timing in Lab-on-a-CD systems and its application in digital chemical analysis, *Chemical Engineering & Technology*, 31(9), 1328–1335, 2008.
106. D. S. Kim, and T. H. Kwon, Modeling, analysis and design of centrifugal force driven transient filling flow into rectangular microchannel, *Microsystem Technologies—Micro- and Nanosystems-Information Storage and Processing Systems*, 12(9), 822–838, 2006.
107. D. S. Kim, and T. H. Kwon, Modeling, analysis and design of centrifugal force-driven transient filling flow into a circular microchannel, *Microfluidics and Nanofluidics*, 2(2), 125–140, 2006.
108. J. Siegrist, M. Amasia, N. Singh et al., Numerical modeling and experimental validation of uniform microchamber filling in centrifugal microfluidics, *Lab on a Chip*, 10(7), 876–886, 2010.
109. J. Kim, H. Kido, R. H. Rangel et al., Passive flow switching valves on a centrifugal microfluidic platform, *Sensors and Actuators B—Chemical*, 128(2), 613–621, 2008.
110. J. Ducree, S. Haeberle, T. Brenner et al., Patterning of flow and mixing in rotating radial microchannels, *Microfluidics and Nanofluidics*, 2(2), 97–105, 2006.
111. M. S. Al-Qahtani, and M. N. Basha, Prediction of flow and heat transfer in narrow rotating rectangular channels using Reynolds stress model, *Heat and Mass Transfer*, 44(5), 505–516, 2008.

112. J. V. Zoval, and M. J. Madou, Centrifuge-based fluidic platforms, *Proceedings of the IEEE*, 92(1), 140–153, 2004.
113. D. D. Nolte, Invited Review Article: Review of centrifugal microfluidic and bio-optical disks, *Review of Scientific Instruments*, 80(10), 101101, 2009.
114. D. Mark, S. Haeberle, G. Roth et al., Microfluidic lab-on-a-chip platforms: Requirements, characteristics and applications, *Chemical Society Reviews*, 39(3), 1153–1182, 2010.
115. X. Y. Peng, and P. C. H. Li, Centrifugal pumping in the equiforce spiral microchannel, *Canadian Journal of Pure and Applied Sciences*, 2(3), 551–556, 2008.
116. J. W. Larson, G. R. Yantz, Q. Zhong et al., Single DNA molecule stretching in sudden mixed shear and elongational microflows, *Lab on a Chip*, 6(9), 1187–1199, 2006.
117. L. Wang, M.-C. Kropinski, and P. C. H. Li, Analysis and modeling of flow in rotating spiral microchannels: towards math-aided design of microfluidic systems using centrifugal pumping, *Lab on a Chip,* 2011, in press.
118. L. Wang and P. C. H. Li, Gold nanoparticle-assisted single base-pair mismatch discrimination on a microfluidic microarray device. *Biomicrofluidics,* 4(3), 32209, 2010.

27 Microfluidic Systems to Study the Biology of Human Diseases and Identify Potential Therapeutic Targets in *Caenorhabditis elegans*

Pouya Rezai, Sangeena Salam, P. Ravi Selvaganapathy, and Bhagwati P. Gupta

CONTENTS

27.1 INTRODUCTION

Drug discovery is the process of identifying drugs for human diseases. Typically, this involves screening for a large number of chemical compounds against certain targets in cells using *in vitro* and *in vivo* disease models [1]. In general, the process includes five stages: target identification and validation, lead screening, optimization, preclinical development, and clinical trials. A protein or biochemical pathway that plays a key role in the origin or progression of the disease is identified in the target identification and validation stage. The lead screening stage involves screening of a large number of chemical compounds against the biomolecular target protein or gene in order to identify candidates with potential therapeutic effect. This is followed by an optimization stage in which small chemical modifications of the initial lead compounds are made and screened to produce an optimal chemical species. The preclinical stage involves testing the candidates in various other animal models for efficacy as well as toxicity, and finally, in the clinical stage, testing is carried out in humans on a smaller scale. If successful, the drug is made commercially available in the market.

The lead screening and optimization in the drug discovery process is frequently carried out by high-throughput screening (HTS) of chemical compounds using *in vitro* assays (e.g., against a protein target present either in solution or in cultured cells). As these approaches ignore the complexity of biological processes in the context of multicellular organisms that involve interactions between different types of cells and tissues, they often fail to produce desired results in subsequent animal and human trials. This results in poor efficacy, nonspecific effects, delay in clinical trials, and a significant increase in the cost of developing new drugs. A better approach would be to use a whole animal model that allows monitoring of various steps in drug screening, such as administration, distribution, metabolism, and toxicity, during the screening phase. Although human subjects are ideal, they cannot be tested due to the enormous complexity of the cellular and molecular processes, as well as the ethical issues associated with subjecting them to experimentation. Therefore, alternative eukaryotic systems (e.g., *Caenorhabditis elegans*) are desired, which are simpler and easier to manipulate yet complex enough to address many of the questions relevant to human biology.

Traditional methods of drug screening and studies of its mode of action in animal models have involved feeding the subjects with chemicals present in food (e.g., on a Petri dish or in a 96-well microtiter plate) while monitoring the effects on various biological processes, and parameters such as growth and fertility, by visual inspection [2]. These methods are time consuming, expensive, tedious, prone to human flaws, and frequently result in failure. It is a significant bottleneck that has forced the use of animal model approaches to later stages of lead optimization. Using them at earlier stages of screening will increase the physiological relevance of drug candidates during the lead identification process as well as reveal potential toxic effects, thereby helping to accelerate the process of drug discovery. This could be achieved by automation and parallelization of screening that will enable low-cost high-throughput analysis in a rapid, sensitive, and accurate manner.

This chapter provides a comprehensive review of HTS and drug discovery-related research in *C. elegans*. It begins with a brief description of leading animal models with an emphasis on *C. elegans*. This is followed by a survey of currently available microfluidic and other robotic systems for various worm applications. The chapter ends with a discussion on tools and approaches needed to facilitate high-throughput microfluidic screens in *C. elegans* for the study of movement behavior and related disorders.

27.2 ANIMAL MODELS TO STUDY HUMAN DISEASES

The ultimate target of most of the ongoing biomedical research is to understand human diseases and develop effective therapeutic treatments. As humans cannot be manipulated in a laboratory due to ethical reasons and are too complex and slow growing, researchers have established alternative models to study disease mechanisms and search for potential drug targets [2–6]. This has involved conducting experiments in unicellular and multicellular animals (the *in vivo* approach) as well as cultured cells (the *in vitro* approach). In addition, computer software is also used to study biological processes by developing mathematical models (the *in silico* approach) and to analyze large experimental datasets.

The *in vivo* approach, involving animals, has traditionally focused on a relatively small set of living entities known as model organisms. Much of our understanding of human biology and diseases has come from studies carried out in these systems. Such models have been immensely useful for the understanding of fundamental biological processes such as cell division and differentiation that occur in all eukaryotes. They provide powerful tools to accelerate studies on diseases without dealing with actual human subjects and free from ethical considerations. By reducing the time needed to study diseases and find cures, they help improve our lives.

27.2.1 CULTURED CELLS AND EUKARYOTES

In vitro cultures of animal cells offer several advantages in biological studies. These cultures mimic many of the cellular and molecular processes observed in live animals, increase the throughput of the experiment, and reduce the space and infrastructure compared to that needed to house animals. A large number of cell cultures, derived from humans and other animals, are currently available for investigation. Many of these are well characterized in terms of growth and differentiation properties. This, together with the relative ease in culturing and obtaining large quantities of pure cell populations, has been valuable for investigating processes in normal and disease conditions [7,8].

Two eukaryotic model organisms that resemble cultured cells in many ways are the baker's yeast *Saccharomyces cerevisiae* (*S. cerevisiae*) and the fission yeast *S. pombe*. Both are rapidly growing micron-size organisms that can be cultured fairly easily and inexpensively in the laboratory. Normally they reproduce asexually (*S. cerevisiae* by budding and *S. pombe* by fission); however, in certain conditions they can also mate and reproduce sexually. The ability to switch between asexual and sexual lifestyles provides many advantages in genetic experiments. Both organisms have been at the forefront of many biological discoveries for decades. They offer a number of powerful genetic, biochemical, and molecular biological tools to accelerate the study of conserved processes (e.g., cell cycle control) [9,10] and human diseases [11,12].

While the cell cultures and unicellular organisms are useful in biological studies, they poorly mimic the three-dimensional environment and complexity observed in multicellular animals. Since live cells communicate with their neighbors as well as the environment, diseases affecting one tissue or cell population often indirectly impact other parts of the body. In this respect whole animal models provide advantages to study the broad range of phenotypes, disease mechanisms, and complex cellular interactions. A number of animal models are available today for experimentation that include vertebrates, such as mouse (*Mus musculus*) and zebrafish (*Danio rerio*), and invertebrates, such as worm (*C. elegans*) and fruitfly (*Drosophila melanogaster*). The main advantages of vertebrates are their higher degree of genetic and physiological similarities to humans. Due to their large size, these animals can be surgically operated to isolate tissues and cells for various experiments. They also offer rich morphological and behavioral features that make them suitable models for many human diseases. However, vertebrates also have several drawbacks that limit their use in the laboratory. These include slow growth, long life span, and high cost of maintenance. Additionally, the large size and slow growth of vertebrates are not suitable for HTS-based studies. In these respects the invertebrate models, *C. elegans* and *D. melanogaster*, possess many features that are particularly appealing. For example, they have a short generation time (few days) and are relatively cheap to maintain and perform experiments on. A number of pioneering discoveries in these organisms have helped improve our understanding of human biology and diseases. Both of these boast a rich history, powerful cellular, molecular, and genomic tools, and extensive literature to undertake detailed investigations of biological problems. However, due to their small size (1–2 mm), one needs microscopes and special tools for handling them. This poses difficulties in studies requiring the examination of a large number of such animals.

27.2.2 The Nematode *C. elegans*

C. elegans is an established model organism to investigate the molecular mechanisms of conserved biological phenomena that occur in all organisms including humans [13]. It is one of the most thoroughly studied multicellular organisms in terms of genetics, development, behavior, and physiology. It offers many experimental advantages including small size (~1 mm), rapid life cycle (Figure 27.1), and the ease of culture conditions. The adult worm has roughly 1000 somatic cells and a transparent body that allows visualization of cellular and molecular events in live animals using fluorescent proteins, such as green fluorescent protein (GFP), without the need for sacrificing the animal. The worm genome is compact (~20 times smaller than the human genome) and is fully sequenced, which greatly facilitates experimental manipulations and the study of gene function.

27.2.2.1 Development and Behavior

The worm contains two sexes, self-fertilizing hermaphrodites and rare males. The hermaphrodites are essentially females except that they initially produce sperm for a few hours before switching to make oocytes. While males are not necessary for reproduction, mating provides opportunities for new genetic material to be introduced. The fertilized embryo goes through four larval stages (L1–L4) to generate an adult animal (Figure 27.1). An adult hermaphrodite contains 959 somatic nuclei that are organized into specialized cell types such as neurons, muscles, and intestine.

Due to its small size and transparent body, *C. elegans* allows the study of biological processes at a single-cell resolution. Through a laser-assisted cell ablation technique researchers have determined the lineage history and function of every cell in the animal. The electron microscope was used in ultrastructural studies, which among other things has revealed interconnections of all neurons (302

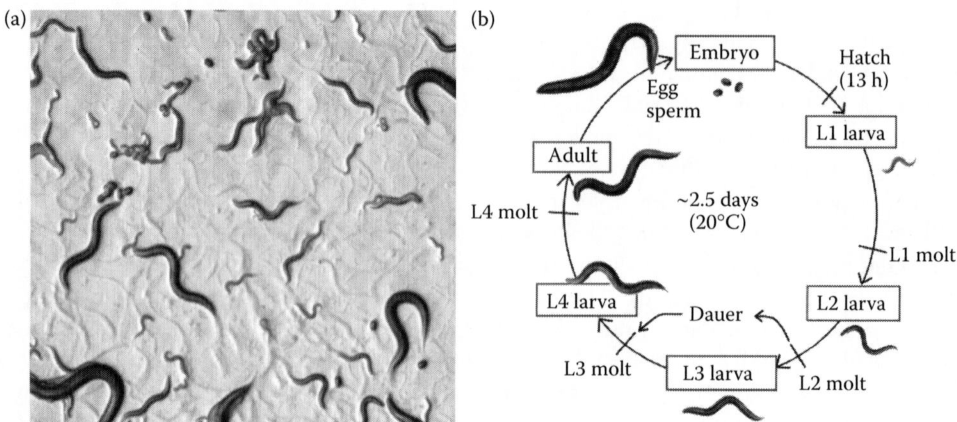

FIGURE 27.1 *C. elegans* and its life cycle. (a) A typical culture on an agar plate. Different stages of animals are visible. (b) Life cycle of *C. elegans* at 20°C. A fertilized embryo goes through four larval stages to give rise to an adult in roughly two-and-a-half days. Dauer is a reversible alternative developmental program that is induced by unfavorable growth conditions.

in total). This serves as an invaluable resource in the study of the development and function of the nervous system.

C. elegans has a well-developed chemosensory system to detect a wide variety of volatile and water-soluble chemicals in the environment. This allows the animal to find food, avoid harmful substances, and modulate physiological conditions such as diapause. All these responses are mediated by certain neurons located primarily in the head and tail regions. Additionally, *C. elegans* contains thermosensory and mechanosensory neurons to sense temperature and external substances (e.g., soil particles) that make physical contacts with the animal in its habitat. While these behaviors have been studied in significant detail and genes and mechanisms are identified, a few others such as responses to light (phototaxis) and electric field (electrotaxis) are poorly characterized.

27.2.2.2 Conservation of Biological Processes

The amenability of *C. elegans* to genetic manipulations has led researchers to study biological processes by means of isolating mutations and characterizing phenotypes. This "forward genetics" approach has been very successful in understanding the development and behavior of the worm and the extent to which molecular mechanisms are conserved in eukaryotes. The availability of the genome sequence of *C. elegans* has further strengthened its utility by enabling large-scale functional genomic approaches to identify genes and understand their *in vivo* function. The findings have revealed that *C. elegans* shares more than half of its genes with humans and utilizes many of the same processes [14]. For example, genetic and molecular studies have identified conserved cellular machinery that control processes such as cell proliferation, cell differentiation, and cell death. It has been demonstrated that these processes utilize similar mechanisms in almost all eukaryotes, supporting the conclusion that results obtained in worms can be successfully translated to other organisms including humans.

In addition to its value in addressing basic questions about animal development and behavior, *C. elegans* has also proven to be an excellent system for studying the biology of human diseases. The worm genome contains many human disease gene orthologs [14,15] that makes it possible to establish worm disease models, study cellular and molecular changes, and develop potential drug targets. This is evident from research on diseases such as cancers, bacterial and fungal infections, obesity, hypertension, and neuronal disorders [3,16–19].

27.3 *C. ELEGANS* AS A MODEL FOR STUDYING NEURODEGENERATIVE AND MOVEMENT DISORDERS AND SCREEN FOR DRUG CANDIDATES

Because of its simpler anatomy and comparatively fewer neuronal and muscle cells, *C. elegans* is an ideal system for studying disorders affecting these cell types. The worm contains just 302 neurons, as compared to over 100 billion in the human brain, thus conferring unparalleled precision and control in the identification and manipulation of neuronal cells. In the case of muscles the most abundant class (somatic, striated type) consists of 95 body wall muscles that are used for locomotion. They are arranged in a stereotypic manner and can be readily visualized under a microscope. Studies in *C. elegans* have revealed that neuronal and muscle cells share many similarities with humans in terms of structure, composition, and function. Furthermore, mutations in human disease gene orthologs that affect these cells can be readily analyzed in worms due to its amenability to genetic analysis and the power to probe gene function at a single-cell level. These and other features described earlier make *C. elegans* a valuable model for gaining insights into movement-related disorders, such as Duchenne's muscular dystrophy (DMD), Alzheimer's disease (AD), Huntington's disease (HD), and Parkinson's disease (PD) [2,20,21]. In addition to learning the basis of these diseases, *C. elegans* is also promising in accelerating the process of drug discovery by helping us to perform high-throughput genetic and chemical screens [22,23] (Table 27.1).

TABLE 27.1
***C. elegans* Disease Models, Candidate Targets, and Potential Drugs that Confer Protection**

Disease Model	Mode of Induction	Genetic and Cellular Target(s)	Protecting Chemicals/Drugs
DMD	*dys-1/dystrophin; hlh-1/MyoD* mutants		Serotonin Prednisone
AD	Ectopic Aβ (1–42) expression	Insulin signaling pathway αB-cystallin Tumor necrosis factor-induced protein 1 Arsenite-inducible protein (AIP-1)	*Ginkgo biloba* extract EGb 761
HD	Ectopic Poly-Q expression		Lithium chloride Mitramycin Trichostatin A
PD	6-OHDA exposure	*dat-1/dat1* Mitochondrial enzyme complex I and IV *egl-1/puma* *cep-1/p53*	GABA NMDA Bromocriptine Quinpirol Acetaminophen
	MPTP exposure	Mitochondrial enzyme complex I	Rofecoxib Modafinil
	Rotenone exposure	Mitochondrial enzyme complex I	D-α-Hydroxybutyrate in combination with Tauroursodeoxycholic acid
	Ectopic α-syn expression	ER-to-Golgi trafficking, mitochondria Aging-associated genes, such as *sir-2.1/SIRT1* and *lagr-1/LASS2* Endocytic pathway genes Cellular trafficking genes	1,2,3,4-Tetrahydroquinolinones
	TH overexpression		Acetaminophen

27.3.1 Muscle Disorders

C. elegans possesses many conserved genes that are involved in muscular dystrophies. One of these, *dystrophin*, is linked to DMD [24]. DMD is an X-linked recessive disorder that is characterized by progressive degeneration of skeletal and cardiac muscles [25]. The presence of dystrophin-like gene *dys-1* in *C. elegans* has been useful for studying the mechanism of muscle degeneration [26–28]. In addition, researchers have carried out pilot screens for candidate drugs that suppress the disease phenotype [29,30] (Table 27.1). These studies illustrate the use of the worm DMD model in understanding the disease mechanism and identifying potential treatments.

27.3.2 Neurodegenerative Diseases

C. elegans neurodegenerative disease models include three major disorders (AD, HD, and PD), all of which cause age-dependent progressive loss of neurons or neural activity. A common feature of these disorders is the accumulation of misfolded protein aggregates. Because of its short life span and other experimental advantages (see Section 27.2.2), *C. elegans* can be used to accelerate the research on disease mechanisms. Researchers have created transgenic worm strains that are valuable in understanding the basis of protein aggregation and neuronal defects, and search for therapeutic targets.

27.3.2.1 Alzheimer's Disease

AD is the most common cause of dementia primarily affecting people over 60 years of age. Its symptoms include memory loss and cognitive decline that become severe with age as neuronal degeneration increases and affects larger areas of the brain. The cellular hallmarks of AD are senile plaques and neurofibrillary tangles consisting mainly of β-amyloid (Aβ) peptide and the microtubule-associated protein tau, respectively [31,32]. In spite of the extensive work from several laboratories, little is understood about factors that trigger the accumulation of misfolded tau and Aβ and the resulting neuronal toxicity. Researchers have generated transgenic *C. elegans* AD models by expressing the toxic human Aβ peptide (Aβ1–42) in body wall muscles [33–35]. The accumulation of the protein interferes with normal muscle function thereby causing paralysis. These models provide a means to identify molecular pathways that induce protein misfolding and facilitate the identification of potential targets to understand the cause of AD [34,36–38] (Table 27.1). When combined with findings in other animal models, the knowledge could prove valuable to understand the disease mechanism in humans, ultimately helping to develop effective treatments.

27.3.2.2 Huntington's Disease

HD is another age-dependent neurodegenerative disorder caused by abnormal expansion of glutamine repeats (polyglutamines or polyQ) in *huntingtin (htn)* [39]. Although *C. elegans* does not carry an *htn* counterpart, it has been shown that forced expression of human *htn-polyQ* in worms causes neurodegeneration similar to that seen in HD patients [40–43]. This suggests that *htn-polyQ*-mediated neuronal toxicity occurs through the disruption of certain cellular processes that are conserved between worms and humans. Therefore, advanced genetics and genomics technologies in *C. elegans* can be harnessed to understand disease mechanisms and discover candidate drugs. This is demonstrated by screens to identify candidate genes and biological processes that are involved in polyQ-mediated neuronal toxicity in a worm HD model [44,45]. In addition, researchers have also used the worm system to find drugs such as resveratrol, mithramycin (MTR), and trichostatin A (TSA) that reduce polyQ toxicity and promote neuronal survival [46,47] (Table 27.1). These studies demonstrate the power of *C. elegans* in understanding the disease mechanism and drug discovery.

27.3.2.3 Parkinson's Disease

PD is one of the common neurodegenerative diseases of elderly people above the age of 65. One of the major causes of PD is the marked loss of dopaminergic (DA) neurons in substantia niagra, a region of the brain that controls balance and movement of the body. Its major symptoms are tremor, bradykinesis (slow movement), stiffness of the limbs and trunks or akinesia (inability to move), and postural instability (impaired balance and coordination). The C. elegans genome contains homologs of most PD-related genes (Table 27.2).

The pathological hallmark of PD is the presence of intracellular inclusions termed Lewy bodies (LBs) in patient brains. The most abundant protein in LBs is α-synuclein (α-syn) that appears to be responsible for DA degeneration. In order to understand the basis of α-syn accumulation and toxicity, researchers have generated transgenic *C. elegans* strains overexpressing human α-syn that show protein accumulation similar to LBs in PD patients [21]. These animals serve as suitable models for molecular dissection of PD and screening of drug candidates. Thus, chemical and genetic screens have been carried out using α-syn-induced neuronal toxicity as an assay [48–52]. These screens have identified components of endocytosis, vesicular trafficking, and lipid metabolism (Table 27.1).

Besides mutations and other genetic modifications, several chemical compounds (e.g., 6-OHDA, MPTP, and pesticides such as rotenone and paraquat) (Table 27.1) have been found to induce PD-like symptoms in humans and other animal models [53–58]. These chemicals cause degeneration of DA neurons by oxidative stress and/or inactivation of mitochondrial complex I [59]. The DA neurons in *C. elegans* are also susceptible to these neurotoxins and give rise to movement defects [60]. Such PD worm models have been valuable in exploring the mechanism of neuronal degeneration and identification of potential neuroprotective compounds [61–64] (Table 27.1).

TABLE 27.2
PD-Related Genes in *C. elegans*

PD Gene	*C. elegans* Ortholog	Protein Family	Details
PARK1	None	α-Synuclein	Possible role in synaptic transmission
PARK2	*pdr-1*	Parkin	RING-type E3 ubiquitin ligase
PARK3	na	na	Specific gene is yet to be identified
PARK5	*ubh-1*	UCHL-1	Ubiquitin carboxy-terminal hydrolase L1
PARK6	*pink-1*	PINK1	PTEN-induced kinase 1 (serine/threonine kinase family)
PARK7	*djr-1.1* and *djr-1.2*	DJ-1	Atypical peroxiredoxin-like peroxidase; acts as a chaperone and a sensor for oxidative stress
PARK8	*lrk-1*	LRRK2	Leucine-rich repeat kinase 2
PARK9	*catp-6*	ATP13A2	P5-type ATPase
PARK10	na	na	Specific gene is yet to be identified
PARK11	na	na	The evidence of PARK11 encoding GIGYF2 (Grb10-interacting GYF protein-2) is contradictory
PARK12	na	na	Specific gene is yet to be identified
PARK13	None	HtrA2	Mitochondrial, antiapoptotic serine protease

Note: na, not applicable; None, ortholog unknown.

27.4 HIGH-THROUGHPUT AND AUTOMATED TECHNIQUES TO MANIPULATE *C. ELEGANS*

Among the various features of *C. elegans*, its small size, rapid growth, and simple food requirements have made it a valuable model organism for high-throughput-based studies to address questions related to basic and applied biology. These include fundamental processes such as cell growth and differentiation and treatment of human diseases by identifying drug candidates [3,60,65–67]. Over the years, several HTS methods have been developed to manipulate worms in a rapid and efficient manner. Typically, these involve cultivating animals in multiwell format plates (either agar or liquid media-based) and screening for morphological and behavioral changes under a microscope. These methods could be semiautomated by the use of robotic and sorting devices. Methods have also been developed to rapidly screen for the viability of animals using fluorescent dyes. In some cases, computer softwares have also been used to accelerate the analysis. In the following, we provide an overview of these technologies and summarize their progress.

27.4.1 Classical Approaches

Being a genetic model system, *C. elegans* is frequently used to screen for mutations that affect development and behavior. The characterization of such mutations has been valuable in understanding how genes function and interact to control cellular activities. Typically, the mutant screening protocols involve growing worms on Petri dishes for about a week and observing animals under a microscope for desired phenotypes. Putative lines are grown and retested to confirm the presence of a mutation before initiating genetic experiments. Such an approach mostly involves working with a very small set of genes and often takes many years of hard work to obtain a reasonable understanding of biological processes.

The discovery of RNA interference (RNAi) phenomenon has accelerated the pace of genetic analysis [68]. Depending on convenience, researchers can carry out RNAi experiments on traditional agar-based culture plates or in liquid media-containing microwell plates. The liquid medium has the advantage of scaling up the volume with less effort compared to the plate culture and is therefore a method of choice for large-scale RNAi studies involving a large number of genes [69]. Several chemical screens have also successfully utilized the liquid media protocol to identify beneficial compounds and to assess the effect of toxic substances on animal health and viability [70,71]. For example, as mentioned in Section 27.3, chemical screens in *C. elegans* disease models have identified several candidates that inhibit neuronal toxicity (Table 27.1).

While the above plate and liquid culture-based protocols are well established, the process is slow, labor intensive, and does not readily scale up. Furthermore, the phenotypic assays (such as movement and growth) are largely manual and therefore prone to error and subjectivity. This limits the use of *C. elegans* in large-scale studies that require rapid, sensitive, and quantitative assessment of phenotypes with very little or no variation in measurements. In order to overcome some of these limitations, a few high-throughput methods have been developed that utilize cutting edge engineering and computer technologies.

27.4.2 Engineering Approach

As mentioned earlier worms are highly suitable for HTS-based studies due to their small size and rapid growth. This, together with other advantages, makes them an excellent model to screen for potential drug candidates and gene targets for human diseases. Drug discovery is a long and multistep process. Typical phases involve initial screening of tens of thousands of chemical compounds by *in vitro* (using mammalian cell cultures) approaches, selected *in vivo* testing in other animal models (e.g., mouse) to identify potential candidates, clinical testing in humans to determine beneficial and side effects, registration of a successful drug, and production for public use. This entire process usually takes more than a decade, of which most of the time is spent in the initial chemical screening phase. Therefore, reducing the time for screening, by using the *C. elegans* model, will greatly accelerate drug discovery, create more opportunities for clinical trials, and ultimately more drugs to treat patients. Additionally, worms could also accelerate the understanding of molecular mechanisms underlying a disease, leading to the development of improved drugs and other therapeutic interventions [2]. Over the years, many protocols and tools have been developed to handle worms in a high-throughput fashion. All of them have shown promise and continue to evolve to meet new challenges and overcome shortcomings. In the remainder of this section we discuss major techniques available today and highlight their uniqueness, advantages, and limitations.

27.4.2.1 Conventional Robotics

The conventional liquid handling robotic systems used in molecular biology experiments have been successfully adopted in worm screening protocols. These systems typically consist of a pipetter, a culture plate-handling unit, a microscope, and a computer. The computer controls various operations such as pipetter movement, volume adjustment, and plate handling. The pipetter can dispense defined volumes of liquid media (containing bacteria and/or chemicals) into microwells of a culture plate (e.g., 96-well or 384-well plate). Worms are grown inside microwells for a desired period of time and their phenotypes are monitored by a microscope on a regular basis. In certain kinds of screens, such as those involving thermal avoidance behavior [72], data collection, and analysis, could be automated by using a computer [73]. The speed, accuracy, and automation afforded by robotic equipment have been valuable in carrying out many high-throughput screens in *C. elegans* (e.g., see [69,74]).

Although useful, a major drawback of conventional robotic systems is their high cost that limits their widespread use. Additionally, the instrumentation cannot be used for certain kinds of HTS-based *C. elegans* studies. For example, one of the key operations in screening worms is to obtain fluorescent and visual images of individual worms that have been fed with RNAi bacteria or treated with chemicals. This operation is difficult to perform in the microwell plate format due to the inherent motion of animals and fluorescent signal distraction. Although it is possible to analyze the speed and shape of moving worms using specialized software [75], the technology is not advanced enough and therefore has not been widely adopted. The robotic systems are also not suitable for screens that require precise measurement of movement-related parameters (e.g., angle of body bends and frequency and amplitudes of sine waves), time course of phenotypic changes, and single-cell observations.

27.4.2.2 Biosorter

Two of the few automated HTS and sorting devices for *C. elegans* research available today are BioSorter and COPAS (Complex Object Parametric Analyzer and Sorter), both made by Union Biometrica (Figure 27.2). These are large particle flow cytometers capable of analyzing, sorting, and dispensing worms, cells, and other micron-sized objects (up to 1500 μm). As the object passes through the flow cell, its optical density, length, and fluorescence are measured with the help of lasers. This information is analyzed by computer software that in turn controls a pneumatic sorting mechanism to dispense the object in a predefined manner. Compared to COPAS, BioSorter is more flexible and has a few additional features that make it suitable for a larger range of applications. Both systems can sort worms into multiwell microtiter plates in a rapid (more than 100 worms per second) and efficient manner. This has facilitated several high-throughput screens using phenotypes such as size, viability, and GFP fluorescence as screening criteria [69,76–79]. These equipment have made significant contributions to *C. elegans* research by making large-scale animal sorting and aliquoting a routine job that was earlier not possible. However, similar to the robotic systems, COPAS and BioSorter have limited applications and cannot be used in screens requiring high-resolution single worm and movement-related analyses.

27.4.2.3 Microfluidic Devices

As reviewed earlier, many protocols are available to manipulate worms on agar plates and in liquid media, but there is virtually none that can efficiently analyze individual animals at high resolution

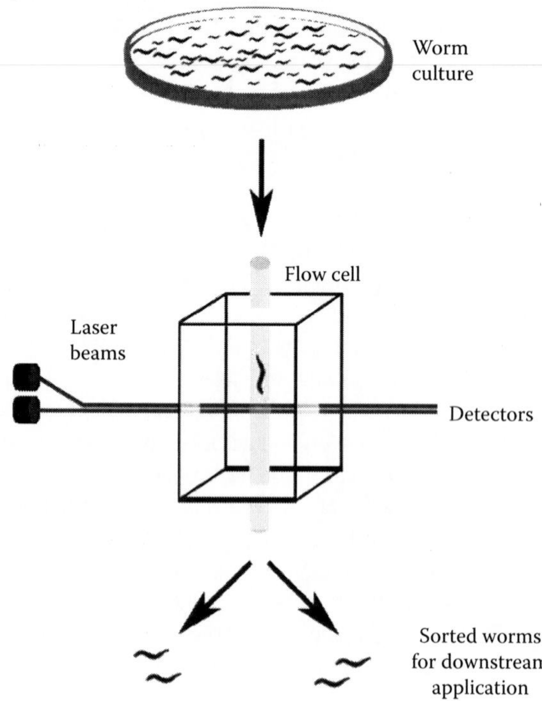

FIGURE 27.2 Principle of BioSorter and COPAS systems. As worms pass through the flow cell, various parameters, such as size and GFP fluorescence, are recorded. Depending on the experiment, animals can be sorted into different categories.

in a rapid, high-throughput, automated, and cost-effective manner. This has been a major impediment in the widespread use of *C. elegans* in drug discovery. Recently, microfluidic techniques have been developed to overcome some of these limitations.

Microfluidics is the science of understanding and controlling fluid flow at a microscale level. It offers numerous advantages over manual and robotic methods such as rapid analysis, reduced chemical consumption, lower cost, and automation. Due to their miniature size, microfluidic structures confer great precision in visualizing and quantifying biological processes in living systems. For example, microfluidics has been used in genetic and proteomic analyses [80,81], cell cytometry [82], cellular biosensors [83], cell chemotaxis [84], and cell culture [85]. Drug discovery is one of the areas where microfluidics is expected to have enormous impact [86–90].

27.5 MICROFLUIDIC AND MINIATURIZED APPROACHES APPLIED TO *C. ELEGANS*

As discussed above, the microfluidic approach offers several advantages over traditional plate-based and macrorobotic methods in *C. elegans* HTS applications. As a result, several worm-specific devices have been developed in recent years for more precise and quantitative analysis of biological processes [91–93]. Due to their tiny size, low cost, and design flexibility, these devices have facilitated a number of experiments related to behavior, *in vivo* imaging of neuronal activity, culturing, sorting and screening, and *in vivo* studies of neuronal regeneration. This section summarizes the current status of microdevices and their applications.

27.5.1 MINIATURIZED FORCE-SENSING DEVICES

Microdevices have been used recently to study physical parameters in live worms as they interact with the environment. One of the setups incorporated a two-axis microstrain gauge-force sensor to measure mechanical interaction forces generated by moving worms [94] (Figure 27.3a and b). The device consisted of an active force-sensing SU8 pillar, located on cantilevers junction center, surrounded by four passive pillars. Using a Wheatstone bridge configuration, four strain sensors at the base of the cantilevers measured the forces generated by a worm, which was found to be in a micro-Newton range (2.5 ± 2.5 μN). In most cases, the contact time between the worm and the pillar was less than 500 ms. Although brief, this interaction was sufficient to evoke a behavioral response demonstrating the efficiency of the neuronal circuit.

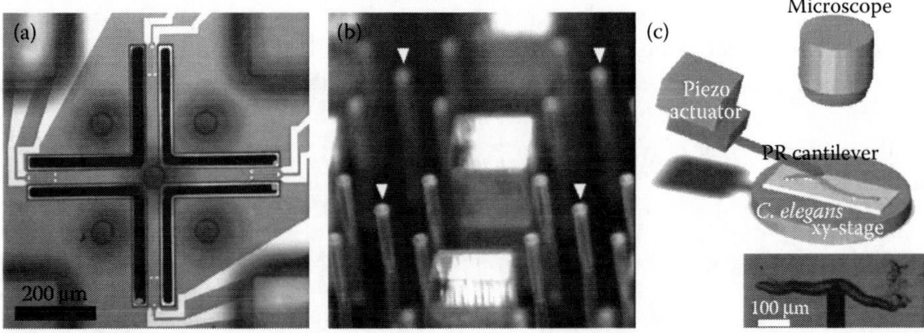

FIGURE 27.3 Force-sensing microdevices for *C. elegans*. (a, b) A MEMS device for measuring locomotion-generated force [94]. (a) A cross-shaped bridge with a fabricated force sensing SU8 pillar at the center (shown by white arrows in (b) and four surrounding passive pillars. Each bridge is connected to a strain gauge at the other end forming a Wheatstone bridge configuration. (c) A piezoresistive cantilever-based sensor [95]. An actual image of a worm under compression beneath the cantilever actuator is shown on the bottom. (Copyright ©, The Royal Society of Chemistry 2009 (a and b) and National Academy of Sciences USA 2007 (c).)

In another study, the mechanical property of the *C. elegans* cuticle was measured by a piezoresistive cantilever (Si) force–displacement sensor [95] (Figure 27.3c). A piezoresistive material exhibits electrical resistance change in response to mechanical stress. The worms were glued at the head and tail just beneath the cantilever tip. Forces were applied through the cantilever tip on the worm cuticle and the stiffness was measured through the electrical resistance change in the piezoresistive material at the root of the cantilever. It was found that the force–displacement curve of the *C. elegans* body is linear that can be modeled as a cylindrical shell with an internal hydrostatic pressure. Using this model, it was estimated that the *C. elegans* cuticle has an effective elastic modulus on the order of 380 MPa. Reducing the internal hydrostatic pressure (by cuticle puncturing using a sharp tip or by hyperosmotic shock) had only a modest influence (~20% reduction) on animals' stiffness, suggesting that the cuticle proteins may also contribute to stiffness of the body. Consistent with this, mutants with altered body shape and cuticle structure had significant effect on stiffness. It was therefore concluded that the overall body stiffness is contributed by both cuticle stiffness and the internal hydrostatic pressure.

27.5.2 Devices Consisting of Microstructured Environments

Unlike in the laboratory where *C. elegans* is grown on a simple agar-based media, the natural habitat of the animal is far more complex that consists of soil, compost, and numerous microorganisms. Therefore, it has evolved a highly sophisticated nervous system to recognize external stimuli and generate an appropriate (attraction and repulsion) response. In order to study such behaviors, researchers have fabricated microdevices that mimic soil-like environments. One of these consisted of agar-based microstructures in the form of an array of squared centered posts or grids [96]. The device was filled with a buffer solution and worms were allowed to swim and crawl in this microenvironment. It was observed that the wild-type worms moved faster in the grid whereas mutants such as *unc-29*, which exhibit abnormal sinusoidal movement, were severely compromised. Additional testing of two mechanosensory mutants, *mec-4* and *mec-10*, revealed defects in movement, thus revealing the role of the mechanosensory neurons in sensing obstacles in the environment and directing the movement of the animal. It is therefore possible to use this device in a genetic screen to identify genes involved in mechanosensation.

Two other microstructured devices were also described that consisted of cylindrical posts and a sinusoidal channel [97]. The cylindrical posts-containing device, called "artificial dirt," had variable post diameters (100–500 μm) and interspacing (60–100 μm). This device was used to study the crawling behavior of the worm. The movement of animals in the device was undulatory with dorsoventral bends, similar to the control model trajectory pattern on the agar surface, although the frequency of sinusoidal body posture was reduced compared to the agar gel. Topographic changes in the artificial dirt device were reported to have minimal effect on animals' crawling behavior (0.14 ± 0.017 mm/s speed in the case of 0.1 mm post diameter and 0.1 mm interspacing compared to 0.2 ± 0.25 mm/s speed on the agar surface). The sinusoidal channel device was used to study the waveform and trajectory of crawling worms, and the amplitude and wavelength of motion were quantified.

27.5.3 Growth-Chamber-Based Devices

Another type of microfluidic design incorporates growth chambers to culture and monitor worms for a longer duration. One such system that was developed earlier had the shape of a compact disc (CD) with enclosed chambers in which worms could be kept alive for more than a week [98]. Since this time period is enough to support growth for 2–3 generations, the device is useful to carry out a broad range of genetic, biochemical, and pharmacological experiments in a precise and controlled manner. The platform contains interconnected cultivation, nutrient, and waste chambers that are arranged in a row in an axial direction of a CD (Figure 27.4a). Upon rotation of the CD, nutrients

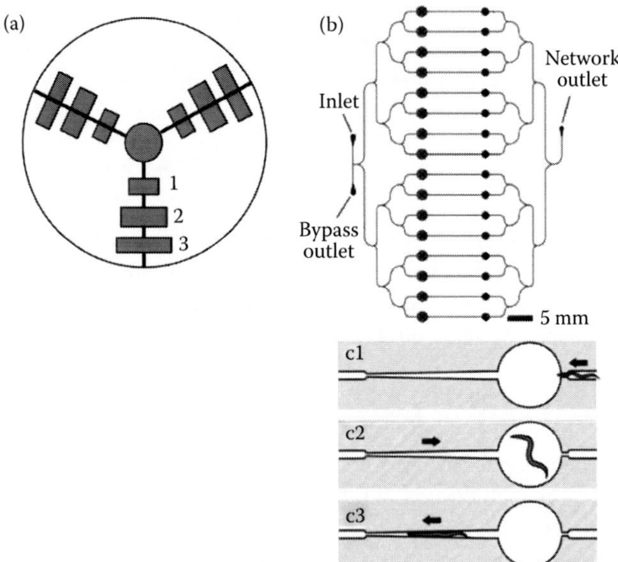

FIGURE 27.4 Microfluidic devices consisting of growth chambers. (a) A CD format device that has three interconnected chambers (1: nutrient, 2: cultivation, and 3: waste). (b, c1–c3) An array format device [99]. (b) The left and right circles represent valves (to control liquid flow from the inlet to the outlets) and microchambers, respectively. (c1) The right end of the channel is just wide enough to allow entry of an early L4 stage animal. (c2) As the worm grows it is unable to escape the chamber. (c3) For observation purposes the worm can be immobilized into the narrow region of the middle channel. The arrows in B2 and B3 mark the direction of the liquid flow. (Copyright ©, The Royal Society of Chemistry 2010 (b, c1–c3).)

are pumped into the cultivation chamber while the waste is ejected to the outer chamber via centrifugal force-driven fluid mechanics. A single hermaphrodite placed in the cultivation chamber was able to reproduce after 3 days. The animals continued to reproduce till day 9 (1100 worms per chamber) indicating that the population was viable and fertile. After day 9, the chambers were saturated and many worms entered into the dauer stage due to the lack of nutrients and overcrowding. The effect of cultivation conditions on worms' health was determined by measuring the body bending frequency. The compact and fully automated design of the device is highly suitable for studies requiring long-term observations of behavior and reproduction.

Hulme et al. [99] recently reported a microfluidic device containing an array of tapered channels for long-term culturing and phenotypic analysis of worms (Figures 27.4b, c1–c3). In this device channels are connected to microchambers at one end to allow individual worms to be cultured over an extended period of time. By directing the worm into the tapered channel (via liquid flow), it could be immobilized for visualization. Reversing the liquid flow forces the animal to return to the growth chamber. The survival and growth of the animal are ensured by a continuous supply of bacterial solution and removal of the waste. In this process, the embryos and newborn worms are also removed, thereby avoiding overcrowding and ensuring that growth chambers contain only adult animals. The parallel design of channels is suitable for HTS of chemicals to study changes in the growth and life span of animals.

In addition to fabricating microdevices of polydimethylsiloxane (PDMS) material as described above, researchers have also used liquid microdroplets as isolated chambers for worms. Due to their tiny size, the droplets provide unparalleled control and sensitivity in biochemical and molecular biological assays while reducing the cost of reagents. In a study focused on the viability and growth, *C. elegans* eggs were compartmentalized in small aqueous culture vessels (plugs) of 660 nL volume within a piece of tubing using perfluorocarbon oil as a carrier [100]. The eggs hatched into larvae in 2 days and within 4 days adults were able to reproduce and survive inside plugs for up to 6 days.

An application of droplet-based growth of worms could be to study the effect of chemicals on neuronal development and behavior. This was demonstrated by the use of MPP+ (an active metabolite of neurotoxin MPTP) in droplets (16–20 nL volume) that were generated by *n*-hexadecane oil as a shearing agent [101]. The effect of MPP+ in humans and other animal models, including *C. elegans*, has been described in detail [59,60,102]. It causes degeneration of dopamine neurons leading to PD-like symptoms (see Section 27.3.2.3). The introduction of MPP+ in droplets affected the activity of animals as measured by stroke frequency (2.6 Hz compared to 3.1 Hz in control animals). Additionally, exposed animals were frequently frozen in omega shape and exhibited reduced movement. Thus, the microdroplet system could be used for chemical screening in worms.

27.5.4 Microfluidic Devices for Immobilization

One of the main challenges in observing worms in liquid environment is their continuous motion. This severely limits high-resolution imaging to analyze cellular processes, perform microsurgery, and characterize certain behavioral processes. The traditional methods of immobilization such as those involving chemicals to paralyze animals or glue to irreversibly bond them to a surface are slow and harmful, and hence not suitable in high-throughput experiments. In contrast, microfluidic systems employ several methods to immobilize worms in a rapid, efficient, and reversible manner to facilitate such experiments. Two of these, vacuum suction channels and the inflatable PDMS membrane layer inside the channel, can physically hold the worms. The other methods include temperature-based control to reduce swimming and body motion, and anesthetic such as carbon dioxide (CO_2). In the following sections we briefly discuss various applications of the immobilization-based approach in carrying out genetic and cell biological studies.

27.5.4.1 Behavioral Studies

The optical transparency of *C. elegans* and its relatively simple nervous system have greatly aided the analysis of neuronal function in mediating behavior. While the traditional plate-based approach is quite successful [103,104], it is not suited for single worm and single neuron-based studies due to the small size of the animals and a lack of spatial and temporal control over stimulus delivery. The microfluidic approach can overcome these limitations. Recently, two microfluidic devices, olfactory and behavior chips [105], were developed to examine the activity of certain neurons that mediate movement and odor sensing (olfaction). The behavior chip, consisting of a simple PDMS microchannel, has wide ends to allow worms to freely enter into the channel. The middle region is only slightly wider than young adults allowing them to squeeze inside but narrow down at one end to prevent them from escaping (Figure 27.5a). Thus, a trapped worm has little room to wiggle its body sideways but the head can move freely. Because of this design, the sinusoidal waves generated by the worm can propagate along its body. This setup was used to measure the activity of a pair of neurons known as AVA that are major command neurons mediating backward locomotion. The findings not only confirmed the role of AVA neurons in reversal behavior but also revealed the precise duration of their activity.

The olfactory chip, also made of PDMS, consisted of a tapered microchannel (wedge shaped) to trap the worm. One end of this trap is just wide enough to allow the worm's head to protrude out of the channel. This configuration allows the nose of a worm to be exposed to chemicals that are supplied through a set of four channels (Figure 27.5b and c). This setup provides spatial and temporal control over chemical exposure that is not possible in a standard plate-based experiment. Additionally, the system allows rapid and efficient recovery of animals. The analysis of ASH neurons (that respond to various stimuli such as mechanical, osmotic, and chemical) in such a setup revealed new roles when exposed to an osmotic stimulus. These results demonstrate the power of microfluidic chips to understand the precise roles of neurons and how neuronal activity modulates behavior.

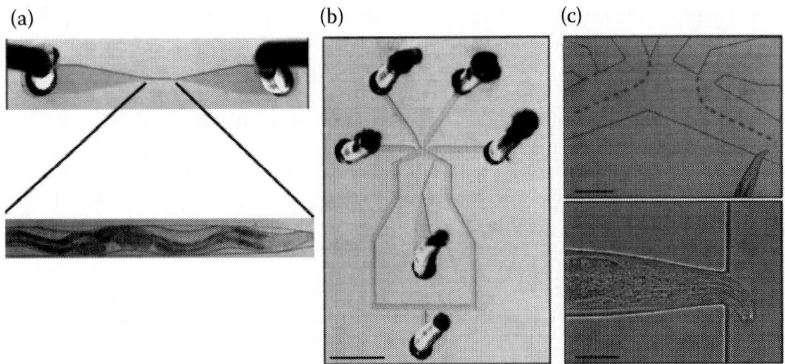

FIGURE 27.5 Microfluidic chips for analyzing behavioral and olfactory responses in *C. elegans*, modified from [105]. (a) The "behavior" chip for studying neuronal activity in locomotion. The worm is trapped in the narrow region in the middle. (b) The "olfactory" chip design. (c) A close-up view of the olfactory chip showing the head region of an immobilized worm. The dotted lines mark the interfaces between the fluids. (Copyright ©, Nature Publishing Group 2007.)

27.5.4.2 Screening and Sorting Worms

Over the years, the methods of phenotyping and mutant screening in *C. elegans* have matured from exclusively using morphological and behavioral criteria to combining them with fluorescent markers, such as GFP, to obtain detailed information on morphologies of cells and subcellular structures. While these approaches provide valuable information, the entire process of screening animals is manual and therefore slow, serial, and subjective. Robotic systems such as Biosorter (see Section 27.4.2.2) provide a good alternative but a number of factors limit their usage. In order to address this, several laboratories are developing microfluidic systems with varying degree of automation and throughput.

A majority of the microfluidic devices that have been described use a pressure-based immobilization approach. One of these consists of suction ports (narrow channels with diameter less than an adult worm) located perpendicular to the main channel that carries worms [106] (Figure 27.6). The application of suction through these ports physically immobilizes an animal. The medium inside the main channel can be exchanged allowing new worms to be introduced into the channel. An advanced version of this setup consists of multiple parallel microchambers each of which is capable of

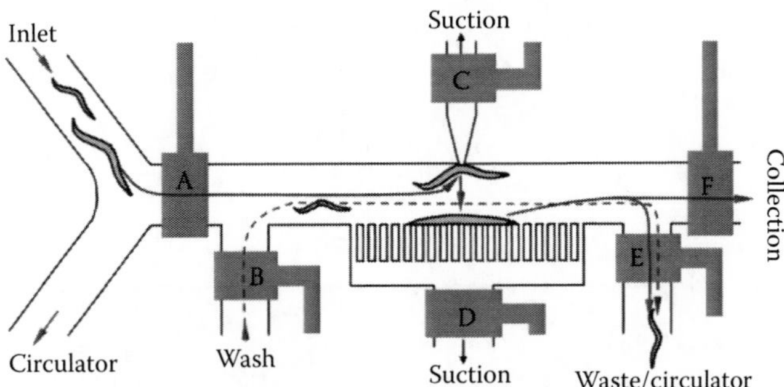

FIGURE 27.6 A microfluidic device to immobilize worms using side suction channels [106]. Worms enter the main channel from the left inlet. A–F mark different valves to direct the flow of worms. For high-resolution imaging, animals are briefly captured in the middle region by pneumatic valves applied suction pressure. The dotted line shows the direction through which worms are flushed during channel washing. (Copyright ©, National Academy of Sciences USA 2007.)

immobilizing worms by suction to facilitate subcellular imaging and sorting. In order to enable screening of chemicals and RNAi libraries, the microchamber device could be connected to an interface chip consisting of an array of aspiration tips. When lowered in a microwell plate, the aspiration tips draw minute quantity of media from individual wells and deliver to worms in microchambers. This integrated system promises to accelerate the screening of a large number of animals and chemicals in a high-throughput manner.

Chung et al. [107] reported a modified version of the above-mentioned suction-based immobilization approach by incorporating a temperature control mechanism to allow high-resolution imaging and screening. The worms were first positioned in the detection zone by suction and then rapidly cooled to 4°C (within ~2 s). The two levels of control proved to be highly effective in complete immobilization of animals, thus allowing detailed examination of neuronal processes. The entire procedure of worm handling and imaging was automated and shown to have a much higher resolution compared to other microfluidic-based screening devices.

The flexibility of the PDMS polymer offers possibilities to immobilize worms in different ways. One such approach involves the use of compressible microchambers in which worms are held in place by physical trapping. Such a microfluidic system typically consists of a bilayered channel that contains pressurized air in the top layer and worms in liquid in the bottom layer. The layers are separated by a thin flexible PDMS membrane that deflects downward as the pressure in the top layer is increased, thus confining the worm to a very small region and effectively trapping it (Figure 27.7). A microfluidic chip consisting of this control mechanism was recently used to screen for mutants in a high-throughput manner [108]. The device had three arms, one of which (main arm) was used to load, immobilize, and image worms. The other two arms were used to collect nonmutant (wild type) and mutant animals. The screening and sorting were aided by a computer to facilitate opening and closing of channel valves to direct worm flow. It was demonstrated that the device could screen worms at a sustained rate of 1500/h.

Another type of pressure-based device, developed by Hulme et al. [109], consisted of a tapered (wedge-shaped) channel that acts as a clamp. The flow of the liquid through the channel (toward the narrow end) forces a worm to move down the channel until it gets physically confined in the narrow region. A device consisting of 128 such parallel channels was shown to distribute and immobilize worms in less than 15 min [109]. The device allows high-resolution imaging of cell morphology using GFP markers and is suitable for HTS of a large number of animals.

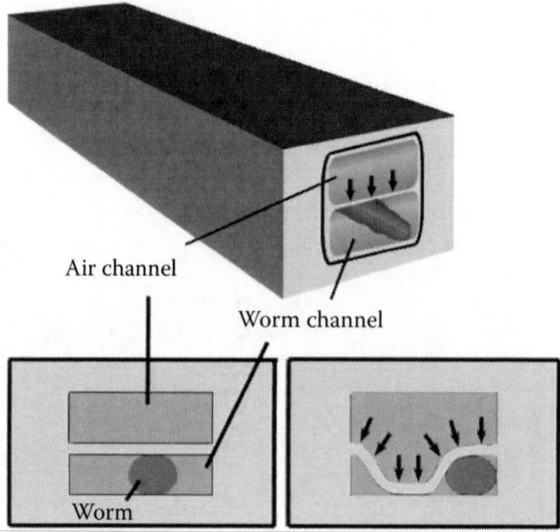

FIGURE 27.7 Schematic drawings of a two-layered microfluidic device for immobilization of *C. elegans*. The middle layer consists of a deflectable PDMS membrane that, in the presence of compressed air in the top channel, bends downward and physically wraps the worm in the bottom channel.

Finally, a different kind of immobilization approach involves the use of an anesthetic CO_2. Unlike the pressure-based approach, which is appropriate for only a short period (few minutes), CO_2 has the advantage of keeping animals immobile for a much longer duration (up to 2.5 h) without any apparent defect in their behavior [110]. Furthermore, it is relatively easy to introduce CO_2 in the PDMS-based channel as it diffuses within 1–2 min and almost completely immobilizes the animals. This makes it an attractive method that could facilitate high-throughput worm screening.

27.5.4.3 Laser-Assisted Microsurgery

Immobilization of *C. elegans* in a microfluidic channel provides a powerful means to perform surgical operations without the need of chemicals and agar gel pad mounting. Because it is possible to recover operated animals and image them in the channel over extended periods of time, the microfluidic approach offers unparalleled flexibility and control to explore subcellular structures and nerve regeneration processes *in vivo* [111].

Nearly all immobilization approaches discussed above (Section 27.5.4.2) have been used to perform laser-assisted ablations of neuronal processes. The suction pressure-based device developed by Rohde et al. [106] was successfully used to sever the axon of a touch neuron and the process of regeneration was monitored subsequently. Guo et al. [112] and Zeng et al. [113] performed similar operations using a bilayered microchannel design consisting of a flexible PDMS middle layer (Figure 27.7). While both approaches appear to work efficiently, the bilayered system may offer a better control as animals are completely surrounded by the membrane and have no room to wiggle.

The tapered channel design, which was earlier developed by Hulme et al. [109] for phenotyping and screening, has also been adopted in surgical experiments. Allen et al. [114] used a variation of this design in a microfluidic chip consisting of several parallel two-stage taper channels, each having a wide region to load worms and a shallow taper to immobilize animals. The worms were recovered after surgery and the process of nerve development was examined by time-lapse imaging.

While the above-mentioned pressure-based devices are quite successful, they can cause physical damage to worms due to excessive compression resulting in death of some of the animals. In order to overcome this limitation, Chung and Lu [115] developed a temperature-based microfluidic system. Their device consisted of two parallel channels that function independently to allow simultaneous worm-loading and exiting. The diameter and length of channels were comparable to the L1 worm (~14 μm and ~190 μm, respectively) to allow precise fit into the channel. A wide temperature control channel located perpendicular to worm channels rapidly cooled the animals such that they were completely immobilized. Specific neurons were ablated using a computer-based automated imaging and laser guiding system. Because of the automation, the setup can perform ablations in a high-throughput manner, something that is not possible with the traditional manual method.

27.5.5 Stimulus-Based Devices

The flexibility of the design, operation, and integration of microfluidic devices has led to new applications in *C. elegans*-related research. One of these deals with the use of stimuli to manipulate the movement of animals for behavioral and physiological studies (e.g., [116]). In spite of having a relatively simple nervous system [117], *C. elegans* responds to a diverse range of stimuli and exhibits both attractive and repulsive responses. The stimuli are detected by amphid sensory neurons in the head region that are exposed to the outside at the base of the lips [103]. Although how environmental cues are processed by these neurons leading to altered movement is not fully understood, movement serves as an important readout to dissect the neuronal network and signaling. Hence, a stimulus-based microfluidic system could serve as a powerful tool to study movement-related neuronal disorders in *C. elegans* disease models.

Chemotaxis studies in worms have identified certain chemicals that elicit robust movement (attractive and repulsive) response. A few other nonchemical agents such as light, temperature, and electric field induce a similar behavior. Thus, one or more of these stimuli may be used to manipulate the movement of worms. In the following, we first summarize the utility of these agents in a microfluidic environment and then discuss one of these, that is, electric field, in detail.

27.5.5.1 Types of Stimuli

Chemicals: *C. elegans* can detect several types of volatile (e.g., alcohols, esters, and aldehydes) and water-soluble (e.g., cations, anions, cyclic nucleotides, and amino acids) chemicals that are associated with food and other sources [103]. Compared to water-soluble chemicals that do not diffuse easily and therefore are likely to be used for short-range chemotaxis, volatile odors rapidly diffuse through air due to their small size and can be detected at a very low concentration range (picomolar) making them suitable for long-range chemotaxis.

In spite of the diversity of chemical compounds detected by *C. elegans*, several factors limit the application of the chemotaxis-based approach to manipulate worm movement in a microfluidic setup. These include a lack of control over chemical gradient, variability in chemosensory response of the animals, and sensory adaptation.

Oxygen: Oxygen is necessary for the development and survival of *C. elegans* [118]. Under aerobic conditions, it is typically required in mitochondria to carry out metabolic function. In the absence of oxygen (anoxia), worms cease movement and any development. This arrested state can last for several hours without any significant damage to tissues and physiological processes and, when supplied with oxygen, the animals resume normal function.

The microfluidics approach has been used to study oxygen sensation and behavioral changes in worms. It has been found that animals strongly avoid lower (<2%) and higher (>12%) oxygen levels and prefer to live within a range of 5–12% concentration [119]. Although potentially useful, oxygen is not suitable as a stimulus to control movement of animals in a microfluidic setup because the response is variable and not fully penetrant.

Light: The response of *C. elegans* to light, known as phototaxis, has been studied in some detail [120,121]. It was found that although *C. elegans* does not possess eyes, it senses light stimulus via ciliated amphid neurons and demonstrates repulsive reactions to it in a dose-dependent manner. Although ultraviolet-A, violet, and blue lights appeared to be most sensitive and induced reversals within few seconds, prolonged exposures (15 min) were detrimental, causing paralysis and death. In comparison, the repulsive response to green light was mild, low penetrant, and no paralysis was observed in 20 min exposure. Thus, while the phototactic response is rapid, because of its lethal effect (in the case of UV-A, violet, and blue lights) and low response (in the case of green light) it does not appear to be suitable to manipulate worm movement in a microfludic setup.

Magnetic field: Magnetic field is another nonchemical agent whose effect has been studied in *C. elegans*. Exposure to both static magnetic fields (SMFs) and alternating current magnetic fields (ACMFs) induces a range of phenotypes. Bessho et al. [122] used ACMFs up to 1.7 Teslas (T) to intermittently expose growing worms and found that it caused a small but significant decrease in the growth and reproduction. The animals also showed reduced pharyngeal pumping and abnormal locomotion but these changes were transient and reversible. Similar to ACMFs, SMFs also have a range of effects on worms. Exposure of worms to 200 mT reduces their life-span and fertility [123]. SMFs have also been shown to affect gene expression as determined by real-time PCR and microarray experiments [123,124], thus linking developmental defects to molecular changes. While these studies highlight the effect of magnetic field on worms, there is no indication that it could serve as a stimulus to guide worms in a microfluidic channel.

Electric field: Electrical potential has long been reported to influence the movement of nematodes [125,126]. In 1978, Sukul and Croll [127] showed for the first time that *C. elegans* exhibits electrotaxis behavior. Subsequent studies showed that worms exposed to a direct current (DC) electric field on the open agar gel surface swam toward the cathode electrode (negative pole) at an angle that was proportional to the field strength (15°–60° range) [128]. Genetic experiments have revealed that electrotaxis is mediated by certain amphid neurons (mainly ASJ and ASH, and to a lesser extent AWB, AWC, and ASK) since their removal abolishes this behavior [128]. Although the mechanism of electric field response is unknown, the signal may mimic external stimuli that excite sensory neurons. This could lead to the generation of an electrical signal that propagates to other neurons and muscles, ultimately affecting movement of the animal. However, why such a response causes cathode-driven movement is unclear. Recently, a DC electric field was tested as a stimulus in a microchannel setup (Figure 27.8a) and was found to be highly effective in inducing movement in worms [129]. In spite of the long exposure of the field (10 min. or more) the animals continued to swim and appeared normal, suggesting that this approach could be useful in movement-based HTS in a microfluidic setup.

27.5.5.2 Electric Field as a Stimulus in a Microfluidic System

Among the stimuli described above, the electric field is the only signal that appears to be harmless to worms at a low voltage yet generates a directional movement response in a microfluidic system. A low-voltage electric field (2–13 V/cm) in the axial direction of the buffer-filled channel (Figure 27.8a) has been shown to stimulate animals to move toward the negative pole (cathode) [129]. This behavior appears to be primarily mediated by neurons, and to some extent muscles, since mutations affecting these cell types failed to show a normal response. Most importantly, the effect is fully penetrant, immediate, and benign.

Further analysis of the electrotactic response in channels revealed that it is exhibited by worms that are L2 stage and older. While the speed of movement increases, as animals grow older, for a given stage it is independent of the electric field strength (Figure 27.8b). Changing the direction of the electric field causes the animals to immediately turn back and resume motion in the reverse orientation. These findings suggest that the electric field could be used as a stimulus in HTS of chemicals and gene targets in *C. elegans* neuronal disease models.

In addition to the DC field, the response of worms to an alternating current (AC) electric field has also been characterized. Interestingly, symmetric square wave AC fields of 1 Hz frequency and higher were found to effectively localize worms in the channel (Figure 27.8c) [130]. Such a property of the AC field offers several attractive possibilities. For example, new kinds of microfluidic devices could be fabricated that combine both DC and AC fields to manipulate the movement of worms as desired.

27.6 MICROFLUIDIC HTS OF CHEMICALS AND GENE TARGETS IN *C. ELEGANS*

As discussed above, the ease and low cost of culturing make *C. elegans* an ideal whole animal model for drug discovery but its widespread use is hampered by a lack of robust automated high-throughput methods to quantify behavioral and cellular changes. Microfluidics offers advantages in overcoming these limitations but more work is needed to develop and test new systems and make them commercially available to end users for routine applications. Because microfluidic devices will be primarily used in HTSs, they need to be robust and working efficiently over hundreds of thousands of cycles without breaking down. Furthermore, in cases where live worms are to be handled, it is necessary that the device must not cause any harm while the worms are being treated and examined (such as microsurgery and genetic screens). In addition, certain types of experiments require following worms over a period of time (e.g., after feeding a chemical), and therefore the device must be capable of keeping them alive, capture images at defined time points, and transfer data to a computer for analysis. This will require development of integrated microfluidic devices that consist of various components to automate culturing of worms, arraying them in a desired manner, dispensing chemicals and other materials at precise concentrations, incubating them in microchambers, and capturing and analyzing data, all in a seamless manner. Some of the automated methods such as those used for accurately dispensing small quantities of chemicals, proteins, and genetic materials could be adopted more or less directly from the existing HTS platform. Additionally,

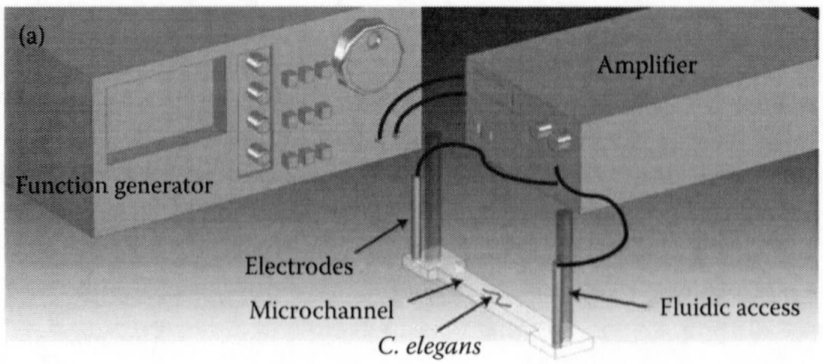

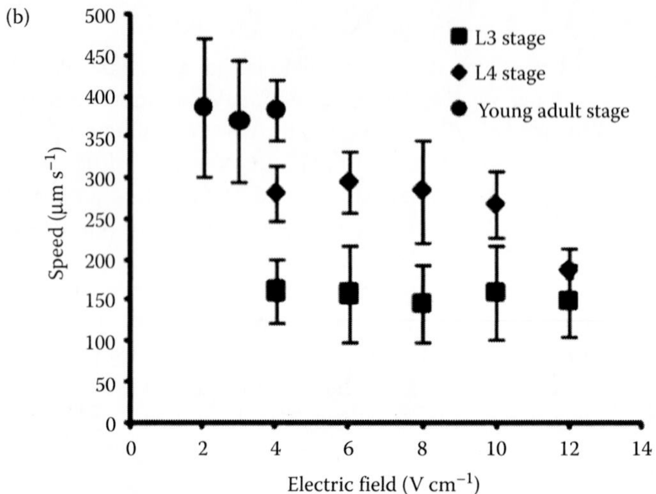

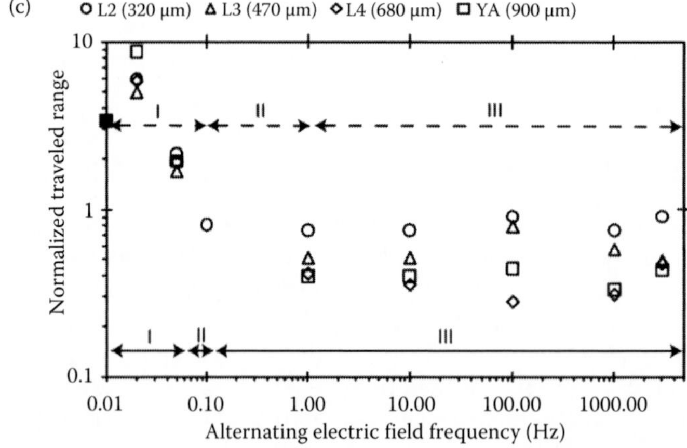

FIGURE 27.8 Electrotactic response of *C. elegans* in a microfluidic channel setup. (a) The device consisting of a function generator connected to an amplifier to set desired output electric fields (DC or AC), a PDMS-embedded microchannel with electrodes, and fluidic access tubes at channel reservoirs. (b) The relationship between the speed of worms and the electric field strength, at different developmental stage [129]. (c) The response of worms in the presence of AC electric fields, modified from [130]. Different stages of wild-type animals are shown. Three regions of response on increase in the frequency are: (1) DC-like responses toward the cathode due to the long duration of each cycle. (2) Unidirectional movement toward the initial direction of swimming. (III) Localization. (Copyrights ©, The Royal Society of Chemistry 2010 (b) and The American Institute of Physics 2010 (c).)

recently developed microfluidic methods to incorporate hundreds of valves and pumps and their individual control could be used to lower the cost of fluid handling automation [131]. The control, transport, immobilization, and dispensing of worms could involve implementation of many of the existing microfluidic techniques [132].

In recent years, several new applications of microfluidics in *C. elegans* have emerged that include phenotypic sorting, cell ablations, drug exposure, and behavioral studies [105–107,109,112]. Because of their focus on imaging cells and/or certain regions of the worm, they rely on pneumatics to immobilize animals. These devices have been successful in automating some steps and providing an increased throughput that is not possible with traditional manual approaches. While advantageous in many applications, they are not suitable to study movement behaviors of worms in the absence of an external force. In this respect, an electric field-based microfluidic approach promises to be useful as it offers a convenient method to control movement [129,130]. Furthermore, since the movement relies on coordinated activities of neurons and muscles, it provides strong support to the idea that a microfluidic device incorporating electric field control mechanism may accelerate the study of movement-related disorders (e.g., HD, PD, and DMD) in worm models. This stimulus-based approach will benefit from a number of factors that favor the use of the electric field in a microfluidic environment. These include easy and inexpensive setup, instantaneous on/off control, no gradient or decay over time, compatibility with liquid culture media, scalability, and the ability to induce movement in a desired direction without sensory adaptation. The ongoing work in our laboratories has shown that the electrotaxis behavior is a highly sensitive measure of the function of neurons and muscles since any defect can be quickly revealed in a microfluidic assay in the form of reduced speed, altered body bends, and sporadic pauses. Therefore, we believe that the microfluidic electrotaxis approach could serve as a powerful tool to facilitate high-throughput study of *C. elegans* disease models, identify molecular changes and genetic pathways, and screen for chemicals/drugs as candidates for potential treatment options.

In order for the electric field-based microfluidic device to facilitate HTS, it will be necessary to automate the analysis of *C. elegans* movement. Currently, this is done by manual examination of captured images. Although some software automation is possible, this process is data intensive, time consuming, and a key bottleneck in increasing the throughput of the experiment. Electrical sensors to quantify position and speed of the worm needs to be developed so that multiplexing technology that is already in existence could be used to parallelize the measurement process. One approach is to implement electrical impedance sensors [133,134] to detect the position of the worm and calculate its velocity. Another method is to use optical wave guiding technology to microfabricate optical sensors [135–137]. Having two sets of position detectors, at the beginning and end of the microchannel, will reveal the presence of the worm at detector locations as it moves in response to an electric field. This information, when fed to a computer, could easily allow determination of the speed of the worm.

Any plan involving development of HTS microfluidic systems cannot afford to ignore the importance of imaging and data processing components. Automated high-resolution image capture and robust analysis is crucial for the success of high-throughput experiments. Although in some cases visual analysis could be done, the power of the system will only be fully utilized if most decisions were performed in an automated manner. This means that the imaging software must be highly trainable to distinguish between broad ranges of phenotypes to be screened and should be capable of performing such operations in real time, mostly in a user-independent manner. Depending on the type of experiments, both bright-field and fluorescent images will require processing. Typically, such images are acquired by a differential interference contrast (DIC) fluorescence microscope connected to a digital or video camera. Currently, there is no real substitute of it, CMOS lensless imaging technology may hold promise in some future microfluidic systems. The main advantages of CMOS sensors are high-speed image acquisition (that lowers the effect of inherent motion in worms), small size, and low cost of design and operation compared to standard microscopes. This has led to the development of a few prototypes in recent years. For example, a miniaturized CMOS video camera device was earlier shown to be capable of acquiring shadow images of worms grown in a liquid media inside polycarbonate microchambers [138]. Another lensless device, termed as optofluidic microscopy (OFM), was also developed for high-resolution on-chip imaging [139,140]. The OFMs incorporated a microflow to deliver worms over a series of microapertures fabricated on a metal-coated CMOS sensor to generate direct projection images. Yet another device was described earlier this year that captures both monochrome and colored images of worms over a field-of-view of more than 24 mm^2 [141]. This was done by recording animals using incoherent in-line holography and digitally reconstructing diffraction holograms to create the entire image. In summary, the CMOS sensor approach appears to work for *C. elegans*, raising the possibility that it could become a viable imaging option in future microfluidic applications.

27.7 CONCLUDING REMARKS

Microfluidic technology offers many advantages to address problems in basic and applied biology. While the field is still evolving, a number of successful applications have emerged that involve cells, microorganisms, and tiny animals such as *C. elegans*. In this review we have highlighted discoveries and novel microfluidic approaches for *C. elegans*. These studies have revealed that one of the key areas where *C. elegans* could make a significant contribution is drug discovery and drug target analysis. As a whole animal model that is amenable to manipulations in a microfluidic setup, *C. elegans* allows HTS of chemicals in a physiologically relevant manner. Given that the worm has many human counterparts, and several of these mediate conserved biological processes, it could accelerate identification of potential drug targets, thereby facilitating testing in higher animal models, and eventually in humans. Furthermore, *C. elegans* offers advanced genetic and genomic tools to identify drug action and potential side effects that could be utilized to accelerate the process of drug discovery.

In recent years, several microfluidic and miniaturized devices have been designed to handle *C. elegans*. All of these have demonstrated the potential to probe worms in a manner that is not feasible by traditional manual protocols. Using these devices the phenotypes of animals could be precisely and quantitatively characterized. Additionally, they provide a suitable format to handle a large number of animals individually and in parallel, thus accelerating the study of biological processes. These advantages make microfluidic devices ideal for high-throughput applications to identify drugs and gene targets in *C. elegans* disease models. The work in our own laboratories has shown that the electric field-based microfluidic system could serve as a powerful tool to manipulate the movement of worms and facilitate the study of movement-related disorders. While this is promising, there are certain challenges that need to be addressed. In this respect it is satisfying to note that several laboratories are making an effort to overcome some of these limitations, and if the progress in the past one decade is any indication, then there is every hope that microfluidic devices will soon be used in *C. elegans*-based drug discovery.

ACKNOWLEDGMENTS

This work is supported by funds from Early Researcher Award (BPG) and National Science and Engineering Research Council and Ontario Centres of Excellence grants (PRS). We thank Sandhya Koushika (NCBS) for critical reading of the manuscript.

ABBREVIATIONS

6-OHDA	6-Hydroxydopamine
α-syn	α-Synuclein
Aβ	β–Amyloid
AC	Alternate current

ACMF	Alternating current magnetic field
AD	Alzheimer's disease
CD	Compact disc
CMOS	Complementary metal oxide semiconductor
CO_2	Carbon dioxide
COPAS	Complex object parametric analyser and sorter
DA	Dopaminergic neurons
DC	Direct current
DIC	Differential interference contrast
DMD	Duchenne's muscular dystrophy
GABA	γ-Aminobutyric acid
GFP	Green fluorescent protein
HD	Huntinton's disease
htn	Huntingtin
HTS	High-throughput screening
LB	Lewy body
MPP^+	1-Methyl-4-phenylpyridinium
MPTP	1-Methyl-4-phenyl-1,2,3,6-tetrahydropyridine
MTR	Mithramycin
NMDA	*N*-methyl-d-aspartic acid
OFM	Optofluidic microscopy
PD	Parkinson's disease
PDMS	Polydimethylsiloxane
Poly-Q	Poly-glutamine
RNAi	RNA interference
SMF	Static magnetic field
TSA	Trichostatin A

REFERENCES

1. Drews, II. 2000. Drug discovery today and tomorrow. *Drug Discov Today* 5: 2–4.
2. Segalat, L. 2007. Invertebrate animal models of diseases as screening tools in drug discovery. *ACS Chem Biol* 2: 231–236.
3. Johnson, J. R., Jenn, R. C., Barclay, J. W., Burgoyne, R. D., Morgan, A. 2010. *Caenorhabditis elegans*: A useful tool to decipher neurodegenerative pathways. *Biochem Soc Trans* 38: 559–563.
4. Walhout, M., Endoh H., Thierry-Mieg, N., Wong, W., Vidal, M. 1998. A model of elegance. *Am J Hum Genet* 63: 955–961.
5. Dooley, K., Zon, L. I. 2000. Zebrafish: A model system for the study of human disease. *Curr Opin Genet Dev* 10: 252–256.
6. Wolfe, J. H. 2009. Gene therapy in large animal models of human genetic diseases. *Introduction. ILAR J* 50: 107–111.
7. Mather, J. P., Roberts, P. E. 1998. *Introduction to Cell and Tissue Culture: Theory and Technique*. New York: Springer. 260pp.
8. Gulati, R., Simari, R. D. 2009. Defining the potential for cell therapy for vascular disease using animal models. *Dis Model Mech* 2: 130–137.
9. Meyer, M., Vilardell, J. 2009. The quest for a message: Budding yeast, a model organism to study the control of pre-mRNA splicing. *Brief Funct Genomic Proteomic* 8: 60–67.
10. Morgan, D. O. 1997. Cyclin-dependent kinases: Engines, clocks, and microprocessors. *Annu Rev Cell Dev Biol* 13: 261–291.
11. Walberg, M. W. 2000. Applicability of yeast genetics to neurologic disease. *Arch Neurol* 57: 1129–1134.
12. Khurana, V., Lindquist, S. 2010. Modelling neurodegeneration in *Saccharomyces cerevisiae*: Why cook with baker's yeast? *Nat Rev Neurosci* 11: 436–449.

13. Antoshechkin, I., Sternberg, P. W. 2007. The versatile worm: Genetic and genomic resources for *Caenorhabditis elegans* research. *Nat Rev Genet* 8: 518–532.
14. Kaletta, T., Hengartner, M. O. 2006. Finding function in novel targets: *C. elegans* as a model organism. *Nat Rev Drug Discov* 5: 387–398.
15. Baumeister, R., Ge, L. 2002. The worm in us—*Caenorhabditis elegans* as a model of human disease. *Trends Biotechnol* 20: 147–148.
16. Ashrafi, K, Chang, F. Y., Watts, J. L., Fraser, A. G., Kamath, R. S., et al. 2003. Genome-wide RNAi analysis of *Caenorhabditis elegans* fat regulatory genes. *Nature* 421: 268–272.
17. Kwok, T. C., Ricker, N., Fraser, R., Chan, A.W., Burns, A., et al. 2006. A small-molecule screen in *C. elegans* yields a new calcium channel antagonist. *Nature* 441: 91–95.
18. Kirienko, N. V., Mani, K., Fay, D. S. 2010. Cancer models in *Caenorhabditis elegans. Dev Dyn* 239: 1413–1448.
19. Irazoqui, J. E., Urbach, J. M., Ausubel, F. M. 2010. Evolution of host innate defence: Insights from *Caenorhabditis elegans* and primitive invertebrates. *Nat Rev Immunol* 10: 47–58.
20. Voisine, C., Hart, A. C. 2004. *Caenorhabditis elegans* as a model system for triplet repeat diseases. *Methods Mol Biol* 277: 141–160.
21. Lakso, M., Vartiainen, S., Moilanen, A. M., Sirvio, J., Thomas, J. H., et al. 2003. Dopaminergic neuronal loss and motor deficits in *Caenorhabditis elegans* overexpressing human alpha-synuclein. *J Neurochem* 86: 165–172.
22. Jones, A. K., Buckingham, S. D., Sattelle, D. B. 2005. Chemistry-to-gene screens in *Caenorhabditis elegans. Nat Rev Drug Discov* 4: 321–330.
23. van Ham, T. J., Breitling, R., Swertz, M. A., Nollen, E. A. 2009. Neurodegenerative diseases: Lessons from genome-wide screens in small model organisms. *EMBO Mol Med* 1: 360–370.
24. Hoffman, E. P., Brown, R. H., Jr., Kunkel, L. M. 1987. Dystrophin: The protein product of the Duchenne muscular dystrophy locus. *Cell* 51: 919–928.
25. Campbell, K. P. 1995. Three muscular dystrophies: Loss of cytoskeleton-extracellular matrix linkage. *Cell* 80: 675–679.
26. Mariol, M. C., Segalat, L. 2001. Muscular degeneration in the absence of dystrophin is a calcium-dependent process. *Curr Biol* 11: 1691–1694.
27. Mariol, M. C., Martin, E., Chambonnier, L., Segalat, L. 2007. Dystrophin-dependent muscle degeneration requires a fully functional contractile machinery to occur in *C. elegans. Neuromuscul Disord* 17: 56–60.
28. Carre-Pierrat, M., Grisoni, K., Gieseler, K., Mariol, M. C., Martin, E., et al. 2006. The SLO-1 BK channel of *Caenorhabditis elegans* is critical for muscle function and is involved in dystrophin-dependent muscle dystrophy. *J Mol Biol* 358: 387–395.
29. Carre-Pierrat, M., Mariol, M. C., Chambonnier, L., Laugraud, A., Heskia, F., et al. 2006. Blocking of striated muscle degeneration by serotonin in *C. elegans. J Muscle Res Cell Motil* 27: 253–258.
30. Gaud, A., Simon, J. M., Witzel, T., Carre-Pierrat, M., Wermuth, C. G., et al. 2004. Prednisone reduces muscle degeneration in dystrophin-deficient *Caenorhabditis elegans. Neuromuscul Disord* 14: 365–370.
31. Glenner, G. G., Wong, C. W. 1984. Alzheimer's disease: Initial report of the purification and characterization of a novel cerebrovascular amyloid protein. *Biochem Biophys Res Commun* 120: 885–890.
32. Kosik, K. S., Joachim, C. L., Selkoe, D. J. 1986. Microtubule-associated protein tau (tau) is a major antigenic component of paired helical filaments in Alzheimer disease. *Proc Natl Acad Sci USA* 83: 4044–4048.
33. Link, C. D. 1995. Expression of human beta-amyloid peptide in transgenic *Caenorhabditis elegans. Proc Natl Acad Sci USA* 92: 9368–9372.
34. Link, C. D., Taft, A., Kapulkin, V., Duke, K., Kim, S., et al. 2003. Gene expression analysis in a transgenic *Caenorhabditis elegans* Alzheimer's disease model. *Neurobiol Aging* 24: 397–413.
35. Fay, D. S., Fluet, A., Johnson, C. J., Link, C. D. 1998. *In vivo* aggregation of beta-amyloid peptide variants. *J Neurochem* 71: 1616–1625.
36. Kraemer, B, C., Burgess, J. K., Chen, J. H., Thomas, J. H., Schellenberg, G. D. 2006. Molecular pathways that influence human tau-induced pathology in *Caenorhabditis elegans. Hum Mol Genet* 15: 1483–1496.
37. Hassan, W. M., Merin, D. A., Fonte, V., Link, C. D. 2009. AIP-1 ameliorates beta-amyloid peptide toxicity in a *Caenorhabditis elegans* Alzheimer's disease model. *Hum Mol Genet* 18: 2739–2747.
38. Fonte, V., Kapulkin, V., Taft, A., Fluet, A., Friedman, D., et al. 2002. Interaction of intracellular beta amyloid peptide with chaperone proteins. *Proc Natl Acad Sci USA* 99: 9439–9444.

39. Gil, J. M., Rego, A. C. 2008. Mechanisms of neurodegeneration in Huntington's disease. *Eur J Neurosci* 27: 2803–2820.
40. Faber, P. W., Alter, J. R., MacDonald, M. E., Hart, A. C. 1999. Polyglutamine-mediated dysfunction and apoptotic death of a *Caenorhabditis elegans* sensory neuron. *Proc Natl Acad Sci USA* 96: 179–184.
41. Morley, J. F., Brignull, H. R., Weyers, J. J., Morimoto, R. I. 2002. The threshold for polyglutamine-expansion protein aggregation and cellular toxicity is dynamic and influenced by aging in *Caenorhabditis elegans*. *Proc Natl Acad Sci USA* 99: 10417–10422.
42. Satyal, S. H., Schmidt, E., Kitagawa, K., Sondheimer, N., Lindquist, S., et al. 2000. Polyglutamine aggregates alter protein folding homeostasis in *Caenorhabditis elegans*. *Proc Natl Acad Sci USA* 97: 5750–5755.
43. Parker, J. A., Connolly, J. B., Wellington, C., Hayden, M., Dausset, J., et al. 2001. Expanded polyglutamines in *Caenorhabditis elegans* cause axonal abnormalities and severe dysfunction of PLM mechanosensory neurons without cell death. *Proc Natl Acad Sci USA* 98: 13318–13323.
44. Faber, P. W., Voisine, C., King, D. C., Bates, E. A., Hart, A. C. 2002. Glutamine/proline-rich PQE-1 proteins protect *Caenorhabditis elegans* neurons from huntingtin polyglutamine neurotoxicity. *Proc Natl Acad Sci USA*, 99: 17131–17136.
45. Nollen, E. A., Garcia, S. M., van Haaften, G., Kim, S., Chavez, A., et al. 2004. Genome-wide RNA interference screen identifies previously undescribed regulators of polyglutamine aggregation. *Proc Natl Acad Sci USA* 101: 6403–6408.
46. Parker, J. A., Arango, M., Abderrahmane, S., Lambert, E., Tourette, C., et al. 2005. Resveratrol rescues mutant polyglutamine cytotoxicity in nematode and mammalian neurons. *Nat Genet* 37: 349–350.
47. Voisine, C., Varma, H., Walker, N., Bates, E. A., Stockwell, B. R., et al. 2007. Identification of potential therapeutic drugs for huntington's disease using *Caenorhabditis elegans*. *PLoS ONE* 2: e504.
48. Kritzer, J. A., Hamamichi, S., McCaffery, J. M., Santagata, S., Naumann, T. A., et al. 2009. Rapid selection of cyclic peptides that reduce alpha-synuclein toxicity in yeast and animal models. *Nat Chem Biol* 5: 655–663.
49. Kuwahara, T., Koyama A., Koyama S., Yoshina S., Ren C. H., et al. 2008. A systematic RNAi screen reveals involvement of endocytic pathway in neuronal dysfunction in alpha-synuclein transgenic *C. elegans*. *Hum Mol Genet* 17: 2997–3009.
50. Su, L. J., Auluck, P. K., Outeiro, T. F., Yeger-Lotem, E., Kritzer, J. A., et al. 2010. Compounds from an unbiased chemical screen reverse both ER-to-Golgi trafficking defects and mitochondrial dysfunction in Parkinson's disease models. *Dis Model Mech* 3: 194–208.
51. Hamamichi, S., Rivas, R. N., Knight, A. L., Cao, S., Caldwell, K. A., et al. 2008. Hypothesis-based RNAi screening identifies neuroprotective genes in a Parkinson's disease model. *Proc Natl Acad Sci USA* 105: 728–733.
52. van Ham, T. J., Thijssen, K. L., Breitling, R., Hofstra, R. M., Plasterk, R. H., et al. 2008. *C. elegans* model identifies genetic modifiers of alpha-synuclein inclusion formation during aging. *PLoS Genet* 4: e1000027.
53. Menegon, A., Board, P. G., Blackburn, A. C., Mellick, G. D., Le, Couteur, D. G. 1998. Parkinson's disease, pesticides, and glutathione transferase polymorphisms. *Lancet* 352: 1344–1346.
54. Betarbet, R., Sherer, T. B., MacKenzie, G., Garcia-Osuna, M., Panov, A. V., et al. 2000. Chronic systemic pesticide exposure reproduces features of Parkinson's disease. *Nat Neurosci* 3: 1301–1306.
55. Langston, J. W., Ballard, P. A., Jr. 1983. Parkinson's disease in a chemist working with 1-methyl-4-phenyl-1,2,5,6-tetrahydropyridine. *N Engl J Med* 309: 310.
56. Langston, J. W., Ballard, P., Tetrud, J. W., Irwin, I. 1983. Chronic Parkinsonism in humans due to a product of meperidine-analog synthesis. *Science* 219: 979–980.
57. Onofrj, M., Ghilardi, M. F. 1990. MPTP induced parkinsonian syndrome: Long term follow-up and neurophysiological study. *Ital J Neurol Sci* 11: 445–458.
58. Bocchetta, A., Corsini, G. U. 1986. Parkinson's disease and pesticides. *Lancet* 2: 1163.
59. Blum, D., Torch, S., Lambeng, N., Nissou, M., Benabid, A. L., et al. 2001. Molecular pathways involved in the neurotoxicity of 6-OHDA, dopamine and MPTP: Contribution to the apoptotic theory in Parkinson's disease. *Prog Neurobiol* 65: 135–172.
60. Harrington, A. J., Hamamichi, S., Caldwell, G. A., Caldwell, K. A. 2010. *C. elegans* as a model organism to investigate molecular pathways involved with Parkinson's disease. *Dev Dyn* 239: 1282–1295.
61. Nass, R., Hall, D. H., Miller, D. M., 3rd, Blakely, R. D. 2002. Neurotoxin-induced degeneration of dopamine neurons in *Caenorhabditis elegans*. *Proc Natl Acad Sci USA* 99: 3264–3269.
62. Nass, R., Hahn, M. K., Jessen, T., McDonald, P. W., Carvelli, L., et al. 2005. A genetic screen in *Caenorhabditis elegans* for dopamine neuron insensitivity to 6-hydroxydopamine identifies dopamine transporter mutants impacting transporter biosynthesis and trafficking. *J Neurochem* 94: 774–785.

63. Marvanova, M., Nichols, C. D. 2007. Identification of neuroprotective compounds of *Caenorhabditis elegans* dopaminergic neurons against 6-OHDA. *J Mol Neurosci* 31: 127–137.
64. Locke, C. J., Fox, S. A., Caldwell, G. A., Caldwell, K. A. 2008. Acetaminophen attenuates dopamine neuron degeneration in animal models of Parkinson's disease. *Neurosci Lett* 439: 129–133.
65. Segalat, L. 2006. Drug discovery: Here comes the worm. *ACS Chem Biol* 1: 277–278.
66. Artal-Sanz, M., de Jong, L., Tavernarakis, N. 2006. *Caenorhabditis elegans*: A versatile platform for drug discovery. *Biotechnol J* 1: 1405–1418.
67. Silverman, G. A., Luke, C. J., Bhatia, S. R., Long, O. S., Vetica, A. C., et al. 2009. Modeling molecular and cellular aspects of human disease using the nematode *Caenorhabditis elegans. Pediatr Res* 65: 10–18.
68. Fire, A., Xu, S., Montgomery, M. K., Kostas, S. A., Driver, S. E., et al. 1998. Potent and specific genetic interference by double-stranded RNA in *Caenorhabditis elegans. Nature* 391: 806–811.
69. O'Rourke, E. J., Conery, A. L., Moy, T. I. 2009. Whole-animal high-throughput screens: The *C. elegans* model. *Methods Mol Biol* 486: 57–75.
70. Moy, T. I., Ball, A. R., Anklesaria, Z., Casadei, G., Lewis, K., et al. 2006. Identification of novel antimicrobials using a live-animal infection model. *Proc Natl Acad Sci USA* 103: 10414–10419.
71. Bischof, L. J., Huffman, D. L., Aroian, R. V. 2006. Assays for toxicity studies in *C. elegans* with Bt crystal proteins. *Methods Mol Biol* 351: 139–154.
72. Wittenburg, N., Baumeister, R. 1999. Thermal avoidance in *Caenorhabditis elegans*: An approach to the study of nociception. *Proc Natl Acad Sci USA* 96: 10477–10482.
73. Hertweck, M., Baumeister, R. 2005. Automated assays to study longevity in *C. elegans. Mech Ageing Dev* 126: 139–145.
74. Breger, J., Fuchs, B. B., Aperis, G., Moy, T. I., Ausubel, F. M., et al. 2007. Antifungal chemical compounds identified using a *C. elegans* pathogenicity assay. *PLoS Pathog* 3: e18.
75. Buckingham, S. D., Sattelle, D. B. 2008. Strategies for automated analysis of *C. elegans* locomotion. *Invert Neurosci* 8: 121–131.
76. Doitsidou, M., Flames, N., Lee, A. C., Boyanov, A., Hobert, O. 2008. Automated screening for mutants affecting dopaminergic-neuron specification in *C. elegans. Nat Methods* 5: 869–872.
77. Boyd, W. A., McBride, S. J., Freedman, J. H. 2007. Effects of genetic mutations and chemical exposures on *Caenorhabditis elegans* feeding: Evaluation of a novel, high-throughput screening assay. *PLoS ONE* 2: e1259.
78. Byrne, A. B., Weirauch, M. T., Wong, V., Koeva, M., Dixon, S. J., et al. 2007. A global analysis of genetic interactions in *Caenorhabditis elegans. J Biol* 6: 8.
79. Dupuy, D., Bertin, N., Hidalgo, C. A., Venkatesan, K., Tu, D., et al. 2007. Genome-scale analysis of *in vivo* spatiotemporal promoter activity in *Caenorhabditis elegans. Nat Biotechnol* 25: 663–668.
80. Easley, C. J., Karlinsey, J. M., Bienvenue, J. M., Legendre, L. A., Roper, M. G., et al. 2006. A fully integrated microfluidic genetic analysis system with sample-in-answer-out capability. *Proc Natl Acad Sci USA* 103: 19272–19277.
81. Navratil, M., Whiting, C. E., Arriaga, E. A. 2007. Microfluidic devices for the analysis of single cells: Leaving no protein uncounted. *Sci STKE* 2007: pe29.
82. Fu, A. Y., Spence, C., Scherer, A., Arnold, F. H., Quake, S. R. 1999. A microfabricated fluorescence-activated cell sorter. *Nat Biotechnol* 17: 1109–1111.
83. Bousse, L. 1996. Whole cell biosensors. *Sens Actuators B: Chem* 34: 270–275.
84. Sinclair, J., Pihl, J., Olofsson, J., Karlsson, M., Jardemark, K., et al. 2002. A cell-based bar code reader for high-throughput screening of ion channel–ligand interactions. *Anal Chem* 74: 6133–6138.
85. Park, T. H., Shuler, M. L. 2003. Integration of cell culture and microfabrication technology. *Biotechnol Prog* 19: 243–253.
86. Dittrich, P. S., Manz, A. 2006. Lab-on-a-chip: Microfluidics in drug discovery. *Nat Rev Drug Discov* 5: 210–218.
87. Kang, L., Chung, B. G., Langer, R., Khademhosseini, A. 2008. Microfluidics for drug discovery and development: From target selection to product lifecycle management. *Drug Discov Today* 13: 1–13.
88. Carstens, C., Elbracht, R., Gärtner, C., Becker, H. 2010. Opportunities and limits of cell-based assay miniaturization in drug discovery. *Expert Opin Drug Discovy* 5: 673–679.
89. Wen, Y., Yang, S.-T. 2008. The future of microfluidic assays in drug development. *Expert Opin Drug Discov* 3: 1237–1253.
90. Fernandes, T. G., Diogo, M. M., Clark, D. S., Dordick, J. S., Cabral, J. M. 2009. High-throughput cellular microarray platforms: Applications in drug discovery, toxicology and stem cell research. *Trends Biotechnol* 27: 342–349.

91. Lockery, S. 2007. Channeling the worm: Microfluidic devices for nematode neurobiology. *Nat Methods* 4: 691–692.
92. Hulme, S. E., Shevkoplyas, S. S., Samuel, A. 2008. Microfluidics: Streamlining discovery in worm biology. *Nat Methods* 5: 589–590.
93. Ben-Yakar, A., Chronis, N., Lu, H. 2009. Microfluidics for the analysis of behavior, nerve regeneration, and neural cell biology in *C. elegans*. *Curr Opin Neurobiol* 19: 561–567.
94. Doll, J. C., Harjee, N., Klejwa, N., Kwon, R., Coulthard, S. M., et al. 2009. SU-8 force sensing pillar arrays for biological measurements. *Lab Chip* 9: 1449–1454.
95. Park, S. J., Goodman, M. B., Pruitt, B. L. 2007. Analysis of nematode mechanics by piezoresistive displacement clamp. *Proc Natl Acad Sci USA* 104: 17376–17381.
96. Park, S., Hwang, H., Nam, S. W., Martinez, F., Austin, R. H., et al. 2008. Enhanced *Caenorhabditis elegans* locomotion in a structured microfluidic environment. *PLoS ONE* 3: e2550.
97. Lockery, S. R., Lawton, K. J., Doll, J. C., Faumont, S., Coulthard, S. M., et al. 2008. Artificial dirt: Microfluidic substrates for nematode neurobiology and behavior. *J Neurophysiol* 99: 3136–3143.
98. Kim, N., Dempsey, C. M., Zoval, J. V., Sze, J. Y., Madou, M. J. 2007. Automated microfluidic compact disc (CD) cultivation system of *Caenorhabditis elegans*. *Sens Actuators B* 122: 511–518.
99. Hulme, S. E., Shevkoplyas, S. S., McGuigan, A. P., Apfeld, J., Fontana, W., et al. 2010. Lifespan-on-a-chip: Microfluidic chambers for performing lifelong observation of *C. elegans*. *Lab Chip* 10: 589–597.
100. Clausell-Tormos, J., Lieber, D., Baret, J. C., El-Harrak, A., Miller, O. J., et al. 2008. Droplet-based microfluidic platforms for the encapsulation and screening of Mammalian cells and multicellular organisms. *Chem Biol* 15: 427–437.
101. Shi, W., Qin, J., Ye, N., Lin, B. 2008. Droplet-based microfluidic system for individual *Caenorhabditis elegans* assay. *Lab Chip* 8: 1432–1435.
102. Przedborski, S., Tieu, K., Perier, C., Vila, M. 2004. MPTP as a mitochondrial neurotoxic model of Parkinson's disease. *J Bioenerg Biomembr* 36: 375–379.
103. Bargmann, C. I. 2006. Chemosensation in *C. elegans*. WormBook ed. The *C. elegans* Research Community, WormBook, doi/10.1895/wormbook.1.123.1, http://www.wormbook.org.
104. Hobert, O. 2006. Specification of the nervous system. WormBook ed. The *C. elegans* Research Community, WormBook, doi/10.1895/wormbook.1.12.1, http://www.wormbook.org.
105. Chronis, N., Zimmer, M., Bargmann, C. I. 2007. Microfluidics for *in vivo* imaging of neuronal and behavioral activity in *Caenorhabditis elegans*. *Nat Methods* 4: 727–731.
106. Rohde, C. B., Zeng, F., Gonzalez-Rubio, R., Angel, M., Yanik, M. F. 2007. Microfluidic system for on-chip high-throughput whole-animal sorting and screening at subcellular resolution. *Proc Natl Acad Sci USA* 104: 13891–13895.
107. Chung, K., Crane, M. M., Lu, H. 2008. Automated on-chip rapid microscopy, phenotyping and sorting of *C. elegans*. *Nat Methods* 5: 637–643.
108. Crane, M. M., Chung, K., Lu, H. 2009. Computer-enhanced high-throughput genetic screens of *C. elegans* in a microfluidic system. *Lab Chip* 9: 38–40.
109. Hulme, S. E., Shevkoplyas, S. S., Apfeld, J., Fontana, W., Whitesides, G. M. 2007. A microfabricated array of clamps for immobilizing and imaging *C. elegans*. *Lab Chip* 7: 1515–1523.
110. Chokshi, T. V., Ben-Yakar, A., Chronis, N. 2009. CO2 and compressive immobilization of *C. elegans* on-chip. *Lab Chip* 9: 151–157.
111. Ben-Yakar, A., Bourgeois, F. 2009. Ultrafast laser nanosurgery in microfluidics for genome-wide screenings. *Curr Opin Biotechnol* 20: 100–105.
112. Guo, S. X., Bourgeois, F., Chokshi, T., Durr, N. J., Hilliard, M. A., et al. 2008. Femtosecond laser nanoaxotomy lab-on-a-chip for *in vivo* nerve regeneration studies. *Nat Methods* 5: 531–533.
113. Zeng, F., Rohde, C. B., Yanik, M. F. 2008. Sub-cellular precision on-chip small-animal immobilization, multi-photon imaging and femtosecond-laser manipulation. *Lab Chip* 8: 653–656.
114. Allen, P. B., Sgro, A. E., Chao, D. L., Doepker, B. E., Scott Edgar, J., et al. 2008. Single-synapse ablation and long-term imaging in live *C. elegans*. *J Neurosci Methods* 173: 20–26.
115. Chung, K., Lu, H. 2009. Automated high-throughput cell microsurgery on-chip. *Lab Chip* 9: 2764–2766.
116. Qin, J., Wheeler, A. R. 2007. Maze exploration and learning in *C. elegans*. *Lab Chip* 7: 186–192.
117. White, J. G., Southgate, E., Thomson, J. N., Brenner, S. 1986. The Structure of the nervous system of the nematode *Caenorhabditis elegans*. *Philos Trans R Soc Lond B, Biol Sci* 314: 1–340.
118. Van Voorhies, W. A., Ward, S. 2000. Broad oxygen tolerance in the nematode *Caenorhabditis elegans*. *J Exp Biol* 203: 2467–2478.

119. Gray, J. M., Karow, D. S., Lu, H., Chang, A. J., Chang, J. S., et al. 2004. Oxygen sensation and social feeding mediated by a *C. elegans* guanylate cyclase homologue. *Nature* 430: 317–322.
120. Ward, A., Liu, J., Feng, Z., Xu, X. Z, 2008. Light-sensitive neurons and channels mediate phototaxis in *C. elegans. Nat Neurosci* 11: 916–922.
121. Burr, A. H. 1985. The photomovement of *Caenorhabditis elegans*, a nematode which lacks ocelli. Proof that the response is to light not radiant heating. *Photochem Photobiol* 41: 577–582.
122. Bessho, K., Yamada, S., Kunitani, T., Nakamura, T., Hashiguchi, T., et al. 1995. Biological responses in *Caenorhabditis elegans* to high magnetic fields. *Experientia* 51: 284–288.
123. Hung, Y. C., Lee, J. H., Chen, H. M., Huang, G. S. 2010. Effects of static magnetic fields on the development and aging of *Caenorhabditis elegans. J Exp Biol* 213: 2079–2085.
124. Kimura, T., Takahashi, K., Suzuki, Y., Konishi, Y., Ota, Y., et al. 2008. The effect of high strength static magnetic fields and ionizing radiation on gene expression and DNA damage in *Caenorhabditis elegans. Bioelectromagnetics* 29: 605–614.
125. Caveness, F. E., Panzer, J. D. 1960. Nemic galvanotaxis. *Proceedings of the Helminthological Society*, Washington 27: 73–74.
126. Gupta, S. P. 1962. Galvanotactic reaction of infective larvae of *Trichostrongylus retortaeformis. Exp Parasitol* 12: 118–119.
127. Sukul, N. C., Croll, N. A. 1978. Influence of potential difference and current on the electrotaxis of *Caenorhaditis elegans. J Nematol* 10: 314–317.
128. Gabel, C. V., Gabel, H., Pavlichin, D., Kao, A., Clark, D. A., et al. 2007. Neural circuits mediate electrosensory behavior in *Caenorhabditis elegans. J Neurosci* 27: 7586–7596.
129. Rezai, P., Siddiqui, A., Selvaganapathy, P. R., Gupta, B. P. 2010. Electrotaxis of *Caenorhabditis elegans* in a microfluidic environment. *Lab Chip* 10: 220–226.
130. Rezai, P., Siddiqui, A., Selvaganapathy, P. R., Gupta, B. P. 2010. Behavior of *Caenorhabditis elegans* in alternating electric field and its application to their localization and control. *Appl Phys Lett* 96: 153702.
131. Whitesides, G. M. 2006. The origins and the future of microfluidics. *Nature* 442: 368–373.
132. Crane, M. M., Chung, K., Stirman, J., Lu, H. 2010. Microfluidics-enabled phenotyping, imaging, and screening of multicellular organisms. *Lab Chip* 10: 1509–1517.
133. Satake, D., Ebi, H., Oku, N., Matsuda, K., Takao, H., et al. 2002. A sensor for blood cell counter using MEMS technology. *Sens Actuators B—Chem* 83: 77–81.
134. Fuller, C. K., Hamilton, J., Ackler, H., Krulevitch, P., Boser, B., et al. 2000. Microfabricated multi-frequency particle impedance characterization system. In: Berg Avd, Olthuis, W., Bergveld, P. (Eds). *Micro Total Analysis Systems 2000, Proceedings. Enschede*, Netherlands: Kluwer Academic Publishers. pp. 265–268.
135. Wang, Z. Y., Kutter, J. P., Wolff, A. 2004. Microchip flow cytometer with integrated polymer optics for fluorescence analysis of cells. In: Laurell, T., Nilsson, J., Jensen, K., Harrison, D. J., Kutter, J. P. (Eds). *Micro Total Analysis Systems 2004, 8th International congress on miniaturized systems in chemistry and life sciences*. Malmo, Sweden: The Royal Society of Chemistry. pp. 460–462.
136. Lin, C. H., Chang, G. L., Lee, G. B. 2002. Micro flow cytometers with buried SU-8/SOG optical waveguides for on-line cell counting. *Intl J Nonlinear Sci Numer Simul* 3: 177–180.
137. Lee, G. B., Lin, C. H., Chang, G. L. 2002. Multi-cell-line micro flow cytometers with buried SU-8/SOG optical waveguide. *Fifteenth IEEE International Conference on Micro Electro Mechanical Systems, Technical Digest*. Las Vegas, Nevada, pp. 503–506.
138. Lange, D., Storment, C. W., Conley, C. A., Kovacs, G. T. A. 2005. A microfluidic shadow imaging system for the study of the nematode *Caenorhabditis elegans* in space. *Sens Actuators B—Chem* 107: 904–914.
139. Heng, X., Erickson, D., Baugh, L. R., Yaqoob, Z., Sternberg, P. W., et al. 2006. Optofluidic microscopy—A method for implementing a high resolution optical microscope on a chip. *Lab Chip* 6: 1274–1276.
140. Cui, X., Lee, L. M., Heng, X., Zhong, W., Sternberg, P. W., et al. 2008. Lensless high-resolution on-chip optofluidic microscopes for *Caenorhabditis elegans* and cell imaging. *Proc Natl Acad Sci USA* 105: 10670–10675.
141. Isikman, S. O., Sencan, I., Mudanyali, O., Bishara, W., Oztoprak, C., et al. 2010. Color and monochrome lensless on-chip imaging of *Caenorhabditis elegans* over a wide field-of-view. *Lab Chip* 10: 1109–1112.

28 III-Nitrides–Based Biosensing

Manijeh Razeghi and Ryan McClintock

CONTENTS

28.1 INTRODUCTION

Many chemical and biological compounds have characteristic florescence in the ultraviolet (UV). This fluorescence signature can be used as a fingerprint to identify unknown agents for biosensing applications. Developing a portable biosensing system based on this approach relies on the availability of compact high-performance UV sources and detectors.

III-Nitrides are a family of wide band-gap III–V semiconductor materials that can be tuned to span the entire UV and visible region. By studying the physics, material growth, and fabrication of III-nitride devices it is possible to realize high-performance UV light-emitting diodes (LEDs) and photodetectors for florescence-based spectroscopy. By combining them together at the chip-level a low-cost portable biosensing system can be developed. One of the most important applications of such a system is bioagent detection.

28.1.1 Biological Agent Detection

Biological weapons pose a significant global threat. If deployed in a major terrorist act or and act of war, biological agents could have devastating effects on public health. The power of biological weapons is amplified due to the current lack of readily available real-time detection systems that allows for a lag-time between the occurrence of the attack and the appearance of symptoms—this delay can allow the agents to be dispersed much more widely than the initial attack.

These agents can be simply manufactured and transported in mass quantities, which makes them a major source of concern for homeland security. Some of these agents, such as anthrax, smallpox, Marburg virus, Ebola virus, pneumonic plague, and tularemia, can cause high rates of mortality if sufficient mitigation procedures are not in place. In addition, some agents are transmissible from person to person, adding to the need for early detection and proper quarantines. It is therefore crucial to develop advanced detection systems to provide early threat warning to identify the contaminated areas and facilitate prompt treatment [1]. Rapid detection may also be instrumental in mitigating the spread of biological agents and thus limiting the quarantine area, and potentially saving more lives, as well as considerable amounts of money and effort.

There are currently two major methods of detecting biological agents: wet chemical and fluorescence based. Wet chemical-based detection includes flow cytometry, which measures both the physical and the chemical characteristics of a cell by taking measurements of cells within a fluid stream as they pass through a testing point, as well as DNA-specific techniques such as immunoassay [1]. Both these wet chemical techniques require time-consuming sample preparation as well as consumable products; in contrast, fluorescence-based detection has the distinct advantages of requiring no consumables and operating in near real time.

In fluorescence-based detection, the characteristic UV fluorescence of biological markers is used to detect the presence of biological agents in the environment. A UV light source illuminates the unknown agent in short pulses. If fluorescent biological markers are present, they will emit light at a characteristic wavelength slightly longer than the absorption wavelengths. This emitted light is then detected by a sensor with a peak detection adjusted to the characteristic fluorescence of the marker. The detected signal is then analyzed for each pulse: threat discrimination is based on spectral fingerprinting and comparison of the signal to the background in order to detect significant changes in bioaerosols.

Current fluorescence-based biological agent detection systems such as BAWS (Biological Agent Warning Sensor), BARTS (Biological Agent Real-Time Sensor), and FLAPS (Fluorescence Aerodynamic Particle Sizer) provide a good solution to the protection of fixed centralized locations. However, these devices are large, expensive, and heavy based on frequency-doubled laser sources. They have very high power consumption and are not easily portable. All this makes them commercially impractical for widespread use and drives the need to develop a compact semiconductor-based approach.

28.1.2 Fluorescence-Based Biodetection

Biodetection targets living cells and viruses that contain various amino acids and proteins that fluoresce when illuminated with UV light of the appropriate wavelength. While there is no straightforward way to use this fluorescence to directly differentiate between different biological materials, the simultaneous use of several wavelengths, as is possible with the small size and low power consumption of semiconductor-based UV optical sources, allows for the development of a spectral fingerprint. This fingerprint can be compared against a database to find a list of possible sources. This can further be combined with historical tracking to sense a sudden increase in biologically active aerosols that can be the basis for providing a timely warning.

UV fluorescence-based biological detection is based on the fluorescence properties of one or more of the following four compounds: tryptophan, tyrosine, phenylalanine, and Nicotinamide Adenine Dingcleotide Hydride (NADH).

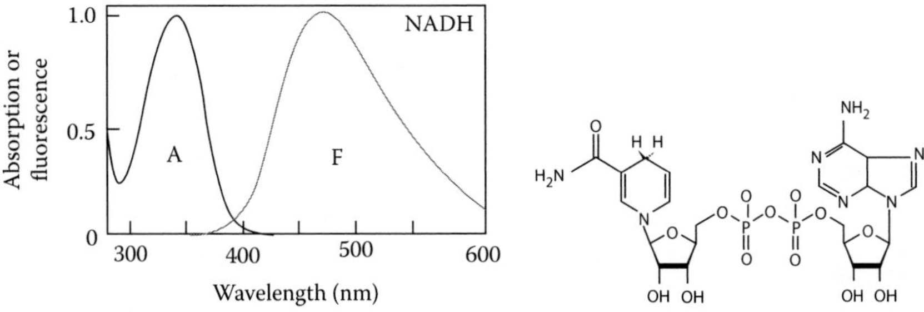

FIGURE 28.1 Absorption and fluorescence spectra of NADH.

NADH is the easiest biological marker to detect because it requires longer-wavelength sources that are more mature (Figure 28.1); however, there are a number of drawbacks to a system that only detects NADH. NADH is a by-product of aerobic cellular respiration and as such is found only in living cells; NADH, unlike the other three compounds mentioned above, is not found in viruses. Despite having a very high absorptivity (number of photons absorbed per incident photon), NADH has a very low quantum yield (number of photons emitted per incident photon), which makes its fluorescence efficiency very low (see Table 28.1).

Unlike NADH, the three fluorescent amino acids (tyrosine, phenylalanine, and tryptophan) are found in the proteins that make up both viruses and bacteria, as well as some protein-based toxins secreted by cells. The absorption wavelengths of these amino acids are shorter than that of NADH (Figure 28.2, Table 28.1), which illustrates the need for shorter-wavelength sources, such as the deep UV LEDs (discussed in Section 28.4). Among these biological markers, tryptophan has the highest fluorescence efficiency due to its high absorptivity and quantum yield. On the other hand, phenylalanine is difficult to detect in the presence of tryptophan and tyrosine. The reason is that the emitted light spectra of phenylalanine (peak $\lambda \sim 280$ nm) overlaps with the absorption spectra of tryptophan and tyrosine, resulting in the reabsorption of the light, or a so-called *resonance energy transfer.* This phenomenon causes phenylalanine to possess the lowest fluorescence efficiency in this set.

28.1.3 III-Nitrides Material System

The nitrides of group-III metal elements or "III-nitrides" are commonly referred to as aluminum nitride (AlN), gallium nitride (GaN), indium nitride (InN), and their alloys, all of which are compounds of nitrogen—the smallest group V element in the Periodic Table and an element with one of the highest values of electronegativity. The III-nitride material system exhibits a direct band-gap energy that can be continuously tuned from 0.7 eV all the way to 6.2 eV, which corresponds to a

TABLE. 28.1
Absorption and Fluorescence Properties of the Biological Markers in Discussion

Biological Marker	Absorption Wavelength (nm)	Fluorescence Wavelength (nm)	Absorptivity (L/mol.cm)	Quantum Yield	Fluorescence Efficiency[a] (cm^{-1})
NADH	340	470	6320	0.02	5.2
Tryptophan	280	356	5600	0.2	46.4
Tyrosine	274	303	1400	0.14	8.1
Phenylalanine	257	280	200	0.04	0.3

[a] Fluorescence efficiency is defined as Absorptivity × Quantum yield/24.15 (cm^{-1}).

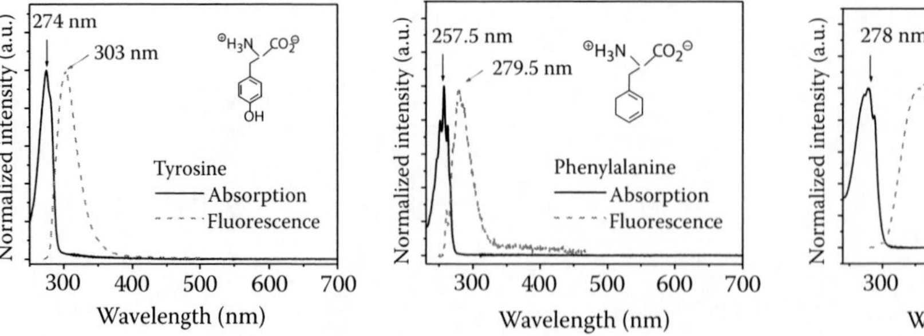

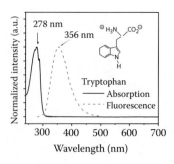

FIGURE 28.2 Absorption and fluorescence spectra of the three fluorescent amino acids: tyrosine, phenylalanine, and tryptophan.

wavelength range from 1.78 μm to 200 nm. This makes it ideally suited toward the realization of sources and detectors for UV florescence-based biodetection.

The first AlN, GaN, and InN compounds were synthesized as early as 1907 [2], 1910 [3], and 1932 [4], respectively; however, the III-nitride material system has been slow to develop. Little significant progress was reported until the end of the 1960s. In the late 1960s and early 1970s, the advent of modern epitaxial growth techniques led to a resurgent interest in III-nitrides [5–8]. However, it was not until the 1980s with the advent of the low-temperature GaN buffer [9,10] that material quality became sufficient for device research to begin in earnest. However, little success had been realized in the area of p-type III-nitrides limiting the prospects for junction device. The critical discovery that catapulted III-nitrides to the forefront of modern semiconductor research was Akasaki's demonstration of p-type GaN films through low-energy electron beam irradiation (LEEBI) in 1989 [11]—this led to a swelling of III-nitride research in the 1990s.

At the beginning of the III-nitride boom in the 1990s there was a great need to develop device quality material growth. This was a difficult task due to the lack of available GaN substrates, and most growth was conducted on Sapphire substrates that led to very large dislocation densities that made device realization difficult. However, Professor Manijeh Razeghi had extensive experience in developing growth in the difficult GaInAsP–InP [12] and GaAs and GaInP [13] material systems that aided her entry into the III-nitride material system. In January 1994, through collaboration between Professor Razeghi and Aixtron, the world's first commercial reactor designed for the growth of GaN, the Aixtron 200–4/ HT, was designed and installed at the Center for Quantum Devices (CQD) at Northwestern University [14]. From there the CQD rapidly demonstrated the capability to grow device quality AlGaN material across the compositional range from AlN to GaN, as shown in Figure 28.3 [15]. Research at the CQD has played a pivotal role in recent development of the first short wavelength UV detectors and sources. CQDs currently represent one of only a few groups with the technology necessary to realize both LEDs and detectors at the strategic wavelengths necessary for UV florescence-based biological detection [2,3].

28.2 BIOSENSING WITH III-NITRIDES

The most promising way of realizing a portable hand-held fluorescence-based biodetector is to develop a system using semiconductor-based optical sources, rather than the bulky, inefficient diode-pumped frequency-quadrupled solid-state lasers currently in use. By combining III-nitride-based short-wavelength UV emitters with III-nitride-based photodetectors, it becomes possible to devise a compact system that can rapidly detect and discriminate among various biological compounds based on their fluorescence signature. For this, UV emitters and detectors at several strategic wavelengths are required. The choice of wavelength is dictated by the specific absorption and fluorescence of the corresponding biological markers (Figure 28.4). The UV light sources are

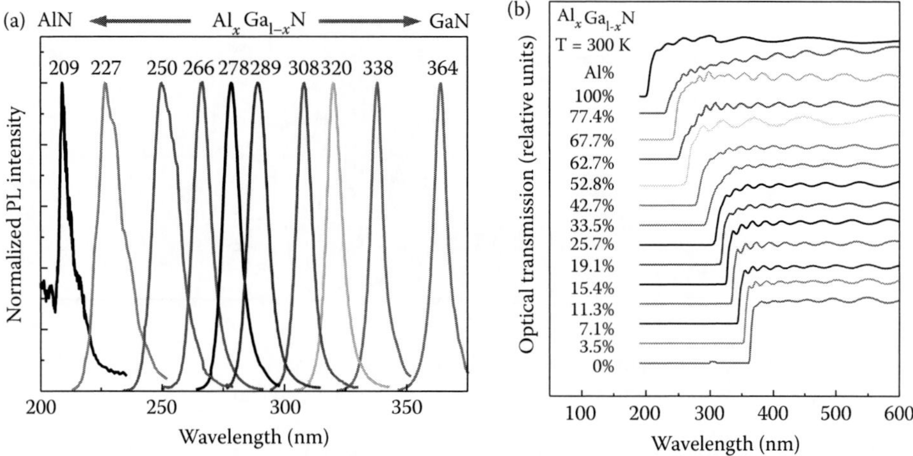

FIGURE 28.3 Optical characterization of AlGaN material grown across the entire compositional range from GaN to AlN: photoluminescence (a). Optical transmission (b).

selected to emit at the peak absorption wavelength of the biomarker in question, for example, at 280 nm for tryptophan, 274 nm for tyrosine, and 257 nm for phenylalanine—the three important amino acids with fluorescence properties—and ~340 nm for NADH. The resulting signal is subsequently collected by a photodetector with a band-pass detection window corresponding to the florescence wavelength of interest. The use of efficient semiconductor-based UV light sources and photodetectors would enable the overall system to be more compact, inexpensive, and portable with lower power consumption than current existing biological and chemical detection systems. Additionally, the reduced size and lower power consumption of the semiconductor UV sources will enable the incorporation of multiple excitation sources at different wavelengths in the same compact enclosure. The use of additional sources is expected to increase the specificity of the biological detection system by simultaneously targeting specific fluorescence excitations from a variety of biological markers.

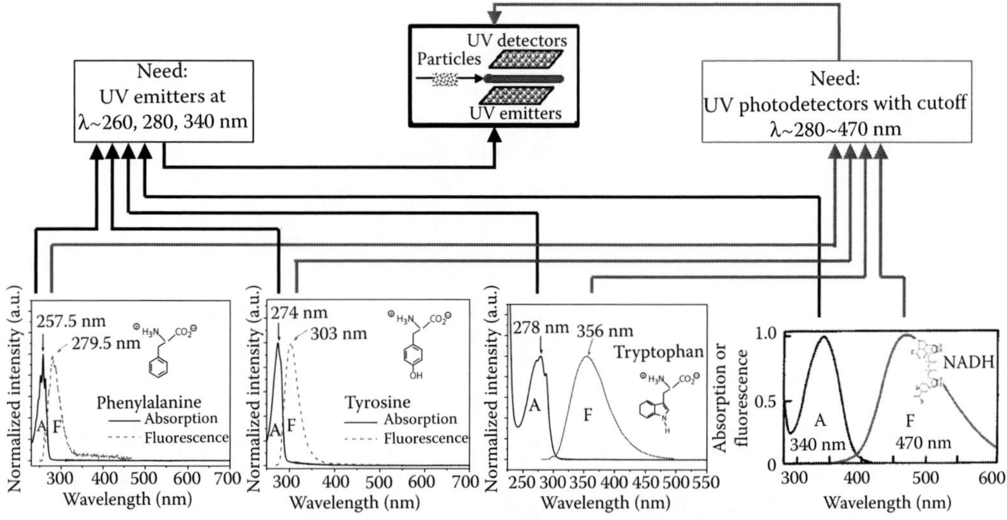

FIGURE 28.4 Absorption and fluorescence of the most important biological markers (phenylalanine, tyrosine, tryptophan, and NADH) along with the requirements for the corresponding UV emitter/detector sets.

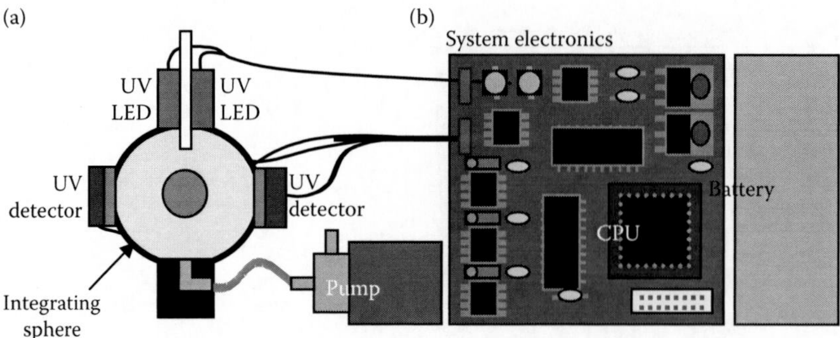

FIGURE 28.5 Schematic diagram of bioagent detection system: (a) Biological agent sensor utilizing Semiconductor UV optical sources and PMTs; (b) support electronics and battery power.

28.2.1 Design of a Biosensor Using Discreet Components

There are several ways that one could envision constructing such a semiconductor-based UV florescence system based on III-nitrides. The most straightforward way would be to adapt an existing flow cell for use with III-nitride sensors and detectors. Such a design would be based around a laminar flow that is drawn through a small integrating sphere via a compact vacuum pump. The various wavelength emitters and UV detectors with various band-pass cutoffs would then be located around the periphery of the integrating sphere to measure the fluorescence. A schematic diagram of such a system is shown in Figure 28.5. The overall system would be about half the size of a shoebox, suitable for hand carrying and easy tabletop deployment.

The system operates by using a small vacuum pump to draw in a sample of air with potential biological contamination. A miniature virtual impact-based aerosol concentrator is used to enhance the concentration of any particulate matter in the incoming air. This concentrated air is then drawn through the center of the integrating sphere. A laminar flow of filtered shield gas surrounds this central column of sample gas to avoid contamination of the interior of the integrating sphere. The various III-nitride sources are placed in a ring coaxial with the sample gas flow. Stray light from the LEDs is captured by an outlet baffle integrated into the gas outlet at the bottom of the sphere. The LEDs are sequentially illuminated for a brief pulse with the corresponding detector's output sampled for any detection events. This sequence repeats until all LED–detector combinations have been tested. The LEDs and detectors are controlled by a CPU/driver board that creates a florescence fingerprint for each sample. These fingerprints are compared against the time-varying background and against a database of calibrated fingerprints to make a determination as to the biological contents of the sampled air. This output can be used to make a qualitative analysis of a sample of unknown gas and can be directly wired to alarm circuits that provide advance warning if any unusual detection event occurs.

28.2.2 Monolithic System Design

Another option would be to use monolithic integration of detectors and photodetectors to create a small integrated sensor module that is less than 1 cm × 1 cm in size. Such a sensor module would only require a very small pump and associated electronics in order to create a fully functional system. By doing away with the large integrating sphere it is not possible to create a pocket-sized sensor system that might resemble a personal data assistant or a cell phone. This would allow for ubiquitous deployment of such sensor systems.

However, such a biodetector module is not easy to fabricate. It requires integrating multiple UV light sources and UV photodetectors with various band-pass-like detection bands—at least six individual devices. The easiest way to achieve this would be to fabricate a single chip consisting of the

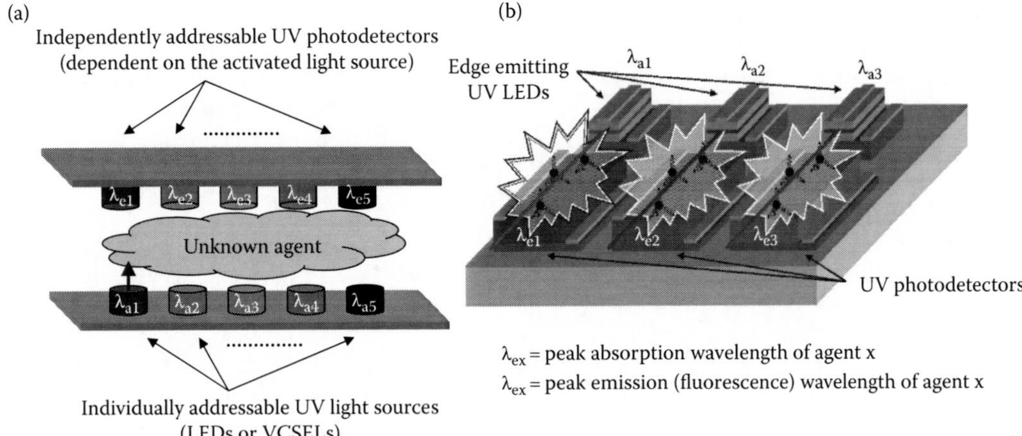

FIGURE 28.6 (a) Biosensor chip utilizing surface-emitting UV light emitters such as LEDs or vertical cavity surface-emitting lasers (VCSELs); (b) alternative design using edge-emitting devices.

various detectors and a separate chip consisting of the emitters. This can be accomplished by processing multiple detectors or emitters from a single multilayered wafer structure, or by mounting single-chip components onto a suitable substrate. The two wafers would then be bonded facing each other to a spacer support forming the optical sampling cavity. A schematic of this layout is shown in Figure 28.6a. The other option would be to fabricate edge emitting LEDs (or laser diodes) and traditional normal incidence detectors and bond both of these onto a single chip (Figure 28.6b).

The UV fluorescence efficiency of the characteristic fluorescent biological markers described in Table 28.1 is low. In the discreet device approach this is overcome by using a large sample volume—nearly the whole length of the integrating sphere. However, as the size of the sensor array is shrunk in the monolithic approaches the sample volume is also decreased dramatically. This results in very low-level signals. In order to maximize sensitivity and reduce the background, the system needs to employ a synchronous detection scheme. This is accomplished using the puling of the various wavelength LED excitation sources. One alternative to further increase the sensitivity is to develop UV Geiger-mode avalanche photodiodes (APDs) capable of single-photon detection.

28.3 III-NITRIDE MATERIAL GROWTH

III-Nitride material is traditionally grown by either metalorganic chemical vapor deposition (MOCVD) of metal beam epitaxy. Unlike many other III–V semiconductors, III-nitrides cannot be grown via Czochralski crystal growth. This means that there is a general lack of commercially available lattice-matched substrates. Instead, most III-nitride growth is conducted on sapphire (Al_2O_3) substrates. Sapphire has the advantage of being transparent in the visible and UV which makes it easy to fabricate back-illuminated or back-emission devices. However, the crystal structure of sapphire is poorly matched to that of III-nitrides. This makes the growth of III-nitride devices challenging.

28.3.1 Low-Temperature AlN Buffer Layers

Due to the large difference between the lattice parameters of Al(In)GaN alloys and sapphire, it is practically impossible to grow high-quality epilayers directly on top of sapphire. In order to address this problem, a low-temperature GaN or AlN layer is generally grown first on top of the sapphire substrate to initiate nucleation [16]. The purpose of this low-temperature buffer layer is to optimize the transition between the sapphire substrate and subsequent high-temperature epilayers. This creates a dislocated interface between the low-temperature buffer layer and the sapphire substrate.

However, the following high-temperature layers will be of high quality and do not have to follow the surface arrangement of the sapphire substrate.

A theoretical model has been suggested for the epitaxial relation between AlN and sapphire [17]. The model is shown in the inset of Figure 28.7. Since the (00.1) surface of sapphire is oxygen terminated, each Al atom will be placed between three oxygen atoms, meaning that the first atomic plane will have the same structure as sapphire. The N atoms from NH_3 combined with Al ions to form a tetrahedron with oxygen. The chemical bonds will then gradually change their nature from ionic to covalent. Lattice mismatch can be calculated from the change of Al–Al atomic distances between AlN and Al_2O_3 and will be about 13%, meaning that roughly every nine Al–Al atomic distance in sapphire corresponds to eight Al–Al atomic distance in AlN:

$$\Delta a = \frac{a_{\text{AlN}} - a_{\text{sapphire}}/\sqrt{3}}{a_{\text{sapphire}}/\sqrt{3}} = \frac{3.112 - 2.747}{2.747} = 13.2\% \tag{28.1}$$

In practice, we have found the exact same behavior as predicted by theory. Figure 28.7 shows a lattice image of an AlN buffer layer grown on top of the sapphire substrate. This image clearly shows the 9:8 relationship predicted by theory. It should be noted that a misfit dislocation appears at the termination of each atomic plane.

28.3.2 Growth of Crack-Free AlGaN Layers

One of the most important aspects of the growth of III-nitrides is the difference in lattice parameters and thermal expansion coefficients of the AlInGaN compounds. For example, the difference between the lattice constants of AlGaN and GaN results in biaxial strain in the top AlGaN layer which together with the difference in the thermal expansion coefficients, can eventually form cracks in the epilayers. For $Al_xGa_{1-x}N$ on GaN, the in-plane stress is of *tensile* type, because the lattice parameter of $Al_xGa_{1-x}N$ is smaller than that of GaN.

One of peculiar property of III-nitrides is the absence of an effective slip system [18], which makes it difficult for dislocations to generate and glide. Brittle relaxation occurs due to the fact that it is not possible to nucleate misfit dislocations by the Matthews–Blakeslee mechanism in

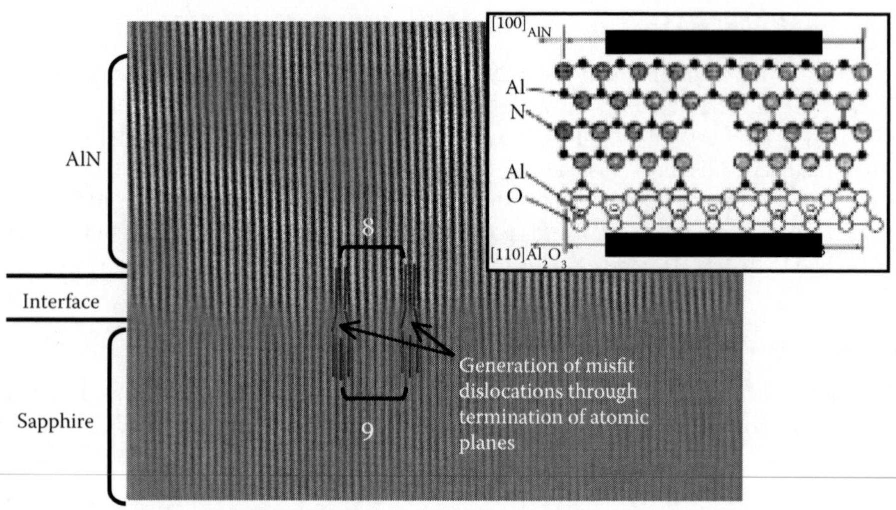

FIGURE 28.7 Lattice image of the AlN/sapphire interface. The inset shows a cross-sectional view of the interfacial atomic structure model of AlN on (00.1) Al_2O_3 showing the formation of an edge-type dislocation.

[00.1]-oriented III-nitrides [19]. The Matthews–Blakeslee theory describes the introduction of a misfit segment by the binding of preexisting dislocations. It also explains the nucleation and glide of dislocations from the surface. However, for hexagonal III-nitrides, these glide systems have not been observed. Consequently, the plastic relaxation of AlGaN layers directly grown on GaN templates occurs through cracking [20].

In order to avoid cracking, the magnitude of tensile strain should be reduced to near zero. This can be achieved through the insertion of an underlying layer that adds a *compressive* strain component such that it cancels out the tensile strain component. It has been reported that $Al_xGa_{1-x}N$ with $x > 0.4$ grown on sapphire is under biaxial compression [21]. Therefore, growth of AlGaN on $Al_xGa_{1-x}N$ with $x > 0.4$ results in a layer that is compressively strained below its critical thickness. This leads to an increased critical thickness of the top $Al_xGa_{1-x}N$ layer that will eventually delay cracking of the material. A similar approach has been employed for AlGaN/GaN heterostructures. Amano et al. [22] employed low-temperature AlN interlayers between GaN and AlGaN for dislocation filtering. They later combined this approach with substrate patterning to obtain crack-free AlGaN layers on GaN [23]. AlN interlayers have been also employed for the growth of thick crack-free AlGaN/GaN distributed Bragg reflectors [24,25]. Similarly, crack-free AlGaN on GaN layers have been successfully grown on Si substrates using AlN interlayers [26]. Strain relief has also been achieved using AlGaN/AlN [27] or AlGaN/GaN superlattices (SLs) [28]. SLs are known to help relieve the strain, caused by the large lattice mismatch between sapphire and III-nitrides as well as among the AlInGaN family itself [29,30]. $Al_xGa_{1-x}N$/AlN SLs can also be used for dislocation filtering purposes [31].

28.3.3 Doping of High Al-Content $Al_xGa_{1-x}N$ Layers

28.3.3.1 n-Type Doping

Silicon is the most common n-type dopant for the III-nitride material system. However, while Si-doping of GaN is not much of an issue, doping of high Al-content AlGaN films seems to be more challenging. At high aluminum concentrations, the electrical conductivity of Si-doped $Al_xGa_{1-x}N$ layers is very low which makes these layers not suitable for optoelectronic devices. Impurities, dislocations, and native defects can form compensation sites with an acceptor-like character leading to reduced n-type conductivity of AlGaN:Si. Oxygen, for instance, can behave as a deep acceptor when it becomes a DX center [32,33]. Carbon also has been speculated to act as an acceptor [34]. Cation vacancies are another acceptor-like compensating source whose formation energy decreases with increasing Al composition [35]. For instance, Wagener et. al. [36] found two mid-gap states arising from the third and second ionization states of the aluminum vacancy that could be responsible for the compensation mechanism. In addition to all these, dislocations may also introduce acceptor-like centers through dangling bonds along the dislocation line [37]. Deepening of the Si impurity level as a function of Al composition is another plausible argument as to why the electrical conductivity decreases [38]. Therefore, either the presence of compensation centers, or the deepening of the Si level, or a combination of both could be responsible for the increase in the resistivity of Si-doped, high Al-content $Al_xGa_{1-x}N$ layers.

Adding a small amount of indium to the Si-doped AlGaN epilayers has been shown to be beneficial. A few groups have reported Si–In codoping of high Al-content AlGaN layers resulting in high carrier concentrations and low resistivities [39,40].

There are a number of hypotheses as to why indium increases the conductivity of Si-doped AlGaN layers. The addition of indium into ternary AlGaN layers results in the reduction of defect density. This improvement in the structural quality can result in higher conductivity through suppression of the dislocation-induced compensation sites. It has also been speculated that indium may counteract the incorporation of defects responsible for self-compensation of high Al-content AlGaN layers, such as DX centers and cation vacancies [41]. Indium may occupy the cation vacancies (V_{III} sites) to inhibit the acceptor formation.

28.3.3.2 p-Type Doping

p-Type doping of GaN and its ternary alloys is one of the most challenging tasks pertaining to the growth of III-nitride materials. The most common p-type dopant is magnesium (Mg); however, Mg doping without postgrowth treatment still results in a compensated material. Amano et al. [42] achieved the first p-type doping by performing a postgrowth LEEBI. Two years after this breakthrough, it was found that thermal annealing of the Mg-doped GaN layer under N_2 could also yield a p-type layer. The annealing temperature is in the range of 800–1000°C. Annealing under NH_3, on the other hand, resulted in a compensated material. Therefore, it was concluded that hydrogen is the compensating agent. In fact, it is suggested that hydrogen passivates Mg [43] and therefore postgrowth treatment is necessary to break the H–Mg bonds and liberate the acceptors.

Magnesium can be considered as a *deep acceptor* since the acceptor level in Mg-doped AlGaN layers lies hundreds of meV above the valence band. The energy difference between the valence band and the acceptor level is called the *activation energy* of the acceptor, which for Mg in AlGaN system increases with increasing Al composition. Figure 28.8 shows the Mg activation energy as a function of Al composition, up to 20% [44] (Data collected from Refs. [45–49]). For AlN:Mg, an activation energy of 510 meV has been measured which means that only a very tiny fraction of the Mg dopants (10^{-9}) contribute free holes at room temperature [50].

One way to tackle the problem of p-type doping is to take advantage of the spontaneous and piezoelectric polarization in AlGaN/GaN heterostructures. III-Nitrides normally have a wurtzite structure which is the structure with the highest symmetry compatible with the existence of spontaneous polarization. Furthermore, the piezoelectric coefficients for wurtzite GaN-based materials are about one order of magnitude higher than other zinc-blende III–V and II–VI semiconductors. These two effects combine to build a huge electric field, on the order of few MV/cm. This large polarization field creates a periodic sawtooth variation in the band structure which results in a periodic lowering of the acceptor level below the Fermi level, thus increasing the fraction of ionized acceptors [51].

28.4 III-NITRIDE-BASED UV SOURCES

The minimum attainable wavelength using $In_xGa_{1-x}N$-based active layers is around 365 nm. For emission at shorter wavelengths, ternary $Al_xGa_{1-x}N$ or quaternary $Al_xIn_yGa_{1-x-y}N$ with low indium

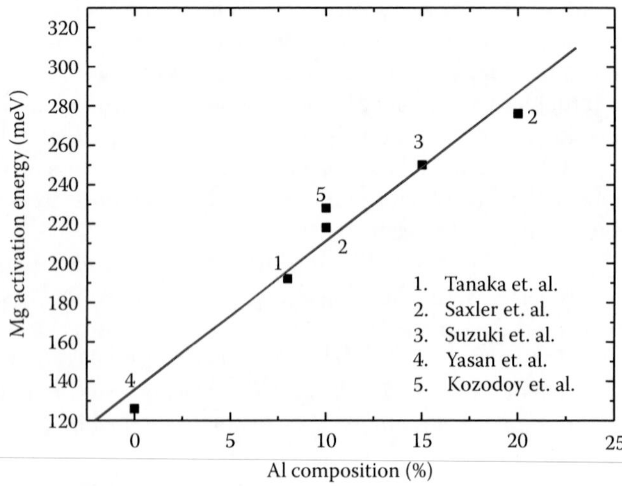

FIGURE 28.8 Activation energy of magnesium in p-type $Al_xGa_{1-x}N$ as a function of aluminum mole fraction. (Data collected from Refs. [45–49].)

composition replaces $In_xGa_{1-x}N$ as the active layer material of choice. There are two possible configurations for LEDs depending on where the light is emitted from: either top- or back-emission. Either device geometry can be used to create a biodetector system.

Top-emission LEDs have the advantage that they can be grown on GaN buffer layers over sapphire, SiC, or freestanding GaN substrates. However, the need for a top contact can severely limit the efficiency of top-emission UV LEDs since the top p-GaN cap layer and the semitransparent p-type ohmic metal contact partially absorb the UV light leading to reduced efficiency of the LED. Only 70% of the light is transmitted through the semitransparent contact layer at the wavelength of 400 nm and this value decreases as the wavelength decreases (~60% at 340 nm and 50% at 280 nm) [52]. In addition, the p-GaN contact layer on the top absorbs the light markedly above its band gap [52]. Despite these problems, top-emission UV LEDs with peak emission wavelengths as short as 280 nm have been demonstrated [53]. However, due to the aforementioned problems, usually the extraction efficiency of top-emission short-wavelength LEDs is very low.

Back-emission devices have a marked advantage over top-emission devices in a sense that the bottom n-type AlGaN layers and the sapphire substrate are completely transparent to the emitted UV light. However, for back-emission UV devices, no GaN template layer can be used prior to the growth of the LED structure, because GaN has a band gap of 3.4 eV which absorbs photons of wavelengths of 364 nm and below. Thus, AlN- or high aluminum composition AlGaN buffer layers and template layers are required under the device. It is worth noting that SiC also cannot be used as a substrate for back-emission short-wavelength UV LEDs because it has a band-gap energy of ~2.9 eV and absorbs the UV light.

28.4.1 Top-Emission 340 nm UV LEDs Grown on GaN Substrates

Native substrates such as GaN are of great interest because they possess low dislocation densities and are lattice matched to epitaxial GaN. In addition, they provide a better heat dissipation due to their large thermal conductivity, which is about five times higher than that of sapphire. The only problem that has prevented GaN substrates from being the substrates of choice is the complicated growth techniques that have made them expensive and luxurious substrates at the present time. The growth of laser diodes on GaN substrates is simpler than the growth on other substrates, because there will no longer be a need for time-consuming processes such as lateral epitaxial overgrowth (LEO) [54–57], pendeo-epitaxy [58], or substrate patterning [59–61] to reduce the dislocation density of the subsequent epitaxial layers.

Characteristics of UV LEDs grown on freestanding GaN substrates were investigated by fabricating 340 nm MQW UV LED structures on sapphire and GaN substrates and comparing their properties [62]. The complete UV LED structure is given in the inset of Figure 28.9. The *I–V* characteristics of the devices are also shown in this figure. The turn-on voltage of both devices is ~4 V. However, the LED grown on GaN substrate shows a sharper turn-on with a differential resistance of 13 Ω. The same LED structure grown on sapphire gives a value of 40 Ω for differential resistance. This indicates that the LED grown on GaN substrate has higher material quality than that of sapphire, due to lower defect density.

In Figure 28.10, we compare the output power of the device grown on a GaN substrate with the one grown on sapphire in pulsed injection mode. An enhancement of more than one order of magnitude has been achieved for the LED grown on the GaN substrate due to higher material quality. The slope efficiency for the LED grown on the GaN substrate is one order of magnitude higher. In addition, GaN substrates provide better heat dissipation, as for the LED grown on sapphire, power saturates at a current of higher than 120 mA in the continuous-wave (CW) injection mode due to heating inside the device. However, for the LED grown on the GaN substrate, the output power in CW injection mode does not saturate for the injection currents up to 350 mA. This is understandable by the fact that the thermal conductivity of GaN is about five times higher than that of sapphire.

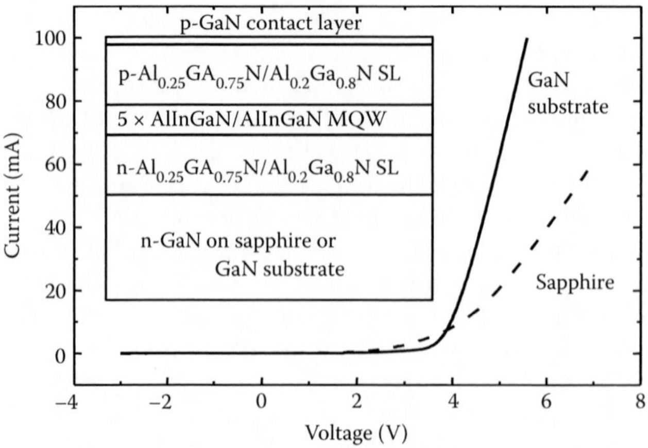

FIGURE 28.9 Current–voltage characteristics of 340 nm UV LED grown on freestanding GaN substrate (solid line) and on sapphire (dashed line); inset shows complete structure of the devices.

28.4.2 Back-Emission AlGaN UV LEDs (λ = 280 nm)

As described earlier, top-emission UV LEDs suffer from optical absorption losses mainly in the p-GaN contact layer and the semitransparent metal contact. It is possible to fabricate a top-emission 280 nm LED [53]; however, the performance is inferior to back-emission designs. The back-emission device structure begins with a 20 nm low-temperature AlN buffer layer grown at ~700°C followed by a 350 nm-thick high-temperature AlN layer and a 30-period $Al_{0.85}Ga_{0.15}N/AlN$ (50 Å/50 Å) SL topped with a 50 nm AlN compliance layer. These layers collectively comprise a high-quality template for the growth of the UV LED structure (as described in detail in Section 28.3.2). This template is not only transparent to wavelengths longer than 230 nm, but also keeps the top layers under compressive strain to avoid cracking of the material. As pointed out before, the SL structure can be used for strain relief as well as dislocation filtering.

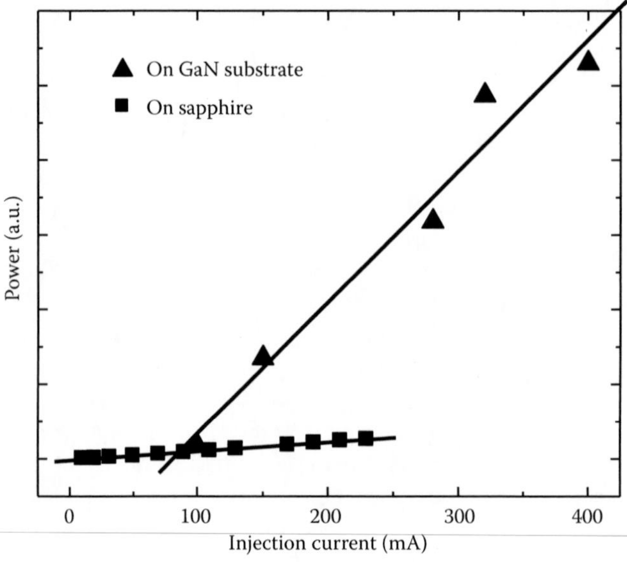

FIGURE 28.10 Comparison between output power of the 340-nm LED grown on GaN substrate (triangles) and on sapphire (squares) in pulsed injection mode (duty cycle = 1%).

On top of this template, 0.8 μm of highly conductive Si–In codoped $Al_{0.5}Ga_{0.5}N$ was deposited forming the n-type contact layer. Hall Effect measurement of this layer shows the resistivity, mobility, and carrier concentration to be 0.04 Ω · cm, 55 $cm^2/V \cdot s$, and 3.1×10^{18} cm^{-3}, respectively. The Si-In codoping scheme was used for increasing the electrical conductivity of this high Al-content AlGaN layers. A 100 nm-thick n-$Al_{0.45}Ga_{0.45}N$ layer was then grown as a confinement layer. The high Al mole fractions of the previous layers are chosen for transparency at 280 nm, so as to allow back-emission. The active region consisted of a 10 nm $Al_{0.4}Ga_{0.6}N$ barrier, after which a 5 nm $Al_{0.36}Ga_{0.64}N$ quantum well (QW) was grown, ending with a second 5 nm $Al_{0.4}Ga_{0.6}N$ barrier. The asymmetric design of the active region is intended to compensate for the lower mobility of holes compared to electrons. This allows more of the injected electrons to recombine in the QW, which in turn increases the efficiency of the LED. A 10 nm $Al_{0.6}Ga_{0.4}N$ current blocking layer was then deposited to help prevent overflow of electrons out of the active region. The structure was then completed with a 50-nm-thick p-$Al_{0.45}Ga_{0.55}N$ layer followed by a 50-nm-thick p-GaN contact layer. After the growth, the sample was examined with both an optical and a scanning electron microscope and was found to be crack free. A cross section of the device structure including the ohmic contacts is shown in Figure 28.11a.

Standard photolithographic processing is used for forming mesa isolated diodes; however, in order to operate the diode under back-emission it is necessary to flip-chip bond it to a submount. The LED wafer was diced into arrays of five devices before bonding to thermally conducting AlN submounts, via Au–Sn solder bumps. The diced die was bonded, epi-down, to the submount using thermocompressive bonding. The back of the submounted LED was then bonded to a copper heatsink using indium. Figure 28.11b shows a schematic cross section of a flip-chip-bonded LED die.

This UV LED has a turn-on voltage of ~4.5 V with a series resistance of 25 Ω. The turn-on voltage is around the expected value obtained from the band gap of the QW layer. Figure 28.12a shows the room-temperature electroluminescense (EL) spectra of the LED at various current injection levels. The dominant peak occurs at ~280 nm with a full-width at half-maximum of ~10 nm. A very small defect-related peak with a very low integrated intensity is also observed in the spectra at $\lambda = 320$ nm, which becomes even less significant as the current increases. The ratio of the primary peak to the secondary peak, the *primary-to-stray light ratio*, is plotted in Figure 28.12b as a function of current with the semilog EL spectra shown as an inset.

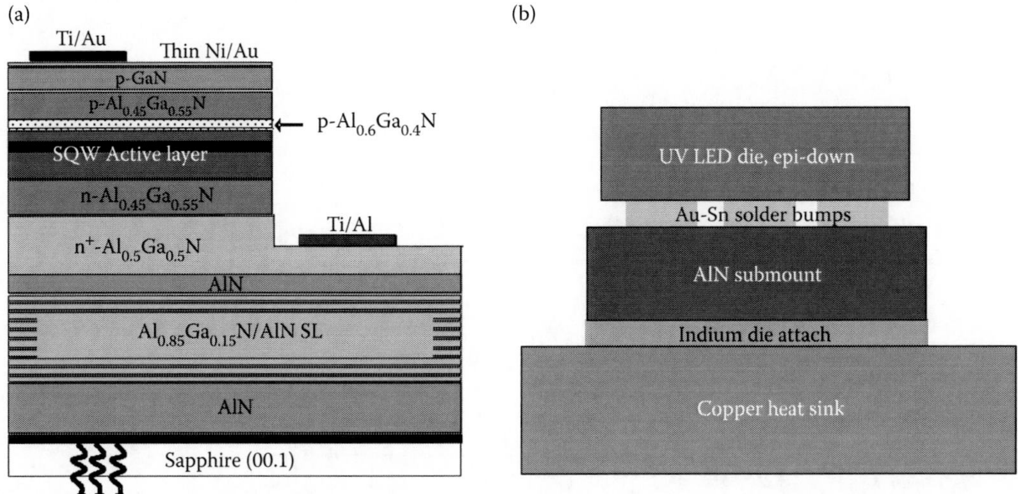

FIGURE 28.11 Structure of the 280 nm UV LED including the metal contacts (a). Schematic of a flip-chip-bonded LED (b).

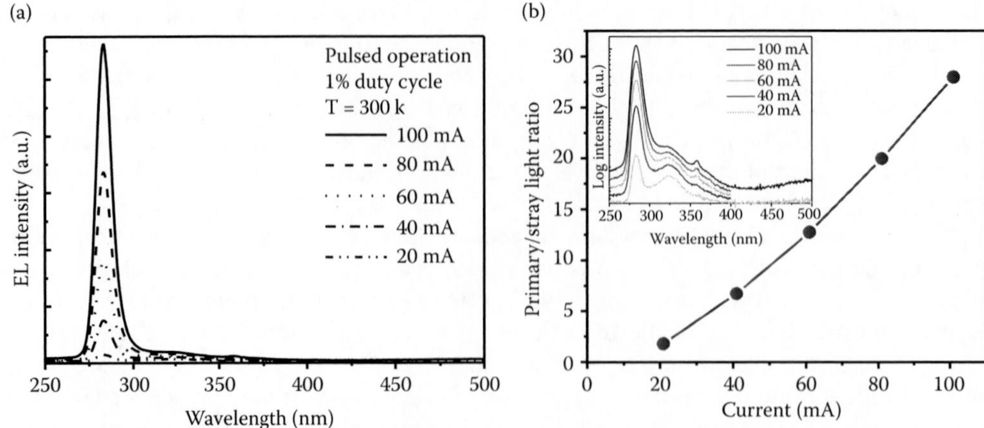

FIGURE 28.12 EL spectra of the 280 nm UV LED at various injection currents at room temperature (a) and the ratio of primary to stray light; the inset shows the EL spectra in semilog scale (b).

Output power of the device was measured inside a calibrated integrating sphere. Figure 28.13 shows the output power of the flip-chip-bonded device in pulsed operation mode (pulse width of 200 ns, frequency of 200 Hz). A high value of 1.8 mW at a current of 400 mA was achieved for the bonded LED. The *P–I* curve deviates from a linear relationship at higher currents due to heating inside the device. The CW power is substantially lower than the pulsed power which shows that removal of the generated heat is one of the major problems that needs to be addressed.

28.4.3 Back-Emission Deep UV LEDs (λ = 265 nm)

Growth of UV LEDs becomes more challenging as we move toward shorter wavelengths. This is due to deteriorated material quality and pronounced problem of the doping of high Al-content $Al_xGa_{1-x}N$ layers. Apart from the increased molar fraction of Al in $Al_xGa_{1-x}N$ layers, the structure of a 265 nm UV LED resembles that of a 280 nm LED. A cross section of the device structure is shown in Figure 28.14.

The *I–V* characteristics of the 265 nm UV LED exhibit a turn-on voltage of ~5.5 V with a series resistance of 72 Ω. The turn-on is sluggish due to the high resistivity of the n- and p-type layers

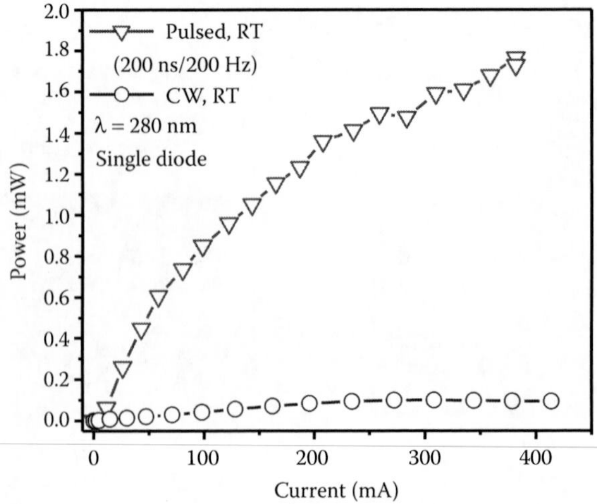

FIGURE 28.13 Power versus current for a single 280 nm UV LED in pulsed and CW mode.

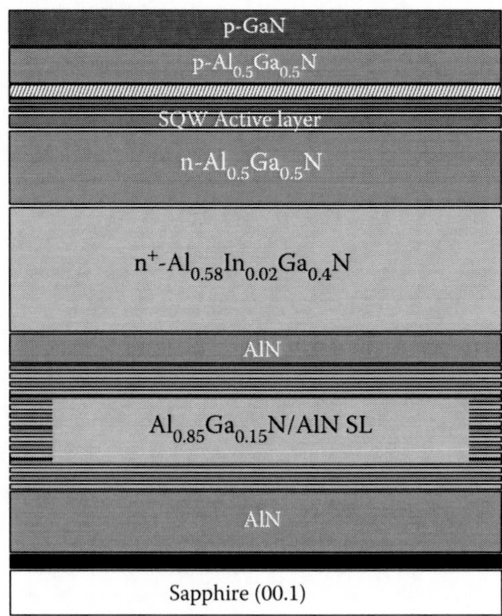

FIGURE 28.14 Structure of a 265 nm UV LED.

arising from the difficulty of doping of $Al_xGa_{1-x}N$ at high Al mole fractions. Figure 28.15 shows the room-temperature EL spectra of the LED at various current injection levels. The dominant peak occurs at 265 nm with a full width at half-maximum of ~9.5 nm. A very small defect-related peak with a very low integrated intensity is also observed in the spectra centered at $\lambda = 310$ nm, which saturates rapidly as the current increases.

Figure 28.16a shows the output power of the flip-chip-bonded device in pulsed operation mode (pulse width of 200 ns, frequency of 200 Hz). A high value of 2.4 mW at a current of only 360 mA was achieved for the bonded LED. The optical power at a pulsed current of 50 mA is as high as 0.5 mW. The *P–I* curve deviates slightly from a linear relationship at higher currents due to heating inside the device. For the same reason, the slope efficiency decreases from 12.8 μW/mA at low injection currents to 4.3 μW/mA at higher injection currents. For an array of four diodes in parallel, the slope efficiency increased from 4.3 to 7.4 μW/mA and the output power increased from 2.4 to

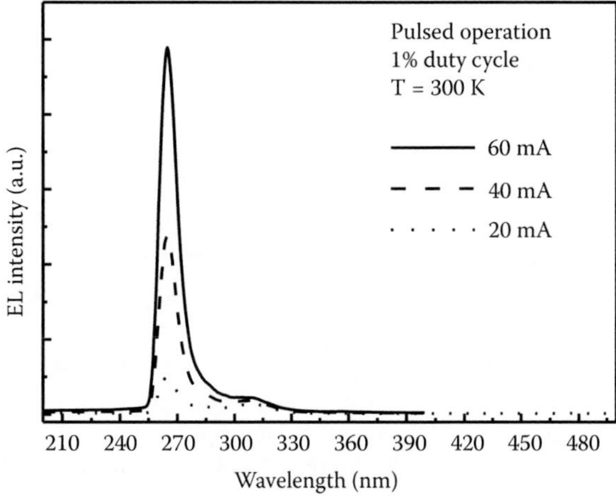

FIGURE 28.15 EL spectra of the 265 nm UV LED at various injection currents.

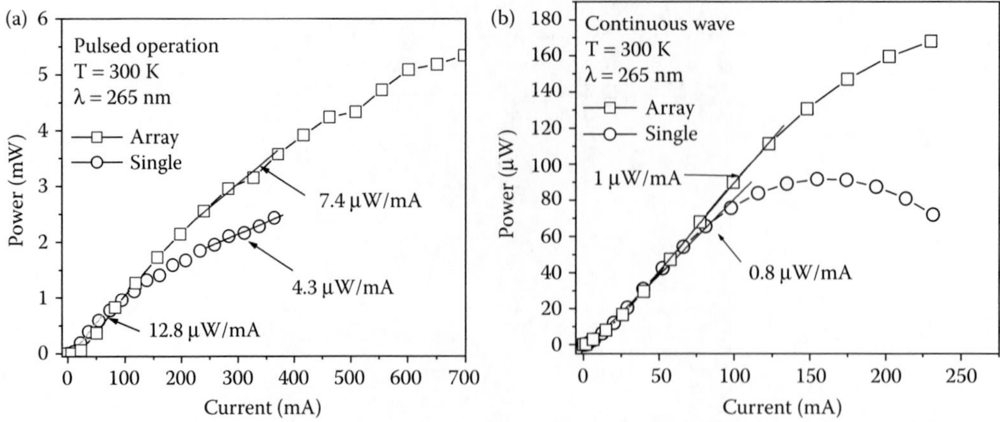

FIGURE 28.16 Output power versus current for the 265 nm UV LEDs under (a) pulsed and (b) CW injection current for a single diode (triangles) and an array of four diodes (circles). Also shown in the figure are the slope efficiencies.

3.5 mW at an injection current of 400 mA. The output power for this packaged array reached a value as high as 5.3 mW at a pulsed injection current of 700 mA.

Figure 28.16b shows the output power of the LED under CW current injection. The *P–I* curve starts to deviate from a linear trend at 100 mA and the power saturates at a current of ~150 mA where it reaches a maximum power of 90 μW. The slope efficiency of the CW power versus current is much lower than that of the pulsed power, even at low currents. This figure also shows the CW output power of an array of four diodes in parallel. The slope efficiency has improved by 20% compared to the single-diode case and power does not roll off until ~250 mA when the power reaches a value of 170 μW.

The external quantum efficiency (η_{ext}) of the LED in pulsed mode, η_{ext} reaches its maximum of ~0.23% at a current of 40 mA, corresponding to a current density of ~44 A/cm^2. The value of η_{ext} starts to decrease with increasing current at a current of 50 mA due to the generated heat. By further improving the material quality, hence reducing nonradiative recombination centers, we expect to achieve higher efficiencies. The value of η_{ext} is much lower under CW injection current and begins to decrease after reaching a maximum value of 0.03%. This again results from excessive heating of the device and will be improved by further optimization of the packaging technology.

28.5 III-NITRIDE-BASED UV DETECTORS

For many decades, the detection of UV light has been accomplished using photomultiplier tubes. These enjoy a high sensitivity to UV photons while being insensitive or "blind" to photons with wavelengths longer than the detector cutoff wavelength. However, they are fragile vacuum tube devices that require bulky high-voltage power sources to operate. This inherent complexity also makes them relatively expensive. A solid-state alternative to photo multiplier tubes (PMTs) is silicon-based photodetectors [63]. However, Si-based devices are not as robust as III-nitride-based photodetectors, and they have considerable sensitivity to photons in the visible and infrared spectral regions in addition to the UV portion of the spectrum. The out-of-band response is commonly addressed by the use of filters, such as a Woods glass optical filter. However, these filters increase the size and weight of the system, and reduce the overall quantum efficiency of the system. Other semiconductor materials besides Si have also been proposed by researchers with more or less success, including Ge, GaAs, and SiC; this is done in the hope of realizing an efficient solid-state UV photodetector that would enjoy the visible blindness of a photomultiplier tube. It is only in the second half of the 1990s that wide band-gap III-nitride semiconductors, and $Al_xGa_{1-x}N$ in particular, have begun to emerge as the most promising material systems for such a device, thanks to their exceptional material properties [63].

28.5.1 AlGaN-Based UV Photoconductors

Photoconductive UV detectors were the first to be demonstrated, as they are the simplest types of detectors. The first solar blind $Al_xGa_{1-x}N$-based detectors demonstrated were photoconductive detectors [64]. Shortly thereafter, $Al_xGa_{1-x}N$ photoconductive detectors were demonstrated across the entire compositional range from GaN to AlN [65]. Single undoped epilayers with thicknesses 0.5–1.5 μm were grown on basal plane sapphire substrates by MOCVD and photoconductors were fabricated with Ti/Au contacts. The photoconductors exhibited sharp cutoff wavelengths from 365 to 200 nm as shown in Figure 28.17. Specifically, the peak responsivity for $x = 0.34$ (λ_{cutoff} ~285 nm) is about 0.6 A/W. This was the first proof that $Al_xGa_{1-x}N$ materials were suitable for deep UV applications.

28.5.2 Front-Illuminated AlGaN-Based p–i–n Photodiodes

The first photovoltaic effects in GaN p–n junctions were reported in a paper published in 1995 [66], in which the modeling of the spectral response allowed determination of the hole diffusion length in n-type GaN to be 1000 Å. A similar modeling later led to an electron diffusion length in p-type GaN of 880 Å. Shortly thereafter, AlGaN-based p–i–n photodetectors across the compositional range were demonstrated, as shown in Figure 28.18. By tuning, the AlGaN composition detectors targeting the specific wavelengths necessary for biodetection can be realized.

28.5.3 Back-Illuminated AlGaN-Based p–i–n Photodiodes

AlGaN-based back-illuminated detectors are of special interest for the same reason that it is advantageous to fabricated back-emission LEDs—mainly higher efficiency. Back illumination also allows the detector to be epi-side down hybridized to a silicon chip that contains additional detector read-out electronics read while still collecting light through the back of the transparent sapphire

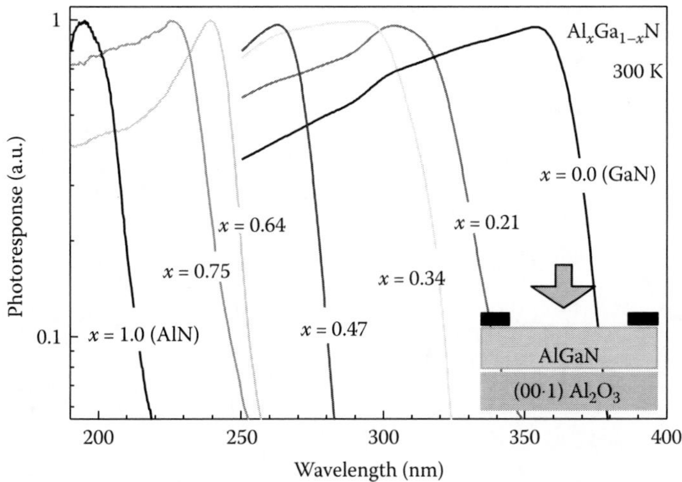

FIGURE 28.17 Room-temperature photoconductive response of AlGaN photoconductors across the entire compositional range from 200 to 365 nm.

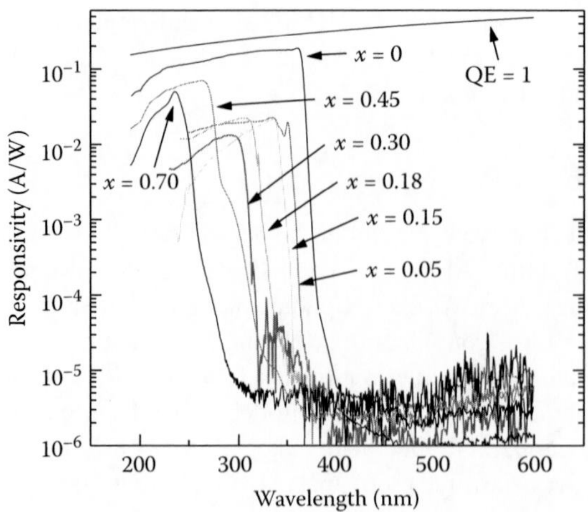

FIGURE 28.18 Spectral response of a wide range of front-illuminated $Al_xGa_{1-x}N$ photodiodes ($0 \leq x \leq 70\%$).

substrate. The biggest advantage for biodetection of using a back-illuminated device is that they inherently have a band-pass spectral shape. By carefully designing the heterojunction it is possible to tailor the band-pass to the fluorescence of the specific biomarkers.

As described in Section 28.3, novel atomic layer epitaxy techniques allow for the realization of very high-quality transparent AlN templates [68]. By using a novel $Al_{0.5}Ga_{0.5}N$ silicon–indium codoped layer as the bottom contact carrier concentrations of $n \sim -5 \times 10^{18}$ cm^{-3} and mobilities of $\mu \sim 60$ cm^2/V s are obtained, corresponding to an electrical conductivity approximately five times higher than conventional singly doped AlGaN of the same aluminum composition. This allowed us to report the highest quantum efficiency back-illuminated AlGaN-based p–i–n photodetectors with a record peak responsivity of 150 mA/W at 280 nm, corresponding to a high external quantum efficiency of 68%, increasing to 74% under 5 V reverse bias [69]. Also, Back-illuminated photodetectors with a peak response as short as 255 nm (Figure 28.19b) have been demonstrated. This device shows an unbiased peak responsivity of 95.7 mA/W at 255 nm with an FWHM of ~7 nm, which corresponds to a value of 46.5% for the external quantum efficiency of the device. The absolute response drops three orders of magnitude from the peak into the near-UV region [70].

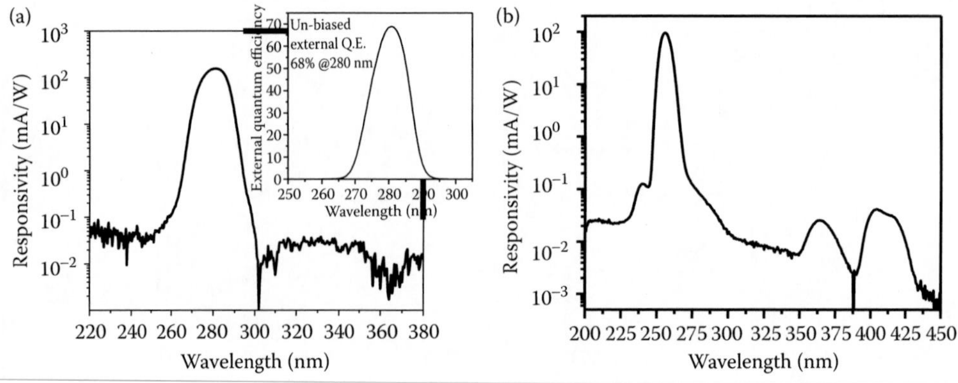

FIGURE 28.19 Responsivity versus wavelength, showing a peak responsivity of 150 mA/W at a wavelength of 280 nm (a); this peak responsivity corresponds to an external quantum efficiency of 68% (inset). (b) Responsivity versus wavelength, showing a peak responsivity of 95.7 mA/W at a wavelength of 255 nm.

28.5.4 Avalanche Photodiodes for Single-Photon Detection

In order for UV III-nitride-based photodetectors to truly compete effectively with the detective performance of PMTs, there is a need to develop photodetectors that take advantage of low-noise avalanche gain. Furthermore, in certain applications with low photon fluxes such as biodetection, it is desirable to obtain UV photon counting performance [71–73]. Most of the early III-nitride-based APD devices reported in the literature were designed for front-illumination operation with photons reaching the p-layer first. This configuration has been used historically because one would get fewer defects by growing a device structure on several-micron-thick *n*-type GaN templates on sapphire or even GaN substrates. However, there is a strong scientific and technological desire to investigate back-illuminated GaN avalanche photodiodes. A back-illuminated p–i–n GaN structure, in which photons reach the n-layer first, allows the device to take advantage of hole-initiated multiplication—this is advantageous since hole impact ionization coefficients are higher than the electron coefficient in GaN [74,75].

By using the same template that allowed for the realization of back-illuminated p–i–n photodiodes it is possible to realize back-illuminated III-nitride-based APDs. Back-illumination maximizes the injection of holes into the multiplication region making it a better approach for III-nitride-based avalanche photodiodes yielding higher gain and significantly reduced excess multiplication noise performance (Figure 28.20).

It is also possible to carefully design the structure to minimize the external bias necessary to reach the critical electric field necessary for breakdown (typically of 3×10^6 V · cm^{-1}). This can be accomplished by reducing the width of the combination absorption/multiplication layer in a traditional p–i–n device structure; however, this also increases the leakage current of the diodes, and thus, the dark count rate (DCR) in Geiger mode. In order to help overcome this, we have developed a novel separate absorption and multiplication APD structure (SAM-APD) [76]. By separating the absorption and multiplication regions using a *p–i–n–i–n* structure it becomes possible to absorb more than 99% of the light in the bottom layers resulting in nearly pure hole-injection into the multiplication region. This maximizes the advantage of the higher hole-ionization coefficient resulting in a device with a maximum linear mode gain of nearly 80,000. This high gain paves the way for the development of single-photon detection.

Geiger-mode operation under gated quenching has been previously demonstrated in front-illuminated GaN APDs with a SPDE of 13% at a DCR of 400 kHz in devices with an area of 1075 μm^2 [77]. Taking advantage of our recent work on back-illuminated GaN APDs we have already demonstrated the first back-illuminated GaN APDs operating in Geiger mode [78]. These

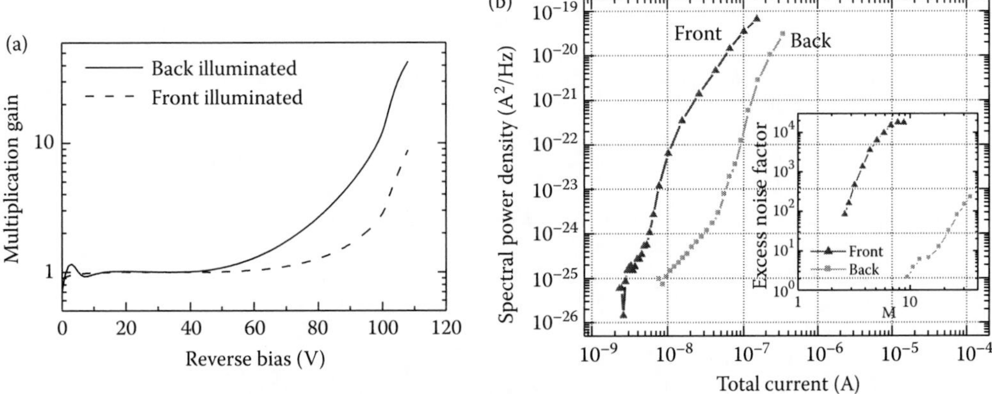

FIGURE 28.20 Comparison of front- and back-illuminated performance of GaN APDs showing that back illumination offers higher gain (a) and lower noise spectral power density and thus a lower excess noise factor (b).

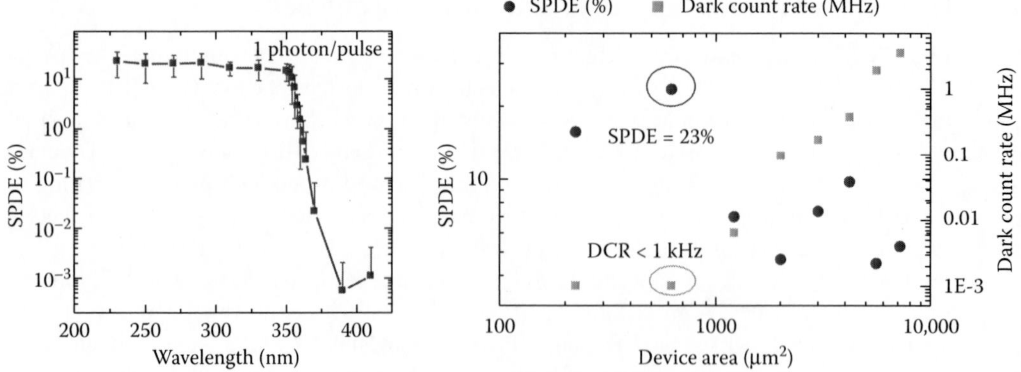

FIGURE 28.21 (a) Single-photon Geiger-mode response spectrum. (b) SPDE and dark count rate (DCR) versus device area.

Geiger-mode APDs operate using gated pulsed-quenching to detect very low UV-light levels. The spectral response shows a flat Geiger-mode response for photon energies above the band gap, and a high visible-light rejection ratio. These devices are capable of single-photon counting. The SPDE of these devices is more than 23%, with DCRs of less than 10 kHz [79] (Figure 28.21).

ACKNOWLEDGMENTS

The authors gratefully acknowledge many contributions of C. Bayram, P. Kung, K. Minder, J. L. Pau, D. Walker, and A. Yasan over the years in developing the study of III-nitride-based emitters and detectors at the CQD, department of Electrical Engineering and Computer Science, Northwestern University, Evanston, IL.

REFERENCES

1. A. A. Fatah, J. A. Barrett, R. D. Arcilesi, Jr., K. J. Ewing, C. H. Lattin, and LTC T. F. Moshier, *NIJ Guide 101–00*, U.S. Department of Justice, Office of Justice Programs, National Institute of Justice, 2001.
2. F. Fichter, Uber aliminiumnitride, *Z. Anorg. Chem.* 54, 322, 1907.
3. F. Fischer and F. Schröter, Berichte der deutschen chemischen gesellschaft, 43, 1465, 1910.
4. V. C. Johnson, J. B. Parsons, and M. C. Crew, Nitrogen Compounds of Gallium. I, II, *J. Phys. Chem.* 36, 2588, 1932.
5. H. P. Maruska and J. J. Tietjen, The preparation and properties of vapor-deposited single-crystalline GaN, *Appl. Phys. Lett.* 15, 327, 1969.
6. H. M. Manasevit, F. M. Erdmann, and W. I. Simpson, The use of metalorganics in the preparation of semiconductor materials. IV. The nitrides of aluminum and gallium, *J. Electrochem. Soc.* 118, 1864, 1971.
7. I. Akasaki et al., MITI Report [in Japanese]; 1974. I. Akasaki and I. Hayashi, [in Japanese] *Ind. Sci. Technol.* 17, 48, 1976.
8. S. Yoshida, S. Misawa, and A. Itoh, Epitaxial growth of aluminum nitride films on sapphire by reactive evaporation, *Appl. Phys. Lett.* 26, 461, 1975.
9. S. Yoshida, S. Misawa, and S. Gonda, Improvements on the electrical and luminescent properties of reactive molecular beam epitaxially grown GaN films by using AlN-coated sapphire substrates, *Appl. Phys. Lett.* 42, 427, 1983.
10. H. Amano, N. Sawaki, I. Akasaki, and Y. Toyoda, Metalorganic vapor phase epitaxial growth of a high quality GaN film using an AlN buffer layer, *Appl. Phys. Lett.* 48, 353, 1986.
11. H. Amano, M. Kito, K. Hiramatsu, and I. Akasaki, P-type conduction in Mg-doped GaN treated with low-energy electron beam irradiation (LEEBI), *Jpn. J. Appl. Phys.* 28, L2112, 1989.
12. M. Razeghi, *The Mocvd Challenge Volume 1: A Survey of GaInAsP-InP for Photonic and Electronic Applications*, Adam Hilger, Bristol and Philadelphia, 1989.

13. M. Razeghi, *The Mocvd Challenge Volume II: A Survey of GaInAsP-GaAs for Photonic and Electronic Device Applications*, Institute of Physics Publishing Bristol and Philadelphia, 1995.
14. Compound Semiconductor.net http://compoundsemiconductor.net/cws/article/magazine/17873/2, 2003.
15. X. Zhang, P. Kung, A. Saxler, D. Walker, T. C. Wang, and M. Razeghi. Growth of AlxGa1 – xN:Ge on sapphire and silicon substrates, *Appl. Phys. Lett.* 67(12), 1745, 1995.
16. K. Hiramatsu, S. Itoh, H. Amano, I. Akasaki, N. Kuwano, T. Shiraishi, and K. Oh, Growth mechanism of GaN grown on sapphire with AlN buffer layer by MOVPE, *J. Cryst. Growth* 115, 628, 1991.
17. C. J. Sun, P. Kung, A. Saxler, H. Ohsato, K. Haritos, and M. Razeghi, A crystallographic model of (00.1) aluminum nitride epitaxial thin film growth on (00.1) sapphire substrate, *J. Appl. Phys.* 75, 3964, 1994.
18. X. J. Ning, F. R. Chien, P. Pirouz, J. W. Yang, and M. Asif Khan, Growth defects in GaN films on sapphire: The probable origin of threading dislocations, *J. Mater. Res.* 11, 580, 1996.
19. B. Jahnen, M. Albrecht, W. Dorsch, S. Christiansen, H. P. Strunk, D. Hanser, and R. F. Davis, Pinholes, dislocations and strain relaxation in InGaN, *MRS Internet J. Nitride Semicond. Res.* 3, 39, 1998.
20. J.-M. Bethoux, P. Vennéguès, F. Natali, E. Feltin, O. Tottereau, G. Nataf, P. De Mierry, and F. Semond, Growth of high quality crack-free AlGaN films on GaN templates using plastic relaxation through buried cracks, *J. Appl. Phys.* 94, 6499, 2003.
21. A. Krost, J. Blasing, F. Schulze, O. Schon, A. Alam, and M. Heuken, Nearly strain-free AlGaN on (00.1) sapphire: X-ray measurements and a new crystallographic growth model, *J. Cryst. Growth* 221, 251, 2000.
22. H. Amano, M. Iwaya, N. Hayashi, T. Kashima, M. Katsuragawa, T. Takeuchi, C. Wetzel, and I. Akasaki, Improvement of crystalline quality of group III-nitrides on sapphire using low temperature interlayers, *MRS Internet J. Nitride Semicond. Res.* 4S1, G10.1, 1999.
23. T. Detchprohm, M. Yano, S. Sano, R. Nakamura, S. Mochiduki, T. Nakamura, H. Amano, and I. Akasaki, Heteroepitaxial lateral overgrowth of GaN on periodically grooved substrates: a new approach for growing low-dislocation-density GaN single crystals, *Jpn. J. Appl. Phys. Part 2* 40, L16, 2001.
24. K. E. Waldrip, J. Han, J. J. Figiel, H. Zhou, E. Makarona, and A. V. Nurmikko, Stress engineering during metalorganic chemical vapor deposition of AlGaN/GaN distributed Bragg reflectors, *Appl. Phys. Lett.* 78, 3205, 2001.
25. F. Natali, D. Byrne, A. Dussaigne, N. Grandjean, J. Massies, and B. Damilano, High-Al-content crack-free AlGaN/GaN Bragg mirrors grown by molecular-beam epitaxy, *Appl. Phys. Lett.* 82, 499, 2003.
26. A. Dadgar, J. Blasing, A. Diez, A. Alam, M. Heuken, and A. Krost, Metalorganic chemical vapor phase epitaxy of crack-free GaN on Si(111) exceeding 1 μm in thickness, *Jpn. J. Appl. Phys.* 39, L1183, 2000.
27. C. Q. Chen, J. P. Zhang, M. E. Gaevski, H. M. Wang, W. H. Sun, R. S. Q. Fareed, J. W. Yang, and M. Asif Khan, AlGaN layers grown on GaN using strain-relief interlayers, *Appl. Phys. Lett.* 81, 4961, 2002.
28. E. Feltin, B. Beaumont, M. La üget, P. De Mierry, P. Vennéguès, H. Lahrèche, M. Leroux, and P. Gibart, Stress control in GaN grown on silicon (111) by metalorganic vapor phase epitaxy, *Appl. Phys. Lett.* 79, 3230, 2001.
29. K. Ito, K. Hiramatsu, H. Amano, and I. Akasaki, Preparation of $Al_xGa_{1-x}N$/GaN heterostructure by MOVPE, *J. Cryst. Growth* 104, 533, 1990.
30. S. Nakamura, M. Senoh, S. Nagahama, N. Iwasa, T. Yamada, T. Matsushita, H. Kiyoku Y. Sugimoto, T. Kozaki, H. U., M. Sano, and K. Chocho, InGaN/GaN/AlGaN-based laser diodes with modulation-doped strained-layer superlattices grown on an epitaxially laterally overgrown GaN substrate, *Appl. Phys. Lett.* 72, 211, 1998.
31. H. M. Wang, J. P. Zhang, C. Q. Chen, Q. Fareed, J. W. Yang, and M. Asif Khan, AlN/AlGaN superlattices as dislocation filter for low-threading-dislocation thick AlGaN layers on sapphire, *Appl. Phys. Lett.* 81, 604, 2002.
32. M. D. McCluskey, N. M. Johnson, C. G. Van de Walle, D. P. Bour, M. Kneissl, and W. Walukiewicz, Metastability of oxygen donors in AlGaN, *Phys. Rev. Lett.* 80, 4008, 1998.
33. S. T. Bradley, S. H. Goss, L. J. Brillson, J. Hwang, and W. J. Schaff, Deep level defects and doping in high Al mole fraction AlGaN, *J. Vac. Sci. Technol. B* 21, 2558, 2003.
34. S. Fisher, C. Wetzel, E. E. Haller, and B. K. Meyer, On p-type doping in GaN—acceptor binding energies, *Appl. Phys. Lett.* 67, 1298, 1995.
35. C. G. Van de Walle, C. Stampfl, J. Neugebauer, M. D. McCluskey, and N. M. Johnson, Doping of AlGaN alloys, *MRS Internet J. Nitride Semicond. Res.* 4S1, G10.4, 1999.
36. M. C. Wagener, G. R. James, and F. Omnès, Intrinsic compensation of silicon-doped AlGaN, *Appl. Phys. Lett.* 83, 4193, 2003.
37. B. Pödör, Electron mobility in plastically deformed germanium, *Phys. Status Solidi* 16, K167, 1966.

38. A. Y. Polyakov, N. B. Smirnov, A. V. Govorkov, M. G. Milidivskii, J. M. Redwing, M. Shin, M. Showronski, D. W. Greve, and R. G. Wilson, Properties of Si donors and persistent photoconductivity in AlGaN, *Solid State Electron*. 42, 627, 1998.
39. P. Cantu, S. Keller, U. Mishra, and S. DenBaars, Metalorganic chemical vapor deposition of highly conductive $Al_{0.65}Ga_{0.35}N$ films, *Appl. Phys. Lett*. 82, 3683, 2003.
40. V. Adivarahan, G. Simin, G. Tamulaitis, R. Srinivasan, J. Yang, A. Khan, M. Shur, and R. Gaska, Indium–silicon co-doping of high-aluminum-content AlGaN for solar blind photodetectors, *Appl. Phys. Lett*. 79, 1903, 2001.
41. C. Stampfl and C. Van de Walle, Doping of $Al_xGa_{1-x}N$, *Appl. Phys. Lett*. 72, 459, 1998.
42. H. Amano, M. Kito, K. Hiramatsu, and I. Akasaki, p-type conduction in Mg-goped GaN treated with low-energy electron beam irradiation (LEEBI), *Jpn. J. Appl. Phys*. 28, L2112, 1989.
43. J. A. Van Vechten, J. D. Zook, R. D. Hornig, and B. Goldenberg, Defeating compensation in wide gap semiconductors by growing in H that is removed by low temperature de-ionizing radiation, *Jpn. J. Appl. Phys*. 31, 3662, 1992.
44. P. Kung, A. Yasan, R. McClintock, S. Darvish, K. Mi, and M. Razeghi, Future of $Al_xGa_{1-x}N$ materials and device technology for ultraviolet photodetectors, In *Photodetector Materials and Devices VII, Proceedings of SPIE 4650*, Eds G. J. Brown and M. Razeghi, p. 199, 2002.
45. T. Tanaka, A. Watanabe, H. Amano, Y. Kobayashi, I. Akasaki, S. Yamazaki, and M. Koike, p-type conduction in Mg-doped GaN and $Al_{0.08}Ga_{0.92}N$ grown by metalorganic vapor phase epitaxy, *Appl. Phys. Lett*. 65, 593, 1994.
46. A. Saxler, W. C. Mitchel, P. Kung, and M. Razeghi, Aluminum gallium nitride short-period superlattices doped with magnesium, *Appl. Phys. Lett*. 74, 2023, 1999.
47. M. Suzuki, J. Nishio, M. Onomura, and C. Hongo, Doping characteristics and electrical properties of Mg-doped AlGaN grown by atmospheric-pressure MOCVD, *J. Cryst. Growth* 189/190, 511, 1998.
48. A. Yasan, R. McClintock, S. R. Darvish, Z. Lin, K. Mi, P. Kung, and M. Razeghi, Characteristics of high-quality p-type $Al_xGa_{1-x}N$/GaN superlattices, *Appl. Phys. Lett*. 80, 2108, 2002.
49. P. Kozodoy, M. Hansen, S. P. DenBaars, and U. K. Mishra, Enhanced Mg doping efficiency in $Al_{0.2}Ga_{0.8}N$/GaN superlattices, *Appl. Phys. Lett*. 74, 3681, 1999.
50. K. B. Nam, M. L. Nakarmi, J. Li, J. Y. Lin, and H. X. Jiang, Mg acceptor level in AlN probed by deep ultraviolet photoluminescence, *Appl. Phys. Lett*. 83, 878, 2003.
51. A. Yasan and M. Razeghi, Very high quality p-type $Al_xGa_{1-x}N$/GaN superlattices, *Solid State Electron*. 47, 303, 2003.
52. A. Yasan, R. McClintock, K. Mayes, S. R. Darvish, P. Kung, M. Razeghi, and R. J. Molnar, 280 nm UV LEDs grown on HVPE GaN substrates*Opto-Elect. Rev*. 10, 287, 2002.
53. A. Yasan, R. McClintock, K. Mayes, S. R. Darvish, P. Kung, and M. Razeghi, Top-emission ultraviolet light-emitting diodes with peak emission at 280 nm, *Appl. Phys. Lett*. 81, 801, 2002.
54. M. Razeghi, P. Kung, D. Walker, M. Hamilton, and J. E. Diaz, High quality LEO growth and characterization of GaN films on Al_2O_3 and Si substrates, *Proc. SPIE Int. Soc. Opt. Eng*. 3725, 14, 1999.
55. S. Nakamura, M. Senoh, and S. Nagahama, N. Iwasa, T. Yamada, T. Matsushita, H. Kiyoku, Y. Sugimoto, T. Kozaki, H. U., M. Sano, and K. Chocho, InGaN/GaN/AlGaN-based laser diodes with modulation-doped strained-layer superlattices grown on an epitaxially laterally overgrown GaN substrate, *Appl. Phys. Lett*. 72, 211, 1998.
56. T. S. Zheleva, O. Nam, M. D. Bremser, T. S. Zheleva, and R. F. Davis, Dislocation density reduction via lateral epitaxy in selectively grown GaN structures, *Appl. Phys. Lett*. 71, 2472, 1997.
57. J. T. Torvik, J. I. Pankove, E. Ilinopoulos, H. M. Ng, and T. D. Moustakas, Optical properties of GaN grown over SiO_2 on SiC substrates by molecular beam epitaxy, *Appl. Phys. Lett*. 72, 244, 1998.
58. T. S. Zheleva, S. A. Smith, D. B. Thomson, T. Gehrke, K. J. Linthicum, P. Rajagopal, E. Carlson, W. M. Ashmawi, and R. F. Davis, Pendeo-epitaxy: A new approach for lateral growth of gallium nitride structures, *MRS Internet J. Semicond. Res*. 4s1, G3.38, 1999.
59. T. Detchprohm, M. Yano, S. Sano, R. Nakamura, S. Mochiduki, T. Nakamura, H. Amano, and I. Akasaki, Heteroepitaxial lateral overgrowth of GaN on periodically grooved substrates: A new approach for growing low-dislocation-density GaN single crystals, *Jpn. J. Appl. Phys. Part 2* 40, L16, 2001.
60. C. I. H. Ashby, C. C. Mitchell, J. Han, N. A. Missert, P. P. Provencio, D. M. Follstaedt, G. M. Peake, and L. Griego, Low-dislocation-density GaN from a single growth on a textured substrate, *Appl. Phys. Lett*. 77, 3233, 2000.
61. T. M. Katona, M. D. Craven, P. T. Fini, J. S. Speck, and S. P. DenBaars, Observation of crystallographic wing tilt in cantilever epitaxy of GaN on silicon carbide and silicon (111) substrates, *Appl. Phys. Lett*. 79, 2907, 2001.

62. A. Yasan, R. McClintock, K. Mayes, S. R. Darvish, H. Zhang, P. Kung, M. Razeghi, S. K. Lee, and J. Y. Han, Comparison of ultraviolet light-emitting diodes with peak emission at 340 nm grown on GaN substrate and sapphire, *Appl. Phys. Lett.* 81, 2151, 2002.
63. M. Razeghi and A. Rogalski, Semiconductor ultraviolet detectors, *J. Appl. Phys.* 79(10), 7433–7473, 1996.
64. D. Walker, X. Zhang, P. Kung, A. Saxler, S. Javadpour, J. Xu, and M. Razeghi, AlGaN ultraviolet photoconductors grown on sapphire, *Appl. Phys. Lett.* 68(15), 2100–2101, 1996.
65. D. Walker, X. Zhang, A. Saxler, P. Kung, J. Xu, and M. Razeghi, $Al_xGa_{1-x}N$ ($0 \leq x \leq 1$) ultraviolet photodetectors grown on sapphire by metal-organic chemical-vapor deposition, *Appl. Phys. Lett.* 70(8), 949–951, 1997.
66. X. Zhang, P. Kung, D. Walker, J. Piotrowski, A. Rogalski, A. Saxler, and M. Razeghi, Photovoltaic effects in GaN structures with p–n junctions, *Appl. Phys. Lett.* 67(14), 2028–2030, 1995.
67. M. Razeghi, Short wavelength solar-blind detectors: Status, prospects, and markets *Proc. IEEE* 90(6), 1006, 2002.
68. R. McClintock, A. Yasan, K. Mayes, D. Shiell, S. Darvish, P. Kung, and M. Razeghi, High quantum efficiency solar-blind photodetectors, *Proc. SPIE* 5359 434, 2004.
69. R. McClintock, A. Yasan, K. Mayes, D. Shiell, S. R. Darvish, P. Kung, and M. Razeghi, High quantum efficiency AlGaN solar-blind photodetectors, *Appl. Phys. Lett.* 84(8), 1248, 2004.
70. R. McClintock, A. Yasan, K. Mayes, P. Kung, and M. Razeghi, Back-illuminated solar-blind photodetectors for imaging applications, *Proc. SPIE* 5359, 434, 2004.
71. P. Kung, A. Yasan, R. McClintock, S. R. Darvish, K. Mi, and M. Razeghi, Future of Al*x*Ga1 − *x*N materials and device technology for ultraviolet photodetectors, *Proc. SPIE* 4650, 199–206, 2002.
72. M. Razeghi, Short-wavelength solar-blind detectors—Status, prospects, and markets, *Proc. IEEE* 90, 1006–1014, 2002.
73. M. Ulmer, M. Razeghi, and E. Bigan, Ultra-violet detectors for astrophysics, present and future, *Proc. SPIE* 2397, 210–216, 1995.
74. I. J. Oguzman, E. Bellotti, K. Brennan, J. Kolnik, R. Wang, and P. Ruden, Theory of hole initiated impact ionization in bulk zincblende and wurtzite GaN, *J. Appl. Phys.* 81, 7827, 1997.
75. R. McClintock, J. L. Pau, K. Minder, C. Bayram, P. Kung, M. Razeghi, *Appl. Phys. Lett.* 90, 1411121, 2007.
76. J. L. Pau, C. Bayram, R. McClintock, M. Razeghi, and D. Silversmith, Back-illuminated separate absorption and multiplication GaN avalanche photodiodes, *Appl. Phys. Lett.* 92(10), 2008.
77. K. A. McIntosh, R. J. Molnar, L. J. Mahoney, K. M. Molvar, N. Efremow, Jr., S. Verghese, *Appl. Phys. Lett.* 76, 3938, 2000.
78. J. L. Pau, R. McClintock, K. Minder, C. Bayram, P. Kung, M. Razeghi, E. Muñoz, and D. Silversmith, Geigermode operation of back-illuminated GaN avalanche photodiodes, *Appl. Phys. Lett.* 91(4), 041104-1, 2007.
79. R. McClintock, J. L. Pau, K. Minder, C. Bayram, and M. Razeghi, III-Nitride photon counting avalanche photodiodes, *Proc. SPIE* 6900, 69000N-1, 2008.

29 Nanotechnology-Derived Orthopedic Implant Sensors

Sirinrath Sirivisoot and Thomas J. Webster

CONTENTS

29.1 INTRODUCTION

Osteoblasts and osteoclasts are located in bone, a natural nanostructured-mineralized organic matrix. While osteoblasts make bone, osteoclasts decompose bone by releasing acid that degrades calcium phosphate-based apatite minerals into an aqueous environment. The synthesis, deposition, and mineralization of this organic matrix, in which osteoblasts proliferate and mineralize (i.e., deposit calcium), require the ordered expression of a number of osteoblast genes. Bone has the ability to self-repair or remodel routinely. However, osteoporosis (unbalanced bone remodeling) and other joint diseases (such as osteoarthritis, rheumatoid arthritis, or traumatic arthritis) can lead to bone fractures. These disabilities associated with bone all lead to difficulties in performing common activities and may require an orthopedic implant. However, the average functional lifetime of, for example, a hip implant (usually composed of titanium) is only 10–15 years. A lack of fixation into surrounding bone eventually loosens the implant and is the most common cause of hip replacement failure.

Approximately 200,000 total and 100,000 partial hip replacements as well as 36,000 revision hip replacement surgeries were performed in the United States in 2003 [1]. Unfortunately, only limited techniques, such as insensitive imaging (through x-rays or bone scans), exist to determine if sufficient bone growth is occurring next to a titanium implant after surgery. Thus, techniques used in orthopedic diagnostics need to more accurately identify musculoskeletal injuries and conditions after implantation. Although there have been improvements in implants to increase bone formation, the clinical diagnosis of new bone growth surrounding implants remains problematic, sometimes significantly increasing hospital stays and decreasing the ability of doctors to quickly prescribe a change in action if new bone growth is insufficient.

Currently, a physical examination (e.g., palpation, or laboratory testing) might be completed before imaging techniques are used to inform a clinician about a patient's health. Although advanced imaging techniques, such as bone scans, computer tomography scans, and radiographs (x-rays) are important in medical diagnosis, each has its own limitations and difficulties. A bone scan is used to identify areas of abnormal active bone formation, such as in arthritis, infection, or bone cancer. However, bone scans require an injection of a radioactive substance (e.g., technetium) and a prolonged delay for absorbance before performing the scan. Computer tomography combines x-rays with computer technology to produce a two-dimensional (2D) cross-sectional image of a body on the computer screen. Although this technique produces more detail than an x-ray, in some cases (e.g., severe trauma to the chest, abdomen, pelvis, or spinal cord), a dye (e.g., barium sulfate) must be injected for improving the clarity of the image. This often causes pain to the patient. Another technique, called electromyography, has been used to analyze/diagnose nerve functions inside body conditions. Thin electrodes are placed in soft tissues to help analyze and record electrical activity in the muscles. However, this electrode technique leads to pain and discomfort for the patient. When the needles are removed, soreness and bruising can occur.

Electrochemical biosensors on the implant itself show promise for medical diagnostics *in situ* to possibly determine new bone growth surrounding the implant. Yet, this technology has not been fully explored. Incorporation of such electrochemical biosensors into current bone implants may be possible through nanotechnology; different types of nanoscale biomaterials have varying abilities to enhance *in vitro/in vivo* bone formation. Carbon nanotubes (CNTs) are macromolecules of carbon, classified either as single-walled carbon nanotubes (SWCNTs) with diameters of 0.4–2 nm or multiwalled carbon nanotubes (MWCNTs) with diameters of 2–100 nm [2,3]. Due to their unique electrical, mechanical, chemical, and biological properties [4–11], CNTs have shown promise for bone implantation. For example, nanocomposites of polylactic acid and MWCNTs increased osteoblast proliferation by 46% and calcium production by greater than 300% when an alternating current was applied *in vitro* [12,13]. In addition, combining MWCNTs with precursor powders improves the mechanical properties of as-aligned hydroxyapatite (HA) composite coatings [9]. MWCNTs, reinforced with HA coatings, promoted human osteoblast proliferation *in vitro*, as observed in the appearance of cells near MWCNT regions [8]. Osteoblasts extended in all directions within the CNT scaffold that formed on polycarbonate membranes [14]. Osteoblasts significantly enhanced their adhesion on vertically aligned MWCNT arrays, according to Giannona et al. [15] by recognizing nanoscaled features. In addition, Zanello et al. (2006) [7] showed that CNTs are suitable for the proliferation of osteosarcoma ROS 17/2.8 cells on SWCNT and MWCNT scaffolds. Human osteoblast-like (Saos2) cells grown on the MWCNT scaffold showed a higher cell density and transforming growth factor-β1 concentration compared with those grown on polystyrene and polycarbonate scaffolds [16].

Our previous studies have shown greater osteoblast differentiation on MWCNT-Ti than on Ti alone [17]. Moreover, MWCNTs are a promising material for electrochemical biosensors because they also possess relatively well-characterized behavior in terms of electron transport [18–21]. Coating CNTs on Ti electrodes also increases the active surface area and enhances direct electron transfer [22,23]. These studies encourage the use of MWCNTs to modify currently used Ti for orthopedic implants. CNTs can be produced by the laser furnace arc and chemical vapor deposition (CVD) methods. Unlike the laser furnace arc, CVD is a scalable and controllable method of obtaining high purity CNTs [24]. A strong mechanical connection between CNTs and the metal is needed for nanosensor applications [25], and the reduced resistance between the Ti and CNTs [26] leads to increased current passage. For example, Sato et al. [27] showed potential for using CNTs in electrochemical biosensors by using CVD to grow MWCNTs with Ti biometallic particles and cobalt (Co) as a catalyst. They revealed that Co has the ability to combine with Ti [27] and since CNTs were grown by using a Co-catalyst in that study, a strong electrical contact between metallic Ti and MWCNTs was possible.

As mentioned, to form a more robust interconnection, CNTs have been anchored in the pores of anodized nanotubular Ti. MWCNTs have then been grown using CVD techniques out of the anodized Ti nanotubes (with diameters of 50–60 nm and depths of 200 nm) as a template. *In vivo*, many cell processes that are important during new bone growth rely on the redox reactions of various biomolecules and ions. The mechanisms of electron transfer reaction and the role of proteins in aiding the electron transfer of redox processes can be examined by electrochemical analysis. In electronic theory, when two different materials come in contact with each other, electron transfer will occur in an attempt to balance Fermi levels, causing the formation of a double layer of electrical charges at the interface. Because, the formation of electric contact between the redox proteins and the electrode surface is the fundamental challenge of electrochemical biosensor devices, in one study, the redox reactions of iron (II/III) and the osteoblast extracellular components at the surface of Ti, anodized Ti, and MWCNT-Ti have been investigated. How to create such novel orthopedic sensors along with the latest data concerning their use is present below.

29.2 MAKING ORTHOPEDIC IMPLANT SENSORS

29.2.1 Step One: Preparation of Nanotubular Anodized Titanium

In order to create orthopedic sensors, currently implanted titanium (Ti) has been modified to have a nanotube-structured thin layer of titanium dioxide (TiO_2) by anodization [17]. Briefly, 99.2% commercially pure Ti sheets (Alfa Aesar) can be cut into squares (1 cm^2) and cleaned with acetone and 70% ethanol under sonication for 10 min each. After rinsing with deionized water, Ti can be etched for 10 s in a solution of 1.5% by weight of nitric acid and 0.5% by weight of hydrofluoric acid to remove the existing oxidized-layer on Ti. Immediately after etching, Ti can be placed as an anode electrode and a high-purity platinum (Pt) mesh (Alfa Aesar) can be used as a cathode. In a Teflon beaker, both electrodes can be immersed in an electrolyte solution of 1.5% by weight of hydrofluoric acid in deionized water. The distance between Ti and the platinum mesh should be around 1 cm. A direct current power supply (3645A; Circuit Specialists) can then be used at 20 V between the anode and cathode for 10 min to create uniform nanotubes of TiO_2 on commercially pure Ti. It is from these uniform titanium nanotubes that electrically active sensing MWCNTs can be grown, as described next.

29.2.2 Step Two: Cobalt-Catalyzed CVD for Growing MWCNTs

Afterward, MWCNTs can be grown out of the nanoporous TiO_2 by CVD. A plasma-enhanced chemical vapor deposition system (Applied Science & Technology Inc.) can be used to grow MWCNTs from the nanotubular anodized Ti. In order to do this, the anodized Ti samples can be soaked in a solution of 5% by weight of Cobaltous Nitrate (Allied Chemical) in methanol for 5 min prior to the CVD process. Then, Cobalt-catalyzed anodized Ti should be rinsed with distilled water and dried with compressed air. The samples can then be placed in the CVD chamber and the air pumped out to a base pressure below 10 mTorr. The samples can be heated to 700°C in a flow of 100 standard cubic centimeters per minute (sccm) hydrogen gas (H_2) for 20 min. The gas composition can be changed to 40 sccm H_2 and 160 sccm acetylene gas (C_2H_2) for 30 min to grow MWCNTs. The MWCNT-Ti should be cooled in a 100 sccm Argon flow. The dense and entangled MWCNTs can form a 3D structure on the Ti surface with exceptional electrical conductivity and surface area. In particular, conventional Ti, shown in Figure 29.1a, exhibits a smooth Ti oxide surface. After anodization, nanopores of Ti oxide are formed on the Ti surface uniformly with diameters of 50–60 nm and depths of 200 nm, as shown in Figure 29.1b. After the CVD process described here, MWCNTs covered the anodized Ti as shown in Figure 29.1c side view and 29.1d top view.

29.3 BIOLOGICAL RESPONSES TO ORTHOPEDIC IMPLANT SENSORS

Importantly, results have shown similar numbers of osteoblasts after 4 h on unanodized Ti, anodized nanotubular Ti without MWCNTs, and anodized nanotubular Ti with MWCNTs (Figure 29.2); all were greater than the carbon nanopaper (used as a chemical control). These initial data were important as they indicated that the MWCNT sensor was not detrimental to osteoblast functions.

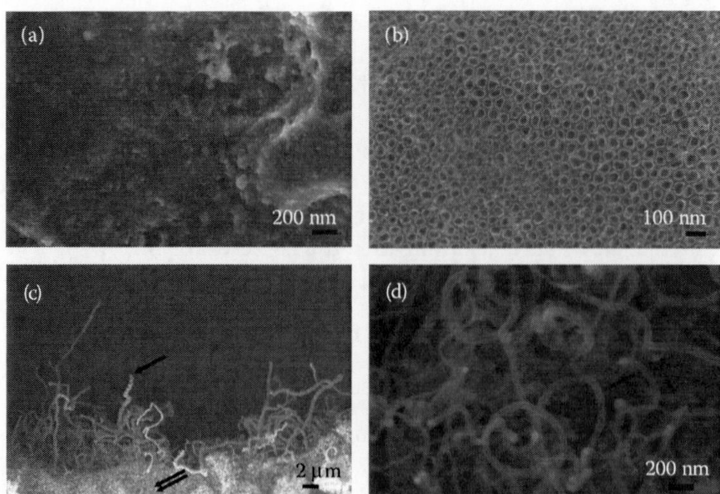

FIGURE 29.1 Scanning electron micrographs (SEM) of the electrode surfaces: (a) conventional Ti; (b) anodized Ti; (c) side view; and (d) top view of MWCNT-Ti. A single arrow shows MWCNTs, whereas double arrow show the anodized Ti template.

Moreover, osteoblasts were observed with cytoplasmatic prolongation on the surfaces of MWCNTs grown out of anodized nanotubular Ti (Figures 29.3c and d), resulting in stronger adhesion (more density of the points of contact) and some might say resembling osteoblast interactions with extracellular matrix proteins [17]. In contrast, osteoblasts on anodized Ti without MWCNTs were not observed to have cytoplasmic prolongation (Figures 29.3a and b). Zanello et al. also observed a thin neurite-like cytoplasmic prolonagation of osteoblasts that reached the nanotube bundles after cell culture for 5 days. More impressively, results have demonstrated that alkaline phosphatase activity and calcium deposition by osteoblasts increased on the MWCNTs grown from anodized nanotubular Ti sensors compared to anodized nanotubular Ti without MWCNTs, unanodized Ti, and carbon nanopaper after 21 days (Figure 29.4). This result suggested even better osteoblast responses on MWCNT sensors than currently used Ti.

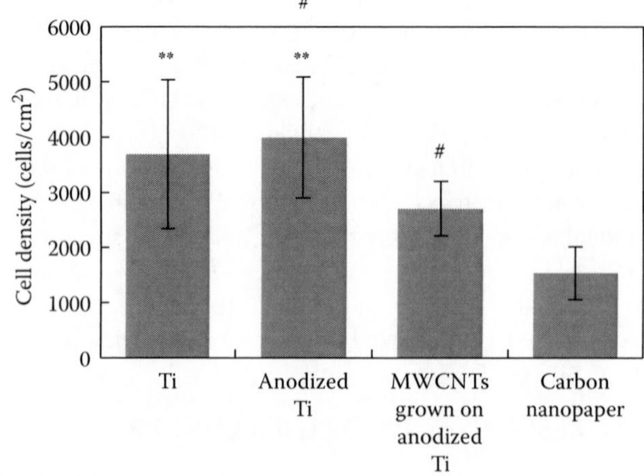

FIGURE 29.2 Osteoblast adhesion for 4 h on Ti, anodized Ti, MWCNTs grown on anodized Ti, and carbon nanopaper. Values are mean ± SEM; $N = 3$; $^{**}p < 0.05$ compared to carbon nanopaper; $\#p < 0.05$ compared to MWCNTs grown on anodized Ti.

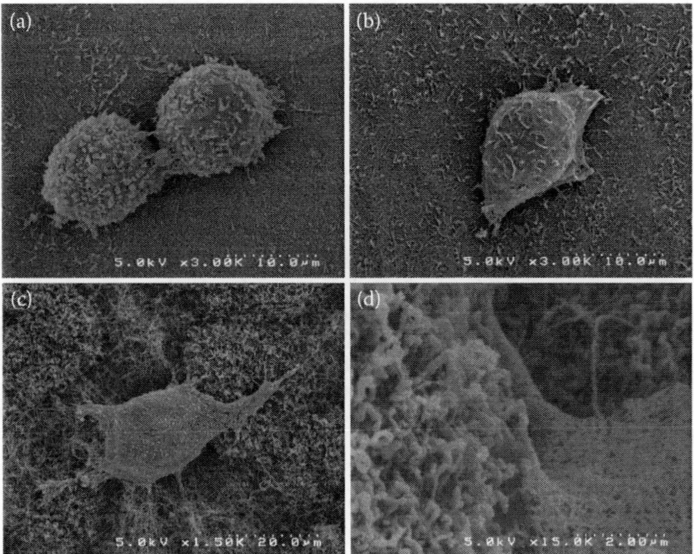

FIGURE 29.3 Osteoblast morphology after 4 h adhesion on: (a, b) anodized Ti (Scale bars = 10 μm). Round-shaped osteoblasts are on the anodized Ti substrate without MWCNTs; and (c, d) MWCNTs grown on anodized Ti (Scale bars = 20 μm left and 2 μm right). The single arrow shows the cytoplasmic prolongations of osteoblasts to MWCNTs. Double arrows show MWCNTs, while triple arrows show the osteoblast membrane.

29.4 SENSING ABILITY OF ORTHOPEDIC IMPLANT SENSORS

Of course, the next question is how well do these MWCNTs sense new bone growth? As a starting point, experiments were conducted with the $Fe(CN)_6^{4-/3-}$ redox system. The $Fe(CN)_6^{4-/3-}$ redox system with an exhibition of heterogeneous one electron transfer ($n = 1$) is one of the most extensively studied redox couples in electrochemistry [28]. It has been performed on the cyclic voltammetry experiments of the $Fe^{2+/3+}$ redox couple by placing MWCNT-Ti in an electrolyte solution of 10 mM $K_3Fe(CN)_6$ and 1 M KNO_3. In potassium ferricyanide ($K_3Fe(CN)_6$), the reduction process is Fe^{3+} ($Fe(CN)_6^{3-} + e^- \rightarrow Fe(CN)_6^{4-}$) followed by the oxidation of Fe^{2+} ($Fe(CN)_6^{4-} \rightarrow Fe(CN)_6^{3-} + e^-$) under a sweeping voltage. In such studies, the iron (II/III) redox couple did not exhibit any observable peaks for bare Ti or anodized Ti electrodes, as shown in Figures 29.7a and b. This implies that the electrochemical reaction is slow on both these electrodes. However, highly directed electron transfer at the MWCNT-Ti sensor electrode was observed as redox peaks, shown in Figure 29.10c. At a scan rate of 100 mV/s in Figure 29.10c, a well-defined redox peak appeared with the anodic (E_{pa}) and cathodic (E_{pc}) potentials at 175 mV and 345 mV, respectively. Moreover, on the inner set of Figure 29.7c, the relationship is linear between the anodic and cathodic peak currents versus the square root of the scan rate, while the ratio of I_{pa}/I_{pc} is about 1, corresponding to the Randles–Sevcik equation 29.1. Because the root scan rate has this linear relation with the peak currents, the mass transport in this process must be by diffusion. Zhang et al. [29] found that the heterogeneous charge-transfer rate constant (k) of the $Fe(CN)_6^{4-/3-}$ complex with H_2O as a solvent is 0.05 cm/s. Since the k value is in the range of 10^{-4}–10^{-1} cm/s and $\Delta E_p > 59/n$ mV (in this case $n = 1$ and $\Delta E_p \sim 170$ mV), this process is quasireversible.

In order to analyze the electrochemical behavior at the surface of the MWCNT-Ti sensor electrode, researchers have used the Randles–Sevcik equation for quasireversible processes, Equation 29.1. Hence, the peak current (I_p) is given by

$$I_p = 2.99 \times 10^5 \mathrm{AD}^{1/2} n (n_a \gamma)^{1/2} C \tag{29.1}$$

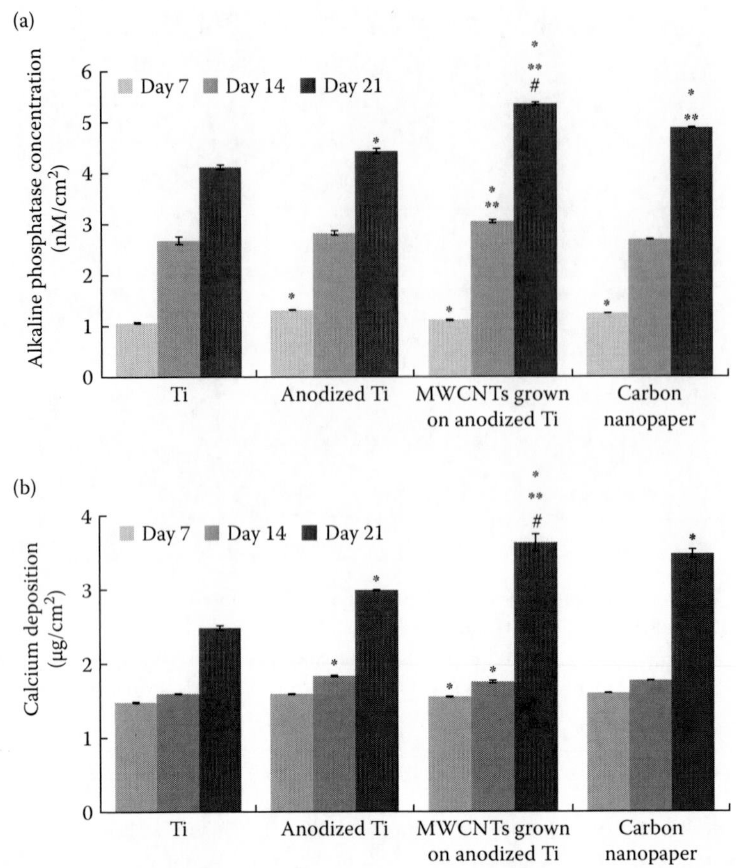

FIGURE 29.4 Osteoblasts long-term functions: (a) alkaline phosphatase activity; values are mean ± SEM; $n = 3$; $*p < 0.05$ compared to Ti; $**p < 0.1$ compared to anodized Ti; and $\#p < 0.1$ compared to carbon nanopaper and (b) calcium deposition; values are mean ± SEM; $N = 3$; $*p < 0.1$ compared to Ti; $**p < 0.1$ compared to anodized Ti; and $\#p < 0.05$ compared to carbon nanopaper.

where n is the number of electrons participating in the redox process, n_a is the number of electrons participating in the charge-transfer step, A is the area of the working electrode (cm^2), D is the diffusion coefficient of the molecules in the electrolyte solution (cm^2/s), C is the concentration of the probe molecule in the bulk solution (molar), and γ is the scan rate of the sweep potential (V/s). When the $Fe(CN)_6^{4-/3-}$ redox system exhibits heterogeneous one-electron transfer ($n = n_a = 1$) and the concentration C is equal to 10 mM, the diffusion coefficient D is equal to $6.7 \pm 0.02 \times 10^{-6}$ cm^2/s [30,31]. Hence, the quasireversible redox of iron (II/III) is truly enhanced by the novel MWCNT sensors.

In order to estimate how such sensors would do for bone growth, osteoblasts were cultured for 21 days and energy-dispersive spectroscopy (EDS) was performed to verify the presence of the various minerals in newly formed bone. Figure 29.5 shows the results of one such study doing this in which the peaks of many inorganic substances, consisting of magnesium (Mg), phosphorus (P), sulfur (S), potassium (K), and calcium (Ca) were detected. The Ca/P weight ratio of minerals deposited by osteoblasts in that study on Ti (1.34) was less than that on a MWCNT-Ti sensor (1.52). However, the Ca/P ratio of HA, the main calcium–phosphate crystallite in bone, is typically about 1.67 [32,33]. This study demonstrated that the minerals deposited by osteoblasts on MWCNT-Ti were more similar to natural bone than the minerals deposited on Ti. X-ray diffraction (XRD) analysis also showed that more HA was deposited on MWCNT-Ti sensors than on both conventional and anodized Ti

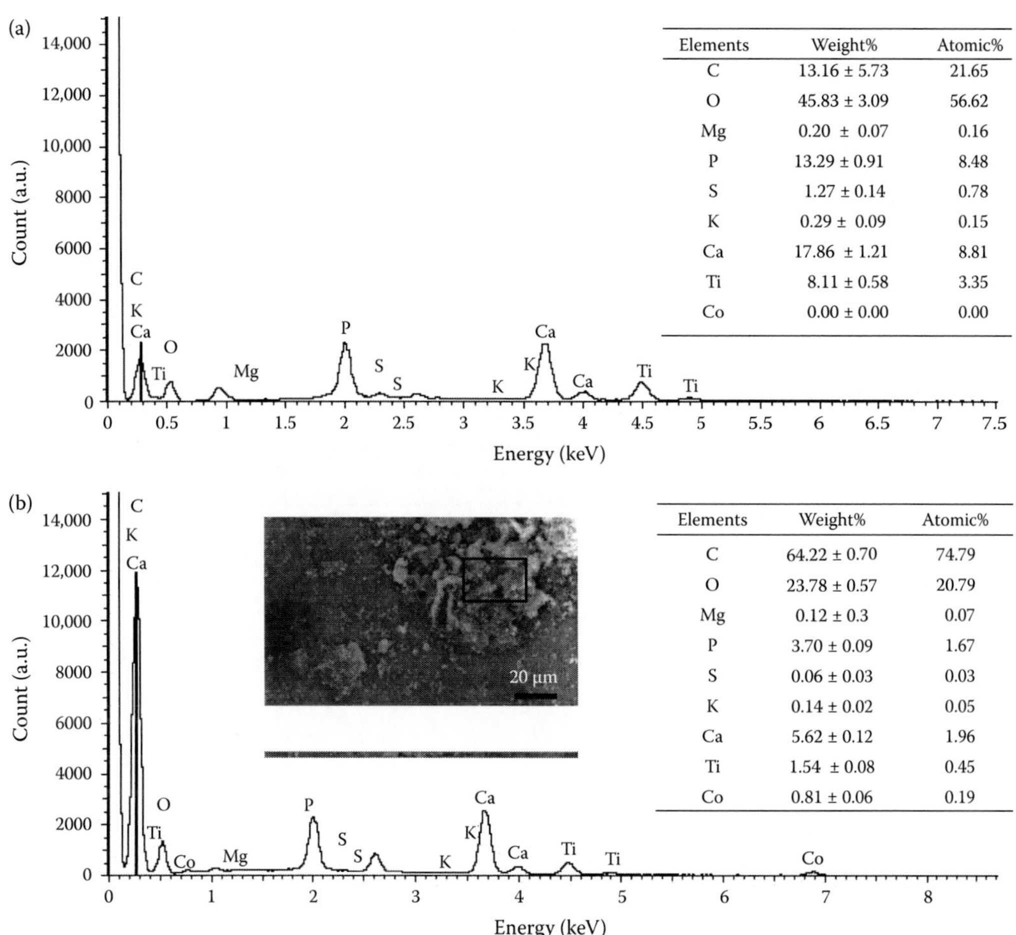

(a)

Elements	Weight%	Atomic%
C	13.16 ± 5.73	21.65
O	45.83 ± 3.09	56.62
Mg	0.20 ± 0.07	0.16
P	13.29 ± 0.91	8.48
S	1.27 ± 0.14	0.78
K	0.29 ± 0.09	0.15
Ca	17.86 ± 1.21	8.81
Ti	8.11 ± 0.58	3.35
Co	0.00 ± 0.00	0.00

(b)

Elements	Weight%	Atomic%
C	64.22 ± 0.70	74.79
O	23.78 ± 0.57	20.79
Mg	0.12 ± 0.3	0.07
P	3.70 ± 0.09	1.67
S	0.06 ± 0.03	0.03
K	0.14 ± 0.02	0.05
Ca	5.62 ± 0.12	1.96
Ti	1.54 ± 0.08	0.45
Co	0.81 ± 0.06	0.19

FIGURE 29.5 EDS analysis of osteoblasts cultured for 21 days on (a) Ti and (b) MWCNT-Ti. The SEM micrograph of inset (b) shows the analyzed area. For the MWCNT-Ti, more Ca and P deposited by osteoblasts were observed. Tables in (a) and (b) show the composition of the mineral deposits after osteoblasts were cultured for 21 days. The Ca/P weight ratio on bare Ti was 1.32 and on MWCNT-Ti was 1.52.

after 21 days of culture, as shown in Figure 29.6. In addition, the amount of calcium deposited by osteoblasts as determined by a calcium quantification assay kit was 1.481 μg/cm^2 for 7 days, 1.597 μg/cm^2 for 14 days, and 2.483 μg/cm^2 for 21 days on conventional Ti, as shown in Figure 29.10b. These results imply a greater deposition of calcium by osteoblasts on MWCNT-Ti sensors than currently implanted Ti.

Bone resorption and remodeling involve the secretion of hydrochloric acid (HCl) by osteoclasts [34]. Osteoclasts dissolve bone mineral by isolating a region of the matrix and then secreting HCl and proteinases at the bone surface, resulting in the bone acting as a reservoir of Ca^{2+}, PO_4^{3-}, and OH^- minerals [35]. This can be the reason that HCl is so prevalent in laboratories to dissolve calcium minerals deposited on osteoblast-seeded scaffolds *in vitro* for further use in a calcium deposition assay. Thus, after dissolving with 0.6 N HCl, it is likely that Ca^{2+}, PO_4^{3-}, and OH^- are contained in the solution of the osteoblast extracellular components.

The formation of bone matrix minerals first depends on achieving a critical concentration of calcium and phosphorus. Then phospholipids, anionic proteins, as well as calcium and phosphorus aggregate in nucleation pores that are in the 35 nm "hole-zone" between collagen molecules [36].

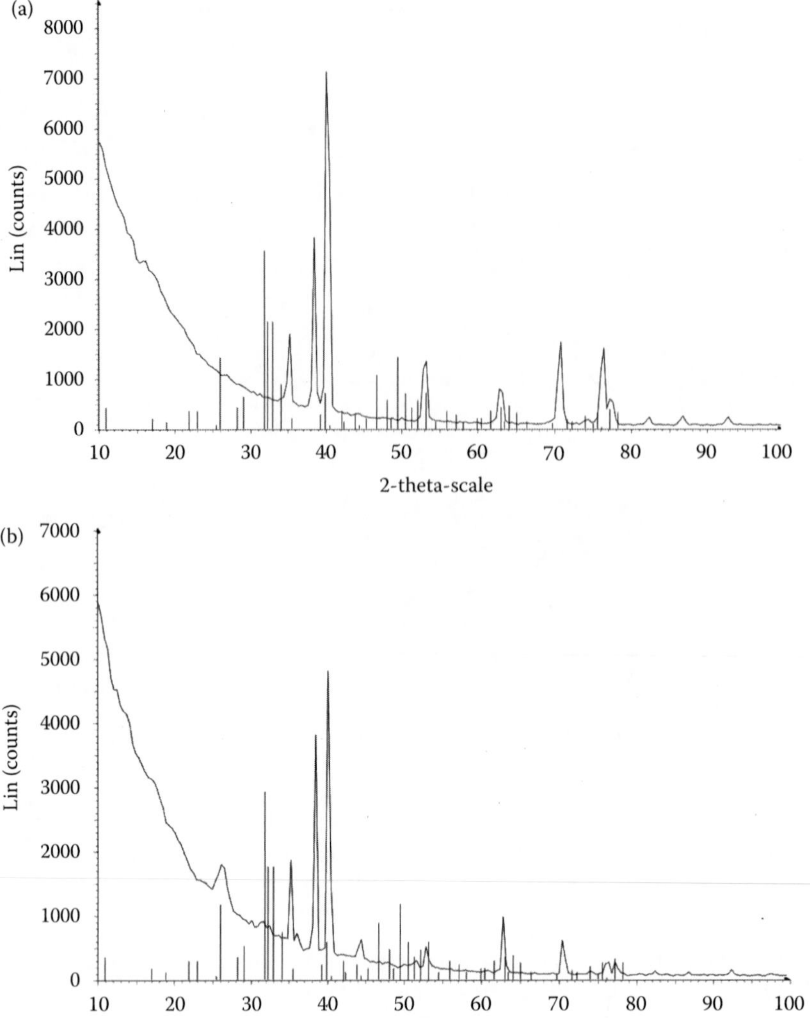

FIGURE 29.6 XRD analysis of HA-like (HA; $Ca_5(PO_4)_3OH$) deposited minerals after osteoblasts were cultured for 21 days on (a) Ti and (b) MWCNT-Ti. The micrographs show that the peak pattern of HA more closely matches that of the mineral deposited by osteoblasts when cultured on MWCNT-Ti than Ti.

The addition of calcium, phosphate, and hydroxyl ions contributes to the growth of crystalline HA. However, the crystals are not pure since they also contain carbonate, sodium, potassium, citrate, and traces of other elements, such as strontium and lead. The imperfection of HA contributes to its minerals' solubility, which plays a role in the ability of osteoclasts to resorb the mineral phases. Although osteoblasts synthesize type I collagen, which is the predominant organic components of bone, type III/V/VI collagen also exists in bone. Moreover, noncollagen proteins of bone (such as growth factors, osteocalcin, osteopontin, and osteonectin) and proteins in serum and other tissues (such as fibronectin, vitronectin, and laminin) are absorbed into the mineral component during bone growth. These components are directly involved in the genesis and maintenance of bone. Thus, not only minerals but also other noncollagenous proteins are broken down after dissolution with HCl. As such, nonspecific proteins may exist in the supernatant of bone formation when cyclic voltammetry is performed with MWCNT-Ti sensors and may contribute to the observed redox process shown in this chapter. On an electrode surface, the native conformation of a protein may be retained (reversible

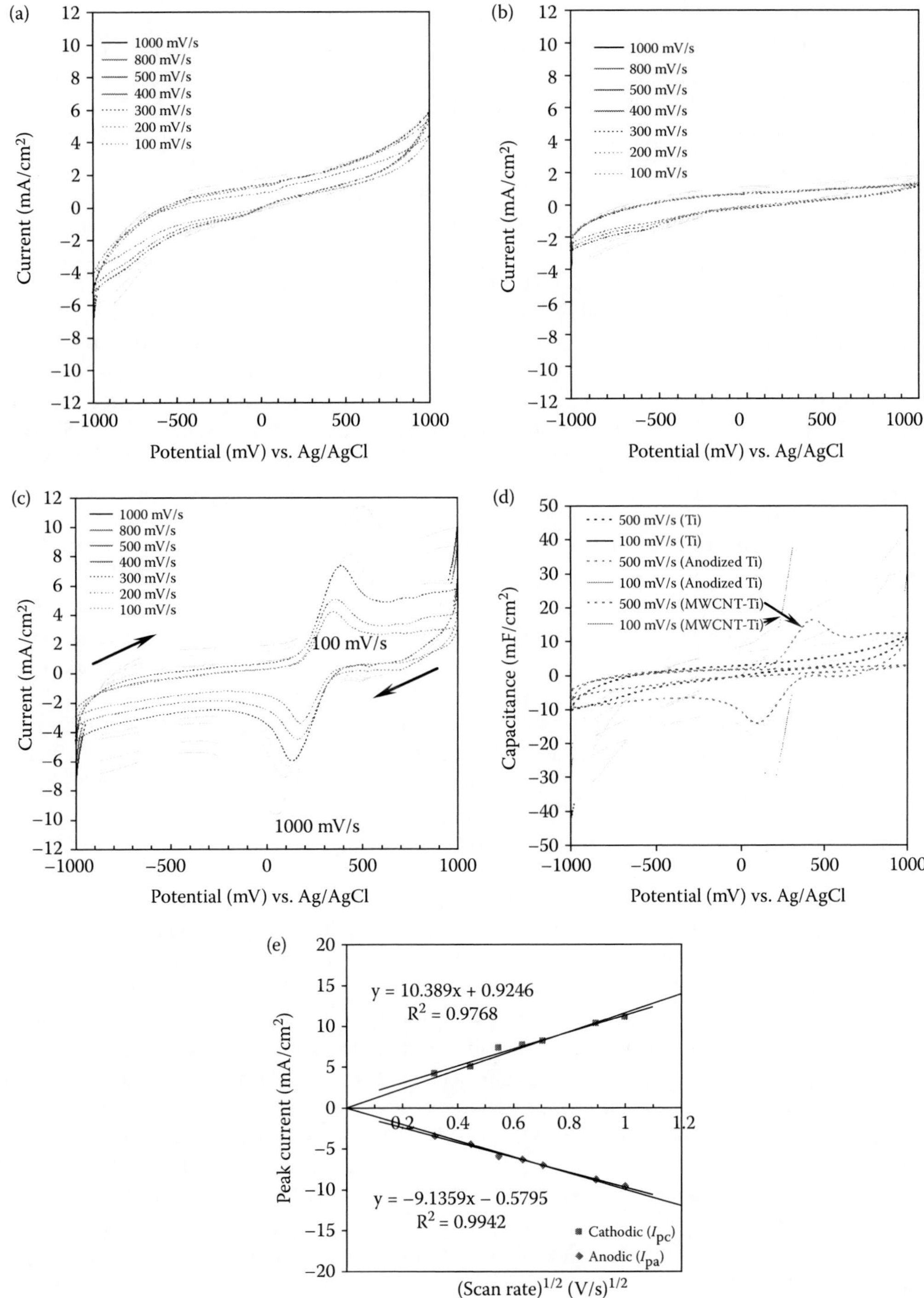

FIGURE 29.7 Cyclic voltammograms (CV) with an electrolyte solution of 10 mM $K_3Fe(CN)_6$ in 1 M KNO_3 for: (a) conventional Ti; (b) anodized Ti; and (c) MWCNT-Ti. (d) The capacitance of all the electrodes in comparison. (e) The plot of the square root of scan rates with anodic peak currents (I_{pa}) and cathodic peak currents (I_{pc}).

or diffusion-controlled) or distorted (irreversible or adsorption-controlled), depending on the extent of the interactions (such as the electrostatic or covalent bonds) between them.

The type of electrolyte is important to the redox reaction because the gained capacitance and scan rate window are dependent on it [37]. Studies to date have not degassed with nitrogen or argon when performing the cyclic voltammetry with MWCNT sensors, and thus, the redox reactions in cyclic voltammograms (CV) are related to the H_2O decomposition, which includes H^+ reduction and OH^- oxidation. The pH of the electrolyte also affects the H_2O decomposition. In the case of a acidic 1 N HCl solution (without other electroactive molecules), the H^+ ions induced the formation of H_2 gas at −0.2 V as a result of the increased reduction current [37]. In the alkaline 1 M KOH solution, OH^- ions resulted in the formation of O_2 gas at 0.7 V by the oxidation process. This fact should be noted because *in vivo*, these decompositions may occur at the interface of the Ti implant due to pH changes and the presence of H_2O and O_2 around the implant.

Other studies have shown promising results when using CNT-modified electrodes in biosensing. Since MWCNTs have good electrochemical characteristics as electron mediators and adsorption matrices [38], they may further enhance applications in biosensor systems. For example, Harrison and Atala [11] showed that CNTs offer a promising method to enhance detection sensitivity because they have high signal-to-noise ratios. The structure-dependent metallic character of CNTs should allow them to promote electron-transfer reactions for redox processes, which can provide the foundation for unique biochemical sensing systems at low overpotentials [19]. The electrolyte–electrode interface barriers are reduced by CNTs because they facilitate double-layer effects [39]. Typically, when the supporting electrolyte is at least a 100-fold greater than the active electrolyte [40], the charge in the electrolyte solution causes the Debye layer to be more compact. Therefore, this compact layer can rapidly exchange electrons between electroactive proteins and the surface of an MWCNT-Ti electrode. This is likely the reason why the sharpened cathodic and anodic peaks in CV have been observed, as shown in Figures 29.7a, 29.7c, 29.8c, and 29.9b.

Although the area of the working electrode is constant in the presence of MWCNTs, the overall surface area and the electroactivity of the surface are increased. The MWCNTs act as a nanobarrier between the titanium oxide layer, which was its growth template, and the electrolyte solution. The surface atoms or molecules of MWCNTs play an important role in determining its bulk properties due to their nanosize effects [41]. A large surface, corresponding to the greater electrocatalytic activity, confers the catalytic role on the MWCNTs in the chemical reaction. Well-defined and persistent redox peaks are shown in Figure 29.7c, confirming the increases of electron transfers and higher electrochemical activities at the MWCNT-Ti surface. Cyclic voltammetry was also performed with a glassy carbon electrode (GCE; Bioanalytical) and a platinum electrode (PTE; Bioanalytical), and it also showed $\Delta E_p > 59/n$ mV (data not shown). Importantly, for the same scan rate, CV of GCE and PTE showed the redox reactions with similar but more widely separated anodic and cathodic peaks, confirming the performance of the MWCNT-Ti electrode.

However, in Figures 29.7a and b, the Ti and anodized Ti did not show any redox peaks. This is likely due to the inert inhibiting property of the titanium oxide on electron transfer. Figures 29.7a and b show that bare Ti has less capacitance than MWCNT-Ti. The capacitance relation is derived from $i = C(dv/dt)$, where dv/dt is a scan rate [28]. Hence, the capacitance between the working and reference electrodes during cyclic voltammetry was calculated by dividing the current in CV with respect to the specific scan rate, as shown in Figures 29.7d and 27.9d. In summary, the electrochemical response of the MWCNT-Ti electrode promoted a higher charge transfer than the Ti and anodized Ti electrodes.

29.5 DISCUSSION

The result from the previous section and study showed the utility of MWCNT-Ti as an electrode for detecting $Fe^{2+/3+}$ redox couples. For biological applications, it is also necessary to show that MWCNT-Ti can detect redox reactions associated with osteoblast differentiation. The extracellular components from osteoblasts in an HCl solution have been used to mimic the biological environment around an orthopedic implant. Figures 29.8a and b show that the bare Ti and anodized Ti electrodes cannot detect any redox process. However, the results in Figure 29.8c confirmed that MWCNTs enhance the direct electron transfer through Ti by adding the high conductivity surface of the MWCNTs.

After decreasing the surface area of the MWCNT-Ti electrode from 1 cm^2 to 1 mm^2, the redox potentials were also decreased as shown in Figures 29.8c and 29.9b. The faradic current of the oxidation process dropped approximately 10 times with respect to the decrease in surface area A, corresponding to Equation 29.1. Corresponding with the Randles–Sevcik equation, the peak current was linearly proportional to the area. When plotting the anodic (I_{pa}) and cathodic peak (I_{pc}) currents of MWCNT-Ti, a linear relationship to the square root of the scan rates was observed, as shown in Figure 29.9c.

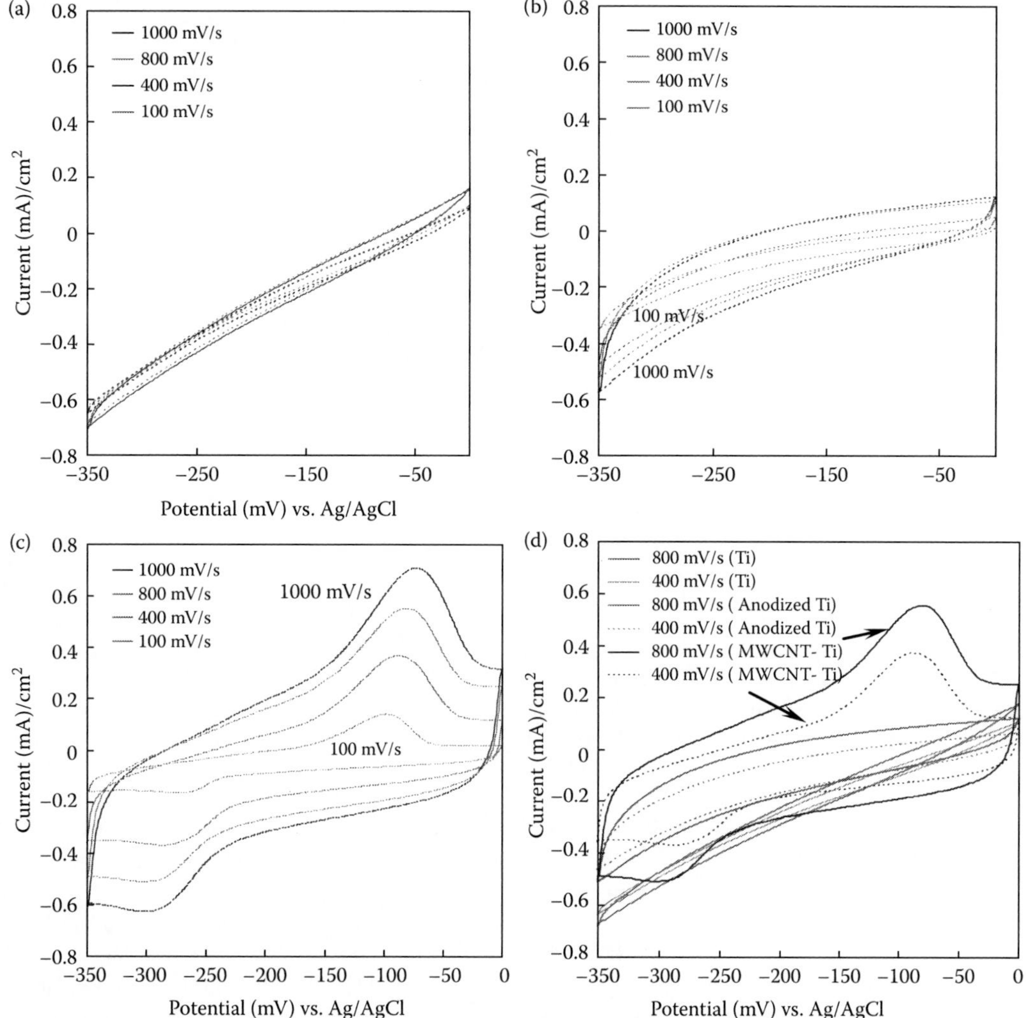

FIGURE 29.8 Cyclic voltammograms (CV) with an electrolyte solution of the extracellular matrix secreted by osteoblasts after 21 days of culture for (a) conventional Ti; (b) anodized Ti; and (c) MWCNT-Ti with a working area of 1 cm^2. (d) CV of all three electrodes in comparison. Only MWCNT-Ti possessed the quasireversible redox potential, while conventional Ti and anodized Ti did not.

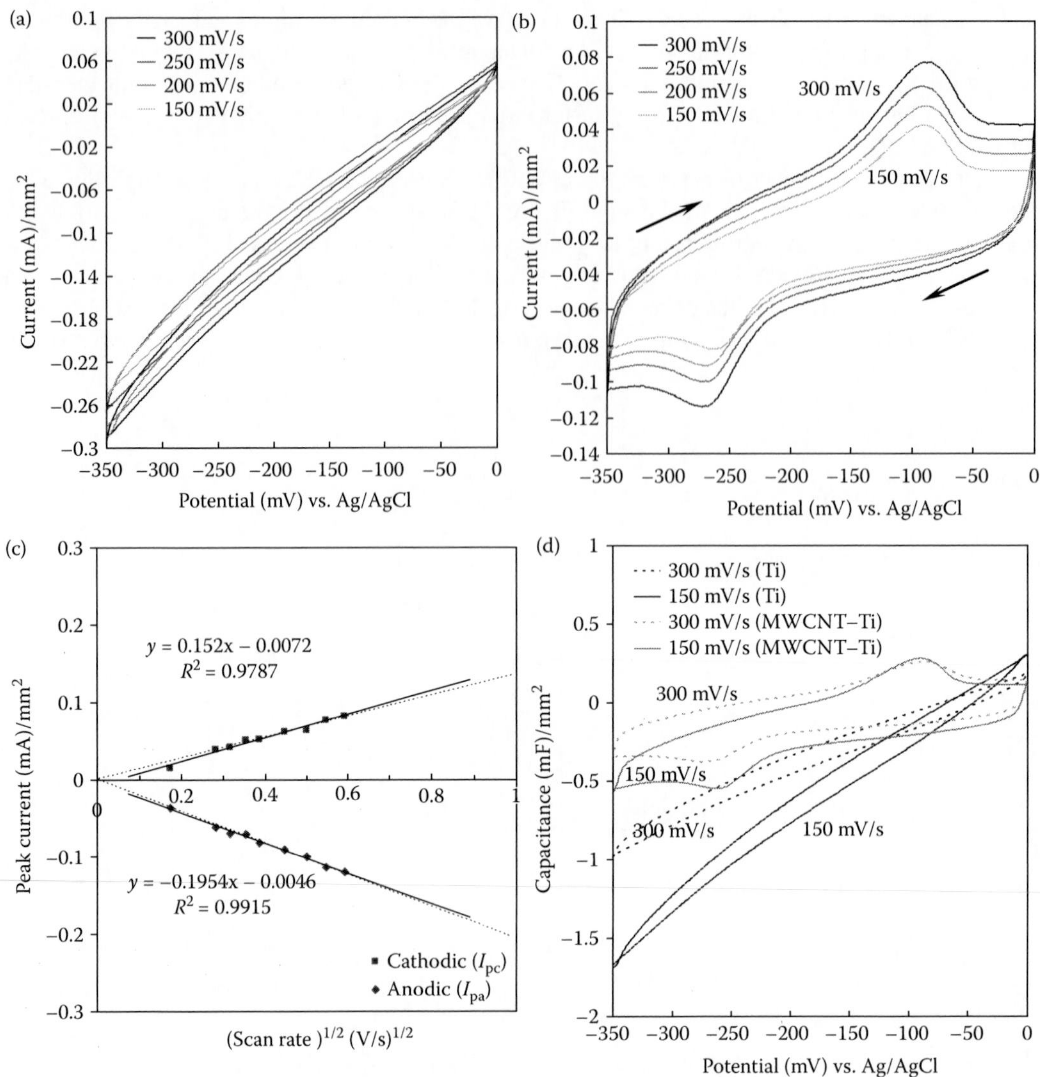

FIGURE 29.9 Cyclic voltammograms (CV) with an electrolyte solution of the extracellular matrix secreted by osteoblasts after 21 days of culture for (a) conventional Ti and (b) MWCNT-Ti with a working area of 1 mm². (c) Plot of the experimental cathodic and anodic peak currents, obtained from (b), versus the square root of the scan rates; and (d) the compared capacitance of MWCNT-Ti and Ti.

The CV showed well-defined redox peaks in the osteoblast supernatants at all concentrations. The peaks detected in the solution at the calcium concentrations of 1.481 μg/cm² (after 7 days), and 1.597 μg/cm² (after 14 days) had less faradic current and *I*–*V* graph area than the concentration of 2.48 μg/cm² (after 21 days), as shown in Figures 29.10a and b. Typically, the more HA deposited and synthesized by osteoblasts, the higher the calcium and protein concentrations. Therefore, it is likely that the supernatant from 21 days had higher protein concentrations than the solutions from 7 and 14 days, leading to the stronger redox reactions and higher capacitance between the electrode surfaces.

In addition, interpretation of CV results must consider other factors. In particular, a measurement of the redox reactions when oxygen was dissolved in the electrolyte solution showed that the peak currents were shifted toward the negative. Furthermore, a change in the pH of the electrolyte solution and the presence of water may also shift the current and affect the potential of the redox peaks.

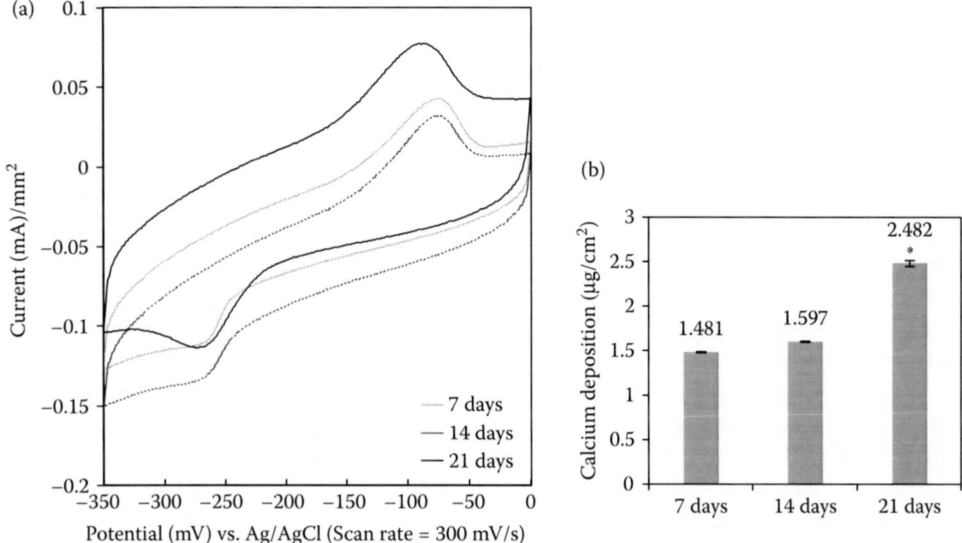

FIGURE 29.10 (a) Cyclic voltammograms (CV) of MWCNT-Ti electrodes in an electrolyte solution of the extracellular matrix secreted by osteoblasts cultured on conventional Ti after 21 days. (b) Results from a calcium deposition assay determined the calcium concentrations in an electrolyte solution of the extracellular matrix secreted by osteoblasts on conventional Ti after 7, 14, and 21 days of culture. Data = mean ± SEM; $n = 3$; $*p < 0.01$ (compared to 7 and 14 days).

Thus, CV with the potential range between –1 and 1 V of MWCNT-Ti was performed in a pure solution of 0.6 N HCl without other proteins or ions. An H^+ reduction peak at a potential between –0.5 and –0.8 V was found (data not shown). Moreover, the H^+ reduction peak still appeared when window ranges from –5 to 5 V and from –0.35 to 0 V were used, confirming that the H_2O decomposition occurred in our CV experiments.

It is clear that the MWCNT-Ti electrodes showed the potential for better performance than commercially available electrodes, such as GCE and PTE. When using the sweep voltage from –1 to –1 V, a set of mixed redox peaks with two oxidations and two reductions appeared (data not shown). These two redox peaks in the CV indicated that the process likely involved more than one electron transfer. For each couple, the amplitude and position of the oxidation peak in CV were unequal to those of the reduction peak. The second oxidation peak (omitted from Figure 29.8c or 29.6b) was observed at 236 mV for the MWCNT-Ti electrode, 405 mV for the GCE, and –33 mV for the PTE, all with the scan rate of 100 mV/s. However, for the GCE and the PTE electrodes, a second reduction did not appear, while the MWCNT-Ti showed two complete and well-defined redox reactions. These two peaks reflected that more than one electron transfers were involved. Since one occured at a positive potential and one at a negative in the CV. Further, the current amplitude for the MWCNT-Ti peaks was noticeably larger than that for GCE and PTE. Thus, it can be concluded that the MWCNT-Ti electrode has higher electron transfer as well.

At first it can be hypothesized that these redox reactions happened due to the redox of inorganics such as Ca or P. In the case of Ca, the reduction of Ca^{2+} to Ca crystal (nucleation) typically is expected with the reduction current for a highly negative potential. A positive feedback IR compensation (IRC) needs to be applied to the CV to drive the oxidation current to dissolve the Ca crystal into Ca^{2+}. For example, an overpotential of more than –1 V, an IRC of 0.771 Ω,a melting temperature of 900°C, and a scan rate of 50 mV/S were required [42]. Without applying IRC in this study, diffusion-controlled behavior, which electrochemically depletes calcium cations near the electrode surface, has been impossible to achieve. In addition, the reduction and oxidation of titanium oxides, which are the reaction counterparts of calcium redox, appeared at a positive potential between 0 and 0.25 V, respectively, which have not appeared in our CV studies. In the case of P, the cyclic voltammetry experiments have been performed further in phosphate-buffered saline (PBS). A final concentration of 1 M PBS, which was prepared in-house, had 137 mM NaCl, 10 mM phosphate, 2.7 mM KCl, and a pH of 7.4. The metal orthophosphate ions exhibited a high stability to reduce from P(V) (such as PO_4^{3-}, PO_4^-) to P(III), or further to P(I). However, no redox peaks appeared in the potential range of −1 to 1 V (data not shown). It is therefore likely that neither the redox reactions of calcium ions nor phosphate occurred due to the absence of the peaks. Instead, it has been hypothesized that the appearance of the redox peaks when using an MWCNT-Ti electrode is likely because of the reduction and oxidation of proteins from the osteoblast supernatant.

The observed quasireversible redox reaction reflected the fact that MWCNT-Ti sensors promote electrochemical reactions. However, an irreversible process can occur at the interface of an electrode due to the denaturation of proteins, or ion reduction. Typically, when the carbon bonds of proteins are changed, irreversible organic reduction or oxidation only happens [43]. While, the configurations of ions (Ca^{2+}, PO_4^{3-}, OH^-) which remain unchanged also can lead the irreversible process due to only its reduction or oxidation. Importantly, without MWCNTs on the Ti surface, nonspecific protein adsorption may readily occur, leading to an electrochemically insulating surface layer. Nevertheless, the redox at MWCNT-Ti did not decrease its oxidation and reduction current after applying the sweep voltage for some time, and so protein adsorption did not occur apparently in significant amounts at the MWCNT-Ti electrode. Indeed, in the osteoblast supernatant, the MWCNT-Ti electrode provides a relatively specific surface to which the proteins can bind reversibly by diffusion while retaining their function. The protein redox is also dependent on the pH of the electrolyte solution (acidic or basic) [44]. This shift appears due to the influence of 0.6 N HCl with H_2O as a solvent that influences proteins, leading the peak shift into the negative potential, as shown in Figures 29.8b, 29.9c, and 29.10a.

It has been hypothesized that the proteins from the solution of osteoblast extracelluar components were involved in these redox reactions at the surface of MWCNT-Ti. If those proteins maintain their function and are detected by the MWCNT-Ti electrode, the excellent electrochemical behavior explained here may show that MWCNT-Ti sensors are superior candidates for biosensor applications. However, investigating the type and size of acidic resistant proteins is still in progress.

As shown here, the electrodic performance of MWCNT-Ti sensors, but not the bare Ti, provides excellent redox reactions. As mentioned, the electrochemical experiments were performed so far without degassing with bubble nitrogen gas. This omission may have resulted in an apparent background signal, which was mixed and appeared in current–voltage curves (CVs). Moreover, the redox reaction at the MWCNT-Ti sensor mentioned here may depend on various ion sources, including reversible protein adsorption, dissolved oxygen, and acidic nature of HCl. However, the redox reactions of iron (II/III) and the osteoblast extracellular components still occurred only when using MWCNT-Ti sensors, and not when using Ti or anodized Ti. Importantly, it was shown that MWCNT sensors performed as the electrocatalysts for the oxidation and reduction of iron (II/III) and of extracellular components, which included various proteins and inorganic substances synthesized and deposited by osteoblasts.

The electrolyte solution of osteoblast extracellular components was composed of inorganic and organic substances. This solution was not classified in terms of the types of molecules in solution, but rather, all components were dissolved together in the acidic solution and used in all cyclic voltammetry studies. Future work needs to classify the type of proteins in such osteoblast supernatants.

However, it is likely that *in vivo* the capacitance and the electroactive surface of Ti will be enhanced after bone tissue is formed without the presence of MWCNTs. After hip implant insertion, blood and body fluids surround the Ti implant, creating a specific capacitance for the Ti electrode in the beginning. Within 1 month, as osteoblasts deposit calcium around the implant, the capacitance of the implant and bone tissue increases. Cell membranes also have electric potentials and perform redox processes [45,46], and it has been found that after 14 days *in vitro* these redox processes at the surface of bare Ti increased.

In vitro, nevertheless, MWCNTs have been used to modify the electrodes to detect other biomolecules and enhance their redox reactions, such as NADH [47], hydrogen peroxide [21,47], glucose [22], putrescine [48], and DNA [49]. Specifically, the growth of MWCNTs from nanoporous metal electrodes can enhance many diverse sensor applications. For example, MWCNTs functionalized with thiol groups have been used for sensing aliphatic hydrocarbons (such as methanol and ethanol), forming unique electrical identifiers [18]. Moreover, MWCNTs grown on silicon substrates enhanced ionic conductivity and have been integrated with unmodified plant cellulose as a film, and used as a cathode electrode in a lithium ion battery, or as a supercapacitor with bioelectrolytes (such as biological fluid and blood) [50]. Interestingly, both supercapacitors and batteries, derived from an MWCNTs-nanocomposite film, can be integrated to build a hybrid, or dual-storage battery-in-supercapacitor device. The cytocompatible MWCNTs-device may be useful to integrate with an orthopedic–implant biosensor as passive energy storage.

Not only can an implanted electronics circuit be powered by an implant battery (fabricated or self-integrated) within the implant material, but it also can be induced by an external power supply. For orthopedic applications, telemetric devices started in 1966 and became imperative as a telemetric orthopedic implant to transmit a signal to an external device [51–56]. For example, Graichen et al. (2007) [57] developed a new 9-channel telemetry transmitter used for *in vivo* load measurements in three patients with shoulder Ti endoprostheses. The low radio frequency (RF) of an external inductive power source generates power transmission through the implanted metal. At the end of the Ti implant, the pacemaker feedthrough rounds a single-loop antenna to transmit the pulse interval signal, which is modulated at a higher RF by the microcontroller, to an external device. Then, the RF receiver of the external device synchronizes with the modulated pulse interval to recover the data stream and report to a clinician. Thus, either an implanted battery or a telemetry system can supply the electrical power to a calcium-detectable chip inside the orthopedic implant for clinical use.

The automatically sensing concept for bone growth juxtaposed to orthopedic implants also can apply for determining infection and scar tissue formation. An energy source energizes a telemetric-implanted circuit, and allows it to transmit data to an external receiver to determine bone growth. Indeed, the electrochemical biosensor may reduce the complexity of imaging techniques and patient difficulties.

29.6 CONCLUSIONS

The capabilities of using Ti as an electrochemical electrode have been increased remarkably by growing MWCNTs out of anodized Ti nanopores (MWCNT-Ti). MWCNTs improved the sensitivity of the bare Ti electrode displaying redox peaks in CVs and interestingly high capacitance. Such results provide evidence that MWCNT-Ti can serve as a novel electrochemical electrode with great electrocatalytic properties due to increased surface area and conductivity. Moreover, MWCNTs were shown to be more highly electroactive in chemical transformations than the metallic (Ti) surface, which typically undergoes electrochemical oxidation or dissolution of metal oxides, but is chemically susceptible to corrosion. MWCNTs promoted a redox reaction by enhancing the direct electron transfer through their electrically conductive surface surrounded by ionic solutions, which contained the electroactive species, herein ferri/ferricyanide and the extracellular components from osteoblasts. Moreover, MWCNTs are cytocompatible, promoted osteoblast differentiation after 21 days, and can be integrated into a supercapacitor or battery to enhance the functionalities of biosensing systems *in vivo*. Therefore, MWCNT-Ti sensors are an exceptional candidate as an electrochemical electrode to determine *in situ* new bone growth surrounding an orthopedic implant. Further, the ability of MWCNT-Ti to sense osteoblast extracellular components by detecting their redox reaction profiles in specific concentrations may improve the diagnosis of orthopedic implant success or failure, and thus improve clinical efficacy.

ACKNOWLEDGMENTS

The authors thank the Coulter Foundation for funding some of the results in this chapter.

REFERENCES

1. Zhan, C., Kaczmarek, R., Loyo-Berrios, N., Sangl, J., Bright, R. A. Incidence and short-term outcomes of primary and revision hip replacement in the United States. *The Journal of Bone and Joint Surgery. American Volume* 2007;89(3):526–533.
2. Iijima, S. Helical microtubules of graphitic carbon. *Nature* 1991;354(6348):56–58.
3. Lin, Y., Taylor, S., Li, H., Fernando, K. A. S., Qu, L., Wang, W. et al. Advances toward bioapplications of carbon nanotubes. *Journal of Materials Chemistry* 2004;14(4):527–541.
4. Webster, T. J., Waid, M. C., McKenzie, J. L., Price, R. L., Ejiofor, J. U. Nano-biotechnology: Carbon nanofibres as improved neural and orthopaedic implants. *Nanotechnology* 2004;15(1):48–54.
5. Smart, S. K., Cassady, A. I., Lu, G. Q., Martin, D. J. The biocompatibility of carbon nanotubes. *Toxicology of Carbon Nanomaterials* 2006;44(6):1034–1047.
6. Zanello, L. P. Electrical properties of osteoblasts cultured on carbon nanotubes. *Micro & Nano Letters* 2006;1(1):19–22.
7. Zanello, L. P., Zhao, B., Hu, H., Haddon, R. C. Bone cell proliferation on carbon nanotubes. *Nano Letters* 2006;6(3):562–567.
8. Balani, K., Anderson, R., Laha, T., Andara, M., Tercero, J., Crumpler, E. et al. Plasma-sprayed carbon nanotube reinforced hydroxyapatite coatings and their interaction with human osteoblasts *in vitro. Biomaterials* 2007;28(4):618–624.
9. Chen, Y., Zhang, T. H., Gan, C. H., Yu, G. Wear studies of hydroxyapatite composite coating reinforced by carbon nanotubes. *Carbon* 2007;45(5):998–1004.
10. Wei, W., Sethuraman, A., Jin, C., Monteiro-Riviere, N. A., Narayan, R. J. Biological properties of carbon nanotubes. *Journal of Nanoscience and Nanotechnology* 2007;7:1284–1297(1214).
11. Harrison, B. S., Atala, A. Carbon nanotube applications for tissue engineering. *Cellular and Molecular Biology Techniques for Biomaterials Evaluation* 2007;28(2):344–353.
12. Supronowicz, P. R., Ajayan, P. M., Ullmann, K. R., Arulanandam, B. P., Metzger, D. W., Bizios, R. Novel current-conducting composite substrates for exposing osteoblasts to alternating current stimulation. *Journal of Biomedical Materials Research* 2002;59(3):499–506.
13. Ciombor, D. M., Aaron, R. K. The role of electrical stimulation in bone repair. *Orthobiologics* 2005;10(4):579–593.
14. Aoki, N., Yokoyama, A., Nodasaka, Y., Akasaka, T., Uo, M., Sato, Y. et al. Cell culture on a carbon nanotube scaffold. *Journal of Biomedical Nanotechnology* 2005;1:402–405(404).
15. Giannona, S., Firkowska, I., Rojas-Chapana, J., Giersig, M. Vertically aligned carbon nanotubes as cytocompatible material for enhanced adhesion and proliferation of osteoblast-like cells. *Journal of Nanoscience and Nanotechnology* 2007;7:1679–1683(1675).
16. Tsuchiya, N., Sato, Y., Aoki, N., Yokoyama, A., Watari, F., Motomiya, K. et al. Evaluation of multi-walled carbon nanotube scaffolds for osteoblast growth. In: *Water Dynamics 4th International Workshop on Water Dynamics*, Tohji, K., Tsuchiya, N., Jeyadevan, B., eds; AIP; 2007, p. 166–169.
17. Sirivisoot, S., Yao, C., Xiao, X., Sheldon, B. W., Webster, T. J. Greater osteoblast functions on multi-walled carbon nanotubes grown from anodized nanotubular titanium for orthopedic applications. *Nanotechnology* 2007;18(36):365102.
18. Padigi, S. K., Reddy, R. K. K., Prasad, S. Carbon nanotube based aliphatic hydrocarbon sensor. *Biosensors and Bioelectronics* 2007;22(6):829–837.
19. Roy, S., Vedala, H., Choi, W. Vertically aligned carbon nanotube probes for monitoring blood cholesterol. *Nanotechnology* 2006;17(4):S14–S18.
20. Tang, H., Chen, J. H., Huang, Z. P., Wang, D. Z., Ren, Z. F., Nie, L. H. et al. High dispersion and electrocatalytic properties of platinum on well-aligned carbon nanotube arrays. *Carbon* 2004;42(1):191–197.
21. Kurusu, F., Koide, S., Karube, I., Gotoh, M. Electrocatalytic activity of bamboo-structured carbon nanotubes paste electrode toward hydrogen peroxide. *Analytical Letters* 2006;39:903–911.
22. Liu, Y., Wang, M., Zhao, F., Xu, Z., Dong, S. The direct electron transfer of glucose oxidase and glucose biosensor based on carbon nanotubes/chitosan matrix. *Biosensors and Bioelectronics* 2005;21(6):984–988.
23. Liu, S., Lin, B., Yang, X., Zhang, Q. Carbon-nanotube-enhanced direct electron-transfer reactivity of hemoglobin immobilized on polyurethane elastomer film. *Journal of Physical Chemistry B* 2007;111(5):1182–1188.

24. Robertson, J. Realistic applications of CNTs. *Materials Today* 2004;7(10):46–52.
25. Talapatra, S., Kar, S., Pal, S. K., Vajtai, R., Ci, L., Victor, P. et al. Direct growth of aligned carbon nanotubes on bulk metals. *Nat Nano* 2006;1:112–116.
26. Ngo, Q., Petranovic, D., Krishnan, S., Cassell, A. M., Ye, Q., Li, J. et al. Electron transport through metal-multiwall carbon nanotube interfaces. *Nanotechnology, IEEE Transactions* 2004;3:311–317.
27. Sato, S., Kawabata, A., Kondo, D., Nihei, M., Awano, Y. Carbon nanotube growth from titanium–cobalt bimetallic particles as a catalyst. *Chemical Physics Letters* 2005;402(1–3):149–154.
28. Tamir, G., Moti, B.-D., Itshak, K., Raya, S., Ze'ev, R. A., Eshel, B.-J. et al. Electro-chemical and biological properties of carbon nanotube based multi-electrode arrays. *Nanotechnology* 2007;3:035201.
29. Zhang, Y., Baer, C. D., Camaioni-Neto, C., O'Brien, P., Sweigart, D. A. Steady-state voltammetry with microelectrodes: Determination of heterogeneous charge transfer rate constants for metalloporphyrin complexes. *Inorganic Chemistry* 1991;30(8):1682–1685.
30. Hrapovic, S., Liu, Y., Male, K. B., Luong, J. H. T. Electrochemical biosensing platforms using platinum nanoparticles and carbon nanotubes. *Analytical Chemistry* 2004;76(4):1083–1088.
31. Hrapovic, S., Luong, J. H. T. Picoamperometric detection of glucose at ultrasmall platinum-ased biosensors: Preparation and characterization. *Analytical Chemistry* 2003;75(14):3308–3315.
32. Calafiori, A., Di Marco, G., Martino, G., Marotta, M. Preparation and characterization of calcium phosphate biomaterials. *Journal of Materials Science: Materials in Medicine* 2007;18:2331–2338.
33. Wang, H., Lee, J.-K., Moursi, A., Lannutti, J. J. Ca/P ratio effects on the degradation of hydroxyapatite *in vitro. Journal of Biomedical Materials Research Part A* 2003;67A(2):599–608.
34. Zaidi, M., Moonga, B. S., Huang, C. L.-H. Calcium sensing and cell signaling processes in the local regulation of osteoclastic bone resorption. *Biological Reviews* 2004;79(01):79–100.
35. Blair, H. C., Zaidi, M., Schlesinger, P. H. Mechanisms balancing skeletal matrix synthesis and degradation. *Biochem J* 2002;364(2):329–341.
36. Bronner, F., Farach-Carson, M. C. *Bone Formation*. New York, NY: Springer, 2003.
37. Hong, M. S., Lee, S. H., Kim, S. W. Use of KCl aqueous electrolyte for 2 V manganese oxide/activated carbon hybrid capacitor. *Electrochemical and Solid-State Letters* 2002;5(10):A227–A230.
38. Sotiropoulou, S., Gavalas, V., Vamvakaki, V., Chaniotakis, N. A. Novel carbon materials in biosensor systems. *Biosensors and Bioelectronics* 2003;18(2–3):211–215.
39. Fang, W. C., Sun, C. L., Huang, J. H., Chen, L. C., Chyan, O., Chen, K. H. et al. Enhanced electrochemical properties of arrayed CNx nanotubes directly grown on Ti-buffered silicon substrates. *Electrochemical and Solid State Letters* 2006;9(3):A175–A178.
40. Christian, G. D. *Analytical Chemistry*. New York, NY: John Wiley & Sons, 1980.
41. Cao, G. *Nanostructures and Nanomaterials: Synthesis, Properties and Applications*. London: Imperial College Press, 2004.
42. Chen, G. Z., Fray, D. J. Voltammetric studies of the oxygen-titanium binary system in molten calcium chloride. *Journal of the Electrochemical Society* 2002;149(11):E455–E467.
43. Schuring, J. *Redox Fundamentals, Processes, and Application*. New York, NY: Springer, 2000.
44. Battistuzzi, G., Loschi, L., Borsari, M., Sola, M. Effects of nonspecific ion-protein interactions on the redox chemistry of cytochrome *c. Journal of Biological Inorganic Chemistry* 1999;4(5):601–607.
45. Jeansonne, B. G., Feagin, F. F., McMinn, R. W., Shoemaker R. L., Rehm W. S. Cell-to-cell communication of osteoblasts. *Journal of dental research* 1979;58(4):1415–1423.
46. Jeansonne, B. G., Feagin, F. F., Shoemaker, R. L., Rehm, W. S. Transmembrane potentials of osteoblasts. *Journal of Dental Research* 1978;57(2):361–364.
47. Lin, Y., Yantasee, W., Wang, J. Carbon nanotubes (CNTs) for the development of electrochemical biosensors. *Frontiers in Bioscience: A Journal and Virtual Library* 2005;10:492–505.
48. Luong, J. H. T., Hrapovic, S., Wang, D. Multiwall carbon nanotube (MWCNT) based electrochemical biosensors for mediatorless detection of putrescine. *Electroanalysis* 2005;17(1):47–53.
49. He, P., Xu, Y., Fang, Y. Applications of carbon nanotubes in electrochemical DNA biosensors. *Microchimica Acta* 2006;152(3):175–186.
50. Pushparaj, V., Shaijumon, M., Kumar, A., Murugesan, S., Ci, L., Vajtai, R. et al. Flexible energy storage devices based on nanocomposite paper. *Proceedings of the National Academy of Sciences* 2007;104(34):13574–13577.
51. Kaufman, K., Kovacevic, N., Irby, S., Colwell, C. Instrumented implant for measuring tibiofemoral forces. *Journal of Biomechanics* 1996 5;29(5):667–671.
52. Bergmann, G., Deuretzbacher, G., Heller, M., Graichen, F., Rohlmann, A., Strauss, J. et al. Hip contact forces and gait patterns from routine activities. *Journal of Biomechanics* 2001;34(7):859–871.

53. Bergmann, G., Graichen, F., Rohlmann, A., Verdonschot, N., van Lenthe, G. H. Frictional heating of total hip implants. Part 1: Measurements in patients. *Journal of Biomechanics* 2001;34(4):421–428.
54. D'Lima, D. D., Townsend, C. P., Arms, S. W., Morris, B. A., Colwell, C. W. An implantable telemetry device to measure intra-articular tibial forces. *Journal of Biomechanics* 2005;38(2):299–304.
55. Graichen, F., Bergmann, G. Four-channel telemetry system for *in vivo* measurement of hip joint forces. *Journal of Biomedical Engineering* 1991;13(5):370–374.
56. Graichen, F., Bergmann, G., Rohlmann, A. Hip endoprosthesis for *in vivo* measurement of joint force and temperature. *Journal of Biomechanics* 1999;32(10):1113–1117.
57. Graichen, F., Arnold, R., Rohlmann, A., Bergmann, G. Implantable 9-channel telemetry system for *in vivo* load measurements with orthopedic implants. *IEEE Transactions on Bio-Medical Engineering* 2007; 54(2):253–261.

30 Engineering Bone Formation with Biologically Inspired Nanomaterials

Esmaiel Jabbari

CONTENTS

30.1 INTRODUCTION

Clinical methods of treating skeletal defects [1] involve bone transplantation or the use of synthetic materials to restore continuity. Autograft tissue is limited by supply and morbidity at the harvest site. Allograft tissue is limited by disease transfer and immunogenic response from the host tissue. Stress shielding and particulate wear are potential concerns with the use of nondegradable polymers such as poly(methyl methacrylate), PMMA. Bioinspired synthetic composites are an attractive option because mechanical properties can be designed independently for each application. In addition, the composite degradation can be designed to coincide with the rate of tissue regeneration for a given application.

The flexibility in the design of polymer composites allows the synthesis of a wide range with varying mechanical, biological, degradation, and rheological properties. For instance, their mechanical and degradation properties can be manipulated by changing the molecular weight during synthesis, and can thus be tailored to fit a particular application. Degradable polymers based on polyhydroxyalkanonates (PHA) have been used as scaffolds for guided regeneration of skeletal tissues in orthopedics [2]. PHA polymers include poly(L-lactic acid) (PLLA), poly(glycolic acid) (PGA), polycaprolactone (PCL), poly(trimethylene carbonate), poly(butylene terephthalate), poly(hydroxybutyrate), poly(hydroxyvalerate), and poly(dioxanone) (PDS) and their copolymers [3–8]. The development of self-reinforced PGA (SR-PGA) and PLLA (SR-PLLA) has expanded the use of PHA in load-bearing orthopedic applications [9,10]. A hybrid of PLGA and collagen has been used for guided bone regeneration to treat periodontesis [11]. A group of poly(anhydrides) consisting of different ratios of sebacic acid (SA) and 1,6-bis(p-carboxyphenoxy) hexane have been developed that degrade by surface erosion while maintaining their bulk mechanical properties [12,13].

In an effort to develop materials for minimally invasive applications, an unsaturated lactide-*co*-glycolide macromer has been synthesized to fabricate scaffolds *in situ* with degradation profile that can be tailored to a particular application [14]. In order to produce a less rigid and faster degrading poly(propylene fumarate) (PPF) macromer [15–17], the propylene glycol in PPF was replaced with low-molecular-weight poly(ε-caprolactone) providing four free rotating carbon–carbon bonds, resulting in poly(ε-caprolactone fumarate) with higher crosslink density and hydrolytic degradation rate [18]. Photopolymerizable arginine-glycine-aspartic acid (RGD) peptide-modified poly(ethylene glycol) (PEG) hydrogels have been used to enhance cytoskeletal reorganization of osteoblasts after encapsulation [19]. Alginate hydrogels grafted with adhesion ligands have also been used for the encapsulation of calvarial osteoblasts [20]. An *in situ* crosslinkable enzymatically degradable poly(lactide-*co*glyoclide ethylene oxide) macromer has been developed for the encapsulation of bone marrow stromal (BMS) cells [21].

Calcium phosphates such as hydroxyapatite (HA) and tricalciumphosphate are biocompatible, osteoconductive, and promote bone ingrowth, but the drawback is their low initial strength, which leads to difficulty in maintaining the composite within the defect. In order to overcome this issue, bioactive ceramics that harden *in vivo* such as calcium-deficient hydroxyapatite have been developed [22,23] that promote bone growth and have compressive strengths higher than that of cancellous bone [24,25]. Potential drawbacks of calcium phosphates are fatigue fractures that limit their use to skeletal tissues that are subject to uniform compressive loading [26]. Natural [27–30] and synthetic [31–37] reinforced with calcium phosphates exhibit compressive strengths in the range of 2–30 MPa, suitable for trabecular bone replacement. The addition of HA to drawn PLLA not only improved biodegradability and strength, but it also increased compatibility with the bone tissue.

Cell-based approaches using osteoblasts [38], bone marrow-derived osteoprogenitor cells [39], and stem cells [40] are attractive for bone reconstruction. The rate of extracellular matrix deposition and mineralization in cell-based systems depends on the presence of soft tissue for blood supply and degradation rate, porosity, pore size, and the extent of pore interconnectivity of the scaffold [41–43]. Although progress is made in developing composites for skeletal tissue regeneration [44,45], these matrices do not provide the cell–substrate interactions for differentiation of progenitor cells into multiple mature phenotypes. Furthermore, these composites are not applicable for reconstruction of load-bearing tissues, because they fail to mimic the bone's natural micro- and nanostructure.

30.2 BONE STRUCTURE

Bone is a composite material consisting of a collagenous and an apatite phase [46]. The inorganic apatite crystals contribute approximately 65% to the wet weight of the bone while the collagenous phase contributes 20% [47]. Glycoproteins and proteoglycans control the water content of the bone to 15% [48]. The collagenous phase gives bone its form and contributes to its ability to resist bending, while the apatite crystals resist compression [49–51]. Bone exhibits many orders of hierarchical structures from macroscopic to microscopic, submicroscopic, nanoscale, and subnanostructure length scales [52]. These levels of organization include the cancellous and cortical macrostructures, the osteons (10–500 μm), the lamellae submicrostructures (1–10 μm), the fibrillar collagen and embedded mineral nanostructures (100–1000 nm), and the molecular structure of the constituent elements [53]. The properties of bone are determined at the nanoscale with nanoapatite calcium phosphate crystals embedded in the soft collagen fibrils. The extended sheets of mineral are positioned along the long axis of collagen molecules and parallel to one another in neighboring collagen layers. The sheets fuse with one another to form a structurally stable composite. The plate-shaped apatite crystals are 2–3 nm thick and tens of nanometers long and wide. The collagen fibers in the matrix have different levels of organization from 1 to 4 nm for fibrils to 50–70 nm for fibers and 150–250 nm for bundles.

The collagenous phase plays a central role in the regulation of mineralization, control of cell division, migration, differentiation, and maturation, and maintenance of matrix integrity, growth factor modulation, and the extent of mineral–collagen interactions [54,55]. Noncollagenous proteins play complex functions during bone formation and remodeling [56]. The collagenous phase facilitates communication with the cellular environment and provides a medium for proteins to maintain their bioactivity [57,58]. For example, osteonectin protein is involved in several functions including linking of the mineral and collagenous phases and regulation of mineralization. An engineered composite should mimic the complexity of the bone's extracellular matrix with nanoscale structures to control cell–matrix interactions.

30.3 COLLAGEN NANOSTRUCTURE AND ITS EFFECT ON CELL DIFFERENTIATION

BMS cells are a heterogeneous population [59] that give rise to a variety of fully differentiated connective tissues of both mesenchymal and nonmesenchymal origin [60–64]. Differentiation of stem cells depends on the growth media components as well as the type of substrate cells that are cultured [65,66]. Since endothelial precursor cells have been identified in the adult bone marrow, BMS cells have the capacity to undergo vasculogenic as well as osteogenic differentiation under appropriate substrate and culture conditions. The effect of substrate on differentiation of progenitor BMS cells was investigated with aligned collagen tubular scaffolds [67,68]. BMS cells were seeded into collagen tubes and cultured in osteogenic media. At each time interval, the cell cultures were assessed by immunofluorescence for the pattern of specific proteins. The staining patterns for bone-related proteins and minerlization are shown in Figure 30.1. BMS cells displayed the distinctive polygonal phenotype with cell aggregates positive for osteopontin (Figure 30.1a), osteocalcin and osteonectin (not shown), and alkaline phosphatase (Figure 30.1b). BMS cells formed multiple foci of multilayered mineralized structures, as a result of coalescing cellular aggregates, positive for Alizarin red (Figure 30.1c).

The gene-expression profile of the BMS cells seeded on the collagen scaffold showed sustained upregulation of osteopontin (an early stage marker) and a marked upregulation of osteocalcin at day 12 which was maintained through day 18. BMS cells cultured showed vessel-like structures positive for Pecam-1, Flk-1, α-SMA, and tomato lectin (see Figure 30.2a). Linear as well as branching tubular structures consisting of endothelial cells with their nuclei arranged in Indian foil appearance and surrounded and wrapped by elongated α-smooth muscle actin positive cells were observed, as shown in Figure 30.2b. In addition, areas of extensive capillaries reminiscent of neovascularization were observed (see Figure 30.2c).

It is well established that type I collagen promotes the osteogenic differentiation of mesenchymal stem cells in conventional two-dimensional (2D) monolayer cultures [69–71]. The extracellular matrix has profound effects on cell behavior, including cell proliferation, migration, and vasculogenesis [72]. Three-dimensional matrices containing collagen and laminin have been shown to promote the formation of tubular structures resembling capillaries in cultured endothelial cells [73]. When BMS cells were cultured on aligned collagen type I scaffold in osteogenic media they showed

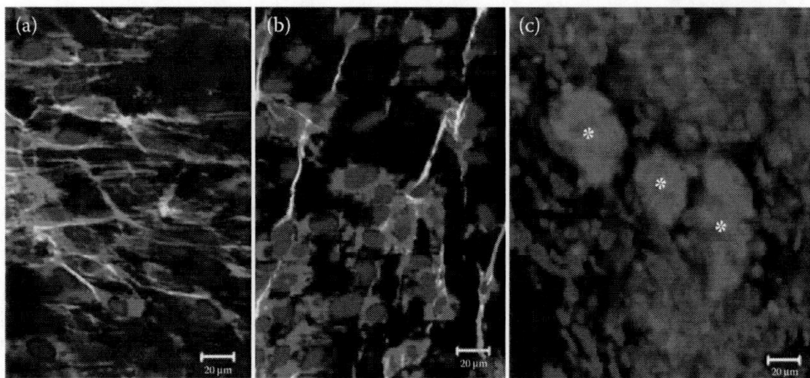

FIGURE 30.1 Expression pattern of various osteogenic markers and pattern of mineralization and nodule formation in the collagen tube showing areas of multilayered cellular aggregates positive for osteopontin (white in a), osteocalcin (white in b), and Alizarin red (diffuse gray in c). Cells were also stained with DAPI (dark gray) for nuclei and Alexa-488 phalloidin (light gray) for actin (scale bars are 20 μm).

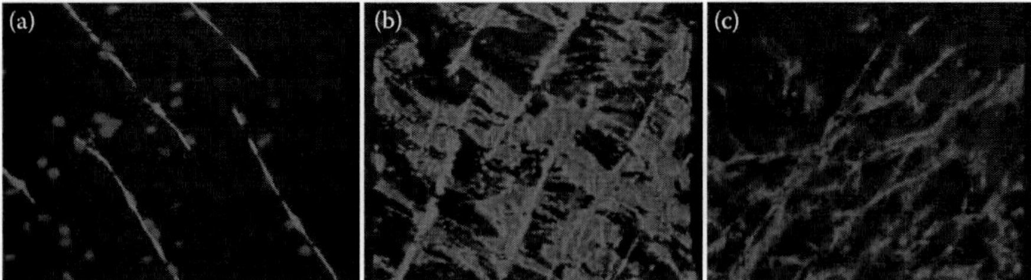

FIGURE 30.2 Expression pattern of vasculogenic markers α-SMA and tomato lectin (TL). Localization of vascular progenitor cells cultured on the collagen tube by confocal microscopy is seen in panels a, b, and c. Sections of the tubes showed capillary-like structures positive for α-SMA (gray streaks in a). Sheets of parallel oriented α-SMA positive cells abutting the vessel-like structures were observed (gray streaks in b). Sprouting and branching tubular structures positive for the endothelial marker tomato lectin were observed (gray web-like structure in c).

vascular morphogenesis. It appears that the subnano-, nano-, and microstructural organization of the 3D scaffold not only enhanced osteoblastic differentiation but also supported the process of generating microvascular structures. The α-SMA positive cells were not only recruited in juxtaposition to the aligned endothelial cells but the endothelial cells evoked the process of wrapping around the cord-like structure to produce the actual neovascularization. These findings demonstrate that the structural organization of the scaffold at the nano- and microscale affects maturation and differentiation of the BMS cells to multiple pathways including osteogenesis and vasculogenesis.

30.4 PEPTIDE-REINFORCED NANOCOMPOSITES

Hydrogels reinforced with calcium phosphate fillers are very attractive for bone tissue regeneration [74,75]. They exhibit the typical mechanical properties of the bone and replicate bone microstructure [76]. Composites with nanoparticles (<100 nm) exhibit a higher stiffness compared to those with microparticles at the same volume fraction [77]. The radius of gyration of the chains in microcomposites is orders of magnitude smaller than the size of the filler particles; therefore, the filler particles do not affect the chain relaxation time. The radius of gyration of the chains in nanocomposites is of the same order of magnitude as the size of the filler particles; therefore, the relaxation time of the chains interacting with multiple filler particles increases. It has been shown that the mechanical performance of the composites is significantly improved by increasing the interfacial adhesion between the polymer and dispersed particle phases [78,79]. While filled systems with large particles (>1 μm) exhibit linear behavior in a wide range of deformations, nonlinearity can emerge even at small strains in nanofilled composites [80,81].

The combination of a hard inorganic nanoparticulate phase and an elastic collagen network provides bone with unique mechanical properties while facilitating communication with the cellular environment [58,82,83]. Unique factors that contribute to the toughness of bone are the presence of nanosize apatite crystals, a dense network of collagen fibers on which the mineral crystals are deposited, and the acidic proteins with the ability to link the calcium-binding apatite crystals to the collagen fibers to form a completely crosslinked network [84,85]. One of the proteins with bone-specific functions is osteonectin or bone connector because it has a strong affinity for both collagen and HA and it is believed to be a nucleator of mineralization [86,87].

It is believed that the first seventeen N-terminal amino acids of osteonectin are responsible for binding to the bone collagen network [88] while a glutamic acid-rich sequence binds to the bone HA nanoparticles [85]. Osteonectin has the highest affinity for calcium ions among all bone proteins [84] and the apatite formed in the presence of osteonectin has the smallest crystal size [89]. These observations suggest that the switch from osteopontin to osteonectin for cells in the ossification front is to limit the size of the apatite crystals and produce a crosslinked composite by linking the collagen network to the mineral phase.

In order to test the effect of interactions between the apatite crystals and collagenous matrix, a glutamic acid-rich peptide (a sequence of six glutamic acids) derived from osteonectin, functionalized with an acrylate group (Ac-Glu6) was synthesized [90]. A similar procedure was used to synthesize the neutral glycine and positively charged lysine peptides with an acrylate group at one chain end (Ac-Gly6 and Ac-Lys6, respectively). The Ac-Glu6 sequence was attached to the surface of HA microparticles (diameter 50 μm) or nanoparticles (diameter 50 nm) by electrostatic interactions, as shown in Figure 30.3a. Next, an *in situ* crosslinkable terpolymer poly(lactide ethylene oxide fumarate) (PLEOF) consisting of low-molecular-weight poly(L-lactide) (LMW PLA) and PEG blocks linked by fumaric acid units was added to the suspension [91–97] and the gelation kinetics was measured with a rheometer.

Figure 30.3a shows the dependence of the composite shear modulus on the size of the HA particles. Nanoapatite composites (treated and untreated) displayed far larger stiffness compared with microcomposites, at the same volume fraction. The modulus of the composites with micron-sized particles did not appreciably change with the addition of Ac-Glu6. The storage modulus of the composites prepared with micron-sized particles can be reasonably predicted by Guth–Smallwood equation [98]. However, the large difference between the experimental and predicted results for composites prepared with nanosize HA implies that the reinforcement cannot be explained solely by the hydrodynamic effect in nanoparticulate systems.

Similar measurements were performed on the composites treated with equal molar concentrations of Ac-Gly6 and Ac-Lys6 in place of Ac-Glu6. In contrast to the Glu6 peptide, Gly6 and Lys6 are neutral and positively charged, respectively, and they have no ionic interactions with HA nanoparticles. HA/Ac-Gly6 and HA/Ac-Lys6 nanocomposites did not show a significant change in shear modulus compared to that without HA surface treatment, as shown in Figure 30.3c. These results demonstrate that the increase in overall viscoelastic response of the nanocomposite is specific to the Ac-Glu6 peptide, and the reinforcement is amplified as the size of the nanoparticles is reduced from 5 μm to 50 nm. The ionic bonds formed by the interaction of Ac-Glu6 with HA have a relatively higher adsorption energy and longer residence time on the particles. Thus, more matrix-filler crosslinks exists in Ac-Glu6-treated samples compared to untreated samples. This gives rise to a higher concentration of (physical) crosslinks in the vicinity of the particles, leading to the higher modulus of the HA/Ac-Glu6 composites. These results demonstrate that one of the factors contributing to the toughness of bone is the crosslinking of the gelatinous and mineral phases, mediated by a specific

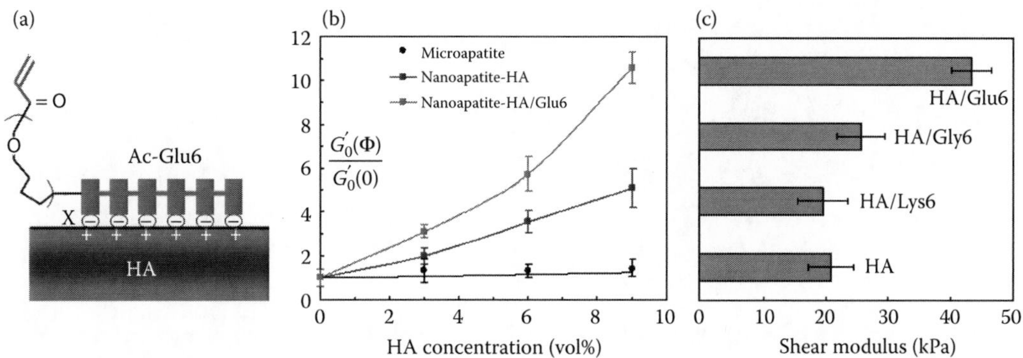

FIGURE 30.3 (a) Schematic diagram showing the binding of the glutamic acid-rich sequence of osteonectin protein to HA nanoparticles; (b) dependence of the shear modulus of the PLEOF/Ac-Glu6/apatite composite on the size of the HA particles; (c) comparison of the modulus of the nanocomposites treated with the Ac-Glu6 peptide with those treated with Ac-Gly6 and Ac-Lys6. Nanoapatite composites (treated and untreated) displayed far larger stiffness compared with microcomposites, at the same volume fraction. The modulus of the composites with micron-sized particles did not appreciably change with the addition of Ac-Glu6. G_0' (0) and G_0' (Φ) are the storage modulus of the gel and that of the composite, respectively, and Φ is the HA volume fraction.

peptide derived from osteonectin. The findings can be used to develop biomimetic composites for bone tissue regeneration in load-bearing applications.

30.5 BONE MIMETIC LAMINATED NANOCOMPOSITES

Bone exhibits hierarchical levels of organization from macroscopic to microscopic to nanoscale [99]. On the microscale, layers of fibrils are glued together by extracellular matrix (ECM) proteins to form laminated structures, called osteons, which make bone elastic and allow diffusion of nutrients and oxygen to cells embedded in the bone matrix [100]. The apatite crystals provide mechanical support in compression, the laminated structure of the osteons confers elasticity, while the hydrophilic ECM proteins allow diffusion of nutrients and oxygen to cells in the bone matrix. The objective of this work was to investigate the effect of lamination on water uptake, modulus, and extent of mineralization of nanofiber-reinforced laminated composite. Sheets of poly(L-lactide) (L-PLA) nanofibers were fabricated by electrospinning. The sheets were dipped in a poly(lactide-*co*-ethylene oxide fumarate) (PLEOF) hydrogel macromer/apatite precursor solution, stacked and pressed together, and allowed to crosslink by photopolymerization to form a fiber-reinforced hydrogel/apatite laminated structure. A one-layer scanning electron microscope (SEM) image of the laminated composite sheet is shown in Figure 30.5a.

The water uptake and modulus of the samples are shown in Figures 30.4b and 4c, respectively. Groups include Gel, L-PLA electrospun fiber mesh (Fiber), L-PLA fiber mesh/Gel laminate (Lam), and laminate with 1% acrylate-terminated glycine-arginine-glycine-aspartic acid (GRGD) and 10% HA (Lam-RGD-HA). The gray area in Figure 30.4b is the range for water content of the collagenous phase of the natural bone excluding the mineral component (bone water content is 15–20% by weight [101] corresponding to 43–50% (0.75–1.0 g/g dry) without the mineral component). The water uptake (g water/g dry sample) of the Gel and fiber mesh were 17.5 ± 3.4 and 4.6 ± 1.3, respectively. Lamination of the fiber mesh with the hydrogel drastically reduced water content to 1.6 ± 0.3. For the laminate, the gel-swelling pressure was counterbalanced by the elastic force of the fiber mesh, resulting in significant reduction in water uptake. With the addition of HA and RGD to the laminate, water uptake reduced from 1.6 ± 0.3 to 1.1 ± 0.3. Lamination of the fiber mesh with the

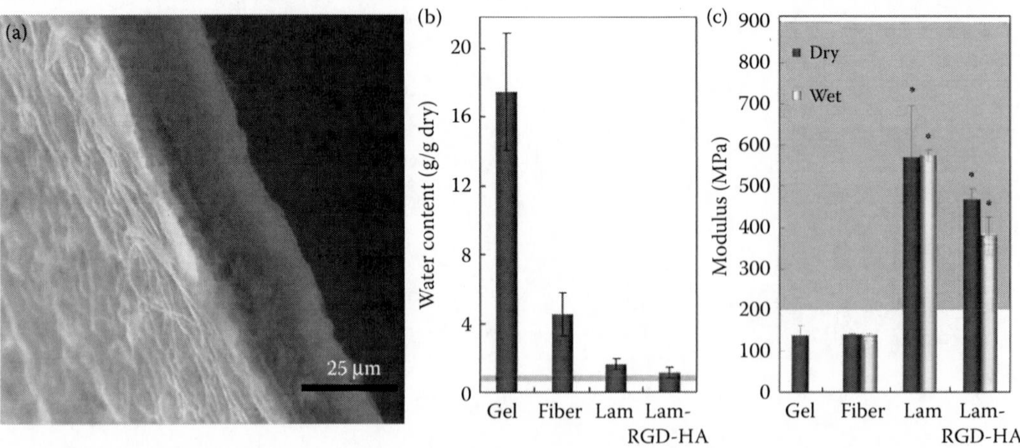

FIGURE 30.4 (a) SEM images of a one-layered fiber mesh; water uptake and (b) and moduli (c) under dry and wet conditions of the laminates; groups include Gel, L-PLA electrospun fiber mesh (Fiber), L-PLA fiber mesh/Gel laminate (Lam), and laminate with 1% Ac-GRGD and 10% HA (Lam-RGD-HA). The gray area in (b) is the range for water content of the natural bone excluding the mineral component. The gray area in (c) is the reported range for Young's modulus of wet human cancellous bone. Error bars correspond to means ± 1 SD for $n = 3$. One star in (c) indicates statistically significant difference between the test group and Gel/Fiber.

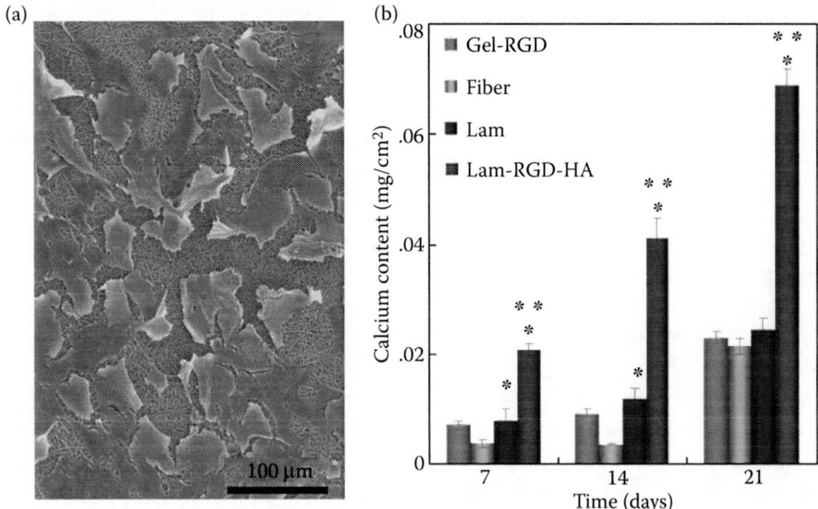

FIGURE 30.5 (a) SEM image of the BMS cells on L-PLA fiber mesh/Gel laminate; (b) calcium content of the BMS cell-seeded samples with incubation time. Groups include RGD-Gel, Fiber, Lam, and Lam-RGD-HA. One star in (b) indicates statistically significant difference between the test group and Fiber. Two stars in (b) indicate statistically significant difference between the test group and other groups for the same incubation time. Error bars correspond to means ± 1 SD for $n = 3$.

gel produced composites with water content similar to that of the collagenous phase of the bone matrix.

The moduli of the laminates under dry and wet conditions are shown in Figure 30.4c. The gray are is the reported range for Young's modulus of wet human cancellous bone [102]. The modulus of the fiber mesh under dry and wet conditions was 140 ± 3 MPa, but modulus of the hydrogel under wet condition was two orders of magnitude lower than that under dry condition (0.50 ± 0.07 versus 139 ± 23 MPa). Lamination of the fiber mesh with PLEOF hydrogel increased modulus dramatically (compared to the fiber mesh or hydrogel) to 570 ± 130 MPa. More importantly, Lam had similar modulus under dry and wet conditions (570 ± 130 for dry and 575 ± 14 MPa for wet). It is interesting to note that all laminates exhibited modulus values within the range for that of wet human cancellous bone (within the gray area) while modulus of the fiber mesh or hydrogel was significantly less than that of cancellous bone. The fiber mesh reinforced and reduced water uptake of the matrix, resulting in a laminated structure with robust mechanical properties under wet and dry conditions. The modulus of Lam-RGD-HA samples under dry and wet conditions was 470 ± 25 and 380 ± 47 MPa, respectively. These results demonstrate that fiber-reinforced laminated composites have the potential to provide structural support to the regenerating region in load-bearing orthopedic applications.

BMS cells were seeded on the laminates and cultured in complete osteogenic media. Surface coverage and morphology of the BMS cells on the laminate is shown in Figure 30.5a that shows the cuboidal to polygonal morphology of the BMS cells on the surface of laminate. It is well established that mechanical factors such as surface hardness and modulus as well as biochemical factors affect cell adhesion and spreading [103,104]. For example, human chondrosarcoma cells spread on high modulus surfaces (0.4 MPa) but they tend to be more rounded on low modulus surfaces (10–50 KPa) [104]. The laminates without RGD, due to nonadherent nature of the gel, had lower cell coverage but adhesion improved by reinforcement with HA, conjugation with RGD, or modification with HA and RGD. Figure 30.5b shows the calcium content of the BMS cells seeded on the samples with incubation time. L-PLA fiber mesh, Gel-RGD, and Lam groups had similar calcium contents ranging between 0.003–0.008 and 0.021–0.026 mg/cm² after 14 and 21 days, respectively. RGD conjugation and HA reinforcement (Lam-RGD-HA) increased the calcium content of the laminates by 2.7-, 3.5-, and 2.8-fold (compared to lam) after 7, 14, and 21 days, respectively. The apatite nanocrystals, suspended in the gel phase, provide an osteoconductive substrate for differentiation and mineralization of BMS cells. For example, BSM cells seeded on the laminates with 10% apatite crystals and conjugated with 1% RGD (Lam-RGD-HA group) had significantly higher calcium content after 21 days, and higher expression of osteogenic markers (data not shown) compared to other laminates, fiber mesh, and gel.

30.6 CONCLUSIONS

In this chapter, we have summarized recent advances in the development of biologically inspired nanomaterials for providing mechanical strength and to support complex cell–matrix interactions in bone regeneration. We demonstrated that surface treatment of HA nanocrystals with a peptide mimicking the terminal region of the osteonectin glycoprotein of bone resulted in an order of magnitude increase in modulus of the apatite-filled composite hydrogel, with the reinforcement effect modulated by the size of the apatite crystals. This interaction was specific to glutamic acid sequence as the addition of a neutral glycine or a positively charged lysine sequence did not reinforce the composite. We further demonstrated that osteon–mimetic composites consisting of L-PLA nanofiber mesh laminated with a hydrogel/apatite precursor solution produces a multifunctional substrate with superior mechanical and biological properties. The fiber layers can provide structural support and dimensional stability to prevent the regenerating region from soft tissue collapse. The hydrogel phase can support diffusion of oxygen and nutrients, solubilization of growth factors, and conjugation of bioactive peptides, as well as providing a matrix with a bimodal degradation profile. The apatite nanocrystals can provide an osteoconductive substrate for differentiation and mineralization of BMS cells. These works demonstrate that novel composites with improved mechanical and biological properties can be developed for load-bearing skeletal tissue regeneration by mimicking the nanoscale morphological and structural features of osseous tissue.

ACKNOWLEDGMENTS

This study was supported by research grants to E. Jabbari from the National Science Foundation under Grant nos. CBET-0756394 and CBET-0931998, the National Institutes of Health under Grant no. R03 DE19180-01A1, and the National Football League Charities.

REFERENCES

1. M. J. Yaszemski, J. B. Oldham, L. Lu, and B. L. Currier, Clinical needs for bone tissue engineering technology, in *Bone Engineering*, J. E. Davis (Ed.), em squared, Toronto, pp. 541–547, 2000.
2. H. Ueda and Y. Tabata, Polyhydroxyalkanonate derivatives in current clinical applications and trials, *Adv. Drug Deliv. Rev*, 55, 501–518, 2003.
3. S. H. Rhee, Bone-like apatite-forming ability and mechanical properties of poly(epsilon-caprolactone)/silica hybrid as a function of poly(epsilon-caprolactone) content, *Biomaterials*, 25, 1167–1175, 2004.
4. H. Suh, M. J. Song, M. Ohata, Y. B. Kang, and S. Tsutsumi, *Ex vivo* mechanical evaluation of carbonate apatite–collagen-grafted porous poly-L-lactic acid membrane in rabbit calvarial bone, *Tissue Eng.*, 9, 635–643, 2003.
5. J. M. Karp, M. S. Shoichet, and J. E. Davies, Bone formation on two-dimensional poly(DL-lactide-*co*-glycolide) (PLGA) films and three-dimensional PLGA tissue engineering scaffolds *in vitro*, *J. Biomed. Mater. Res.*, 64A, 388–396, 2003.
6. F. Kandziora, G. Schmidmaier, G. Schollmeier, H. Bail, R. Pflugmacher, T. Gorke, M. Wagner, M. Raschke, T. Mittlmeier, and N. P. Haas, IGF-I and TGF-beta1 application by a poly-(D,L-lactide)-coated cage promotes intervertebral bone matrix formation in the sheep cervical spine, *Spine*, 27, 1710–1723, 2002.

7. C. G. Simon Jr., C. A. Khatri, S. A. Wight, and F. W. Wang, Preliminary report on the biocompatibility of a moldable, resorbable, composite bone graft consisting of calcium phosphate cement and poly(lactide-*co*-glycolide) microspheres, *J. Orthop. Res.*, 20, 473–482, 2002.
8. K. Matsuzak, F. Walboomers, A. de Ruijter, and J. A. Jansen, Effect of microgrooved poly-L-lactic (PLA) surfaces on proliferation, cytoskeletal organization, and mineralized matrix formation of rat bone marrow cells, *Clin. Oral Implants Res.*, 11, 325–333, 2000.
9. S. Leinonen, J. Tiainen, M. Kellomaki, P. Tormala, T. Waris, M. Ninkovic, and N. Ashammakhi, Holding power of bioabsorbable self-reinforced poly-L/DL-lactide 70/30 tacks and miniscrews in human cadaver bone, *J. Craniofac. Surg.*, 14, 171–175, 2003.
10. P. Nordstrom, T. Pohjonen, P. Tormala, and P. Rokkanen, Shear-load carrying capacity of cancellous bone after implantation of self-reinforced polyglycolic acid and poly-L-lactic acid pins: Experimental study on rats, *Biomaterials*, 22, 2557–2561, 2001.
11. G. Chen, T. Sato, T. Ushida, R. Hirochika, and T. Tateishi, Redifferentiation of dedifferentiated bovine chondrocytes when cultured *in vitro* in a PLGA-collagen hybrid mesh, *FEBS Lett.*, 542(1–3), 95–999, 2003.
12. A. K. Poshusta, J. A. Burdick, D. J. Mortisen, R. F. Padera, D. Ruehlman, M. J. Yaszemski, and K. S. Anseth, Histocompatibility of photocrosslinked polyanhydrides: A novel *in situ* forming orthopaedic biomaterial, *J. Biomed. Mater. Res.*, 64(1), 62–69, 2003.
13. K. S. Anseth, V. R. Shastri, and R. Langer, Photopolymerizable degradable polyanhydrides with osteocompatibility, *Nat. Biotech*, 17, 156–159, 1999.
14. E. Jabbari and X. He, Synthesis and material properties of functionalized lactide oligomers as *in situ* crosslinkable scaffolds for tissue regeneration, *Polym. Prepr.*, 47(2), 353–354, 2006.
15. J. P. Fisher, J. W. Vehof, D. Dean, J. P. van der Waerden, T. A. Holland, A. G. Mikos, and J. A. Jansen, Soft and hard tissue response to photocrosslinked poly(propylene fumarate) scaffolds in a rabbit model, *J. Biomed. Mater. Res.*, 59, 547–556, 2002.
16. D. D. Frazier, V. K. Lathi, T. N. Gerhart, and W. C. Hayes, *Ex vivo* degradation of a poly(propylene glycol-fumarate) biodegradable particulate composite bone cement, *J. Biomed. Mater. Res.*, 35, 383–389, 1997.
17. M. J. Yaszemski, R. G. Payne, W. C. Hayes, R. S. Langer, and A. G. Mikos, *In vitro* degradation of a poly(propylene fumarate)-based composite material, *Biomaterials*, 17(22), 2127–2130, 2006.
18. E. Jabbari, S. Wang, L. Lu, J. A. Gruetzmacher, S. Ameenuddin, T. E. Hefferan, B. L. Currier, A. J. Windebank, and M. J. Yaszemski, Synthesis, material properties and biocompatibility of a novel self-crosslinkable poly(caprolactone fumarate) as an injectable tissue engineering scaffold, *Biomacromolecules*, 6, 2503–2511, 2005.
19. J. Elisseeff, K. S. Anseth, D. Sims, W. McIntosh, M. Randolph, and R. Langer, Transdermal photopolymerization for minimally invasive implantation, *Proc. Natl. Acad. Sci.*, 96, 3104–3107, 1999.
20. E. Alsberg, K. W. Anderson, A. Albeiruti, R. T. Franceschi, and D. J. Mooney, Cell-interactive alginate hydrogels for bone tissue engineering, *J. Dent. Res.*, 80(11), 2025–2029, 2001.
21. X. He and E. Jabbari, Material properties and cytocompatibility of injectable MMP degradable poly(lactide ethylene oxide fumarate) hydrogel as a carrier for marrow stromal cells, *Biomacromolecules*, 8, 780–792, 2007.
22. K. Fujimura, K. Bessho, Y. Okubo, N. Segami, and T. Iizuka, A bioactive bone cement containing Bis-GMA resin and A-W glass–ceramic as an augmentation graft material on mandibular bone, *Clin. Oral Implan. Res.*, 14, 659–667, 2003.
23. J. van den Dolder, J. G. Wolke, and J. A. Jansen, The cytocompatibility and early osteogenic characteristics of an injectable calcium phosphate cement, *Tissue Eng.*, 13(3), 493–500, 2007.
24. S. A. Hutchens, R. S. Benson, B. R. Evans, H. M. O'Neill, and C. J. Rawn, Biomimetic synthesis of calcium-deficient hydroxyapatite in a natural hydrogel, *Biomaterials*, 27(26), 4661–4670, 2006.
25. P. Kasten, J. Vogel, R. Luginbuhl, P. Niemeyer, M. Tonak, H. Lorenz, L. Helbig, S. Weiss, J. Fellenberg, A. Leo, H. G. Simank, and W. Richter, Ectopic bone formation associated with mesenchymal stem cells in a resorbable calcium deficient hydroxyapatite carrier, *Biomaterials*, 26(29), 5879–5889, 2005.
26. B. R. Constantz, I. C. Ison, M. T. Fulmer, R. D. Poser, S. T. Smith, M. VanWagoner, J. Ross, S. A. Goldstein, J. B. Jupiter, and D. I. Rosenthal, Skeletal repair by *in situ* formation of the mineral phase of bone, *Science*, 267, 1796–1799, 1995.
27. L. Liu, L. Zhang, B. Ren, F. Wang, and Q. Zhang, Preparation and characterization of collagen–hydroxyapatite composite used for bone tissue engineering scaffold, *Artif. Cells Blood Substit. Immobil. Biotechnol.*, 31(4), 435–448, 2003.

28. C. V. Rodrigues, P. Serricella, A. B. Linhares, R. M. Guerdes, R. Borojevic, M. A. Rossi, M. E. Duarte, and M. Farina, Characterization of a bovine collagen–hydroxyapatite composite scaffold for bone tissue engineering, *Biomaterials*, 24(27), 4987–4997, 2003.
29. J. M. Oliveira, M. T. Rodrigues, S. S. Silva, P. B. Malafaya, M. E. Gomes, C. A. Viegas, I. R. Dias, J. T. Azevedo, J. F. Mano, and R. L. Reis, Novel hydroxyapatite/chitosan bilayered scaffold for osteochondral tissue-engineering applications: Scaffold design and its performance when seeded with goat bone marrow stromal cells, *Biomaterials*, 27(36), 6123–6137, 2006.
30. T. Furuzono, S. Yasuda, T. Kimura, S. Kyotani, J. Tanaka, and A. Kishida, Nano-scaled hydroxyapatite/polymer composite IV. Fabrication and cell adhesion properties of a three-dimensional scaffold made of composite material with a silk fibroin substrate to develop a percutaneous device, *J. Artif. Organs*, 7(3), 137–144, 2004.
31. Z. Ajdukovic, S. Najman, L. J. Dordevic, V. Savic, D. Mihailovic, D. Petrovic, N. Ignjatovic, and D. Uskokovic, Repair of bone tissue affected by osteoporosis with hydroxyapatite-poly-L-lactide (HAp-PLLA) with and without blood plasma, *J. Biomater. Appl.*, 20(2), 179–190, 2005.
32. Y. Shikinami and M. Okuno, Bioresorbable devices made of forged composites of hydroxyapatite (HA) particles and poly L-lactide (PLLA). Part II: Practical properties of miniscrews and miniplates, *Biomaterials*, 22(23), 3197–211, 2001.
33. Y. Shikinami and M. Okuno, Bioresorbable devices made of forged composites of hydroxyapatite (HA) particles and poly-L-lactide (PLLA): Part I. Basic characteristics, *Biomaterials*, 20(9), 859–877, 1999.
34. S. S. Kim, K. M. Ahn, M. S. Park, J. H. Lee, C. Y. Choi, and B. S. Kim, A poly(lactide-*co*-glycolide)/hydroxyapatite composite scaffold with enhanced osteoconductivity, *J. Biomed. Mater. Res.*, 80A(1), 206–215, 2007.
35. D. Hakimimehr, D. M. Liu, and T. Troczynski, *In-situ* preparation of poly(propylene fumarate)/hydroxyapatite composite, *Biomaterials*, 26(35), 7297–303, 2005.
36. F. E. Wiria, K. F. Leong, C. K. Chua, and Y. Liu, Poly(ε-caprolactone)/hydroxyapatite for tissue engineering scaffold fabrication via selective laser sintering, *Acta Biomater.*, 3(1), 1–12, 2007.
37. Y. Hu, C. Zhang, S. Zhang, Z. Xiong, and J. Xu, Development of a porous poly(L-lactic acid)/hydroxyapatite/collagen scaffold as a BMP delivery system and its use in healing canine segmental bone defect, *J. Biomed. Mater. Res.*, 67A(2), 591–598, 2003.
38. M. C. Kruyt, W. J. Dhert, F. C. Oner, C. A. van Blitterswijk, A. J. Verbout, and J. D. de Bruijn, Analysis of ectopic and orthotopic bone formation in cell-based tissue-engineered constructs in goats, *Biomaterials*, 28(10), 1798–805, 2007.
39. S. L. Hall, K. H. Lau, S. T. Chen, J. C. Felt, D. S. Gridley, J. K. Yee, and D. J. Baylink, An improved mouse Sca-1+ cell-based bone marrow transplantation model for use in gene- and cell-based therapeutic studies, *Acta Haematol.*, 117(1), 24–33, 2007.
40. G. Pelled, K. Tai, D. Sheyn, Y. Zilberman, S. Kumbar, L. S. Nair, C. T. Laurencin, D. Gazit, and C. Ortiz, Structural and nanoindentation studies of stem cell-based tissue-engineered bone, *J. Biomech.*, 40(2), 399–411, 2007.
41. U. Meyer, H. P. Wiesmann, K. Berr, N. R. Kubler, and J. Handschel, Cell-based bone reconstruction therapies-principles of clinical approaches, *Int. J. Oral Maxillofac. Implants*, 21(6), 899–906, 2006.
42. J. Handschel, H. P. Wiesmann, R. Depprich, N. R. Kubler, and U. Meyer, Cell-based bone reconstruction therapies: Cell sources, *Int. J. Oral Maxillofac. Implants*, 21(6), 890–898, 2006.
43. M. C. Kruyt, C. E. Wilson, J. D. de Bruijn, C. A. van Blitterswijk, C. F. Oner, A. J. Verbout, and W. J. Dhert, The effect of cell-based bone tissue engineering in a goat transverse process model, *Biomaterials*, 27(29), 5099–5106, 2006.
44. E. Jabbari, L. Lu, and M. J. Yaszemski, Synthesis and characterization of injectable and biodegradable composites for orthopedic applications, in *Handbook of Biodegradable Polymeric Materials and Their Applications*, S. K. Mallapragada and B. Narasimhan (Eds), American Scientific Publishers, Stevenson Ranch, CA, 2, 2004.
45. E. Jabbari, L. Lu, B. L. Currier, A. G. Mikos, and M. J. Yaszemski, Injectable polymers and hydrogels for orthopedic and dental applications, in *Tissue Engineering in Musculoskeletal Clinical Practice*, L. J. Sandell and A. J. Grodzinsky (Eds), American Academy of Orthopaedic Surgeons, Rosemont, IL, Chapter 32, 2004.
46. M. J. Glimcher, The nature of the mineral component of bone and the mechanisms of calcification, in D*isorders of bone and mineral metabolism*, F. L. Coe and M. J. Favus (Eds), Raven Press, New York, NY, pp. 265–286, 1992.
47. G. M. Herring, Methods for the study of glycoproteins and proteoglycans of bone using bacterial collagenase: Determination of bone sialoprotein and chondroitin sulfate, *Calcif. Tissue Res.*, 24, 29–36, 1977.

48. M. A. Fernández-seara, S. L. Wehrli, M. Takahashi, and F. W. Wehrli, Water content measured by proton–deuteron exchange NMR predicts bone mineral density and mechanical properties, *J. Bone Miner. Res.*, 19, 289–296, 2004.
49. A. J. Bailey and L. Knott, Molecular changes in bone collagen in osteoporosis and osteoarthritis in the elderly, *Exp. Gerontol.*, 34, 337–351, 1999.
50. M. C. Summitt and K.D. Reisinger, Characterization of the mechanical properties of demineralized bone, *J. Biomed. Mater. Res.*, 67A, 742–750, 2003.
51. S. P. Kotha, W. R. Walsh, Y. Pan, and N. Guzelsu, Varying the mechanical properties of bone tissue by changing the amount of its structurally effective bone mineral content, *Biomed. Mater. Eng.*, 8, 321–334, 1998.
52. W. J. Landis, The strength of a calcified tissue depends in part on the molecular structure and organization of its constituent mineral crystals in their organic matrix, *Bone*, 16(5), 533–544, 1995.
53. J.-Y. Rho, L. Kuhn-Spearing, and P. Zioupos, Mechanical properties and the hierarchical structure of bone, *Med. Eng. Phys.*, 20, 92–102, 1998.
54. J. A. Buckwalter and R. R. Cooper, Bone biology Part II: Formation, form, modeling, remodeling, and regulation of cell function, *J. Bone Joint Surg.*, 77A, 1276–1289, 1995.
55. R. Fujisawa, Y. Wada, Y. Nodasaka, and Y. Kuboki, Acidic amino acid-rich sequences as binding sites of osteonectin to hydroxyapatite crystals, *Biochim. Biophys. Acta.*, 1292(1), 53–60, 1996.
56. V. I. Sikavitsas, J. S. Temenoff, and A. G. Mikos, Biomaterials and bone mechanotransduction. *Biomaterials*, 22, 2581–2593, 2001.
57. Y. Tabata, Tissue regeneration based on growth factor release, *Tissue Eng*, 9(Suppl. 1), S5–S15, 2003.
58. M. F. Young, Bone matrix proteins: Their function, regulation, and relationship to osteoporosis, *Osteoporos. Int.*, 14(Suppl. 3), S35–S42, 2003.
59. P. Bianco, M. Riminucci, S. Gronthos, and P. G. Robey, Bone marrow stromal stem cells: Nature, biology, and potential applications, *Stem Cells*, 19, 180–192, 2001.
60. A. J. Friedenstein, I. I. Shapiro-Piatetzky, and K. V. Petrakova, Osteogenesis in transplants of bone marrow cells, *J. Embryol. Exp. Morphol.*, 16, 381–390, 1966.
61. M. Owen, Marrow stromal stem cells, *J. Cell Sci.*, 3S, 393–403, 1988.
62. S. Makino, K. Fukuda, and S. Miyoshi, Cardiomyocytes can be generated from marrow stromal cells *in vitro*, *J. Clin. Invest.*, 103, 697–705, 1999.
63. S. Wakitani, T. Saito, and A. Caplan, Myogenic cells derived from rat bone marrow mesenchymal stem cells exposed to 5-azacytidine, *Muscle Nerve*, 18, 1417–1426, 1995.
64. D. Woodbury, E. J. Schwarz, D. J. Prockop, and I. B. Black, Adult rat and human bone marrow stromal cells differentiate into neurons, *J. Neurosci. Res.*, 61, 364–370, 2000.
65. P. Carmeliet and A. Luttun, The emerging role of the bone marrow-derived stem cells in (therapeutic) angiogenesis, *Thromb. Haemost.*, 68, 289–297, 2001.
66. C. Maniatopoulos, J. Sodek, and A. H. Melcher, Bone formation *in vitro* by stromal cells obtained from bone marrow of young adult rats, *Cell tissue Res.*, 254, 317–330, 1988.
67. M. J. Yost, C. F. Baicu, C. E. Stonerock, R. L. Goodwin, R. L. Price, J. M. Davis, H. Evans, et al., A novel tubular scaffold for cardiovascular tissue engineering, *Tissue Eng.*, 10(1–2), 273–284, 2004.
68. J. A. Henderson, X. He, and E. Jabbari, Concurrent differentiation of marrow stromal cells to osteogenic and vasculogenic lineages, *Macromol. Biosci.*, 8(6), 499–507, 2008.
69. S. Shi, M. Kirk, and A. J. Kahn, The role of type I collagen in the regulation of the osteoblast phenotype, *J. Bone Miner. Res.*, 11, 1139–1145, 1996.
70. C. W. Lan and Y. J. Wang, Collagen as an immobilization vehicle for bone marrow stromal cells enriched with osteogenic potential, *Artif. Cells Blood Substit. Immobil. Biotechnol.*, 31, 59–68, 2003.
71. M. Taira, S. Toyosawa, and N. Ijyuin, Studies on osteogenic differentiation of rat bone marrow stromal cells cultured in type I collagen gel by RT-PCR analysis, *J. Oral. Rehabil.*, 30, 802–807, 2003.
72. D. J. Carey, Control of growth and differentiation of vascular cells by extracellular matrix proteins, *Annu. Rev. Physiol.*, 53, 161–177, 1991.
73. D. S. Grant, K. Tashiro, R. B. Segui-Real, Y. Yamada, G. R. Martin, H. K. Kleinman, Two different laminin domains mediate the differentiation of human endothelial cells into capillary-like structures *in vitro*, *Cell*, 58, 933–943, 1989.
74. S. Ramakrishna, J. Mayer, E. Wintermantel, and K. W. Leong, Biomedical applications of polymer–composite materials: A review, *Comp. Sci. Tech.*, 61, 1189–1224, 2001.
75. J. F. Mano, R. A. Sousa, L. F. Boesel, N. M. Neves, and R. L. Reis, Bioinert, biodegradable and injectable polymeric matrix composites for hard tissue replacement: State of art and recent developments, *Comp. Sci. Tech.*, 64, 789–817, 2004.

76. M. J. Yaszemski, R. G. Payne, W. C. Hayes, R. Langer, and A. G. Mikos, Evolution of bone transplantation: Molecular, cellular and tissue strategies to engineer human bone, *Biomaterials*, 17, 175–185, 1996.
77. S. N. Nazhat, R. Joseph, M. Wang, R. Smith, K. E. Tanner, and W. Bonfield, Dynamic mechanical characterisation of hydroxyapatite reinforced polyethylene: Effect of particle size, *J. Mater. Sci. Mater. Med.*, 11, 621–628, 2000.
78. S. Deb, M. Wang, K. E. Tanner, and W. Bonfield, Hydroxyapatite polyethylene composites: Effect of grafting and surface treatment of Hydroxyapatite, *J. Mater. Sci. Mater. Med.*, 7, 191–197, 1996.
79. M. Wang and W. Bonfield, Chemically coupled hydroxyapatite polyethylene composites: Structure and properties, *Biomaterials*, 22, 1311–1320, 2001.
80. X. Wang and C. G. Robertson, Strain-induced nonlinearity of filled rubbers, *Phys. Rev.*, 72E, 031406–031409, 2005.
81. A. S. Sarvestani, X. He, and E. Jabbari, The effect of osteonectin-derived peptide on the viscoelasticity of hydrogel/apatite nanocomposite scaffolds, *Biopolymers*, 85(4), 370–378, 2007.
82. G. E. Fantner, H. Birkedal, J. H. Kindt, T. Hassenkam, J. C. Weaver, J. A. Cutroni, B. L. Bosma et al., Influence of the degradation of the organic matrix on the microscopic fracture behavior of trabecular bone, *Bone*, 35, 1013–1022, 2004.
83. K. A. Athanasiou, C. F. Zhu, D. R. Lanctot, C. M. Agrawal, and X. Wang, Fundamentals of biomechanics in tissue engineering of bone, *Tissue Eng.*, 6, 361–381, 2000.
84. A. L. Boskey, Mineral–matrix interactions in bone and cartilage: Clinical orthopedics and related research, *Clin. Orthop. Relat. Res.*, 281, 244–274, 1992.
85. J. D. Termine, H. K. Kleinman, S. W. Whitson, K. M. Conn, M. L. McGarvey, and G. R. Martin, Osteonectin, a bone-specific protein linking mineral to collagen, *Cell*, 26, 99–105, 1981.
86. T. Nakase, M. Sugimoto, M. Sato, M. Kaneko, T. Tomita, K. Sugamoto, S. Nomura et al., Switch of osteonectin and osteopontin mRNA expression in the process of cartilage-to-bone transition during fracture repair, *Acta Histochem.*, 100, 287–295, 1998.
87. J. Sodek, B. Zhu, M. H. Huynh, T. J. Brown, and M. Ringuette, Novel functions of the matricellular proteins osteopontin and osteonectin, *Connect. Tissue Res.*, 43, 308–319, 2002.
88. R.-L. Xie and G. L. Long, Elements within the first 17 amino acids of human osteonectin are responsible for binding to type V collagen, *J. Biol. Chem.*, 271, 8121–8125, 1996.
89. A. L. Boskey, D. J. Moore, M. Amling, E. Canalis, and A. M. Delany, Infrared analysis of the mineral and matrix in bones of osteonectin-null mice and their wildtype controls, *J. Bone Miner. Res.*, 8, 1005–1011, 2003.
90. X. He and E. Jabbari, Solid-phase synthesis of reactive peptide crosslinker by selective deprotection, *Prot. Pept. Lett.*, 13, 715–718, 2006.
91. A. S. Sarvestani, X. He, E. Jabbari, The role of filler–matrix interaction on viscoelastic response of biomimetic nanocomposite hydrogels. in special issue: Nanostructured materials for biomedical applications, *J. Nanomater.*, article #126803, 2008.
92. A. S. Sarvestani and E. Jabbari, A model for the viscoelastic behavior of nanofilled hydrogel composites under oscillatory shear loading, *Polym. Compos.*, 29, 326–336, 2008.
93. A.S. Sarvestani, X. He, and E. Jabbari, Osteonectin-derived peptide increases the modulus of a bone–mimetic nanocomposite, *Euro. Biophys. J. Biophys. Lett.*, 37(2), 229–234, 2007.
94. A. S. Sarvestani, W. Xu, X. He, and E. Jabbari, Gelation and degradation characteristics of *in-situ* photo-crosslinked poly(L-lactide-*co*-ethylene oxide-*co*-fumarate) hydrogels, *Polymer*, 48, 7113–7120, 2007.
95. A. S. Sarvestani, X. He, and E. Jabbari, Effect of composition on gelation kinetics of unfilled and nano-apatite-filled poly(lactide-ethylene oxide-fumarate) hydrogels, *Mater. Lett.*, 16, 5278–5281, 2007.
96. A. S. Sarvestani, X. He, and E. Jabbari, Viscoelastic characterization and modeling of gelation kinetics of injectable *in situ* crosslinkable poly(lactide-ethylene oxide-fumarate) hydrogels, *Biomacromolecules*, 8(2), 406–415, 2007.
97. A. S. Sarvestani and E. Jabbari, Modeling and experimental investigation of rheological properties of injectable poly(lactide ethylene oxide fumarate)/hydroxyapatite nanocomposites, *Biomacromoelcules*, 7, 1573–1580, 2006.
98. E. J. Guth, Theory of filler reinforcement, *J. Appl. Phys.*, 16, 20–25, 1945.
99. J. A. Buckwalter and R. R. Cooper, Bone structure and function, *Instr. Course Lect.*, 36, 27–48, 1987.
100. S. Weiner, W. Traub, and H. D. Wagner, Lamellar bone: Structure-function relations, *J. Struct. Biol.*, 126(3), 241–255, 1999.

101. M. A. Fernandez-Seara, S. L. Wehrli, M. Takahashi, and F. W. Wehrli, Water content measured by proton–deuteron exchange NMR predicts bone mineral density and mechanical properties, *J. Bone Miner. Res.*, 19(2), 289–296, 2004.
102. K. A. Athanasiou, C. Zhu, D. R. Lanctot, C. M. Agrawal, X., and Wang X, Fundamentals of biomechanics in tissue engineering of bone, *Tissue Eng.*, 6(4), 361–381, 2000.
103. M. T. Thompson, M. C. Berg, I. S. Tobias, M. F. Rubner, and K. J. Van Vliet, Tuning compliance of nanoscale polyelectrolyte multilayers to modulate cell adhesion, *Biomaterials*, 26(34), 6836–6845, 2005.
104. A. Schneider, G. Francius, R. Obeid, P. Schwinté, J. Hemmerlé, B. Frisch, P. Schaaf, J.-C. Voegel, B. Senger, and C. Picart, Polyelectrolyte multilayers with a tunable Young's modulus: Influence of film stiffness on cell adhesion, *Langmuir*, 22(3), 1193–1200, 2006.

31 Resonance for Multitransducer Systems

Behraad Bahreyni

CONTENTS

31.1 INTRODUCTION

In many engineering applications, resonance is undesired and avoided. In large-scale civil and mechanical engineering applications, the amplified displacements at resonance often cause excessive noise, accelerated aging, and even destruction of a device. Micromachined resonators, on the other hand, can undergo sustained resonance for extended duration that often exceeds their designed lifetime. This operation longevity is a consequence of the small structural volumes of these devices and the fact that they are made of materials such as crystalline silicon that have very small defect densities.

Many linear physical systems exhibit an amplified response to their input at particular frequencies. In many cases, the peaks in the frequency response of a system of order n can be attributed to the existence of complex conjugate poles among the eigenvalues of the system. Figure 31.1 illustrates an example of the response of such a system. The equation of motion for displacements of the mass of a second-order mass–damper–spring system, as shown in Figure 31.2, is

$$M_{\text{eff}} \frac{d^2x}{dt^2} \xi \frac{dx}{dt} + K_{\text{eff}} x = F \tag{31.1}$$

where M_{eff} is the *effective* mass of the object, K_{eff} is the *effective* spring constant, and ζ represents all the damping mechanisms in the system, which are assumed to be proportional to the velocity of the moving body. Defining $\omega_0^2 = K/M$ and $Q = M\omega_0/\xi$, the eigenvalues of the system are given by $\lambda_{1,2} = (\omega_0/2Q) \pm j\omega_0\sqrt{1-1/4Q^2}$. For a resonant system, Q is a measure of damping and is referred to as the *quality factor*. For large values of Q (i.e., larger than ~10), the eigenvalues of the system approach $\pm j\omega_0$ on the imaginary axis, where ω_0 is called the *undamped natural frequency* of the system. Parameters ω_0 and Q are the primary factors when describing the operation of resonators.

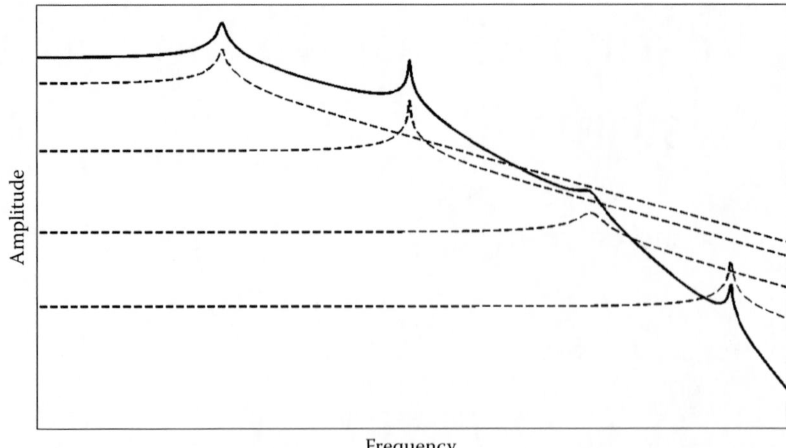

FIGURE 31.1 An example of the frequency response of a system with multiple resonant frequencies. The dashed lines represent the response of the approximate second-order systems around each peak.

Figure 31.3 illustrates how these two parameters can be estimated from the time or frequency response of a high-Q second-order system. If the complex conjugate eigenvalues of a high-Q system are found through numerical analysis, the resonant frequency can be approximated by $\omega_{ri} = \text{Im}\{\lambda_i\}$ and the quality factor is found from

$$Q = -\frac{\text{Im}\{\lambda_i\}}{2\,\text{Re}\{\lambda_i\}} \tag{31.2}$$

When a system has several underdamped complex conjugate eigenvalues (infinite in case of continuous structures), the system response around each of the resonant peaks can be approximated by that of an underdamped second-order system (dashed lines in Figure 31.1) with a proper gain factor that accounts for the DC gain of that second-order system. The overall behavior of the system can then be approximated as the superimposition of these lower-order resonators, allowing the investigator to use much of the results from the analysis of second-order systems [1].

31.2 TRANSDUCTION MECHANISMS

Resonance is used for sensing, actuation, or signal processing at micro- and nanoscales. In all these cases, it is needed to employ proper transduction mechanisms to convert signals from an electrical

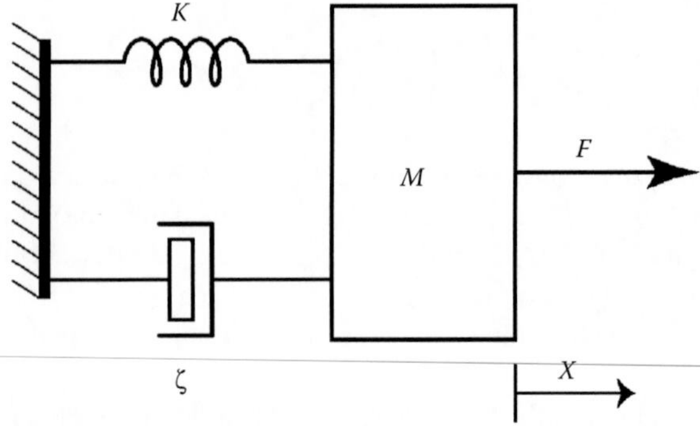

FIGURE 31.2 A damped mass–spring system.

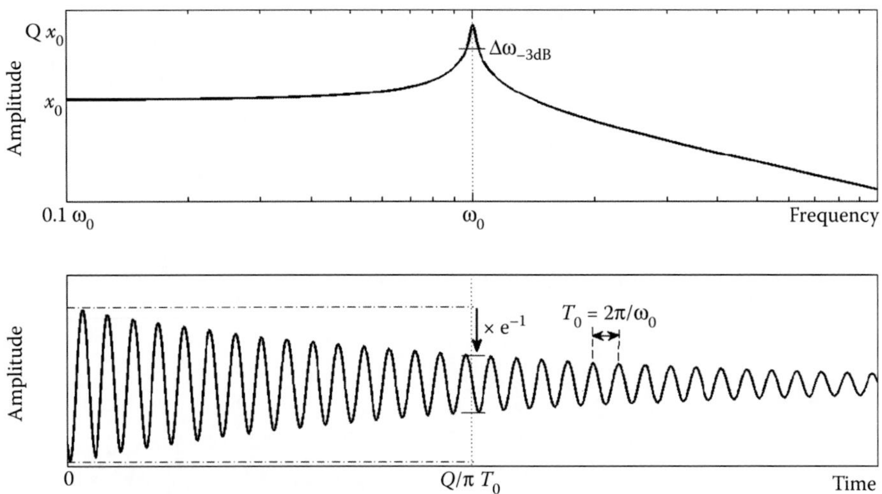

FIGURE 31.3 Responses of a high-Q resonator to a constant-amplitude input signal (top) and to a step input (bottom). The quality factor can be estimated from the ratio of the resonant frequency, ω_0 to the −3 dB bandwidth of the resonance peak (i.e., $\omega_0/\Delta\omega_{-3dB}$). Q can be estimated from the step response of the resonator by noticing that the oscillations amplitude drops by about 63% after Q/π cycles. (From B. Bahreyni, *Fabrication and Design of Resonant Microdevices*. New York, NY: William Andrew Publishing, 2008. With permission.)

domain to mechanical at the input port of the device, and often, from a mechanical domain to electrical at an output port. At micro- and nanoscales, transduction mechanisms for actuation include electrostatic [2,3], piezoelectric [4,5], thermal [6–8], magnetic [9], and optical [10]. Due to the ease of fabrication and low power consumption, most commercialized resonant devices use electrostatics for both sensing and actuation. If C_{in} is the capacitance between the two electrodes of the input port of a device, the exerted force on the structure is given by

$$F = -\frac{1}{2}\nabla C_{in} V_{in}^2 \tag{31.3}$$

where V_{in} is the applied potential between the electrodes. It is noteworthy that the mechanism of generating a force through electrostatic actuation (and similarly for the thermal actuation) is inherently nonlinear and the generated force will have higher harmonics of the drive signal.

Sensing of resonance is also achieved through a variety of techniques such as electrostatic [11,12], piezoelectric [13,14], piezoresistive [15,16], and optical [17]. Electrostatics is again the most commonly used sensing technique. The output current from a capacitor C_{out} at the output port of a resonator is

$$i_{out} = \frac{dQ_{out}}{dt} = C_{out}\frac{dV_{out}}{dt} + V_{out}\left(\nabla C_{out} \cdot \frac{d\vec{r}}{dt}\right) \tag{31.4}$$

where V_{out} is the bias voltage, often DC, on the output capacitor and $\vec{r}$ is the vector for the relative displacements of the electrodes. As can be seen from Equations 31.3 and 31.4, the efficiency of energy coupling between electrical and mechanical domains for electrostatic actuators and sensors strongly depend on the rate of changes of the transducer capacitance with displacements.

Piezoelectricity is the other common actuation and sensing mechanism. The energy conversion efficiencies between the mechanical and electrical domains are higher for piezoelectric transducers than electrostatic devices. This leads to the lower losses of piezoelectric resonators compared to electrostatic resonators should the other resonator parameters, such as quality factor and resonant frequency, be on the same order. However, process flow integration is more challenging for piezoelectric transducers as there are few piezoelectric materials, such as aluminum nitride, that are permitted in a general fabrication process. Furthermore, the performance of piezoelectric transducers depends on the thickness and quality of the piezoelectric film or substrate, which is difficult to accurately maintain across large–area wafers. Therefore, piezoelectric transducers are employed when there are significant incentives to minimize the losses through a resonator, as is the case for filters, for example.

Piezoresistivity is another sensing mechanism that has been employed for sensing of the resonator displacements. Typically, piezoresistors are used when they can be easily placed on the structure without adding to the fabrication complexity [18,19].

31.3 MODELING

There are three basic resonance modes that are utilized in micro- and nanoresonator design. The difference between these modes is in how the acoustic waves are affecting the structure that can be any of the flexural (or bending), bulk, or surface resonant modes. Complete analytical analysis of these resonators is often too complicated to provide insight, and therefore, numerical analysis is usually employed to study the details of device behavior. Nevertheless, even a highly simplified analytical model is extremely valuable during the initial phases of the device design. Furthermore, it is often possible to breakdown a complex structure into subsystems, such as beams and rectangular or circular plates, which are easier to analyze.

The dynamic behavior of many resonators can be estimated from their static behavior. For example, if $\psi(x)$ describes beam shape under a given static load, $\psi(x)\, e^{j\omega t}$ is a good estimate for the bending of the beam under a harmonic load that is applied to the structure similar to the static one. Euler's equation is used to model the bending of long slender beams under a continuous normal load of $F(x,t)$:

$$EI\frac{\partial^4\psi}{\partial x^4} - P\frac{\partial^2\psi}{\partial x^2} + \rho A_b\frac{\partial^2\psi}{\partial t^2} + \zeta\frac{\partial\psi}{\partial t} = F(x,t) \tag{31.5}$$

where E and ρ are Young's modulus and density of the material, A_b is the cross-sectional area of the beam, P is the axial load on the beam, ζ is the damping coefficient, and F is the point load applied normally to the beam axis [20,21]. As can be expected, the equations for bending of thin plates are extensions of the above equation to two dimensions [22,23]. Figure 31.4 illustrates some basic flexural and bulk modes of beams and plates.

Several approximate techniques exist for estimation of the resonant frequencies and mode shapes of simple resonant structures, among which Rayleigh's method is probably better known and more often used [20,24,25]. For an undamped device, the maxima for kinetic and potential energies at resonance are equal, or $T_{max} \equiv \frac{1}{2}[\dot{\vec{x}}_{max}][M_{eff}][\dot{\vec{x}}_{max}] = 1/[\vec{x}_{max}][K_{eff}][\vec{x}_{max}] \equiv U_{max}$, where $[\vec{x}]$ is the displacement vector for oscillations and $[M_{eff}]$ and $[K_{eff}]$ are the effective mass and stiffness matrices for the system. However, for linear harmonic vibrations we have $[\dot{\vec{x}}] = j\omega[\vec{x}]$, and therefore, the resonance frequency can be estimated from

$$\omega_0^2 = \left|\frac{U_{max}}{T_{max}}\right| = \left|\frac{[\vec{x}_{max}][K_{eff}][\vec{x}_{max}]}{[\vec{x}_{max}][M_{eff}][\vec{x}_{max}]}\right| \tag{31.6}$$

Device displacements can be estimated from the shape of the particular resonant mode that is being studied [24]. Rayleigh's method often gives an upper bond for the resonant frequency as the calculated kinetic energy is often limited to a few of the dominant modes.

Electrical resonance is frequently encountered during the design of electrical systems and circuits and is often modeled as a series or parallel RLC network. It is also common practice to use an

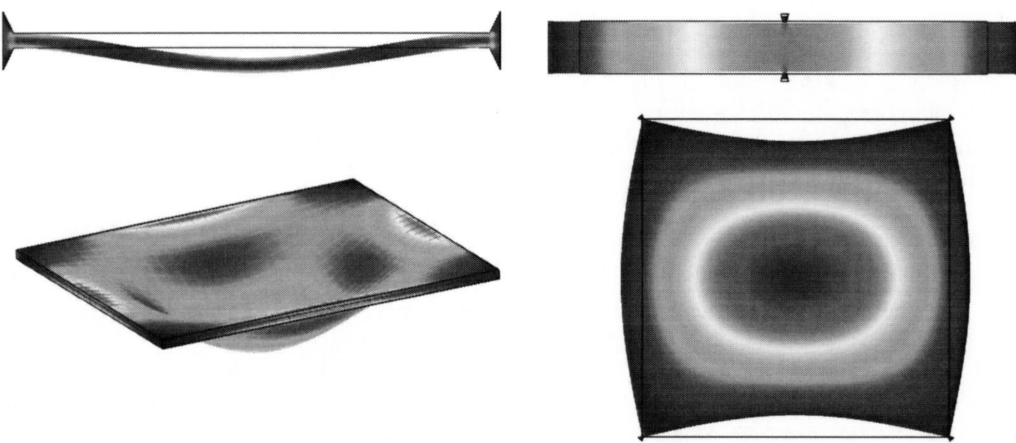

FIGURE 31.4 Flexural (left) and bulk (right) modes of a slender beam and a square plate.

equivalent electrical network to represent the operation of a mechanical resonator [25,26]. The reason for this conversion, besides its familiar presentation to electrical engineers, is that the resonator model can then be used in circuit simulators along with the interface electronics for that system, and hence, performing a more comprehensive analysis of the system. Table 31.1 illustrates the correspondence between the equivalent electrical and mechanical models of a resonator. When the resonator is modeled around its resonant frequency, the equivalent electrical models are called motional resistance, motional inductance, and motional capacitance. The motional resistance, R_m, is particularly important as it represents the resonator losses.

31.4 APPLICATIONS OF MICRORESONATORS

Resonant devices are used in several applications for sensing, actuation, or signal processing. The resonant frequency, ω_0, of a resonant sensor changes in response to the measurand. Resonant actuators take advantage of the amplified response of the structure to the excitation signal at resonance to improve the displacements by a factor of $\sim Q$. For signal processing applications, the resonator is essentially used to filter out unwanted signals and provide high selectivity using one or a number of coupled resonators. We will discuss these applications in more detail in the following sections.

31.4.1 Signal Processing

Resonators have long been used for signal processing applications due to their highly selective frequency response [27–29]. Two of the major application areas have been in realization of high-frequency bandpass filters and low-phase noise oscillators. For both applications, the resonators

TABLE 31.1

Mechanical Parameter	Electrical Equivalent
Force, F	Voltage, v
Displacement, x	Charge, q
Velocity, $\dot{x}$	Current, i
Momentum, p	Magnetic flux linkage, λ
Mass, M	Inductance, L
Compliance, K^{-1}	Capacitance, C
Viscous resistance, ζ	Resistance, R

must have low losses and high Qs and be able to handle large amounts of electrical/mechanical power (e.g., as high as 2 W for filters at the output of mobile handsets).

Micromachined resonators can be used to fabricate integrated filters for multiple frequency bands and potentially replace several passive, off-chip components [30,31]. Resonator-based filters use multiple resonators that are coupled electrically or mechanically. Besides the requirements for passband and the rejection of signals outside the passband, the primary design objectives are reduction of insertion losses, increasing Q for narrow band filters, and avoiding resonator nonlinearities [20,32–34]. Power handling has been the most significant challenge in the design of filters based on microresonators. These resonators have small volumes, and therefore, the mechanical energy that they can contain is limited, which leads to mechanical nonlinearities when excited by large signals. The other source of nonlinearity is the selected transduction mechanism.

At high frequencies, the impedance of the filter should be on the same order of the rest of the system so that simple impedance matching techniques could be employed. This can be very difficult to achieve, as the operating frequency increases, the dimensions of the resonators need to become smaller. This often leads to a smaller transduction factor, and hence, increasing the motional resistance of the resonator. For these reasons, filters based on micromachined resonators often employ bulk or surface resonant modes of piezoelectric resonators.

Precision time and frequency references are often made with high-Q and low-loss resonators that are placed within the feedback loop of a linear or nonlinear circuit [35–40]. It can be shown that the phase noise of a simple linear oscillator, as shown in Figure 31.5, at the offset frequency f_m is given by [41]

$$\mathcal{L}(f_m) = 10 \cdot \log\left[\frac{4K_BTR_{gain}}{\vec{v}_{out}^2}\left(1+\left(\frac{f_0}{2Q_l f_m}\right)^2\right)+\frac{4K_BTR_m}{\vec{v}_{out}^2}\left(\frac{f_0}{2Q_l f_m}\right)^2\right] \tag{31.7}$$

where K_B is the Boltzmann constant, T is the temperature, and Q_l is the loaded Q of the resonator with a resonant frequency f_0. The noise term with R_{gain} is due to the electronic noise and the term with R_m is from the mechanical losses of the resonator. The oscillation criterion requires that $R_{gain} = R_m$ in order to have a loop gain of exactly 1 at the oscillations frequency. This equation clearly illustrates that in order to make a low-phase noise oscillator, one needs to reduce the resonator losses and increase its quality factor and power-handling capability. As an example, the motional resistance of an electrostatic resonator with parallel electrodes, separated with a gap g, at resonance is given by [20]

$$R_m = \frac{g^4\sqrt{K_{eff}M_{eff}}}{Q\in^2 A^2V^2} \tag{31.8}$$

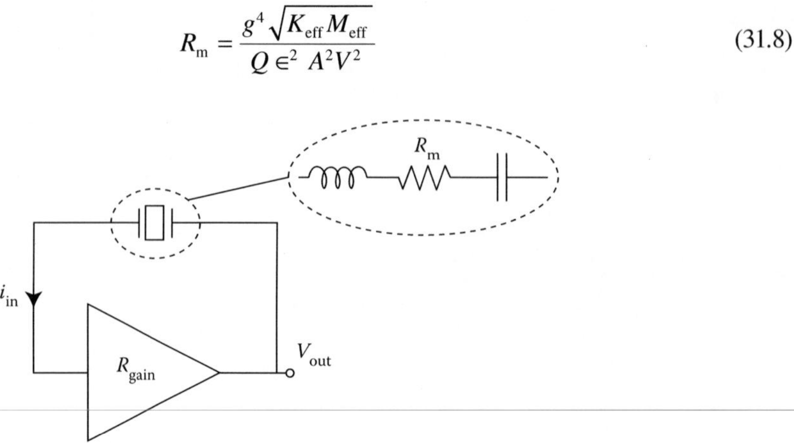

FIGURE 31.5 Schematic of a simple linear oscillator using a linear transimpedance amplifier and a resonator.

where ε is the dielectric constant of the medium, A is the effective area of the electrodes, and V is the bias voltage between the electrodes. Typical values of R_m for electrostatic resonators are in the 100 kΩ to 100 MΩ range, depending on the gap, resonant frequency, and quality factor of the device. On the other hand, the amount of signal power that an electrostatic resonator can handle before exhibiting electrostatic nonlinearities is also proportional to the gap (e.g., to $g^{5/2}$ for parallel plate actuation electrodes) [20]. Considering the power-handling requirements for signal processing applications, the challenge to make low-loss electrostatic resonators for applications that require high power-handling capability is obvious. It is noteworthy that the motional resistance of similar piezoelectric resonators is typically in the range of 100 Ω to 10 kΩ.

In addition to phase noise requirements, the timing resonators are often needed to be extremely stable against temperature variations. This poses a serious challenge in using micromachined silicon resonators, as the typical temperature coefficient of $\Delta f_0/f_0$ for these resonators is between −15 to −25 ppm/°C, or about two orders of magnitude larger than temperature-compensated quartz oscillators. Consequently, a variety of electronic, mechanical, and material engineering techniques are employed to compensate for temperature variations and improve the oscillator stability [42–45].

Another challenge for commercialization of resonators for signal processing applications is the requirement for hermetic packaging to isolate the device from variations in ambient pressure, humidity, and so on. Most micromachined resonators need to operate at low vacuum to reduce air damping and have large quality factors. The need for vacuum further complicates packaging of these devices. The typical solution is to fabricate the resonator separately from the electronics, cap the MEMS chip with another wafer, and place it next to the electronic circuitry in one package. In order to save space, some designs use the electronics chip to cap the MEMS chip. A particularly interesting packaging solution was proposed by Candler et al. [46] where fabricated devices where coated with a capping layer and released afterward through etch-holes. If the capping layer is an epitaxial silicon layer, it can be used to fabricate the complementary metal-oxide-semiconductor (CMOS) interface electronics directly on top of the resonator.

All the basic resonant modes of structures have been employed for signal processing applications. At low frequencies (i.e., 1 kHz to 10 MHz), beam-based flexural resonators are typically used. At higher operating frequencies (i.e., 1 MHz to 1 GHz), bulk resonators based on simple plate geometries offer lower losses and higher quality factors compared to flexural resonators. Surface resonant modes have had widespread applications in the design of bandpass filters for the 100 MHz to 2 GHz frequency range. Figure 31.4 illustrates how a rectangular beam or a square plate can be used in their flexural or bulk modes.

31.4.2 Sensing

The output signal from a resonant sensor is a change in frequency, which is more robust against noise and interferences compared to a typical voltage or current signal. On the other hand, time and frequency are quantities that can be easily measured with a very high level of accuracy and precision. For example, it is routine to have a 1 ppb resolution in frequency measurements (or control) with a simple setup in laboratories while achieving a similar level of measurement precision for a voltage or current signal is extremely challenging, if not impossible. Therefore, resonant sensors typically have a superior resolution and noise performance within a given family of sensors. Recalling that $\omega_0 = \sqrt{K_{\text{eff}}/M_{\text{eff}}}$, it can be seen that a shift in the resonant frequency of a structure is a consequence of a change in either its effective mass or its effective spring constant:

$$\Delta\omega_0 = \frac{\omega_0}{2}\left(\frac{\Delta K_{\text{eff}}}{K_{\text{eff}}} - \frac{\Delta M_{\text{eff}}}{M_{\text{eff}}}\right) \tag{31.9}$$

The effective mass of the structure can change from binding or deposition of target particles onto the surface or a change in mass distribution in the resonator structure. Changes in the effective spring constant are often caused by an axial or shear stress on the structure. In addition to fabrication and signal processing issues, realization of micromachined resonant sensors requires design of mechanical elements for proper coupling of the desired measurand to the resonator while avoiding interference from unwanted sources such as packaging stresses. These technical challenges have led to a significant amount of research on the design, modeling, and fabrication of resonant sensors. Some of the developed devices include mass [47,48], strain [49,50], pressure [51,52], charge [53,54], magnetic field [12,55], acceleration [6], and chemical sensors [11,56].

A resonant magnetic field sensor is shown in Figure 31.6 [12]. The main body of the sensor is a flexural electrostatic comb-drive resonator. During the sensor operation, a DC current flows through the two vertical crossbars in opposite directions. When inside a magnetic field, the produced Lorentz force on the crossbars is axially transferred to the beam springs of the resonator, modifying the resonant frequency of the structure. The sensor was used within a nonlinear oscillator circuit and the variations in the resonant frequency of the device were processed using a sensitive frequency-shift-to-voltage converter.

The operation of a small number of resonant sensors is based on a change in the quality factor or other parameters of the resonant device [57,58]. However, it is difficult to accurately control the absolute value of the quality factor of resonators and such sensors have limited application.

31.4.3 Actuation

Resonant actuators have an amplified response to their excitation around the resonant frequency of the structure by a factor that can be as high as Q times their DC response. For a low-loss resonator, this allows using input signals that are orders of magnitude smaller than the off-resonance excitations for the same amount of displacement. Resonant actuators are often used as part of a sensor structure to either reduce the interference from input signals or to amplify the influence of the measurand on the sensor performance [8].

Micromachined vibratory gyroscopes are the most widely available sensors in this category [59,60]. In vibratory gyroscopes, a resonator body is kept under continuous oscillations at one of its

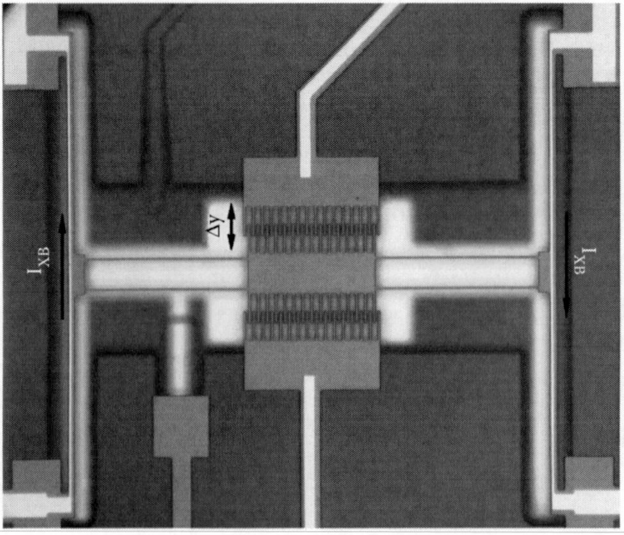

FIGURE 31.6 A resonant magnetic field sensor. A magnetic field normal to the plane of the resonator produces a Lorentz force on the current carrying corssbars, which is axially transferred to the beam springs of the electrostatic resonator, causing a shift in the resonant frequency of the structure.

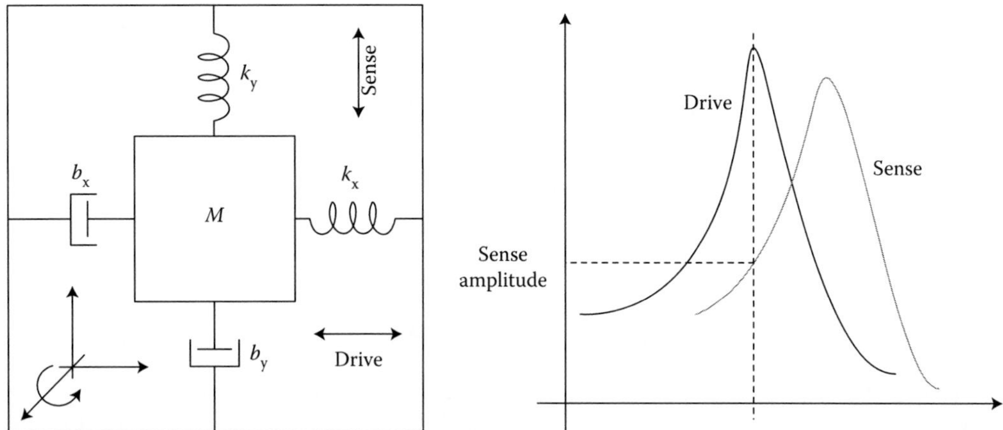

FIGURE 31.7 Illustration of the principle of operation for a vibratory gyroscope. The resonator body is driven at its resonant frequency in the sense direction. An external Coriolis force couples energy into a normal (sense) mode and causes vibrations in the sense direction at the drive frequency. Coupling of the energy between the modes is amplified by bringing the drive and sense resonant frequencies close to each other.

resonant modes (see Figure 31.7). The Coriolis effect leads to the coupling of energy into orthogonal modes whose displacements are then sensed as a function of the rotation rate. Proper mechanical design and electrical tuning of the structure ensures that the resonant frequencies of the excitation and sense modes are close to each other in order to take advantage of the displacement amplification around the resonant frequency of the orthogonal modes.

31.5 INTERFACE CIRCUITS

Typically, a resonant sensor is placed inside the feedback loop of an electronic circuit to form an oscillator circuit. For timing resonators, the oscillator produces the required stable reference signal that will be used by other system components. In case of resonant sensors, the variations in the oscillator frequency are used to extract information about the measurand. Finally, the role of the oscillator circuit for resonant actuators is to ensure that the actuator is excited at exactly its resonant frequency for optimum electrical to mechanical conversion of energy. However, design of high-performance oscillator circuits for microresonators is quite challenging due to the small electrical signals from these devices, existence of parasitic elements, and the interference from the drive signal [48,54,61]. For example, unlike timing resonators, the resonators for sensing applications may not be designed for high power handling. Therefore, the signal amplitudes within the oscillator loop need to be accurately controlled to avoid nonlinearities and signal degradation. On the other hand, resonant sensors may require additional circuitry to detect the variations in the resonant frequency of the device due to the measurand, and at the same, isolate parasitic effects such as temperature variations. For multitransducer systems, mixing and multiplexing circuits will also be needed and should be included in the design process. Considering the aforementioned issues, interface circuit design should be an integral component of research on resonant sensors.

31.6 RESONANCE FOR MULTITRANSDUCER SYSTEMS

Resonance is a promising candidate as the transduction mechanism for the realization of single-chip, multitransducer systems. Often, these systems need to communicate the collected data to some external inquiring device. Therefore, filters and reference oscillators are often needed and can be fabricated with the on-chip resonators. Moreover, using resonance allows a simple combination of signals from multiple transducers as long as the dynamic ranges of these transducers do not

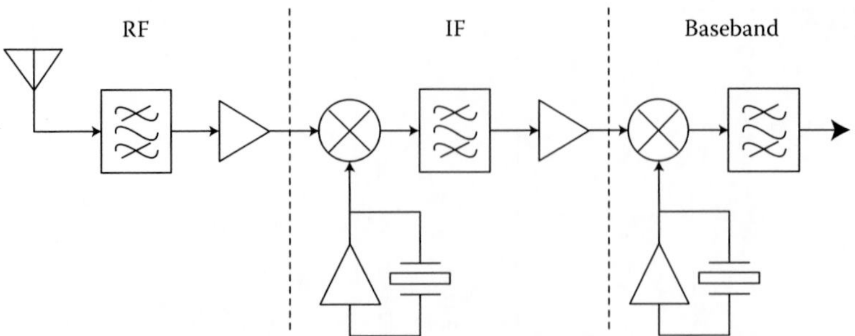

FIGURE 31.8 Different stages of a typical receiver with a superheterodyne architecture.

overlap. It is often possible to also use resonant transducers for many of the remaining transducers. Therefore, the emphasis will be placed on the design of the transducers and their interface circuits rather than the development of fabrication processes for individual devices.

Portable communication devices, such as mobile phones, are examples of systems that can greatly benefit from integration of multiple resonators on one chip [3]. In a typical telecommunication system, the radio-frequency (RF) signal from the antenna is filtered to remove image channels and amplified at the input stage of the receiver (see Figure 31.8). The signal is then down-converted to an intermediate frequency using a local oscillator and filtered again. After some processing, the signal can then be down-converted into baseband frequencies using another local oscillator. In modern telecommunication systems, the signal from intermediate frequency (IF) is demodulated into two orthogonal signals using phase-shifted signals from an oscillator and then the information is digitally processed. In either case, it can be seen that several resonators are needed throughout the receiver chain. A similar scenario applies to the transmitter chain. Therefore, significant cost and space savings can be achieved if one could integrate these resonant elements on one chip. Since most modern devices operate at multiple frequency bands and support several communication standards, the benefits multiply.

31.7 CONCLUSIONS

An overview of resonance and its applications in sensor, actuator, and signal processor design were briefly discussed. The challenges of designing resonant transducers make the field a rather interesting area of research. It is believed that we will witness numerous commercialized resonant transducers in future as we understand their short- and long-term behavior more deeply.

REFERENCES

1. D. Ewins, *Modal Testing*. Great Britain: John Wiley & Sons, 2000.
2. W. C. Tang, Electrostatic comb drive for resonant sensor and actuator applications, PhD dissertation, Department of Electrical Engineering and Computer Sciences, University of California, Berkeley, USA, 1992.
3. C. T.-C. Nguyen, Frequency-selective MEMS for miniaturized low-power communication devices, *IEEE Transactions on Microwave Theory and Techniques*, 47(8), 1486–1503, 1999.
4. D. DeVoe and A. Pisano, Surface micromachined piezoelectric accelerometers (PiXLs), *IEEE Journal of Microelectromechanical Systems*, 10(2), 180–186, 2001.
5. G. Piazza, R. Abdolvand, G. K. Ho, and F. Ayazi, Voltage-tunable piezoelectrically-transduced single-crystal silicon micromechanical resonators, *Sensors and Actuators A: Physical*, 111(1), 71–78, 2004.
6. M. Aikele, K. Bauer, W. Ficker, F. Neubauer, U. Prechtel, J. Schalk, and H. Seidel, Resonant accelerometer with self-test, *Sensors and Actuators A: Physical*, 92(1–3), 161–167, 2001.
7. A. M. Leung, Rotation sensing apparatus and methods, USA Patent 61/226160, 2009.
8. B. Bahreyni, G. Wijeweera, C. Shafai, and A. Rajapakse, Analysis and design of a micromachined electric field sensor, *IEEE Journal of Microelectromechanical Systems*, 17(1), 31–36, 2008.

9. X. Huang, X. Feng, C. Zorman, M. Mehregany, and M. Roukes, VHF, UHF and microwave frequency nanomechanical resonators, *New Journal of Physics*, 7, 247, 2005.
10. L. Hao, J. C. Gallop, and D. Cox, Excitation, detection, and passive cooling of a micromechanical cantilever using near-field of a microwave resonator, *Applied Physics Letters*, 95(11), 113501, 2009.
11. R. Howe and R. Muller, Resonant-microbridge vapor sensor, *IEEE Transactions on Electron Devices*, 33(4), 499–506, 1986.
12. B. Bahreyni and C. Shafai, A resonant micromachined magnetic field sensor, *IEEE Sensors Journal*, 7 (9), 1326–1334, 2007.
13. R. M. White, Acoustic sensors for physical, chemical and biochemical applications, in *Proceedings of the 1998 IEEE International Frequency Control Symposium*, May 1998, pp. 587–594.
14. G. Piazza and A. P. Pisano, Two-port stacked piezoelectric aluminum nitride contour-mode resonant MEMS, *Sensors and Actuators A: Physical*, 136(2), 638–645, 2007.
15. D. Jin, X. Li, J. Liu, G. Zuo, Y. Wang, M. Liu, and H. Yu, High-mode resonant piezoresistive cantilever sensors for tens-femtogram resoluble mass sensing in air, *Journal of Micromechanics and Microengineering*, 16(5), 1017–1023, 2006.
16. K. Phan, J. van Beek, and G. Koops, Piezoresistive ring-shaped MEMS resonator, in *Digest of Technical Papers of the International Conference on Solid State Sensors and Actuators, Transducers '09*, Denver, CO, June 2009, pp. 1413–1416.
17. O. Holmgren, K. Kokkonen, V. Kaajakari, A. Oja, and J. V. Knuuttila, Direct optical measurement of the Q values of RF-MEMS resonators, in *Proceedings of the IEEE Ultrasonics Symposium*, Vol 4, Rotterdam, Netherlands, September 2005, pp. 2112–2115.
18. B. Bahreyni, F. Najafi, and C. Shafai, Piezoresistive sensing with twin-beam structures in standard MEMS foundry processes, *Sensors and Actuators A: Physical*, 127(2), 325–331, 2006.
19. J. van Beek, P. Steeneken, and B. Giesbers, A 10MHz piezoresistive MEMS resonator with high Q, in *IEEE International Frequency Control Symposium*, Miami, USA, June 2006, pp. 475–480.
20. B. Bahreyni, *Fabrication and Design of Resonant Microdevices*. New York, NY: William Andrew Publishing, 2008.
21. S. Timoshenko, D. Young, and W. Weaver, *Vibration Problems in Engineering*. New York, NY: John Wiley & Sons, 1974.
22. L. Landau and E. Lifshitz, *Mechanics*, 3rd edn., ser. *Course of Theoretical Physics*. Oxford, UK: Butterworth Heinemann, 1976, Vol. 1, translated by J.B. Sykes and J.S. Bell.
23. L. Meirovitch, *Analytical Methods in Vibrations*. New York, NY: MacMillan, 1967.
24. W. T. Thomson, *Theory of vibration with applications*, 2nd edn., Englewood Cliffs, NJ: Prentice-Hall, 1981.
25. S. D. Senturia, *Microsystem design*. Boston, MA: Kluwer Academic Publishers, 2000.
26. H. A. Tilmans, Equivalent circuit representation of electromechanical transducers: I. lumped-parameter systems, *Journal of Micromechanics and Microengineering*, 6(1), 157–176, 1996.
27. C. W. Hansell, Filter, USA Patent 2005083, 1927.
28. L. Rohde, Piezoelectric crystal filter, USA Patent 2262966, 1939.
29. A. Warner, High-frequency crystal units for primary frequency standards, *Proceedings of the IRE*, 40(9), 1030–1033, 1952.
30. G. Piazza, P. J. Stephanou, and A. P. Pisano, Single-chip multiple-frequency AlN MEMS filters based on contour-mode piezoelectric resonators, *IEEE Journal of Microelectromechanical Systems*, 16(2), 319–328, 2007.
31. S. Li, Y. Lin, Z. Ren, and C. Nguyen, An MSI micromechanical differential disk-array filter, in *Digest of Technical Papers of the International Conference on Solid State Sensors and Actuators, Transducers '07*, Lyon, France, June 2007, pp. 307–311.
32. S. A. Bhave, D. Gao, R. Maboudian, and R. T. Howe, Fully differential SiC Lamé mode resonator and checkerboard filter, in *IEEE Micro Electro Mechanical Systems Conference*, Miami, FL, February 2005, pp. 223–226.
33. F. Bannon, J. Clark, and C.-C. Nguyen, High-Q HF microelectromechanical filters, *IEEE Journal of Solid-State Circuits*, 35(4), 512–526, 2000.
34. D. Galayko, A. Kaiser, B. Legrand, L. Buchaillot, C. Combi, and D. Collard, Coupled-resonator micromechanical filters with voltage tuneable bandpass characteristic in thick-film polysilicon technology, *Sensors and Actuators A: Physical*, 126(1), 227–240, 2006.
35. E. Rubiola, *Phase Noise and Frequency Stability in Oscillators*. Cambridge: Cambridge University Press, 2009.
36. C. T.-C. Nguyen and R. T. Howe, An integrated CMOS micromechanical resonator high-Q oscillator, *IEEE Journal of Solid-State Circuits*, 34(4), 440–455, 1999.

37. T. Mattila, O. Jaakkola, J. Kiihamäki, J. Karttunen, T. Lamminmäki, P. Rantakari, A. Oja, H. Seppä, H. Kattelus, and I. Tittonen, 14 MHz micromechanical oscillator, *Sensors and Actuators A: Physical*, 97–98, 497–502, 2002.
38. Y.-W. Lin, S. Lee, S.-S. Li, Y. Xie, Z. Ren, and C. T.-C. Nguyen, Series-resonant VHF micromechanical resonator reference oscillators, *IEEE Journal of Solid-State Circuits*, 39(12), 2477–2491, 2004.
39. L. Seungbae and C.-C. Nguyen, Mechanically-coupled micromechanical resonator arrays for improved phase noise, in *Proceedings of the IEEE International Frequency Control Symposium and Exposition*, Montreal, Canada, August 2004, pp. 144–150.
40. J.-Y. Lee, B. Bahreyni, Y. Zhu, and A. Seshia, A single-crystal-silicon bulk-acoustic-mode microresonator oscillator, *IEEE Electron Device Letters*, 29(7), 701–703, 2008.
41. A. Seshia, A linear model for phase noise in silicon micro-electro-mechanical resonator oscillators, in *Proceedings of the 6th Conference on MEMS for Millimeter-Wave Communications*, Lausanne, Switzerland, 2005.
42. R. Abdolvand, H. Mirilavasani, and F. Ayazi, A low-voltage temperature-stable micromechanical piezoelectric oscillator, in *Digest of Technical Papers of the International Conference on Solid State Sensors and Actuators, Transducers '07*, Lyon, France, June 2007, pp. 53–56.
43. G. Ho, K. Sundaresan, S. Pourkamali, and F. Ayazi, Low-motional-impedance highly-tunable I^2 resonators for temperature-compensated reference oscillators, in *Proceedings of the 18th IEEE Micro Electro Mechanical Systems Conference, MEMS '05*, Miami, FL, January 2005, pp. 116–120.
44. H. Jianqiang, Z. Changchun, L. Junhua, and L. Peng, A novel temperature-compensating structure for micromechanical bridge resonator, *Journal of Micromechanics and Microengineering*, 15(4), 702–705, 2005.
45. B. Kim, R. Melamud, M. A. Hopcroft, S. A. Chandorkar, G. Bahl, M. Messana, R. N. Candler, G. Yama, and T. Kenny, Si–SiO_2 composite MEMS resonators in CMOS compatible wafer-scale thin-film encapsulation, in *Proceedings of the International IEEE Frequency Control Symposium*, Geneva, Switzerland, May 2007, pp. 1214–1219.
46. R. Candler, W.-T. Park, H. Li, G. Yama, A. Partridge, M. Lutz, and T. Kenny, Single wafer encapsulation of MEMS devices, *IEEE Transactions on Advanced Packaging*, 26(3), 227–232, 2003.
47. R. Abdolvand, Z. Hao, and F. Ayazi, A temperature-compensated ZnO-on-diamond resonant mass sensor, in *Proceedings of the 5th IEEE Conference on Sensors*, Daegu, Korea, October 2007, pp. 1297–1300.
48. J.-Y. Lee, B. Bahreyni, Y. Zhu, and A. Seshia, Ultrasensitive mass balance based on a bulk acoustic mode single-crystal silicon resonator, *Applied Physics Letters*, 91(23), 234103:1–3, 2007.
49. R. G. Azevedo, D. G. Jones, A. V. Jog, B. Jamshidi, D. R. Myers, L. Chen, X. an Fu, M. Mehregany, M. B. J. Wijesundara, and A. P. Pisano, A SiC MEMS resonant strain sensor for harsh environment applications, *IEEE Sensors Journal*, 7(4), 568–576, 2007.
50. K. Wojciechowski, B. Boser, and A. Pisano, A MEMS resonant strain sensor operated in air, in *Proceedings of the 17th IEEE Micro Electro Mechanical Systems Conference, MEMS '04*, Maastricht, The Netherlands, January 2004, pp. 841–845.
51. J. C. Greenwood, Etched silicon vibrating sensor, *Journal of Physics E: Scientific Instruments*, 17(8), 650–652, 1984.
52. K. Ikeda, H. Kuwayama, T. Kobayashi, T. Watanabe, T. Nishikawa, T. Yoshida, and K. Harada, Silicon pressure sensor integrates resonant strain gauge on diaphragm, *Sensors and Actuators A: Physical*, 21, (1–3), 146–150, 1990.
53. P. Riehl, K. Scott, R. Muller, R. Howe, and J. Yasaitis, Electrostatic charge and field sensors based on micromechanical resonators, *IEEE Journal of Microelectromechanical Systems*, 12(5), 577–589, 2003.
54. J. E.-Y. Lee, B. Bahreyni, and A. A. Seshia, An axial strain modulated double-ended tuning fork electrometer, *Sensors and Actuators A: Physical*, 148(2), 395–400, 2008.
55. R. Sunier, T. Vancura, Y. Li, K.-U. Kirstein, H. Baltes, and O. Brand, Resonant magnetic field sensor with frequency output, *IEEE Journal of Microelectromechanical Systems*, 15(5), 1098–1107, 2006.
56. I. Voiculescu, M. Zaghloul, R. McGill, E. Houser, and G. Fedder, Electrostatically actuated resonant microcantilever beam in CMOS technology for the detection of chemical weapons, *IEEE Sensors Journal*, 5(4), 641–647, 2005.
57. P. Thiruvenkatanathan, J. Yan, J. Woodhouse, and A. Seshia, Enhancing parametric sensitivity in electrically coupled MEMS resonators, *IEEE Journal of Microelectromechanical Systems*, 18(5), 1077–1086, 2009.
58. J. Lu, T. Ikehara, Y. Zhang, T. Mihara, and R. Maeda, Mechanical quality factor of microcantilevers for mass sensing applications, in *Proceedings of SPIE*, H. H. Tan, J.-C. Chiao, L. Faraone, C. Jagadish, J. Williams, and A. R. Wilson, Eds., vol. 6800 no. 1. SPIE, 2007, p. 68001Y.

59. C. Acar and A. Shkel, *MEMS Vibratory Gyroscopes: Structural Approaches to Improve Robustness*, ser. *MEMS Reference Shelf*. New York: Springer, 2009.
60. F. Ayazi and K. Najafi, A HARPSS polysilicon vibrating ring gyroscope, *IEEE Journal of Microelectromechanical Systems*, 10(2), 169–179, 2001.
61. B. Bahreyni and C. Shafai, Oscillator and frequency-shift measurement circuit topologies for micromachined resonant devices, *Sensors and Actuators A: Physical*, 137(1), 74–80, 2007.

32 Piezoelectric Thin Films for MEMS Applications

Isaku Kanno

CONTENTS

32.1 INTRODUCTION

Microelectromechanical systems (MEMS) technologies have attracted considerable attention for the development of next-generation functional microdevices. Generally, the functionality of MEMS devices originates from complicated microstructures fabricated by Si microfabrication technologies; therefore the materials used have been usually limited in Si-based materials, or conducting metals and specific organic materials. On the other hand, functional materials, such as ferroelectric materials, have gradually been integrated into MEMS and they can give new functionality on simple microstructures. Among them, piezoelectricity is very attractive for the application of microsensors and actuators. Piezoelectricity has two characteristics: one is piezoelectric effect, which means the charge generation by external stress or strain, and the other is inverse piezoelectric effect, that is, force generation by external electric field. These characteristics imply that the piezoelectric materials are inherently sensors and actuators. Therefore, if we integrate piezoelectric materials into MEMS, it enables unique functionality, especially in simple microstructures [1–3].

For integration of piezoelectric materials into MEMS, the piezoelectric materials should be prepared in thin-film form to be microfabricated by photolithography. The most popular piezoelectric materials are $Pb(Zr,Ti)O_3$ (PZT), and the deposition and characterization of PZT thin films have been intensively studied. Recently, some of piezoelectric MEMS composed of PZT films have been developed as commercial products. However, several issues remain; deposition of the well-crystallized films, and precise measurement of piezoelectric properties of thin films.

In this chapter, I describe the fabrication process of PZT thin films and the evaluation method of the piezoelectric characteristics of the thin films from the viewpoint of MEMS applications. In addition, the progress of the lead-free piezoelectric thin films and fundamental examples of microfabricated piezoelectric MEMS actuators were also introduced.

32.2 PREPARATION OF PIEZOELECTRIC THIN FILMS

32.2.1 Deposition of PZT Thin Films for MEMS

For the deposition of the piezoelectric materials, especially PZT-based perovskite thin films, several methods have been studied: chemical solution deposition (CSD; sol–gel deposition) [4], chemical vapor deposition (CVD) [5,6], pulsed laser deposition (PLD) [7], and sputtering [8]. Those three methods can produce well-crystallized PZT thin films; however, each of them has both advantages and disadvantages from the viewpoint of piezoelectric MEMS, respectively. The CSD method can produce PZT thin films without expensive deposition apparatus based on the vacuum system, and it is relatively easy to prepare PZT thin films with perovskite structure. However, the thickness of the layer by the single spin coating process is typically as thin as ~0.1 μm, and the thick PZT films more than 1 μm, which is usually required in order to obtain sufficient piezoelectric actuation or sensing, have to be prepared by the multispin coating process. Therefore, the repetition of the spin coating and drying processes needs a long time to accomplish the total deposition.

On the other hand, CVD is another candidate for PZT deposition. This method has the advantage of the excellent step coverage, which is strongly required for semiconductor memories (FeRAM). However, the source materials of PZT are relatively expensive so that it is not suitable for the deposition of micrometer-thick PZT films. Therefore, CVD is rarely used for the PZT deposition in MEMS. PLD is also a popular method for high-quality PZT deposition; however, the area with uniform thickness is so small that it is not suitable for the device fabrication as commercial products.

For the piezoelectric MEMS, radio-frequency (RF)-magnetron sputtering is a practical deposition method of PZT films. By sputtering deposition, PZT films can be formed on a variety of substrates with high deposition rates, more than 1 μm/h. In addition, commercial products such as inkjet printer heads and gyro sensors have adopted the sputtering method for the PZT deposition [9] because of its stable growth conditions as well as cost-effective process compared with the other methods.

32.2.2 Sputtering Deposition

The RF-magnetron sputtering is a useful deposition technique, especially for thin films composed of complicated chemical composition, and it is often used for the deposition of the piezoelectric PZT thin films. Typical sputtering conditions of the PZT thin films are listed in Table 32.1. The sputtering is performed under Ar/O_2 mixed gas atmosphere of 0.3–0.5 Pa, where the substrates were heated to about 600°C to grow the PZT films with perovskite structure. Postannealing with a temperature around 600°C is also effective in crystallizing PZT films deposited under low substrate temperature. However, postannealing often involves fatal damage such as cracking or peeling off of the films, especially for the thick PZT films due to a large thermal stress. On the other hand, sintered ceramics are usually used as target materials to stabilize film composition. It is well known that the morphotropic phase boundary (MPB) exists at the Zr/Ti ratio of 52/48, where dielectric and piezoelectric properties show a maximum. Therefore, the PZT ceramic target with the MPB composition is usually used for the piezoelectric PZT films. Furthermore, since Pb and PbO are easy to reevaporate from the deposited films during the deposition, excess PbO was often added to the target to maintain the stoichiometry of the resulting film.

TABLE 32.1
Sputtering Conditions of PZT Thin-Film

Substrate	(001)Pt/MgO, (111)Pt/Ti/SiO2/Si
Target	[Pb(Zr0.53,Ti0.47)O3]0.8+[PbO]0.2
Substrate temperature	600°C
Gas composition	Ar(19.5SCCM)+O2(0.5SCCM)
Gas pressure	0.3–0.5 Pa
Post annealing (as needed)	600°C/30 min

32.2.3 Crystal Structure of PZT Thin Films

Since piezoelectricity originates from asymmetry of the crystal structure, control of the crystal structure is the most important factor to determine piezoelectric properties. Usually, PZT films were grown on the Pt-coated Si substrates with Ti adhesive layer at the interface of Si [10]. For Si substrates, oxide layer is deposited on the Si surface by thermal oxidation. The x-ray diffraction (XRD) patterns of PZT films deposited on Pt/Ti/SiO_2/Si substrates are shown in Figure 32.1a. The clear diffraction peaks from perovskite PZT can be observed without the other phases such as pyrochlore. Furthermore, the films were preferentially oriented along the ⟨111⟩ direction, since the Pt bottom electrode on Si is oriented along ⟨111⟩ due to the closest packing of the fcc crystal structure. A cross-sectional scanning electron microscopy (SEM) image is shown in Figure 32.1b. Clear columnar grain can be observed, indicating that the PZT films are of polycrystalline structure.

On the other hand, epitaxial substrates such as MgO and $SrTiO_3$ enable epitaxial growth of PZT films by RF-sputtering, PLD, or CVD [5–7,11]. Epitaxial substrates can control the orientation and domain structure of the PZT films so that the electrical properties including piezoelectricity can be enhanced by perfect alignment of the polar direction. Figure 32.2 shows the XRD pattern and the cross-sectional SEM image of the PZT films on Pt-coated MgO substrates. PZT films were perfectly

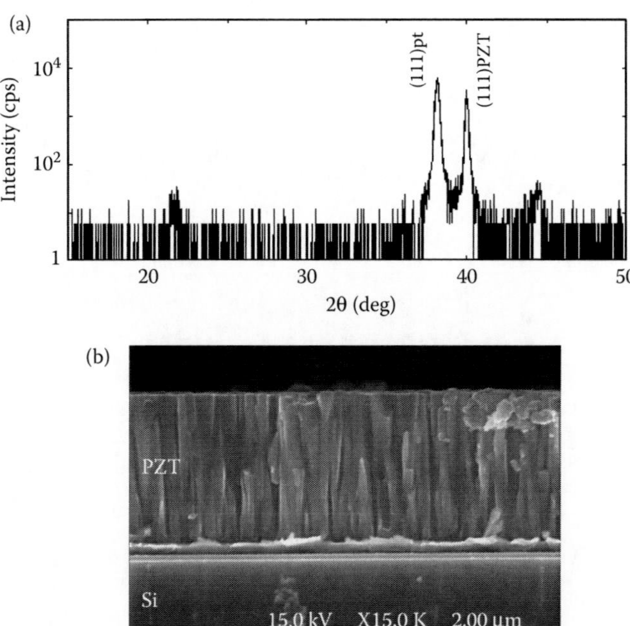

FIGURE 32.1 Crystal structure of PZT thin films on Pt/Ti/SiO_2/Si substrates: (a) XRD pattern and (b) cross-sectional SEM image.

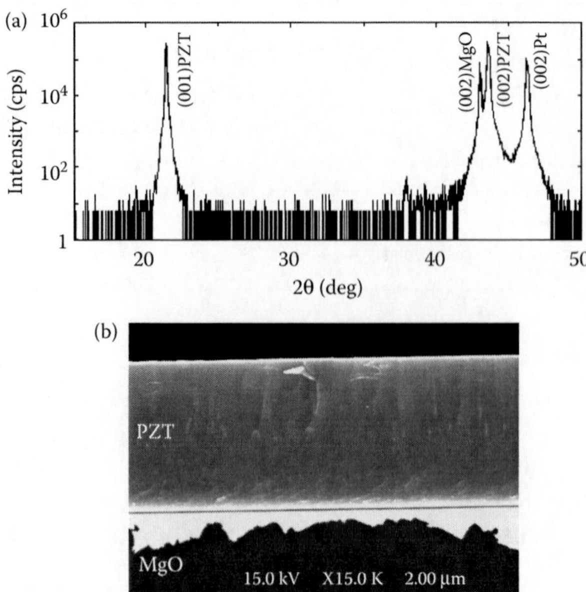

FIGURE 32.2 Crystal structure of *c*-axis-oriented epitaxial PZT thin films on Pt/MgO substrates: (a) XRD pattern and (b) cross-sectional SEM image.

oriented along the *c*–axis, which is the polarization direction of tetragonal PZT. A Pt electrode is also epitaxially grown on the MgO or $SrTiO_3$ substrates.

By sputtering deposition, a PZT film can be directly deposited on Pt-coated metal substrates, for example, stainless steel and titanium [12,13]. As mentioned later, direct deposition of PZT on metal substrates is advantageous for the practical applications of piezoelectric MEMS. Figures 32.3a and b show the XRD patterns of the PZT films deposited on Pt-coated stainless-steel and titanium metal substrates, respectively. The diffraction peaks of perovskite PZT were clearly observed for both substrates. The films are of polycrystalline structure, although the orientation of the PZT film on each substrate is different and depends on the sputtering conditions. The deposition of PZT films on metals by CSD or CVD has not been reported; thus sputtering deposition mitigates the limitation of substrates for PZT deposition.

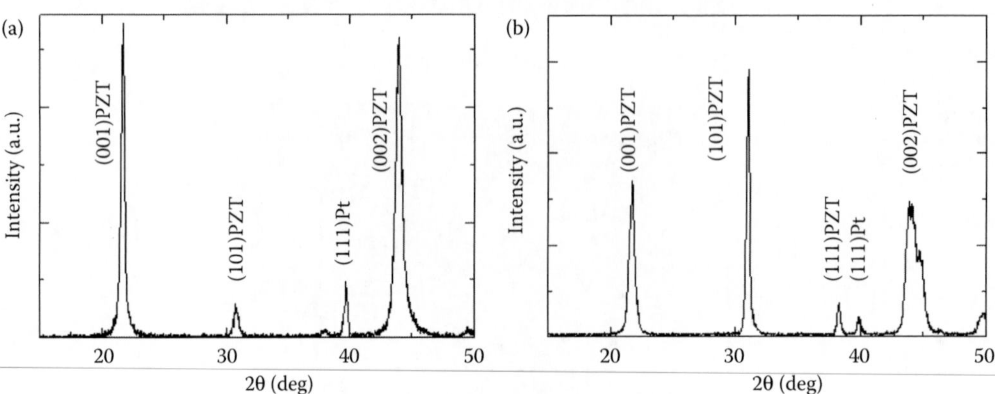

FIGURE 32.3 XRD patterns of the PZT films on Pt-coated meal substrates deposited by RF-magnetron sputtering: (a) stainless-steel and (b) titanium metal substrates.

32.3 EVALUATION OF PIEZOELECTRIC PROPERTIES FOR THIN FILMS

32.3.1 Dielectric and Ferroelectric Properties

Since PZT is a typical ferroelectric material, it shows a variety of functionality such as large spontaneous polarization and dielectric constant, pyroelectric coefficient, and piezoelectricity. However, these properties are closely related to each other; therefore dielectric and ferroelectric properties, which are easy to measure, are generally measured to evaluate the quality of the PZT films.

Dielectric properties are measured by an impedance analyzer. From the measurement of capacitance between the top and bottom electrodes, relative dielectric constants ε_r are estimated. The typical relative dielectric coefficient ε_r of the polycrystalline PZT films with MPB composition is around 1000; however, the *c*-axis-oriented epitaxial PZT films show a lower relative dielectric constant, around 200 [10].

Ferroelectric materials have spontaneous polarization, which can be reversed by the external electric field. Ferroelectric properties can be evaluated from the polarization–electric field (*P–E*) hysteresis curves taken by the Sowyer–Tower circuit. Figures 32.4a and b show the *P–E* hysteresis curves of the PZT films deposited on (001)Pt/MgO and (111)Pt/Ti/Si, respectively. It can be confirmed that both of the PZT films have clear ferroelectric properties. The *P–E* hysteresis loop of the epitaxial PZT film on Pt/MgO shows a clear square shape, indicating that the polarization reversal abruptly occurred at the coercive electric field (E_c) because the *c*-axis orientation is the polarization direction of the tetragonal PZT. On the other hand, the P-E hysteresis loop of the polycrystalline PZT film on Pt/Ti/Si has almost the same characteristics as PZT bulk ceramics, as shown in Figure 32.4b. Compared with Figure 32.4a, polarization reversal gradually occurred with the applied electric field. This result suggests the contribution of the off-axis polar domain, which corresponds to the nonlinear piezoelectric characteristics of the polycrystalline PZT films.

32.3.2 Modeling Piezoelectric Unimorph Actuators

In order to design micropiezoelectric devices, it is necessary to identify precise piezoelectric properties of PZT films. Since piezoelectric films are clamped by substrates, piezoelectric measurements of thin films are not easy. Several attempts have been reported to evaluate the piezoelectric coefficient of the thin films [14]. One of the most popular methods is the measurement of the thickness change using an atomic force microscope or a laser interferometer to measure the longitudinal piezoelectric effect [15,16]. This method is popular due to ease of measurement of the effective longitudinal piezoelectric strain. However, from the viewpoint of device design of piezoelectric MEMS, the transverse piezoelectric coefficient d_{31} has indispensable properties rather than the longitudinal piezoelectric coefficient d_{33}, since a long lateral dimension can generate large output deformation or electric charge. Several methods have been reported to measure the d_{31} of piezoelectric

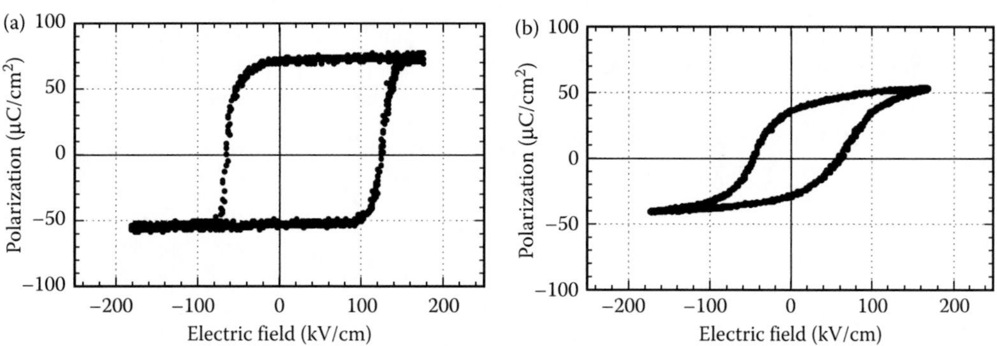

FIGURE 32.4 *P–E* hysteresis curves of PZT films: (a) (001)Pt/MgO and (b) (111)Pt/Ti/Si substrates.

thin films, such as observing the piezoelectric response of a microcantilever made of PZT films or the measurement of the electric charge generated by the laterally deformed PZT film on Si wafer [8,17–19]. However, standard methods for the evaluation of the proper transverse piezoelectric coefficient d_{31} have not yet been established.

The most practical method to evaluate the transverse piezoelectric properties of thin films is the measurement of cantilever displacement. The piezoelectric properties of *d*- and *e*-forms are expressed by the following equations:

$$T_i = c_{ij}^{E} S_j - e_{ki} E_k, \tag{32.1}$$

$$S_i = s_{ij}^{E} T_j - d_{ki} E_k, \tag{32.2}$$

where $k = 1, 2, 3$ and $i, j = 1, 2, 3, 4, 5, 6$. T_i, S_j, and E_k are the stress, strain, and electric field components, c_{ij}^{E} and S_{ij}^{E} are constant-electric-field elastic stiffness components and elastic compliance components, and e_{ki} and d_{ki} are piezoelectric coefficients, respectively. In the case of piezoelectric thin films on the substrate, we can neglect out of plane and shear strains. If we apply an external electric field along thickness, the transverse piezoelectric coefficient e_{31} is written as

$$e_{31} = \frac{c_{13}^{E} S_3 - T_1}{E_3} = \frac{c_{13}^{E} S_3}{E_3} + \frac{d_{31}}{s_{11}^{E} + s_{12}^{E}}. \tag{32.3}$$

The effective transverse piezoelectric coefficient $e_{31,f}$ is defined as $e_{31,f} = d_{31}/(S_{11}^{E} + S_{12}^{E})$ [20], and then Equation 32.3 is expressed as

$$e_{31} = e_{31,f} + \frac{c_{13}^{E}}{c_{33}^{E}} e_{33}. \tag{32.4}$$

On the other hand, the tip displacement of the unimorph cantilever is expressed as

$$\begin{aligned} d_{31} &= -\frac{\delta K}{3 s_{11,p}^{E} s_{11,s} h_s \left(h_s + h_p\right) V L^2}, \\ K &= 4 s_{11,p}^{E} s_{11,s} h_s \left(h_p\right)^3 + 4 s_{11,p}^{E} s_{11,s} \left(h_s\right)^3 h_p + \left(s_{11,p}^{E}\right)^2 \left(h_s\right)^4 \\ &\quad + \left(s_{11,s}^{E}\right)^2 \left(h_p\right)^4 + 6 s_{11,p}^{E} s_{11,s} \left(h_s\right)^2 \left(h_p\right)^2, \end{aligned} \tag{32.5}$$

where h, s_{11}, L, V, and δ are the thickness, the elastic compliance, the length of the cantilever, the applied voltage, and the tip displacement, respectively [21]. The subscripts "s" and "p" denote the substrate and the PZT thin film, respectively. In the case of the unimorph cantilever composed of a piezoelectric thin film and a thick substrate, the transverse piezoelectric coefficient d_{31} can be approximated as

$$d_{31} \cong -\frac{h_s^2}{3L^2} \frac{s_{11,p}^{E}}{s_{11,s}} \frac{\delta}{V}. \tag{32.6}$$

The mechanical properties of the thin films depend on the deposition process and the substrate. Therefore it is inevitably necessary to measure the elastic properties of the PZT thin films precisely to obtain the transverse piezoelectric coefficient d_{31}, although they are difficult to evaluate. On the other hand, the simplified transverse piezoelectric coefficient was defined to eliminate the ambiguous mechanical properties of the thin films [10],

$$e_{31}^{*} = \frac{d_{31}}{s_{11,p}^{E}} \cong -\frac{h_s^2}{3s_{11,s}L^2V}\delta. \tag{32.7}$$

The simplified transverse piezoelectric coefficient e_{31}^{*} can be easily obtained from the tip displacement of a unimorph cantilever and it is useful to evaluate the transverse piezoelectric property as a kind of figure of merit.

32.3.3 Transverse Piezoelectric Properties of PZT Thin Films on Si and MgO Substrates

The measurement setup of the piezoelectric thin films is shown in Figure 32.5. For the measurement of piezoelectric properties of the PZT films on MgO or Si substrates, we cleaved the substrates into beam shape with a size of around 15 × 2.5 mm^2. Then the thin Au or Pt top electrode was evaporated over the surface of the PZT films. Finally, the edge of the beam was clamped using a vise and unimorph cantilevers composed of PZT film and substrate were prepared. The dimension of the cantilevers is listed in Table 32.2. Piezoelectric vibration is generated by means of applying sine wave voltage between upper and bottom electrodes, and the tip displacement was measured using a laser Doppler vibrometer. The electric contact of the bottom electrode was obtained from the clamped edge, whereas the upper electrode was connected to a fine lead line using silver paste not to disturb the piezoelectric actuation. From the tip displacement of the cantilever, the transverse piezoelectric properties of the PZT films were evaluated.

To evaluate the transverse piezoelectric properties, the tip displacements of the cantilevers were measured by applying unipolar sine wave voltage. The frequency of the input sine wave signal should be lower than the mechanical resonant frequency of the cantilevers. For the sputtered PZT films, it is not necessary to conduct compulsory poling treatments since the intrinsic self-polarization is usually induced from the bottom to the top electrodes [8]. This is advantageous for the sensor or actuator application to obtain stable piezoelectric output. The maximum displacement of the MgO and Si cantilevers is plotted in Figures 32.6a and b as a function of peak-to-peak voltage. In the case of the unimorph cantilever composed of the PZT film on the MgO substrate, tip displacement exhibits an excellent proportional relationship with applied voltage, as shown in Figure 32.6a.

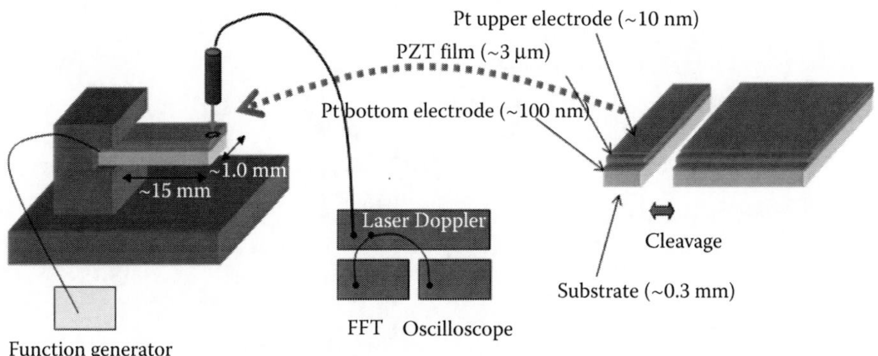

FIGURE 32.5 Measurement setup of transverse piezoelectric properties of piezoelectric thin films. Tip displacement of unimorph cantilever composed of piezoelectric thin films and substrates is measured by a laser Doppler vibrometer.

TABLE 32.2
Dimension of Unimorph Cantilevers

PZT/MgO	
Thickness	
MgO substrate	310 μm
PZT films	2.9 μm
Pt bottom electrode	0.1 μm
Length	15.2 mm
Width	2.5 mm
Orientation along the length	<100>MgO
PZT/Si	
Thickness	
Si substrate	212 μm
PZT films	2.4 μm
Pt/Ti bottom electrode	0.2 μm
Length	14.9 mm
Width	2.5 mm
Orientation along the length	<110>Si

This result indicates that the piezoelectric strain of the PZT film on Pt/MgO is caused by intrinsic lattice motion of elongation and shrinkage since the PZT films on MgO show perfect *c*-axis orientation, which is the polarization axis of the tetragonal PZT. On the other hand, the PZT/Si cantilever shows obvious nonlinear displacement and it is enhanced at the higher applied voltage as shown in Figure 32.6b. The PZT films on Pt/Ti/Si substrates have polycrystalline structure with preferential (111) orientation, and this result suggests that extrinsic domain motions were superimposed on the

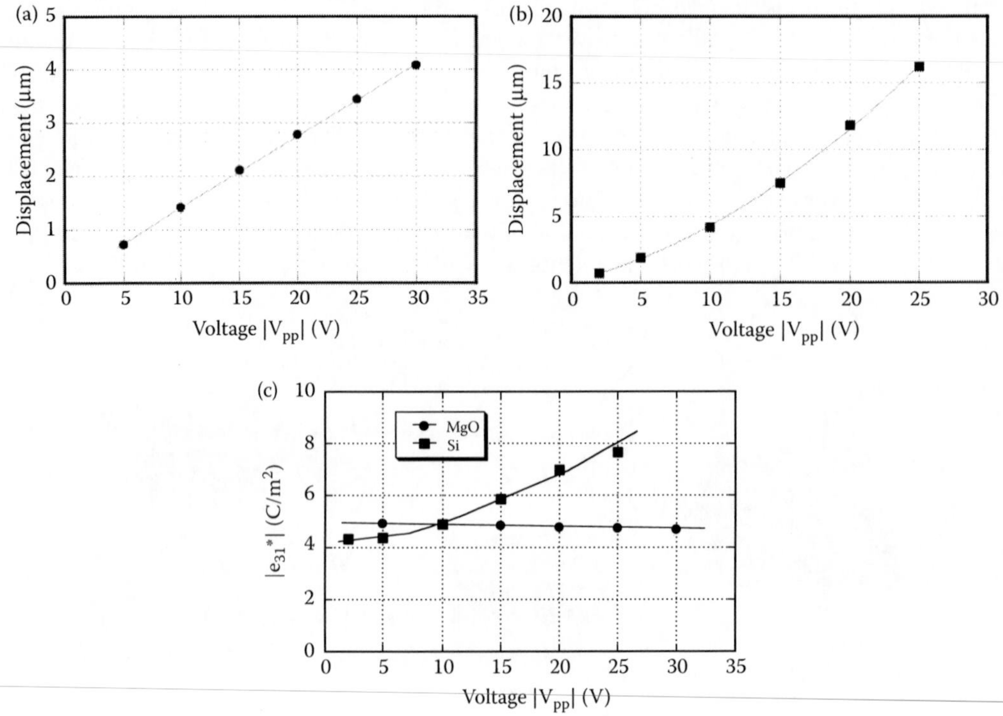

FIGURE 32.6 Tip displacement of unimorph cantilevers for (a) PZT on MgO, (b) PZT on Si substrates, and (c) e_{31}^* of the PZT films on MgO and Si substrates as a function of the applied voltage.

intrinsic lattice motion of the PZT films, especially under high applied voltage. The simplified transverse piezoelectric coefficient e_{31}^* was evaluated from Equation 32.7 and the result is shown in Figure 32.6c. Both films show an excellent e_{31}^* of −4.7 to −4.9 C/m^2 for PZT/MgO and −4.3 to −7.7 C/m^2 for PZT/Si, respectively. It should be noted that the absolute value of e_{31}^* of the PZT films on Si is higher than those on MgO, especially at high applied voltage, while the PZT films on Si show strong dependence on applied voltage. On the other hand, the PZT films on MgO substrate show almost constant values of e_{31}^* which is independent of the applied voltage. These results indicate that *c*-axis-oriented epitaxial PZT films on MgO have stable transverse piezoelectric properties since their piezoelectricity is caused only by the intrinsic lattice motion. For the polycrystalline PZT films on Si, large e_{31}^* is attributed to extrinsic effects such as reorientation of off-axis polarization such as 90° domains and it is superimposed on the intrinsic lattice motion.

The domain motion was also observed by applying bipolar sine wave voltage on the unimorph cantilevers and the results are shown in Figures 32.7a and b. Tip displacement is measured by using the laser interferometer, which can measure the precise deflection at low frequency, and butterfly displacement curves caused by domain rotation can be easily observed. Figure 32.7a shows the tip deflection of the cantilever made of *c*-axis-oriented PZT film on MgO substrate. The deflection curve is the ideal butterfly loop with clear 180° polarization rotation (domain switching) at +29 V and −17 V, corresponding to the coercive electric field. Furthermore, the unimorph cantilever shows excellent linearity due to the perfect *c*-axis orientation of the PZT films. On the other hand, the deflection curve of the cantilever made of polycrystalline PZT film on Si substrates was different from that of PZT/MgO and showed large displacement hysteresis as shown in Figure 32.7b. This curve has almost the same characteristics as the transverse strain curve of bulk PZT, indicating that the piezoelectric strain of the polycrystalline PZT films originates not only from the lattice motion but also from the off-axis domain motion like reorientation of 90° domains. These results correspond to the results of Figure 32.6.

32.3.4 Piezoelectric PZT Thin Films on Metal Substrates

Single-crystal silicone substrate is usually used for the PZT deposition because of the ease of three-dimensional microfabrication by surface or bulk micromachining techniques in various geometries such as membranes, bridges, and cantilevers. However, the brittleness of the silicone is often problematic for the fabrication and practical use of the device. As mentioned before, sputtering deposition enables PZT thin films to be formed on the metal substrates such as stainless steel or titanium. Because metals have excellent mechanical elasticity and strong fracture toughness compared with Si, a thin metal-based microcantilever or membrane has sufficient toughness and flexibility even at small thicknesses less than 100 μm. Furthermore, if we can deposit PZT films directly on a microfabricated metal sheet, it can simplify the fabrication process such as the etching of PZT, electrodes, and substrates that is usually

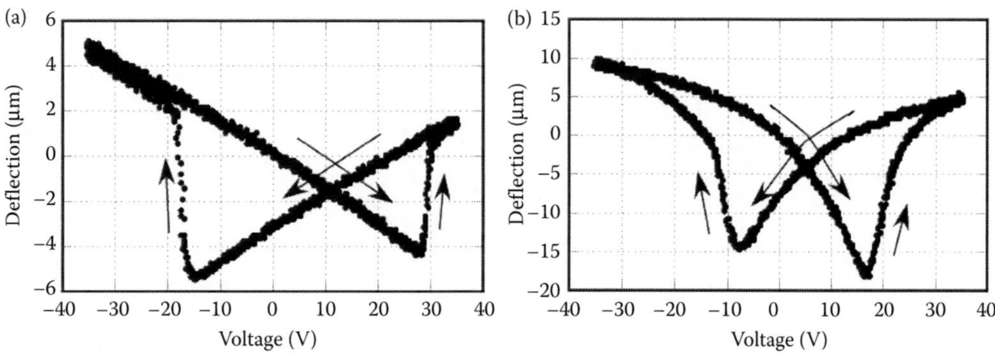

FIGURE 32.7 Hysteresis of tip displacement (butterfly curves) of the unimorph cantilevers: (a) PZT on MgO and (b) PZT on Si substrates.

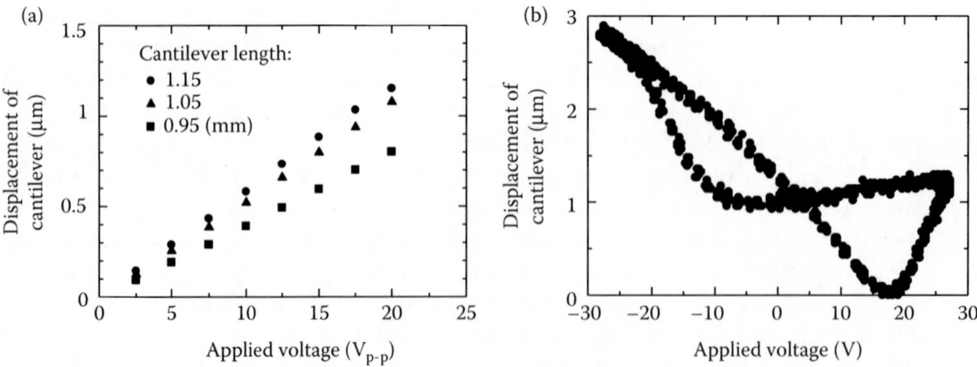

FIGURE 32.8 Transverse piezoelectric properties of the PZT films deposited on Ti: (a) relationship between the tip displacements of the cantilevers with 0.95, 1.05, and 1.15 length and the applied voltage and (b) tip deflection hysteresis curves (butterfly curves) of a PZT/Ti unimorph cantilever.

conducted after PZT deposition. Furthermore, metal sheets usually cost lower than Si; thus the sputtering deposition of PZT on metal substrates is advantageous to commercialize piezoelectric MEMS.

The PZT thin films were deposited on 50-μm-thick Ti sheets which were preliminarily microfabricated into the shape of cantilever array, and the piezoelectric properties were investigated. The length of the cantilever ranged from 0.7 to 1.25 mm and the width was 0.2 mm. After deposition of Au/Cr top electrodes, the actuator characteristics were evaluated by measuring the tip displacement of the cantilever. The relationship between the tip displacements of the cantilevers with the lengths of 0.95, 1.05, and 1.15 mm was measured by applying a unipolar sine wave signal at a frequency of 1 kHz and the results are shown in Figure 32.8a. The tip displacement proportionally increased with the applied voltage. The hysteresis of tip deflection of the unimorph cantilever was also observed by applying bipolar sine wave voltage and the result is shown in Figure 32.8b. A clear butterfly-shaped curve was observed with polarization reversals at the electric fields of +20 and −10 kV/cm, indicating that displacement is caused by typical transverse piezoelectric actuation of the PZT films on Ti cantilevers.

The simplified transverse piezoelectric coefficient e_{31}^* was evaluated from the result of Figure 32.8a. Figure 32.9 shows the e_{31}^* of the PZT films on Ti substrates as a function of applied voltage. The e_{31}^* of the PZT films on Ti was calculated to be −3.6 to −4.3 C/m^2, which is slightly smaller than that of Si substrates. However, it is almost constant against the external electric field due to the linear relationship between applied voltage and displacement.

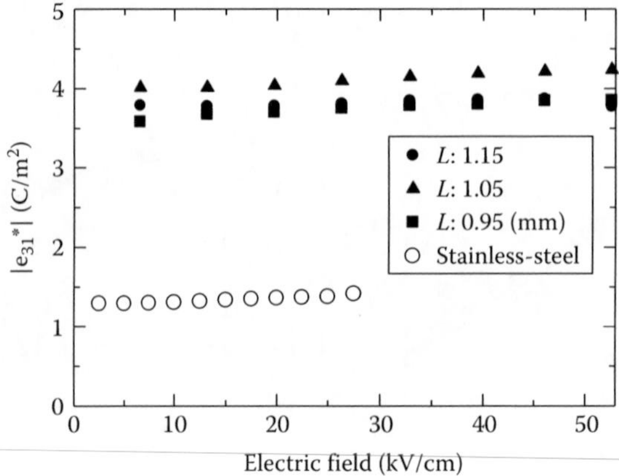

FIGURE 32.9 Transverse piezoelectric coefficient e_{31}^* of the PZT films on Ti and stainless-steel (SUS304) substrates as a function of the applied voltage.

The same measurement was performed for the PZT films on a stainless-steel sheet (SUS304), and clear piezoelectric deflection could also be observed. However, the e_{31}^* of the PZT films on stainless steel was about three times smaller than that on Ti substrates as shown in Figure 32.9. Better piezoelectricity for the PZT film on Ti is attributed to the compatibility of the thermal expansion coefficient. Another reason is compositional affinity; Ti is one of the components of the PZT, indicating that it would be harmless against the diffusion of the Ti atoms from the substrate to the PZT films.

32.4 LEAD-FREE PIEZOELECTRIC THIN FILMS

The alkali niobate-based ferroelectric perovskite materials have attracted attention as promising substitutes for lead-based piezoelectric materials. Among the alkali-based perovskite materials, it is known that the bulk solid solution of $KNbO_3$ and $NaNbO_3$, $(K_xNa_{1-x})NbO_3$ (hereafter referred to as KNN), shows a high electromechanical coupling at around $x = 0.5$ [22,23]. Furthermore, it has been reported that the doping of Li, Ta, and/or Sb as well as the orientation control leads to further enhancement of the piezoelectricity [24]. On the other hand, KNN thin films are useful not only for the environmental friendly piezoelectric MEMS. Several deposition processes have been employed for the growth of the KNN films including sputtering [25], CVD [26], and PLD [27,28]. Among these processes, RF-magnetron sputtering can produce high-quality KNN thin films by using almost the same sputtering conditions as PZT. Shibata [29,30] reported that he successfully fabricated the KNN thin films by RF-magnetron sputtering, and confirmed excellent piezoelectric properties compatible with PZT.

Figure 32.10 shows the XRD patterns of the KNN thin films on (001)Pt/MgO and (111)Pt/Ti/SiO_2/Si substrates, respectively. KNN films on both substrates were grown with the perovskite structure by RF-magnetron sputtering. The transverse piezoelectric properties were evaluated from the tip displacement of unimorph cantilevers by the same system as shown in Figure 32.5. Figure 32.11 shows the tip displacement and e_{31}^* of the KNN/MgO or KNN/Si unimorph cantilever as a function of the applied voltage. The tip displacement proportionally increased with the applied voltage. The e_{31}^* of the KNN films on MgO and Si substrates were calculated to be $-3.6\ C/m^2$ and $-5.5\ C/m^2$, respectively. The characteristics of the KNN films on MgO and Si are almost compatible with those of PZT films, although the piezoelectric coefficients are slightly smaller than those of PZT films. However, lead-free piezoelectric thin films are strongly required for practical applications, and piezoelectric MEMS of lead-free thin films will be commercialized in the near future.

32.5 FABRICATION OF MICROACTUATORS USING PIEZOELECTRIC THIN FILMS

A variety of piezoelectric MEMS devices have been reported using piezoelectric thin films as microsensors and actuators. In this section, I introduce typical microfabrication process for the piezoelectric microcantilevers, and some examples of piezoelectric MEMS devices.

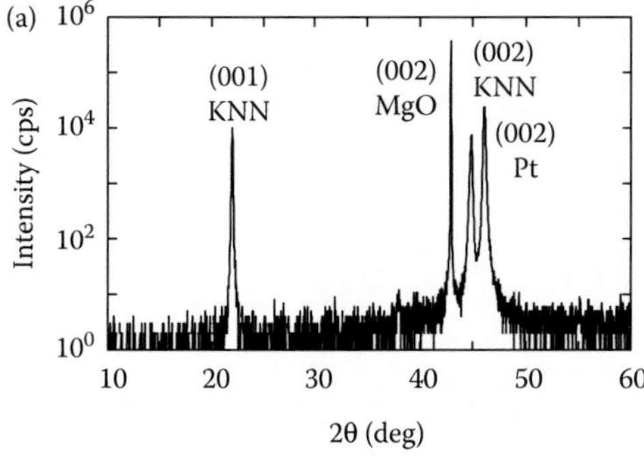

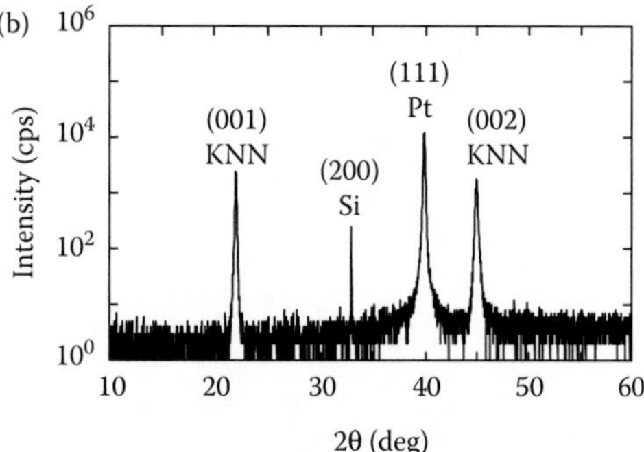

FIGURE 32.10 XRD patterns of KNN thin films on (a) (001)Pt/MgO and (b) (111)Pt/Ti/SiO_2/Si substrates.

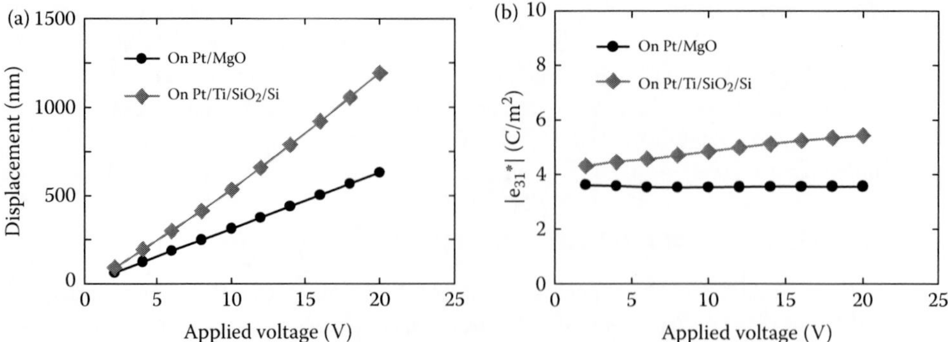

FIGURE 32.11 Transverse piezoelectric properties of KNN thin films: (a) tip displacement of the KNN/MgO or KNN/Si unimorph cantilevers and (b) transverse piezoelectric coefficient e_{31}^* of the KNN films as a function of the applied voltage.

32.5.1 Microfabrication of Piezoelectric Cantilevers

A microcantilever is a fundamental structure for the application of piezoelectric sensors and actuators [31–33]. By using photolithography, piezoelectric thin films on Si substrates can be fabricated into microcantilevers. Figure 32.12 shows the typical microfabrication process of the unimorph cantilevers composed of PZT thin films on Si substrates. The process sequence is as follows:

1. Sputtering deposition of a Ti adhesive layer (~20 nm)
2. Sputtering deposition of a Pt bottom electrode (~100 nm)
3. Sputtering deposition of PZT thin films (2–3 μm)
4. Spin coat and photolithograph of lift-off resist
5. Deposition of Al top electrode (~1 μm)

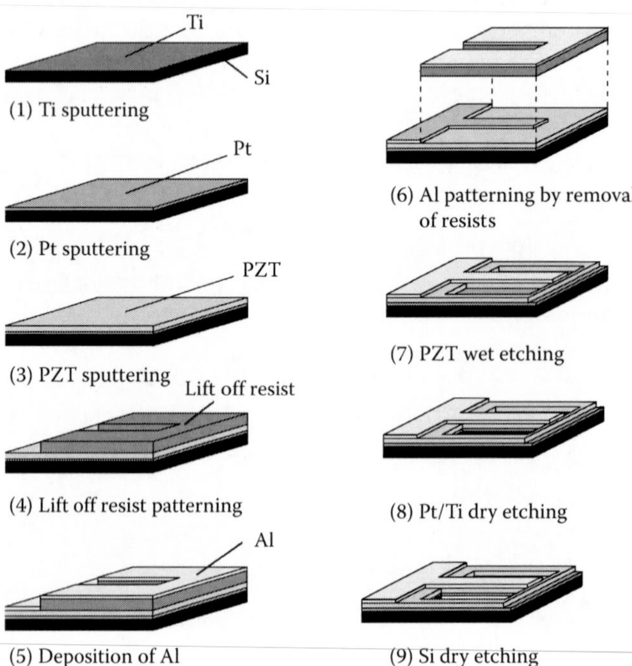

FIGURE 32.12 Typical microfabrication process of piezoelectric unimorph cantilevers composed of PZT thin films on Si substrates.

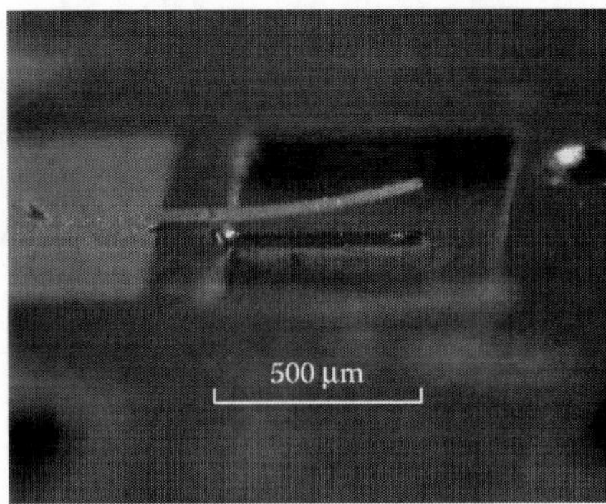

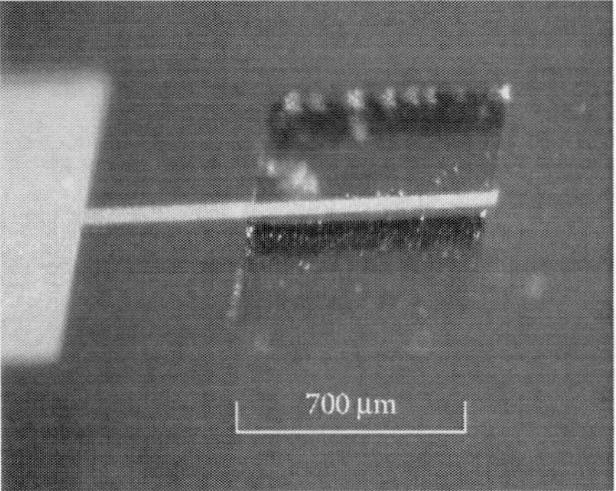

FIGURE 32.13 A piezoelectric microcantilever and the fixed–fixed beam of the unimorph structure composed of PZT thin films on the Si substrate.

6. List-off of Al electrode
7. PZT wet etching
8. Pt/Ti dry etching
9. Si isotropic etching

Patterning of PZT thin films is possible using HNO_3 + HF solution. At the end of the process, the Si substrate underneath the cantilever beam is etched out by isotropic dry etching of SF_6, or back etching by deep-reactive ion etching to release the cantilever. Figure 32.13 shows the simple micro-cantilever and fixed–fixed beam fabricated by the aforementioned process. In this case, a thick Cr layer is used as the top electrode, and it also acts as the vibrating layer for the unimorph structure. As shown in Figure 32.13, the cantilever beam is initially bent by the residual stress because of the mismatch of the thermal expansion coefficient, and the control of the internal stress of each layer is an important issue to obtain the flat beam structure.

32.5.2 Piezoelectric MEMS Switches

Micromechanical switches called MEMS switches are promising devices for RF communications, especially in the millimeter wave band. Compared to conventional semiconductor devices, RF-MEMS switches have the advantage of not only high isolation and low insertion loss, but also low power consumption [34]. An electrostatic microactuator has generally been used for the driving force of the switch due to the ease of microfabrication using well-established semiconductor-integrated circuit (IC) technologies. Considering compatibility of MEMS switches with the ICs, a low-voltage operation of the switch is strongly required because the typical operation voltage of ICs is as low as 5 V; however, electrostatic MEMS switches need a relatively large operation voltage, more than 30 V. On the other hand, the piezoelectric actuator can generate a larger force originating from the deformation of the volume, which is advantageous for a low-voltage drive. Recently, piezoelectric MEMS switches have been developed and low-voltage actuation as well as excellent switching performance was reported [33]. As mentioned before, for the MEMS switch with simple cantilever structure, large initial bending due to the mismatch of thermal stress of the multilayerd films is observed, while for the fixed–fixed beam, insufficient displacement due to the restriction of the beam motion by holding both ends of the beam is observed. To solve these problems, the unique structure of a piezoelectric microactuator has been reported, such as two connected cantilevers.

The illustration and SEM photograph of the resulting actuator are shown in Figure 32.14 [35]. The piezoelectric PZT films of 2.5 μm thickness are deposited on Pt/Ti-coated Si substrates using RF-sputtering, and successively, a 0.8-μm-thick Cr elastic layer is deposited onto the PZT films. The length and the width of the beam are 800 and 200 μm, respectively. In this configuration, the flat

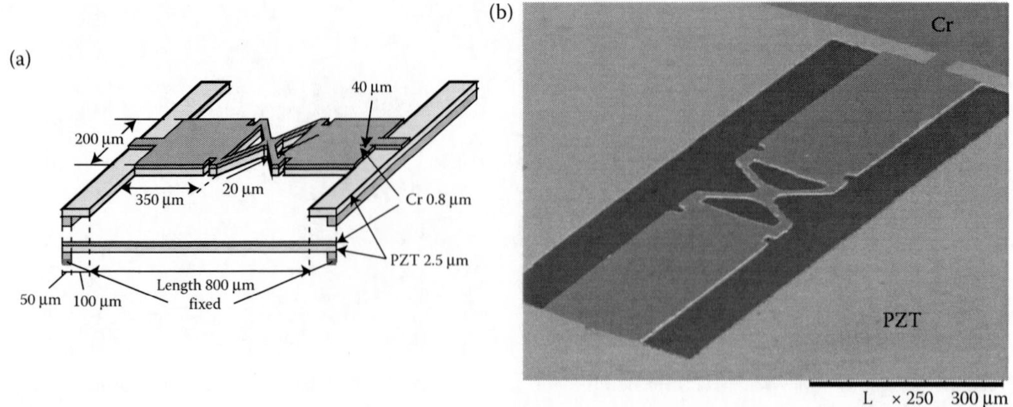

FIGURE 32.14 Illustration and SEM image of the piezoelectric unimorph microactuator with the X-shaped connector fabricated from PZT thin films on Si substrates.

beam structure could be prepared, indicating that the X-shaped connector is effective in mitigating the initial bending of a simple cantilever. Furthermore, the X-shaped connector is flexible not to suppress the piezoelectric motion like the conventional fixed–fixed beam structure. The displacement increases with the applied voltage and it reaches 0.5 μm/5 V. Although the displacement is relatively small, the flat shape of the actuator is very important for applications such as microswitches.

32.5.3 Piezoelectric Micropumps

In recent years, microfluidic systems have attracted considerable attention in a variety of applications, especially for micro-total analysis systems (μTAS). The general components of microfluidic systems are flow sensors, micromixers, microvalves, and micropumps. Among them, micropumps are significant devices and a variety of pumping systems have been studied for downsizing, integration, and high efficiency [36,37]. At microscale, the flow field is generated typically by piezoelectric actuators that are equipped with a pressure chamber for generating a pressure difference between the inlet and the outlet. The piezoelectric micropumps can transport a variety of liquids at a high flow rate and with excellent controllability; however, further miniaturization is not easy because of the difficulty in integrating the rectification system in microchannels to control the flow direction such as diffusers or check valves. On the other hand, the flexural plate wave (FPW) has been proposed as a valveless micropump [38,39]. It consists of piezoelectric thin films on a Si membrane with an interdigital transducer electrode. The FPW is advantageous for microfluidic systems because of its simple structure. Liquid flow is induced by generating plate waves on the membrane; however, the displacement is as small as a few nanometers; thus the maximum flow velocity is localized a few micrometers below the membrane [39]. On the other hand, a new mechanical micropumping device has been reported for the microfluidic system that uses a piezoelectric vibrating channel wall [40]. The vibrating wall has a unimorph structure of piezoelectric PZT thin films directly deposited on the ceiling of the microchannel. In this configuration, there is no need to prepare a pressure chamber and microvalves; thus it is advantageous to integrate the mechanical pumping system on a chip.

Schematics of the microchannel and the photographs are shown in Figure 32.15. The top ceiling walls of the microchannels were composed of Si and buried SiO_2 (BOX) layers of silicon-on-insulator (SOI) wafer whose surface was covered by piezoelectric PZT thin films. Nine separate top electrodes were arranged on the microchannel, and the traveling wave was induced beneath the ceiling wall by applying sinusoidal voltages with a phase difference of $2\pi/3$. The liquid beneath the wall moves along an elliptic curve when a channel wall oscillates in the form of a traveling wave as shown in Figure 32.16 [41]. After a period of oscillation, the fluid moves slightly forward from the initial position due to its viscosity. The transportation of the liquid by a traveling wave is controlled

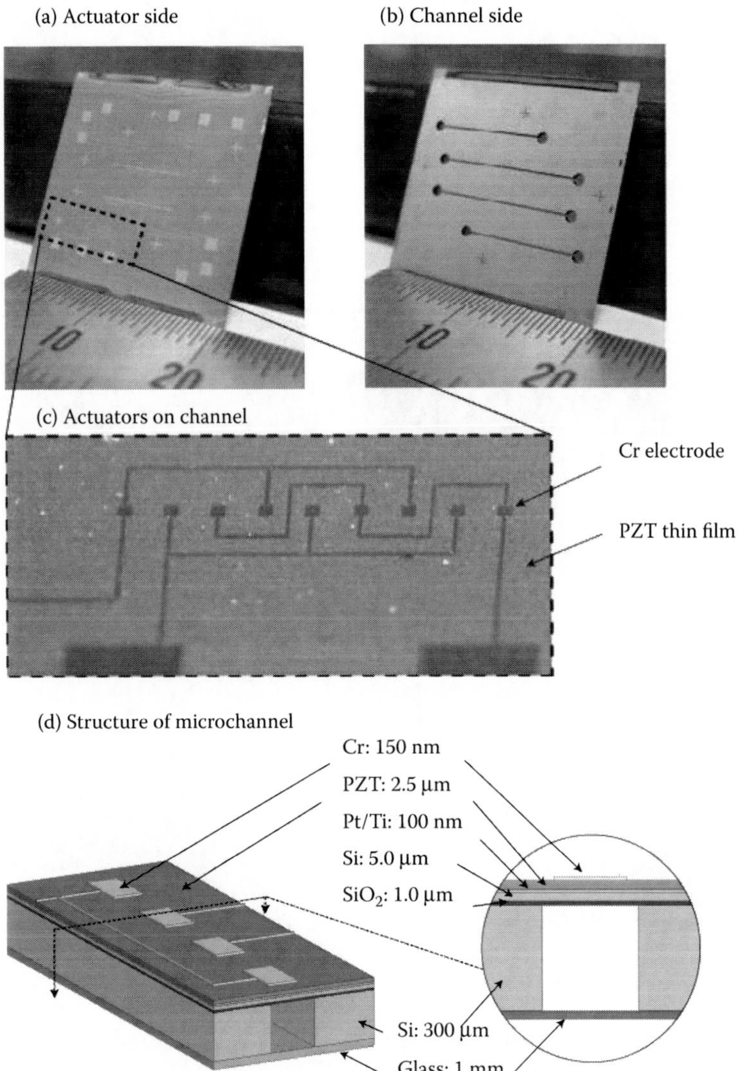

FIGURE 32.15 Photographs and schematic illustration of micropumps composed of PZT thin films; (a) PZT thin-film microactuator array, (b) microchannels, (c) electrode pattern prepared on the microchannel, and (d) structure of the micropumps.

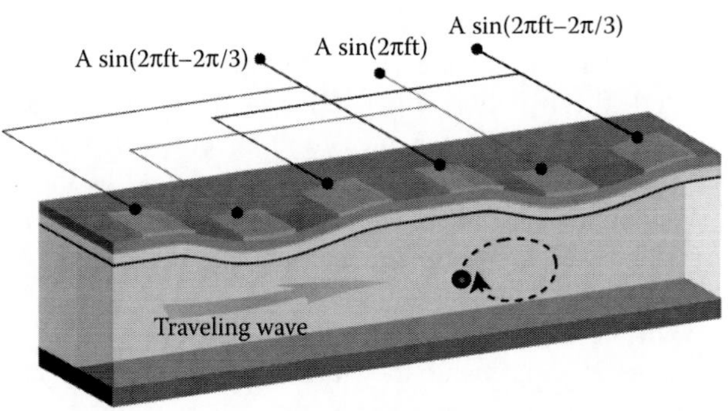

FIGURE 32.16 Liquid flow in microchannel induced by the traveling wave.

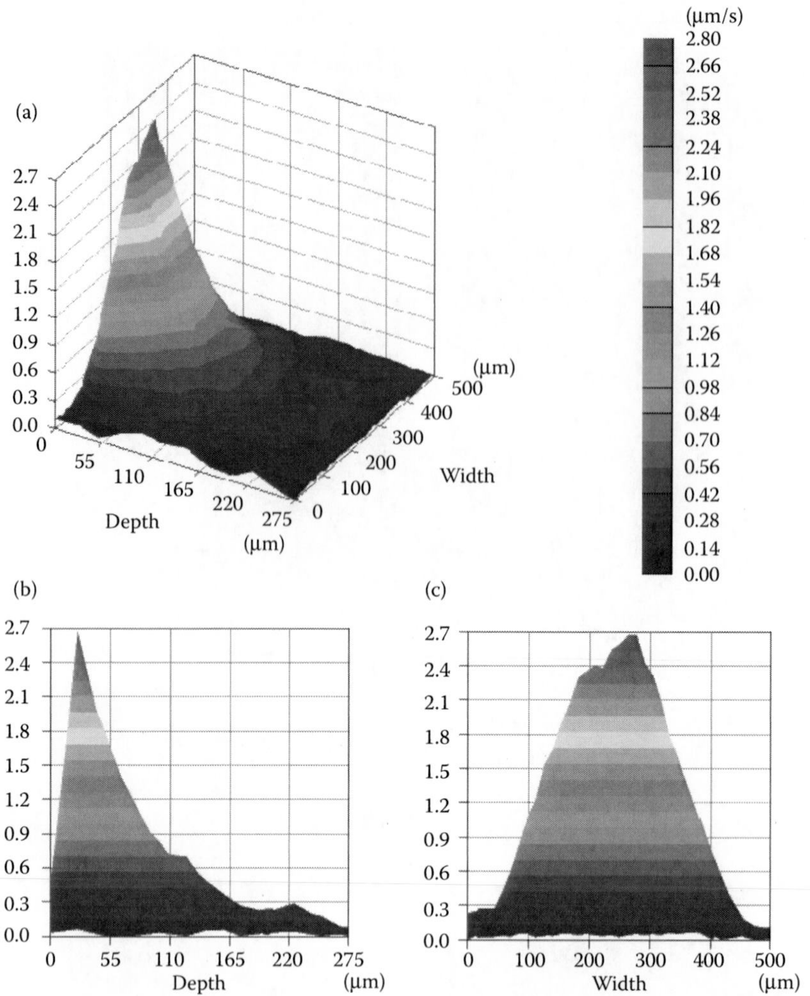

FIGURE 32.17 Flow profile of a 500-μm-wide channel measured by a confocal micro-PIV system.

by the magnitude and frequency of the piezoelectric vibration, and the flow direction can be changed by altering the direction of the traveling wave.

The flow velocity was measured by micro-particle image velocimetry (micro-PIV). Fluorescent microbeads with a diameter of 1 μm and a density of 1.05 g/cm^3 were dispersed in the water and the motion of the microbeads was observed. A traveling wave was generated beneath the channel wall when a sinusoidal voltage was applied with a phase difference of $2\pi/3$. The mean flow velocity proportionally increased with the square of the voltage applied to each actuator. This result is consistent with the theoretical calculation of peristaltic pumping phenomena [41]. The flow velocity profile of the 500-μm-wide channel was measured under the actuator array with a confocal micro-PIV system, by changing the observation height. Figure 32.17 shows the velocity profiles along with the width and height of the channel at 10 V_{pp} and a frequency of 80 kHz. The velocity profile in the width direction was approximately parabolic, indicating the generation of Poiseulle flow. On the other hand, the flow profile along the height direction was Couette-like flow. These results are consistent with the flow profile generated by the FPW [39]. Although the maximum velocity was located at about 25 μm beneath the vibrating wall, it was larger than that of FPW flow (~5 μm). This is attributed to the large displacement of the traveling waves induced beneath the channel wall in our pumping device.

32.5.4 Optical MEMS using Piezoelectric Thin-Film Actuators

Adaptive Optics (AO) is a significant technique to compensate for optical aberration caused by atmospheric turbulence [42], which has been used in astronomical research to obtain high-resolution images. In the AO system, a deformable mirror (DM) is commonly used as a wave front corrector by adjusting the deflection of the mirror surface to the aberration. Recently, the application area of AO has been expanded to industrial and medical optics, and in particular, *in vivo* high-resolution human retinal imaging has attracted attention in AO [43–45]. To achieve small and low-cost DMs, MEMS DMs have successfully been developed and manufactured as commercial products [46]. The MEMS DMs are commonly actuated by an electrostatic force; however, for practical use, several issues still remain unsolved: the large driving voltage of more than 100 V and the vibration noise of the mirror membrane owing to its very small thickness. Furthermore, since an electrostatic actuator only generates an attractive force and its magnitude is not large, there is a limitation on the control of the mirror deformation.

On the other hand, large-scale DMs are commonly actuated by bulk piezoelectric actuator arrays, and recently bimorph DMs have been developed for low-cost AO systems [47]. A piezoelectric actuator can generate a large force and its response is very fast. In addition, concave and convex deformation can be generated by just changing the polarity of the applied voltage. In order to produce small piezoelectric DMs, the mirror membrane should be actuated by piezoelectric thin films because of the microfabrication of the piezoelectric actuators. To realize small, low-cost DMs, especially for human retinal imaging, simple MEMS DMs actuated by piezoelectric PZT thin films have been proposed [48].

The piezoelectric MEMS DM consists of a continuous membrane mirror on the back of which piezoelectric PZT films are deposited on an SOI substrate. The piezoelectric actuator array consists of a unimoph structure of PZT film and a Si device layer, and the structure is shown in Figure 32.18. The application of the voltage induces a transverse strain, which is converted into the vertical deflection due to the restriction of the Si elastic layer. Both concave and convex deformations are possible by just changing the polarity of the applied voltage. Compared to conventional electrostatic MEMS DMs, the thickness of the membrane can be greater because the piezoelectric force is generally larger than the electrostatic one. The photographs of the piezoelectric MEMS DMs are shown in

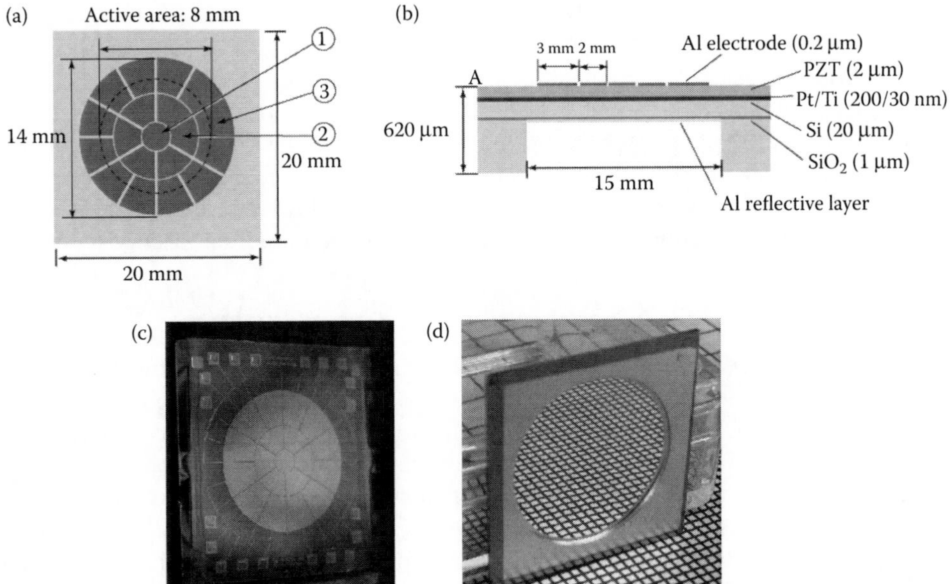

FIGURE 32.18 Schematic illustration and photographs of piezoelectric MEMS DMs; (a) top view, (b) cross-sectional view, and photos of (c) actuator side, (d) mirror side, respectively.

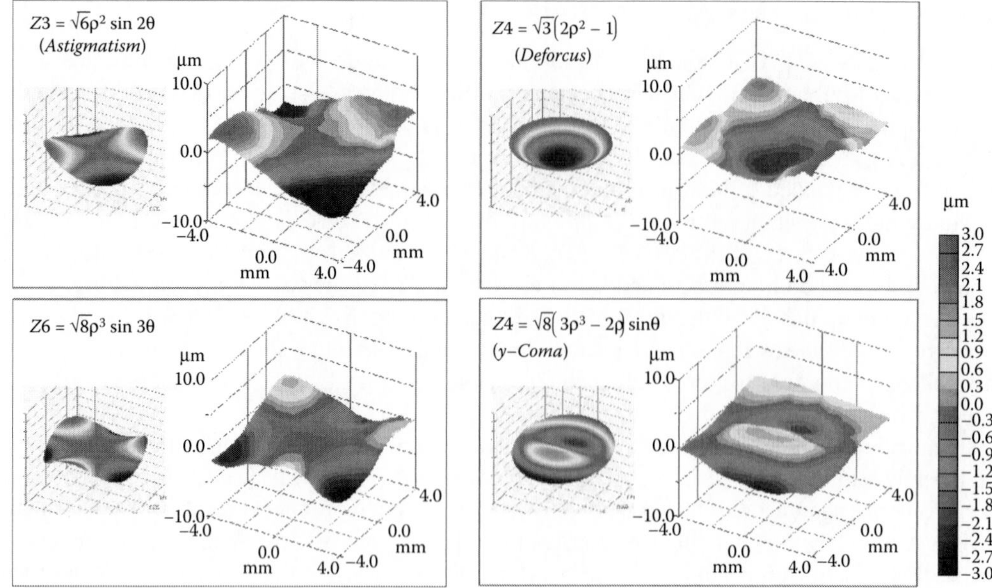

FIGURE 32.19 Ideal and measured surface profiles that correspond with Zernike modes of Z3, Z4, Z6, and Z7.

Figures 32.18c and d. The 19-actuator array is prepared on the Si device layer of SOI, while the back of the SOI was etched out to prepare a diaphragm structure and the buried oxide (BOX) layer acted as a stopping layer for Si etching by the dry etching process of SF_6. The Al layer was deposited on the exposed BOX layer as a mirror surface.

In order to evaluate the applicability of piezoelectric MEMS DMs to the AO system, deformation of the mirror corresponding to the Zernike mode was produced. The Zernike polynomials are commonly used to express the deformation of a circular plane by a complete set of orthogonal polynomials [49]. If the optical wave front is represented by the Zernike polynomials, aberration can be corrected by producing deformation of the Zernike mode by the DMs. Figure 32.19 shows both the ideal and reproduced Zernike modes of Z3, Z4, Z6, and Z7, respectively. The Zernike modes of Z3, Z4, and Z7 are known as the aberrations of astigmatism, defocus, and coma-aberration, respectively. Although some deviations still remain between the ideal and observed deformations, it was confirmed that the piezoelectric MEMS DMs can reproduce low-order Zernike modes by low-voltage operation. For the practical use of the piezoelectric MEMS DMs to AO, it is necessary to increase the number of individual electrodes in order to correct the higher-order aberration. However, piezoelectric MEMS DMs composed of PZT films are promising devices for the low-voltage wave front generator in AO.

32.6 SUMMARY

In this chapter, the outline of MEMS technologies integrated with piezoelectric thin films was introduced. Ferroelectric materials have a variety of functionality including piezoelectricity, and integration of piezoelectric materials on MEMS causes enhancement of the function of the devices even in the simple microstructures. For the development of piezoelectric MEMS, deposition, evaluation, and microfabrication of piezoelectric thin films should be established. PZT is the most popular piezoelectric material and for the MEMS applications, the deposition of PZT thin film with the thickness of a few micrometers is required. RF-magnetron sputtering is a suitable method for the deposition of piezoelectric PZT films. Transverse piezoelectric properties of the thin films are indispensable to design the piezoelectric MEMS, and they can be evaluated from the actuator properties of unimorph cantilevers of a PZT film and a substrate. On the other hand, lead-free piezoelectric thin films has been investigated as environment-friendly materials, and it was reported that the KNN thin films show large piezoelectric properties almost compatible with that of PZT films. Recently, piezoelectric MEMS have been fabricated by photolithographic techniques of PZT films and some of them have been produced as commercial products. Because of attractive functionality of the piezoelectric thin films, piezoelectric MEMS will play an important role in the development of next-generation microdevices.

REFERENCES

1. P. Muralt, Recent progress in materials issues for piezoelectric MEMS, *J. Am. Ceram. Soc.* 91, 2008, 1385–1396.
2. P. Muralt, Ferroelectric thin films for micro-sensors and actuators: A review, *J. Micromech. Microeng.* 10, 2000, 136–146.
3. S. Trolier-McKinstry, P. Muralt, Thin film piezoelectrics for MEMS, *J. Electroceram.*, 12, 2004, 7–17.
4. B. Piekarski, M. Dubey, E. Zakar, R. Polcawich, D. DeVoe, D. Wickenden, Sol–gel PZT for MEMS applications, *Integr. Ferroelectr.* 42, 2002, 25–37.
5. Y. K. Kim, H. Morioka, H. Funakubo, Domain structures in highly (100)-oriented epitaxial $Pb(Zr_{0.35},Ti_{0.65})O_3$ thin films, *J. Appl. Phys.* 101, 2007, 064112.
6. C. M. Foster, G. R. Bai, R. Csencsits, J. Vetrone, R. Jammy, L. A. Wills, E, Carr, J. Amano, Single-crystal $Pb(Zr_x,Ti_{1-x})O_3$ thin films prepared by metal–organic chemical vapor deposition: Systematic compositional variation of electronic and optical properties, *J. Appl. Phys.*, 81, 1997, 2349–2357.
7. I. Vrejoiu, G. Le Rhun, L. Pintilie, D. Hesse, M. Alexe, U. Gösele, Intrinsic ferroelectric properties of strained tetragonal $PbZr_{0.2}Ti_{0.8}O_3$ obtained on layer–by–layer grown, defect–free single–crystalline films, *Adv. Mater.* 18,, 2006, 1657–1661.
8. I. Kanno, S. Fujii, T. Kamada, R. Takayama, Piezoelectric properties of *c*-axis oriented $Pb(Zr,Ti)O_3$ thin films, *Appl. Phys. Lett.* 70, 1997, 1378–1380.
9. E. Fujii, R. Takayama, K. Nomura, A. Murata, T. Hirasawa, A. Tomozawa, S. Fujii, T. Kamada, and H. Torii Preparation of (001)-oriented $Pb(Zr,Ti)O_3$ thin films and their piezoelectric applications, *IEEE Trans. Ultrason. Ferroelectr. Freq. Control* 54, 2007, 2431–2438
10. I. Kanno, H. Kotera, K. Wasa, Measurement of transverse piezoelectric properties of PZT thin films, *Sens. Actuators A* 107, 2003, 68–74.
11. I. Kanno, H. Kotera, K. Wasa, T. Matsunaga, T. Kamada, R. Takayama, Crystallographic characterization of epitaxial $Pb(Zr,Ti)O_3$ films with different Zr/Ti ratio grown by radio-frequency-magnetron sputtering, *J. Appl. Phys.* 93, 2003,4091–4096.
12. T. Suzuki, I. Kanno, J. J. Loverich, H. Kotera, K. Wasa, Characterization of $Pb(Zr, Ti)O_3$ thin films deposited on stainless steel substrates by RF-magnetron sputtering for MEMS applications, *Sens. Actuators A* 125, 2006, 382–386.
13. K. Kanda, I. Kanno, H. Kotera, K. Wasa, Simple fabrication of metal-based piezoelectric MEMS by direct deposition of $Pb(Zr,Ti)O_3$ thin-films on titanium substrates, *J. Microelectromech. Syst.* 18, 2009, 610–615.
14. J.-M. Liu, B. Pan, H. L. W. Chan, S. N. Zhu, Y. Y. Zhu, Z. G. Liu, Piezoelectric coefficient measurement of piezoelectric thin films: An overview, *Mater. Chem. Phys.* 75, 2002, 12–18.
15. G. Zavala, J. H. Fendler, S. T. McKinstry, Characterization of ferroelectric lead zirconate titanate films by scanning force microscopy, *J. Appl. Phys.* 81, 1997, 7480–7491.
16. A. L. Kholkin, C. Wutchrich, D. V. Taylor, N. Setter, Interferometric measurements of electric field-induced displacements in piezoelectric thin films, *Rev. Sci. Instrum.* 67, 1996, 1935–1941.
17. I. Kanno, S. Fujii, T. Kamada, R. Takayama, Piezoelectric characteristics of *c*-axis oriented $Pb(Zr,Ti)O_3$ thin films, *J. Korean Phys. Soc.* 32, 1998, S1481–S1484.
18. J. F. Shepard Jr., P. J. Moses, S. T. McKinstry, The wafer flexure technique for the determination of the transverse piezoelectric coefficient (d_{31}) of PZT thin films, *Sens. Actuators A* 71, 1998, 133–138.
19. J. F. Shepard Jr., F. Chu, I. Kanno, S. T. McKinstry, Characterization and aging response of the d_{31} piezoelectric coefficient of lead zirconate titanate thin films, *J. Appl. Phys.* 85, 1999, 6711–6716.
20. M. A. Dubois, P. Muralt, Measurement of the effective transverse piezoelectric coefficient $e_{31,f}$ of AlN and $Pb(Zr_x,Ti_{1-x})O_3$ thin films, *Sens. Actuators A* 77, 1999, 106–112.
21. J. G. Smits, W. Choi, The constituent equations of piezoelectric heterogeneous bimorphs, *IEEE Trans. Ultrason. Ferroelectr. Freq. Control*, 38, 1991, 256–270.

22. G. Shirane, R. Newnham, R. Pepinsky, Dielectric properties and phase transitions of $NaNbO_3$ and (Na, K)NbO_3, *Phys. Rev.* 96, 1954, 581–588.
23. G. H. Haertling, Properties of hot-pressed ferroelectric alkali niobate ceramics, *J. Am. Ceram. Soc.* 50, 1967, 329–330.
24. Y. Saito, H. Takao, T. Tani, T. Nonoyama, K. Takatori, T. Homma, T. Nagaya, M. Nakamura, Lead-free piezoceramics, *Nature* 432, 2004, 84–87.
25. X. Wang, U. Helmersson, S. Olafsson, S. Rudner, L. Wernlund, S. Gevorgian, Growth and field dependent dielectric properties of epitaxial $Na_{0.5}K_{0.5}NbO_3$ thin films, *Appl. Phys. Lett.* 73, 1998, 927–929.
26. A. Onoe, A. Yoshida, K. Chikuma, Heteroepitaxial growth of $KNbO_3$ single-crystal films on $SrTiO_3$ by metalorganic chemical vapor deposition, *Appl. Phys. Lett.* 69, 1996, 167–169.
27. S. I. Khartsev, M. A. Grishin, A. M. Grishin, Characterization of heteroepitaxial $Na_{0.5}K_{0.5}NbO_3$/$La_{0.5}Sr_{0.5}CoO_3$ electro-optical cell, *Appl. Phys. Lett.* 86, 2005, 062901.
28. T. Saito, T. Wada, H. Adachi, I. Kanno, Pulsed laser deposition of high-quality (K,Na)NbO_3 thin films on $SrTiO_3$ substrate using high-density ceramic targets, *Jpn. J. Appl. Phys.* 43, 2004, 6627–6631.
29. K. Shibata, F. Oka, A. Ohishi, T. Mishima, I. Kanno, Piezoelectric properties of (K,Na)NbO_3 films deposited by RF magnetron sputtering, *Appl. Phys. Express* 1, 2008, 11501.
30. K. Shibata, F. Oka, A. Nomoto, T. Mishima, I. Kanno, Crystalline structure of highly piezoelectric (K,Na)NbO_3 films deposited by RF magnetron sputtering, *Jpn. J. Appl. Phys.* 47, 2008, 8909–8913.
31. Y. Lee, G. Lim, W. Moon, A piezoelectric micro-cantilever bio-sensor using the mass-micro-balancing technique with self-excitation, *Microsyst. Technol.* 13, 2007, 563–567.
32. M. Renaud, K. Karakaya, T. Sterken, P. Fiorini, C. Van Hoof, R. Puers, Fabrication, modelling and characterization of MEMS piezoelectric vibration harvesters, *Sens. Actuators A* 145–146, 2008, 380–386.
33. H. C. Lee, J. Y. Park, Piezoelectrically actuated RF MEMS DC contact switches with low voltage operation, *IEEE MicroWirel. Compon. Lett.* 15, 2005, 202–204.
34. G. Reveiz, J. Muldavin, RF MEMS switches and switch circuits, *IEEE Microwave Mag.* 2, 2001, 59–71.
35. I. Kanno, Y. Tazawa, T. Suzuki, H. Kotera, Piezoelectric unimorph miroactuators with X-shaped structure composed of PZT thin films, *Microsyst. Technol.* 13, 2007, 825–829.
36. N. T. Nguyen, X. Huang, T. K. Chuan, MEMS-micropumps: A review, *J. Fluids Eng.* 124, 2002, 384–392.
37. D. J. Laser, J. G. Santiago, A review of micropumps, *J. Micromech. Microeng.* 14, 2004, R35–R64.
38. R. M. Moroney, R. M. White, R. T. Howe, Microtransport induced by ultrasonic Lamb waves, *Appl. Phys. Lett.* 59, 1991, 774–776.
39. N. T. Nguyen, R. M. White, Design and optimization of an ultrasonic flexural plate wave micropump using numerical simulation, *Sens. Actuators A* 77, 1999, 229–236.
40. J. Ogawa, I. Kanno, H. Kotera, K. Wasa, T. Suzuki, Development of liquid pumping devices using vibrating microchannel walls, *Sens. Actuators A* 152, 2009, 211–218.
41. F. C. P. Yin, Y. C. Fung, Comparison of theory and experiment in peristaltic transport, *J. Fluid Mech.* 47, 1971, 93–112.
42. J. W. Hardy, J. E. Lefebvre, C. L. Koliopoulos, Real-time atmospheric compensation, *J. Opt. Soc. Am.* 67, 1977, 360–369.
43. J. Liang, D. R. Williams, D. T. Miller, Supernormal vision and high-resolution retinal imaging through adaptive optics, *J. Opt. Soc. Am. A.* 14, 1997, 2884.
44. H. Hofer, L. Chen, G. Y. Yoon, B. Singer, Y. Yamauchi, D. R. Williams, Improvement in retinal image quality with dynamic correction of the eye's aberrations, *Opt. Express* 8, 2001, 631–643.
45. N. Doble, G. Yoon, L. Chen, P. Bierden, B. Singer, S. Olivier, D. R. Williams, Use of a microelectromechanical mirror for adaptive optics in the human eye, *Opt. Lett.* 27, 2002, 1537–1539.
46. J. A. Perreault, T. G. Bifano, B. M. Levine, M. N. Horenstein, Adaptive optic correction using microelectromechanical deformable mirrors, *Opt. Eng.* 41, 2002, 561–566.
47. E. Dalimier C. Dainty, Comparative analysis of deformable mirrors for ocular adaptive optics, *Opt. Express* 13, 2005, 4275–4285.
48. I. Kanno, T. Kunisawa, T. Suzuki, H. Kotera, Development of deformable mirror composed of piezoelectric thin films for adaptive optics, *IEEE J. Select. Top. Quantum Electron.* 13, 2007, 155–161.
49. L. Zhu, P.-C. Sun, D.-U. Bartsch, W. R. Freeman, Y. Fainman, Wave-front generation of Zernike polynomial modes with a micromachined membrane deformable mirror, *Appl. Opt.* 38, 1999, 6019–6026.

33 HfO_2 Thin Film for Microelectromechanical Systems Application

Bing Miao and Alton B. Horsfall

CONTENTS

33.1 INTRODUCTION

From the time when integrated circuit (IC) was invented, continuous reduction in the charge required for logic storage and operations has resulted in a steady increase in the density of logic gates and memory cells on a single chip. The scaling trend of IC, as described by Moore in 1975, is that on-chip logic density has doubled about every 24 months for decades [1]. The semiconductor industry accepted this trend as a roadmap and continuously pursuit a device size shrinking. However, passive devices (inductors, resistors, and capacitors) for these applications have not shrunk in size as rapidly as active devices due to the consideration of impedance levels and signal path properties. Meanwhile an increasing number of passive devices are required in modern wireless applications where the larger fraction of analog signals are involved [2]. Therefore, thin film integrated passive are applied as an alternative to discrete passives in the effort to save board space and improve electrical performance and system reliability.

Three types of capacitors are developed to meet the requirements for reduced board-level components: metal-oxide-semiconductor (MOS) capacitors, poly-insulator-poly capacitors, and metal–insulator–metal (MIM) capacitors. The MIM structures physically distance the devices from the relatively low-resistivity substrate and the planar back-end-of-line topology in order to build in high reliability [3]. These capacitors gain benefit from advantageous performance such as high Q at high frequency, excellent matching and the fabrication process with less heat that is important for submicron transistors. Thick metal plates offer lower series resistance and much lower parasitic capacitance resulting in much better voltage linearity. These features suggest the suitability of integrating high-density MIM capacitors in submicron CMOS for both mixed-signal and radio frequency (RF) process technologies.

Increasing the capacitance density, while maintaining a minimal thickness to preserve low leakage currents, a high breakdown voltage, and precision analog performance, requires the use of dielectrics with a high dielectric constant (high-k). The need for high-k gate dielectrics has been emphasized in numerous scientific reports. As the dielectric constant increases the band gap decreases, and high-k dielectric materials face challenges of leakage current and reliability issues. Thus, it is imperative to understand the electronic structure of defects such as C, H, and Si impurities, which can be incorporated into high-k dielectric materials in the growth process. Various C-, H-, and Si-related defects exist in high-k dielectrics; these defects will cause charge trapping and detrapping, according to gate voltages, which induce the threshold voltage instability in MOS devices. However, effects of the impurities on MIM device performance are not well understood.

Furthermore, a typical hostile environment includes radiation environment where intense radiation doses could easily damage the electronic circuitries [4]. Various types of radiation including electrons, protons, neutrons, and heavy ions in radiation environments cause transient and permanent changes in the devices used in complex ICs. The failure of a particular IC is owing to the basic material, device parameter changes, and the circuit environment in which the device is located. The effects of radiation in some advanced technologies are poorly understood, and extensive researches are needed to ensure the reliability of the advanced technologies in radiation environment. In addition, highly scaled devices may be sensitive to the naturally occurring radiation at the earth's surface, even though the atmosphere provides significant protection. The studies on the radiation tolerance combined with heavy-ion-induced breakdown of high-k dielectric/SiO_2 stacks were observed to be more resistant to radiation induced degradation. Thus, high-k dielectrics could be more suitable for being introduced into future technologies for space applications. Moreover, before these materials can be used for space applications, it is important to understand their radiation response.

In this chapter, we investigate the influence of carbon contamination on MIM capacitor performance. Besides, we have begun to develop an understanding of the physical nature of HfO_2-based MIM device radiation damage.

33.2 FABRICATION OF HFO_2 THIN FILM

33.2.1 Different Deposition Techniques

An ever-growing interest has been emerging concerning the application of high-k dielectric materials in the gate stack of the aggressively scaled semiconductor devices including transistors, capacitors, and so on. The introduction of these new materials is expected to improve capacitance density, reduce the leakage of future devices, and reduce corresponding power dissipation. The characteristics of high-k film depend on the deposition technologies due to the contamination, impurity density, interface issues, and so on.

As HfO_2 is the primary choice of semiconductor industry, various methods are used to deposit HfO_2: sputtering [5,6], e-beam evaporation [7], atomic layer deposition (ALD) [8,9], and metal-organic chemical vapor deposition (MOCVD) [10] have been reported for depositing HfO_2 on silicon. Each deposition method has its own strengths and weaknesses in achieving good electronic properties in layers deposited and excellence in layer uniformity.

The surface damage inherent in a sputtering PVD process and device morphology inherent to the scaling process generally rule out PVD deposition approaches. Within all the manufacturing options, chemical vapor deposition-based methods, ALD and MOCVD, draw the highest industrial interest for deposition of high-k dielectrics. ALD approaches appear to be promising, because of its precision in layer growth and high layer uniformity in large deposition areas such as 300 mm wafer technology. However, the generation of polycrystalline dielectrics in the manufacturing environment may cause high leakage currents and a possible diffusion path for dopants along its grain boundaries. Another major disadvantage of ALD is the long processing time, which makes it an expensive tool to operate. Besides, the demand for complex precursors decreases its flexibility for using in material research. The other technique is MOCVD, because of its good film conformality and control on deposition rates. However, choice of the precursor, deposition temperature, and incorporation of carbon impurities are major concerns in this technique.

On the other hand, Tan et al. reported that the HfO_2 prepared by thermal oxidation from Hf metal film has a denser HfO_2 top layer and a thinner interface of Hf-rich silicates compared with the HfO_2 deposited by reactive sputtering [11]. Although oxidation is not an industrial option for the deposition of high-k gate dielectrics because of growth kinetics/high-temperature deposition, it is a powerful tool for understanding the properties of high-k oxides.

33.2.2 Thermally Grown HfO_2

In this chapter, the MIM capacitors with HfO_2 high-k dielectric films were fabricated on 100–300 nm SiO_2 layer grown on a silicon substrate. A 65–70-nm Pt layer with a 5-nm Ti flash layer was deposited on the SiO_2 as the bottom electrode by means of E-beam evaporation. Subsequently, HfO_2 films were grown by evaporating metallic Hf (30–35 nm in thickness) in an electron-beam deposition system at a base pressure of 1×10^{-6} mbar, followed by thermal oxidation in dry O_2 ambient at 500°C. Then, 100 nm Al or 5 nm Cr/100 nm Au was deposited and patterned for top electrodes using contact photolithography followed by reactive ion etching. The areas of the capacitors are defined to be 1.02×10^{-3}, 6.15×10^{-4}, and 3.14×10^{-4} cm^2. The typical structure of the fabricated MIM capacitors in this chapter is shown in Figure 33.1.

The capacitance density at 0 MV/cm, ranging from 5.21 to 5.48 fF/μm^2, is obtained from the fabricated capacitor measuring from 1 M to 10 kHz. The capacitance density obtained is around five times higher than current SiO_2- or Si_3N_4-based MIM capacitors of 30 nm thickness [12]. The frequency-dependent shifts in dielectric constant is measured using capacitance–frequency measurement, the result shows that the dielectric constant increases slightly from 20.6 to 20 over the

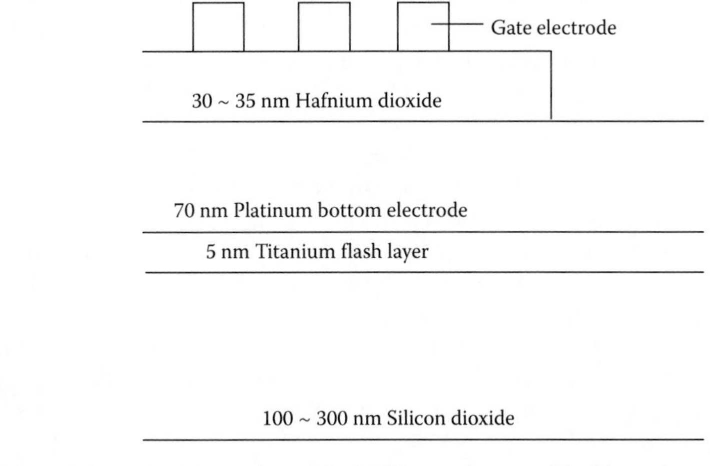

FIGURE 33.1 Schematic cross section of the MIM capacitors used in this study.

frequency range from 10 kHz to 1 MHz. This dispersion behavior is believed to relate with bulk HfO_2 traps. These traps are located within a tunneling distance of the oxide/metal interface such that they are capable of modulating the total capacitance with different time constants [13]. The effect is similar to that observed in MOS capacitors that may be modeled by a bulk capacitance term in parallel with an interface capacitance term.

The sensitivity of capacitors to temperature is another important parameter that enables precision analog design. The result from the measurement of 1 MHz capacitance as a function of electric field at different temperatures indicates a temperature coefficient of capacitance (TCC) of 244 ppm/°C at 1.0 MHz measured up to 200°C.

Temperature-dependent leakage current is observed for HfO_2 films, temperature ranging from room temperature to 350°C. It is also observed that, compared with positive gate bias, a slightly higher leakage current is observed under negative gate bias. This is believed to be due to the smaller band gap and barrier height of HfO_2/Al than Pt/HfO_2. It can be noted that, at low bias (<0.5 MV/cm) and temperature (room temperature to 150°C), the leakage current density of HfO_2 capacitor is lower than 10 nA cm^{-2}.

In summary, the MIM capacitor with thermally grown HfO_2 shows a high-capacitance density of 5.21 fF/μm^2 at 1 MHz, which can meet the requirement of the International Technology Roadmap for Semiconductor (ITRS), and leakage current of 1×10^{-7} A cm^{-2} at low bias (<0.5 MV/cm) and temperature (room temperature to 150°C). It is comparable with the MIM capacitors using HfO_2 fabricated by other deposition technologies [14].

33.3 INTERFACE CONTAMINATION

33.3.1 Carbon Contamination

High-k dielectric materials are being actively perused as a replacement for SiO_2 as the insulating layer for the capacitor technology. However, numerous issues, such as thermal stability, high densities of oxide charge and traps, and voltage linearity, must be resolved before any of them can be implemented. In order to overcome these problems, it is imperative to understand the performance degradation caused by defects such as C, H, and Si impurities, which can be incorporated into high-k dielectric materials in the growth process.

The high-k oxides are not materials with a low intrinsic defect concentration, because their bonding cannot relax as easily as SiO_2. The oxygen vacancy concentration in HfO_2 is much higher than that in SiO_2. Recent studies show that the higher concentration of oxygen vacancies leads to the formation of electron leakage paths, via hopping between the oxygen vacancies [15]. In accordance with the work on MOS capacitors, carbon can form complexes with oxygen vacancies to form C/O-complex single donors, which are much shallower than the native double oxygen vacancy donors [15]. These donors can cause a severe performance degradation of the capacitor such as flat-band shift, low capacitance, and high leakage current. The influence of carbon contamination on MIM capacitor performance is investigated in this section.

Two experimental groups of MIM capacitor with thermally grown HfO_2 are prepared to compare their electrical characteristics. The deposition of hafnium is performed with different sweeping areas of the electron beam in the electron beam deposition system. Using a larger sweeping area, the edge between the hafnium source and the graphite crucible may be heated and melted, and hence this batch of hafnium will have higher carbon concentration. The carbon concentrations in the dielectric films were qualified using Auger electron spectroscopy (AES) analysis. The compositional depth profile obtained from SiO_2/Ti/Pt/HfO_2 (~30 nm)/Al (S-1) structure and SiO_2/Ti/Pt/HfO_2 (~35 nm)/Cr/Au (S-2) structure were evaluated from the top electrodes to the silicon substrate using Ar ion etching. The scanning electron microscopy (SEM) measurements were performed on the top of the HfO_2 thin film and the Pt bottom electrode to evaluate roughness of HfO_2 and SiO_2/Ti/Pt after oxidation.

A typical Auger depth profile for sample S-2 is shown in Figure 33.2. Carbon peaks can be observed at the top and bottom interfaces between the metal and HfO_2. The carbon contaminations in these two peaks are calculated to be 9.1% and 3.6%, respectively. Similarly, the carbon contents of 0.3% and 1.3% are observed at the top and bottom interfaces of capacitor S-1, respectively. These impurities are most likely to be incorporated from the crucible during the deposition process. It has also been observed that a low level of oxygen diffuses through into the Pt bottom layer and the Ti buffer layer. According to other works, the Si/SiO_2/Ti/Pt system undergoes chemical and microstructural change after oxidation in O_2 in the temperature range 500–800°C; the top surface of the Pt film was found to be totally encapsulated by an amorphous titanium oxide film, and so the surface morphology of the Pt became rough, and the appearance of Pt hillocks is observed in SEM morphology. By comparing the profiles of AES and SEM for the two capacitors, the carbon contamination at the metal–oxide interfaces are of great interest, since the performance of the MIM capacitor significantly depends on the nature of the electrode and metal–oxide interface properties.

33.3.2 Changes in Electrical Parameters

The capacitance–voltage measurements were conducted on the MIM capacitors with HfO_2 dielectric at 1 MHz and room temperature. The zero-biased capacitance density ($C_{density}$) of 5.21 and 4.05 fF/μm^2 yields dielectric constants of $k = 17$ and 16 for samples S-1 and S-2, respectively. It is observed that the voltages at which the lowest value of capacitance is obtained are −0.5 and −1.0 V for S-1 and S-2, respectively. These voltage differences are due to oxide fixed charges similar to those in thermally grown SiO_2, which causes the flat-band shift in the high-frequency C–V curve of a MOS capacitor. The higher voltage shift is observed in sample S-2, which is due to the higher carbon contamination in the HfO_2 film as observed by AES.

From Figure 33.3, the temperature dependence of the capacitance–voltage characteristics provides further evidence. The relative variation of capacitance as a function of electric field for capacitors S-1 and S-2 at different temperatures is given by [15]

$$\frac{\Delta C}{C_0} = \frac{C(V) - C_0}{C_0} = \alpha V^2 + \beta V \tag{33.1}$$

where C_0 is the zero-bias capacitance at 1 MHz, ΔC the relative variations of capacitance to the zero-bias capacitance, and α and β are the quadratic and linear voltage coefficients, respectively. It is noticed that MIM capacitor S-2 with higher carbon contamination shows the strongest voltage

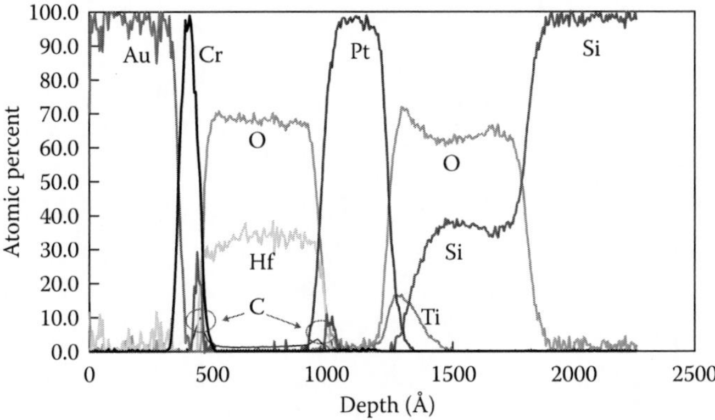

FIGURE 33.2 Profile of AES of the SiO_2/Ti/Pt/HfO_2 (~35 nm)/Al (S-2) MIM capacitor structure.

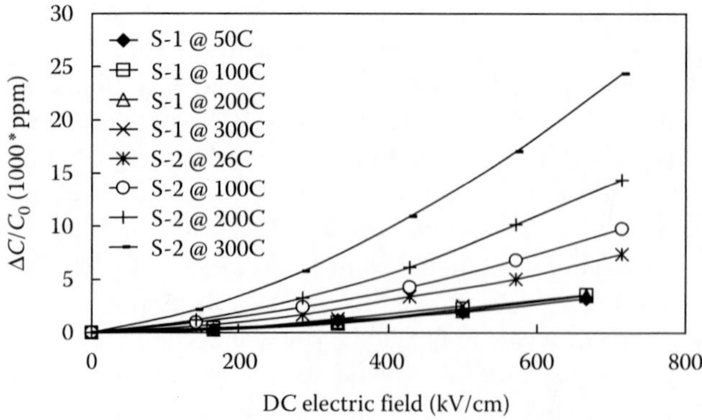

FIGURE 33.3 $\Delta C/C_0$ as a function of the DC electric field at 1 MHz and different temperatures.

dispersion. The values of quadratic and linear capacitance voltage linearity (voltage coefficient of capacitance (VCC)) are 236 ppm/V^2 and 1700 ppm/V for S-1 and 662 ppm/V^2 and 1880 ppm/V for S-2 at room temperature, respectively, and the voltage dispersion becomes more obvious with increasing temperature. The relationship between the voltage nonlinearity and oxide thicknesses (αt_{ox}^2) is constant for capacitors fabricated using the same top and bottom electrodes [15]. But, the effect of the electrodes cannot be ignored for capacitors with different metal electrodes [16]. In general, the voltage nonlinearity improves as the work function of metal increases. It is known that $\phi_{Al} = 4.1$ eV [13], $\phi_{Cr} = 4.5$ eV [17], $\phi_{Au} = 5.1$ eV [13], and $\phi_{Pt} = 5.4$ eV [17]; therefore, the relationship of voltage nonlinearity between capacitors S-1 and S-2 should be $\alpha_{S\text{-}2} < \alpha_{S\text{-}1}$. However, our experimental results are not consistent with this trend. Therefore, this difference in voltage nonlinearity comes mainly from the interface properties. The stronger voltage dependence for capacitor S-2 with Cr and Pt electrodes indicates a higher interface trap density, which produces a distortion in the shape of the *C–V* curve. These interface traps are due to structural defects such as the presence of carbon impurities as observed in the AES spectra.

The frequency-dependent capacitance for capacitors S-1 and S-2 are shown in Figure 33.4. The stronger frequency dependence is observed in capacitor S-2 with higher carbon contamination. This frequency dispersion is believed to relate to the existence of bulk-dielectric traps near the metal–oxide interface. Different traps will induce charges with different time constants and strongly modulate capacitor charge at certain frequencies [12]. As the frequency decreases, the induced charges will easily follow the AC signal, and therefore a higher capacitance is observed. A reduction in capacitance

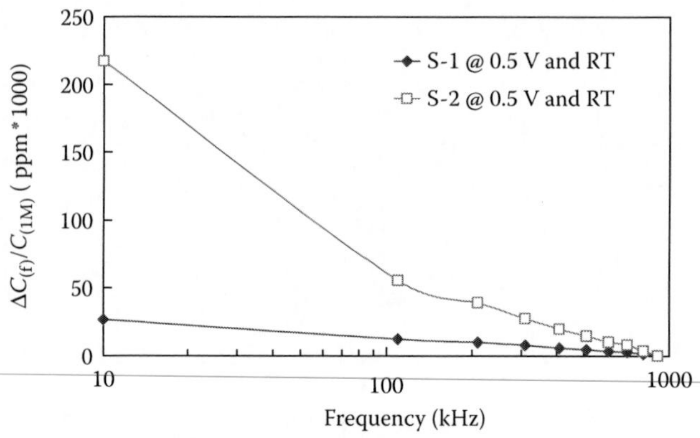

FIGURE 33.4 $\Delta C/C_0$ as a function of frequency at 0.5 V and room temperature.

of 2.5% is obtained between the frequency range of 10 k and 1 MHz for capacitor S-1, while, capacitor S-2 shows a reduction of 17.8%. This frequency-dependent behavior is dominated by the properties of the interface and is consistent with the previous voltage-dependence analysis. The higher carbon contamination present at the metal–oxide interface is believed to be the main cause of the higher interface trap density that leads to the poorer performance of capacitor S-2.

The TCC at 1 MHz are 232 and 409 ppm/°C for S-1 and S-2, respectively. Compared to the TCC of 232 ppm/°C at 1 MHz in the MIM capacitor with low carbon contamination, the HfO_2 MIM capacitor with carbon contamination shows comparable TCC.

Studies on the conduction mechanisms have been performed by measuring current–voltage (*J*–*V*) characteristics at room temperature. Capacitor S-2 with carbon contamination gives a current two orders of magnitude higher than S-1 for the range of electrical fields studied. Therefore, the interface properties and bulk traps degraded by carbon contamination are responsible for this difference in conduction behavior.

33.3.3 Analysis of Defect Density Using Electrode Polarization Model

In order to quantify the effects of carbon contamination, the interface barrier heights are extracted using the recently proposed model based on electrode polarization mechanism, which is successfully used to fit the experimental results of other MIM capacitors using HfO_2 thin films [17]. Electrode polarization is a mechanism in which mobile carriers form an accumulation layer at electrodes leading to a voltage-dependent double-layer capacitance. The mobile carriers involved in the formation of the double layer were appealed to be free electrons that are injected at electrodes or to be oxygen vacancies that are inherently created during oxide growth [18]. As oxygen vacancies are the energetically favored intrinsic defects in HfO_2 [19] and carbon contamination can complex with these oxygen vacancies to form C/O complex [19], this model which is based on the fact that oxygen vacancies are at the origin of a double-layer capacitance is suitable for our experimental results. This model is expressed as [17]

$$C = C_{\mathrm{m}}\left(1+\frac{A'}{1+\omega^{2n}\tau^{2n}}\right) \tag{33.2}$$

where C_{m} is the capacitance in the absence of electrode polarization, $C_{\mathrm{m}} = \varepsilon_0\varepsilon_r A/t_{\mathrm{ox}}$, A, the electrode area, n, an exponent introduced for a Jonscher response, and t_{ox}, the film thickness. Parameters A' and τ are given by

$$A' = \frac{2}{(2+\rho)^2}\frac{t_{\mathrm{ox}}}{L_{\mathrm{D}}}, \quad \tau = \tau_0\frac{1}{2+\rho}\frac{t_{\mathrm{ox}}}{L_{\mathrm{D}}} \tag{33.3}$$

where parameter ρ is the blocking parameter that accounts for electrode transparency and L_{D} is the Debye length, expressed as

$$L_{\mathrm{D}} = \sqrt{\frac{\varepsilon\varepsilon_0 k_{\mathrm{B}}T}{Nq^2}} \tag{33.4}$$

where N is the density of mobile charges. For Ohmic contacts, which are strongly injecting contacts in AC, ρ approaches infinity, $A' \approx 0$, and $C \approx C_{\mathrm{m}}$, which indicates that there is no space charge formation at the metal–oxide interface. On the contrary, for the blocking contacts, there is no charge transfer at the electrodes for AC, ρ is small, A' reaches a saturation value *of* ($t_{\mathrm{ox}}/L_{\mathrm{D}}$), which depends on the oxide thickness and Debye length, and the effect of space charge is important. By approximating $C \approx C_m$ [20] the relative variation of capacitance is given by

$$\frac{\Delta C}{C_0} = \frac{2}{(\varepsilon\varepsilon_0)^{2n}}\left(\frac{L}{L_D}\right)^{1-2n} \frac{1}{(\rho+2)^{2(1-n)}}\frac{1}{\omega^{2n}}\sigma_0^{2n} \cdot \left[\exp\left(\frac{nqEs}{k_B T}\right) - 1\right] \tag{33.5}$$

According to Equations 33.2 and 33.5, the $\Delta C(f)/C_0$ decreases as frequency increases (ω^{-2n}, $0 < n < 0.5$). The capacitance at constant voltage is plotted as a function of frequency ($\ln \Delta C(f)/C_0 \sim \ln f$). The slope of the curve gives the value of $2n$, which is 0.35 and 0.6 for S-1 and S-2, respectively. An exponential fit to $\Delta C/C_0$ gives the exponential factor $nqEs/k_BT$, and the hopping distance (s) is calculated using the value of "n." The obtained hopping distance shown in Table 33.1 is much higher than the interatomic distance, which suggests that the mobile charges calculated from this model are electronic in nature [20]. The density of defects may be estimated from $N \approx 1/s^3$ and the Debye length is calculated using Equation 33.4. DC conductivity experiments (J–E characteristics) give σ at a given field and we set the electric field value of 1 MV/cm to estimate the conductivity in our samples. In this way, the blocking parameter ρ is the only adjustable parameter in Equation 33.5. Given the parameters in Equation 33.5, the relative variations of capacitance for both capacitors with HfO_2 thin films have been calculated as shown by solid lines in Figure 33.5. It is observed that the electrode polarization model fits the experimental data for both capacitors well at room temperature. Beaumont and Jacobs [21] expressed ρ as

$$\rho = av\left(\frac{L}{D}\right)\exp\left(\frac{-\varphi_i}{kT}\right) \tag{33.6}$$

where a is the jumping distance from bulk to the interface, v the jumping frequency from bulk to the interface, ϕ_i the interface energy barrier height, and D the bulk diffusion coefficient, expressed as $D = \sigma k_B T/Nq$. The same value of $v \approx 10^{12}$ Hz for HfO_2 as used in the previous work [9] has been taken in our calculation.

TABLE 33.1
Comparison of Parameters Describing the Voltage Dependence of MIM Capacitors S-1 and S-2

Parameters	56 nm HfO_2 [13]	S-1	S-2
Deposition method	ALD	Thermally grown	Thermally grown
t_{ox} (nm)	56	30	35
$C_{density}$ (fF/μm^2)	—	5.21	4.05
VCC (ppm/V^2)	—	236	662
$2n$	0.15	0.35	0.62
s (Å)	52	58	28
N (cm^{-3})	7.0×10^{18}	7.7×10^{18}	4.6×10^{19}
σ (S cm^{-1})	3.7×10^{-15}	9.0×10^{-11}	1.1×10^{-9}
σ_0 (S cm^{-1})	4.4×10^{-14}	8.8×10^{-11}	1.1×10^{-9}
K	18.5	17	22.2
L_D (nm)	1.9	1.8	0.8
w (kHz)	10	10	10
P	42.2	6	31
ϕ_i (AC) (eV)	0.9	0.95	0.58
$J_{density}$ (A cm^{-2})	—	1.3×10^{-7}	1.1×10^{-3}
ϕ_B (DC) (eV)	—	1.1	0.26

Source: Adapted from F. El Kamel, P. Gonon, and C. Vallée, *Applied Physics Letter*, 91, 172909, 2007.

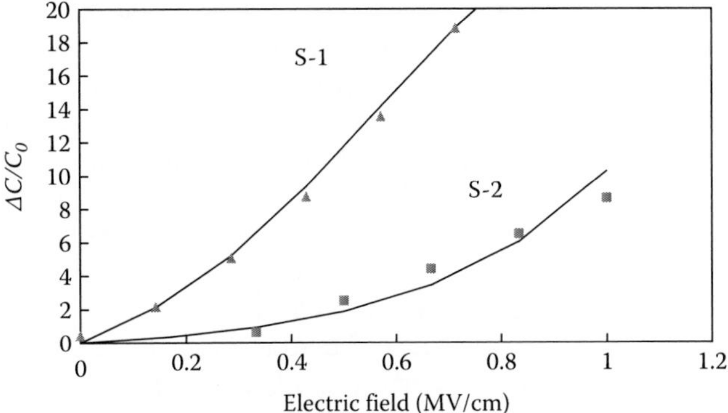

FIGURE 33.5 Relative variation of capacitance as a function of the electric field and their calculated values using the electrode polarization model.

The energy barriers at the metal–oxide interface are obtained for both capacitors, as shown in Table 33.1, which are 0.95 eV for capacitor S-1 and 0.58 eV for capacitor S-2. The lower barrier heights for the MIM capacitor (S-2) may be due to higher carbon contamination at the interface as observed by AES. The defect density for S-2 device is found to be one order of magnitude larger than S-1 which suggests that contamination-induced defects are the main reason for the observed reduction in barrier height, decrease in voltage nonlinearity with frequency and temperature for the MIM capacitor.

33.4 RADIATION TESTING

Microelectromechanical systems (MEMS) are receiving great interest for being used in the space system. However, in space, the electronics are exposed to various forms of radiation including electrons, protons, neutrons, and heavy ions. The radiation may cause long-term degradation in electronics [22]. To date, few radiation tests have been performed on MEMS devices. MIM capacitors are passive components used in RF MEMS switches. The capacitance stability (the voltage nonlinearity of the capacitance) is the key issue to evaluate the reliability of the device. Despite the large amount of ongoing research into alternative dielectrics, very little work has been done to understand the radiation responses of these materials. In this section, MIM structures were employed and radiation-introduced defects in HfO_2 dielectric layer have been investigated. The effects on the performance and reliability of these devices are also discussed.

33.4.1 Defects in Pre-irradiated HfO_2-Based Device

The MIM capacitors with HfO_2 high-*k* dielectric films and 100 nm Au/5 nm Cr top electrodes were fabricated on a 300-nm SiO_2 layer thermally grown on a silicon substrate by the same process described in Section 33.2.2. The areas of the capacitors were defined to be, 6.15×10^{-4}, 3.14×10^{-4} cm^2, and 7.85×10^{-5} cm^2, respectively.

33.4.1.1 *C–V* Characteristics

The capacitance–voltage measurement of MIM capacitors before irradiation was conducted at room temperature. The capacitance was measured with the DC bias swept from −3–3 V with an AC signal of 10 kHz, 100 kHz, and 1 MHz, respectively. These characteristics follow the well-known parabolic voltage behavior of MIM capacitor structures. Since the dielectrics involved in MIM capacitors comprise polar molecules, this leads to a dielectric permittivity that depends on the electric field (*E*). The variation of capacitance with bias voltage may be described by Equation 33.1.

The zero-biased capacitance density ($C_{density}$) of 4.05 fF/μm^2 yields dielectric constants of $k = 16$ at 1 MHz for these capacitors. The extracted voltage nonlinearities give two different values for the forward and reverse C–V curves (α_1, forward voltage linearity; α_2, reverse voltage linearity). Reports in the literature state that the voltage nonlinearity is dependent on the work function of metal contacts and improves as the work function of metal increases. From Figure 33.6, the α values are 822 ppm/V^2 and 1503 ppm/V^2 at 1 MHz for the Pt bottom contact and Au/Cr top gate, respectively. A voltage linearity at 1 MHz of 1000 ppm/V^2 meets the ITRS requirement for a bypass capacitor in RF applications.

From Figure 33.6, it can also be seen that the voltage linearity of capacitance increases with decreasing frequency. This dispersive behavior of the MIM capacitor with HfO_2 dielectric is believed to relate to the existence of bulk-dielectric traps near the dielectric–metal interface [14]. Different traps will capture and generate carriers with different time constants and hence strongly modulate the capacitance at certain frequencies. When the frequency is decreased, a greater number of the traps will be able to follow the AC signal, and therefore a higher VCC is observed.

The tendency of dielectric constant with increasing frequency is studied. The result shows that the dielectric constant decreases monotonically from 19.4 to 16 as the frequency increases from 10 k Hz to 1 MHz. The dependence of capacitance on both voltage and frequency indicates the existence of interface states and bulk defects. These traps, which are located near the dielectric–metal interface reduces interface barrier height between the electrode and the dielectric film and result in higher voltage and frequency dispersion.

In order to explain these voltage-dependent capacitance variations, the C–V characteristics of HfO_2 capacitors are modeled with the electrode polarization model. This model offers a high-quality fit to our experimental results of HfO_2 MIM capacitors as mentioned in Section 33.3.3. It considers the mobile charge carriers that create the electrode polarization and relate these to oxygen vacancy-type defects in the dielectric, as oxygen vacancies are the dominant intrinsic defect in the bulk of many transition metal oxides [23]. According to Equations 33.2 and 33.5, $\Delta C/C_0$ decreases as frequency increases (ω^{-2m} with $0 < m < 0.5$). The slope of capacitance at constant voltage as a function of frequency ($\ln\Delta C/C_0 \sim \ln f$) has been calculated. This slope gives the value of 2m, which is 0.40 for the as-fabricated capacitor.

An exponential fit to $\Delta C/C_0$ gives the exponential factor $mqEs/k_BT$ (4.9), and hence the hopping distance (s) can be evaluated using the value $m = 0.20$. The obtained hopping distance (shown in Table 33.1) is greater than the interatomic distance, which indicates that the mobile charges used in this model are electronic in nature [18]. The density of defects in the dielectric film may be then

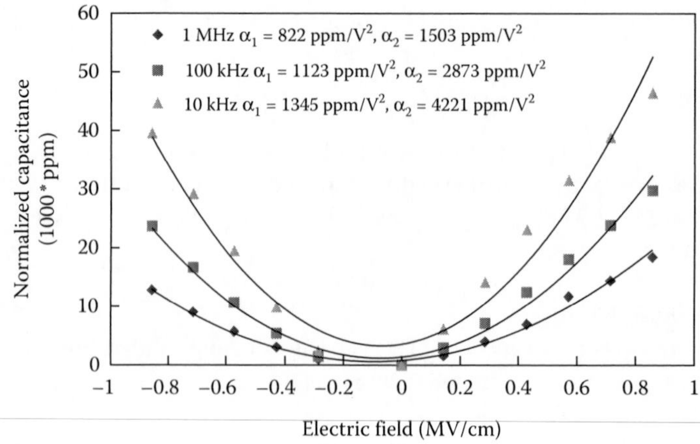

FIGURE 33.6 DC bias dependence of normalized capacitance ($\Delta C/C_0$) at 1 MHz, 100 k, and 10 k for the MIM capacitor without radiation.

extracted using $N \approx 1/s^3$ and then the Debye length is calculated using Equation 33.5. DC conductivity experiments (*J–E* characteristics) give σ as a function of electric field and we set the electric field to 1 MV/cm to calculate the conductivity in our devices.

Given the parameters in Equation 33.5, the relative variations of capacitance for the as-fabricated capacitors with HfO_2 thin films are calculated. According to Equation 33.6, the value of $\nu \approx 10^{12}$ Hz for HfO_2 as used in Section 33.3.3. Taking $L = 35$ nm, $a \approx s = 34 \pm 0.8$ Å, $\nu = 10^{12}$ Hz, $\sigma = 4.1 \times 10^{-11}$ S cm^{-1}, $N = (2.53 \pm 0.18) \times 10^{19}$ cm^{-3}, and $\rho = 9.8 \pm 0.3$, we obtain $\phi_i \sim 0.69$ eV that can be viewed as the effective barrier at the electrode for AC charge transfer. It should be pointed out that the relatively high density of mobile charges (N) indicates the high density of preexisting trapping states, which is suggested to be $>3 \times 10^{19}$ cm^{-3} in HfO_2 [24]. This trapping state is expected to be significantly enhanced by oxygen vacancies and/or interstitials that are clustered potentially at the grain boundaries. Oxygen vacancy defect states have been known to lie in the upper half of the forbidden band gap within 2 eV of the conduction band-gap edge; on the other hand, oxygen interstitial defect states are located in the lower half of the bandgap, within about 1–2 eV of the valence band edge. These preexisting defects serve as precursors to the defects in irradiated films, such as electron centers.

A control experiment was performed out on devices fabricated in the same batch as those studied. In the control experiment, the capacitance–voltage (*C–V*) measurement at 10, 100, and 1000 kHz and capacitance–frequency (*C–f*) measurements between 10 and 1000 kHz were performed 20 times on each capacitor. The results show a change in the capacitance that is less than 0.9%. There is no detectable tendency to fail with the voltage levels used in the tests over the period of the investigations.

33.4.1.2 *I–V* Characteristics

The DC conduction mechanisms have been studied by measuring current–voltage (*J–V*) characteristics on the as-fabricated capacitor at temperatures between room temperature and 125°C. A significant temperature dependence of the current–voltage characteristics for capacitors suggests that Poole–Frenkel emission is responsible for the observed data [25]. The current from the Poole–Frenkel effect can be expressed as

$$J = \sigma_0 E \exp\left(-\frac{q}{kT}\left(\varphi_t - \sqrt{\frac{qE_m}{\pi\varepsilon_0\varepsilon_{op}}}\right)\right) \tag{33.7}$$

where ϕ_t is the energy separation between the trap and the conduction band, E_m the maximum electric field at the interface, σ_0 the zero bias conductivity, and ε_{op} the dynamic high-frequency dielectric constant. The dynamic high-frequency dielectric constant is extracted from the barrier lowering by means of $\Delta\phi_{PF}$,

$$\Delta\varphi_{PF} = \sqrt{\frac{q^3 E_m}{\pi\varepsilon_0\varepsilon_{op}}} = \beta_{PF} E^{1/2} \tag{33.8}$$

The Poole–Frenkel effect is caused by the field-enhanced emission of carriers from traps in the dielectric. This is a bulk-limited current and is controlled by the existence of defects in the bulk of insulator [26].

A plot of ln(*J/E*) versus $E^{1/2}/kT$ results in a straight line with a gradient of β_{PF}. Using the experimental data, the dynamic dielectric constant ε_{op} can be extracted and is then used to calculate the refractive index (n) of the dielectric by equating $\varepsilon_{op} = n^2$ [25]. The extracted refractive index is in the range of 2–3 for the as-fabricated capacitors, which is close to the theoretical value of the dynamic dielectric constant for HfO_2 (2.9–3.6) [27]. This result indicates that the conductivity for the as-fabricated devices is bulk-limited.

Further, Figure 33.7 shows that the plot of ln J versus $1/T$ is fitted with a straight line at different electric fields for the as-fabricated capacitors [28], which confirms that the leakage current density in MIM capacitors is dominated by Poole–Frankel conduction mechanisms. Hence, the leakage current is controlled by existing defects in the bulk of the HfO_2. The magnitude of the leakage current depends on the possibility and amount of the carriers that can detrap from the trap centers (defects) to the conduction band. Using $\varepsilon_{op} = 4$, the calculated trap level energy is 0.39–0.46 eV for the as-fabricated capacitor structures.

33.4.2 Radiation-Induced Changes in Electrical Parameters

Irradiations were performed at the dose of 10, 100, and 1000 krad, incrementally, using a ^{60}Co gamma-ray source. A total of 21 capacitors were irradiated and all of these capacitors were measured before and after every irradiation. All these capacitors experienced the total dose of 1110 krad radiation dose. Each time after the irradiation, the capacitance–voltage measurements (C–V) were performed on these capacitors at frequencies varied from 10 kHz to 1 MHz. The leakage current measurement was performed before and after total-dose radiation at room temperature. After irradiation, some of the devices showed little change, whereas some showed characteristics of failure.

33.4.2.1 Good Devices

The values of capacitance–voltage linearity VCC increase on irradiation. For the capacitor that was operational after 1000 krad total dose, the preirradiation VCC of $\alpha_{pre} = 822$ ppm/V^2 (forward) and 1503 ppm/V^2 (reverse) rises to $\alpha_{post} = 1013$ ppm/V^2 (forward) and 1582 ppm/V^2 (reverse) at 1 MHz. The capacitance density decreases by 3.5% in comparison with the preirradiated values for frequencies between 10 kHz and 1 MHz.

In order to quantify the effects of irradiation, the defect concentration and interface barrier heights for the irradiated capacitors are extracted using the electrode polarization model, which is detailed in Section 33.3.3. The capacitance as a function of the electric field has been calculated for as-fabricated and 1000 krad postirradiation, as shown by the solid lines in Figure 33.8. It can be observed from Figure 33.8 that both data sets can be fitted using the electrode polarization model. As listed in Table 33.2, the energy barriers at the metal–dielectric interface are 0.69 eV (as-fabricated) and 0.61 eV (postirradiation). The energy blocking parameter (ρ) for the contacts is 9.8 before and 18 after irradiation at a total dose of 1000 krad. The small change in barrier height suggests that the radiation changes the interface trapping properties of the dielectric at the interface with the metal contacts. The observed variation in the extracted bulk diffusion coefficient (D) is

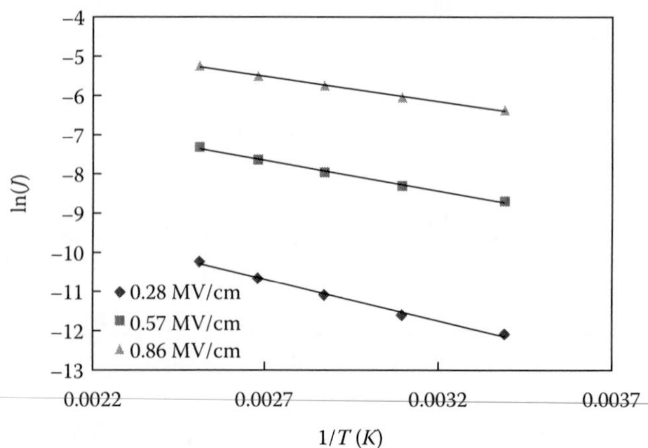

FIGURE 33.7 The logarithmic leakage current density as a function of $1/T$.

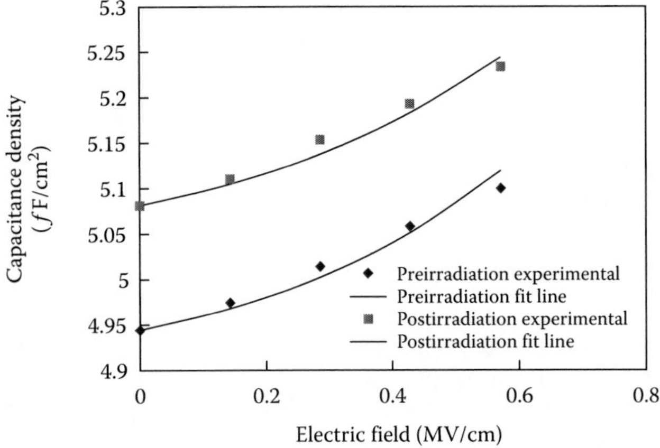

FIGURE 33.8 Capacitance density as a function of the electric field and their calculated values using the electrode polarization model.

three times higher than the value extracted from the as-fabricated devices. During irradiation, a greater number of unrecombined charge carriers become trapped near the metal–oxide interface and these carriers are known to be linked to the radiation-introduced interface trap formation in devices with HfO_2 as the dielectric [29].

The leakage current densities as a function of temperature of the MIM capacitors pre- and postirradiation at a total dose of 1000 krad are compared. It has been observed that the leakage current density is only slightly influenced by gamma radiation. After irradiation, the leakage current density of the HfO_2 film was observed to be higher than that of the as-fabricated devices by less than one order of magnitude. It is found that the temperature-dependent current for the postirradiated

TABLE 33.2
Comparison of Parameters Describing the Voltage Dependence of MIM Capacitor Preirradiation and Postirradiation

Parameters	Preirradiation	Postirradiation at Total Dose of 1000 krad	Failure at Total Dose of 10 krad	Failure at Total Dose of 100 krad	Failure at Total Dose of 1000 krad
T_{ox} (nm)	35	35	35	35	35
$C_{density}$ (fF μm^{-2})	4.94	5.08	1.73	1.66	1.72
VCC_{IM} (ppm V^{-2})	822	1503	38100	8100	14100
Frequency (kHz)	10	10	1000	1000	1000
2m	0.40 ± 0.01	0.46 ± 0.03	1.9 ± 0.01	2.1 ± 0.08	2.0 ± 0.1
N (cm^{-3})	$(2.53 \pm 0.18) \times 10^{19}$	$(3.8 \pm 0.7) \times 10^{19}$	$(2.01 \pm 0.3) \times 10^{21}$	$(1.24 \pm 0.7) \times 10^{21}$	$(4.68 \pm 0.8) \times 10^{20}$
σ (S cm^{-1})	4.1×10^{-11}	2.0×10^{-10}	1.1×10^{-4}	4.7×10^{-5}	2.2×10^{-5}
σ_o (S cm^{-1})	4.1×10^{-11}	2.0×10^{-10}	1.1×10^{-4}	4.7×10^{-5}	2.3×10^{-5}
K	20	21	6.85	6.55	6.80
L_D (nm)	1.08	0.89 ± 0.09	0.07 ± 0.004	0.12 ± 0.007	0.14 ± 0.01
s (Å)	34 ± 0.8	29.8 ± 0.2	0.89 ± 0.001	0.93 ± 0.04	1.29 ± 0.06
ρ	9.8 ± 0.3	12.8 ± 1.3	34 ± 0.5	55 ± 3	53 ± 3
ϕ_i (AC) (eV)	0.69 ± 0.002	0.61 ± 0.007	0.35 ± 0.001	0.35 ± 0.001	0.36 ± 0.002
$J_{density}$ (A cm^{-2})	5×10^{-6}	3.5×10^{-5}	109	47	22
ϕ_i (DC) (eV)	0.39–0.46	0.37–0.44	—	—	—

capacitors is dominated by Poole–Frankel emission as well. From the experimental data, the extracted refractive indexes are in the range of 1.7–2 for the postirradiated capacitors, compared with 2–3 for the as-fabricated capacitors preirradiated over the temperature range studied. The increase in leakage current is caused by defects in the dielectric generated during the irradiation process. The calculated trap level energy is 0.37–0.44 eV for the capacitor after irradiation. This result is in good agreement with our *C–V* results, the slight reductions of both AC and DC barrier heights after radiation suggests the generation of more defects by radiation near the metal–oxide interface.

33.4.2.2 Failed Devices

Not all the devices investigated in this study were fully operational after the radiation exposure. Of the 21 devices tested, six showed no failure after 1000 krad, whereas five showed failure after 10 krad, five after 100 krad, and a further five after 1000 krad. For the failed devices, the capacitance density decreases by 85–35%, when the conductance increases to 10^{-2} S, which is 100 times greater than its initial value. This is due to the degradation of an MIM capacitor caused by the gamma radiation, which produces Frenkel pairs in the dielectric. The capacitance measured by the Agilent 4284A is influenced by the dramatic increase in the conductivity, according to [30]

$$C_{\mathrm{m}} = \frac{C_{\mathrm{t}}}{\left(G_{\mathrm{t}}R_{\mathrm{s}}+1\right)^2 + w^2C_{\mathrm{t}}^2R_{\mathrm{s}}^2} \tag{33.9}$$

where C_t is the true capacitance of the device, C_m the measured result, G_t the conductance, and R_s the series resistance. When G_t becomes large (as is observed in the failed devices), the effect of the series resistance is amplified and so the value of C_m decreases and becomes more voltage dependent [31]. Because the value of the conductivity is limited by the capabilities of the system we have not attempted to calculate the corrected capacitance for these devices, only to use the substantial decrease as a metric to observe failure.

Recently reported results on HfO_2-based MOS structure state that there are atomic scale differences between radiation damage in conventional Si/SiO_2 devices and the new Si/dielectric devices based on HfO_2 [23]. There are three defects responsible for the postirradiation variation: interface trapping centers, an O^{2-}/hafnium ion trap in the HfO_2 (which is an electron trap), and oxygen vacancies. Both the O^{2-} /hafnium ion trapping centers and oxygen vacancies are intrinsic defects [32].

The defect density for the capacitor preirradiated, postirradiated and failed is estimated using the electrode polarization model mentioned earlier (Equations 33.2 through 33.5). As discussed previously, the key assumption to describe the *C–V* nonlinearity using the electrode polarization model is to consider the shift of relaxation time (τ) toward high frequencies as the bias increases. The value of the carrier lifetime (τ) used in the equations is proportional to conductivity and so the observed increase in conductivity with bias results in the rise in relaxation time. The electrode polarization model is built on the assumption that under the influence of an AC field, an excess charge density accumulates at the electrodes [18] and that the charge transfer rate is low in comparison with the excitation frequency. This is a reasonable assumption as the charge transfer is controlled by tunneling injection, which is a relatively slow process.

The carrier relaxation frequency is related to the relaxation time constant, using $f_c = 1/2\pi\tau$; hence, the injection process is slow and only the AC space charge builds up at electrodes at the high frequencies used in the measurements. Considering carrier tunneling distances around 20 Å [21], we calculate the relaxation frequency to be 1 kHz (corresponding to a relaxation time constant of 6.28×10^{-3} s) which is lower than the frequencies used [13]. However, with an increase in relaxation frequency in the failed capacitors, the validity of the ($f > f_c$) condition may change, and so we evaluate the relaxation frequency by normalizing the capacitance to that measured at 10 kHz and using Equation 33.2. The corresponding relaxation frequencies are 1.2 kHz for capacitors without failure and 10 kHz for capacitors after failure. We compare the defect densities extracted using the electrode polarization model at 1 M, 100 k and 10 kHz and these are shown in Figure 33.9. From the data in given in this figure, we can see that the capacitor fails when the defect density exceeds 10^{20} cm^{-3}. It should be noted that the trap concentration at a frequency of 10 kHz after failure is lower than this threshold. For the capacitors that showed failure at a dose of 10 and 1000 krad, the calculated trap concentrations are around 5×10^{19} cm^{-3}, much lower than the concentration estimated at higher frequencies, which is in excess of 10^{20} cm^{-3}. As more traps are generated during the irradiation, the Debye length and hopping distance both reduce and so the relaxation frequency increases to 10 kHz. Thus, the electrode polarization model is no longer able to accurately calculate the defect density at low frequencies and so the extracted values shown in Figure 33.9 are lower than those for higher frequencies.

The hopping distances extracted from the before and after data for all capacitors studied are much higher than interatomic distances, which implies that the mobile charges are electronic in nature [14] even for devices showing failure. It is worth noting that the mechanisms of HfO_2 charge build up in the oxide appears to be different than that observed in SiO_2-based dielectrics and the relationship between oxide charge trapping and failure is still not clear.

The leakage current densities at room temperature for the capacitors that showed failure at different total radiation dose are studied. There is no significant difference in the leakage current densities for different failure doses. All capacitors that failed show high leakage current density in comparison with the capacitor without failure, which gives a low leakage current density even after irradiation. The observed change in leakage current density after radiation indicates an increase in the density of traps generated during the radiation exposure.

The increase in trap density in the dielectric is responsible for the increased conduction. Once the density exceeds a critical value, carriers can hop between proximate traps and a conductive path forms between the electrodes. This conduction through a series of conducting pathways is consistent with a percolation-type behavior [33,34]. The observed behavior may be explained by the fact that the traps have to be located close together to form a percolative path between the capacitor electrodes. Analysis of ultrathin oxides suggests that distance between adjacent traps is of the order 0.4 nm [33]; however, in our case with substantially thicker oxides, we found that the traps are separated by around 2 nm, based on the extracted trap density and the hopping distances listed in Table 33.1. The distribution of the charge to failure (and hence early failures of some of the devices) is consistent with the statistical nature of this failure mechanism [35] and the random distribution of defects from the fabrication process.

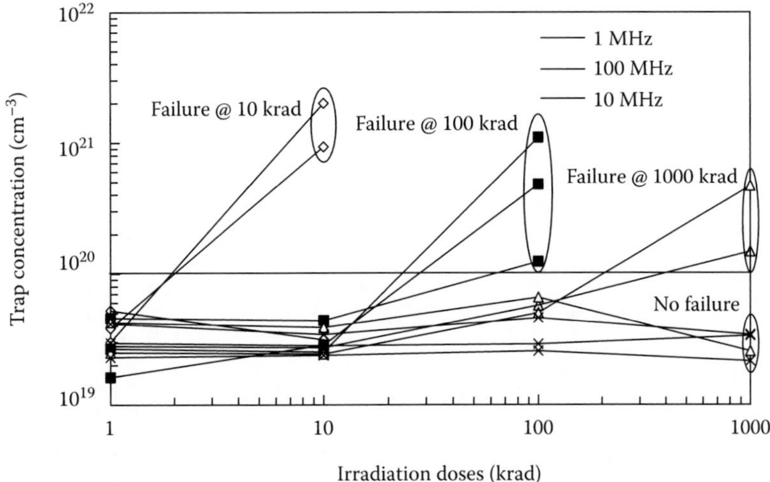

FIGURE 33.9 Defect densities as a function of dose at 1 M, 100 k, and 10 kHz, respectively.

33.4.3 Annealing Studies

Following irradiation, the annealing characteristics of the 35 nm HfO_2 MIM devices were measured at room temperature. The annealing process was carried out after irradiation at 1000 krad. Samples were annealed under air atmosphere at 400°C for 30 min. It is found that compared to the capacitances after 1000 krad irradiation the capacitance density are decreased by annealing. The annealing leads to a shift in the direction of original position. Compared to the as-fabricated capacitance, it is believed that a great part of the defects induced by irradiation can be annihilated by annealing processes. However, to reach the original values at 100 k and 1 MHz, longer time and higher annealing temperature are necessary [36].

The voltage-dependent capacitance of good capacitors as-fabricated, as-irradiated, and annealed can be modeled and explained by electrode polarization mechanism. Based on the electrode polarization mechanism, the capacitance–voltage nonlinearity originates from the mobility of hopping carriers, and the increment of defects concentration leads to the reduction in the mean free path and results in a higher polarization at the cathode on biasing [21,37]. Therefore, after irradiation, these induced defects cause higher capacitance–voltage nonlinearity. This is supported by the defect concentration and interface barrier heights extracted using the electrode polarization model, which shows that the energy barrier at the metal–dielectric interface is reduced from 0.69 (as-fabricated) to 0.61 eV (postirradiation) while the concentration of mobile charges is increased from 2.53×10^{18} cm^{-3} to 3.81×10^{19} cm^{-3} as shown in Table 33.2. After annealing, an increase in the parameters (N, σ, VCC, J) of the irradiated device, compared to the non-irradiated device, reflects the increase in the induced trapped charge density. This increase is of importance since it constitutes a direct evidence of radiation-induced damage. It also can be observed from Figure 33.10 that the capacitance–voltage nonlinearity is improved and the experimental data set can be fitted using the electrode polarization model. As listed in Table 33.3, the energy barrier at the metal–dielectric interface is 0.62 eV and the concentration of mobile charges is 2.8×10^{19} cm^{-3}. The restoration of the device with HfO_2 as the dielectric is confirmed by the shift of the energy barrier and mobile charge density in the direction to the as-fabricated values. Furthermore, the current density at 1 MV clearly illustrates that the annealing process reduces irradiation-induced defects, compared to the irradiated result.

33.5 SUMMARY AND FUTURE TRENDS

The HfO_2 prepared by thermal oxidation from metallic Hf film is used in our MIM capacitors. As a fabrication process study, the carbon contamination-induced degradation characteristics in HfO_2

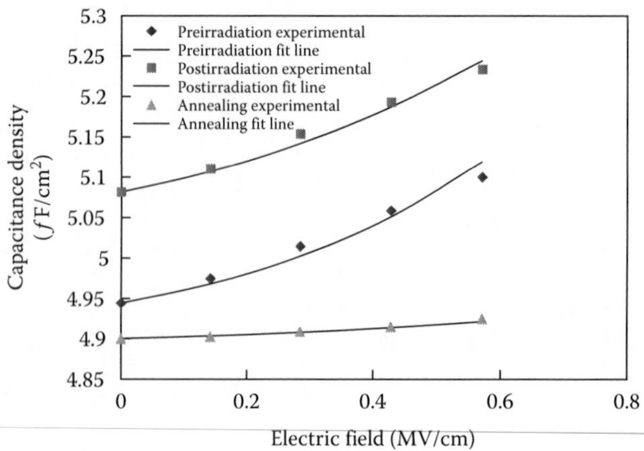

FIGURE 33.10 Capacitance density as a function of the electric field and their calculated values using the electrode polarization model before and after annealing.

TABLE 33.3
Comparison of Parameters Describing the Voltage Dependence of MIM Capacitor Preirradiation and Postirradiation and after Postirradiation Annealing

Parameters	Preirradiation	Postirradiation at Total Dose of 1000 krad	After Annealing
T_{ox} (nm)	35	35	35
$C_{density}$ (fF μm^{-2})	4.94	5.08	4.90
VCC_{IM} (ppm V^{-2})	822	1503	1180
Frequency (kHz)	10	10	10
2m	0.40 ± 0.01	0.46 ± 0.03	0.41 ± 0.01
N (cm^{-3})	$(2.53 \pm 0.18) \times 10^{19}$	$(3.8 \pm 0.7) \times 10^{19}$	$(2.81 \pm 0.7) \times 10^{19}$
σ (S cm^{-1})	4.1×10^{-11}	2.0×10^{-10}	3.0×10^{-10}
σ_o (S cm^{-1})	4.1×10^{-11}	2.0×10^{-10}	3.0×10^{-10}
K	20	21	19.8
L_D (nm)	1.08	0.89 ± 0.09	1.15 ± 0.9
s (Å)	34 ± 0.8	29.8 ± 0.2	32.9 ± 1.8
ρ	9.8 ± 0.3	12.8 ± 1.3	21 ± 1.0
ϕ_i (AC) (eV)	0.69 ± 0.002	0.61 ± 0.007	0.62 ± 0.04
$J_{density}$ (A cm^{-2})	5×10^{-6}	3.5×10^{-5}	2.0×10^{-5}

dielectric MIM capacitors were investigated. The electrical characteristics with dependency in frequency, voltage, and temperature provided insight into contamination-enhanced charge trapping in HfO_2 high-k dielectric. Different current transportation mechanisms of leakage current are addressed, Poole–Frenkel emission for the dielectric with low carbon contamination and Schottky for the other with high carbon contamination. Both the AC and DC barrier heights were found to be reduced by the carbon impurity existing at the metal–oxide interface. The overall high performance achieved by the HfO_2 film with lower carbon contamination suggested that an attention should be given to minimize the carbon contamination during the fabrication of MIM capacitor.

The effects of gamma-ray radiation on the HfO_2-based MIM capacitors have been discussed. The MIM capacitors using HfO_2 dielectric showed promising radiation tolerance, for the devices which were still operable after a total dose of 1 Mrad, the parameters describing the behavior of the capacitors showed only a small change to those for the as-fabricated devices. However, a number of devices showed a dramatic decrease in capacitance in conjunction with a large rise in leakage current after exposure to radiation, which we consider to be a sign of failure for the device. The previous works on MOS devices suggest that high-k device fabrication will likely be a major concern for radiation response of future devices which incorporate alternative gate dielectrics and the trapped charge density is very sensitive to the oxide growth process. Therefore, the further oxide charges and interface traps due to gamma radiation led to the failure behavior. We explain this change in behavior by means of a percolation model and suggest that the failure behavior may occur once the mobile charge density exceeds 10^{20} cm^{-3}. Additionally, the investigation of improvement in device characteristics after 400°C annealing for 30 min further agrees with the radiation-introduced defects, which cause the degradation of the device. The energy barrier at the metal–dielectric interface increased slightly back to the as-fabricated value and the concentration of mobile charges reduced to 2.8×10^{19} cm^{-3}. Further recovery of radiation-induced damage in the dielectric would be necessary to apply a higher annealing temperature and/or a longer annealing time. In addition, further optimization to reduce oxide charges in the dielectric would be necessary for the application of MIM capacitors using advanced high-k dielectric in hostile environments.

In future, the capacitance of gate dielectric needs to be continuously increased. The effects of radiation bias, film thickness, and device processing conditions on the radiation response of high-k

alternative dielectric stacks need further investigation. The variation in radiation response with processing could be the result of change in either the hole or the electron-trapping properties of these materials. Currently, no well-defined standard processes for making devices with alternative gate dielectrics exists; therefore, it is important to continue to research these materials and determine how variations in processing and device design affect radiation response.

ACKNOWLEDGMENT

The authors acknowledge the financial support from the Innovative electronics Manufacturing Research Council and Richard Jenkinsand Jon Silvie from BAE Systems for the irradiation of capacitors.

REFERENCES

1. G. E. Moore, Progress in digital integrated electronics, *Electron Devices Meeting*, Washington, DC, 1975.
2. J. S. Dunn, D. C. Ahlgren, D. D. Coolbaugh, N. B. Feilchenfeld, G. Freeman, D. R. Greenberg, R. A. Groves et al., Foundation of RF CMOS and SiGe BiCMOS technologies, *IBM Journal of Research and Development*, 47, 2003.
3. A. Farcy, J. Torres, V. Arnal, M. Fayolle, H. Feldis, F. Jourdan, M. Assous, J. L. Di Maria, and V. Vidal, A new damascene architecture for high-performance metal–insulator–metal capacitors integration, *Microelectronic Engineering*, 70, 368–372, 2003.
4. J. R. Hauser and S. E. Kerns, Circuit related issues due to radiation in hostile environments, *Journal of Electronic Materials*, 19, 671–688, 1990.
5. L. Pereira, A. Marques, N. Aguas, N. Nedev, S. Georgiev, E. Fortunato, and R. Martins, Performances of hafnium oxide produced by radio frequency sputtering for gate dielectric application, *Materials Science and Engineering* B, 89, 89–93, 2004.
6. F. Gourbilleau, L. Khomenkova, C. Dufour, P.-E Coulon, and C. Bonafos, HfO_2-based thin films deposited by magnetron sputtering, *MRS*, 2009 Spring, Symposium H, Strasbourg, 2009.
7. D. Y. Cho, K. S. Park, B. H. Choi, S. J. Oh, Y. J. Chang, D. H. Kim, T. W. Noh, R. Jung, J.-C. Lee, and S. D. Bu, Control of silicidation in HfO_2/Si(100) interfaces, *Applied Physics Letters*, 86, 041913, 2005.
8. S. Duenas, H. Castan, H. Garcia, J. Barbolla, K. Kukli, M. Ritala, and M. Leskela, The electrical-interface quality of as-grown atomic-layer-deposited disordered HfO_2 on p- and n-type silicon, *Thin Solid Films*, 474, 1141–1148, 2005.
9. E. P. Gusev, C. D'emic, S. Zafar, and A. Kumar, Ultrathin HfO_2 films grown on silicon by atomic layer deposition for advanced gate dielectrics applications, *Microelectronic Engineering*, 69, 145–151, 2003.
10. A. C. Jones, H. C. Aspinall, and P. R. Chalker, Molecular design of improved precursors for the MOCVD of oxides used in microelectronics *Surface and Coatings Technology*, 201, 9046–9054, 2007.
11. R. Q. Tan, Y. Azuma, T. Fujimoto, J. W. Fan, and I. Kojima, Preparation of ultrathin HfO_2 films and comparison of HfO_2/SiO_2/Si interfacial structures, *Surface and Interface Analysis*, 36, 1007–1010, 2004.
12. J. A. Babcock, S. G. Balster, A. Pinto, C. Dirnecker, P. Steinmann, R. Jumpertz, and B. El-Kareh, Analog characteristics of metal–insulator–metal capacitors using PECVD nitride dielectrics, *IEEE Electron Device Letter*, 22, 230–232, 2001.
13. F. El Kamel, P. Gonon, and C. Vallée, Experimental evidence for the role of electrodes and oxygen vacancies in voltage nonlinearities observed in high-*k* metal–insulator–metal capacitors *Applied Physics Letter*, 91, 172909, 2007.
14. H. Hu, C. Zhu, Y. F. Lu, M. F. Li, B. J. Cho, and W. K. Choi, A high performance MIM capacitor using HfO_2 dielectrics, *IEEE Electron Device Letters*, 23, 514–516, 2002.
15. W. S. Lau, L. L. Leong, T. Han, and N. P. Sandler, Detection of oxygen vacancy defect states in capacitors with ultrathin Ta_2O_5 films by zero-bias thermally stimulated current spectroscopy, *Applied Physics Letter*, 83, 2835, 2003.
16. S. J. Ding, H. Hu, H. F. Lim, S. J. Kim, X. F. Yu, C. Zhu, M. F. Li, and B. J. Cho, Evidence and understanding of ALD HfO_2-Al_2O_3 laminate MIM capacitors outperforming sandwich counterparts, *IEEE Electron Device Letter*, 25, 681–683, 2004.
17. S. Krishnan, E. Stefanakos, and S. Bhansali, Effects of dielectric thickness and contact area on current–voltage characteristics of thin film metal–insulator–metal diodes, *Thin Solid Films*, 516, 2244–2250, 2008.

18. K. Xiong and J. Robertson, Point defects in HfO_2 high-*k* gate oxide, *Microelectronic Engineering*, 80, 408–411, 2005.
19. W. S. Lau, T. S. Tan, and P. Babu, Mechanism of leakage current reduction of tantalum oxide capacitors by titanium doping, *Applied Physics Letter*, 90, 112903, 2007.
20. P. Gonon and C. Vallée, Modeling of nonlinearities in the capacitance–voltage characteristics of high-*k* metal–insulator–metal capacitors, *Applied Physics Letter*, 2007.
21. J. H. Beaumont, and P. W. M. Jacobs, Polarization in potassium chloride crystals, *Journal of Physics and Chemistry of Solids*, 28, 1967.
22. M. D. Greenbelt, E. G. Stassinopoulos, and J. P. Raymond, The space radiation environment for electronics, *Proceedings of the IEEE*, 76, 1423–1442, 1988.
23. J. T. Ryan, P. M. Lenahan, A. Y. Kang, J. F. Conley, Jr., G. Bersuker, and P. Laysaght, Identification of the atomic scale defects involved in radiation damage in HfO_2 based MOS devices, *IEEE Transactions on Nuclear Science*, 52, 2272–2275, 2005.
24. G. Lucovsky, D. M. Fleetwood, S. Lee, H. Seo, R. D. Schrimpf, J. A. Felix, J. Lüning, L. B. Fleming, M. Ulrich, and D. E. Aspnes, Differences between charge trapping states in irradiated nano-crystalline HfO_2 and non-crystalline Hf silicates, *IEEE Transactions on Nuclear Science*, 53, 3644–3648, 2006.
25. B. Miao, R. Mahapatra, N. G. Wright, and A. B. Horsfall, The role of carbon contamination in voltage linearities and leakage current in high-*k* metal–insulator–metal capacitors, *Journal of Applied Physics*, 104, 054510, 2008.
26. P. Zubko, D. J. Jung, and F. Scott, Electrical characterization of $PbZr_{0.4}Ti_{0.6}O_3$ capacitors, *Journal of Applied Physics*, 100, 114113, 2006.
27. Y. Wang, Z. Lin, X. Chenc, H. Ziao, F. Zhang, and S. Zou, Study of HfO_2 thin films prepared by electron bam evaporation, *Applied Surface Science*, 228, 93–99, 2004.
28. S. Pan, S.-J. Ding, Y. Huang, Y-J Huang, D. W. Zhang, L-K. Wang, and R. Liu, High temperature conduction behaviour of HfO_2/Tan-based metal–insulator–metal capacitors, *Journal of Applied Physics*, 102, 073706, 2007.
29. M. R. Shaneyfelt, J. R. Schwank, D. M. Fleetwood, P. S. Winokur, K. L. Hughes, and F. W. Sexton, Field dependence of interface-trap buildup in polysilican and metal gate MOS devices, *IEEE Transactions on Nuclear Science*, 37, 1632–1640, 1990.
30. C.-H. Choi, Y. Wu, J.-S. Goo, Z. Yu, and R. W. Dutton, Capacitance reconstruction from measured *C–V* in high leakage, nitride/oxide MOS, *IEEE Transactions on Electron Devices*, 47, 1843–1850, 2000.
31. E. M. Vogel, W. K. Henson, C. A. Richter, and J. S. Suehle, Limitations of conductance to the measurement of the interface state density of MOS capacitors with tunneling gate dielectrics, *IEEE Transactions on Electron Devices*, 47, 601–608, 2000.
32. A. B. Pakhomov, S. K. Wong, X. Yan, and X. X. Zhang, Low frequency divergence of the dielectric constant in metal–insulator nanocomposites with tunneling, *Physical Review* B, 58, R13373, 1998.
33. M. Houssa, T. Nigram, P. W. Mertens, and M. M. Heyns, Soft breakdown in ultrathin gate oxides: Correlation with the percolation theory of non linear conductors, *Applied Physics Letters*, 73, 514–516, 1998.
34. S. W. Kenkel and J. P. Straley, Percolation theory of non linear circuit elements, *Physical Review Letters*, 49, 767–770, 1982.
35. R. Degraeve, G. Groeseneken, R. Bellens, M. Depas, and H. E. Maes, A consistent model for the thickness dependence of intrinsic breakdown in ultra thin oxides, *Proceedings of IEDM, 12,* 863–866, 1995.
36. A. Kraft and K.-H. Heckner, Neutron irradiation induced changes of the electrochemical properties of *n*-GaAs, *Journal of Electroanalytical Chemistry*, 393, 29–33, 1995.
37. C. Bonnelle, Charge trapping in dielectrics, *Microscopy and Microanalysis*, 10, 691–696, 2004.

Index

A

B

C

F

I

J

K

L

M

N

Q

U

V